Clinical Approach to Infection in the Compromised Host

Second Edition

Clinical Approach to Infection in the Compromised Host

Second Edition

Edited by
ROBERT H. RUBIN, M.D.
Infectious Disease and Transplantation Units
Massachusetts General Hospital
and Department of Medicine
Harvard Medical School
Boston, Massachusetts

and

LOWELL S. YOUNG, M.D.
Kuzell Institute for Arthritis and Infectious Diseases
Division of Infectious Diseases
Pacific Presbyterian Medical Center
San Francisco, California

With a Foreword by
J. KLASTERSKY, M.D.
Professor and Chief of Medicine
Jules Bordet Institute
Brussels, Belgium

SPRINGER SCIENCE+BUSINESS MEDIA, LLC

Library of Congress Cataloging in Publication Data

Clinical approach to infection in the compromised host.

Includes bibliographies and index.
1. Communicable diseases. 2. Immunological deficiency syndromes—Complications and sequelae. I. Rubin, Robert H., date. II. Young, Lowell S. [DNLM: 1. Communicable Diseases—immunology. 2. Immunity. 3. Immunologic Deficiency Syndromes—complications. WC 100 C641]
RC112.C59 1987   616.9′0479   87-30036
ISBN 978-1-4615-6647-2   ISBN 978-1-4615-6645-8 (eBook)
DOI 10.1007/978-1-4615-6645-8

© 1988 Springer Science+Business Media New York
Originally published by Plenum Publishing Corporation in 1988
Softcover reprint of the hardcover 1st edition 1988
233 Spring Street, New York, N.Y. 10013

Contributors

Neil M. Ampel • Department of Medicine, Section of Infectious Diseases, Veterans Administration Medical Center, Arizona Health Sciences Center, Tucson, Arizona 85724

Donald Armstrong • Department of Medicine, Infectious Disease Service and Microbiology Laboratory, Memorial Sloan-Kettering Cancer Center, Cornell University Medical College, New York, New York 10021

A. Benedict Cosimi • Department of Surgery, Massachusetts General Hospital, Boston, Massachusetts 02114

Jules L. Dienstag • Gastrointestinal Unit, Medical Services, Massachusetts General Hospital; and Department of Medicine, Harvard Medical School, Boston, Massachusetts 02114

Layne O. Gentry • Infectious Disease Section, St. Luke's Episcopal Hospital, Houston, Texas 77030

Michael S. Gottlieb • Department of Medicine, University of California–Los Angeles, Los Angeles, California 90024

Reginald Greene • Chest Division, Radiology Service, Massachusetts General Hospital; and Department of Radiology, Harvard Medical School, Boston, Massachusetts 02114

Harry R. Hill • Departments of Pediatrics and Pathology, Division of Clinical Immunology and Allergy, University of Utah School of Medicine, Salt Lake City, Utah 84132

Martin S. Hirsch • Infectious Disease Unit, Massachusetts General Hospital; and Department of Medicine, Harvard Medical School, Boston, Massachusetts 02114

Françoise Meunier • Department of Internal Medicine and Henri Tagnon Laboratory of Clinical Investigation, Section of Microbiology and Infectious Diseases Unit, Jules Bordet Institute, 1000 Brussels, Belgium

Joel D. Meyers • Fred Hutchinson Cancer Research Center; and Department of Medicine, University of Washington School of Medicine, Seattle, Washington 98104

Donald G. Payan • Divisions of Allergy–Immunology and Infectious Diseases, University of California, San Francisco, California 94143

Philip A. Pizzo • Pediatric Branch, Clinical Oncology Program, Division of Cancer Treatment, National Cancer Institute, Bethesda, Maryland 20892

Bruce Polsky • Department of Medicine, Infectious Disease Service, Memorial Sloan-Kettering Cancer Center, Cornell University Medical College, New York, New York 10021

Robert H. Rubin • Infectious Disease and Transplantation Units, Massachusetts General Hospital; and Department of Medicine, Harvard Medical School, Boston, Massachusetts 02114

Joel Ruskin • Department of Medicine, Infectious Diseases Service, Kaiser Permanente Medical Center, Los Angeles, California 90027; and University of California–Los Angeles School of Medicine, Los Angeles, California 90024

Stephen C. Schimpff • University of Maryland Cancer Center, Section of Infectious Diseases and Microbiology, Division of Oncology and Infectious Diseases, University of Maryland

School of Medicine, Baltimore, Maryland 21201

Robert T. Schooley • Infectious Disease Unit, Massachusetts General Hospital; and Harvard Medical School, Boston, Massachusetts 02114

Harvey B. Simon • Infectious Disease Unit, Massachusetts General Hospital; and Department of Medicine, Harvard Medical School, Boston, Massachusetts 02114

Arthur J. Sober • Dermatology Service, Massachusetts General Hospital; and Department of Dermatology, Harvard Medical School, Boston, Massachusetts 02114

E. Donnall Thomas • Fred Hutchinson Cancer Research Center; and Department of Medicine, University of Washington School of Medicine, Seattle, Washington 98104

Jos W. M. van der Meer • Department of Infectious Diseases, University Hospital, 2300 RC Leiden, The Netherlands

James C. Wade • University of Maryland Cancer Center, Section of Infectious Diseases and Microbiology, Division of Oncology and Infectious Diseases, University of Maryland School of Medicine, Baltimore, Maryland 21201

Edward J. Wing • Department of Medicine, Division of Infectious Diseases, Montefiore Hospital, University of Pittsburgh School of Medicine, Pittsburgh, Pennsylvania 15213

John S. Wolfson • Infectious Disease Unit, Medical Services, Massachusetts General Hospital; and Department of Medicine, Harvard Medical School, Boston, Massachusetts 02114

Lowell S. Young • Kuzell Institute for Arthritis and Infectious Disease, Division of Infectious Diseases, Pacific Presbyterian Medical Center, San Francisco, California 94115

Barry Zeluff • Infectious Disease Section, St. Luke's Episcopal Hospital, Houston, Texas 77030

Foreword

"Infection in the Compromised Host" has become a classic chapter in textbooks devoted to infectious diseases and internal medicine. The numbers of compromised hosts are increasing in the era of modern medicine because of our expanded capabilities to deal with difficult diseases, especially neoplasms. As a consequence, microbiologic complications related to the intensive care administered to these patients are increasing as well. Under these circumstances, not only does the underlying illness create conditions favorable for the development of unusual infections, but often the therapy contributes to the acquisition of potential pathogens that turn into agents responsible for severe and frequently fatal disease.

Granulocytopenia and immunosuppression have been the two key factors in predisposing patients with cancer and other serious diseases to severe bacterial infections. Colonization by hospital-acquired pathogens and breaks in the anatomic barriers—as a result of disease or medical intervention—have contributed to the high incidence of infectious diseases in these patients. Although there is some overlap between the types of infection in granulocytopenic and immunosuppressed hosts, each of these clinical entities has distinctive features that justify considering them separately, reserving the term *immunocompromised hosts* only when referring to patients who are predisposed to opportunistic infections.

For about two decades, infections in granulocytopenic patients have attracted the attention of clinicians because they represent a model for the study of antimicrobial drugs in hosts deprived of an essential element of defense against bacterial infection, that is, an adequate number of normally functioning granulocytes.

Infection in granulocytopenic patients has been, and still is, caused predominantly by gram-negative pathogens. *Pseudomonas aeruginosa* is particularly important because of its aggressiveness and relative resistance to antimicrobial therapy. However, the spectrum of infection in the granulocytopenic patient is changing. Gram-positive infections, especially those due to *Staphylococcus epidermidis*, have become more common. Although less rapidly lethal than gram-negative bacillary infections, they are associated with substantial morbidity and numerous complications. The multiresistant nature of these pathogens has led to the need for novel antimicrobial approaches and new drugs.

Infections in immunocompromised hosts are those found particularly in transplant recipients, in patients receiving immunosuppressive therapy for collagen disease, chronic active hepatitis, inflammatory bowel disease, and so forth, and in those suffering from the acquired immunodeficiency syndrome (AIDS). Fungal, viral, and protozoan pathogens are common problems requiring special skills for diagnosis and new concepts for therapy, since antifungal and antiviral treatments are still at their initial stages mainly because of the persisting lack of effective drugs.

Correction of the underlying defect—granulocytopenia or immunosuppression—remains the ultimate goal for successful therapy for infections in the patients afflicted with these conditions. As far as granulocytopenia is concerned, transfusions of granulocytes have not

vii

been as rewarding as initially thought, mainly because of many cumbersome aspects of their realization and the numerous side effects related to their use. Correction of immunosuppression is still in its earliest stages and no convincing approaches have yet been proposed; a major investigational effort is needed. Although still of minimal efficacy, the specific correction of the basic defect of the host's mechanisms of defense against infection would provide the optimal means of protecting the patient against complicating infections. Even today, it can be achieved to some degree by curing the underlying disease of the host (effective antineoplastic therapy or successful bone marrow transplantation) or by decreasing the amount of exogenous immunosuppressive therapy being administered.

Prophylaxis, that is, prevention of infection, has become a crucial aspect of our approach to the management of infections in the compromised host. The frequency of infections in the granulocytopenic patient can be substantially decreased by eradication from the host of hospital-acquired pathogens; this is optimally achieved within a protective environment such as the laminar airflow room. The elimination of pathogenic gastrointestinal flora achieves significant protection against bacterial (and possibly fungal) infections in the granulocytopenic patient; the optimal regimens to achieve this are still to be found, although the concept of *selective decontamination* offers a potential basis for research to be conducted in that area. Prevention might be even more important for infections against which no active or only little effective therapy exists. This is particularly the case in viral infections, namely cytomegalovirus infections, for which no therapy has existed, although we appear to be entering a new era of effective antiviral chemotherapy, as exemplified by ganciclovir. Passive immunization has some efficacy, and more specific antiviral approaches, such as those using ganciclovir, interferon, and other drugs, remain to be more fully investigated.

Prevention of fungal infections, especially those caused by *Aspergillus* sp., deserves a special effort, since therapy of these complications is still unsatisfactory. At this point, it is important to underline that control of the infectious complications of the compromised host lies mostly in the hands of those who are fighting the underlying disease itself. More effective antineoplastic agents, or novel approaches and a better understanding of what immunosuppression is are likely answers to the problem of infections in the compromised host. Until these new routes are discovered, the clinician will continue to face the management of increased numbers of patients for whom prevention of infection has failed.

Therapy of gram-negative infections has reached a sort of plateau during the past decade. Combinations of antibiotics (β-lactams plus aminoglycosides or combinations of β-lactams) have achieved a standard rate of cure of febrile granulocytopenic patients that is close to 70%. There is no clear indication that the new antibiotics will alter these results in a very significant way. Perhaps newer approaches using early immunotherapy directed against the toxic aspects of infections will improve mortality. As far as gram-positive infections are concerned, it is likely that better attention to the sites of infection (indwelling catheters) and new antibiotics, some of which are already in sight, will achieve a substantial improvement in the clinical course of these complications.

Therapy of fungal infections remains a field for much improvement; we have essentially only one active drug (amphotericin B) available, and its use still leaves ample room for improvement. As far as viral infections are concerned, acyclovir has solved many problems related to herpes simplex virus infections but leaves us without action against cytomegalovirus infection, which represents the most important problem in transplanted patients. New developments in the 1980s will undoubtedly take place in that field.

It can be feared that the ultimate answer to the infectious problems of the compromised host will appear only when the basic understanding of the underlying condition is achieved. There is no question that our efforts in preventing and treating infections of the compromised host represent an important contribution to present medical science. However, I believe that it is still in the range of supportive care. The ultimate answer lies in the better management of the underlying disease of the compromised host. Until this goal is achieved, the prevention and therapy of the complicated infections of the compromised host will require the efforts and the imagination of many dedicated physicians. Without attacking the evil itself, these physicians play an obscure and effective role in making our patients more comfortable and provide them with a better chance to enjoy a reasonably satisfactory life a bit longer.

It is hoped that this book will aid in helping us to understand and deal with the problems as they exist today and target the areas for intensive research for tomorrow. As one compares this second edition with the previous edition of this volume, one can only be impressed with the progress that has been made—from the discovery of the etiology and pathogenesis of AIDS to the effective control of herpes simplex and varicella–zoster virus infections with acyclovir and from the increasing success of bone marrow transplantation to the great promise of hyperimmune globulin therapies in a variety of clinical problems of the compromised host. Although the road taken is long and arduous, it is paved with many rewards—the survival of individual patients who might otherwise have succumbed and the effective therapy of a whole group of patients with certain forms of infection. This book provides the state-of-the-art information necessary to take this journey—the prevention and therapy of infection in the compromised host.

J. Klastersky, M.D.
Professor and Chief of Medicine
Jules Bordet Institute
Brussels, Belgium

Preface

Somewhat more than half a decade ago, several groups of authors—including ourselves—decided to publish books on the subject of infections in immunocompromised hosts. This occurred at a time when there was already a substantial literature to review on the subject of the management of infectious complications following cancer chemotherapy, organ transplantation, and the use of immunosuppressive drugs for a variety of medical and surgical disorders. Much of this material was highly controversial and in need of clarification by good clinical studies. Since then, the world's literature has grown exponentially on this broad subject. In addition, the advent of the acquired immunodeficiency syndrome (AIDS), unknown when the first edition of this book was sent to press, has made the subject of infection in the immunocompromised host a common feature, not only in every medical journal, no matter what the medical specialty, but also in daily newspapers, television news, and weekly newsmagazines.

For both these reasons, it is clear that interest in this field has increased logarithmically since 1981, and we have been asked to prepare a second edition. Our effort to comply with this request is more than an attempt simply to update the English language literature on the ever-growing complex and controversial aspects of clinical management in this field. Indeed, there is so much new information in this area that we have been obliged to produce a second edition that is considerably augmented in subject matter and breadth—some 40% larger than the original volume. We are excited that the expansion in this field has necessitated and justified such an increase in material.

As we reflect on the events of the past decade—from the time we just began to plan the first edition at an Epidemic Intelligence Service Conference of the Centers for Disease Control in the spring of 1977 to the present—we are impressed by two observations: The explosion in interest and scientific research into the problems associated with infection in the immunocompromised host has been accompanied by an increasing demand from doctor and patient alike for practical clinical advice based on firm scientific principles. With all the medical conferences, newsletters, cassettes, videotapes, and other multimedia attempts to convey medical information, there remains a compelling need for the clinician to have access in the dead of night or the heat of day to well-written, sage advice from veterans of battles similar to those they are now undertaking. This book attempts to fulfill these needs. We have previously stated that the best way to learn is to sit at the feet of a master for several years—like Mark Hopkins and The Log. It is our hope that we have been able to bring together a group of Mark Hopkinses, all veterans of these battles and distinguished contributors to the field, with this book serving as a Log for all those with a need to know. All credit for achieving these objectives is owed to our contributors. We accept responsibility for any inadequacies.

As before, a special debt of thanks is due to several groups of very special people: to Nina, Matilda, and our families, who have supported this work and allowed us to steal time from them so that this work might be completed late at night, on weekends, and during ''vacation time''; to our teachers and colleagues, who continue to lead by example and to provide a model of devotion to patients; and to the immunocompromised patients whose courage has inspired us all to go on in this field. Finally, a special word of gratitude must be expressed to Mrs. Janice Stern of Plenum Publishing Corporation, whose encouragement, patience, and support played a major role in bringing this second edition to fruition.

Robert H. Rubin
Lowell S. Young

Boston and San Francisco

Preface to the First Edition

The science and practice of infectious disease cut across all medical disciplines, from medicine to surgery, and from cardiology to neurology. Because of the diverse nature of infection and the clinical settings in which it occurs, the acquisition of the skills needed to become expert in clinical infectious diseases has usually required a lengthy apprenticeship. As one of us has noted, ''The practice of infectious disease is akin to many primitive arts, being handed down by oral traditions from generation to generation. The best way to learn is to sit at the feet of a master for several years, asking, observing, and studying—the medical equivalent of Mark Hopkins and the Log.''

However, increasingly it has become apparent that a more efficient means of communicating the art and science of clinical infectious disease to the general medical community is necessary. The infections themselves, the potential therapeutic modalities, the clinical settings in which they occur, and the occurrence of such infections far away from the academic medical center—all these have put a new emphasis on disseminating the most up-to-date information available to diagnose and treat clinical infection. This is particularly true when one considers the gamut of infections which afflict the patient with a defect in host defense. Those of us with a particular interest in this area of medicine and infectious diseases are painfully aware of the special nature of these patients and their problems and the rather extended apprenticeship we have served in learning to deal with these problems. We have been impressed that although great strides had been taken in general infectious disease in moving beyond the Log and the oral tradition, in this area of infectious disease such efforts are just beginning. Thus, the idea for this book was conceived to attempt to meld the scientific advances in this area with the experience that we had had in dealing with such patients to construct a useful, practical guide to the problem of infection in the compromised host. We wanted to share the fruits of our apprenticeship with the rest of the medical community who increasingly are being called upon to deal with these clinical problems.

The next step was to find out whether a publisher would be interested. Ms. Hilary Evans of Plenum was quickly recruited to the effort. She has been a bulwark of strength and encouragement during the lengthy gestation period. Finally, there comes the recruitment of the other contributors. Perhaps the most pleasant surprise in this whole experience was the enthusiasm with which our contributors brought their expertise to the endeavor—all of us agreeing that a need existed for a practical guide to patient management in the immunosuppressed host that was based upon firm scientific data whenever this was available and on the art and judgment of medicine when such data was unavailable. With admiration and gratitude we thank our contributors, who have taught us so much in the preparation of this book.

Finally, it is fitting that we express our gratitude to three different groups of individuals who have made this book possible—our teachers, Mort Swartz, Louis Weinstein, Alex Langmuir, Don Armstrong, and Don Louria, who have served as our models in their ability to blend the sciences of microbiology, immunology, and epidemiology with the art of clinical medicine; our families, who have supported us in this effort and whose time has been stolen to prepare this work; and, perhaps most of all, our patients, the immunocompromised patients with life-threatening infections who continue to teach us and inspire us with their courage and faith as we painfully learn how best to deal with infection in the compromised host.

Robert H. Rubin
Lowell S. Young

Boston and Los Angeles

Contents

1 Introduction..1
   LOWELL S. YOUNG and ROBERT H. RUBIN

2 Epidemiology and Prevention of Infection
   in the Compromised Host 5
   JAMES C. WADE and STEPHEN C. SCHIMPFF

   1. Infection As It Relates to Defects in Host Defense 5
      1.1. Granulocytopenia 5
      1.2. Cellular Immune Dysfunction 6
      1.3. Humoral Immune Dysfunction 7
      1.4. Obstruction to Natural Body Passages 7
      1.5. Breech of Body Barriers 7
   2. Origin of Infecting Organisms 8
      2.1. Shifts in Microbial Flora 9
      2.2. Sources of Acquisition of Exogenous Organisms 11
   3. Infection Prevention: Effective but Complex Techniques 13
      3.1. Reverse Isolation in Laminar Airflow Rooms or Other Forms of Complete
           Barrier Isolation 13
      3.2. Microbial Suppression with Oral Nonabsorbable Antibiotics 13
      3.3. Combined Use of Laminar Airflow Room or Similar Isolation plus
           Microbial Suppression with Oral Nonabsorbable Antibiotics 14
      3.4. Prophylactic Granulocyte Transfusions 15
   4. Ineffective Techniques of Infection Prevention 16
   5. "Simplified" and Effective Techniques of Infection Prevention 16
   6. Suppression of Potential Pathogens 18
      6.1. Granulocytopenia 18
      6.2. Prophylactic Trials 19
      6.3. Other Prophylactic Trials Using Trimethoprim–Sulfamethoxazole 23
      6.4. Disadvantages of Selective Microbial Modulation 24
      6.5. Fungal Prophylaxis 25
      6.6. Oral Antifungal Agents (Nonabsorbable) 26
      6.7. Skin 30
      6.8. Dental Hygiene 31
   7. Cellular Immune Dysfunction 31
      7.1. Tuberculosis 31
      7.2. *Pneumocystis carinii* 31

xv

7.3. Varicella–Zoster Virus 32
7.4. Herpes Simplex Virus 32
8. Humoral Immune Dysfunction 33
9. Relief of Obstruction 34
10. Care in the Breeching of Body Barriers 34
11. Staff Education 34
12. Patient Education 34
    References 34

3   Defects in Host-Defense Mechanisms 41

JOS W. M. VAN DER MEER

1. Colonization 41
2. The First Line of Defense 41
   2.1. The Skin 41
   2.2. The Mucosa 41
3. The Second Line of Defense 42
   3.1. Humoral Defense Mechanisms 42
   3.2. Cellular Defense Mechanisms 46
4. Factors Influencing the Quality of Host Defense 54
   4.1. Genetic Control of Host Defense against Infection 54
   4.2. Nutritional Status 54
   4.3. Age and Host Defense 55
   4.4. Body Temperature and Host Defense 55
5. Diseases Affecting Host Defense 56
   5.1. Leukemia and Lymphoma 56
   5.2. Splenectomy 56
   5.3. Sickle Cell Anemia 57
   5.4. Diabetes Mellitus 57
   5.5. Chronic Renal Failure 58
   5.6. Alcoholism and Hepatic Cirrhosis 58
   5.7. Systemic Lupus Erythematosus, Rheumatoid Arthritis,
        and Felty Syndrome 59
   5.8. Infections 59
6. Immunosuppressive Drugs 60
   6.1. Glucocorticosteroids 60
   6.2. Other Immunosuppressive Agents 60
7. Radiation 61
8. Attempts to Strengthen Host Defense 62
   References 63

4   Fever and Septicemia 75

LOWELL S. YOUNG

1. Introduction 75
2. Criteria for Fever, Fever of Undetermined Origin, and Septicemia 75
3. Pathogenesis of Fever 76
4. Syndrome-Oriented Approach to Fever and Suspected Infection:
   Differential Diagnosis 78

5. Some Emerging Pathogens in the Immunocompromised Host 84
6. Clinical Approach to Fever: History and Physical Examination 85
7. Interaction between the Clinician and the Microbiology Laboratory 87
8. Specific Laboratory Studies 87
9. Diagnosis of Infection: Antibody Measurements and Skin Tests 89
10. Noninvasive Diagnostic Procedures 89
11. Invasive Diagnostic Procedures 90
12. Diagnostic Tests of Limited Usefulness 91
13. Persistent or Recurrent Fever in the Patient with Negative Cultures:
    Diagnostic Considerations 91
14. Findings Suggestive of Microbial Infection Rather Than Fever Secondary
    to Underlying Disease 94
15. Initial or Empirical Antimicrobial Therapy: Indications for Treatment 95
16. Relationship of Antimicrobial Therapy and Underlying Disease
    to Outcome of Infection 96
17. Factors Underlying Recommendation of Initial or Empirical Antimicrobial
    Therapy Regimens 96
18. Antimicrobial Agents 100
    18.1. Aminoglycosides 100
    18.2. Antipseudomonal Penicillins 101
    18.3. Cephalosporins 101
    18.4. Antistaphylococcal Semisynthetic Penicillins 103
19. Is Specific Antistaphylococcal Therapy Necessary? 103
20. Alteration of Empirical Therapy after Documentation of Bacterial Infection 103
21. Role of Other Antibacterial Agents in Therapy 104
22. Therapeutic Drug Monitoring 105
23. Management of Catheter-Associated Infection 105
24. Should Fever Be Suppressed? 106
25. Therapy of Underlying Disease during Documented Infection 107
26. Duration of Antimicrobial Therapy in Documented Infection 107
27. Undocumented Infection and the Decision to Continue or Withhold
    Antimicrobial Agents 107
28. Recommendations for Continuing or Discontinuing Antimicrobial Therapy
    and Initiating Empirical Antifungal Therapy 109
    References 111

5 Dermatologic Manifestations of Infection in the Compromised Host 115

JOHN S. WOLFSON and ARTHUR J. SOBER

1. Introduction 115
2. Skin as a Barrier to Infection 115
3. Types of Skin Infection 117
    3.1. Primary Skin Infection with Common Pathogens 117
    3.2. Unusually Widespread Cutaneous Infection 117
    3.3. Opportunistic Primary Cutaneous Infection 120
    3.4. Systemic Infection Metastatic to Cutaneous and Subcutaneous Sites 121
4. Dermatologic Lesions Associated with AIDS 125
5. Diagnostic Considerations of Skin Infections in the Compromised Patient 125
    References 126

6 Etiology and Management of the Compromised Patient with Fever and Pulmonary Infiltrates 131
ROBERT H. RUBIN and REGINALD GREENE

1. Febrile Pneumonitis Syndrome and Its Importance 131
2. Epidemiologic Clues to the Diagnosis of Pulmonary Infection 134
3. Clinical Clues to the Diagnosis of Pulmonary Infection 138
4. Clinical Clues to the Diagnosis of Noninfectious Causes of Febrile Pneumonitis
   Syndrome 140
   4.1. Radiation Pneumonitis 140
   4.2. Drug-Induced Pneumonitis 141
   4.3. Neoplastic Pulmonary Invasion 144
   4.4. Other Noninfectious Causes of Febrile Pneumonitis Syndrome 145
5. Radiologic Clues to the Diagnosis of Febrile Pneumonitis Syndrome 147
6. Definitive Diagnosis 149
   6.1. Immunologic Techniques 150
   6.2. Conventional Sputum Examination 150
   6.3. Transtracheal Aspiration 151
   6.4. Invasive Diagnostic Techniques 152
7. Pulmonary Infiltrates in the Patient with AIDS 155
8. Superinfection 156
   References 157

7 Central Nervous System Infections in the Compromised Host 165
DONALD ARMSTRONG and BRUCE POLSKY

1. Introduction 165
2. Microorganisms 166
   2.1. Bacteria 166
   2.2. Fungi 174
   2.3. Parasites 181
   2.4. Viral Infections 182
3. Clinical Presentation: The Approach to the Patient 184
   3.1. Meningitis 185
   3.2. CNS Infections Complicating AIDS 185
   References 188

8 Fungal Infections in the Compromised Host 193
FRANÇOISE MEUNIER

1. Introduction 193
2. Diagnostic Approach: A General Overview 193
   2.1. Histology 194
   2.2. Cultures 194
   2.3. Serology 194
3. Candidiasis 195
   3.1. *Candida* Species 195
   3.2. Clinical Presentation 196
4. Aspergillosis 199

5. Mucormycosis 203
  5.1. Mucoraceae 203
  5.2. Clinical Presentation 203
6. Cryptococcosis 204
  6.1. *Cryptococcus neoformans* 204
  6.2. Clinical Presentation 204
7. Coccidioidomycosis 205
  7.1. *Coccidioides immitis* 205
  7.2. Clinical Presentation 205
8. Histoplasmosis 206
  8.1. *Histoplasma capsulatum* 206
  8.2. Clinical Presentation 206
9. Other Fungal Infections 207
10. Prevention of Opportunistic Fungal Infection 207
  10.1. General Considerations 207
  10.2. Chemoprophylaxis 207
  10.3. Isolation 208
11. Antifungal Therapy 209
  11.1. Antifungal Agents 209
  11.2. Current Controversies in the Management of Fungal Infections
    in the Immunocompromised Host 210
12. Perspectives for the Future 212
  References 212

9 Mycobacterial and Nocardial Infections in the Compromised Host 221
HARVEY B. SIMON

1. Introduction 221
2. Mycobacteria 221
  2.1. Classification and Microbiology 221
  2.2. Host Defenses 223
  2.3. Skin Testing 223
  2.4. Pathogenesis 224
  2.5. Epidemiology 226
  2.6. Clinical Features 229
  2.7. Management of Mycobacterial Infections 238
3. *Nocardia* 243
  3.1. Classification and Microbiology 243
  3.2. Epidemiology and Pathogenesis 244
  3.3. Clinical Features and Diagnosis 244
  3.4. Therapy 247
  3.5. Infection Caused by Related Organisms 247
  References 248

10 Parasitic Diseases in the Compromised Host 253
JOEL RUSKIN

1. Introduction 253
2. *Pneumocystis carinii* Pneumonia 253
  2.1. Historic Perspective 254

2.2. The Organism 254
2.3. Histopathology 257
2.4. Conditions Associated with Pneumocystosis in Humans and Animals 257
2.5. Predisposing Factors and Host-Defense Mechanisms 258
2.6. Epidemiology and Transmission 258
2.7. Clinical Features (Non-AIDS Related) 259
2.8. Radiologic Findings 261
2.9. Diagnostic Approaches to Suspected *Pneumocystis carinii* Infection 263
2.10. Treatment 266
2.11. Patient Isolation and Prophylaxis of *Pneumocystis* Infection 271
2.12. Postinfection Fibrosis 272
2.13. Overview of Therapeutic and Prophylactic Approaches 275
3. Babesiosis 275
3.1. Clinical Features 276
3.2. Laboratory Diagnosis 277
3.3. Treatment 278
4. Giardiasis 279
4.1. The Organism 279
4.2. Epidemiology 280
4.3. Pathogenesis 280
4.4. Clinical Manifestations 281
4.5. Giardiasis in the Compromised Host 281
4.6. Diagnosis 281
4.7. Treatment 282
5. Toxoplasmosis 282
5.1. History 283
5.2. The Organism 283
5.3. Pathogenesis 285
5.4. Signs and Symptoms of Toxoplasmosis in Immunologically Intact Patients   286
5.5. Toxoplasmosis in the Compromised Host 287
5.6. Toxoplasmosis in AIDS Patients 288
5.7. Diagnosis 289
5.8. Summary of Diagnostic Approach to Possible CNS Toxoplasmosis 290
5.9. Therapy 291
5.10. Prevention 292
6. Coccidial Infections 292
7. Strongyloidiasis 295
7.1. The Organism 295
7.2. Clinical Manifestations 295
7.3. Diagnosis 297
7.4. Treatment 297
References 298

11 Legionellosis in the Compromised Host 305

NEIL M. AMPEL and EDWARD J. WING

1. Introduction 305
2. Microbiology 305
2.1. Classification 305
2.2. Morphology 306
2.3. Cultural and Biochemical Characteristics 306

   3. Pathology, Pathogenesis, and Immunology 307
      3.1. Pathology and Pathogenesis 307
      3.2. Immunology 308
   4. Epidemiology 309
      4.1. General Considerations 309
      4.2. Ecology 309
      4.3. Nosocomial Legionellosis 309
   5. Clinical Manifestations 310
      5.1. Symptoms 310
      5.2. Signs 311
      5.3. Laboratory Findings 311
      5.4. Radiographic Findings 311
      5.5. Extrapulmonary Complications 313
   6. Diagnosis 314
      6.1. Differential Diagnosis 314
      6.2. Dual Infection 315
      6.3. Specific Diagnosis 315
      6.4. Diagnostic Approach 316
   7. Treatment 317
      7.1. Retrospective Studies 317
      7.2. Animal Studies 317
      7.3. Factors Determining Antimicrobial Efficacy 318
      7.4. Recommendations 318
      7.5. Course 318
   8. Prevention and Control 319
      References 319

12   Viral Hepatitis in the Compromised Host 325

JULES L. DIENSTAG

   1. Introduction 325
   2. Role of Immunologic Mechanisms in the Pathogenesis of Viral Hepatitis 326
      2.1. Hepatitis B 326
      2.2. Non-A, Non-B Hepatitis 327
   3. Viral Hepatitis in the Immunocompromised Host 327
      3.1. Hemodialyzed Patients with Chronic Renal Failure 329
      3.2. Hepatitis in Recipients of Organ Transplants 330
      3.3. Hepatitis in Oncology Patients 335
   4. Prevention 338
   5. Summary 340
      References 341

13   Herpes Group Virus Infections in the Compromised Host 347

MARTIN S. HIRSCH

   1. Introduction 347
   2. Herpes Simplex Virus 347
      2.1. Clinical Epidemiology and Patterns of Infection 348

2.2. Pathogenesis 350
2.3. Diagnosis and Therapy 351
3. Varicella–Zoster Virus 351
   3.1. Clinical Epidemiology and Patterns of Infection 352
   3.2. Pathogenesis 354
   3.3. Diagnosis and Therapy 355
4. Cytomegalovirus 356
   4.1. Clinical Epidemiology and Patterns of Infection 356
   4.2. Pathogenesis 358
   4.3. Diagnosis and Therapy 359
5. Epstein–Barr Virus 359
   5.1. Clinical Epidemiology and Patterns of Infection 360
   5.2. Pathogenesis 360
   5.3. Diagnosis and Therapy 361
6. Other Human Herpesviruses 362
References 362

14   Morbidity in Compromised Patients Due to Viruses Other Than Herpes Group and Hepatitis Viruses 367

ROBERT T. SCHOOLEY

1. Introduction 367
2. DNA Viruses 367
   2.1. Adenoviruses 367
   2.2. Papovaviruses 369
   2.3. Vaccinia 372
3. RNA Viruses 373
   3.1. Picornaviruses 373
   3.2. Paramyxoviruses 374
   3.3. Rotaviruses 375
   3.4. Human T-Lymphotropic Viruses 376
References 376

15   Acquired Immunodeficiency Syndrome 381

MICHAEL S. GOTTLIEB

1. Introduction 381
2. Epidemiology 381
   2.1. Case Definition 381
   2.2. AIDS in the United States and Europe 382
   2.3. AIDS in Africa and the Caribbean 383
3. Etiology and Pathogenesis 384
   3.1. Human T-Lymphotropic Retroviruses 384
   3.2. Immunologic Features 386
4. Risk Groups for AIDS and HIV Infection 387
5. Clinical Features 388
   5.1. General 388
   5.2. Clinical Approach to Fever in AIDS and in Population Groups at Increased Risk 389

6. Laboratory Studies in AIDS and HIV-Related Syndromes 391
  6.1. Routine Diagnostic Studies 391
  6.2. Specific Serologic and Immunologic Tests 391
  6.3. Cultures 392
  6.4. Other Studies 392
7. Differential Diagnosis 392
  7.1. General 392
  7.2. Homosexual and Bisexual Males 392
  7.3. Women 393
  7.4. Intravenous Drug Users 393
  7.5. Blood Product and Organ Transplant Recipients 393
  7.6. Pediatric Age Group 394
8. Therapy 395
  8.1. General Approach 395
  8.2. Management of Infection 395
  8.3. Presentation and Management of Common Opportunistic Infections 395
  8.4. Immunotherapy and Antiretroviral Therapy 400
9. Hospital Infection Control and Protection of Health Workers 400
10. Appendix 400
  References 401

16 Infections Complicating Congenital Immunodeficiency Syndromes 407

HARRY R. HILL

1. Introduction 407
2. Aim of Therapy in Congenital Immunodeficiency Diseases 410
  2.1. Treatment of Life-Threatening Infections 410
  2.2. Minimizing the Effects of Less Severe Acute Infections 414
  2.3. Prevention of Chronic Infections and Their Sequelae 416
3. Specific Infections in Immunodeficiency Syndromes 419
  3.1. Combined B- and T-Cell Defects 419
  3.2. Pure T-Cell Congenital Immunodeficiencies 422
  3.3. B-Cell Immunodeficiency 423
  3.4. Complement Component Deficiencies 425
  3.5. Phagocyte Abnormalities 427
  References 432

17 Diagnosis and Management of Infectious Disease Problems in the Child with Malignant Disease 439

PHILIP A. PIZZO

1. Cancers of Childhood 439
2. Interface between Cancer and Infection 441
3. Perturbations of Host Defenses That Contribute to the Risk of Infection
  in Children with Cancer 442
4. Fever in Childhood Cancer 442
5. Primary Causes of Fever and Infection in the Granulocytopenic Child 443
  5.1. Bacteria 443
  5.2. Viruses 444

5.3. Fungi 445
5.4. Protozoa 445
6. Diagnostic Evaluation of the Febrile Child with Cancer 445
7. Is There a Correct Starting Regimen for Granulocytopenic Children
   Who Become Febrile? 448
8. When Is It Appropriate to Modify the Initial Empirical Antibiotic Regimen? ... 453
9. If a Microbial Isolate Is Identified and the Antibiotic Sensitivities Are Known,
   Should the Antibiotic Spectrum Be Narrowed? 454
10. If the Patient Has a Bacteremia and Also Has an Indwelling Catheter,
    Are Additional Modifications of Therapy Necessary? 455
11. Do the Principles Gleaned from the Management of Intravascular Catheters
    Apply to Other Types of Foreign Bodies? 457
12. What Is the Role of Invasive Diagnostic Procedures in the Evaluation
    and Management of the Febrile Child with Cancer? 459
13. Are There Situations in Which Surgery Should be Incorporated into the
    Management Plan, Even if the Patient is Profoundly Granulocytopenic? 462
14. How Long Should Antibiotic Therapy Be Continued, and How Should It Be
    Modified When the Clinical and Microbiologic Evaluation Has Failed
    to Reveal an Infectious Etiology for Fever? 463
15. Summary 464
    References 464

18   Management of Infections in Leukemia and Lymphoma

.... 467

LOWELL S. YOUNG

1. Introduction 467
2. Host Defenses against Infection in Leukemias and Lymphomas 468
3. The Role of Infection in Mortality from Leukemia and Lymphoma 471
4. Problems with the Interpretation of Fever and Infection Incidence Data
   in Neutropenic States 473
5. Causes of Fever in Leukemia and Lymphoma 474
6. Site of Involvement and the Nature of the Microbial Pathogen(s) 477
7. Synthesis 482
8. Summary of Recommended Therapeutic Strategies 486
   8.1. Different Approaches to Leukemia and Lymphoma 486
   8.2. Environmental Considerations 486
   8.3. Prophylactic Antibiotics 487
   8.4. Systemic Antimicrobial Agents 488
9. Approach to the Splenectomized Patient 489
10. Neutrophil Transfusions in the Treatment and Prophylaxis of Infection 490
11. Immunoprophylaxis and Immunotherapy of Infection 494
    11.1. Childhood Immunizations 494
    11.2. Passive Antibody 494
    11.3. Influenza Immunization 494
    11.4. Pneumococcal Immunization 494
    References 497

19 Evaluation and Management of Infections in Patients with Collagen Vascular Disease 503
DONALD G. PAYAN

1. Introduction 503
2. Novel Features of Host–Microorganism Interactions in CVD 503
3. Morbidity and Mortality Caused by Infections in Patients with CVD 505
4. Host Abnormalities as Potential Contributing Factors to Infections in Patients with CVD 507
5. Role of Immunosuppressive Therapy in Predisposing Patients with CVD to Infections 509
6. Spectrum of Infection in Patients with CVD 511
7. Unique Clinical Features of Infection in Patients with CVD 514
8. Clinical Examples of Infection and Their Management 515
   8.1. Altered Mental Status in a Patient with SLE 515
   8.2. Pleuritic Chest Pain and Fever in a Patient with SLE 516
   8.3. Abdominal Pain in a Patient with SLE 518
   8.4. Painful Knee in a Patient with Rheumatoid Arthritis 519
9. Conclusions 520
   References 521

20 Infection Complicating Bone Marrow Transplantation 525
JOEL D. MEYERS and E. DONNALL THOMAS

1. Introduction 525
2. Recovery of Host Defenses 526
3. Phases of Infection after Marrow Transplantation 527
4. Phase I: Early Infections 527
   4.1. Bacteremia 527
   4.2. Bacterial Pneumonia 528
   4.3. Use of Surveillance Cultures 529
   4.4. Hyperalimentation Lines 533
   4.5. Antibiotic Treatment 533
   4.6. Therapeutic Granulocyte Transfusions 534
   4.7. Infection Control Programs 534
   4.8. Fungal Infections 536
5. Phase II: Infections to Day 100 541
   5.1. Interstitial Pneumonia 541
   5.2. Cytomegalovirus-Associated Pneumonia 544
   5.3. *Pneumocystis carinii* Pneumonia 546
   5.4. Idiopathic Interstitial Pneumonia 547
   5.5. Other Manifestations of Cytomegalovirus Infection 548
   5.6. Herpes Simplex Virus Infection 549
   5.7. Other Protozoan Infections 550
6. Phase III: After 100 Days 550
   6.1. Varicella–Zoster Virus Infection 550
   6.2. Late Infections in Patients with Graft-versus-Host Disease 551

7. Future Considerations 552
   References 553

21   Infection in the Renal and Liver Transplant
Patient 557

ROBERT H. RUBIN

1. Introduction 557
2. Timetable of Infection in the Renal Transplant Patient 560
3. Infection in the First Month following Renal Transplantation 562
   3.1. Preexisting Infection in the Allograft Recipient 562
   3.2. Infection from the Donor 564
   3.3. Wound Infection 566
   3.4. Other Causes of Infection in the First Month 568
4. Infection 1–6 Months Post-transplant 569
   4.1. Cytomegalovirus Infection in the Renal Transplant Patient 569
   4.2. Other Viruses 582
   4.3. Urinary Tract Infection in the Renal Transplant Patient 588
   4.4. Liver Disease in the Renal Transplant Patient 591
5. Infection in Renal Transplant Patients More than 6 Months Post-transplant 594
6. Infectious Disease Problems of Particular Importance 595
   6.1. Central Nervous System Infection in the Renal Transplant Patient 595
   6.2. Bacteremia in the Renal Transplant Patient 597
   6.3. Fungal Infection in the Renal Transplant Patient 599
   6.4. Tuberculosis and Atypical Mycobacterial Infection
        in the Renal Transplant Patient 599
   6.5. Dermatologic Manifestations of Infection in the Renal Transplant Patient .. 600
7. Infection in the Liver Transplant Patient 603
   7.1. Infection Related to Pre-Liver Transplant Events 603
   7.2. Infection in the First Month Post-Liver Transplant 605
   7.3. Infection Beyond 1 Month Post-transplant 607
8. Summary and Prospects for the Future 608
   References 609

22   Infection in the Cardiac Transplant Patient 623

LAYNE O. GENTRY and BARRY ZELUFF

1. Introduction 623
2. Infection in the First Month Post-transplant 624
   2.1. Bacteremia 625
   2.2. Urinary Tract Infection 626
   2.3. Pneumonia 626
3. Infection 1–6 Months Post-Cardiac Transplant 629
   3.1. Cytomegalovirus Infection in Cardiac Transplant Recipients 630
   3.2. Infectious Disease Syndromes Produced by Cytomegalovirus 631
   3.3. Superinfection Associated with Cytomegalovirus Infection 632
   3.4. Management of Cytomegalovirus Infection 633
   3.5. Herpes Group Viruses Other Than Cytomegalovirus 633
4. *Pneumocystis carinii* Infection in Cardiac Transplant Patients 635

5. *Legionella* Infections 636
6. Fungal Infections in the Cardiac Transplant Patient 637
  6.1. *Aspergillus* Infection in the Cardiac Transplant Patient 638
  6.2. *Candida* Infection in the Cardiac Transplant Patient 639
  6.3. *Cryptococcus* Infection in the Cardiac Transplant Patient 640
7. Nocardial and Mycobacterial Infection in the Transplant Patient 641
8. Toxoplasmosis in the Cardiac Transplant Patient 642
9. General Surgical Considerations in the Cardiac Transplant Patient 643
10. Special Infectious Disease Problems of Patients Undergoing
    Heart–Lung Transplants 644
    References 644

23   Surgical Aspects of Infection in the Compromised Host 649

A. BENEDICT COSIMI

1. Introduction 649
2. Diagnostic Approach 649
  2.1. Pneumonia in the Immunocompromised Host 649
  2.2. Colonic Complications of the Immunosuppressed State 650
  2.3. Occult Intraabdominal Sources of Fever and Infection 652
3. Preoperative Preparation 653
  3.1. Infection and Adrenal Insufficiency 653
  3.2. Infection and Ketoacidosis 654
  3.3. Infection and Malnutrition 654
  3.4. Preoperative Antibiotics 655
4. Intraoperative Considerations 656
  4.1. Choice of Anesthesia and Patient-Monitoring Techniques 656
  4.2. Surgical Technique 657
5. Postoperative Management 659
  5.1. Respiratory Management in the Immunocompromised Patient 659
  5.2. General Postoperative Care in the Immunocompromised Patient 661
  5.3. Management of the Burn or Trauma Patient 661
  5.4. Gastrointestinal Bleeding in the Immunocompromised Patient 663
  5.5. Sepsis following Splenectomy 665
6. Conclusions 665
  References 666

Index 669

Index 669

Clinical Approach to Infection in the Compromised Host

Second Edition

1

Introduction

LOWELL S. YOUNG and ROBERT H. RUBIN

One need not look far in the contemporary literature of internal medicine, surgery, or pediatrics to find the term *immunocompromised host* or some variant of this expression used to connote the patient with impaired host defenses who is at risk of developing an opportunistic infection. Depressingly, this in part reflects the increasing public, medical, and scientific concern with the unprecedented epidemic of opportunistic infection and malignancy, the acquired immunodeficiency syndrome (AIDS), which is spreading throughout the world. More optimistically, this in part reflects major advances in the use of immunosuppressive therapy for organ transplantation, in the treatment of a variety of autoimmune conditions, and in the management of malignant disease. Because of these advances, there is an increasing population of patients who are no longer succumbing quickly to their primary disease (be it chronic renal failure, intractable heart failure, cancer, aplastic anemia, or collagen disease) and who now have the potential for many years of productive life. The price for their survival has been the creation of large numbers of patients with major defects in host defense. For many of these patients, infection—not their primary illness—has become the major cause of mortality.

As the numbers of these patients have increased,

responsibility for their care has spread from the academic medical center to practitioners at every level—the primary care physician, the general internist and surgeon, as well as the subspecialist. It is incumbent upon all of us to become familiar both with the unusual infectious disease problems that occur in these patients—the prevention, diagnosis, and treatment of these problems—and with the ways in which underlying disease and/or its therapy can modify the clinical presentation and management of common conditions. For example, we have too often seen the diagnosis of a perforated abdominal viscus in a patient on immunosuppressive therapy missed, and the patient succumb, because of the absence of the classic signs of an acute abdomen in such patients.

This book was conceived as an attempt to deal with this problem—to summarize directly and succinctly the major issues and controversies involving the medical and surgical management of immunocompromised patients. We hope that the dominant characteristics of this assembly of views are candor and the presentation of a particular approach to the clinical management of infection in the compromised host. The contributors have been asked to meet the important issues "head on" and to identify those areas in which useful knowledge does or does not exist. After giving a fair summary of the published literature, they elaborate on their views about the most expeditious, economically sound, logical approach to the challenging manifestations of infection in what are likely to be very ill patients. Where data are insufficient to enable one to choose among several clinical alternatives, they have said so, thereby distinguishing fact from opinion. This effort is not intended as an encyclopedic compendium of the re-

LOWELL S. YOUNG • Kuzell Institute for Arthritis and Infectious Disease, Division of Infectious Diseases, Pacific Presbyterian Medical Center, San Francisco, California 94115. ROBERT H. RUBIN • Infectious Disease and Transplantation Units, Massachusetts General Hospital; and Department of Medicine, Harvard Medical School, Boston, Massachusetts 02114.

cent medical knowledge on this complicated subject but, rather, as a practical guide to clinical decision making.

The guiding theme of this book is to identify the epidemiologic, pathophysiologic, and clinical clues that will lead to early diagnosis and effective therapy or, better yet, prevention, rather than to discuss the way a disease looks at the autopsy table. This treatise has been purposely organized with this perspective in mind. On the one hand there are detailed chapters on host defenses, epidemiology, and prevention of infection, as well as particular infections (e.g., herpes viruses, fungi, parasites). On the other hand, since the patient does not present with a label stating the name of the infection, other chapters are devoted to particular organ system infections (septicemia, skin, lung, and central nervous system) and infection is in particular patient groups (e.g., transplant patients, cancer patients, AIDS patients). The clinician needs both kinds of information—an approach to the patient with pneumonia as well as detailed analysis of what to do and what to anticipate once the diagnosis of the cause of the pneumonia in this particular patient population has been made. Although such a multifaceted approach results in some repetition of material, we believe that such repetition is both warranted and useful. Throughout the book, great reliance has been placed on actual case examples to illustrate important clinical points.

When we wrote the introduction to the first edition, we believed that there were some major areas of controversy in the clinical management of the immunocompromised patient that clinicians of the 1970s faced; we voiced optimism that some of these issues would be satisfactorily addressed in the ensuing years. Although many of these issues persist, and Table 1 has been accordingly modified and brought up to date, we have seen many positive developments in these areas:

1. The introduction into clinical practice of many new antimicrobial agents of increased potency and broader spectrum, which has made a definite contribution to empirical and directed therapy.
2. An improved understanding of host-defense mechanisms and particularly our ability to quantify specific components of the immune response such as the helper and suppressor

TABLE 1. Areas of Controversy in the Management of Infection in the Immunocompromised Host

1. Empirical antimicrobial therapy for suspected bacterial sepsis: monotherapy versus synergistic therapy; double β-lactam versus β-lactam plus aminoglycoside
2. Indications for starting and stopping empirical antifungal therapy
3. Value of noninvasive techniques for diagnosing invasive fungal disease
4. Indications for continued empirical antibacterial therapy in the culture-negative but persistently febrile neutropenic patient
5. What elements of protected environments, antibiotic prophylaxis, and selective microbial decontamination are most useful in preventing infection in compromised hosts
6. Comparative yield and risk of invasive procedures for diagnosing pulmonary infection
7. Clinical indications for prophylactic antibiotics
8. Passive immunoprophylaxis and treatment (as an adjunct to antibiotics) of gram-negative bacterial infection with antibiotics directed against "core" endotoxin moieties
9. Management of asymptomatic carriers of the human immunodeficiency virus (the AIDS virus)
10. Infection prophylaxis in patients with AIDS and the AIDS-related complex (ARC)

lymphocytes identified by modern biotechnologic techniques. Indeed, this development has paved the way for better understanding of the immunopathology of AIDS, which coincidentally appeared with the advent of this new monoclonal antibody technology.
3. The publication of controlled clinical trials which have established the limited benefits from prophylactic and therapeutic granulocyte transfusions.
4. Continued studies on the prophylaxis of infection whether via chemotherapy or barrier isolation techniques which have clearly emphasized the limitations of these approaches. However, these studies provide the foundation for new approaches using such new drugs as the hydroxyquinolones for bacterial prophylaxis and cyclic nucleotide analogues for viral prophylaxis.

As we look back at the past half-decade, we can say that there has not been a really important new opportunistic pathogen identified as a major cause of localized infection in immunocompromised hosts. In other words, there is no recent equivalent of the Legionnaire's bacillus for the world to become cognizant of—an infecting agent that was heretofore unrecognized but simply missed because we lacked the ability to identify that pathogen in clinical specimens. On the other hand, one can hardly overlook the most dramatic development within the past few years; namely, the description, etiologic determination, and understanding of the disturbing new syndrome that is the basis for a worldwide pandemic of life-threatening disease—AIDS. When the first edition was being prepared, the first human cases of AIDS were being recognized by Gottlieb and colleagues at UCLA. The snowballing number of human patients and the untold suffering that has occurred has been paralleled by the extraordinary insights into the biology of an entirely new virus and the havoc it has raised on the immune system that predispose to lethal opportunistic infections of a magnitude that we have never seen before. One need only visit the wards of major teaching hospitals in the United States and Europe to see the protean manifestations of such pathogens as the atypical mycobacteria. AIDS hangs over the entire immunocompromised host field like a specter. Not only must we be alert to this problem in any patient presenting with fever, lung infiltrates, or unexplained inanition, but we must consider that through the vehicle of blood transfusions this lethal infection has been transmitted to cancer patients, recipients of transplants, and any patient receiving blood products. The one positive side of the AIDS pandemic is that knowledge gained in the care of these patients is applicable to the other immunocompromised patients with less complex forms of similar infections.

Aside from the way that AIDS has affected the way we attempt to diagnose and practice medicine, two major developments have certainly affected the practice of medicine in the United States and Europe. One development is the governmental and societal pressures for the implementation of cost-effective measures in clinical practice. How we define *cost effective* per se is controversial. Anyone, however, who treats patients is aware of the increased consciousness relating to reducing unnecessary tests, the use of less expensive antimicrobial agents, and the desire to discharge patients early following chemotherapy or pharmacologic therapy with many persisting side effects. One would hope that much of these cost-cutting measures have been of benefit. In certain situations, however, they may limit our ability to understand fully the complexities of the biological phenomena which are occurring in our more complicated immunosuppressed patients. Clinically, early discharge may spell early readmission. It is likely that the trend emphasizing economics will persist for some time and many of the changes in this text are aimed at providing the clinician with useful guidelines that will enable the practice of first-rate medicine without cutting back on absolutely essential diagnostic studies and therapy.

The second but more optimistic development that we perceive that will have enormous influence in the years ahead is the expanding application of the tools of modern biotechnology. The availability of monoclonal antibody staining came just about the time the first cases of AIDS appeared. The idea of helper and suppressor lymphocytes has now become familiar to neophyte students of medicine. But biotechnology has far greater potential; several examples include recombinant DNA techniques for rapid diagnosis of infection and the tremendous proliferation of additional diagnostic studies using monoclonal antibody technology. On the horizon, and now certainly in use in the research setting, are far greater applications and these can only be briefly summarized: the use of monoclonal antibodies for treating graft-versus-host disease, the use of antibodies of diverse specificities to treat cancer, and passively administered antibodies as adjunctive therapy in various infectious processes seem obvious future applications. Biotechnology has made possible the production of recombinant pharmacologic agents that almost surely will revolutionize the clinical practice of medicine. Heretofore scarce quantities of biologically active complex molecules such as interferons, interleukins, and other cytokines will greatly increase the complexity of pharmacologic therapy, as well as induce a set of complicating problems of their own, since many of these substances have paradoxical effects on biologic systems. It is perhaps through the application of biotechnology that we will be able to confront the paramount problem of our time—AIDS. Clearly, it is going to take every resource to develop strategies for manipulating the immune system and antiviral therapy to deal with AIDS. The next few years for clinicians and scientists who work in the field of immunosuppression are likely to be exciting as the secrets of the immune system are unlocked, and specific strategies developed for dealing with one of the most impressive challenges that medical science and clinicians have yet faced.

It should be emphasized, however, that this is not a book about the management of AIDS. Rather, it is hoped that the material included will lead to a useful approach to the patient with this and other syndromes where immunosuppression sets the stage for opportunistic infection. This book is primarily an attempt to summarize the many developments that have occurred in a rapidly evolving field and to direct the thoughts of investigators to where major opportunities lie.

2

Epidemiology and Prevention of Infection in the Compromised Host

JAMES C. WADE and STEPHEN C. SCHIMPFF

1. Infection As It Relates to Defects in Host Defense

A useful approach to the study of infection in the immunocompromised host is to first consider what factors make such a patient a compromised host. Knowledge regarding the major compromising factors then allows one to focus on diagnostic, therapeutic and preventative measures specific for that patient's specific infection risks. These dysfunctions of host-defense mechanisms or factors that predispose to infection are discussed together with the types of infections with which they are most commonly associated.

1.1. Granulocytopenia

Infection is related to the absolute level of circulating granulocytes (polymorphonuclear leukocytes; band forms and metamyelocytes).[1] The frequency of infection begins to rise as the granulocyte count drops below $500/\mu l$ with a dramatic increase as the granulocyte count approaches zero. The more severe infections and gram-negative bacteremias are more likely to occur when the granulocyte count is less than $100/\mu l$.[2] The exact level of granulocytopenia is a very useful index of infection

JAMES C. WADE and STEPHEN C. SCHIMPFF • University of Maryland Cancer Center, Section of Infectious Diseases and Microbiology, Division of Oncology and Infectious Diseases, University of Maryland School of Medicine, Baltimore, Maryland 21201.

risk, but the granulocyte count alone does not adequately portray the dynamics associated with granulocyte functions. For example, a rapidly dropping granulocyte count is much more likely to be associated with an increased risk of infection than is either the slow decline observed with syndromes such as cyclic neutropenia or the stable granulocytopenia often seen with some cases of chronic stable aplastic anemia, or benign idiopathic neutropenia.[3] Defects in granulocyte function such as leukocyte mobilization, chemotaxis, phagocytosis, and microbial killing often accompany conditions that produce granulocytopenia. Nevertheless, the absolute level of granulocytopenia, even in the absence of other data, is a reliable indicator of the infection risk.

Granulocytopenia usually follows the administration of chemotherapy or radiation therapy and is present frequently with damage to other host defense mechanisms. The patient who has undergone a renal transplant or the patient with a collegan vascular disease may experience myelosuppression while receiving azathioprine or cyclophosphamide. Together with corticosteroids, this combination produces a pronounced deficit in immune function. The patient with acute leukemia who receives remission-induction chemotherapy usually has concurrent alimentary canal and respiratory tract mucosal damage that serves as a potential portal of entry for the infecting organisms. Thus, one of the most common sites of infection will be the alimentary tract including the oral cavity, esophagus, colon, and rectum.[4] Underlying periodontal disease or herpes virus reactivation may be a cofactor in the development of oral infections.[5] Drug-induced vomiting with stomach acid reflux may help explain the increased risk of infection in the distal third of the esophagus although direct viral reactivation may occur at this site as well. The high pressure generated during defecation in association with frequent bowel movements and preexisting hemorrhoidal damage to the anal mucosa probably account for the frequent rectal infections. Finally, concurrent damage to ciliary function and tracheobronchial mucosa may explain the high frequency of pneumonia and sinusitis in such patients with granulocytopenia. In the absence of adequate numbers of circulating or functional granulocytes, organisms that colonize the mucosa and that are normally considered nonpathogenic in the normal host can penetrate and establish local infection. These infections will rapidly progress and will frequently be associated with a secondary bacteremia.

The organisms that colonize the lower alimentary canal are gram-negative bacilli such as *Escherichia coli, Klebsiella pneumoniae,* and occasionally *Pseudomonas aeruginosa.* These are three of the most common pathogens causing infection in the patient who is granulocytopenic.[6] In the upper respiratory tract, *Staphylococcus aureus* is a common nasopharyngeal colonizer and a frequent cause of infection in the pharynx and lung. There are dramatic microbial flora shifts in individuals who are ill. These changes allow gram-negative bacilli to colonize the upper alimentary canal and respiratory tract and frequently produce infections in the pharynx, esophagus, and lung. Under the added pressure of broad-spectrum antibiotics, the opportunity for overgrowth by yeasts such as *Candida species* and *Torulopsis glabrata* is enhanced. Pharyngitis, esophagitis, and enterocolitis caused by these yeasts and primary pneumonitis caused by *Torulopsis* may ensue. Broad-spectrum antibiotics can also suppress the normal microbial flora of the upper airways. This allows for the growth of filamentous fungi such as *Aspergillus,* which may cause infection either locally in the nose and sinuses or in the lower respiratory tract.[7] Coagulase-negative staphylococci are now frequent pathogens among patients with cancer.[8,9] This organism, a normal skin flora component, has become more prominent because of an increase in the use of long-term indwelling central venous catheters (e.g., Hickman catheters) and as the result of antibiotic induced microbial flora shifts. These changes in flora result in the occurrence of pneumonias, esophagitis, enterocolitis and bacteremias due to these organisms. The frequent difficulty in differentiating a pathogen from contaminant and the high degree of antibiotic resistance of these organisms has made therapy of such infections a difficult challenge.

The patient who is granulocytopenic is also the patient who often has substantial skin damage from long-term central venous catheters, chemotherapy infusions, venipunctures, bone marrow aspirations, and other iatrogenic procedures that damage the skin. Even minor skin trauma such as that caused by axillary shaving, especially when accentuated by occlusive antiperspirants, predisposes to local invasion followed by systemic dissemination of locally colonizing organisms.

1.2. Cellular Immune Dysfunction

Patients such as those with Hodgkins or non-Hodgkin lymphoma or the acquired immunodeficiency syndrome (AIDS) have an inherent abnormality in cellular immune function.[10,11] Alternatively a dysfunction of cellular immune mechanisms may develop as a result of drug or irradiation therapy (e.g. treatment for lymphoma or vasculitis) or the immunosuppression associated with organ transplantation (e.g., marrow, renal, cardiac, liver). A relatively few species of microorganisms tend to cause infection in these settings. These pathogenic agents are more or less common, depending on the specific predisposed host. Most of these organisms are intracellular parasites and include five types of bacteria; e.g., *Listeria monocytogenes, Salmonella* other than *S. typhosa, Nocardia asteroides,* and mycobacteria (both *M. tuberculosis* and the atypical forms, e.g., *avium-intracellulare*), and *Legionella;* one yeast, e.g., *Cryptococcus neoformans,* plus reactivated *Histoplasma capsulatum* and *Coccidioides immitis;* five viruses, e.g., varicella-zoster virus (VZV), cytomegalovirus (CMV), Epstein–Barr virus (EBV), herpes simplex virus (HSV), and adenovirus; three protozoa, e.g., *Pneumocystis carinii, Toxoplasma gondii,* and *Cryptosporidium;* and one helminth, e.g., *Strongyloides stercoralis.*

It is important to emphasize that, although relatively rare, these infections should always be considered in the patient with cellular immune dysfunction. Many of these infections represent reactivation of a latent or dorman organism. *Mycobacterium tuberculosis* is perhaps the best-known example in which immunosuppression is associated with reactivation and development of either local or widespread infection. In a manner similar to *M. tuberculosis, Histoplasma capsulatum, Toxoplasma gondii,* and *Listeria monocytogenes* may be reactivated from macrophages, VZV from the dorsal root ganglia, HSV from sensory root ganglia, *Pneumocystis carinii* from the lung, and CMV from a number of possible dormant foci, including neutrophils, marrow, and renal allografts. These infections may represent new infection following primary or repeat exposure but because of the deficit in host defense, these infections both primary and recurrent will be more severe, and often involve more organ systems than in the normal host.

1.3. Humoral Immune Dysfunction

Certain disease states have an associated abnormality of the humoral immune system. Patients with multiple myeloma are hypogammaglobulinemic but produce an abnormal monoclonal protein that does not possess opsonizing ability against *Streptococcus pneumoniae* or *Hemophilus influezae*. It is interesting that the patient with myeloma may have either no infections with *Pneumococcus* or may have recurrent infections with the same serotype.[12] In the former instance, either effective antibody was produced or exposure did not occur. In the latter, antibody to specific serotypes was not produced, or, for some reason, exposure to the same serotype occurred without adequate antibody production.

1.4. Obstruction to Natural Body Passages

Partial obstruction of a body orifice or passage will lead to infection because of the stasis of body fluids and overgrowth of organisms that may be colonizing nearby. Among the most common forms of obstruction are those of the urinary tract caused by prostatic, ovarian, cervical, or rectal carcinoma leading to urinary tract infection and primary or metastatic tumor of the lung predisposing to postobstructive pneumonia. Other examples are ascending colangitis secondary to obstruction of the biliary tree by lymphoma or pancreatic tumor or otitis media secondary to auditory tube blockage by adenoidal

tissue in lymphocytic leukemia, or non-Hodgkin lymphoma.

1.5. Breech of Body Barriers

These common events predispose to infection in many medical or surgical patients and deserve brief reemphasis here as a reminder that the immunocompromised patient is the same patient who is most likely to have a urinary, venous, or arterial catheter or to suffer skin or periosteum damage by procedures such as venipuncture or bone marrow aspirations.

Consideration of these iatrogenic predisposing factors assists in identifying or providing the explanation for the site of infection. The patient with granulocytopenia who has concurrent alimentary tract mucosal damage is likely to develop infection in the oral cavity, esophagus, lower colon or perianum. Chemotherapeutic effects on the mucociliary escalator are important in the pathogenesis of infection within the lung. Skin infections can be expected if patients who are granulocytopenic are subjected to venipunctures, marrow aspirations, and finger sticks. The multiple blood product transfusions necessary for the support of these patients are associated with viral hepatitis. The patient with a solid tumor, either local or disseminated, is a more likely candidate for infection related to obstruction; the patient with lymphoma, AIDS, or renal transplant is more likely to develop an infection associated with cellular immune dysfunction. The patient with myeloma or chronic lymphocytic leukemia often will have abnormalities of humoral immune function and is more likely to develop a pneumococcal bacteremia, whereas the patient with acute leukemia is most likely to develop infections secondary to granulocytopenia. The patient undergoing marrow transplantation is unique. They suffer serial immune deficiencies which predisposes them to different pathogenic organisms based on the specific post-transplant period. The major predisposing factors during the initial 4–6 weeks after transplant are granulocytopenia, iatrogenic procedures, and disruption of the mucosal barrier.[13] The risk of infections due to pathogens controlled by cellular immunity increases (with the exception of HSV infections) from weeks four to twelve, although graft-versus-host disease will cause further mucosal disruption and may slow the reconstitution of cellular immunity.[14] Humoral dysfunction is most prominent during weeks 10–50.[13]

2. Origin of Infecting Organisms

Eighty percent of infections are caused by organisms that have colonized at or near the site where infection ultimately develops. This has been shown for the patient with acute leukemia through the use of repetitive surveillance culturing (weekly or twice weekly culturing of the nose, gingiva, rectum, and axillae with complete identification of all morphologically distinct colonial isolates) during the period of hospitalization.[4,15] For example, a perianal cellulitis and bacteremia caused by *Pseudomonas aeruginosa* usually can be shown to have been preceded by rectal colonization by this organism. Similarly, a bacterial pneumonia usually will have been preceeded by oral or nasal colonization with the infecting organism. Most staphylococcal skin lesions occurring at sites of skin trauma tend to occur in patients who have nasal colonization with this organism. *Candida* pharyngitis and esophagitis occur more frequently in patients heavily colonized with *Candida* species in the oral cavity,[16] and some cases of *Aspergillus flavus* pneumonia have been found to be preceded by upper airway or nasal colonization.[7]

Thus, surveillance culturing, although expensive, can in some settings be useful in the patient at high risk of infection; e.g., the patient with acute nonlymphocytic leukemia receiving induction chemotherapy. This serial information allows the physician to better select empirical antibiotic therapy should fever develop during granulocytopenia. Even greater accuracy in selection of empirical antimicrobial therapy is possible if antibiotic susceptibility tests have been performed on surveillance culture isolates of those organisms that commonly cause infection. For example, a patient heavily colonized with *Klebsiella pneumoniae* could be treated with a combination of a cephalosporin plus an aminoglycoside, whereas a patient heavily colonized with *Pseudomonas aeruginosa* should be treated empirically with an antipseudonomal penicillin and an aminoglycoside. Knowledge of the antibiotic susceptibilities of colonizing organisms allows one to make empirical antibiotic choices that take the presence of antibiotic resistance into account.

Serial surveillance cultures have also been helpful in defining the degree to which patients become infected with their own endogenous organisms or with organisms that have been acquired during hospitalization. Comprehensive information is available for patients with acute leukemia or those undergoing marrow transplantation.[17–19] In these patients housed in a standard hospital setting, it has been found that organisms are acquired at a relatively steady rate throughout therapy and are frequently the common enteric gram-negative bacilli (e.g., *E. coli*, *K. pneumoniae*, *P. aeruginosa*), coagulase-positive and -negative staphylococci, yeasts (*C. species* and *T. glabrata*), and to a lesser degree, filamentous fungi (*Aspergillus* and Rhizopus). All these organisms have the potential to cause infection in the patient who is granulocytopenic.

In a series of 48 consecutive patients with acute nonlymphocytic leukemia, 87 organisms were isolated from 34 microbiologically documented infections of which about 40 (~ 50%) had an associated bacteremia. Nearly all infections occurred during periods of granulocytopenia and two-thirds were caused by gram-negative bacilli. Surveillance culturing demonstrated that of 29 patients colonized with *Pseudomonas aeruginosa*, 16 subsequently developed a bacteremia.[4] Similarly, of 42 patients colonized with *Klebsiella* species, only six developed bacteremia. Three of the 42 patients colonized with *E. coli*, two of 26 colonized with *S. aureus*, and nine of 29 colonized with *Pseudomonas* species other than *P. aeruginosa* were bacteremic. These data indicate that not only do most infections in these patients occur at levels of profound granulocytopenia but most infections develop from among some, but not all, of those organisms that colonize the patient at or near the site of ultimate infection. Among the most threatening for these patients has been *P. aeruginosa*, for which colonization has had a high predictive value for the development of infection and bacteremia.[4,19]

Overall, 17 organisms isolated from bacteremias and 23 from nonbacteremic, mirobiologically documented infections (total of 40) were the same as those isolated from surveillance cultures during the first week of hospitalization, suggesting that these 40 infections arose from the patient's endogenous flora. Twenty-two bacteremias plus 13 nonbacteremic microbiologically documented infections (total of 35) arose from the 285 organisms that had been previously shown by surveillance cultures to have been acquired during hospitalization. Therefore, not only do these patients acquire multiple organisms from the hospital environment, but nearly one-half of the microbiologically documented infections will be caused by these hospital-acquired organisms.[4,20–23] The use of serial surveillance cultures remains controversial, with some studies demonstrating a poor positive predictive value for many organisms.[24] Yet *P. aeruginosa, K. pneumonia, C. tropicalis,* and *T. glabrata* have routinely been found to have a significant correlation with colonization and the eventual development of infection. The positive predictive values for these organisms had ranged from 0.40 to 0.75, with negative predictive values approaching 1.00.[4,16,19,25] Certainly, the mode by which surveillance cultures are obtained and processed is important but, short of research purposes, surveillance cultures are not necessary for every patient with cancer. However, for those patients at significant risk of infection, e.g., acute leukemia undergoing induction chemotherapy, serial surveillance cultures of nose, gingiva, and rectum can be helpful. Cultures of the nose, gingiva, and rectum should be obtained prior to the patient entering the period of granulocytopenia and continued weekly through the period of risk. All organisms with a high likelihood of causing infection: enteric gram-negative bacilli, *Staphylococcus* species, yeast, filamentous fungi, or organisms isolated in pure growth should be identified, with specific antimicrobial susceptibilities determined.

The epidemiology of the origin of infection is important to the clinician in designing an approach to infection prevention. Recognizing that one-half of all pathogenic organisms will be acquired while the patient is hospitalized emphasizes the need to employ measures to reduce the acquisition of new organisms by this patient population. Similarly, the recognition that one-half of the infections are caused by organisms already colonizing the patient, especially along the alimentary canal, supports the logic of attempting to suppress the pathogenic, colonizing, alimentary canal organisms. The recognition that most *Staphylococcus aureus* infections are preceded by nasal colonization suggests that attempts to eradicate the nasal carrier state at least during periods of granulocytopenia may be helpful. It is important to emphasize that these concepts relate specifically to the infections that occur in the setting of granulocytopenia and particularly in patients with acute leukemia or those undergoing marrow transplantation. Very few data regarding colonization by potentially infecting organisms are available for patients who have cellular immune or humoral immune dysfunction, although a recent observation among patients with AIDS suggests that the presence of oral candidiasis is highly predictive of the presence of invasive candida esophagitis.

2.1. Shifts in Microbial Flora

At least three factors can lead to major shifts in microbial flora: the underlying disease, invasive techniques employed, and the use of antibiotics. The underlying disease itself, for reasons not fully understood, can lead to substantial changes in the organisms colonizing at a given site.

In a simple but elegant study by Johanson et al.[26] throat cultures were obtained from normal volunteers (firemen), patients hospitalized on a psychiatric ward, patients hospitalized on an orthopedic ward, patients on a medical ward with major illnesses such as myocardial infarction, and patients on a medical ward with major illnesses who were receiving antimicrobial therapy. Among firemen and psychiatric ward patients, the throat cultures showed normal flora. However, 16% of the orthopedic ward patients harbored gram-negative bacilli in their throat cultures, as did 57% of the medical patients and 80% of patients receiving antimicrobial therapy.

These data suggest that hospitalization per se does not necessarily lead to shifts in the microbial flora of the throat but that illness does cause a shift of microbial populations so that with increasing degrees of medical or surgical illness the pharynx will become colonized with gram-negative bacilli. The addition of antimicrobial therapy to the seriously ill individual further encourages colonization of the hypopharynx with gram-negative bacilli. In further studies by Johanson and others, changes in the squamous epithelial cells of the buccal mucosa were shown during illness to allow stronger attachment of gram-negative bacilli with the partial exclusion of normal flora such as hemolytic streptococci.

At the Baltimore Cancer Research Center (BCRC), now the University of Maryland Cancer

Center (UMCC), serial surveillance cultures of the axillae have shown that patients at the time of admission are usually colonized with organisms such as *Staphylococcus epidermidis* and *Corynebacterium* species. As the patient's illness progresses the flora begins to shift toward gram-negative bacilli. The severely ill patient's local flora will be composed primarily of gram-negative bacilli and occasionally of yeasts such as *Candida albicans*. The mechanism for these flora shifts is unknown, but it is not simply a manifestation of reduced hygiene. Patients with mycosis fungoides are a population in which the skin in heavily colonized with *Staphylococcus aureus*. This skin colonization is related presumably to skin abnormalities with multiple lesions and dead or dying skin which serve as a satisfactory vehicle for *Staphylococcus aureus*. As a result, the most common cause of infectious death in these patients is staphylococcal bacteremia.

Invasive procedures can also lead to shifts of microbial flora. Insertion of a urinary catheter or intravenous catheter creates a pathway along which organisms that are normally excluded can enter. Recent evaluations of pneumonias in patients with tracheostomies have shown that the pharynx and larynx in such patients will become colonized with gram-negative bacilli within a few days after the insertion of such prosthestic devices. Should pneumonia develop in these patients, it generally is caused by the same type of gram-negative bacilli that colonized the hypopharynx.[27]

Antibiotics notoriously produce a shift in microbial flora. In an evaluation by van der Waaij, 10 patients were monitored with surveillance cultures while receiving ampicillin for 3 weeks.[28] The oropharynx of these patients rapidly became colonized with gram-negative bacilli. Many of these isolates were multiply antibiotic-resistant strains; by the end of the 3 weeks, 9 of the 10 patients had become colonized by ampicillin-resistant Enterobacteriaceae. The concurrent control group who did not receive antibiotics had only one patient acquire a multiresistant bacteria during the study period.

The University of Maryland Cancer Center has used gentamicin, vancomycin, and nystatin (GVN) to suppress alimentary canal microbial flora.[29] This has been clinically effective, but the acquisition of gentamicin-resistant gram-negative bacilli has remained a problem. Among 87 consecutive patient trials on study for a mean of 94 days (of which 71% were days on which the absolute granulocyte count was less than $1000/\mu l$, and 40% were days with less than $100/\mu l$), a total of 274 potential pathogens were acquired.[30] This represents a rather low rate of acquisition with a mean frequency of 3.1 new organisms per patient or approximately one new potential pathogen every 30 days. Yet, 16 of these patients became colonized with 31 gentamicin-resistant gram-negative bacilli. These organisms represent 12% of the total acquired potential pathogens and 30% of the 104 acquired gram-negative bacilli. Twenty-eight of these 31 gentamicin-resistant gram-negative bacilli were resistant at the time of acquisition. Therefore, resistance did not emerge, but rather the microbial vacuum created by the oral nonabsorbable antibiotic regimen allowed for the acquisition and subsequent colonization by gentamicin-resistant gram-negative bacilli from the hospital environment. Concurrently, other patients at the UMCC/BCRC not ingesting the GVN regimen and not receiving other systemic or oral antibiotics only occasionally acquired gentamicin-resistant gram-negative bacilli.

A concept known as colonization resistance has been described by van der Waaij and colleagues as an outgrowth of studies of gnotobiotic animals.[28,31] These investigators noted that the anaerobic flora of the alimentary canal in association with "other factors" help to prevent colonization by new organisms. Animals with their own normal aerobic and anaerobic microbial flora resist intestinal colonization by an aerobic gram-negative bacillus given orally at very high inocula (10^7), whereas germfree animals can be colonized when fed as few as 10–100 organisms. If germfree animals are colonized first with a normal anaerobic flora, these animals then resist colonization almost as well as the animals with a completely normal alimentary tract flora composed of both aerobes and anaerobes.

Other factors affecting colonization resistance include the degree of peristalsis, formation of volatile fatty acids, damage to the mucosal lining of the gastrointestinal tract, and probably dysfunction of local lymphoid tissue and its production of mucosal immunoglobulins. In patients, the use of antibiotics that suppress the anaerobic flora may alter the degree of colonization resistance, so that those organisms acquired from the hospital setting can rapidly colonize the alimentary canal. Concurrently, if the mucosa are damaged, certain colonizing organisms such as *Pseudomonas aeruginosa* can then penetrate, produce a local infection and because of the absence of effective numbers of granulocytes may rapidly progress to bacteremia.

The recognition that these types of shifts in microbial flora occur can be helpful in predicting the types of infection that may occur and in designing approaches to infection prevention. The potential importance of the concept of colonization resistance will be discussed further as a technique for preventing infection.

2.2. Sources of Acquisition of Exogenous Organisms

Of the five Fs (food, fingers, feces, flies, and fomites) traditionally taught to be the source of bacterial spread within a population, food undoubtedly remains one of the most important. The ingestion of microorganisms by an immunocompromised host whose gut flora may have been temporarily suppressed by antimicrobial therapy provides an ideal setting for enhancing the colonization with organisms from exogenous sources. The extended suppression of enteric flora through the use of oral nonabsorbable antibiotics sets the stage for colonization of the gut by microorganisms resistant to the antibiotics used.

A number of ubiquitous gram-negative organisms are uncommonly found in the GI of man but are present in soil and water and on plants and thus appear frequently in fresh foods. *P. aeruginosa* is an opportunistic pathogen for both plants and animals. *Enterobacter, Klebsiella, Citrobacter,* and *Serratia* are among the gram-negative rods often found on vegetables. Mixed salads prepared from such vegetables often contain a wide variety of microorganisms, e.g., a not-unusual chicken salad from our hospital kitchen yielded *S. faecalis, P. aeruginosa, P. fluorescens, K. oxytoca, P. mirabilis,* and *E. agglomerans,* in quantities over 2×10^5 cfu/g, as well as α-hemolytic streptococci, *Bacillus* spp., diphtheroids, and rare colonies of *Aspergillus flavus* and *Candida krusei.*

Although the utilization of cooked foods eliminates these sources of contamination, experience teaches that food presented to patients must be monitored with vigilance. The sudden switch of the hospital supplier of fruit juices to an unpasturized brand that contained large numbers of several varieties of *Candida* as well as occasional colonies of *Serratia* and *Enterobacter*; whipped topping that contained *K. pneumoniae, E. cloacae,* and *Actinobacter*; cream of chicken soup with *E. cloacae, E. coli,* and *P. fluorescens,* and snack sandwiches with large numbers of *Aspergillus* spores are a few examples of unexpected microbial contamination that we have encountered. High bacterial counts will also develop rapidly in outdated milk and milk products.

The microorganisms that are present on plants may colonize man not only through the ingestion of fresh foods as described but also by means of flowers, especially African violets and chrysanthemums,[32] and their vases or containers.[33] In one study, counts of gentamicin-resistant bacteria in flower vases on a surgical ward reached 8×10^6 cfu/ml H_2O.[33] Water from such vases which is changed and discarded into hand basins or toilets with its accompanying splash will heavily contaminate the surrounding area.

Microbes generally do not survive in the environment in the absence of moisture or the protection of proteinaceous covering unless they produce spores, possess larger amounts of lipid in their cell walls, or resist the effects of drying by some other means. Water not only serves as a reservoir for bacteria, but it also promotes transmission of many organisms. Distilled water is often used to store cultures of *P. aeruginosa* because they will remain viable in it for many months. Some atypical mycobacteria are capable of multiplication in distilled water and from this source may contaminate hemodialysis or pharmaceutical preparations.[34] Tap water generally contains only a few viable bacteria, but because of the danger of contamination by *Pseudomonas* or *Flavobacterium,* particularly in the presence of faucet aerators, it is not safe for patient use without sterilization.[35] Similarly, ice machines or ice contaminated by improper handling can be a source of exogenous organisms. A minor outbreak of *P. aeruginosa* at the University of Maryland Cancer Center was traced to a contaminated ice machine, and disappearance of the organism from the patient population coincided with decontamination of this dispenser.

Microorganisms present in the air have two basic sources, man and the environment. Individuals with a cough because of respiratory infection, smoking, or bronchiectasis project many bacteria-containing particles into the air. Traditionally, viruses that cause upper respiratory infection and *S. pneumoniae, K. pneumoniae, S. aureus,* and *Mycobacterium* are known to spread in this manner. Ill patients will also be colonized with gram-negative bacilli and yeasts so that these, too, may be spread by their coughing. Whether these organisms will become a source of exogenous spread is dependent on their concentration in the air and on the size of the particles in which they are contained. Particles larger than 15 μm in diameter fall to the floor fairly promptly, from where they may become airborne again if disturbed. Droplets of the smallest size range, less than 5 μm, remain suspended almost indefinitely and tend to penetrate the respiratory tract most deeply.[36] Nebulizers and humidifiers that become contaminated can be a source of a large number of contaminated air-borne particles.

Another important exogenous air-borne organisms are the *Aspergillus* ssp. *Aspergillus* is second only to *Candida,* causing fungal infections among patients who are immunosuppressed. Although *Aspergillus* spores are ubiquitous and present in great abundance in the outside air during the fall season when leaves are decomposing, they have also been found to have caused an unusually large number of infections among granulocytopenic leukemia patients when they were being hospitalized in a new hospital building where fireproofing material was contaminated with *Aspergillus* spores.[38]

Legionnaires' disease is another infection that has a high case fatality rate among immunosuppressed patients and is spread via air-borne routes. Cases relating to construction where soil was disturbed, contamination of cooling tower water or shower head faucets with *Legionella* species have all been reported.[39,40]

The skin is also a frequent site colonized by exogenous organisms. Persons with dermatologic conditions such as acne, eczema, or seborrhea are often colonized by *Staphylococcus aureus.* These persistent carriers will frequently disseminate the organism.[41] A patient with an underlying disease with cutaneous manifestations (e.g., mycosis fungoides) that becomes colonized with *S. aureus* sheds skin fragments containing large numbers of organisms into the environment. We have been able to trace the movement of such patients down corridors, in and out of rooms, and to detect the chairs in which they were seated by the presence of their particular phage type of *S. aureus.* Hurst and Sutter,[42] studied the survival of *P. aeruginosa* in burn eschar. They showed that the bacterial counts of mop water from hospital floors where burned patients had been hospitalized decreased from 12×10^5 cfu/ml at 5 days after discharge to none by week 8. However, pieces of burned eschar collected from the floor at 8 weeks still contained 3.7×10^6 cfu/cm^3 of *P. aeruginosa.* Crevices and corners of the floor not easily cleansed by standard mopping may provide a nidus where microorganisms survive for long periods.

The skin of the hands has been known to be a source of microorganisms since Semmelweis (1818–1865) first attributed the spread of puerperal fever to the contaminated hands of attending physicians. Although the skin of the hands generally is colonized only by *S. epidermidis* and diptheroids, unscrubbed nail beds may become colonized with alpha streptococci or other bacteria. However, the concern is that hands will be a conveyor of organisms. Organisms from the mouth, nose, or other colonized sites are transferred by hand contact to other paramedical persons or patients.

A source of exogenous organisms that can cause skin contamination and/or colonization is cosmetics. Although most commercial products contain bacteriostatic substances, under certain conditions lotions or cosmetics may become heavily contaminated. Morse and Schonbeck reported finding a variety of gram-negative bacilli from hand creams after the initial discovery that an outbreak of *K. pneumoniae* septicemia had been caused by contaminated lanolin hand cream.[43] In our experience, lotions used for body massage were often found to have $>10^5$ colony forming units of *S. marcescens* per milliliter. Investigation determined that the producer had eliminated the bacteriostatic agent without informing the pharmacy. Such unexpected events may allow the sudden spread of exogenous organisms if not detected early.

Other sources of exogenous organisms are instruments such as endoscopes that may be inadequately decontaminated between patient use.[45] Whirlpools, nebulizers, and oxygen equipment can be readily contaminated with organisms, particularly with *P. aeruginosa.*[46] Splash from sink drains may contain a variety of pseudomonads or other organisms that have contaminated the drain trap.[47] In the same fashion, the flushing action of toilets may cause aerosols that contain fecal organisms (S. C. Schimpff and J. C. Wade, unpublished data). Survival rates of gram-negative bacteria on surfaces such as floors or tables are directly related to relative humidity.[48] Disinfectants used for decontamination may also contain organisms resistant to the disinfectant.[49–5)] Liquid soaps and antiseptic creams have been reported to be contaminated with *P. aeruginosa*.

Occasionally, materials used for intravenous infusions have also been contaminated with organisms such as *Enterobacter, E. agglomerans,* and *Serratia.* Blood products in particular are carriers of microorganisms present in the donor. The development of hepatitis B, non-A, non-B hepatitis, CMV infections, and acquired immunodeficiency syndrome are well-recognized complications of blood product infusion.

3. Infection Prevention: Effective but Complex Techniques

3.1. Reverse Isolation in Laminar Airflow Rooms or Other Forms of Complete Barrier Isolation

The simplest yet most efficient system for total reverse isolation is the laminar airflow room, in which an entire wall is composed of high-efficiency particulate air (HEPA) filters through which air is forced in a laminar or at least unidirectional pattern. The filters remove all particles greater than $0.3/\mu m$ and thus eliminate all bacteria, fungi and even some of the larger viruses. Through brownian movement, smaller viral particles may also be removed. This results in a room with essentially sterile air that is being constantly renewed and that can exit only at points at the end of the room opposite to the filter bank.[52]

Bodey and Johnston[53] have shown that a standard hospital room may have about 3000 potential pathogens per 1000 ft^3 of air. A laminar airflow room has almost sterile air, with most samples showing no organisms, but on occasion may have as many as 15 organisms per 1000 ft^3 of air detected during patient occupancy. Not only is the air entering the room sterile, but the constant movement of air tends to

remove any organisms within the patient's environment. In order for this technique to be useful, it is essential that all items brought into the room be sterile or nearly sterile so that the patient is truly in complete reverse isolation. Therefore, all medical and personal items plus water and food must be either sterile or harbor low counts of microorganisms. Many rooms are built with "glove ports," so that the patient can be examined without the examiner actually entering the room; alternatively, medical personnel or visitors must don sterile gloves, gown, mask, cap, and shoe covers before entering the room.

Since about one-half of all infections in the patient with acute leukemia who is granulocytopenic are caused by acquired organisms, the use of laminar air flow rooms predictably should reduce the infection rate by about 50%. Unfortunately, few evaluations of reverse isolation in laminar airflow in the absence of concurrent microbial suppression have been performed. Nevertheless, there is evidence that this form of total reverse isolation does reduce the acquisition of potential pathogens and that infections are decreased by about 50% compared with concurrent randomly allocated control groups.[54,55]

3.2. Microbial Suppression with Oral Nonabsorbable Antibiotics

Microbial suppression can be directed only toward suppression of the alimentary tract organisms with agents such as oral nonabsorbable antibiotics, or it may be attempted intensively using oral nonabsorbable antibiotics, topical and orificial antibiotic sprays, creams, or ointments, and antimicrobial soaps. Among the more frequently used oral nonabsorbable antibiotic regimens have been combinations of gentamicin, vancomycin, and nystatin (GVN), and framycetin or neomycin, colistin, and nystatin (FRACON or NEOCON). Amphotericin B has been substituted for nystatin in certain regimens. Ointments or gels have been prepared for application to anterior nares, gingiva, auditory canals, vagina, and rectum. Antimicrobial soaps have included hexachlorophene, povidone–iodine, and chlorhexadine. Povidone–iodine products have been used as mouthwashes or vaginal douches or as wipettes for axillae, perineum, and perianum. Chlorhexadine has been used in similar fashion.

Four prospective randomized trails have evaluated oral nonabsorbable antibiotics with or without some of these additional techniques of microbial suppression in comparison to an untreated control group.[29,55–57] Two did and two did not detect a reduction in infection in the groups taking the oral nonabsorbable antibiotics. The reason for these disparities is not entirely clear; our own belief is that these agents are effective in substantially reducing the infection rate if liquid preparations are used, if the patient ingests them regularly, and if the patient is at maximum risk of infection because of granulocyte counts of less than $100/\mu l$ that persist for at least 10–14 days.

The liquid preparation is useful because it helps to suppress the oral flora and hence should reduce pharyngitis, esophagitis, and pneumonitis. Regular ingestion is essential because discontinuation will allow for the rapid regrowth of the pathogenic microbial flora. It has been clearly established by these evaluations that oral nonabsorbable antibiotics exert their maximum benefit when the granulocyte count is less than $100/\mu l$, i.e., that period when the patient is at the greatest risk of developing infection. These patients usually have also received very intensive cytotoxic chemotherapy and hence have sustained mucosal damage which further predisposes them to infection along the damaged alimentary canal. Yet there is no advantage in using oral nonabsorbable antibiotics if the period of granulocytopenia will be only a few days or if the degree of granulocytopenia is not profound. Restated, the indications for oral nonabsorbable antibiotics are limited but, in the face of profound persistent granulocytopenia and significant mucosal disruption, these agents can be useful.

There are other disadvantages to the use of oral nonabsorbable antibiotics. The cost of oral gentamicin, vancomycin, and nystatin (GVN) is about $110/day. Malabsorption of glucose, xylose, methotrexate, and other compounds and drugs is a common accompaniment and can be a potential problem, especially if the patient remains granulocytopenic for prolonged periods of time.[58,59] All these agents, especially vancomycin, are distasteful and may lead to nausea and vomiting. This results in poor patient compliance unless the medical and nursing staff insures regular ingestion. If ingestion is discontinued during granulocytopenia, the resultant rapid repopulation of the alimentary canal by aerobic gram-negative bacilli can lead to overwhelming infection.[29] However, it is our belief that in the appropriate patient the benefits outweigh these risks, but a program of surveillance culturing is absolutely essential so that the antibiotic regimen can be adjusted should a resistant organism be acquired. The utilization of oral nonabsorbable antibiotics cannot be considered lightly; it must be instituted only within a setting of appropriate facilities, staff education, and enthusiasm.

3.3. Combined Use of Laminar Airflow Room or Similar Isolation plus Microbial Suppression with Oral Nonabsorbable Antibiotics

Seven prospective randomly controlled evaluations of a laminar airflow room or similar isolation facility plus oral nonabsorbable antibiotics have been conducted in which a control group without reverse isolation or oral nonabsorbable antibiotics administration was included.[29,54–56,60–62] In summary, each of these studies showed a substantial reduction in the number of total and severe infections for patients treated in sterile environments. The acquisition of potential pathogens and the frequency of gram-negative bacteremias were markedly reduced as was the occurrence of pneumonias, perianal lesions, pharyngitis, esophagitis, and colitis. The utility of the air-filtration system was further demonstrated by the finding of no pneumonias caused by *Aspergillus* in any patient treated continuously in a laminar airflow facility.[63,64]

Given the recognized effectiveness of this technology in reducing infection, one must then evaluate the cost versus benefit of such techniques in terms of money, psychological deprivation for the patient, problems of taste and compliance, malabsorption, and acquisition of resistant organisms. Long-term benefit must also be considered (i.e., increased complete remission rates or improved or increased duration of survival) for treatment rendered in these complex settings. The laminar airflow rooms themselves are expensive, although a relatively simple arrangement that encompasses a single patient bed in a plastic tentlike device with HEPA filters constituting one end of the facility can be purchased for about

$10,000. A more comfortable roomlike arrangement costs $40,000–45,000. Other capital expenses include the equipment for sterilizing large numbers of supplies and a system for the production of sterile water. The nursing, clerical, housekeeping, dietary, pharmacy, and microbiology personnel needs are substantially increased by such isolation techniques. To this must be added the cost of the oral nonabsorbable antibiotics. A daily patient cost of about $1,000–1,500/day, excluding the cost of therapeutic antibiotics, would probably be realistic, with the average length of isolation being approximately 30 days.

Psychologically the patients tend to do well. Often patients feel that the isolation technology represents a special attempt to treat them as individuals, adding to their hope for a successful outcome of therapy. Nevertheless, the physical separation will lead to increasing problems once the projected period of isolation is exceeded or if the patient develops additional medical problems.[29,62,65] The problems of patient compliance with the oral nonabsorbable antibiotics remains a problem, but for the isolated patient it is often easier because the laminar airflow room itself acts as a constant reminder of the importance of infection-prevention techniques.[29]

Nevertheless, the complete remission rate for patients with acute leukemia has not improved substantially with the use of these procedures.[64] Most reports have failed to show a reduction in the frequency of graft-versus-host disease or interstitial pneumonitis in patients with bone marrow transplantation.[61,66] A more recent review of infection prophylaxis techniques employed in patients undergoing marrow transplantation at the Fred Hutchinson Cancer Research Center has been more encouraging. Isolation in laminar airflow rooms, with the administration of oral nonabsorbable antibiotics, was found to delay the occurrence of graft-versus-host disease for patients with aplastic anemia who were undergoing marrow transplantation. The incidence of grades II to IV acute graft-versus-host was less for such isolated patients. However, this association was not found for patients with acute leukemia.[66]

Is there, then, any logic in placing patients into such a facility, or should all patients be treated in a standard fashion in a regular hospital room? The answer to this question is not clearcut. The reduction of infection related morbidity and mortality more than outweighs the disadvantages of psychological deprivation for the patient who achieves a complete remission within the usual 30–40 days. Thus, given an available laminar airflow room, it would be logical to use it. On the other hand, the advantages are hard to justify on a cost–benefit basis when one is contemplating the installation of new rooms in nonresearch settings. We would suggest that the studies that have been performed have clearly shown that the concepts of complete reverse isolation and microbial suppression as means of infection prevention are individually and jointly very effective. Additional research is essential to improve the effectiveness while reducing the complexity, cost, and disadvantages of these techniques. With improved yet simplified and less costly means of infection prevention, the question regarding improved remission rates will vanish. Concurrently, when improved approaches to therapy of acute leukemia become available, the means to use that improved therapy with limited infection risk will then be in place.

3.4. Prophylactic Granulocyte Transfusions

For the patient with granulocytopenia, it would seem that the replacement of granulocytes by transfusion should reduce the incidence of infection. Unfortunately, there are major technologic problems in developing a simple and effective program for granulocyte transfusion. Most important, the number of granulocytes that can be produced by the normal bone marrow under the stress of infection cannot be collected even with the present generation of apheresis equipment and pretreatment of donors with agents such as high-dose corticosteroids. Second, the transfusion of granulocytes from a non-HLA-identical donor can lead to rapid alloimmunization of the patient, making platelet transfusion support more difficult.[68]

A number of studies of prophylactic granulocyte transfusions have been published. In two trials, granulocytes were transfused on a daily basis; in both trials, infections were shown to be reduced compared with an appropriate control.[69,70] Three other trials have used intermittent schedules of transfusion, generally every other day, with one suggesting a possible reduction of infection and two being inconclusive.[68,71,72] In a study by Clift and colleagues,[69] granulocytes from HLA-identical relatives were transfused on a daily basis following bone marrow transplantation until marrow engraftment had occurred. The technological problems were substantial, including the need for arteriovenous shunts in the donors, and the development of a significant degree of anemia among the donors. The mean number of granulocytes per transfusion was 15.7×10^9, with an average of 12 transfusions per patient. The 29 transfused patients had a total of two infections, whereas 40 control patients had a total of 17 infections ($p < 0.05$). No septicemias occurred in the transfused group, but 10 occurred in the control group ($p < 0.005$). Winston et al.[73] also employed daily prophylactic granulocyte transfusions in a group of uninfected marrow transplant patients. These workers found no benefit for transfused patients with regard to the number of febrile days, days on antibiotics, or the frequency of infection. This study, and a later evaluation from the Seattle marrow transplant group, however, noted a substantial increase in the frequency of CMV infections among the recipients of granulocyte transfusions.[73,74]

In the study by Schiffer et al.,[68] noninfected adults receiving their initial remission-induction chemotherapy for ANLL were randomized to receive either platelet transfusions alone or platelet transfusions plus prophylactic granulocyte transfusions on an every-other-day schedule. Granulocytes were obtained by intermittent centrifugation; each patient received an average dose of 1.5×10^{10} granulocytes. These Baltimore Cancer Research Center patients were receiving concurrent oral nonabsorbable antibiotics. Before the study had progressed far enough to evaluate this method of infection prevention adequately, it was recognized that the transfused patients who received granulocytes were developing significantly more transfusion reactions and that infusion related fever and chills were common. Alloimmunization was common and apparently related to the use of random donors rather than HLA-matched donors for leukophoresis. This high incidence of alloimmunization clearly indicated that any attempt at prophylactic granulocyte transfusions must be done with HLA-identical donors to prevent this complication. In effect, this negates the possibility of prophylactic granulocyte transfusions except in the difficult-to-achieve setting where all donors are HLA matched.

4. Ineffective Techniques of Infection Prevention

"Standard" Reverse Isolation

Illogical procedures have been used for years as infection prevention techniques for the patient who is granulocytopenic. The most common of these is the initiation of reverse isolation in a regular patient room once the patient's granulocyte count drops below $1000/\mu l$. Assuming first that this type of reverse isolation would be useful, it makes relatively little sense to place the patient in isolation only after the granulocyte count has reached its low point. Until this time, the patient has had ample opportunity to become colonized with potential pathogens from the hospital environment, and these pathogens can cause infection once the granulocyte count decreases. If reverse isolation is to be effective, it would have to be instituted at the time the patient is first brought into the hospital. Moreover, most single-room reverse isolation procedures do not interfere with the major routes of acquisition of the potential pathogens that cause infection in the granulocytopenic patients. Although staff members are required to wear gowns, gloves, masks, and booties, which will reduce the transfer of organisms from staff to patients, little or no attention is paid to supplies in the room that may be contaminated, nor is attention paid to food and water, two of the most common sources of potential pathogens.[75]

5. "Simplified" and Effective Techniques of Infection Prevention

The effectiveness of oral nonabsorbable antibiotics, of reverse isolation in laminar airflow rooms, of the combined use of both techniques and of prophylactic granulocyte transfusions has been inconsistent. Each of these techniques has provided variable degrees of infection reduction, but each has major disadvantages. What is needed, then, are some simple infection-prevention techniques that can be used by any physician, in any hospital, at reasonable expense and with minimal negative effect upon the patient. These types of measures are important and should not be ignored even if more extensive prophylactic techniques (e.g., prophylactic antibiotics) are employed.

Reduction of the Acquisition of New Organisms

A low microbial diet is important in reducing the number of new organisms acquired during the hospital stay (Table 1). All foods with few exceptions should be thoroughly cooked, placed on sterile dishes and trays, and covered during delivery to the patient. Filtered sterile water or bottled water should be used for drinking purposes, and ice used to cool beverages should be prepared from this sterile water, and ice making machines should be screened for microbial contaminants.

The quality of air relative to its microbial content is directly related to the air-handling system and the effectiveness of the housekeeping cleaning procedures. Positive air pressure should be maintained in all patients' rooms to prevent air-borne bacteria and spores from entering the rooms from more highly contaminated hallways. Air-conditioning filters should be changed or decontaminated on a regularly scheduled basis whether central or room air conditioners are used. Housekeeping equipment that tends to redisperse microorganisms into the air, such as brooms and brushes, are to be avoided, and wet versus damp-mopping procedures using a double-bucket system to kill and remove microorganisms that have settled to the floor should be employed.

Dirty linens must never be shaken but should be carefully folded when removed from the bed. One should be aware that dirty linen laundry chutes may create currents of air with high numbers of microorganisms that can contaminate adjacent areas unexpectedly. Dust generally contains large numbers of bacteria and, occasionally, fungal spores. The presence of lint or minute fibers often permits survival of microorganisms or spores for a longer than the usual time. It follows that clutter should be avoided to permit proper cleaning and decontamination procedures. Phenolic disinfectants have been found to be most effective for decontamination of floors and surfaces in our experience. But the purpose of the disinfectant will be defeated if it is not used in the concentration recommended or if mopheads, buckets, and other equipment are not kept clean and in order.

Also of importance in the reduction of acquisi-

TABLE 1. Cooked Food Diet

Food item	Foods allowed	Foods not allowed
Soups	Cooked hot soups, homemade or canned, canned cold consomme	Cold soups from fresh vegetables
Meat, fish, poultry	Cooked, well-done gravies and sauces, well-cooked bacon, sausage	Raw meat; meat or fish salads
Cheese	Slices, processed American cheese	Natural cheeses
Eggs	Cooked any style	Uncooked eggs
Breads	All bread, rolls, crackers in wrappers	
Cereals	Cooked or boxed cold	
Vegetables	Cooked any style	Raw vegetables; salads
Fruits	Canned, cooked thick-skinned fruits (e g., bananas, decontaminated and peeled under aseptic conditions)	Fresh, frozen, and dried fruits
Desserts and other sweets	All cooked or baked goods; Jell-O, honey, syrup, sugar, ice cream and sherbet made from sterile or pasteurized products	Whipped topping, cream-filled candy
Beverages	Coffee, decaffeinated coffee, hot tea, canned or bottled carbonated beverages, canned fruit juices, pasteurized milk, buttermilk	Instant iced tea
Miscellaneous	Salt, vinegar, catsup, mustard, autoclaved pepper, pickles, gelatin, pasteurized yogurt	Uncooked herbs and spices; black pepper

tion of microorganisms is the proper decontamination of inanimate objects and surfaces such as thermometers and instruments used in patient care. Thermometers should remain in the patient's room and be disinfected with 70% ethyl alcohol or isopropyl alcohol with 0.2% iodine. Used instruments must be thoroughly cleaned to remove organic debris prior to gas sterilization for sterility to be achieved by this technique.

Perhaps of most importance is handwashing before and after contact with each patient. During handwashing, dirt and contaminating microorganisms are mechanically removed by sudsing, friction, and flushing with running water. Hand disinfectant foams and creams are also available and can be effective in destroying bacteria on the hands of hospital personnel between patient contacts if sinks are not readily available. These disinfectants generally have a buildup effect so that after several days' usage, very few microorganisms can be isolated from cultures of the individual hands. Contamination of the hands and skin by the use of contaminated hand lotions and creams can be avoided through the use of proper bacteriostatic agents and of a system of unit aliquots of the material provided for each patient.

The patient who receives chemotherapy that results in severe suppression of platelets and granulocytes is placed at potential risk of developing a variety of infections agents through transfusions of blood and blood products.[76] Viral hepatitis caused by hepatitis B virus or non-A, non-B hepatitis virus are two of the major hazards posed by transfusions, although with the advent of marrow and organ transplantation cytomegalovirus has become of equal concern.

Prior to the advent of sensitive serological techniques to detect hepatitis B viral antigen in the blood of prospective blood donors, infection caused by transfusions of infected blood was a common event. All prospective blood donors are presently screened by the sensitive radioimmunassay (RIA) technique. By eliminating the risk of hepatitis B viral antigen in the blood of prospective blood donors, infection caused by this virus has diminished. Commercial sources of blood, blood plasma, and blood platelets that use a number of donors still afford considerable risk of hepatitis caused by a virus that is neither hepatitis A nor B.[76] A lesser risk is posed by a volunteer blood donor pool. Body fluids, secretions, or excretions of a person infected with type B hepatitis virus contain the virus and parenteral and percutaneous modes of transmission involving minor abrasions of skin or mucous membranes occur.[39] Favero et al.[77] demonstrated that hepatitis B surface antigen

(HBsAg) present in the environment is remarkably stable. In areas where blood is handled extensively, the antigen has been detected on such varied objects as clamps, scissors, telephones, walls, centrifuge, and cups.[78] Particular attention in areas where blood or blood products are handled must be given to adequate disinfection of spillage and of contaminated instruments and surfaces. Appropriate isolation techniques must be instituted for the infected patient.

Cytomegalovirus can also be transmitted by blood transfusions, and, although the prevalence of rising antibody titers in many of the cancer patients may represent reactivation of latent infection, the importance of blood products as a source of disease should not be overlooked.[73,74] Blood donors for high-risk patients such as those undergoing organ or marrow transplantation should be selected who are seronegative for CMV antibody.

Other microorganisms that potentially (but rarely) can be transferred by blood or blood products are *Salmonella* sp. and the parasite *Toxoplasma gondii*. Although both of these organisms are more frequently acquired by the ingestion of improperly or uncooked food (*T. gondii* through meat products), the serological screening of white blood cell donors for *T. gondii* will eliminate this source of infection. Adequate cooking of the food and the use of the cooked-food diet will eliminate food as an avenue of infection by these agents.

6. Suppression of Potential Pathogens

6.1. Granulocytopenia

The approach to microbial suppression in the granulocytopenic patient includes suppression of the alimentary tract organisms most likely to cause infection, suppression of the organisms on the skin that reside in areas such as the axillae and are frequently associated with infection, suppression or possibly elimination of the staphylococcal nasal carrier state, suppression of filamentous fungi colonizing the upper airways, and periodontal prophylaxis to prevent acute gingival infections.

Consideration of van der Waaij's concept of colonization resistance suggests the usefulness of an approach that would suppress the potentially pathogenic gram-negative bacilli and yeast along the alimentary canal that are the most common causes of infection in the granulocytopenic patient while preserving most of the anaerobic flora and thus reducing the acquisition and subsequent colonization by other organisms with which the patient comes into contact. Urinary antiseptics such as nalidixic acid, oxolinic acid, and pipemidic acid and the antibiotic combination of trimethoprim–sulfamethoxazole, and the new orally absorbed quinolone derivatives, norfloxacin and ciprofloxacin have the capacity to suppress Enterobacteriaceae (norfloxacin, ciprofloxacin, and pipemidic acid will also suppress *Pseudomonas aeruginosa*) along the alimentary canal without reducing the anaerobic flora.[79-81] The experience with long-term administration of some of these agents, e.g., nalidixic acid, trimethoprim–sulfamethoxazole (TMP–SMZ), and norfloxacin, suggests that they are safe and nontoxic, that they do suppress the aerobic Enterobacteriaceae, and that they do not suppress the anaerobes.[80,82]

Hughes et al.,[83] while evaluating the prophylactic potential of TMP–SMZ for *Pneumocystis carinii*, noted that the patients receiving TMP–SMZ, like those receiving placebo, were not at an increased risk or did not become colonized with organisms normally resistant to TMP–SMZ such as *Pseudomonas aeruginosa* or *Candida* species.[83] This suggested that the resistance to colonization remained intact despite the use of this antibiotic combination. In addition, the frequency of bacterial infections in pa-

tients treated with TMP–SMZ was reduced compared with the placebo-treated controls. However, for those patients receiving TMP–SMZ, the frequency of oral candidiasis and disseminated candida infections was increased, confirming the importance of administering an appropriate antifungal agent in combination with such prophylactic antibacterial therapy.

6.2. Prophylactic Trials

6.2.1. Comparison of Trimethoprim–Sulfamethoxazole and a Control Group

Since the initial observations of Hughes and colleagues, there have been nine studies in which trimethoprim–sulfamethoxazole has been compared to either an untreated or placebo-treated group.[84-92] Seven studies have used a study population that included primarily patients with acute leukemia who were undergoing induction chemotherapy (Table 2). The study performed by Gualtieri was a double-blind randomized trial,[85] while the other six were prospective and randomized in design.[84,86-90]

A significant proportion of the on-study time in these trials was spent at a granulocyte count of less than 100/μl and this profound granulocytopenia persisted for approximately ten to 14 days in all the studies except in the two reported by Dekker et al., and Estey et al., where the mean study duration of

TABLE 2. Prophylactic Trials Comparing
Trimethoprim–Sulfamethoxazole with Control

Investigators	Disease	Granulocyte level[a]	Infections TMP–SMX (N)	Control (N)	Benefit
Gurwith et al.[84]	Cancer	12/26	15[c,e]	35	Yes
Gualtieri et al.[85]	Cancer	13/21	7[b,c,e]	15	Yes
Kauffmann et al.[86]	Cancer	14/34	7[c,d]	28	Yes
EORTC[87]	Cancer	14/23	46[e]	64	Yes
Sleijfer et al.[88]	Leukemia	11/27	9[f]	38	Yes
Dekker et al.[89]	Leukemia	28/39	9[f]	20	Yes
Estey et al.[90]	Leukemia	22/47	41[c,e]	74	Yes

[a]Days at 100 μl per total study days
[b]No concomitant antifungal therapy
[c]Decrease in the frequency of bacteremias compared with the control group
[d]160/800 mg/day
[e]320/1600 mg/day
[f]480/2400 mg/day

profound granulocytopenia was 28 and 22 days, respectively. All seven studies showed a decrease in the incidence of microbiologically documented infections, and prophylaxis was deemed by the respective authors to have been beneficial. The most dramatic results occurred in the study conducted by Gurwith et al., in which the use of trimethoprim–sulfamethoxazole totally eliminated the occurrence of bacteremias. The studies of Gualtieri et al.,[85] Kauffman et al.[8] and Estey et al.[90] also showed a significant decrease in the occurrence of bacteremias among patients receiving trimethoprim–sulfamethoxazole; (3 versus 9, 2 versus 11, and 16 versus 30 respectively. Riben et al.[93] have reported that the use of prophylactic trimethoprim–sulfamethoxazole decreased the occurrence of deaths due to gram-negative bacillus infections among patients who were granulocytopenic (TMP–SMZ 2/29; control 8/24) and that this effect was most pronounced among patients with acute leukemia; (TMP–SMX 2/24, control 7/12).

Dekker et al.[89] performed one of the better of the nine studies that have compared trimethoprim–sulfamethoxazole-treated patients with a control group. Fifty-two patients were included in this trial. All study patients had acute leukemia, all received identical chemotherapeutic regimens, and all were randomized to receive trimethoprim–sulfamethoxazole plus oral amphotericin B or to receive nothing. The trimethoprim–sulfamethoxazole treated patients experienced fewer total infections (16 versus 31), fewer microbiologically documented infections (9 versus 20), and fewer alimentary tract, skin, and urinary tract infections. Thirteen of 26 antibiotic-treated patients did not acquire an infection during the study, as compared with only three of 26 control patients. Among the microbiologically documented pathogens, the prevalence of gram negative bacilli was less for the trimethoprim–sulfamethoxazole treated patients (7 versus 13), although for these patients the acquisition of and infection due to trimethoprim–sulfamethoxazole resistant organisms was greater. Despite the acquisition of resistant organisms, an increased colonization or infection rate with *P. aeruginosa* was not noted.

It seems from the studies, that for patients with acute leukemia, undergoing induction chemotherapy, who will experience prolonged durations (>10 days) of profound granulocytopenia (<100/μl), that prophylaxis with trimethoprim–sulfamethoxazole is beneficial in

reducing the occurrence of bacterial infection, especially those due to gram-negative bacilli.

There are two other reported trials which have compared trimethoprim–sulfamethoxazole to a control group.[91,92] Each of these studies has involved a somewhat different patient population. The first study was performed at the Memorial Sloan Kettering Cancer Center by Weiser et al.[91] They evaluated selective antimicrobial modulation with trimethoprim–sulfamethoxazole among patients with acute leukemia in remission, who were receiving maintenance therapy. This study showed no benefit for antibiotic prophylaxis. The second study, conducted in Baltimore by deJongh and colleagues, compared trimethoprim–sulfamethoxazole prophylaxis with placebo among patients with small cell carcinoma of the lung who were to receive intensive induction chemotherapy. A beneficial result was reported. However, the important point of these two studies relate to the fact that in both reports the patient groups had a very limited period of infection risk. In the study reported by Weiser, fewer than one-half their patients had granulocyte counts that even nadired at a level of less than 100/μl, while in the Baltimore study a mean of three of 32 on-study days were spent with a granulocyte count of less than 100/μl. This limited period of risk may well have been responsible for the inability of the study of patients in remission undergoing maintenance therapy to show a benefit with trimethoprim–sulfamethoxazole prophylaxis. The benefit demonstrated among patients with small cell carcinoma of the lung treated with trimethoprim–sulfamethoxazole was due primarily to a decrease in the frequency of pneumonias (postobstructive) and periodontal (poor dental hygiene) infections. This benefit appears not to be totally prophylactic, but rather in part therapeutic, and would suggest a role for early therapy of mild to moderate infections in such patients prior to the time they become granulocytopenic.

6.2.2. Comparison of Trimethoprim–Sulfamethoxazole and Oral Nonabsorbable Antibiotics

The next series of studies in the evolution of selective antimicrobial modulation compared trimethoprim–sulfamethoxazole with an oral nonabsorbable antibiotic regimen used outside of the confines of a protective environment. To date, two of

TABLE 3. Prophylactic Trials Comparing Trimethoprim–Sulfamethoxazole
with Oral Nonabsorbable Antibiotics

| Investigators | Disease | Granulocyte levels[a] | Infection (N) | | Benefit |
			TMP–SMX[b]	Other agent	
Watson et al.[94]	Leukemia	13/29	16 ($p = 0.02$)	37[c]	Yes
Wade et al [95]	Leukemia	26/44	22	26[d]	Equivalent

[a]Days at 100 μl per total study days
[b]Trimethoprim–sulfamethoxazole (320/1600 mg/day plus antifungal agent)
[c]Neocon (Neomycin, Colistin, and Nystatin)
[d]GN (Gentamicin plus nystatin)

these trials have been published (Table 3). Watson and colleagues from London compared trimethoprim–sulfamethoxazole plus nystatin to NEOCON, or neomycin, colistin and nystatin.[94] Randomized patients had all received induction therapy for acute leukemia or preparation for allogeneic marrow transplantation. The average study duration of profound granulocytopenia ($<100/\mu$l) was 12 days for trimethoprim–sulfamethoxazole recipients, and 14 days for the NEOCON-treated patients. Prophylaxis with trimethoprim–sulfamethoxazole decreased the incidence of infection (1.26/100 study days versus 3.06/100 study days) and bacteremia (0.84/100 study days versus 1.14/100 study days). Localized alimentary canal, respiratory tract and skin infections were less common among trimethoprim–sulfamethoxazole recipients. More than 50% (22 of 41) of the trimethoprim–sulfamethoxazole treated patients were able to complete the on-study time without developing an infection, while less than 30% (12 of 41) of NEOCON recipients were able to do so. Infections due to gram-negative bacilli were infrequent in both groups, but four *Pseudomonas* species infections occurred among the NEOCON group compared with only one among the trimethoprim–sulfamethoxazole-treated patients.

The second study, performed in Baltimore, compared trimethoprim–sulfamethoxazole plus nystatin with the oral nonabsorbable antibiotic regimen of gentamicin and nystatin.[95] The study population was composed exclusively of patients who were being readmitted to the University of Maryland Cancer Center for treatment of their relapsed acute leukemia. All patients were afebrile and uninfected and were not receiving other therapeutic antibiotics. These patients were specifically chosen for study be-

cause they were to receive intensive therapy, were expected to experience prolonged periods of profound granulocytopenia, and therefore would maximize the risk of infection. Each patient group spent greater than 60% of their on-study time at a granulocyte count of less than $100/\mu$l. The incidence of bacteremia and infection were equivalent for both groups, and seven patients in each treatment group completed their course of reinduction chemotherapy without contracting an infection. Patients given trimethoprim–sulfamethoxazole went a median of 19 days before requiring systemic antibiotics compared to 16 days for gentamicin and nystatin recipients. The sites of infection were similar for both groups except that upper alimentary tract (mouth, pharynx, esophagus) sites were more frequently observed among trimethoprim–sulfamethoxazole recipients (15 versus 5), and skin infections were more frequent among patients receiving the oral nonabsorbable antibiotics (1 versus 6). Infecting pathogens were less likely to be gram-negative bacilli if the patient was receiving trimethoprim–sulfamethoxazole (4/22 versus 10/26) with 5 of the 10 pathogenic gram-negative bacilli recovered from the gentamicin-treated group being resistant to gentamicin and causing infections that subsequently resulted in the death of the patient. One of the four pathogenic gram-negative bacilli isolated from patients receiving trimethoprim–sulfamethoxazole was resistant to gentamicin and was the cause of death for this patient.

6.2.3. Comparison of Different Selective Microbial Modulation Regimens

The third and most recent group of prophylactic studies employing trimethoprim–sulfamethoxazole have compared it to another antibiotic which possesses the ability to suppress potentially pathogenic colonic aerobes while preserving colonic anaerobes. The University of Maryland Cancer Center group evaluated adults with a diagnosis of acute leukemia who were afebrile, had no obvious source of infection, were not receiving therapeutic antibiotics but were to receive cytotoxic chemotherapy for remission induction.[96] Patients were stratified according to whether they were receiving initial induction therapy for newly diagnosed leukemia or reinduction therapy for relapsed leukemia. Both groups were then randomized to receive either trimethoprim–sulfamethoxazole or nalidixic acid. Concomitant oral nystatin was administered to all study patients. The regimen of trimethoprim–sulfamethoxazole plus nystatin was superior to nalidixic acid plus nystatin as prophylaxis of bacterial infections. Patients receiving trimethoprim–sulfamethoxazole had a median time to first documented infection of 17 days, which was significantly longer than the median of 8 days for patients receiving nalidixic acid (Fig. 1). The total incidence of infection for both groups was equivalent, with the majority of infections occurring while the granulocyte count was less than $100/\mu l$. Patients receiving trimethoprim–sulfamethoxazole experienced 1.24 bacteremias and 3.85 total infections per 100 days at a granulocyte count of $<100/\mu l$ compared with 2.17 bacteremias and 7.18 total infections for patients treated with nalidixic acid. Twelve of 34 patients treated with trimethoprim–sulfamethoxazole were able to undergo induction or reinduction chemotherapy without a documented infection, compared with only 4 of 28 patients given nalidixic acid. Upper alimentary tract site infections were more common in the nalidixic acid treated group as were infections caused by gram-negative bacilli. A similar designed trial was recently completed in Winnipeg, Canada. Trimethoprim–sulfamethoxazole (320/1600 mg/day) was compared with nalidixic acid (4 g/day). Not all patients had similar diagnoses or received identical chemotherapy. Trimethoprim–sulfamethoxazole prophylaxis was associated with fewer infections per 100 neutropenic days and pro-

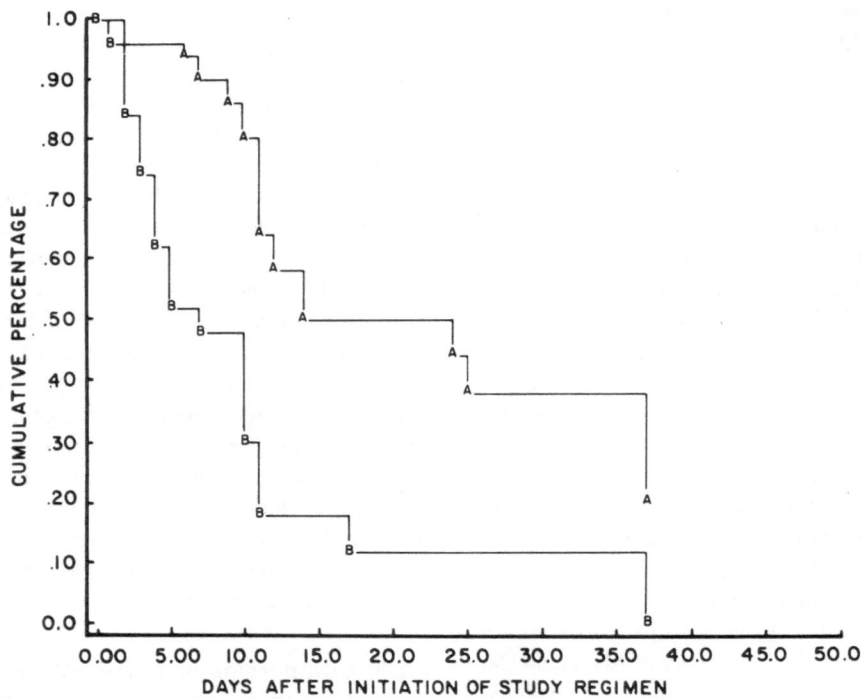

FIGURE 1. The probability of developing an infection following the initiation of prophylactic antibiotics among patients with acute leukemia undergoing induction therapy. A, trimethoprim–sulfamethoxazole plus nystatin, B, nalidixic acid plus nystatin $p = 0.0002$.

vided a longer infection-free period. Gram-negative bacillus infections were uncommon in both groups, while colonization with *Aspergillus* was more frequent among trimethoprim–sulfamethoxazole-treated patients.[96]

6.3. Other Prophylactic Trials Using Trimethoprim–Sulfamethoxazole

Bow et al.[97] reported a trial that compared trimethoprim–sulfamethoxazole with trimethoprim alone. While the overall incidence of infection was similar, trimethoprim appeared to have less protection against the development of infection during periods of profound granulocytopenia ($<100/\mu$l). Patients receiving trimethoprim–sulfamethoxazole cleared aerobic gram-negative bacilli from stool-surveillance cultures more often, and the acquisition of potentially pathogenic gram-negative bacilli was less frequent than for those patients receiving trimethoprim alone. These observations suggest that trimethoprim alone may not be optimal for preventing colonization and infection in patients who are granulocytopenic and that the combination of trimethoprim–sulfamethoxazole is preferred.

Two studies have employed varying combinations of trimethoprim–sulfamethoxazole and of framycetin, colistin, and nystatin (FRACON) as infection prophylaxis for patients with acute leukemia.[98,99] Enno et al.[98] compared FRACON with FRACON plus trimethoprim–sulfamethoxazole. Patients given the trimethoprim–sulfamethoxazole containing regimen had an infection frequency of 57% (8 of 14) compared with 94% (15 of 16) for the group treated with FRACON alone. The combination of trimethoprim–sulfamethoxazole and FRACON delayed the average time to initiation of therapeutic antibiotics from 2 days of neutropenia to 12 days. Starke and associates compared trimethoprim–sulfamethoxazole with FRACON plus trimethoprim–sulfamethoxazole and found equivalency between the regimens.[99] These studies again support a role for the prophylactic use of trimethoprim–sulfamethoxazole but do not lend support to the use of a prophylactic antibiotic combination which contains both trimethoprim–sulfamethoxazole and an oral nonabsorbable antibiotic combination.

More recently Pizzo et al.[100] reported on the combination of trimethoprim–sulfamethoxazole and erythromycin. This study was designed with a placebo control group. Pizzo found that compliance was a critical factor in the assessment of the overall benefit of the prophylactic antibiotic regimen. For those patients who received trimethoprim–sulfamethoxazole plus erythromycin and maintained excellent compliance (took all doses of medication) the incidence of infection and fever was significantly decreased (18.1% versus 32.2%), as was the incidence of bacterial infections (3.8% versus 11.9%) and the incidence of unexplained fever (10.5% versus 19.6%. A decrease in compliance was associated with a loss of benefit from the antibiotic prophylaxis. A similar study by the same group of workers again showed that for those patients with excellent compliance, the incidence of microbiologically and clinically documented infections was lower for the group receiving trimethoprim–sulfamethoxazole plus erythromycin (4 of 18 versus 11 of 17) than for the patients given placebo.[101] Yet, the authors of this study reported a very high level of adverse reactions (65%), most of which were GI in origin. The lack of more substantial efficacy in this latter study may reflect the large number of study patients with solid tumors as an underlying disease (21/29), and the limited infection risk with a median on-study time at a granulocyte count of $<100/\mu$l of only 6.5 days. The high frequency of adverse reactions may well have been due to the trimethoprim–sulfamethoxazole, but it is much more likely that the lack of tolerance to this regimen was due to the orally administered erthromycin.

The efficacy as infection prophylaxis for patients with acute leukemia of two of the new orally administered quinolones, norfloxacin and ciprofloxacin, is now being studied. In a double-blind placebo-controlled trial, Karp et al.[102] showed that norfloxacin prophylaxis significantly decreases the frequency of gram-negative sepsis (1 of 17 versus 7 of 15 patients, $p<0.015$) among adult patients with acute leukemia. Norfloxacin (120 mg/day) or trimethoprim-sulfamethoxazole (480/2400 mg/day), with oral amphotericin-B as the concomitant antifungal therapy have been compared at the University of Maryland Cancer Center.[104] Preliminary analysis has shown equivalence between the two regimens with only one documented gram-negative rod infection occurring among norfloxacin recipients. Winston et al.[103] compared norfloxacin plus nystatin to polymyxin, vancomycin and nystatin. Eighty-three percent of patients were highly compliant with the norfloxacin regimen. The total number of infections were similar between groups although 5 gram-negative bacteremias occurred among polymyxin plus vancomycin recipients, while the norfloxacin recipients were free of gram-negative bacteremias. However, gram-positive bacteremias were common for both treatment regimens. This prophylactic benefit of norfloxacin against gram-negative bacilli has also been observed by investigators from Winnipeg, Canada, although they have suggested that trimethoprim/sulfamethoxazole prophylaxis may be more effective for prevention of infections due to gram-positive pathogens.

Ciprofloxacin is another orally administered quinolone with broad-spectrum gram-negative rod activity and improved gram-positive coverage, but anaerobe-sparing characteristics that make it potentially suitable as an agent for infection prophylaxis.[81] An ongoing trial in the Netherlands, comparing ciprofloxacin with trimethoprim–sulfamethoxazole plus colistin has shown encouraging preliminary results.[106] Bacteriologically documented infections and bacteremias have been less frequent for ciprofloxacin recipients and the acquisition of antibiotic resistant gram-negative bacilli uncommon. Concomitant oral amphotericinB is being administered to both treatment groups, but yeast acquisition has been equivalent.

6.4. Disadvantages of Selective Microbial Modulation

Published trials to date have demonstrated benefit for the use of selective microbial modulation with such antibiotics as trimethoprim–sulfamethoxazole, norfloxacin and possibly ciprofloxacin as infection prophylaxis for a select group of patients. The toxicities seen with oral nonabsorbable antibiotics have in large part been overcome with regimens such as trimethoprim–sulfamethoxazole and norfloxacin. The daily cost of such treatment, even when an antifungal antibiotic such as nystatin is added, is less than $5.00; also, the taste and the compliance with selective antimicrobial modulating regimens are superb. The experience reported in the studies from Baltimore show that greater than 90% compliance can be maintained, and Pizzo reported that even when oral

erythromycin is added that 100% compliance can be maintained in at least 60% of treated patients.[95,96,100] Yet despite the apparent clinical benefits and improved tolerance there are a number of real and potential disadvantages associated with this therapy. Rash will occur in 5–8% of patients with cancer treated with trimethoprim–sulfamethoxazole and will often require discontinuation of therapy. There also appears to be the increased potential for the development of fungal infections. In their study, Hughes et al.[83] noted an increase in the episodes of oral candidiasis among patients receiving trimethoprim–sulfamethoxazole, and warned of a potential increase in disseminated infections in such patients. Gualtierei et al.[85] administered trimethoprim–sulfamethoxazole without concomitant antifungal antibiotics, and noted that yeast colonization as well as the frequency of disseminated candidiasis, candidemia and esophagitis (of presumed fungal etiology) was more frequent among trimethoprim–sulfamethoxazole treated patients. Most of the other reported studies, except for those of Gurwith et al.[84] and Pizzo et al.[100] and Karp et al.,[102] have used a concomitant oral antifungal antibiotic and have not reported a significant increase in yeast colonization or infection. This suggests that the use of an associated antifungal agent is important and that it should be a routine procedure.

The University of Maryland Cancer Center has reported an increase in invasive Aspergillus infections among trimethoprim–sulfamethoxazole recipients. In their study, which compared trimethoprim–sulfamethoxazole with high-dose nalidixic acid, seven *Aspergillus* infections were documented among patients receiving trimethoprim–sulfamethoxazole, five of which were fatal. This compares to only one *Aspergillus* infection among patients given nalidizic acid. To date this increase in the occurrence of *Aspergillus* infections has been reported only in the study performed at the University of Maryland Cancer Center, but an increase in *Aspergillus* nasal colonization was noted in trimethoprim–sulfamethoxazole recipients, in a yet unpublished trial from Winnipeg, suggesting the potential for an increase risk with this infection. Thus this complication must be kept in mind if this type of therapy is to be utilized.

A second potential disadvantage is the development or acquisition of resistant organisms. The occurrence of *P. aeruginosa* colonization, an organism naturally resistant to trimethoprim–sulfamethoxazole has been limited, however the acquisition of other trimethoprim–sulfamethoxazole resistant organisms has not been uncommon. Dekker et al.[89] reported that among 26 patients receiving trimethoprim–sulfamethoxazole, 20 acquired trimethoprim–sulfamethoxazole resistant gram-negative bacilli during the study period and six were responsible for infection. Our experience in Baltimore has been that approximately 15–20% of patients treated with trimethoprim–sulfamethoxazole will acquire a trimethoprim–sulfamethoxazole resistant gram-negative bacillus.[95] These organisms have rarely caused infection and have not been heterotypically resistant as has been reported by others.[107,108] It has also been our observation that the acquisition of trimethoprim–sulfamethoxazole resistant organisms is much more frequent during periods when broad-spectrum therapeutic antibiotics are concomitantly being administered.[95,96]

The last major disadvantage is the potential for marrow suppression with trimethoprim–sulfamethoxazole. Until recently this had not been clinically reported, and many of the early prophylactic trials including the first trial from Baltimore failed to show increased marrow suppression among trimethoprim–sulfamethoxazole recipients.[95] However, the Baltimore trial, which compared trimethoprim–sulfamethoxazole with malidixic acid, showed a significantly prolonged period of profound

($<100/\mu$l) granulocytopenia—24 days versus 16 days, respectively.[96] Further analysis showed this prolongation of profound granulocytopenia to be present only among patients undergoing initial induction therapy; a homogeneous group of patients with similar disease status, who were given similar chemotherapy (Table 4). The lack of this prolongation among patients with relapsed acute leukemia suggests that the marrow suppression due to trimethoprim–sulfamethoxazole may have been hidden by the heterogeneity of the disease status, administered chemotherapy, and antileukemic response. The etiology of the marrow suppression, be that a direct toxic effect, folate antagonism, or suppression of the gut flora necessary for the formation of colony-stimulating factor, remains to be clarified.

6.5. Fungal Prophylaxis

The frequent occurrence of *Candida* species in the normal human flora, particularly of the alimentary tract (e.g., mouth to rectum), and recognizing that the gastrointestinal tract, primarily the esophagus, is the major portal of invasion, have suggested that the suppression of endogenous *Candida* spp. may decrease the occurrence of such infections.[109–113] A number of approaches have been employed, using most of the available antifungal agents. Yet, in general they have capitalized on local effects of nonabsorbable agents, or systemic effects of oral or intravenously administered antifungal agents.

TABLE 4. Duration of Granulocytopenia[a]

	Prophylactic regimen			
	Initial induction		Relapse	
Granulocyte count (per μl)	Trimethoprim–sulfamethoxazole plus nystatin ($N = 17$)	Nalidixic acid plus nystatin ($N = 15$)	Trimethoprim–sulfamethoxazole plus nystatin ($N = 17$)	Nalidixic acid plus nystatin ($N = 13$)
100	22 6 ± 3.3[b]	13.6 ± 2 2[b]	24.7 ± 4.3[c]	19.7 ± 3 73[c]
100–499	6.9	8 6	6 0	8 9
500–999	4.4	4 6	3 4	6.6
1000	6.8	7.4	2 5	5.7
Total	40.7 ± 4 2	34 2 ± 2.9	38.8 ± 4.7	40.9 ± 5.1

[a]Data represent the mean (±SE) number of days on study during which patients had the indicated granulocyte counts
[b]Difference was statistically significant ($p = 0.007$)
[c]Difference was not statistically significant

6.6. Oral Antifungal Agents (Nonabsorbable)

6.6.1. Nystatin, Amphotericin B, and Clotrimazole

Nystatin and amphotericin B are polyene antibiotics with antifungal activity that is dependent on their binding to the sterol moiety, primarily ergosterol, present in the membrane of sensitive fungi.[114] This interaction increases the permeability of the cell membrane, allowing the leakage of a variety of small molecules. Oral nystatin has been the mainstay, until recently, for the treatment of superficial *Candida* infections. Its broad anticandidal spectrum, low cost, tolerability, and lack of oral absorption has made it the most frquently used oral antifungal agent. Stone et al.[112] evaluated hospitalized patients for the presence of alimentary tract *Candida*. They found an initial colonization rate of 20% but, with the use of oral nystatin, the occurrence of rectal colonization with yeast after 3 weeks of hospitalization decreased to only 4%. When nystatin was not used, the frequency of isolation dramatically rose to 56%. This ability of nystatin to suppress alimentary tract yeast continued even for patients who were receiving systemic antibiotics.

Nystatin has been evaluated further in patients with hematologic illnesses during periods of chemotherapy (Table 5). The studies using mystatin without an associated oral antibacterial regimen have frequently used a retrospective study design and have come to variable conclusions. The colonization data presented by Carpenteri et al.[115] and Pizzuto et al.[116]

suggest that the use of daily dosages of nystatin as low as 4×10^5 units markedly lowered the incidence of colonization. Both studies were retrospective in design but suggested that nystatin was effective in decreasing "major" fungal infections. Yet DeGregoria et al.[117] found that using nystatin at a dose of 1.2×10^6 units/day had no effect on the development of minor and major yeast infections. They concluded that it was the development of oropharyngeal candidiasis in patients with severe prolonged leukopenia who had received broad-spectrum antibiotics that led to the development of disseminated disease, and that the administration of nystatin played a minimal role in preventing that process. Williams et al.[118] are the only group to evaluate nystatin prospectively as oral candida prophylaxis. They used doses of 1.2×10^6 units/day in patients with acute leukemia and concluded that prophylactic nystatin treatment was of no value and should be reserved until there is clinical evidence of infection. These four studies are difficult to interpret, for they are in general poorly designed and have soft response criteria. They do suggest however that the effectiveness of nystatin as prophylaxis against disseminated candidiasis is minimal.

Nystatin has frequently been used in combination with other nonabsorbable antibiotics, e.g., GVN (gentamicin, vancomycin, nystatin), FRACON (framycetin, colistin, nystatin), and BKPN (bacitracin, kanamycin, polymyxin, nystatin), in an attempt to provide total suppression of the alimentary tract microbial flora.[88,22] The primary emphasis in most of these studies has been the bacterial infections, and consequently the data regarding fungal colonization

TABLE 5. Nystatin Prophylaxis of Candida Infections

Investigators	Study groups	Patient number	Dosage[a] ($\times 10^6$ units)	Colonization[b]	Major infection[c]
Carpenteri et al.[115]	Nystatin	94	0 4	4	3
	Control	14		48	14
Williams et al.[118]	Nystatin	13	1 2	NA[c]	Equiv
	Control	28			
DeGregoria et al.[117]	Nystatin	55	2	NA[c]	6
	Control	38			8
Pizzuto et al.[116]	Nystatin	284	3 4	2	5
	Control	170		65	54

[a]Dosage daily nystatin dose administered
[b]Percentage of patients colonized with *Candida* sp
[c]NA, not available
[d]Major fungemia, disseminated disease, visceral invasion

TABLE 6. Amphotericin B Prophylaxis of *Candida* Infections

Investigators	Study groups[a]	Patient number	Dosage[b]	Colonization	Infection[d] Major	Minor
Ezdınlı et al [120]	Ampho B	39	200	NA	2	
	Control	33			8	
Dekker et al [89]	TMP–SMX + Ampho B	26	800	NA	2	
	Ampho B	26			5	

[a] Ampho B, amphotericin B; TMP–SMX, trimethoprim–sulfamethoxazole
[b] Daily dose of nystatin administered
[c] Percentage of patients colonized with *Candida* sp
[d] Major fungemia, disseminated disease, visceral infection, minor superficial (oral candidiasis)

and infection have been limited. The study conducted by Levine and colleagues found that to obtain the maximal suppression of yeast growth required not only an orally administered antifungal agent (nystatin) but also a sterile environment, e.g., sterile food, water, and air.[56] This suggests that to adequately suppress alimentary-tract candida, one needs not only to suppress endogenous yeast by administering an antifungal agent but also to limit the patient's acquisition of yeast by decreasing the exposure to exogenous *Candida*. Despite the decreased colonization, Levine et al. were unable to show a significant decrease in *Candida* sp. infections. Although not reporting fungal colonization data, Schimpff et al.[88] and Buckner et al.[22] were able to show a significant decrease in fungal infections. Patients in these trials received oral nystatin and were housed in laminar-airflow environments during their therapy. Using historic controls and nystatin doses of 30×10^6 units/day, Hahn et al.[30] were able to show the most significant decrease in the incidence of candida infections when patients were given nystatin as part of the oral nonabsorbable antibiotic regimen. Nystatin has also been used in combination with selective decontaminating agents such as trimethoprim–sulfamethoxazole, nalidixic acid, or norfloxacin. In two consecutive studies from the University of Maryland Cancer Center, yeast colonization was found in one-fourth of all participants.[95,96] The first study comparing trimethoprim–sulfamethoxazole plus nystatin (4×10^6 units/day) to oral gentamicin plus nystatin (30×10^6 units/day), found similar colonization for both groups and despite the marked difference in daily nystatin doses the occurrence of fungal infections was similar. This suggests that the increased

dose of nystatin is unnecessary or that the mechanism of action of agents such as trimethoprim–sulfamethoxazole and gentamicin (e.g., persistence or suppression of anaerobes) on the colonic bacterial flora is an important variable in the development of invasive yeast infection.

The value of nystatin in combination with oral nonabsorbable or selective decontaminating antibacterial antibiotics appears to be more important than in the setting of no antibacterial prophylaxis. This increased need must in part be modulated through the suppression of the competing bacterial gut flora. Nystatin appears to be only partially successful in suppressing alimentary tract yeast. The use of nystatin prophylaxis for the prevention of major yeast infections is a more difficult question and is still unresolved. Yet, the recommendation to add an antifungal agent to a regimen of oral antibacterial antibiotics appears justified, but it seems that nystatin is not the optimal agent to be used.

The lack of consistent antifungal efficacy with nystatin has led to the use of oral amphotericin B.[89,119,120] While the use of such therapy has been widespread in Europe, the lack of a U.S. Food and Drug Administration (FDA)-approved preparation has led to limited use in the United States. Two studies have been reported and suggest that amphotericin B has some activity when utilized in a prophylactic manner but, despite daily doses of 800 mg, *Candida* infections have not been totally eliminated (Table 6). When one compares the occurrence of invasive yeast infections in the study of Dekker et al.,[89] where amphotericin B was employed, to the two studies from the University of Maryland Cancer Center where nystatin was used[95,96] one finds no major advantage for amphotericin B prophylaxis (2 of 26 versus 9 of 61 patients, respectively, developed an invasive yeast infection).

Clotrimazole troches have been studied in a double-blind placebo-controlled trial. This prophylactic approach was beneficial for renal transplant recipients, and for patients with solid tumors, but ineffective for patients with acute leukemia.[121] The prophylactic role for clotrimazole remains unclear.

6.6.2. Miconazole, Ketoconazole, and Amphotericin B

The variable and often disappointing results with oral nystatin and amphotericin B prophylaxis of *Candida* infections has led to the use of newer systemic imidazoles, such as miconazole or ketoconazole. The antifungal effect of the imidazoles, much like the polyene antibiotics, appears also to be mediated by an interference with ergosterol synthesis.

Miconazole has been marketed in the United States only as an intravenous preparation, yet in Denmark, Brincker[122] used oral miconazole in a double-blind trial as prophylaxis for patients highly predisposed to fungal infections. Thirty patients were randomized to receive either miconazole (500 mg, four times daily) or placebo. The incidence of fungal colonization was equivalent; 4 of 15 patients in each group had positive oral cultures, while 5 of 15 miconazole-treated patients and 2 of 15 placebo-treated patients had positive rectal cultures. Three of the six miconazole patients with initially negative surveillance cultures remained negative during therapy, while only 1 of 11 placebo-treated patients with initial negative cultures remained negative. Miconazole was ineffective in clearing oral and rectal cultures of yeast when initial cultures were positive. Two patients receiving miconazole developed fungal infections: one had oral candidiasis and one developed aspergillosis. Seven placebo patients experienced fungal infections, six with oral candidiasis and one with aspergillosis. The time to the development of infection was also significantly longer for the miconazole patients. This trial evaluated only a small number of patients, but suggests a potential role for oral miconazole as prophylaxis against *Candida* infections. Interestingly, despite a lower incidence of infection, miconazole had only a minor effect on the acquisition or suppression of alimentary tract yeast. This suggests that the benefit of miconazole was mediated primarily through a systemic effect.

It is the feature of systemic absorption and systemic broad-spectrum antifungal activity that has led to a number of trials investigating the utility of ketoconazole for prophylaxis of *Candida* infections (Table 7). The first five studies utilized placebo controls and variable ketoconazole doses ranging from 200 to 400 mg/day.[91,123–126] Ketoconazole therapy did not suppress alimentary tract *Candida* colonization. Brincker[124] was able to show a significant decrease in candida infections for ketoconazole recipients. The marrow transplant patients that Siegel et al[126] studied and the patients with leukemia reported by Estey et al. showed a decrease in the episodes of minor *Candida* infections (stomatitis) if given ketoconazole. Neither study group experienced invasive or disseminated disease, and therapy was well tolerated. Acuna et al.[123] from the University of California, using a placebo-controlled format similar to that of Siegel et al., found no difference in the frequency of colonization. Fungal infections in this trial were not reduced among ketoconazole recipients; rather, all major fungal infections occurred in ketoconazole patients, and the infecting organisms were Aspergillus and *Torulopsis glabrata,* both inherently resistant to ketoconazole. These results were the first indication that superinfections with fungi resistant to ketoconazole may be a major potential problem when ketoconazole prophylaxis is used. When ketoconazole has been used prophylactically and is compared with other antifungal agents, the results have been inconsistent. Hann et al.[127] and Meunier-Carpentier[128] were able to show a significant decrease in minor fungal infections for ketoconazole recipients. However, the other three trials have shown no advantage for ketoconazole over nystatin or oral amphotericin B. de Jongh et al[129] at the University of Maryland Cancer Center evaluated nystatin or ketoconazole in 51 patients. These agents at the doses administered failed to prevent fungal colonization or infection, but the use of ketoconazole was associated with more frequent colonization with *T. glabrata* (11 of 25 versus 4 of 26). Again, this confirmed the concern regarding the potential for resistant fungal colonization and superinfection.

In summary, an oral medication, infrequent administration, and broad antifungal spectrum are in-

TABLE 7. Ketoconazole Prophylaxis of *Candida* Infections

Investigators	Study groups[a]	Patient number	Dosage[b] (mg)	Concomitant medications[e]	Colonization	Infection[d] Major	Minor
Brincker[124]	Keto	19	400	No	Equiv	2	
	Placebo	19				9	
Acuna et al [123]	Keto	28	200	No	75	3	
	Placebo	24			66	0	
Maksymiuk et al. [125]	Keto	30	400	TMP–SMX	82		
	Control	27			80		
Siegel et al [126]	Keto	12	200	No	58	0	1
	Placebo	13			46	0	8
Estey et al.[90]	Keto	32	400		NA[f]	0	0
	Control	38				1	3
Hann et al [127]	Keto	37	400	Neco	14	0	11
	Nystatin + ampho B	35		TMP–SMX	46	2	25
De Jongh et al [129]	Keto	25	400	TMP–SMX	96	5	
	Nystatin	26			88	5	
Meunier-Carpentier et al. [128]	Keto	21	600	No	3	0	
	Ampho B	22			6	2	
	Placebo	17			17	1	

[a]Keto, ketoconazole, ampho B, amphotericin B
[b]Daily ketoconazole dosage administered
[c]Percentage of patients colonized with *candida* sp
[d]Major fungemia, disseminated, visceral infection, minor superficial (oral candidiasis)
[e]NECO, neomycin and colistin, TMP–SMX, trimethoprim–sulfamethoxazole
[f]NA, not available

triguing, but to date ketoconazole has not shown a consistent or significant effect used as prophylaxis against *Candida* infections. Moreover, there are now a number of studies that have suggested that ketoconazole use will be associated with the potential problem of colonization with ketoconazole-resistant fungi, e.g., *T. glabrata* and *Aspergillus* sp. Thus, ketoconazole at the dose employed is not ideal as fungal prophylaxis and is not significantly better than oral nystatin or amphoetricin B. Greater care must be used in institutions where fungal isolates of *T. glabrata* or *Aspergillus* sp. are common if ketoconazole is to be used clinically for prophylaxis or therapy.

The use of an oral antifungal agent as prophylaxis has many potential benefits, including ease of administration, low toxicity, and not requiring in-hospital stay. Yet the results with oral nystatin, amphotericin B, miconazole, and ketoconazole have been inconclusive, inconsistent, and difficult to reproduce. The continued frequency of disseminated *Candida* infections has led investigators to use intravenous antifungal regimens for prophylaxis.

Miconazole and amphotericin B are the two agents that have been tested. They have been used in two settings: as part of an empirical antibiotic regimen for neutropenic patients with fever and as therapeutic adjustments for patients who remain febrile despite empiric antibacterial therapy.

Vaughan and Saral and associates[130] reported on the use of intravenous miconazole as part of an empirical antibiotic regimen. The trial design was prospective, double blind, and placebo controlled; 208 patients with fever and neutropenia were started on antibacterial therapy with an aminoglycoside (gentamicin or tobramycin) plus ticarcillin; at the time antibacterial antibiotics were started, the patients were randomly assigned to receive miconazole (5 mg/kg q8h) or placebo. The frequency of fungal sepsis was significantly decreased for miconazole recipients, although the frequency of use of amphotericin B for both groups was similar. Vaughan and Saral and co-workers concluded that toxicity was minimal and that the use of miconazole prophylaxis and early empiric amphotericin B significantly reduced the incidence of fungal sepsis.

Fainstein et al.[131] used intravenous miconazole somewhat differently. They randomly assigned patients who had failed to respond to initial empiric antibacterial therapy to receive trimethoprim–sulfamethoxazole with or without intravenous miconazole (1800 mg/day). Among the 47 patients randomly chosen to receive miconazole, 8 failed due to fungal infections; 4 of these infections were due to *Candida* spp. Major and minor toxicity was seen with miconazole, and the authors concluded that miconazole was not therapeutically helpful. Pizzo and colleagues took the concept further by randomizing patients who remained neutropenic and febrile by day 7 of empirical antibiotic therapy into one of three groups.[132] Patients had their broad-spectrum antibiotics discontinued or had their antibiotics continued, or had amphotericin B added empirically to their antibiotic regimen. Five of the 16 patients who continued their empirical antibacterial antibiotics developed fungal infections, 4 due to *Candida* spp. Among the 18 patients who received empirical amphotericin B only one developed a fungal infection, that being caused by an amphotericin B-resistant organism, *Petriellidium boydii*. Pizzo concluded from his data that the empirical use of amphotericin B is effective therapy for preventing fungal superinfections or treating those infections that are clinically undetectable. While the empirical data of Pizzo's study were encouraging, they have not been confirmed in adults studied by the EORTC (unpublished data). Patients with clinically documented (clinical evidence of infection with identified site but not microbiologically confirmed) or possible (clinical evidence of infection without an identified site or organism) infections who remained granulocytopenic and febrile after four days of broad-spectrum antibiotics were randomized to receive or not to receive intravenous amphotericin B. The administration of amphotericin B was associated with a significantly greater chance of being afebrile 5 days later, but the occurrence of documented invasive fungal infections, or likelihood of still being alive 21 days after randomization was similar between treatment groups. The use of intravenous antifungal therapy as prophylaxis against the development of *Candida* infections is intriguing, but not yet substantiated. One must remember that the number of patients studied to date is small, and, while Pizzo reported minimal toxicity among his patients with a median age of 17, the toxicity of amphotericin B when used empirically in an older population is often a more significant problem.

It has been recognized that some patients who develop *Aspergillus* pneumonitis or sinusitis can be found to harbor locally invasive *Aspergillus flavus* or occasionally *Aspergillus fumigatus* high on the nasal septum or turbinates. This finding is related in part to a combination of the presence of the organism in the ambient air, granulocytopenia, cortiscosteroid administration, and the use of broad-spectrum antibacterial antibiotics that suppress the normal bacterial flora of the nose, thus creating a microbial vacuum. An untested prophylactic approach might be the use of a nasal spray with amphotericin B in high-risk granulocytopenic patients whose initial nose cultures show no growth of bacteria. Preliminary results from an open trial conducted in Belgium suggests that this technique is of benefit (F. M. Carpentier, unpublished results). We are investigating such prophylaxis in a double-blind placebo-controlled trial.

6.7. Skin

Skin infections are relatively common in the patient with marked granulocytopenia. They are presumably related to damage to the integument as a result of either disease per se or procedures such as venipunctures and bone marrow aspirations. Many of these sites of damage become infected with *Staphylococcus aureus* if this organism colonizes the nose or with gram-negative bacilli that colonize the mouth and colon. For example, the patient who has a blood sample obtained by finger stick and who then picks his nose before initial healing may inoculate *S. aureus* into the wound. Similarly, an iliac crest bone marrow aspiration may become contaminated with stool flora such as *E. Coli*. Another common site of infection in these patients is the axillae. The pathogenesis is not fully elucidated, although it may be related to a combination of moisture, axillary shaving (trauma), and occlusive antiperspirants. Infections in the axillae are caused by locally colonizing bacteria such as *Staphylococcus aureus*, gram-negative bacilli, or normal skin bacteria such as diphtheroids and *Staph epidermidis*. A very simple approach to reducing axillary infections has been to swab the axillae with povidone–iodine three times per day during the period of granulocytopenia.[133] At the University of Maryland Cancer Center, this approach has almost eradicated this once very common infection. In fact, the only patients who have developed axillary infections in the past years have been those patients who discontinued the use of the povidone–iodine swabs before the reappearance of circulating granulocytes.

In addition to these specialized skin problems of finger sticks, venipunctures, bone marrow aspirations, and axillary lesions, it is important to remove the transient potential pathogens on the skin by the use of sound skin hygiene. Many compounds have been utilized in the past such as hexachlorophene or povidone–iodine; even vigorous washing with regular soap will remove most transient organisms. Currently, we prefer chlorhexidine for both a complete daily shower (if a bed bath must be given, it is essential that the nurse do a complete and thorough bathing procedure) along with a three times-weekly chlorhexidine shampoo. Total suppression of the normal skin flora without laminar airflow isolation will probably lead to more rapid colonization by common pathogens. Therefore, the intent is not to sterilize the skin but to remove the acquired potentially pathogenic gram-negative bacilli, *S. aureus,* and yeasts.

As noted previously, most patients with granulocytopenia who develop a *S. aureus* infection can be shown to be nasal carriers. Nasal carrier states have been notoriously difficult to eradicate, but one potentially useful approach is the combination of an oral antistaphylococcal agent such as cloxacillin given with rifampin.[134,135] Cloxacillin or similar agents used alone will usually not eradicate the carrier state but will substantially decrease the total numbers of staphylococci on the nasal mucosa. The addition of rifampin, an antibiotic that is capable of cell penetration, can be useful in eradicating those remaining organisms not affected by the antistaphylococcal antibiotics that cannot penetrate these same cells. Rifampin alone should not be used because of the rapid development of resistant organisms. Among the University of Maryland Cancer Center patients with acute nonlymphocytic leukemia who were *S. aureus* carriers, this approach has been effective in eradicating the carrier state in about 70% of patients at least for the period of remission-induction chemotherapy.[135] Cloxacillin (500 mg) is given four times each day. and rifampin (600 mg) once a day, both for 5 consecutive days. This approach also has been utilized, with variable results, for patients

with mycosis fungoides who are heavily colonized on their skin and mucous membranes with *S. aureus* and whose ultimate cause of death is often staphylococcal bacteremia.

6.8. Dental Hygiene

Most adults have some degree of periodontal disease that serves as a nidus of infection during periods of chemotherapy-induced myelosuppression. The proper approach has been a matter of controversy. Our ongoing randomized controlled trial suggests in the preliminary analysis that a careful dental prophylaxis with plaque removal, repair of any caries, removal of teeth with obvious periapical abscesses (all under broad-spectrum antimicrobial coverage), followed by an intensive daily program of oral hygiene is preferred and not associated with an increased risk of infection or bleeding.[5]

7. Cellular Immune Dysfunction

7.1. Tuberculosis

Any patient receiving relatively long-term immunosuppressive therapy who has not been previously treated for tuberculosis, but is known to be or to have been positive with regard to purified protein derivative (PPD) or who has a Ghon complex on radiography should receive isoniazid, 300 mg/day po. It should be emphasized that the finding of a negative PPD is not sufficient to negate the need for IHN; a current chest radiograph should always be reviewed.

7.2. *Pneumocystis carinii*

Some groups of immunosuppressed patients have been shown to be at high risk of developing *P. carinii* pneumonitis. This has been most thoroughly studied at St. Jude Children's Research Center in Memphis, Tennessee, where Hughes et al.[136] showed that increasing degrees of immunosuppression during maintenance therapy led to an increase in frequency of *P. carinii* pneumonia in children with acute lymphocytic leukemia. In the group with the greatest degree of immunosuppression, the infection rate approached 50%. When these high-risk patients were randomly and blindly allocated to received either placebo or trimethoprim–sulfamethoxazole, a 20% incidence of pneumocystis infection occurred in the placebo-treated group, whereas the TMP–SMZ group was free of the disease.[83] This same benefit has been found for patients undergoing marrow transplantation.[137,138] Since trimethoprim–sulfamethoxazole has associated side effects such as sulfa-related rashes, fever, and neutropenia, this drug combination should only be given when the risk of *P. carinii* infection outweights the disadvantages of drug therapy. This type of prophylaxis has also been shown to be effective for patients with the acquired immunodeficiency syndrome where the frequency of *P. carinii* pneumonia approximates 60%.[139] However, this group of patients appear unusually susceptible to the adverse reactions of trimethoprim–sulfamethosazole.[140]

7.3. Varicella-Zoster Virus

Varicella–zoster virus infections are common in patients with Hodgkin disease and marrow transplant recipients. Herpes zoster tends to occur in the first year following completion of radiation therapy or marrow transplantation, while the patient's cellular immune function is maximally depressed.[141–146]

A live, attenuated VZV vaccine has been produced and is now widely used in immunosuppressed and normal children in Japan.[147–153] Neutralizing, complement fixing, and fluorescent antibodies to membrane antigens are induced by this vaccination. The vaccine has had extensive clinical trials in children with malignancy, and if chemotherapy was temporarily suspended, there was minimal immediate vaccination risk and protection against subsequent exposure was demonstrated. Recently, Brunell et al.[151] administered the live VZV vaccine to 23 children with acute lymphocytic leukemia or non-Hodgkin lymphoma. Seroconversion was noted in all, mild varicella developed in one, and a sibling of one of the vaccinated children seroconverted, but had no clinical evidence of varicella. If further studies confirm these results, the VZV vaccine will be a valuable addition to the antiviral armamentarium for the immunosuppressed child or previously uninfected adult with a hematologic malignancy. However, the use of live virus vaccines remains of significant concern for the patient who has undergone

marrow transplantation and cannot be recommended at this time.

Prophylaxis of VZV infections has relied, to date, on the use of passive immunization.[154–160] A number of trials have substantiated the protective value of zoster immune globulin, and immunosuppressed patients without a history of varicella should receive varicella-zoster immune globulin (VZIG) if exposed to either chickenpox or herpes zoster. Gershon et al.[157] found that for immunosuppressed children, the administration of VZIG significantly ameliorated the clinical infection; and more recently, Zaia et al.,[160] in a double-blind randomized trial, reported that varicella zoster immune globulin protected immunosuppressed children against the development of severe chickenpox. However for VZIG to be maximally effective, it must be administered soon after exposure (72 hr).[161] The current dose regimen is 1.25 ml/kg of body weight, with a maximum dose of 6.25 ml. A single dose is protective for approximately 4 weeks. Commercial immune serum globulin, however is ineffective for prophylaxis. The role of prophylactic oral or intravenous acyclovir for varicella-zoster virus infections is presently being investigated.

7.4. Herpes Simplex Virus

Herpes simplex virus infections that occur in immunocompromised hosts frequently will be localized, self-limited, and may differ little from the infections that occur in patients with intact immune defenses.[162] However, depending on the specific underlying illness, the disease activity, and the temporal relationship to recent cytotoxic or immunosuppressive therapy, infections that are almost exclusively recurrent in origin may be more frequent, severe, and protracted in their course. Patients receiving marrow transplants for aplastic anemia or hematologic malignancies who are seropositive for antibody to HSV before transplant have an 80% chance of experiencing a reactivation of their herpes simplex virus infection within the first 5 weeks after transplantation.[162] Saral et al.[163] evaluated seropositive patients with acute leukemia who were undergoing induction chemotherapy with cytarabine and daunorubicin. Twenty-five percent of their patients experienced a reactivation of HSV during their induction period. These results have been confirmed by Lam et al.[164] in a similar prospective study of patients with acute myelosgenous leukemia. When Saral reanalyzed the occurrence of infection among patients with complement-fixing antibody titers of 1 : 16 or greater, however, he found that 61% of this cohort of patients reactivated a median of 18 days after the initiation of induction chemotherapy.[163] This later analysis suggests that, as in normal hosts, the higher the circulating serum antibody titer, the greater the risk of recurrent infection.[165]

Muller et al.[166] were among the early investigators to suggest that for patients with hematologic malignancies, HSV infections were not only more frequent, but also more severe. The majority of their reported patients experienced multiple, large, chronic, mucocutaneous ulcers (herpes phagenda) that persisted for weeks to months at both nasolabial and genital mucosal sites. The severity and prolonged period required for the healing of HSV infections has also been noted in the marrow transplant recipient. Patients who participated in the recently completed acyclovir treatment trials and were randomized to receive placebo experienced pain at the site of their mucocutaneous lesions for a median of 23 days and required a median of 35 days to heal completely, with many patients having signs of an active infection that persisted for weeks beyond the median time to complete healing.[167–169] These viral infections have been associated with a more severe form of mucositis and its associated morbidity of increased pain and decreased oral mutritional intake. Left untreated, these infections heal slowly; for patients undergoing marrow transplantation or remission-induction chemotherapy for acute leukemia, the healing is often delayed until the circulating neutrophils recover.

Intravenous acyclovir has not only been effective therapeutically, but also prophylactically against HSV infections.[163,170,171] Saral et al.[171] have shown in marrow transplant recipients who are seropositive for antibody to HSV that the reactivation of HSV can be completely suppressed with intravenous acyclovir. This prophylactic effect has also been noted for patients with acute nonlymphocytic leukemia undergoing remission-induction chemotherapy.[163] Saral administered acyclovir to patients with acute nonlymphocytic leukemia undergoing induction therapy, beginning 4 days after initiation of chemotherapy, and continuing for 1 month. None of the 14 acyclovir recipients, compared with 11 of the 15

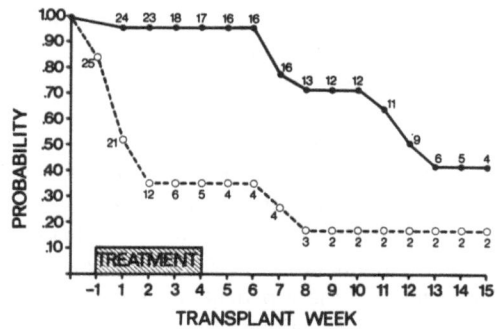

FIGURE 2. Oral acyclovir prophylaxis of herpes simplex virus infections after marrow transplantation. (●) acyclovir, (○) placebo $p = 0.0002$.

placebo recipients, sustained a recurrent HSV infection. Although quantification was difficult, the investigators believed that the observed mucositis, presumably due to the intensive chemotherapy, was less severe for acyclovir recipients.

An oral formulation of acyclovir is now available. Among immunologically competent hosts, oral acyclovir has been effective against primary and recurrent genital herpes simplex virus infections.[172–175] Treatment results in immunocompromised hosts have been published. The Seattle Marrow Transplant Group have used oral acyclovir as prophylaxis against the development of mococutaneous HSV infections after marrow transplantation. Oral acyclovir was 96% virologically and 100% clinically effective in preventing viral recurrence among those patients who maintained a compliance rate of at least 40% of the prescribed drug dosage (400 mg, five times per day) (Fig. 2).[176] This prophylactic activity of oral acyclovir has been confirmed.[177]

The use of acyclovir at doses employed for the therapy or prophylaxis of mucocutaneous herpes simplex virus infections has been well tolerated and not associated with delays in marrow regeneration or engraftment.[167,169,176]

8. Humoral Immune Dysfunction

Pneumococcal Vaccine

Certain patients, such as those with multiple myeloma, have an increased risk of developing pneumococcal infection. No large-scale trials have been conducted with pneumococcal vaccine, but one would predict that it would not be effective for the patient with myeloma who is unable to produce normal antibody. Patients with Hodgkin disease who have had a splenectomy may develop the overwhelming pneumococcal sepsis syndrome that, although relatively more common in splenectomized children under the age of seven, is rare in adults including those with lymphoma.[142,178,179] The evidence to date indicates that these patients do not respond to pneumococcal vaccination with normal antibody production,[180] so administration of the vaccine should not give the physician a false sense of security in this setting.

9. Relief of Obstruction

An obstructive lesion in a natural body passage will ultimately lead to infection. It is therefore important to attempt relief of obstruction as promptly as possible, whether it caused by tumor, by fibrosis following surgery, or other factors. For example, the patient with a lung carcinoma and a postobstructive pneumonitis probably will not clear that infection until radiation or drug therapy relieves the obstruction.

10. Care in the Breeching of Body Barriers

Intravenous catheters should be avoided whenever possible, with butterfly-type needles used instead. These needles should be inserted as aseptically as possible and should be changed frequently, at least every 24 hr, as it has been shown with other indwelling needles that 32% of 74 needles in place longer than 24 hr were contaminated.[181] Venipunctures and finger sticks for blood samples should be done with care, including smooth insertion and withdrawal and application of pressure for several minutes or more if necessary after the procedure to minimize hematoma formation as a nidus of infection. Similar care should be exercised for bone marrow aspirations, lumbar punctures, or other invasive procedures.

11. Staff Education

Often the professional and nonprofessional staff is not fully cognizant of the sources of organisms or of the predisposing factors to infection in these types of patients. A program of education is essential, not only for physicians and nurses but also for the many other individuals, blood-drawing or intravenous fluid insertion team members, respiratory therapists, dietary staff, radiology technicians, and others who come to the patient's bedside on an occasional basis. The housekeeping staff needs to understand its role; in our experience, a well-informed housekeeper takes care and pride in the knowledge that what he or she is doing is of substantial importance to the patient's personal welfare.

12. Patient Education

The education of the patient is also of critical importance. The patient should be instructed in matters of personal hygiene, including proper bathing techniques, oral hygiene, handwashing following bowel movements and urination, and the importance of frequent shampoos. The patient should be instructed not to get out of bed without using slippers, not to place his feet on a pillow where his face will rest later, and to accept and eat only those low-microbial foods that have been approved (assuming that the patient is granulocytopenic and on a cooked food diet). The patient is often his own best "policeman" and should be instructed not to allow anyone to sit on his bed, to draw blood, or perform examinations, without first washing his hands. The patient should be instructed to insist that relatives do the same. Finally, he should be instructed to notify the nurse or physician if there is any change in status that suggests an impending infection.

Infection risks for the immunocompromised host remain substantial. The epidemiology of such infections is now becoming clear, and the need for prevention paramount. However, prevention should begin with education and simple reproducible measures that can be easily enforced. Programs of antimicrobial prophylaxis without the institution of other more basic measures may be hazardous and doomed to failure at outset unless a complete patient and staff preventative program is considered and developed.

References

1 Bodey GP, Buckley M, Sathe YS, et al Quantitative relationships between circulating leukocytes and infection in

patients with acute leukemia. *Ann Intern Med* **64:**328–340, 1966.

2. Schimpff SC, Hahn DM, Brouillet MD, et al. Infection prevention in acute leukemia: Comparison of basic infection prevention techniques, with standard room reverse isolation or with reverse isolation plus added air filtration *Leuk Res* **2:**231–240, 1978.

3. Dale DC, Guerry D, Wewerka IV Jr, et al: Chronic neutropenia *Medicine (Baltimore)* **58:**128–144, 1979.

4. Schimpff SC, Young VM, Greene WH, et al: Origin of infection in acute nonlymphocytic leukemia Significance of hospital acquisition of potential pathogens. *Ann Intern Med* **77:**707–714, 1972.

5 Overholser CD, Peterson DE, Williams LT, et al: Periodontal infections in patients with acute nonlymphocytic leukemia. Prevalence of acute exacerbations. *Arch Intern Med* **142:**551–554, 1982.

6. Levine AS, Schimpff SC, Graw RG Jr, et al: Hematologic malignancies and other marrow failure states: Progress in the management of complicating infections. *Semin Hematol* **11:**141–202, 1974.

7. Aisner, J, Murillo J, Schimpff SC, et al: Invasive aspergillosis in acute leukemia: Correlation with nose cultures and antibiotic use. *Ann Intern Med* **90:**4–9, 1979.

8 Wade JC, Schimpff SC, Newman KA, et al. Staphylococcus epidermidis: An increasingly but frequently unrecognized cause of infection in granulocytopenic patients *Ann Intern Med* **97:**503–508, 1982.

9. Winston DW, Dudnick DV, Chapin M, et al. Coagulase-negative staphylococcal bacteremia in patients receiving immunosuppressive therapy. *Arch Intern Med* **143:**32–36, 1983.

10. Young RC, Corder MP, Haynes HA, et al. Delayed hypersensitivity in Hodgkin's disease A study of 103 untreated patients. *Am J Med* **52:**63–72, 1972.

11. Seligmann M, Chess L, Fahey JL, et al: AIDS—An immunologic reevaluation *N Engl J Med* **311:**1286–1292, 1984.

12 Fahey JL, Scoggins R, Utz JP, et al. Infection, antibody response and gamma blogulin components in multiple myeloma and macroglobulinemia *Am J Med* **35:**698707, 1963

13. Winston DJ, Gale RP, Meyer DV, et al: Infectious complications of human bone marrow transplantation. *Medicine (Baltimore)* **58:**1–31, 1979.

14. Meyers JD, Flournoy N, Thomas ED: Non-bacterial pneumonia after allogeneic marrow transplantation: A review of ten year's experience. *Rev Infect Dis* **4:**1119–1132, 1982

15. Schimpff SC, Aisner J, Wiemik PH. Infection in acute nonlymphocytic leukaemia. The alimentary canal as a major source of pathogens. In van der Waaij D, Verhoef J (eds). *New Criteria for Antimicrobial Therapy Maintenance of Digestive Tract Colonization Resistance*. Excerpta Medica, Amsterdam, 1979, pp 12–29.

16 Schimpff SC, Moody MM, Young VM· Relationship of colonization with *Pseudomonas aeruginosa* to development of *Pseudomonas* bacteremia in cancer patients. *Antimicrob Ag Chemother* **10:**240–244, 1970.

17 Schimpff SC. Surveillance cultures. *J Infect Dis* **144:**81–84, 1981.

18. Newman KA. Schimpff SC, Young VM. et al. Lessons learned from surveillance cultures from patients with acute nonlymphocytic leukemia: Usefulness for epidemiologic

preventive and therapeutic research. *Am J Med* **70:**423–431, 1981

19. Cohen ML, Murphy MT, Counts GW, et al: Prediction by surveillance cultures of bacteremia among neutropenic patients treated in a protective environment. *J Infect Dis* **147:**489–793, 1984

20. Bodey GP: Epidemiological studies of *Pseudomonas* sepsis in patients with leukemia. *Am J Med Sci* **260:**82–89, 1970.

21 Selden R, Lee S, Want WLL, et al: Nosocomial *Klebsiella* infections. Intestinal colonization as a reservoir. *Ann Intern Med* **74:**675–664, 1971

22 van der Waaij D, Tielemans-Speltie TM, Roeck-Houben AJ· Infection by and distribution of biotypes of Enterobacteriaceae species in leukemic patients treated under ward conditions and in units for protective isolation in seven hospitals in Europe. *Infection* **3:**188–194, 1977.

23. Kramer BS, Pizzo PA, Robichaud KJ, et al: Role of serial microbiologic surveillance and clinical evaluation in the management of cancer patients with fever and granulocytopenia *Am J Med* **72:**561–568, 1982

24. Aisner J, Schimpff SC, Sutherland JC, et al· *Torulopsis glabrata* infections in patients with cancer: Increasing incidence and relationship to colonization. *Am J Med* **61:**23–28, 1976.

26 Johanson WG, Pierce AK, Sanford JP: Changing pharyngael bacterial flora of hospitalized patients Emergence of gram-negative bacilli. *N Engl J Med* **281:**1137–1140, 1969.

27. Schwartz SN, Dowling JN, Benkovic C, et al: Sources of gram-negative bacilli colonizing the tracheae of intubated patients, *J Infec Dis* **138:**227–231, 1978

28. van der Waaij D The colonization resistance of the digestive tract in man and animals. Presented at the *Sixth International Symposium for Gnotobiology, Ulm, Germany, June 1978*

29. Schimpff SC, Greene WH, Young VM, et al. Infection prevention in acute nonlymphocytic leukemia. Laminar air flow room reverse isolation with oral, nonabsorbable antibiotic prophylaxis. *Ann Intern Med* **82:**351–358, 1975.

30. Hahn Dm, Schimpff SC, Fortner CL, et al. Infection in acute leukemia patients receiving oral nonabsorbable antibiotics. *Antimicrob Agents Chemother* **13:**958–964, 1978.

31 van der Waaij D, de Vries JM, Lekkerkerk JEC: Colonization resistance of the digestive tract in conventional and antibiotic-treated mice. *J Hyg (Camb)* **69:**405–411, 1971

32. Schroth MN, Cho JJ, Green SK, et al Epidemiology of Pseudomonas aeruginosa in agricultural areas. In Young VM (ed): *Pseudomonas aeruginosa Ecological Aspects and Patient Colonization*. Raven, New York, 1977, pp 1–29.

32 Springmeyer SC, Silvestri RC, Sale GE, et al: The role of transbronchial biopsy for the diagnosis of diffuse pneumonias in immunocompromised marrow transplant recipients *Am Rev Respir Dis* **26:**763, 1982

33. Taplin D, Mertz PM. Flower vases in hospitals as reservoirs of pathogens *Lancet* **2:**1279–1281 1973.

33. McDonald GB, Sharma P, Sale G, et al. Infectious esophagitis in immunosuppressed patients after marrow transplantation. *Gastroenterology* **88:**1111–1117, 1985.

34. Carson LA, Peterson NJ, Favero MS, et al Growth characteristics of atypical mycobacteria in water and their comparative resistance to disinfectants. *Appl Environ Microbiol* **36:**839–846, 1978.

35. Cross DF, Benchimol A, Diamond EG: The faucet aerator—A source of pseudomonas infection. *N Engl J Med* **274**:1430–1431, 1966.

36. Knight V: Instruments and infection. *Hosp Pract* **2**:82–95, 1967.

37. Edmondson EG, Reinarz JA. Pierce AK, et al: Nebulization equipment. A potential source of infection in gram-negative pneumonias. *Am J Dis Child* **111**:357–360, 1966.

38. Aisner J, Schimpff SC. Bennett JE, et al: Aspergillus infections in cancer patients: Association with fireproofing materials in a new hospital. *JAMA* **235**:411–412, 1976.

39. Eickhoff TC: Epidemiology of Legionnaire's disease. *Ann Intern Med* **90**:499–502, 1979.

40. Kirby BD, Snyder KM, Meyer RD, et al: Legionnaire's disease: Report of sixty-five nosocomially acquired cases and review of the literature. *Medicine (Baltimore)* **59**:188–205, 1980.

41. Fekety FR: The epidemiology and prevention of staphylococcal infection. *Medicine (Baltimore)* **43**:593–613, 1964.

42. Hurst V, Sutter VL: Survival of *Pseudomonas aeruginosa* in the hospital environment. *J Infect Dis* **116**:151–154, 1966.

43. Morse LJ, Schonbeck LE: Hand lotions—A potential nosocomial hazard. *N Engl J Med* **278**:364–369, 1968.

44. Mellow MH, Lewis RJ: Endoscopy related bacteremia. *Arch Intern Med* **136**:667–669, 1976.

45. Greene WH, Moody M, Hartley R, et al: Esophagoscopy as a source of *Pseudomonas aeruginosa* sepsis in patients with acute leukemia: The need for sterilization of endoscopes. *Gastroenterology* **67**:912–919, 1974.

46. Phillips I: *Pseudomonas aeruginosa* respiratory tract infections in patients receiving mechanical ventilation. *J Hyg (Camb)* **65**:229–235, 1967

47. Holder IA: Epidemiology of *Pseudomonas aeruginosa* in a burns hospital. In Young VM (ed): *Pseudomonas aeruginosa. Ecological Aspects and Patient Colonization.* Raven, New York, 1977, pp. 86–89

48. McDade JJ, Hall LB: Survival of gram-negative bacteria in the environment. I. Effect of relative humidity on surface exposed organisms. *Am J Hyg* **80**:192–204, 1964.

49. Plotkin SA, Austrian R: Bacteremias caused by *Pseudomonas* sp. following the use of materials stored in solutions of a cationic surface active agent. *Am J Med Sci* **235**:621–627, 1958. ·

50. Malizia WF, Gangarosa EJ, Goley AF: Benzalkonium chloride as a source of infection. *N Engl J Med* **263**:800–802, 1960.

51. Newman KA, Tenney JH, Oken HA, et al: Persistent isolation of an unusual *Pseudomonas* sp. from a phenolic disinfectant system for laminar air flow rooms. *Infect Cont* **5**:219–222, 1984.

52. Perry S, Penland WZ: The portable laminar flow isolator: New Unit for patient protection in a germ-free environment. In Mathe G (ed): *Recent Results in Cancer Research.* Springer-Verlag, New York, 1970, pp. 34–40.

53. Bodey GP, Johnson D: Microbiological evaluation of protected environments during patient occupancy. *Appl Microbiol* **22**:828–836, 1971.

54. Dietrich M, Gaus W, Vossen J, et al: Protective isolation and

antimicrobial decontamination in patients with high susceptibility to infection. A prospective cooperative study of gnotobiotic care in acute leukemia patients. I. Clinical results. *Infection* **5**:3–10, 1977.

55. Yates JW, Holland JF: A controlled study of isolation and endogenous microbial suppression in acute myelocytic leukemia patients. *Cancer* **32**:1490–1498, 1973.

56. Levine AS, Siegel SE, Schreiber AD, et al: Protected environments and prophylactic antibiotis. A prospective controlled study of their utility in the therapy of acute leukemia *N Engl J Med* **288**:477–483, 1973.

57. Storring RA, Jameson B, McElwain TJ, et al: Oral nonabsorbable antibiotics prevent infection in acute non-lymphoblastic leukemia. *Lancet* **2**:837–840, 1977.

58. Dietrich M, Rasche H, Rommel K. et al: Antimicrobial therapy as part of the decontamination procedures for patients with acute leukemia. *Eur J Cancer* **9**:443–447, 1973.

59. Cohen MH, Creaven PJ, Fosseick BE Jr, et al: Effect of oral prophylactic broad spectrum nonabsorbable antibiotics on the gastrointestinal absorption of nutrients and methotrexate in small cell bronchogenic carcinoma patients. *Cancer* **38**:1556–1559, 1976.

60. Klastersky J, Debusscher L, Weerts D, et al: Use of oral antibiotics in protected units environment: Clinical effectiveness and role in the emergence of antibiotic-resistant strains. *Pathol Biol* **22**:5–12, 1973

61. Buckner CD, Clift RA, Sanders JE, et al: Protective environment for marrow transplant recipients. A prospective study. *Ann Intern Med* **89**:893–901, 1978

62. Bodey GP, Gehan EA, Frereich J, et al: Protected environment—prophylactic antibiotic program in the chemotherapy of acute leukemia. *Am J Med Sci* **262**:138–151, 1971.

63. Schimpff SC: Infection prevention during granulocytopenia. In Remington JS, Schwartz MN (eds): *Current Clinical Topics in Infectious Diseases.* McGraw-Hill, New York, 1980, pp. 85–106.

64. Pizzo PA, Levine AS: The utility of protected-environment regimens for the compromised host: A critical assessment. In Brown EB (ed): *Progress in Hematology.* Grune & Stratton, New York, 1977, pp 311–332.

65. Holland J, Plumb M, Yates J, et al: Psychological response of patients with acute leukemia to germ-free environments. *Cancer* **40**:871–879, 1977.

66. Buckner CD, Clift RA, Thomas ED, et al: Prophylaxis of infections in patients with acute leukemia receiving allogeneic marrow transplants. *Infection* **11**:243–250, 1983.

67. Navari, RM, Buckner CD, Clift RA, et al: Prophylaxis of infection in patients with aplastic anemia receiving allogeneic marrow transplants. *Am J Med* **76**:564–572, 1984.

68. Schiffer CA, Aisner J, Daly PA, et al: Alloimmunization following prophylactic granulocyte transfusions. *Blood* **54**:766–774, 1979.

69. Clift RA, Sanders JE, Thomas ED, et al: Granulocyte transfusions for the prevention of infection in patients receiving bone marrow transplantation. *N Engl J Med* **298**:1052–1057, 1978.

70. Mannoni P, Martine R, Radeau E, et al: Granulocyte transfusion: Efficiency of prophylactic granulocyte transfusions in care of patients with acute leukemia. In Hogman CS, Lin-

dahl-Kiessling K, Wigzell H (eds): *Blood Leucocytes. Function and Use in Therapy.* Almquist and Wiksell, Stockholm, 1977, pp. 72–80.

71. Ford JM, Cullen MH: Prophylactic granulocyte transfusions. *Exp Hematol (Suppl)* **5**:65–72, 1977.

72. Cooper MR, Heise E. Richards F, et al: A prospective study of histocompatible leucocyte and platelet transfusion during chemotherapeutic induction of acute myeloblastic leukemia. In Goldman JM, Lowenstein RM (eds): *Leukocytes: Separation, Collection and Transfusion.* Academic, New York, 1975, pp. 436–449.

73. Winston DJ, Winston GH, Howell CL, et al: Cytomegalovirus infections associated with leukocyte transfusions *Ann Intern Med* **93**:671–675, 1980

74. Hersman J, Meyers JD, Thomas ED, et al: The effect of granulocyte transfusions on the incidence of cytomegalovirus infection after allogeneic marrow transplantation *Ann Intern Med* **96**:149–152, 1982.

75. Nausef WM, Maki DG: A study of the value of simple protective isolation in patients with granulocytopenia. *N Engl J Med* **304**:448–453, 1981.

76. Wade JC, McGaffey M, Wiernik, PH, et al: Hepatitis among patients with acute nonlymphocytic leukemia. *Am J Med* **75**:413–422, 1983.

77. Favero MS, Maynard JE, Peterson NJ, et al: Hepatitis B antigen on environmental surfaces. *Lancet* **2**:1455. 1973.

78. Centers for Disease Control: *Hepatitis. Control Measure for Hepatitis B in Dialysis Centers.* HEW Publication No. (CDC) 78:8358, Atlanta, Georgia 30333, 1978.

79. Hargadon MT, Young VM, Schimpff SC, et al: Selective suppression of alimentary tract microbial flora as prophylaxis during granulocytopenia. *Antimicrob Agents Chemother* **20**:620–624, 1981.

80. Wade JC, Joshi J, Devlin A, Moody MC: Alterations in stool anaerobes following antimicrobial therapy. Abst. 955. *In Twenty-fifth Interscience Conference on Antimicrobial Agents and Chemotherapy and Infectious Diseases Society of America, Minneapolis, Minnesota, September 1985.*

81. Rozenberg-Arska M, Dekker AW, Verhoef J: Ciprofloxacin for selective decontamination of the alimentary tract in patients with acute leukemia during remission induction treatment: The effect on fecal flora. *J Infect Dis* **152**:104–107, 1985.

82. Knothe H: The effect of a combined preparation of trimethoprim–sulfamethoxazole following short-term and long-term administration on the flora of the human gut. *Chemotherapy* **18**:285–296, 1973.

83. Hughes WT, Kuhn S, Chaudhary S, et al: Successful chemoprophylaxis for *Pneumocystis carinii* pneumonitis. *N Engl J Med* **297**:1419–1426, 1977.

84. Gurwith MJ, Brunton JL, Lank BA, et al: A prospective controlled investigation of prophylactic trimethoprim–sulfamethoxazole in hospitalized granulocytopenic patients *Am J Med* **66**:248–254, 1979

85. Gualtieri RJ, Donowitz GR, Kaiser DL, et al: Double-blind randomized study of prophylactic trimethoprim–sulfamethoxazole in granulocytopenic patients with hematologic malignancies. *Am J Med* **74**:934–940, 1983.

86. Kauffman CA, Liepman MK, Bergman AG, et al: Trimethoprim–sulfamethoxazole prophylaxis in neutropenic patients. *Am J Med* **74**:599–608, 1983

87. Zinner SH, Schimpff SC, Klastersky J, et al: Trimethoprim–sulfamethoxazole in the prevention of infection in neutropenic patients. Abstr 795. *In Twenty-first Interscience Conference on Antimicrobial Agents and Chemotherapy, Chicago, 1981.*

88. Sleijfer DTH, Mulder NH, de Vries-Hospers, et al: Infection prevention in granulocytopenic patients by selective decontamination of the digestive tract. *Eur J Cancer* **16**:859–869, 1980.

89. Dekker AW, Rozenberg-Arska M, Sixma JJ, et al: Prevention of infection by trimethoprim–sulfamethoxazole plus amphotericin-B in patients with acute nonlymphocytic leukaemia. *Ann Intern Med* **95**:555–559, 1981.

90. Estey E, Maksymiuk A, Smith T, et al: Infection prophylaxis in acute leukemia: Comparative effectiveness of sulfamethoxazole and trimethoprim, ketoconazole, and a combination of the two. *Arch Intern Med* **144**:1562–1568, 1984.

91. Weiser B, Lange M, Fialk MA, et al: Prophylactic trimethoprim–sulfamethoxazole during consolidation chemotherapy for acute leukemia: A controlled trial. *Ann Intern Med* **95**:436–438, 1981.

92. de Jongh CA, Wade JC, Finley RS, et al: Trimethoprim–sulfamethoxazole versus placebo: A double-blind comparison of infection prophylaxis in patients with small cell carcinoma of the lung. *J Clin Oncol* **1**:302–307, 1983.

93. Riben PD, Louie TJ, Lank BA, et al: Reduction in mortality from gram-negative sepsis in neutropenic patients receiving trimethoprim–sulfamethoxazole therapy. *Cancer* **51**:1587–1592, 1983.

94. Watson JG, Powles RL, Lawson, et al. Co-trimexazole versus non-absorbable antibiotics in acute leukaemia. *Lancet* **1**:6–9. 1982.

95. Wade JC, Schimpff SC, Hargadon MT, et al: A comparison of trimethoprim–sulfamethoxazole plus nystatin with gentamicin plus nystatin in the prevention of infections in acute leukemia. *N Engl J Med* **304**:1057–1061, 1981.

96. Wade JC, de Jongh CA, Newman KA, et al: Selective antimicrobial modulation as prophylaxis against infection during granulocytopenia: Trimethoprim–sulfamethoxazole vs. naladixic acid. *J Infect Dis* **147**:624–634, 1983.

97. Bow EJ, Louis TJ, Riben PD, et al: Randomized controlled trial comparing trimethoprim–sulfamethoxazole and trimethoprim for infection prophylaxis in hospitalized granulocytopenic patients. *Am J Med* **76**:223–233, 1984.

98. Enno A, Darrell J, Hows J, et al: Co-trimoxazole for prevention of infection in acute leukaemia. *Lancet* **1**:395–397, 1978.

99. Starke ID, Catowsky D, Johnson SA, et al: Co-trimaxazole alone for prevention of bacterial infection in patients with acute leukaemia. *Lancet* **1**:5–6, 1982.

100. Pizzo PA, Robichaud KJ, Edwards BK, et al. Oral antibiotic prophylaxis in patients with cancer: A double-blind randomized placebo-controlled trial. *J Pediatr* **102**:125–133, 1983.

101. Kramer BS, Carr DJ, Rand KH, et al: Prophylaxis of fever and infection in adult cancer patients. A placebo-controlled

trial of oral trimethoprim–sulfamethoxazole plus erythromycin *Cancer* **53:**329–335, 1984.

102 Karp JE, Hendricksen C, Redden T, et al. Double-blind randomized trial of oral prophylactic norfloxacin on infection in acute leukemia. Abst 149. *In Twenty-fifth Interscience Conference on Antimicrobial Agents and Chemotherapy, Minneapolis, Minnesota, 1985*

103. Winston DJ, Ho WG, Nakao SI, et al: Norfloxacin versus vancomycin/polymixin for prevention of infections in granulocytopenic patients Abst. 386 *In Twenty-fourth Interscience Conference on Antimicrobial Agents and Chemotherapy, Washington, DC, 1984*

104. Joshi JH, Finley RS, Tenney, JH, et al: A comparison of the efficacy and safety of norfloxacin plus amphotericin-B and cotrimaxazole plus amphotericin-B for infection prophylaxis in patients with granulocytopenia SS 4 6/9, 38/46-38/50 In *Thirteenth International Congress of Chemotherapy, Vienna, Austria, 1983.*

105. Bow EJ, Louie TJ, Rayner E, et al: Norfloxacin (N) versus trimethoprim–sulfamethoxazole (T/S) for infection prevention in patients (pts) with acute leukemia (AL). Abs. 150 In *Twenty-fifth Interscience Conference on Antimicrobial Agents and Chemotherapy, Minneapolis, Minnesota, 1985*

106. Roenberg-Arska M, Dekker AW, Verhoef J: A comparison of ciprofloxacin (CF) to trimethoprim/sulfamethoxazole plus colistin (T/S+C) for infection prevention in patients (pts) with acute leukemia during remission induction treatment. Abst. 151. In *Twenty-fifth Interscience Conference on Antimicrobial Agents and Chemotherapy, Minneapolis, Minnesota, 1985.*

107. Wilson JM, Guiney DG· Failure of oral trimethoprim-sulfamethoxazole prophylaxis in acute leukemia. Isolation of resistant plasmids from stains of Enterobactericeae causing bacteremia. *N Engl J Med* **306:**16–20, 1982

108. Jacoby GA: Perils of prophylaxis. *N Engl J Med* **306:**43–44, 1982

109. Fainsein V, Rodriguez V, Turck M, et al Patterns of oropharyngeal and fecal flora in patients with acute leukemia. *J Infect Dis* **144:**10–18, 1981

110. Kostiala I, Kostiala AAI, Kahanpaa A: Acute fungal stomatitis in patients with hematologic malignancies. Quantity and species of fungi. *J Infect Dis* **202:**1476–1479, 1982

111. Sandford GR, Merz W, Wingard JR, et al: The value of fungal surveillance cultures as predictors of systemic fungal infections. *J Infect Dis* **142:**503–509, 1980.

112. Stone HH, Geheber CE, Kolk LD, et al. Alimentary tract colonization by *Candida albicans J Surg Res* **14:**273–276, 1973

113 Wingard JR, Merz WG, Saral R: *Candida tropicalis.* A major pathogen in immunocompromised patients. *Ann Intern Med* **91:**539–543, 1979

114 Witten VH, Katz SI: Nystatin. *Med Clin North Am* **54:**1329–1337. 1970

115. Carpenteri U, Haggard ME, Lockhart LH, et al. Clinical experience in prevention of candidiasis by nystatin in children with acute lymphocytic leukemia *J Pediatr* **92:**593–595, 1978.

116. Pizzuto J, Conte G, Aviles A, et al: Centro Medico National Hospital General. Nystatin prophylaxis in leukemia and lymphoma *N Engl J Med* **299:**661–662, 1978

117. DeGregoria MW, Lee WMF, Ries CA: Candida infections in patients with acute leukemia. Ineffectiveness of nystatin prophylaxis and relationship between oropharyngeal and systemic candidiasis. *Cancer* **50:**2780–2784, 1982.

118 Williams C, Whitehous JMA, Lister TA, et al. Oral anticandidal prophylaxis in patients undergoing chemotherapy for acute leukemia. *Med Pediatr Oncol* **3:**275–280, 1977

119 Sleijfer DT, Mulder NH, de Vries-Hospers HG, et al: Infection prevention in granulocytopenic patients by selective decontamination of the digestive tract *Eur J Cancer* **16:**859–869, 1980

120 Ezdinli EZ, O'Sullivan DD, Wasser LP, et al Oral amphotericin for candidiasis in patients with hematologic neoplasms: An autopsy study *JAMA* **24:**258–260, 1979

121. Owens NJ, Nightingale CH, Schweizer RT, et al: Prophylaxis of oral candidiasis with clortimazole troches. *Arch Intern Med* **144:**290–193, 1984

122 Brincker H: Prophylactic treatment with miconazole in patients highly predisposed to fungal infection *Acta Med Scand* **204:**123–128, 1978.

123. Acuna G, Winston DJ, Young LS. Ketoconazole prophylaxis of fungal infections in the granulocytopenic patient: A double-blind, randomized controlled trial Abst. 852. In *Twenty-first Interscience Conference on Antimicrobial Agents and Chemotherapy, Chicago, Illinois, November 1981.*

124. Brincker H Prevention of mycosis in granulocytopenic leukemia patients with prophylactic ketoconazole treatment Abst. 850 In *Twenty-first Interscience Conference on Antimicrobial Agents and Chemotherapy, Chicago, Illinois, November 1981*

125 Maksymiuk AW, Estey W, Keating MJ, et al: Infection prophylaxis during remission induction therapy of acute leukemia. Abst C327 In *Seventeenth Annual Meeting of the American Society of Clinical Oncology, Washington, DC, April 1981*

126 Siegel M, Murphy M, Counts GW, et al. Prophylactic ketoconazole for the prevention of fungal infection in bone marrow transplant patients. Abst. 166. In *Twenty-second Interscience Conference on Antimicrobial Agents and Chemotherapy, Miami, Florida, October 1982.*

127 Hann IM, Corringham, R, Keaney M, et al Ketoconazole versus nystatin plus amphotericin-B for fungal prophylaxis in severely immunocompromised patients *Lancet* **1:**826–829, 1982

128. Meunier-Carpentier F, Snoeck R, Klastersky J. Oral antifungal prophylaxis in neutropenic cancer patients (pts) Abstract 10. In *Program and Abstracts of the Twenty-second Interscience Conference on Antimicrobial Agents and Chemotherapy, Miami, Florida, October 1982*

129 de Jongh C, Finley R, Joshi, et al A comparison of ketoconazole to nysatin. Prophylaxis of fungal infection in neutropenic patients. Abstract 497. In *Program and Abstracts of the Twenty-second Interscience Conference on Antimicrobial Agents and Chemotherapy, Miami, Florida, October 1982*

130. Vaughan WP, Saral R, Wingard JR, et al: Miconazole (M) prophylaxis against fungal sepsis (FS) complicating empiric antibiotics during chemotherapy induced aplasia. Abstract C726. In *Eighteenth Annual Meeting of the American Society of Clinical Oncology, St. Louis, Missouri, April 1982*

131. Fainstein V, Elting L, Bodey GP: Treatment for antibiotic resistant fever with trimethoprim–sulfamethoxazole ± miconazole in cancer patients Abstract 797 In *Program and Abstracts of the Twenty-first Interscience Conference on Antimicrobial Agents and Chemotherapy, Chicago, Illinois, November 1981.*

132. Pizzo PA, Robichaud KJ, Gill FA, et al: Empiric antibiotic and antifungal therapy for cancer patients with prolonged fever and granulocytopenia. *Am J Med* **72**:101–111, 1987.

133 Murillo J, Schimpff SC, Broullet MD: Axillary lesions in patients with acute leukemia. Evaluation of a preventive program *Cancer* **43**:1493–1496, 1979.

134 Sande MA, Mandell GL: Effect of rifampin on nasal carriage of *Staphylococcus aureus Antimicrob Agents Chemother* **7**:294–297, 1975.

135. Finley RC, Schimpff SC, Fortner CL, et al.. Rifampin and cloxacillin in the reduction of *Staphylococcus aureus* colonization *Clin Pharm* **1**:370–372, 1982.

136 Hughes WT, Feldman S, Aur RJA, et al. Intensity of immunosuppressive therapy and the incidence of *Pneumocystis carinii* pneumonitis. *Cancer* **36**:2004–2009, 1975.

137 Winston DJ, Williams KL, Gale RP and Young LW. Trimethoprim–sulfamethoxazole for the treatment of *Pneumocystic carinii* pneumonia. *Ann Intern Med* **92**:762–769, 1980.

138 Meyers JD, Pifer LL, Sale GE, et al: The value of *Pneumocystis carinii* antibody and antigen detection for diagnosis of *Pneumocystic carinii* pneumonia after marrow transplantation. *Am Rev Respir Dis* **120**:1283–1287, 1979.

139. Fischl MA, Dickinson GM. Trimethoprim–sulfamethoxazole prophylaxis of *Pneumocystis carinii* pneumonia in the acquired immunodeficiency syndrome. Abstract 436. In *Twenty-fifth Interscience Conference on Antimicrobial Agents and Chemotherapy, Miami, Florida, October 1982.*

140 Kovacs JA, Hiemenz JW, Macher AM, et al. *Pneumocystis carinii* pneumonia A comparison between patients with the acquired immunodeficiency syndrome and patients with other immunodeficiencies *Ann Intern Med* **100**:663–671, 1984

141 Schimpff SC, Serpick A, Block J, et al. Varicella zoster infection in patients with cancer *Ann Intern Med* **76**:241–254, 1972

142. Schimpff SC, O'Connell MJ, Greene WH, et al. Infections in 92 splenectomized patients with Hodgkin's disease. A clinical review. *Am J Med* **59**:695–701, 1975.

143. Ruckdeschel JC, Schimpff SC, Smyth AC, et al: Herpes zoster and impaired cell-associated immunity to the varicella-zoster virus in patients with Hodgkin's disease. *Am J Med* **62**:77–85, 1977.

144 Atkinson K, Meyers JD, Storb R, et al. Varicella-zoster virus infection after marrow transplantation for aplastic anemia or leukemia *Transplantation* **29**:47, 1980.

145 Clift RA, Buckner CD, Fefer A, et al Infectious complica-

tions of marrow transplantation *Transplant Proc* **6**:389–393, 1974.

146. Winston DJ, Gale RO, Meyer DW, et al. Infectious complications of human bone marrow transplantation. *Medicine (Baltimore)* **58**:1–31, 1979.

147. Asano Y, Nakayama H, Yazaki T, et al: Protective efficacy of vaccination in children in four episodes of natural varicella and zoster in the ward. *Pediatrics* **59**:8–12, 1977.

148 Asano Y, Nakayama H, Yazaki T, et al. Protection against varicella in family contacts by immediate inoculation with live varicella vaccine *Pediatrics* **59**:3–7, 1977.

149. Asano Y, Takahashi M: Clinical and serologic testing of a live varicella vaccine and two-year follow-up for immunity of the vaccinated children. *Pediatrics* **60**:810–814, 1977.

150. Asano Y, Yazaki T, Miyata T, et al. Application of a live attenuated varicella vaccine to hospitalized children and its protective effect on spread of varicella infection. *Biken J* **18**:35–40, 1975

151. Brunell PA, Geiser C, Sheheb Z, Waugh JE: Administration of live varicella vaccine to children with leukaemia. *Lancet* **2**:1019, 1982

152. Izawa T, Ihara T, Hattori A, et al: Application of a live varicella vaccine in children with acute leukemia or other malignant diseases. *Pediatrics* **60**:805–809, 1977.

153. Takahishi M, Otsuka T, Ojuno Y, et al: Live vaccine used to prevent the spread of varicella in children in hospital. *Lancet* **2**:1288, 1974.

154. Brunell PA, Gershon AA: Passive immunization against varicella-zoster infections and other modes of therapy *J Infect Dis* **127**:415–423, 1973.

155. Brunell PA, Ross A, Miller LH, Juo B: Prevention of varicella by zoster immunoglobulin. *N Engl Med* **280**:1191–1194, 1969.

156 Geiser CF, Bishop Y, Myers M, et al. Prophylaxis of varicella in children with neoplastic disease: Comparative results with zoster immune plasma and gammaglobulin *Cancer* **35**:1027–1030, 1975.

157 Gershon AA, Steinberg S, Brunell PA: Zoster immune globulin A further assessment. *N Engl J Med* **290**:243–245, 1974.

158 Crenstein WA, Heymann DLL, Ellis RJ, et al: Prophylaxis of varicella in high-risk children. Dose-response effect of zoster immune globulin *J Pediatr* **98**:368–373, 1981.

159 Ross AH, Klein SW, McKennett B, et al. Zoster immune globulin *NY State J Med* **74**:1367–1372, 1974.

160 Zaia JA, Levin MJ, Preblud SR, et al: Evaluation of varicella-zoster immune globulin: Protection of immunosuppressed children after household exposure to varicella. *J Infect Dis* **147**:737–743, 1983.

161. Anonymous: Varicella-zoster immune globulin—United States. *MMWR* **30**:15–16, 21, 1981

162 Meyers JD, Fluornoy N, Thomas ED. Infection with herpes simplex virus and cell mediated immunity after marrow transplant *J Infect Dis* **142**:338–346, 1980.

163. Saral R, Ambinder RF, Burns WH, et al Acyclovir prophylaxis against recrudescent herpes simplex virus infections in leukemia patients. A randomized, double-blind placebo controlled study *Ann Intern Med* **96**:11–14, 1982.

164. Lam MT, Pazın GJ, Armstrong JA, et al: Herpes simplex infection in acute myelogenous leukemia and other hematologic malignancies: A prospective study. *Cancer* **48:**2168–2171, 1981.

165. Reeves WC, Corey L, Adams HG, et al: Risk of recurrence after first episodes of genital herpes. Relation to HSV type and antibody response. *N Engl J Med* **305:**315–319, 1981.

166. Muller SA, Herrman EC Jr, Winkelmann RK: Herpes simplex infections in hematologic malignancies. *Am J Med* **52:**102–114, 1972.

167. Meyers JD, Wade JC, Mitchell CD, et al: Multicenter collaborative trial of intravenous acyclovir for the treatment of mucocutaneous herpes simplex virus infection in the immunocompromised host. *Am J Med* **73A:**229–235, 1982.

168. Mitchell CD, Gentry SR, Boen JR, et al: Acyclovir therapy for mucocutaneous herpes simplex infections in immunocompromised patients. *Lancet* **2:**1389–1392, 1981

169. Wade, JC, Newton B, McLaren C, et al: Treatment of mucocutaneous herpes simplex virus infection after marrow transplantation with intravenous acyclovir. A double-blind trial. *Ann Intern Med* **96:**265–269, 1982.

170. Hann IM, Prentice HG, Blacklock HA, et al: Acyclovir prophylaxis against herpes-virus infections in severely immunocompromised patients: randomized double blind trial. *Br Med J* **287:**384, 1983.

171. Saral R, Bums WH, Laskin OL, et al. Acyclovir prophylaxis of herpes-simplex-virus infections: A randomized, double-blind, controlled trial in bone-marrow-transplant recipients. *N Engl J Med* **305:**63–67, 1981.

172. Bryson YJ, Dillon M, Lovett M, et al: Treatment of first episodes of genital herpes simplex virus infection with oral acyclovir. A randomized double-blind controlled trial in normal subjects *N Engl J Med* **308:**916–921, 1983.

173. Nilsen AE, Aasen T, Halsos AM, et al. Efficacy of oral acyclovir in the treatment of initial and recurrent genital herpes. *Lancet* **2:**571, 1982.

174. Douglas JM, Critchlow C, Benedetti J, et al: A double-blind study of oral acyclovir for suppression of recurrences of genital herpes simplex virus infection *N Engl J Med* **310:**1551–1556, 1984.

175. Strauss SE, Takiff HE, Seidlin M, et al. Suppression of frequently recurring genital herpes: A placebo-controlled double-blind trial of oral acyclovir. *N Engl J Med* **310:**1545–1550, 1984.

176. Wade JC, Newton B, Flournoy N, et al: Oral acyclovir prophylaxis of herpes simplex virus infection after marrow transplant *Ann Intern Med* **100:**823–828, 1984.

177. Gluckman E, Devergie A, Melo R, et al: Prophylaxis of herpes infections after bone marrow transplantation by oral acyclovir. *Lancet* **2:**706, 1983.

178. Bisno AL: Hyposplenism and overwhelming pneumococcal infection: A reappraisal. *Am J Med Sci* **262:**101–107, 1971.

179. Desser RK, Ultmann JE: Risk of severe infection in patients with Hodgkin's disease or lymphoma after diagnostic laparotomy and splenectomy *Ann Intern Med* **77:**143–146, 1972

180. Siber GR, Weitzman SA, Aisenberg AC, et al. Impaired antibody response to pneumococcal vaccine after treatment for Hodgkin's disease *N Engl J Med* **299:**442–448, 1978.

181. Lowenbraun S, Young V, Kenton D, Serpick A: Infection from intravenous "scalp-vein" needles in a susceptible population. *JAMA* **212:**45–453, 1970

3

Defects in Host-Defense Mechanisms

JOS W. M. VAN DER MEER

1. Colonization

Under normal conditions, large areas of the human body surfaces are colonized with microorganisms. The skin and the mucous membranes of the oropharynx, nasopharynx, intestinal tract, and parts of the genital tract each have their own microflora.[1] These patterns of colonization are determined by microbial factors, exogenous factors, and host factors.

An important microbial factor is adhesion to epithelial cells, often with distinct specificity for a certain type of epithelial cell.[2] Microorganisms can also influence the patterns of colonization by producing bacteriocins and other products that inhibit the growth of other microorganisms[3] or by competing for essential nutrients.[4] By means of such mechanisms, colonizing microorganisms form a barrier against microorganisms from the outside world. This type of barrier has been designated as *colonization resistance*.[5] In the nose[6] diphtheroids hamper the local growth of *Staphylococcus aureus,* whereas in the gastrointestinal (GI) tract anaerobic microorganisms inhibit the colonization and outgrowth of aerobic gram-negative rods.[4,5] By contrast, certain pathogenic microorganisms (e.g., respiratory viruses) facilitate bacterial colonization.[7,8] Of the exogenous factors that influence the normal flora, diet [1,9] and more importantly disinfectants and antimicrobial drugs[10] should be mentioned.

The host factors that play a role in colonization are rather complex. The adherence of bacteria to epithelial cells is dependent on specific receptors on

somatic cells.[2,11] Interindividual differences in bacterial adherence to epithelial cells may be based on certain blood group glycoproteins[12] or HLA types[13] that are expressed on epithelial cells and serve as receptors. The precise mechanisms by which race,[14] pregnancy,[15] alcoholism,[16] and underlying diseases such as cancer[17-19] and diabetes[16] alter colonization are unknown. Several other factors considered part of the host defense in a stricter sense (Table 1) also influence colonization of the body surfaces.

2. The First Line of Defense

2.1. The Skin

Normal skin is not very hospitable to most microorganisms.[20] By desquamation of the horny layer, bacteria are constantly eliminated from the skin. Dependent on their chemical structure, skin surface lipids produced by the sebaceous glands as well as keratinocytes either inhibit the growth of bacteria, such as streptococci, or promote the growth of diphtheroids.[20] The lactic acid in sweat can be used as a source of energy by staphylococci, although inhibition of growth occurs at higher concentrations.[21] When the skin is humid and the pH increases, higher bacterial counts are found.[22]

2.2. The Mucosa

At the mucosal level, a number of effective mechanisms are encountered. Ciliary motion, ventilation, and coughing maintain sterile airways below the vocal cords in the healthy human being.[23] Gastric

JOS W. M. VAN DER MEER • Department of Infectious Diseases, University Hospital, 2300 RC Leiden, The Netherlands

TABLE 1. Host-Defense Mechanisms

	Nonspecific	Specific
Surface (skin, mucous membranes)	Mechanical barrier	Immunoglobulins
	Secretory barrier	
	Ciliary motion	
	Movement	
Humoral defense	Lysozyme and lactoferrin	Immunoglobulins
	Complement system	
	Fibronectin	
	Interferon	
	Tuftsin	
Cellular defense	Phagocytic cells	
	Neutrophilic granulocytes	
	Eosinophilic granulocytes	
	Mononuclear phagocytes	
	Natural killer cells	Cell-mediated immunity (T lymphocytes and macrophages)

acid is an effective barrier against bacteria from outside; thus, hypochlorhydria (e.g., as induced by H_2-receptor antagonists) is associated with colonization of the stomach and even intestinal infections.[24] Unconjugated bile has antibacterial properties and probably helps restrict the number of bacteria in the small intestine.[25] Intestinal motility also inhibits bacterial outgrowth. Colonization of the urinary tract is largely prevented by regular voiding.[26] In the female genital tract, glycogen stored in vaginal epithelium, which is under hormonal control, is converted to lactic acid by the commensal flora, creating an acid environment that is hostile to many pathogens.

Lysozyme and lactoferrin in tears and saliva display antibacterial activity—lysozyme through inhibition of the cell wall synthesis of gram-positive bacteria and lactoferrin through interference with bacterial iron metabolism[27,28] (see Section 3.1). Probably more important are the immunoglobulins, especially secretory IgA, on these surfaces; by coating microorganisms, secretory IgA prevents adherence to mucosal cells (see Section 3.1.5).

Symbiosis of the host with colonizing microflora depends in the first instance on the integrity of the mechanical barrier of skin and mucous membranes. Damage to this first line of defense, even by trivial injuries such as a puncture, can turn colonizing microorganisms into pathogens that impose great demands on the other defense mechanisms. Moreover, pathogens from the outside world may then gain entrance and cause infection. At this point, it should be stressed that a number of microorganisms are capable of penetrating intact epithelia. If the microorganisms succeed in passing the first line of defense, the second line of defense, consisting of humoral and cellular defense mechanisms (Table 1), is needed for elimination of the invaders.

3. The Second Line of Defense

The second line of defense is made up of humoral and cellular defense mechanisms (Table 1) acting in close cooperation. Thus, separation of the discussions on humoral and cellular defense mechanisms is somewhat artificial. However, for reasons of clarity and because quite a number of pathologic states involve either the humoral or the cellular defense mechanisms, these mechanisms are dealt with separately.

3.1. Humoral Defense Mechanisms

The humoral defense system consists of a number of nonspecific and specific factors that interact with microorganisms (Table 1).

3.1.1. Lysozyme and Lactoferrin

Lysozyme, one of the nonspecific factors (see also Section 2.2), is an enzyme found in many body fluids. It is present in high concentrations in the azurophilic and specific granules of polymorphonuclear leukocytes and is constitutively secreted by mononuclear phagocytes.[29] By cleaving the linkage between N-acetyl-glucosamine and N-acetyl-muramic acid, lysozyme interferes with cell-wall synthesis, especially that of gram-positive bacteria[27]; it also markedly amplifies the effector mechanism of the complement cascade[30] (Section 3.1.2). Lactoferrin is an iron-binding protein that, when not fully saturated with iron, inhibits the growth of microorganisms, such as gram-negative and gram-positive bacteria and various *Candida* species.[28] It then acts as an iron-chelating agent, thereby depriving the microorganisms of the iron necessary for their growth. It is an important enzyme of neutrophil specific granules (Section 3.2.1h).

3.1.2. Complement

More important in the humoral host defense is the complement system, consisting of at least 18 plasma proteins that are able to react in a cascade.[30,31] This cascade has four essential elements: (1) classic activation, (2) alternative activation, (3) amplification, and (4) the effector mechanism (Fig. 1). Antigen–antibody complexes can bind the first component of the complement system C1 at the exposed Fc portion of the antibody; in this way, classic activation is initiated. Activated C1 then activates C4 and C2; the next step is activation of C3, which is converted into C3a and C3b. Bacterial products, especially those lacking sialic acid,[31] can activate the alternative route via factors B, P, and D̄. When C3b, formed by either the classic or the alternative route, reacts with factors B, D̄, and P, complement activation may be amplified. The effector mechanism is then initiated by the conversion of C5 into C5b and C5a and subsequent formation of the multimolecular complex C5b6789.

A number of inhibitors, also part of the complement system, regulate the system. For a more detailed account of these factors, the reader is referred to the reviews by Joiner et al.[30] and Fearon and Austen.[31] The biologic effects of complement are essentially as follows. Factors C3a and C5a are able to liberate histamine and serotonin from mast cells and basophils, thereby increasing vascular permeability.

Factors C5a, Ba, and C5b67, and to a much lesser extent C3a have a chemotactic effect on leukocytes (Section 3.2). Since C3b-bound complexes can bind to C3b receptors on granulocytes and monocytes/macrophages, C3b acts as an opsonin (Section 3.2.1e) and promotes phagocytosis. The effector complex C5b6789 is able to penetrate cell membranes leading to lysis of the microorganisms as well as erythrocytes and tumor cells.

Thus, the complement system provides us with a potent host-defense system against microorganisms that operates via the alternative pathway even before a specific immune response has developed and is also effective via the classic route once there is a specific antibody response. Moreover, it appears that certain antibodies also amplify the alternative route. From the deficiencies of individual complement components in humans, the relative role and importance of these factors in host defense can be assessed. Recurrent bacterial infections have been reported in patients lacking C3.[33,34] Deficiency of C5 is associated with an impaired capacity to generate chemotactic activity in serum and recurrent pyogenic infections.[35] Leiner's syndrome (eczema, diarrhea, and recurrent gram-negative bacteremia) has been qualified as a C5 dysfunction syndrome; generation of chemotactic factors is defective and there is a concomitant, as yet unexplained, opsonic defect.[36,37] Among those with a deficiency of one of the terminal components (C5–C8), a high incidence of chronic or recurrent *Neisseria* infections has been found.[38,39]

Deficiencies in alternative pathway proteins are rare. A combined deficiency of factors B and C2 predisposes to serious infections with encapsulated bacteria.[40] Similar infectious conditions occur in the event of factor D̄ deficiency[41] and also in C3B-inac-

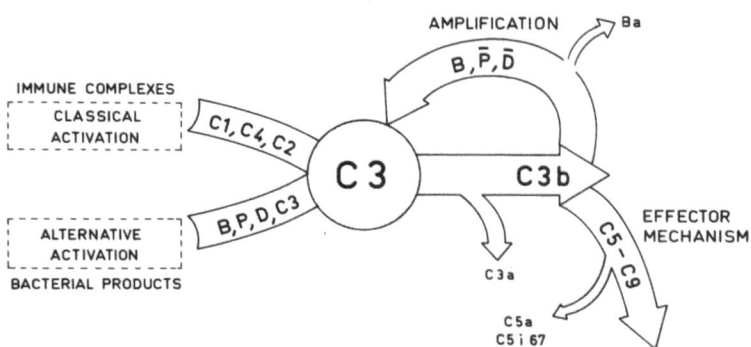

FIGURE 1. Schematic representation of the complement system. (From Daha.[32])

tivator deficiency.[42] In sickle cell disease (Section 5.3) reduced activation of alternative pathway factors leads to impaired opsonization of pneumococci and salmonellae[43,44] Interestingly, a number of complement factor deficiencies are not associated with increased susceptibility to infections (e.g., C1r, C4, C9). A more detailed discussion of the primary complement deficiencies is given in Chapter 16.

During various disease states, such as gram-negative or gram-positive bacteremia, massive complement activation may occur in association with hypotension, respiratory distress syndrome, and disseminated intravascular coagulation (DIC).[45] Under these circumstances, acquired complement deficiency can develop, leading to an inability to cope with infectious agents.[46,47] Acquired complement deficiency, as in systemic lupus erythymatosus (SLE), has been reported to be associated with meningococcal infection.[39,48,49] In Felty's syndrome, acquired hypocomplementemia appears to predispose to serious infectious conditions [50] (Section 5.7).

That virus infections are not an overt problem in complement deficiency states does not mean that complement does not play a role in the defense against viruses. In fact, there is considerable evidence for a central role for the complement system, as reviewed by Lachmann.[51]

3.1.3. Fibronectin

Fibronectin was originally described as cold-insoluble globulin in fibrinogen-rich plasma. It has a molecular weight of 440,000 and is detectable in normal plasma at a concentration of about 0.3 g/liter.[52] It is antigenically related to cell-associated fibronectin. In experimental animal studies, plasma fibronectin has been shown to promote clearance of injected particles.[52] Although mononuclear phagocytes have receptors for fibronectin,[53] it is questionable as to whether it should be regarded as an opsonin,[54–57] i.e., a ligand between a particle and a phagocyte that mediates ingestion (see Section 3.2.1). It is more likely that fibronectin acts by inducing more receptors for endocytosis on phagocytic cells.[57]

Deficiency of fibronectin has been reported in DIC, septicemia, trauma, and shock,[52,58] but the value of fibronectin-rich cryoprecipitate infusions requires further study.[59,60] Congenital fibronectin deficiency does not seem to be associated with impaired host defense.[60a]

The relationship between circulating fibronectin and the fibronectin associated with fibroblasts, endothelial cells, and mononuclear phagocytes has not yet been fully elucidated.[61] Cell-surface-associated fibronectin plays an important role in cell adhesion and cellular interactions.[63]

3.1.4. The Interferons

The interferons (IFNs) are a group of species-specific glycoproteins that exert a wide array of biologic effects. Three main classes of IFN are now distinguished on the basis of their antigenic specificities: α-interferon, β-interferon, and γ-interferon.[64] αIFN, formerly called leukocyte interferon, is highly heterogeneous: there are about a dozen genes that code for human αIFN.[65,66] βIFN, formerly called fibroblast interferon, exists as two subtypes, whereas only one type of γIFN (formerly called immune interferon or acid-labile interferon) is known. Most of the investigations on the biologic effects of IFN were performed before human IFNs, prepared with recombinant DNA techniques, were available. Therefore, the precise biologic effects of the three separate types are not yet fully understood. Generally speaking, αIFN and βIFN act mainly as antiviral agents, whereas γIFN is more active as an immunomodulator. The overall effects of the IFNs are shown schematically in Fig. 2. The antiviral effects are not virus specific. They are mediated partly by intracellular changes leading to inhibition of viral replication in a number of ways.[67] In vivo, the antiviral effects also seem to be mediated by stimulation of host-defense mechanisms, especially natural killer cells (Section 3.2.2) and macrophages (Section 3.2.3c).[65,68] The major lymphokine seems to be γIFN, and as such it is an important activator of macrophages (Section 3.2.3c). The production of γIFN by T cells has been shown to be stimulated by interleukin-2 (IL-2).[69]

It is very likely that the IFNs are designed to work at short range, mainly at the site of the infection. Nevertheless, serum IFN activity can be measured during viral infections such as influenza.[70] An important question with therapeutic implications is

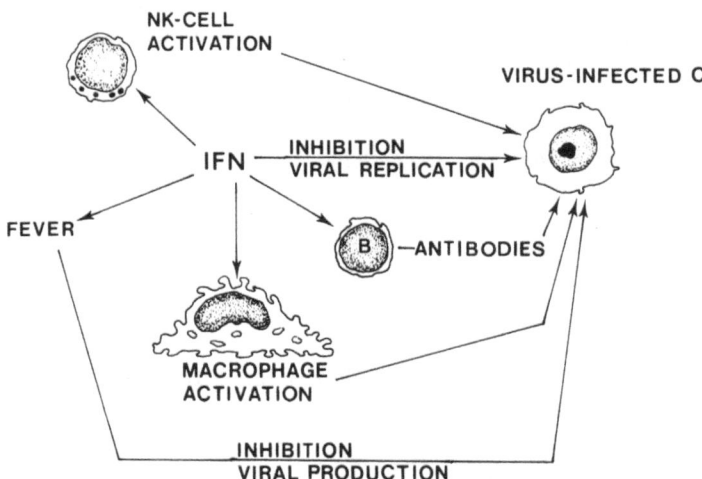

FIGURE 2. Schematic representation of the actions of the interferons (IFN) (modified after a model proposed by Dr. H. Schellekens). No efforts are undertaken to separate the functions of the various type of interferon.

whether there is ever a deficiency of IFNs, e.g., at the cellular level. Such deficiencies have indeed been reported for γIFN in newborns[71] and in patients with primary immunodeficiencies[72-74] and the acquired immunodeficiency syndrome (AIDS).[75,76] For allograft recipients, deficient production of both αIFN and γIFN has been reported.[77,78] By contrast, circulating IFN (probably γIFN) has been demonstrated in bone marrow transplant recipients.[79] More investigations are needed to define the precise indications for the use of the IFNs, which have recently become available on a larger scale, to treat infections in the compromised host.

3.1.5. Tuftsin

The tetrapeptide tuftsin (Thr-Lys-Pro-Arg) binds covalently to the Fc portion of immunoglobulin G (IgG).[80] Its principal function is thought to be activation of phagocytes. To do this, tuftsin must first be freed from the Ig by the action of a splenic enzyme (tuftsin endocarboxypeptidase) and by the enzyme leukokinase, which is bound to the membrane of a neutrophil or mononuclear phagocyte. Its biological relevance is suggested by the occurrence of a congenital deficiency state associated with recurrent infections of the respiratory tract, skin, and lymph nodes.[80] The infectious conditions associated with splenectomy can be explained in part by a failure to free tuftsin from its carrier, the immunoglobulin (Section 5.2).

3.1.6. The Immunoglobulins

The immunoglobulins, which make up the specific humoral response, are products of the B-lymphocyte system. During the development of the pre-B cells, clonal diversity is generated as a consequence of a series of gene rearrangements.[81] In this way, the potential to generate millions of B-cell clones is created. Upon encounter with an antigen, certain B-cell clones expand to produce specific antibodies. Early in this response, IgM is secreted; during differentiation to the plasma cell stage, recombination or deletion of DNA may occur so that the other Ig classes (IgG, IgA, IgE, IgD) are produced and finally secreted. The functioning of B lymphocytes is regulated by regulator T cells (Section 3.2.3b.) and humoral factors such as IL-1 (Section 3.2.3a).

Some B cells do not differentiate into plasma cells but become long-lived memory B cells, which enable the body to produce an immediate antibody response to secondary exposure to the antigen.

Immunoglobulins carry out their functions by means of antigen binding at the Fab sites on the Ig molecule. These functions include neutralization and agglutination of the antigen, complement activation and binding (Section 3.1.2), prevention of epithelial attachment of the antigen, and mediation of endocytosis, i.e., opsonization (Section 3.2.1e). Not all the different classes and subclasses of Ig carry out all these functions to the same extent.

IgM is not in itself an opsonin; only when combined with complement factor C3b is this complex opsonic. Because of its pentameric structure, IgM is very efficient as an agglutinin.

There are four IgG subclasses in humans; of these, IgG1 and IgG3 bind C3b and are especially important as opsonins (Section 3.2.1e). IgG2 and possibly IgG4 seem to play a role as agglutinating antibodies against microbial polysaccharides, e.g., those of the capsules of type B *Hemophilus influenzae* and *Streptococcus pneumoniae*.[82,83]

The IgA found on mucosal surfaces consists of equal amounts of the two subclasses IgA1 and IgA2, produced locally by plasma cells in the mucosa; this secretory IgA is a dimer of two IgA molecules coupled by a small polypeptide, the J chain, with a secretory component that is a polypeptide produced by epithelial cells.[84] Secretory IgA is not opsonic; it prevents adherence of bacteria to the mucosal surface, inhibits the motility of bacteria, may agglutinate bacteria, and neutralizes enterotoxins and viruses.[84] Of the two subclasses of IgA on the mucosa, only IgA1 is cleaved by the IgA proteases produced by such bacteria as *Neisseria gonorrhoeae, Neisseria meningitidis, Hemophilus influenzae, Streptococcus pneumoniae,* and *Streptococcus sanguis*.[84] About 90% of the IgA in serum, which is produced by plasma cells in bone marrow and peripheral blood, is of the IgA1 subclass.[85] The few IgA2-producing B lymphocytes in peripheral blood are probably on their way to the mucosal surfaces. The role of circulating IgA in host defense is unclear.

IgE is normally present in the circulation in very low concentrations.[86] This Ig plays a role in acute allergic reactions and helminthic infestation. When antigen combines with IgE on mast cells and basophils, these cells degranulate and subsequently release a variety of amines (e.g., histamine). These products are responsible for increased vascular permeability and the influx of eosinophils. IgE also acts as a ligand for the killing of schistosomes by macrophages[87]; the ligand for the killing of these organisms by eosinophils is not IgE but IgG and complement.[88]

The role of circulating IgD is unclear. As an Ig on the surface of B cells (like membrane-bound IgM), it serves as a receptor for antigens.[89]

Clearly, the various Ig classes and subclasses play different roles in the handling of antigens. Therefore, a deficiency of all Igs, i.e., hypogam-

maglobulinemia, is associated with undue susceptibility not only to encapsulated bacteria, such as *Streptococcus pneumoniae* and *Hemophilus influenzae* (both of which exhibit tropism in the respiratory tract), but to enteric pathogens such as species of *Salmonella* and *Campylobacter* as well.[90–92] In addition, susceptibility to protozoa such as *Giardia lamblia* and possibly also *Pneumocystis carinii* is enhanced.[93,94] These patients also find it difficult to cope with viruses such as poliovirus, echovirus, and rotavirus.[95–98] Severe *Mycoplasma* infections have also been reported.[99]

Patients with selective IgA deficiency may suffer from recurrent respiratory infections and protracted giardiasis.[100,101] Those with IgG subclass deficiencies, which may be associated with an IgA deficiency, exhibit a relatively high incidence of *H. influenzae* infections.[82,102] Patients with IgM deficiency are especially at risk for meningococcal infections.[103] Strangely enough, not all cases of pronounced Ig deficiencies are associated with repeated infections; many IgA-deficient persons are asymptomatic;[100,101] for instance, an asymptomatic familial complete deficiency of IgA1, IgG1, IgG2, and IgG4 has also been reported.[104]

Primary Ig deficiency states are due to B-cell defects (as in X-linked hypogammaglobulinemia), to abnormalities of T-cell subpopulations or macrophages (as in some cases of late-onset hypogammaglobulinemia),[105,106] or to mechanisms that have not yet been elucidated.

A more detailed account of the primary Ig deficiency states and their treatment is given in Chapter 16. Secondary Ig deficiencies are defined as (1) disorders in which Ig synthesis is decreased, as occurs in chronic lymphocytic leukemia, multiple myeloma, and other lymphoproliferative diseases and to some extent after splenectomy (Section 5.2); or (2) disorders with increased Ig catabolism associated with severe burns, protein-losing enteropathies, and nephrotic syndrome. Administration of Ig to treat disorders with Ig losses is not beneficial in most cases.[88]

3.2. Cellular Defense Mechanisms

3.2.1. Phagocytic Cells

Phagocytic cells are the cells of the granulocytic series (neutrophilic granulocytes and eosinophilic granulocytes) and the mononuclear phagocytes. The development of these cells is shown in Fig. 3.

3.2.1a. Kinetics of Neutrophilic Granulocytes.

In the neutrophilic granulocyte series it takes approximately 6 days for metamyelocytes to form by sequential division and another 6 days for the metamyelocytes to mature into polymorphonuclear granulocytes.[107] A large number of neutrophils (approximately 10 times the circulating population) remain in the bone marrow as a reserve that can be released into the circulation when there is an inflammatory stimulus. The neutrophils that enter the circulation are distributed over two compartments, namely one consisting of free circulating neutrophils (circulating pool) and one of neutrophils that adhere loosely to the vascular endothelium (marginating pool). Under normal circumstances, the two pools are of approximately equal size and in dynamic equilibrium. Several factors can influence the pool sizes by disturbing adherence to the endothelium. Epinephrine and the glucocorticosteroids are potent inhibitors of margination.[108]

There is considerable evidence that the chemotactically active cleavage product of complement factor C5, C5a, plays a key role in the margination of polymorphs.[109-112] An adhesion-promoting glycoprotein is expressed to a greater extent under the influence of C5a.[113] The transient neutropenia that occurs during hemodialysis is the result of complement activation by the dialyzer membrane and subsequent neutrophil margination and sequestration in the pulmonary circulation.[110,112] Since endotoxin also activates complement, the transient neutropenia produced by endotoxin can also be explained by this mechanism.[111]

Neutrophils disappear randomly from the circulation into the tissues with a half-life of approximately 6 hr; in the tissues, they are estimated to survive approximately 1–3 days.[107]

3.2.1b. Kinetics of Eosinophils.

The eosinophilic granulocytes most probably develop from their own committed stem cells (Fig. 3).[113] The time needed for proliferation, maturation, and circulation seems to be similar to that described for neutrophils.[115]

3.2.1c. Kinetics of Mononuclear Phagocytes.

Mononuclear phagocytes also derive from the bone marrow.[116] Monoblasts[117,118] divide to form promonocytes, which divide and form monocytes. Without further maturation, the monocytes enter the circulation, which they leave again with a half-life of approximately 70 hr.[119] In the tissues where these cells differentiate into one of the various types of macrophages, they survive for several weeks.[120] The macrophages together with their precursor cells form the mononuclear phagocyte system (MPS),[121,122] depicted in Fig. 4. The reticuloendothelial system (RES), a grouping of macrophages, reticulum cells, fibroblasts, endothelial cells, and other cells of divergent origin proposed by Aschoff, is considered an outdated concept.

3.2.1d. Kinetics of Phagocytes during Inflammation.

During an acute inflammation, an increase in phagocytes is observed at the site of inflammation. Neutrophils and sometimes eosinophils first appear in the inflammatory field, followed by an increasing number of macrophages. The formation of this inflammatory exudate is the result of various mechanisms. Activation of several inflammatory humoral factors (e.g., kinins, prostaglandins, complement factors), will lead to increased local blood flow and increased vascular permeability. Humoral factors (especially C5a, leukotriene B, and bacterial products) will attract neutrophils and mononuclear phagocytes (chemotaxis).[111,124] In the blood, neutrophilia develops as a result of the release of the marrow reserve as well as increased granulocytopoiesis. Several humoral factors (e.g., the monokine IL-1) seem to play a role in the induction of this granulocytosis.[125,126] Monocytopoiesis is also stimulated; in experimental animals, factor-increasing monocytopoiesis (FIM), produced by tissue macrophages, has been shown to be responsible.[127] Generally, eosinopenia is observed initially during the inflammatory response.[115]

3.2.1e. Endocytosis.

Endocytosis is the cellular uptake of materials, such as microorganisms, debris, immune complexes, effete RBCs and tumor cells by engulfment via the cell membrane. It can be subdivided into (1) pinocytosis (drinking by cells) and (2) phagocytosis (eating by cells). Pinocytosis is the uptake of small particles in small vacuoles. For the uptake of many kinds of molecules, pinocytosis is a receptor-mediated process. Monocytes and macrophages, fibroblasts, endothelial cells, hepatocytes,

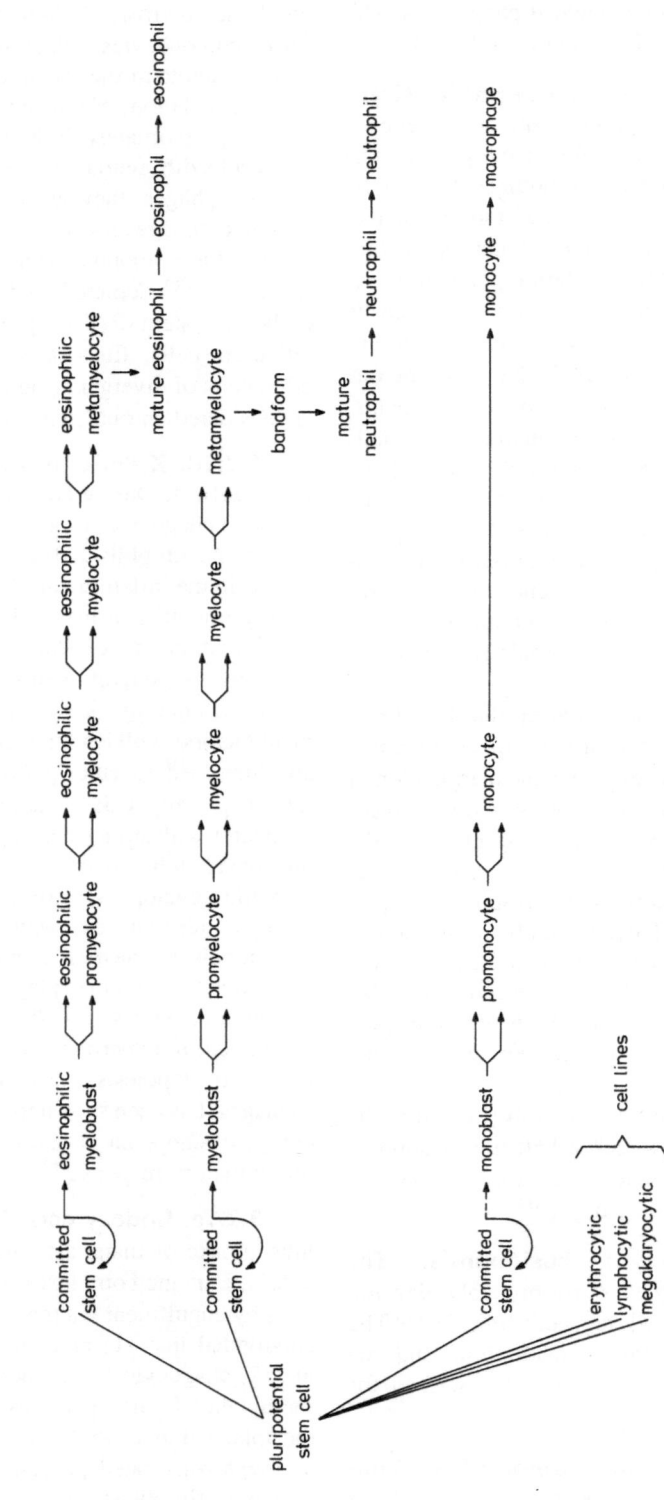

FIGURE 3. Development of the phagocytic cells.

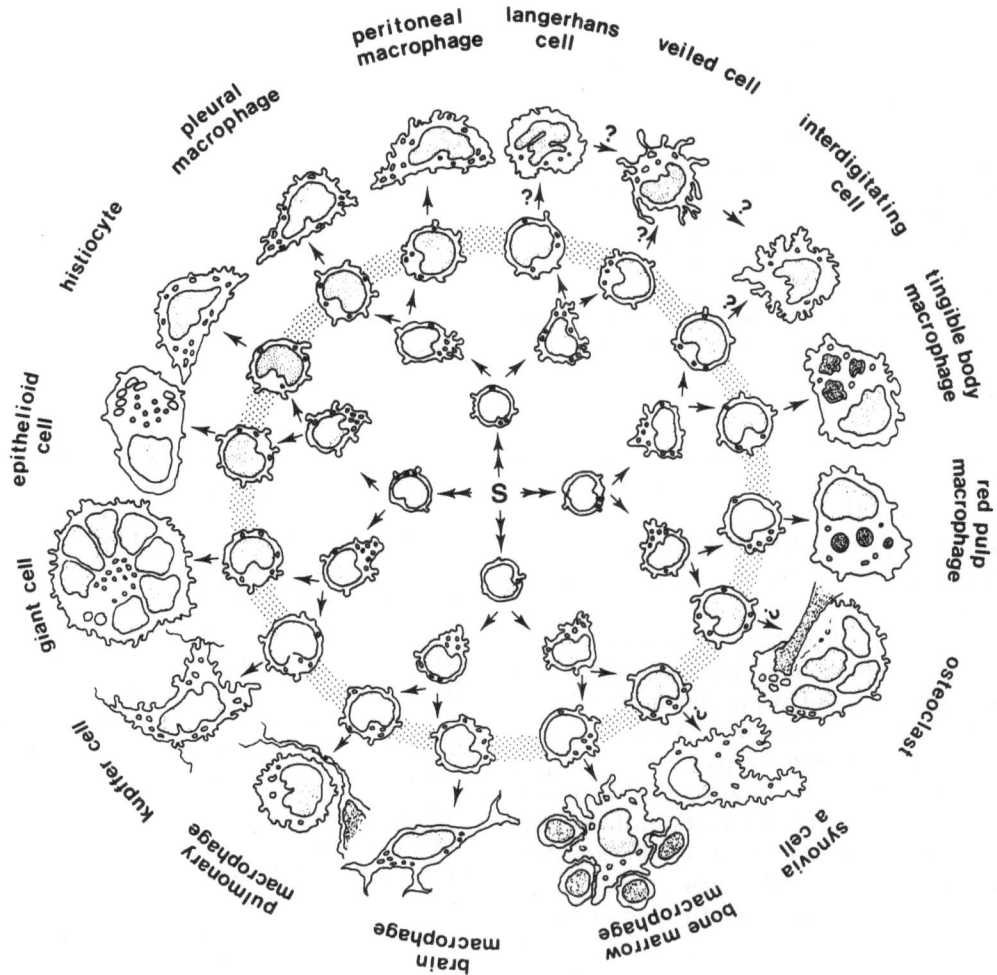

FIGURE 4. The mononuclear phagocyte system (MPS).[121,122] The hematopoietic stem cell (S) is the precursor for the monoblasts (cells that form the inner ring) By division of monoblasts, promonocytes (second ring) are formed, that then form monocytes that enter the bloodstream (shaded area). Monocytes differentiate into macrophages, which have different names in different tissues (outer ring). Those cells for which the evidence to include them in the MPS is inconclusive are indicated with a question mark Based on experiments in the mouse, the monocyte is not considered a precursor of the osteoclast.[123] (Design and drawing by Jos W M. van der Meer.)

and various other cells are able to perform pinocytosis; granulocytes are believed incapable of pinocytosis.

Phagocytosis is the uptake of particles larger than 1 μm. It is a receptor-mediated process, which means that the particles that are taken up bind either directly or by means of ligands to receptors on the cell membrane. The most efficient uptake takes place via the Fcγ receptor and the C3b receptor with IgG1, IgG3, and C3b as ligands or opsonins (Fig. 5). Thus, the first step is the binding of the opsonins to the

particle. IgM is not in itself an opsonin, since there are no receptors for the Fc portion of IgM on phagocytic cells (Section 3.1.6). However, C3b can bind to IgM and then to the C3b receptors on the phagocyte, thereby mediating endocytosis. Fibronectin may be an opsonin as well (Section 3.1.3). Binding of the opsonins to a series of receptors in a zipperlike fashion[128] leads to engulfment of the particle (Fig. 5). The pseudopods of the cell close around the particle until it is enclosed in a vacuole, the phagosome. The rate of ingestion by neutrophils is greater than

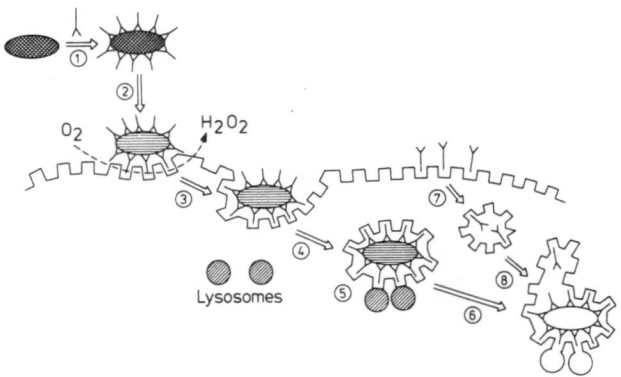

FIGURE 5. Phagocytosis and intracellular killing A particle is opsonized (1) by opsonins (⨏). The next step is recognition and binding (2) of the opsonins to a series of receptors in the membrane of the phagocytic cell. This binding triggers an oxidase in the membrane to activate oxygen-dependent microbicidal mechanisms Meantime, the particle is engulfed by the cell membrane in a zipperlike fashion (3), and a phagosome is formed (4) Lysosomes fuse with the phagosome and pour their enzymes into the phagosome (5). Effective intracellular killing requires extracellular stimulation of the cell membrane by serum factors (6–8).

that of monocytes and macrophages.[129] Eosinophils are also slower phagocytes than neutrophils.[115]

3.2.1f. Intracellular Killing. As soon as the particle (or the opsonins) makes contact with the cell membrane, oxidases in the membrane are triggered to activate oxygen-dependent microbicidal mechanisms.[130,131] Substances such as superoxide (O_2^-), hydrogen peroxide, and hydroxyl radical ($\cdot OH$) will be formed. During and after ingestion, the lysosomes (granules) will fuse with the phagosome and pour their enzymes into the vacuole (degranulation) (Fig. 5). The lysosomal enzymes[132] react with the ingested particle. The lysosomal enzyme, myeloperoxidase, triggers the reaction of H_2O_2 with chloride, which will yield the potent microbicidal product hypochlorite. For effective intracellular killing, extracellular stimulation of the phagocyte membrane by serum factors (IgG and complement factors) is necessary.[133]

During the process of phagocytosis and intracellular killing of microorganisms, neutrophils usually die and are taken up by macrophages. The latter cells have a greater ability to survive and digest much of the endocytosed material enzymatically. Certain microorganisms are not readily killed by normal macrophages but can be digested when the latter are activated by products of stimulated T lymphocytes. These mechanisms are discussed in Section 3.2.3c.

Eosinophils are able to kill several species of metazoa. This is largely an extracellular event.[134] After attachment of the eosinophil to the parasite, a process mediated by Ig and probably also by complement, the parasite will be damaged by exocytosed products of the eosinophil (in particular major basic protein and eosinophil peroxidase).[134]

3.2.1g. Clearance of Particles from the Bloodstream. In the foregoing, phagocyte function in the inflammatory field was described. However, an important question is: What happens to foreign particles (e.g., bacteria) that have gained access to the bloodstream? Circulating neutrophils and monocytes do not seem to play an important role in the elimination of such substances; macrophages in the liver (Kupffer cells) and spleen are especially important, however, for the uptake of this material.[135] The rate of clearance by these macrophages is dependent on the nature of the material, i.e., their charge and chemical composition, which determine binding to macrophage receptors or ligands (opsonins). In addition, the availability of opsonins and the functional state of the macrophages are important for the rate of clearance.[136,137] Opsonins not only increase the rate of clearance but determine the site of uptake as well; particles opsonized by IgG are taken up mainly in the spleen, whereas C3b causes binding by Kupffer cells.[135,138]

3.2.1h. Other Functions of Phagocytes. Neutrophils contain two types of lysosome, i.e., primary (azurophilic) granules and secondary (specific) granules, both of which contain different enzymes.[132] The primary granules tend to fuse with phagosomes (Section 3.2.1f). Degranulation of specific granules, however, occurs earlier at the time of nonspecific surface contact (e.g., during diapedesis), and the enzymes (e.g., lysozyme, lactoferrin, and vitamin B_{12}-binding protein) are released extracellularly by exocytosis.[132] The neutrophil should thus be considered a secretory cell.[132] The secretory capacity of macrophages is much greater. In addition to the lysosomal enzymes, IL-1,[126] tumor necrosis factor (cachectin),[138a] procoagulant factor, various complement factors, prostaglandins (PGs) and other arachidonate metabolites, growth factors, and many other substances are secretory products of macrophages.[139] Apart from this secretory function, macrophages play an important role in the processing and presentation of antigen to T cells.[140]

3.2.1i. Deficient Phagocyte Function. The phagocytic cells constitute such a major defense system against infections that when there is a numerical or functional deficiency of these cells, bacterial or fungal infections are almost inevitable. A shortage of circulating neutrophils, as in idiopathic neutropenia, aplastic anemia, drug-induced agranulocytosis, and leukemia, predisposes to bacterial and fungal infections. There is a quantitative relationship between the number of circulating neutrophils and the incidence of infection[141,142]: at concentrations below 500 granulocytes/mm^3, and even more so below 100 granulocytes/mm^3, there is a high risk for these infections among patients with leukemia and aplastic anemia and, to a lesser extent, idiopathic granulocytopenia.[143] This difference in susceptibility to infection can probably be explained by damaged mucosa as a result of cytotoxic therapy for leukemia, which contributes to infection. In idiopathic granulocytopenic patients, the normal or even elevated monocyte counts also may compensate for the defect. In neutropenia, infectious complications usually arise insidiously, with little or no inflammatory signs and without formation of pus. Such infections usually run a fulminant course (see Chapter 18).

Qualitative defects can affect the various steps of the phagocytic process (Fig. 5), each of which can be assessed in the laboratory.[112,144] A deficiency of chemotactic factors (as in C3 or C5 deficiency) and defective chemotaxis (either congenital or acquired) are also associated with recurrent bacterial and fungal infections. The congenital defects are more extensively reviewed in Chapter 16; the acquired defects are discussed in Sections 4, 5, and 6.

During the late 1950s, it was shown that a delay in the migration of neutrophils of no more than 2 hr has a devastating effect on experimental infections.[145] In patients with defective chemotaxis purulent infections of the skin, subcutaneous tissues, lymph nodes, and lungs are commonly encountered, whereas septicemia is a rare event. *Staphylococcus, Streptococcus, Candida* species and *Escherichia coli* are the major pathogens.

Opsonization of *Streptococcus pneumoniae* and *H. influenzae* in particular is impaired in hypogammaglobulinemia (Section 3.1.5). C3 deficiency also leads to impaired opsonization and clinically to purulent infections caused by gram-positive and gram-negative bacteria as well as fungi. Similar opsonic defects may develop during massive complement consumption (Section 3.1.2). Whether low plasma concentrations of fibronectin, as observed in shock, septicemia, and trauma, should be considered indicative of a hypo-opsonic state is controversial (Section 3.1.3).

Primary defects of endocytosis by granulocytes and mononuclear phagocytes are rare, but a number of disease states and drugs have been reported to affect endocytosis (Sections 4–7). Moreover, it has been well established in in vivo experiments that the uptake of particles from the circulation by macrophages can easily become saturated.[137] Patients with SLE and other diseases in which circulating immune complexes are present[146–149] exhibit impaired clearance, probably due to saturation of receptors by the circulating complexes. Certain histocompatibility antigens (especially HLA B8/DR$_3$ and DR$_2$ haplotypes) have been associated with an Fc receptor defect.[150,151] In primary biliary cirrhosis, defective C3b-mediated clearance has been demonstrated.[152] Impaired clearance of injected material (e.g., labeled aggregated albumin) has been described in alcoholic liver cirrhosis.[153–155] Fat emulsions administered intravenously (Intralipid) have been shown to suppress bacterial clearance in mice.[156] Although controversial in other species,[157] it is conceivable that a mononuclear phagocyte blockade would lead to greater susceptibility to generalized infection and possibly to a poor outcome of infection as well. Similarly, it is of some concern that intravenous gammaglobulin preparations may block Fc receptors in idiopathic thrombocytopenic purpura.[158] Such a mechanism could have a negative impact in compromised hosts receiving such preparations (e.g., hypogammaglobulinemic patients and bone marrow transplant recipients).

Defects of intracellular killing may be congenital or acquired; the congenital abnormalities such as chronic granulomatous disease are discussed in Chapter 16. Some of the acquired abnormalities of intracellular killing are discussed in Sections 4–7.

3.2.2. Natural Killer Cells

Natural killer (NK) cells, which originate in bone marrow and probably belong to the lymphocyte series, are able to kill certain virus-infected cells as well as tumor cells.[159,159a] These cells are not phagocytic and can carry out their cytotoxic function without previous sensitization and in the absence of antibody and complement. Phenotypically they are described as large granular lymphocytes (LGL).[160] Although the precise mechanism of killing has not yet been elucidated, the contents of these granules play an essential role.[161] The relative role of NK cells in host defense in vivo is not precisely known, but it is thought that susceptibility to certain viruses (e.g., herpes simplex virus, cytomegalovirus) can be correlated with NK cell activity.[162,163] Among the immunologic abnormalities that occur in AIDS (Chapter 13), some weight is given to deficient NK cell function.[164]

An important interaction is that between the interferons and NK cells, in which the activity of the latter is enhanced.[65,159] Since these killer cells have receptors for IgG, they may also function as killer cells in the presence of antibody, i.e., antibody-dependent cellular cytotoxicity (ADCC).[159]

3.2.3. Cellular Immunity

Cellular immunity consists of a number of effector mechanisms in which T lymphocytes and macrophages interact.

3.2.3a. Initiation of Cellular Immune Response. It is currently believed that in order to initiate an immune response in T lymphocytes (and B lymphocytes) (Section 3.1.5), most antigens have to be processed and presented by accessory cells.[140] Mononuclear phagocytes act as accessory cells; in addition, dendritic cells[165] and Langerhans cells in the skin[166] also present antigen efficiently. Whether

the latter two cell types belong to the mononuclear phagocyte system is unknown.[122] T cells of the helper-inducer type only recognize antigen when it is presented on the membrane of the antigen-presenting cell together with an HLA-class II [HLA-D(R), HLA-DP, HLA-DQ] molecule (Fig. 6). For the activation and proliferation of T cells that respond specifically to a certain antigen, a number of antigen-nonspecific peptides are required. For instance, macrophages stimulated by antigen release IL-1, which triggers the activation and proliferation of T lymphocytes[167] and also plays a key role in the induction of

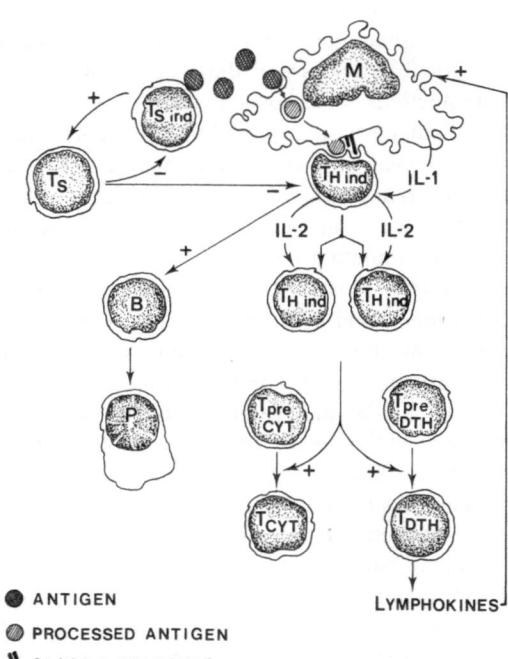

● ANTIGEN
◍ PROCESSED ANTIGEN
❮ CLASS II MOLECULE

FIGURE 6. Macrophage–T lymphocyte interaction The macrophage (M) ingests the antigen; the antigen is then processed and presented on the cell membrane together with a class II molecule of the major histocompatibility complex The presented antigen and the class II molecule are recognized by a T-helper-inducer lymphocyte (TH ind). The latter cell is activated by interleukin-1 (IL-1) secreted by the macrophage stimulated by the antigen The T lymphocyte produces IL-2, proliferates, stimulates B cells, and induces differentiation of effector T cells. The latter consist of cytotoxic T cells and T cells that play a role in delayed-type hypersensitivity (DTH) and their precursors The T DTH will produce lymphokines (mainly γ interferon), which activates the macrophage Suppressor–inducer cells (TS ind) respond to soluble antigen and induce suppressor T lymphocytes (TS), which in turn will inhibit T-helper-inducer cells. (Designed by B J. M. Zegers and J. W M van der Meer)

fever and the acute-phase response.[126,168] Once triggered by antigen and IL-1, T lymphocytes produce a peptide, IL-2,[169] which induces clonal expansion of activated T lymphocytes that respond to that specific antigen (Fig. 6).

3.2.3b. T Lymphocytes.

T lymphocytes can be divided into effector T cells and regulator T cells[170,171] (Fig. 6). Of the effector T cells, only the cytotoxic T cells have been well characterized. These cells are able to kill virus-infected cells and tumor cells in the absence of antibody.[161] For recognition of the target by cytotoxic T cells, class I (HLA-A, HLA-B, HLA-C) molecules must appear together with the antigen.[172] Since HLA class I molecules are expressed on every nucleated cell, this effector mechanism could be operational against all kinds of virus-infected cells. Another effector T cell is the T cell that plays a role in delayed-type hypersensitivity (DTH) reactions and produces lymphokines that activate macrophages.

Regulator T cells can be subdivided into T helper-inducer cells (syn. T helper cells) and suppressor T cells.[170,171] The helper-inducer cells regulate the proliferation and differentiation of not only effector T cells but B cells as well (Fig. 6). During differentiation, T lymphocytes express phenotypically stable antigens that are easily recognizable with commercially available monoclonal antibodies (e.g., OKT). However, it should be kept in mind that these phenotypes cannot be directly associated with function. For example, the T4 population contains not only helper cells but also effector cells as well as suppressor-inducer cells.[173,173a]

3.2.3c. Activated Macrophages.

With the microbicidal systems (Section 3.2.1f), normal macrophages will not be able to kill a number of microorganisms. These microorganisms, which include protozoa (*Toxoplasma gondii, Leishmania* spp., *Trypanosoma* spp., *Pneumocystis* spp.), fungi (*Histoplasma capsulatum, Cryptococcus neoformans*); bacteria (*Mycobacteria, Listeria monocytogenes, Salmonella* spp., *Brucella* spp., *Legionella* spp.), *Chlamydia,* and viruses, survive and even replicate inside the macrophages of a nonimmune individual.[174,175] When T-cell immunity arises, activated T-helper cells will produce lymphokines, such as γIFN (Section 3.1.4) that activate the macrophages (Fig. 6). Upon activation, several events

take place in the macrophages;[176,177] the oxygen-dependent microbicidal mechanisms in particular become fully activated, leading to killing of the intracellular pathogens.[177]

3.2.3d. Defective Cellular Immunity.

All components of the cellular immune system are crucial to optimal functioning. Thus, abnormalities of, or even an imbalance among, regulatory T cells, effector T-cell deficiencies, and macrophage dysfunction may lead to decreased cellular immunity. However, not all disturbances of this delicate network necessarily lead to a state of cellular immunodeficiency. In some instances, Ig deficiency (Section 3.1.6) can be ascribed to the presence of an excess of suppressor T cells or to a deficit of helper T cells.[105,178] In severe chronic inflammatory disease states (e.g., sarcoidosis[179]) an imbalance among regulatory T cells has been demonstrated. In some immunodeficiency states (congenital as well as acquired disorders), both the cellular and humoral immunities are defective. The quality of cellular immunity in patients can be measured to some extent with both in vitro and in vivo tests. The most important in vitro test is still the lymphocyte transformation study using mitogens and antigens. To sort out the nature of a defect, more sophisticated tests can be performed. Lymphokine production can be measured with biologic assays for IL-2 and γIFN, with radioimmunoassays (RIAs) for γIFN and a migration inhibition factor test; the latter test has lost much of its popularity and is not routinely performed in most immunology laboratories. Measurement of macrophage activation in patient material is difficult, and no standard test is currently available. In vivo tests include measurement of delayed-type hypersensitivity skin reactions to recall antigens such as tuberculin, varidase, trichophyton antigen, *Candida* antigen and mumps antigen, as well as a primary antigen such as dinitrochlorobenzene after sensitization. A person who does not respond to the antigens is called anergic.

In the face of true cellular immunodeficiency, infections caused by viruses and the intracellular pathogens (Section 3.2.3c) may ensue. The relative importance of these pathogens is reflected by the fact that many are discussed in separate chapters of this book.

The congenital immunodeficiency diseases with

major cell-mediated immune disorders are discussed in detail in Chapter 16. Acquired disturbances of cellular immunity occur as a result of (1) malignant diseases involving the lymphoid system or the mononuclear phagocyte system e.g., Hodgkin disease and non-Hodgkin lymphoma (Section 5.1); (2) treatment with immunosuppressive drugs, e.g., glucocorticosteroids, azathioprine, cyclophosphamide, and cyclosporin A (Section 6.2); (3) viral infections, such as cytomegalovirus infection, Epstein-Barr virus (EBV) infection, probably non-A, non-B hepatitis, and especially AIDS (Section 5.8); (4) pregnancy[180]; (5) protein energy malnutrition (Section 4.2); and (6) aging (Section 4.3). The mechanisms behind these states of cellular immunodeficiency are rather complex and differ in the various conditions mentioned, since they may involve either regulator T cells, effector T cells, macrophages, or combinations thereof.

4. Factors Influencing the Quality of Host Defense

4.1. Genetic Control of Host Defense against Infection

The quality of the defense against a variety of microorganisms appears to be under genetic control. From animal experiments it is known that genetic susceptibility and resistance involves various aspects of the humoral and cellular immune responses.[181,182] In humans, the degree of the antibody response to a series of antigens has been shown to be associated with HLA and also with certain Ig allotypes (i.e., genetically variable markers within Ig molecules[182]). Moreover, the degradation of antigen by macrophages is affected by both these allotypes and the HLA system.[183] The genetic control of the Fc receptor function of phagocytic cells by HLA haplotypes is discussed in Section 3.2.1i. There is circumstantial evidence that survival during epidemics is under control of the HLA system.[184] Another example of genetic surveillance of immune reactivity is encountered in leprosy, where the HLA type seems to determine the type of leprosy to develop.[185] Our knowledge of the genetic control of host defense is still too limited to be taken into account clinically.[187]

4.2. Nutritional Status

Quantitatively inadequate protein-energy nutrition is an important problem in the world, not only for inhabitants of developing countries but also in many patients with a severe underlying illness requiring intensive treatment. In these patients, host-defense mechanisms may deteriorate further, because malnutrition has an important impact on host defense and may lead to infectious complications. Chandra[188] provides an impressive list of infections that are definitely influenced by nutritional status. Of these, tuberculosis, bacterial diarrhea, bacterial and viral respiratory infections, *Pneumocystis carinii* infection, candidiasis, and aspergillosis should be mentioned. The defects in host defense that are produced by protein-energy malnutrition are dependent on the degree of malnutrition and can be summarized from the vast amount of literature as follows:[188,189]

1. The skin and mucous membrane barriers may become somewhat impaired by thinning of the mucosa with a low lysozyme concentration and decreased secretory IgA levels.
2. Both pathways of the complement system are invariably impaired, which affects chemotaxis and especially opsonization.
3. Apart from the previously mentioned decrease in secretory IgA, the Ig levels and the antibody response to most protein antigens are normal.
4. Although the microbicidal function of neutrophils has been reported to be reduced, it is doubtful whether this contributes to the increased susceptibility to infection.
5. Depressed NK cell activity has been found in malnourished children.[190]
6. Distorted thymic morphology, deficiency of some thymic factors, and an insufficiency of regulatory T cells (especially helper T cells) are probably responsible for the observed cell-mediated immune disorder.

A shortage of some vitamins may affect cell-mediated immunity.[188] Deficiencies of trace elements may also further impair host defense in already compromised patients. Zinc deficiency produces disturbed T-cell function, at least in experimental animals, and increases their susceptibility to *Listeria* and *Salmonella* species.[191] It is important to remember that zinc deficiency has been reported during total parenteral nutrition[192] and in sickle cell disease (Section 5.3). By contrast, supplements of zinc have been shown to affect the functions of phagocytic cells as well as T cells.[191] In iron deficiency, the microbicidal capacity of neutrophils is reduced and T-lymphocyte function is impaired,[193,194] but the development of increased susceptibility to infection in the event of iron deficiency has not been established in humans. On the contrary, iron repletion may lead to an increased susceptibility to infections (such as tuberculosis and brucellosis) and can have a deleterious effect on the course of infections.[195] The latter phenomenon had already been observed by Trousseau in the nineteenth century (cited by Murray et al.[195]). Iron overloading (as in hemochromatosis) has been reported to be associated with listeriosis and septic yersiniosis;[196,197] it is possible that these infections should be traced back to a direct interaction between iron and the microorganism.

A phosphate deficit, which may occur during intravenous hyperalimentation, is associated with a decrease in the chemotactic, phagocytic, and microbicidal functions of granulocytes and clinically with fungal and bacterial infections.[198] The possible effect of intravenous fat emulsions on the mononuclear phagocyte system is discussed in Section 3.2.1g.

4.3. Age and Host Defense

At the two extremes of life, human beings are most susceptible to infection. Neonates can be considered compromised hosts, since they have an important route of entry for microorganisms (i.e., the umbilicus), a blood–cerebrospinal fluid (CSF) barrier that allows bacteria easy access to the meninges, and immature host-defense mechanisms. Of the latter, the initial absence of IgM and IgA, the weak antibody response to polysaccharide antigens,[199] the lower levels of complement factors (especially factors of the alternative pathway[200,201]), and the inadequate functioning of the phagocytic cells[202–205] are crucial. The chemotactic activity of both polymorphs and monocytes is low.[206,207] Cord blood serum does not provide optimal opsonization of those microorganisms requiring activation of the alternative pathway of complement (e.g., *E. coli*).[201] Phagocy-

tosis is generally normal, with the exception of the phagocytosis of group B streptococci by neonatal monocytes.[205] The microbicidal function of granulocytes and monocytes in newborns is a controversial subject. Recently Marodi et al.[205] showed normal killing of *E. coli, S. aureus,* and group B streptococcus by neonatal granulocytes; for monocytes they found defective killing of *S. aureus* and group B streptococcus and normal killing of *E. coli.* The relative importance of abnormal antigen presentation by monocytes, defective γIFN production, and NK cell function in neonates is difficult to assess.[71,208,210]

In the elderly, the decline in the quality of the first line of defense (i.e., atrophy and dryness of skin and mucous membranes), reduced vitality and increased risk for trauma, together with retardation of the repair process, should probably be regarded as the major causes of increased susceptibility to infections. In addition, the primary and secondary humoral responses[211,212] have been reported to be reduced and cell-mediated immunity is suboptimal, probably due to impaired T-cell function (reviewed by Gardner[213]).

4.4. Body Temperature and Host Defense

Elevated body temperature directly affects the susceptibility to infection. First, the replication of certain viruses and bacteria is inhibited at higher temperatures.[214] Microorganisms may require more iron for growth at elevated temperatures.[192] Antibody synthesis as well as T-cell proliferation and function increases at higher temperatures.[213,216] These effects are explained by the greater efficacy of IL 1, the macrophage product that induces fever and an acute-phase response,[168] at higher temperatures. By contrast, NK cell activity seems to be impaired at higher temperatures, as is the production of βIFN.[217,218] The effects of elevated temperatures on the functions of phagocytic cells are less straightforward, but in general phagocytosis and intracellular killing are more efficient at higher temperatures.[127,130] From the foregoing it will be clear that it is difficult to judge whether fever is beneficial; the answer most likely depends to a great extent on the type of infection. Appropriate management of body temperature could be important for compromised hosts, but our knowledge in this respect is still too limited.

5. Diseases Affecting Host Defense

Throughout this chapter, diseases affecting the particular host-defense mechanisms have been mentioned. In this section a number of disease states associated with suppressed host-defense mechanisms are discussed.

5.1. Leukemia and Lymphoma

The number of granulocytes is not the only factor that determines the susceptibility to infection in acute leukemia (Section 3.2.1i); other factors include mucosal damage due to cytotoxic therapy, concomitant monocytopenia and lymphopenia, tissue infiltration by leukemic cells, and leukostasis in the vasculature.

Bone marrow transplantation (BMT), a relatively new therapeutic approach to acute leukemia—as well as aplastic anemia, severe combined immunodeficiencies, and a number of inborn errors of metabolism—is accompanied by a series of infectious complications, depending on the phase of the BMT procedure.[219] Soon after BMT, there are infections associated with granulocytopenia and indwelling catheters; herpes simplex infections may also occur. If graft-versus-host disease of the intestinal tract develops, bacteremia and fungemia may arise in the gut. After BMT there is a state of severe T-cell dysfunction,[220] during which cytomegalovirus (CMV) and varicella-zoster virus (VZV) infections are frequently encountered. Since the B-cell function is suboptimal[220] and there is little humoral immunity left after BMT, severe pneumococcal infections may develop after the patient is released from the hospital. A more detailed account of these infectious conditions and the management of such patients is given in Chapter 20.

In chronic lymphocytic leukemia, hypogammaglobulinemia may become so severe that recurrent infections caused by *Pneumococcus* and *Hemophilus influenzae* develop (Section 3.1.5). Ig substitution may be necessary in these cases (Chapter 16). Similar problems may be encountered in other B-cell malignancies, such as myeloma. In Hodgkin disease, T-cell function is disturbed because of an excess of T-suppressor cells, particularly in the advanced stages and certain histologic types of the disease.[221] T-cell dysfunction decreases cell-mediated immunity, which can be measured both in vitro and in vivo. Infections with intracellular microorganisms, especially VZV, can thus be explained. In Hodgkin disease, the significance of a circulating inhibitor of chemotaxis[222] for the susceptibility to infection is unclear. Radiotherapy and chemotherapy cause not only impairment of T-cell function (Section 6) but also a decrease in the ability to mount specific antibodies against *H. influenzae* B.[223] In addition, splenectomy may enhance the risk of fulminating pneumococcal and *H. influenzae* infections (Section 5.2). Although not yet studied as extensively, the host-defense defects in other lymphoproliferative disorders are very likely to be quite similar to those found in Hodgkin disease.

5.2. Splenectomy

For patients undergoing splenectomy during a staging procedure for hematologic malignancy or for treatment of acquired hemolytic anemia or thalassemia, the risk that they will develop overwhelming septicemia sometime during their life is approximately 5%.[224–226] This risk is much lower after splenectomy due to traumatic rupture of the spleen. The septicemia is caused mainly by *S. pneumoniae* and *H. influenzae*, but the presence of such microorganisms as *Meningococcus, Staphylococcus,* and the DF2 bacillus has also been reported.[224–227] The reasons for this increased susceptibility seem to be manifold. First, the architecture of the spleen is such that it can be considered as a sieve, in which macrophages are present at strategic positions. It is the most important organ for the removal of particles that are not opsonized by complement (Section 3.2.1g). In fact, an increased amount of antibody has been found to be necessary for efficient clearance of opsonized particles after splenectomy.[228] The spleen also plays an important role in the humoral response: the primary Ig response takes place in the spleen,[229] and low levels of IgM have been observed after splenectomy in children.[230] Impaired antipneumococcal antibody production against pneumococcal and other thymus independent antigens has been reported in splenectomized adults.[231,231a] A reduced level of the complement factor properdin has been demonstrated after splenectomy,[232] which could lead to suboptimal opsonization. Furthermore, the decrease in functional tuftsin (Section 3.1.5) described after splenectomy may also be important.[80]

Because of the risk of pneumococcal infection after splenectomy, immunization with polyvalent pneumococcal vaccine is recommended. Although vaccination has been shown to be effective, infection may still occur, especially in patients with underlying disease and small children.[233] Thus, penicillin prophylaxis is still recommended for small children. For patients undergoing elective splenectomy, it is good practice administering the vaccine before the splenectomy in order to obtain a better immune response.

5.3. Sickle Cell Anemia

Infections, especially pneumococcal septicemia, meningitis, and *Salmonella* osteomyelitis, are a major cause of morbidity and mortality in patients with sickle cell anemia.[234] The risk of infectious complications is highest for children with a palpable spleen before 6 months of age. Functional splenectomy, the result of repeated splenic infarctions, appears to be an important host-defense defect. Johnston et al.[43] demonstrated deficient opsonization due to a defect in the alternative pathway of complement. These defective host-defense mechanisms enchance the chance of pneumococcal complications. Susceptibility to Salmonella infections can be explained at least in part by a similar mechanism.[44] Recently, suppressed cell-mediated immunity with zinc deficiency and decreased nucleoside phosphorylase activity was described in sickle cell disease.[235] The efficacy of the pneumococcal vaccine in patients with sickle cell disease has been demonstrated, but pneumococcal infections still occur [233,236] (see also Section 5.2).

5.4. Diabetes Mellitus

Because of the assumption that diabetes is associated with an increased susceptibility to infection, many investigators have studied host defense in this disease. A comprehensive review of this research is given by Allen,[237] who also discusses whether diabetics should be regarded as truly compromised

hosts. Breaches in the first line of defense due to injections, diabetic vascular disease, and neuropathy are important determinants of infections. High concentrations of glucose in urine and secretions may promote colonization by *Candida* species and other microorganisms. Still, it is difficult to explain in this manner the association of diabetes mellitus with, for instance, rhinocerebral mucormycosis[238] or malignant external otitis (caused by *Pseudomonas aeruginosa*).[239] Abnormalities in the second line of defense in diabetics can be summarized as follows:

1. Complement activity and Ig response appear to be normal in diabetic patients.
2. In a series of studies the chemotactic activity of granulocytes was shown to be impaired[240,242]; these abnormalities are not associated with ketoacidosis. The chemotactic responsiveness of monocytes has been found to be depressed, possibly as a consequence of auto-oxidative cell damage.[243] The delayed inflammatory response already noted in experimental diabetic animals many years ago can thus be explained.[244]
3. Phagocytic adherence and phagocytosis have been shown to be reduced at high glucose concentrations, high osmolarity, and low pH.[245,246] Abnormalities of the bactericidal function of granulocytes have also been described[247,248]; the impaired glucose metabolism of the phagocytes could well be the basis of the observed abnormalities.
4. Clearance studies with aggregated albumin demonstrate no abnormalities in patients with diabetes.[249]
5. The T-cell function can be considered normal in diabetic patients, with the possible exception of patients with poorly controlled diabetes.[250,251] Animal experiments have provided some evidence for altered cell-mediated immunity,[252] but the consequences for host defense in diabetic patients are unclear.

An interesting observation is the high frequency of diabetes among patients with myeloperoxidase deficiency and serious fungal infections.[253,254] Thus, when diabetic patients develop severe infections, the myeloperoxidase activity in their leukocytes should be determined.

5.5. Chronic Renal Failure

Patients with chronic renal failure are said to be at increased risk for bacterial infection,[255] but it is questionable whether the chronic renal failure itself is an important factor.[256] Chronic renal failure per se does not seem to impair humoral defense mechanisms. However, discrete abnormalities of the cellular defense mechanisms have been reported. A decreased bone marrow pool reserve of granulocytes has been found in uremic patients.[257] Diminished neutrophil accumulation in vivo[258] and impaired neutrophil chemotaxis in vitro have been observed.[259] These defects can be attributed largely to impaired generation of chemotactic factors in uremic serum and are partially corrected by peritoneal dialysis but not hemodialysis.[259] Both granulocytic function, as measured by surface adherence, phagocytosis and intracellular killing, and opsonization were shown to be normal in chronic renal failure.[260] Phagocytosis by mononuclear phagocytes appears to be abnormal both in vitro [261] and in vivo.[262] Cell-mediated immunity, as measured by the delayed-type hypersensitivity skin reaction, is diminished in chronic renal failure and does not improve with hemodialysis.[263] Lymphocytopenia, which occurs in uremia, and suppression of the proliferative response by uremic serum are in agreement with this observation.[264] In vitro, the mitogenic and antigenic responses of lymphocytes from uremic patients were found to be normal by some investigators and abnormal by others.[265,266]

The situation becomes different when a treatment such as hemodialysis is taken into account. The first line of defense is damaged by multiple punctures, which may lead to intravascular infection—especially when prosthetic material is present. The effects of hemodialysis on complement activation and neutrophil kinetics are discussed in Section 3.2.1a. The fact that antibody response is abnormal in hemodialysis patients was demonstrated by hepatitis B vaccine trials.[267–270] It is of interest, however, that a ninefold increase in the dose of heat-inactivated hepatitis B vaccine gave a high seroconversion rate.[270] In addition, abnormal cell-mediated immu-

nity has also been observed in patients on hemodialysis.[271–273]

In patients on chronic ambulatory peritoneal dialysis (CAPD), peritonitis is the most frequently encountered infectious complication[274] and gram-positive microorganisms (especially *Staphylococcus epidermidis*) the most common microorganism. Exogenous contamination, the catheter, and intestinal disease (such as diverticulitis) play an important role in the pathogenesis. The phagocytic and microbicidal functions of peritoneal macrophages from CAPD patients appear to be adequate, whereas a serious deficiency of opsonins (IgG as well as C3) has been found in the peritoneal dialysis effluent.[275,276] In a prospective study, low-heat stable opsonic activity correlated with a high incidence of *S. epidermidis* peritonitis.[276] Interestingly, diabetic CAPD patients are not at increased risk for peritonitis,[277] and their peritoneal effluent exhibits high opsonic activity.[276]

5.6. Alcoholism and Hepatic Cirrhosis

Alcoholism is associated with a number of infectious complications, such as pneumonia and tuberculosis. In alcoholism, the first line of defense may easily become severely compromised. Repeated aspiration of stomach contents, a depressed cough reflex, reduced glottal closure, trauma, and life-style play a role in the pathogenesis of infections. Disorders are also present in the second line of defense. The antibody response is normal, but the depressed complement activity sometimes found in alcoholics may be responsible for decreased chemotactic responsiveness.[240] Whether an inhibition of granulocyte adherence can be attributed to alcohol is questionable.[278,279] Leukopenia and a blunted granulocyte response to bacterial infection have often been noted. Phagocytosis and the microbicidal function of granulocytes are generally considered normal,[240] whereas cell-mediated immunity has been found to be depressed in severe alcoholism.[280] Fewer T cells and a reduced mitogenic responsiveness have also been described.[281] In vitro, the addition of alcohol has a direct inhibitory effect on lymphocyte proliferation.[282] In alcoholism, other factors usually contribute to the increased susceptibility to infection; often there will be a concomitant protein-energy malnutrition and vitamin deficiency (Section 4.2) as well as liver cirrhosis.

In alcoholic liver cirrhosis, serum has been shown to be less chemotactic for neutrophils than normal serum, probably due to the presence of a specific inhibitor.[283,284] Reduced complement activity and abnormal opsonization have been observed in some patients with alcoholic cirrhosis but are usually normal.[284,285] Phagocytosis and intracellular killing by granulocytes and monocytes are normal.[284] Clearance of particles from the bloodstream is impaired partly as the result of a diminished hepatic blood flow.[153–154] Furthermore, the T-cell responses in cirrhosis may be depressed.[286] The relative roles of the reported abnormalities as well as their relevance for clinical practice are unclear.

5.7. Systemic Lupus Erythematosus, Rheumatoid Arthritis, and Felty Syndrome

It is uncertain whether SLE per se predisposes to infection.[287,288] Such factors as immunosuppressive therapy may well account for the clinical impression of increased susceptibility to infection.[289] Herpes zoster, fungal, and CMV infections are not rare in SLE patients on immunosuppressive therapy.[290] A number of host-defense defects have been found in SLE. Acquired complement deficiencies with defective generation of chemotactic factors and poor opsonization as well as a C5a inhibitor have been reported in SLE.[291–293] A serum inhibitor of both phagocytosis and degranulation could explain the decreased particle uptake in vitro,[294] while immune complexes are probably responsible for impaired particle clearance in vivo[146] (Section 3.2.1g). Furthermore, granulocytopenia and possibly a decreased granulocyte reserve[295] could further contribute to defective host defense. The same holds for the frequently occurring lymphopenia (both T and B cells) and depressed cellular immunity, which leads to anergy.[296]

Whether there is increased susceptibility to infection in rheumatoid arthritis is even more questionable, although a case can be made for infectious arthritis,[288] which may develop as a hematogenous infection or as a complication of intraarticular injections. Hypocomplementemia, the presence of immune complexes and rheumatoid factor, an impaired chemotactic response,[297] and depression of the bactericidal function of monocytes[298] have been suggested as explanations for increased susceptibility to infection. Local defense in joints may be impaired; in synovial fluid a factor that impedes phagocytosis has been found.[299]

The frequent infections encountered in Felty syndrome (rheumatoid arthritis with splenomegaly and granulocytopenia) cannot be related solely to the degree of granulocytopenia.[300,301,301a] The cause of the granulocytopenia is still controversial; impaired granulocytopoiesis, decreased granulocyte reserve, excessive margination, and increased neutrophil destruction have all been suggested.[288] The defects in the host-defense mechanisms are similar to those seen in rheumatoid arthritis.[288] Severe hypocomplementemia may be a major factor in the susceptibility to infection in Felty patients.[50,301a] There is no consensus regarding the therapeutic value of splenectomy in Felty syndrome, but the risk of postsplenectomy septicemia should be taken into account (Section 5.2).

5.8. Infections

Many microorganisms are able to diminish the resistance of the host, thus opening a route for infection with secondary pathogens. Via numerous mechanisms, microorganisms are able to compromise the first line of defense as well as humoral and cellular defense mechanisms (extensively reviewed by Mackowiak[302] and O'Grady and Smith.[303] Hypocomplementemia and blockading of the mononuclear phagocyte system are dealt with in Sections 3.1.2 and 3.2.1i. Whether the function of neutrophils and monocytes is impaired by viral or bacterial infection is a controversial subject.[304,305] An interesting pathogen in this respect is *Capnocytophaga,* a dental microorganism that may cause infection in the compromised host.[306] This bacterium has been reported to be able to induce a disorder of neutrophil migration in vivo.[307]

Impairment of cell-mediated immunity during the infectious disease (by affecting either the macrophages or T-cell function) also seems to be important. Viruses that are able to weaken cellular immunity include CMV, EBV, non-A, non-B hepatitis virus, and human immunodeficiency virus (HIV; Section 3.2.3d). It is well known that CMV infection (which is more extensively discussed in Chapter 13) is accompanied by secondary infections with bacteria, fungi, and protozoa.[308–310] A low level of helper T cells and an increased number of suppressor T cells, as seen in CMV mononucleosis, may be an explanation.[311] However, others have found that such T-cell abnormalities are not produced by CMV in recipients of renal transplants treated with low-dose immunosuppressives.[312] Recently, the association of non-A, non-B hepatitis with prolonged kidney graft survival and increased susceptibility to infection, suggesting impairment of cell-mediated immunity, was reported.[313] The lysis of helper T cells, which occurs in AIDS (Chapter 13), is most probably the major cause of the severe immunodeficiency in this syndrome.

6. Immunosuppressive Drugs

6.1. Glucocorticosteroids

Although there is a consensus that glucocorticosteroids lead to increased susceptibility to infection, the magnitude of this problem for the individual patient is unpredictable.[314] The glucocorticosteroids are able to affect many aspects of the host defense. The skin and mucous membrane barriers suffer relatively little damage, although atrophy and delayed healing after injury may play a role in the pathogenesis of infections. Of the humoral defense mechanisms, the complement system does not seem to be affected, whereas some changes in Ig levels have been observed.[315,316] The major problems involve the cellular defense mechanisms. Although granulocytopoiesis seems to be enhanced by glucocorticosteroids[317] and the marrow pool reserve is mobilized by these drugs,[318] the negative effects on neutrophilic granulocytes seem to outweigh these advantages. At the site of inflammation there is reduced accumulation of neutrophils as a result of impaired margination—probably due to reduced stickiness of the granulocytes—and diminished chemotactic activity.[278,319,320] Glucocorticosteroids only affect phagocytosis and intracellular killing by neutrophils at very high concentrations; most investigators therefore agree that these effects are not of clinical impor-

tance. A fall in the number of eosinophils in the blood is seen after glucocorticosteroid administration.[115]

The mononuclear phagocyte system is also affected by glucocorticosteroids. First, profound monocytopenia occurs after administration of these drugs.[319,321,322] Monocyte chemotaxis may become impaired,[323] but the effects on intracellular killing by mononuclear phagocytes are controversial.[322–325] The clearance of particles from the bloodstream has been shown to be reduced.[326] The production of a number of macrophage products is inhibited by glucocorticosteroids.[327,328] The reduced production of IL-1 may have important consequences for T-cell function, febrile response, and other aspects of the acute-phase response.[168,328] Finally, macrophage activation is impaired, mainly by inhibition of the response to lymphokines.[329] Glucocorticosteroids also have effects on T lymphocytes (reviewed by Cupps and Fauci[330]). Within hours after administration of glucocorticosteroids, a profound lymphocytopenia (also involving B cells to some extent) occurs, due to redistribution of these cells.[314] In contrast to mice, rats, and rabbits, lymphocytolysis is not an important mechanism in humans.[314] The redistribution of lymphocytes as well as the effects on the mononuclear phagocyte system are thought to be the major reasons for altered functioning of lymphocytes during corticosteroid medication.[330]

From the foregoing, the antiinflammatory and immunosuppressive effects of glucocorticosteroids are clear and the consequences for susceptibility to infection can be understood. These effects may even become enhanced by their influence on vascular permeability, wound healing, and a number of metabolic processes. The infections that occur are those associated with impaired phagocyte function (such as infections caused by staphylococci, gram-negative, and *Candida* species) as well as with suppressed cell-mediated immunity (Sections 3.2.3c and 3.2.3d).

To avoid infectious complications, patients who need chronic glucocorticosteroid treatment should be converted to a single alternate-day dose whenever possible.[314,319]

6.2. Other Immunosuppressive Agents

6.2.1. Cytotoxic Drugs

Cytotoxic drugs such as cyclophosphamide, azathioprine, and methotrexate interfere with host defense mainly through their effects on cell proliferation. Thus by inducing neutropenia, monocytopenia, and lymphocytopenia (the degree depending on the drug given), they may give rise to infectious complications. Cyclophosphamide is a potent lymphocytotoxic drug; by interference with the B-cell system, it is able to suppress especially the primary but also the secondary antibody responses[331] and by inhibition of the T-cell response, the drug impairs cell-mediated immunity.[332,333] Azathioprine produces moderate suppression of both the humoral and cellular immune responses.[334-336] Azathioprine and methotrexate act mainly on the primary immune response.[334] For methotrexate, inhibition of phagocytosis and intracellular killing by granulocytes has been shown.[337]

The combination of immunosuppressive cytotoxic agents and glucocorticosteroids greatly affects the susceptibility to infections as well as the outcome of these infections.[338,339]

6.2.2. Cyclosporin A

Cyclosporin A is a potent immunosuppressive drug that is now widely used in transplantation medicine. Its main site of action is the T helper/inducer lymphocyte subpopulation; it has no direct effect on the functions of B cells, macrophages, neutrophils, and NK cells.[346] The drug inhibits production of IL-2 (Section 3.2.3) and lymphokines such as γIFN[341] (Section 3.1.4). Despite its potency, clinical data so far suggest that in transplant recipients cyclosporin A therapy is not associated with a higher incidence of bacterial or viral infections than the conventional immunosuppressive agents (reviewed by Cohen et al.[340]). Whether the incidence of interstitial pneumonitis after bone marrow transplantation decreases with cyclosporin A treatment is controversial.[340] A discussion of the side effects of cyclosporin A and its numerous interactions with other drugs is beyond the scope of this chapter.

6.2.3. Other Drugs

In vitro studies have shown that numerous pharmacologic agents, e.g., antimicrobial drugs (reviewed by Hauser and Remington[342]) interfere with the function of cells involved in the defense against

microorganisms. The clinical significance of these findings is doubtful.

6.2.4. Antilymphocyte Antibodies

Through the destruction of T lymphocytes, antithymocyte globulin (ATG) leads to lymphocytopenia and suppression of cell-mediated immunity, and thus to increased susceptibility to infections (e.g., CMV infections).[338,343] The polyclonal ATG products also act on non-T cells (depending on brand and batch), which may further depress host defenses.[343] Studies are being carried out to evaluate the use of monoclonal antilymphocyte antibodies for immunosuppression.[344]

6.2.5. Blood Products

The immunosuppressive effects of blood products have lately received much attention for two reasons: (1) survival of renal transplants is enhanced when a blood transfusion is given prior to transplantation, and (2) immunologic abnormalities occur in hemophiliacs receiving repeated doses of plasma protein concentrates.[149,345,346] A detailed discussion of these observations goes beyond the scope of this chapter. Suffice it to say that depressed cellular immunity has been observed in HIV-negative hemophiliacs (abnormal T-cell subsets, defective NK cell activity) and in patients who have received multiple blood transfusions (reduced NK cell activity).[347] The significance for susceptibility to infection is unknown. Transmission by transfusion of infectious agents that modulate the immune response (e.g., CMV) should also be taken into account (Section 5.8).

7. Radiation

Radiation damages both proliferating and nonproliferating cells in a dose-dependent fashion. Thus, host-defense mechanisms may be affected in a number of ways. The effects are not only dependent on the dose but on the time course and the radiosensitivity of the cells in that area of the body receiving radiation as well. At the level of the first line of defense, the epithelial barrier may be damaged; the rapidly proliferating epithelium of the gastrointestinal (GI) tract in particular is highly sensitive to radiation injury, and invasion by intestinal bacteria may ensue.

When B cells are irradiated, the primary antibody response is depressed for several weeks.[348] Secondary antibody response is much less sensitive to radiation damage, while plasma cells that produce antibody are relatively radioresistant. Cellular defense may be affected because of the radiosensitivity of the hematopoietic tissues. Granulocytopenia, which occurs after destruction of the mitotic pool and after depletion of the marrow pool reserve (i.e., not until 48–72 hr after total-body irradiation), is the major factor leading to infectious complications. After meningeal irradiation for acute lymphocytic leukemia, neutrophils acquire a transient microbicidal defect that probably reflects damage to the granulocyte precursors.[349] Mononuclear phagocyte precursors in bone marrow are also radiosensitive, whereas monocytes and macrophages are not. Since the latter cells are relatively long-lived, a deficiency of mononuclear phagocytes (e.g., in cell-mediated immunity) may not be immediately apparent. Of the counterpart in cellular immunity, the T cells, it is known that thymocytes are radiosensitive, whereas mature T cells are radioresistant.[348] Cell-mediated immunity may become suppressed when radiation precedes exposure to the antigen, whereas existing cellular immunity reactions are not hampered until large dosages are given.[350] Relapses of infections caused by dormant intracellular pathogens (e.g., *Mycobacterium tuberculosis,* VZV) may occur, especially when the focus of infection is within the area that received radiation. Total lymphoid irradiation,[351] which has been a part of the treatment of Hodgkin disease and non-Hodgkin lymphoma for more than two decades, is not accompanied by significant infectious complications. Nevertheless, there is profound and sustained immunosuppression,[351] which has also been exploited for the treatment of nonhematologic diseases.

8. Attempts to Strengthen Host Defense

When a patient exhibits a defective host-defense response, the prevention of infection is the main concern, followed by optimal treatment once infection has developed. Prevention of both damage to the first line of defense and colonization that could lead to infection with (multiresistant) microorganisms as well as the prevention and control of the adverse effects of treatment are important. The modalities available for the replacement of host-defense defects or even the strengthening of certain defense mechanisms are exceedingly limited. Such measures as physiotherapy, improvement of nutritional status and immunization may be crucial. The nonspecific but largely theoretical therapeutic modalities are reviewed briefly below. Very little can be done to improve the first line of defense, although we can find some pointers in the treatment of burns, which involves not only creams such as silver sulfadiazine to strengthen the barriers but also skin grafting and even covering with in vitro cultured epithelium.[352]

To overcome defects in the humoral defense, a number of options are available. Substitution with cryoprecipitates in fibronectin deficiency is still in the experimental stage (Section 3.1.3). Prophylaxis and treatment with IFNs may help in a number of clinical conditions (e.g., CMV infections)[353] and for selected defects of cell-mediated immunity, but further trials with the newer interferon preparations are needed.

In primary complement deficiency states, fresh plasma or supplementation of individual complement components are worthwhile.[42] There are few data available to support the value of plasma exchange in secondary complement deficiency states such as that encountered in fulminating infection.[354,355]

IgG substitution, either intramuscular, subcutaneous,[356] or intravenous,[357] is indicated in severe hypogammaglobulinemia (see Chapter 16). High-titered specific antibody preparations played an important role in the treatment of varicella infections in immunocompromised children before acyclovir became available.[358] Nowadays anti-CMV IgG is given to prevent CMV pneumonitis after bone marrow transplantation (see Chapter 20). A recent development in the treatment of gram-negative infection is passive immunization with a human antiserum against endotoxin core; the antibody protected against death in gram-negative septicemia in a controlled trial.[359] The protection by active immunization with the core glycolipid of endotoxin has been investigated in experimental animals. Vaccines used in the compromised host are hepatitis B vaccine (Section 5.5) and pneumococcal polysaccharide vaccine (Section 5.2).

Lithium treatment has been shown to accelerate granulocyte recovery after chemotherapy[360] but has apparently not gained much acceptance. In severely granulocytopenic patients with bacterial infection, granulocyte transfusions may be given as an adjunct to antimicrobial therapy (see Chapter 18). Much of the enthusiasm for this approach has waned in recent years for cost–benefit as well as risk–benefit reasons.[361] If granulocyte transfusions are administered to neutropenic patients, it is important to consider plasma supplementation as well, since a deficiency of opsonins has been noted in such patients.[358,362] For some patients with phagocyte dysfunction (as in chronic granulomatous disease), granulocyte transfusions have been beneficial (reviewed by van der Meer and van den Broek[363]). Transfusions of monocytes, which have a longer life-span, have not yet been given; Buescher and Gallin[364] found functional donor monocytes in a patient with chronic granulomatous disease for at least 2 days after white cell transfusions. For treatment of phagocyte disorders, quite a number of drugs (e.g.. ascorbic acid, levamisole, cimetidine) have been tried, most without success.[363] Bone marrow transplantation cannot be considered first-line treatment for these disorders.[363]

In order to restore T-cell function, thymus transplantation[365] or the administration of either thymic hormones[366] or (antigen-specific) transfer factor[367] has been undertaken in selected patients. Lymphocyte transfusions, which are not a common form of treatment, so far have not been successful in AIDS patients.[165] Therapy with IL-2 is still highly experimental and currently under investigation for AIDS patients. Enzymes such as purine nucleoside phosphorylase have been replaced by means of RBC transfusions in patients with severe T-cell immunodeficiency due to deficiency of that enzyme.[368] For severe combined immunodeficiency and Wiskott-Aldrich syndrome, bone marrow transplantation has been shown to be a solution (see Chapter 16).

In animal experiments, cell-mediated immunity has been enhanced by immunologic adjuvants such as *Corynebacterium parvum,* bacille Calmette-Guérin (BCG), and BCG-derived products (e.g., muramyl dipeptide). In humans the success of such agents in cancer patients has been limited, making the options for treatment of infections highly restricted. Live BCG has been reported to be associated with serious side effects.[369,370] The use of γIFN to strengthen cell-mediated immunity is still highly experimental.

ACKNOWLEDGMENTS. I am indebted to Dr. Ralph van Furth, Dr. René de Vries, Dr. Ben J.M. Zegers, and Dr. Mohamed R. Daha for their advice, to Ms. Liesbeth Loovens for typing the manuscript, to Ms. Gail Bieger-Smith for correction of the English, and to Gert Goris for his help with the references.

References

1. Mackowiak PA: The normal microbial flora *N Engl J Med* **307**:83–93, 1982.
2. Abraham SN, Beachy EH: Host defenses against adhesion of bacteria to mucosal surfaces. In Gallin JI, Fauci AS (eds): *Advances in Host Defense Mechanisms*. Raven, New York, 1985, pp. 63–88.
3. Savage DC: Colonization by and survival of pathogenic bacteria on intestinal mucosal surfaces. In Britton G, Marschall KC (eds). *Adsorption of Micro-organisms to Surfaces* Wiley, New York, 1980, pp. 175–206
4. Guiot HFL. Role of competition for substrate in bacterial antagonism in the gut. *Infect Immun* **38**:887–892, 1982.
5. van der Waay D, Berghuis-de Vries JM, Lekkerkerk-van der Wees JEC: Colonization resistance of the digestive tract and the spread of bacteria to the lymphatic organs in mice *J Hyg (Camb)* **70**:335–342, 1972.
6. Heczko PB, Pryjma J, Kasprowicz J, et al: Influence of host and parasite factors on the nasal carriage of Staphylococci. In Jeljaszawicz J (ed): *Staphylococci and Staphylococcal Infection*. S. Karger, Basel, 1973, pp. 581–594
7. Young LS, LaForce FM, Head JJ, et al: A simultaneous outbreak of meningococcal and influenza infections, *N Engl J Med* **287**:5–9, 1972.
8. Sanford BA, Shelokov A, Ramsay MA Bacterial adherence to virus infected cells A culture model of bacterial superinfection *J Infect Dis* **137**:176–181, 1978
9. Komanis SD, Copeland CE, Grosiak B, et al. Introduction of Pseudomonas aeruginosa into a hospital via vegetables *Appl Microbiol* **24**:567–570, 1972
10 Pollack M, Charache P, Nieman RE: Factors influencing colonisation and antibiotic-resistance pathogens of gram-negative bacteria in hospital patients *Lancet* **2**:668–671, 1972
11 Beachy EH. Bacterial adherence: Adhesin–receptor inter-

actions mediating the attachment of bacteria to mucosal surfaces. *J Infect Dis* **143**:325–345, 1981.

12. Svanborg Edén C, Hagberg L, Leffler H, et al: Recent progress in the understanding of the role of bacterial adhesion in the pathogenesis of urinary tract infection. *Infection* **10**:327–333, 1982.

13. Kinsman OS, McKenna R, Noble WC: Association between histocompatibility antigens and nasal carriage of Staphylococcus aureus. *J Med Microbiol* **16**:215–220, 1983.

14. Noble WC: Carriage of Staphylococcus aureus and betahemolytic streptococci in relation to race. *Acta Derm Venerol (Stockh)* **54**:403–405, 1974.

15. Thadepalli H, Chan WH, Maidman JE, et al: Microflora of the cervix during normal labor and the puerperium. *J Infect Dis* **137**:568–572, 1978.

16. Mackowiak PA, Martin RM, Smith JW: The role of bacterial interference in the increased prevalence of oropharyngeal gram negative bacilli among alcoholics and diabetics, *Am Rev Respir Dis* **120**:589–593, 1979.

17. Klein RS, Recco RA, Cataland MT, et al: Association of Streptococcus bovis with carcinoma of the colon, *N Engl J Med* **297**:800–802, 1977.

18. Alpern RJ, Dowell VR Jr: Clostridium septicum. Infections and malignancy. *JAMA* **209**:385–388, 1969.

19. Black PH, Kunz LJ, Swartz MN: Salmonellosis—A review of some unusual aspects, *N Engl J Med* **262**:811–927, 1960.

20. Reichert U, Saint Leger D, Schaeffer H: Skin surface chemistry and microbial infection, *Semin Dermatol* **1**:91–100, 1982.

21. Smith RF: Lactic acid utilization by the cutaneous Micrococcaceae. *Microbiology* **21**:777–779, 1971.

22. Blank I, Oawes RK: The water content of stratum corneum The importance of water in promoting bacterial multiplication on cornified epithelium. *J Invest Dermatol* **31**:141–145, 1958.

23. Newhouse M, Sanchis J, Bienenstock J: Lung defense mechanisms. *N Engl J Med* **295**:990–1320, 1976.

24. Giannella RA, Broitman SA, Zamcheck N: Influence of gastric acidity on bacterial and parasite enteric infections *Ann Intern Med* **78**:271–276, 1973.

25. Binder HJ, Filburn B, Floch M: Bile acid inhibition of intestinal anaerobic organisms. *Am J Clin Nutr* **28**:119–125, 1974.

26. Hinman F Jr, Cox, CE: The voiding vesical defense mechanism: The mathematical effect of residual urine, voiding interval and volume on bacteriuria. *J Urol* **96**:491–498, 1966.

27. Strominger JL, Tipper DJ: Structure of bacterial cell walls. The lysozyme substrate. In Osserman E, Canfield W, et al (eds): *Lysozyme.* Academic, New York, 1974, pp. 169–184.

28. Masson PL, Heremans JF, Schonne E. Lactoferrin, an iron binding protein in neutrophilc leukocytes. *J Exp Med* **130**:643–658, 1969.

29. McClelland DBL, van Furth R: In vitro synthesis of lysozyme by human and mouse tissues and leucocytes. *Immunology* **28**:1099–1114, 1975.

30. Joiner KA, Brown EJ, Frank MM: Complement and bacteria: Chemistry and biology in host defense. *Annu Rev Immunol* **2**:461–491, 1984.

31. Fearon DT, Austen KF. The alternative pathway of complement—A system for host resistance to microbial infection. *N Engl J Med* **303**:259–263, 1980

32. Daha MR: Biological properties of immune complexes. *Neth J Med* **27**:375–379, 1984.

33. Alper CA, Colten HR, Gear JSS, et al: Homozygous human C3 deficiency. *J Clin Invest* **57**:222–229, 1976.

34. Roord JJ, Daha MR, Kuis W, et al: Inherited deficiency of the third component of complement associated with recurrent pyogenic infections, circulating immune complexes and vasculitis in a Dutch family *Pediatrics* **71**:81–89, 1983.

35. Snyderman R, Durack DT, McCarthey GA: Deficiency of the fifth component of complement in human subjects. *Am J Med* **67**:638–645, 1979.

36. Miller ME, Nilson UR: A familial deficiency of the phagocytosis-enhancing activity of serum related to a dysfunction of the fifth component of complement (C5). *N Engl J Med* **282**:354–358, 1970.

37. Miller ME, Koblenzer PT: Leiner's disease and deficiency of C5, *J Pediatr* **80**:879–880, 1972.

38. Ross SC, Densen P: Complement deficiency states and infection: Epidemiology, pathogenesis and consequence of Neisserial and other infections in an immune deficiency. *Medicine (Baltimore)* **63**:243–273, 1984

39. Ellison RT, Kohler PF, Curd JG: Prevalence of congenital or acquired complement deficiency in patients with sporadic meningococcal disease *N Engl J Med* **308**:913–916, 1983.

40. Newman SL, Vogler LB, Feigin RD, et al: Recurrent septicemia associated with congenital deficiency of C2 and partial deficiency of factor B of the alternative complement pathway. *N Engl J Med* **299**:290–292, 1978.

41. Kluin-Nelemans H, van Velzen-Blad H, van Helden HPT, et al: Functional deficiency of complement factor D in a monozygous twin, *Clin Exp Immunol* **58**:724–730, 1984

42 Ziegler JB, Alper CA, Rosen FS, et al: Restoration by purified C3b inactivator of complement-mediated functions in vivo in a patient with C3b inactivator deficiency, *J Clin Invest* **55**:668–672, 1975.

43. Johnston RB Jr, Newman LS, Struth AG: An abnormality of the alternate pathway of complement activation in sickle cell disease. *N Engl J Med* **288**:803–808, 1973.

44 Hand WL, King NL· Serum opsonization of Salmonella in sickle cell anemia. *Am J Med* **64**:388–395, 1978.

45. Fearon DT, Ruddy S, Schur PH, et al: Activation of the properdin pathway of complement in patients with gram negative bacteremia. *N Engl J Med* **292**:937–940, 1975

46. Rytel MW, Dee TH, Ferstenfeld JE, et al: Possible pathogenic role of capsular antigens in fulminant pneumococcal disease with disseminated intravascular coagulation *Am J Med* **57**:889–896, 1974.

47. Greenwood BM, Brueton MJ: Complement activation and meningococcal infection. *Br Med J* **1**:797–799, 1976

48. Dance DAB, Smith CL: Complement deficiency and sporadic meningococcal disease. *N Engl J Med* **309**:615, 1983.

49. Lehman TJH, Bernstein B, Hanson V, et al. Meningococcal infection complicating systemic lupus erythematosus. *J Pediatr* **99**:94–96, 1981

50 Breedveld FC, van den Barselaar MT, Leijh PCJ, et al.

Phagocytosis and intracellular killing by polymorphonuclear cells from patients with rheumatoid arthritis and Felty's syndrome. *Arthritis Rheum* **29:**166–173, 1986.

51. Lachmann PJ: Antibody and complement in viral infections. *Br Med Bull* **41:**3–6, 1985.

52. Saba TM, Niehaus GD, Dillon BC: Reticuloendothelial response to shock and trauma: Its relationship to disturbances in fibronectin and cardiopulmonary function. In Altura BM, Saba TM (eds): *Pathophysiology of the Reticuloendothelial System* Raven, New York, 1981, pp. 131–157.

53. Bevilacqua M, Amrani D, Mosesson MW, et al: Receptors for cold-insoluble globulin (plasma fibronectin) on human monocytes. *J Exp Med* **153:**42–60, 1981.

54. Verbrugh HA, Peterson PK, Smith DE, et al. Human fibronectin binding to staphylococcal surface protein and its relative inefficiency in promoting phagocytosis by human polymorphonuclear leucocytes, monocytes, and alveolar macrophages. *Infect Immun* **33:**811–819, 1981

55. Pommier CG, Inada S, Fries LF, et al: Plasma fibronectin enhances phagocytosis of opsonized particles by human peripheral blood monocytes *J Exp Med* **157:**1844–1854, 1983.

56. Wright SD, Craigmyle LS, Silverstein SC: Fibronectin and serum amyloid P component stimulate C3b- and C3bi-mediated phagocytosis in cultured monocytes *J Exp Med* **158:**1338–1343, 1983.

57. Hosein B, Mosesson MW, Bianco CS: Monocyte receptors for fibronectin. In van Furth (ed): *Mononuclear Phagocytes. Characteristics, Physiology and Function.* Martinus Nijhoff, Boston, Lancaster, 1985, pp. 723–730.

58. Mosher DF, Williams EM: Fibronectin concentration is decreased in plasma of severely ill patients with disseminated intravascular coagulation. *J Lab Clin Med* **91:**729–735, 1978.

59. Saba TM, Blumenstock FA, Shah DM, et al: Reversal of fibronectin and opsonic deficiency in patients. *Ann Surg* **199:**87–96, 1984.

60. Brown RA: Failure of fibronectin as an opsonin in the host defence system: A case of competitive self inhibition. *Lancet* **2:**1058–1060, 1983.

60a. Shirakami A, Shigekiyo T, Hirai Y: Plasma fibronectin deficiency in eight members of one family, *Lancet* **1:**473–475, 1986.

61. Hayashi M, Yamada KM: Differences in domain structure between plasma and cellular fibronectins. *J Biol Chem* **256:**11292–11300, 1981.

62 Tamkun JW, Hynes RO: Plasma fibronectin is synthesized and secreted by hepatocytes. *J Biol Chem* **258:**4641–4647, 1983.

63. Hynes RO: Fibronectin and its relationship to cellular structure and behavior. In Hay ED (ed). *Cell Biology of Extracellular Matrix* Plenum, New York, 1981, pp 295–333.

64. Steward WE II: Interferon nomenclature. *Nature* (Lond) **286:**110, 1980.

65. Rager Zisman B, Bloom BR: Interferons and natural killer cells. *Br Med Bull* **41:**22–27, 1985

66. Stiehm ER, Kronenberg LH, Rosenblatt HM, et al: Interferon: Immunobiology and clinical significance. *Ann Intern Med* **96:**80–93, 1982.

67 Joklik WK: The molecular basis of the antiviral activity of interferons. *Ann NY Acad Sci* **350:**432–440, 1980

68. Schellekens H, Weimar W, Cantell K, et al: Antiviral effect of interferon in vivo may be mediated by the host. *Nature (Lond)* **278:**742, 1979.

69. Kasahara T, Hooks JJ, Dougherty SF, et al. Interleukin 2-mediated immune interferon (IFN-γ) production by human T cells and T cell subsets. *J Immunol* **130:**1784–1789, 1983.

70. Ennis FA, Beare AS, Riley D, et al: Interferon induction and increased natural killer cell activity in influenza infections in man. *Lancet* **2:**891–893, 1981.

71. Bryson YJ, Winter HS, Gard SE, et al: Deficiency of immune interferon production by leucocytes of normal newborns. *Cell Immunol* **55:**191–200, 1980.

72. Epstein LB, Ammon AJ: Evaluation of T lymphocyte effector function in immunodeficiency diseases: Abnormality in mitogen-stimulated interferon in patients with selective IgA deficiency. *J Immunol* **112:**617–626, 1974.

73. Lipinski M, Virelizier JL, Tursz T, et al: Natural killer cell activities in patients with primary immunodeficiencies or defects in immune interferon production. *Eur J Immunol* **10:**246–249, 1980.

74. Virelizier JL, Lenoir G, Griscelli C: Persistent Epstein–Barr virus infection in a child with hypergammaglobulinemia and immunoblastic proliferation associated with selective defect in immune interferon secretion. *Lancet* **2:**231–234, 1978.

75. Murray HW, Rubin BY, Masur H, et al: Impaired production of lymphokines and immune (gamma) interferon in the acquired immunodeficiency syndrome. *N Engl J Med* **310:**883–889, 1984.

76. Buimovici-Klein E, Lange M, Ramey WG, et al: Cell-mediated immune responses in AIDS. *N Engl J Med* **311:**328–329, 1984.

77 Rytel MW, Balay J: Impaired production of interferon in lymphocytes from immunosuppressed patients. *J Infect Dis* **127:**445–449, 1973.

78. Weimar W, van Ruyven CM, Geerlings W, et al: Gamma interferon production capacity after renal transplantation. *Transplant Proc* **15:**421–423, 1983.

79. Rhodes-Feuillette A, Canivet M, Devergie A, et al: Circulating interferon after marrow transplant in cytomegalovirus infection. *Lancet* **1:**1217, 1981.

80. Najjar VA, Fridkin M (eds): Antineoplastic, immunogenic and other effects of the tetrapeptide tuftsin. A natural macrophage activator. *Ann NY Acad Sci.* **419:**1–273, 1983

81. Tonegawa S: Somatic generation of antibody diversity. *Nature (Lond)* **302:**575–581, 1983.

82. Oxelius VA. Chronic infections in a family with hereditary deficiency of IgG2 and IgG4. *Clin Exp Immunol* **17:**19–27, 1974.

83. Siber GR, Schur PH, Aisenberg AC, et al: Correlation between serum IgG2-concentrations and the antibody response to bacterial polysaccharide antigens. *N Engl J Med* **303:**178–182, 1980.

84. Tomasi TB, Plaut AG: Humoral aspects of mucosal immunity. In Gallin JI, Fauci AS (eds): *Advances in Host Defense Mechanisms.* Vol. 4 Raven, New York, 1985, pp. 31–61.

85. André C, André F, Fargier MC: Distribution of IgA1 and IgA2 plasma cells in various normal human tissues and in the

jejunum of plasma IgA deficient patients. *Clin Exp Immunol* **33:**327–331, 1978.

86. Buckley RH, Becker WG: Abnormalities in the regulation of human IgE synthesis. *Immunol Rev* **41:**288–314, 1978.

87. Dessiant JP, Capron A, Joseph M. Interaction of schistosomiasis and macrophages. In van Furth R (ed). *Mononuclear Phagocytes, Characteristics, Physiology and Function.* Martinus Nijhoff, Boston, 1985, pp. 593–598.

88. Vadas MA, Butterworth AE, Colley DG, et al Interactions between human eosinophils and schistosomula of Schistosoma mansoni I Stable and irreversible antibody-dependent adherence. *J Immunol* **124:**1441–1448, 1980.

89. Thorbecke GJ, Leski GA. Immunoglobulin D: Structure and function. *Ann NY Acad Sci* **399:**1–410, 1982

90. Rosen FS, Cooper MD, Wedgewood RJP: The primary immunodeficiencies. *N Engl J Med* **311:**235–310, 1984

91. Melamed I, Bujanover U, Igra VS, et al: Campylobacter enteritis in normal and immunodeficient children. *Am J Dis Child* **137:**752–753, 1983.

92. van der Meer JWM, Mouton RP, Daha MR, et al: Campylobacter jejuni bacteraemia as a cause of recurrent fever in a patient with hypogammaglubulinemia *J Infect* **12:**235–239, 1986.

93. Ochs HD, Ament ME, Davis SD. Giardiasis with malabsorption in X-linked agammaglobulinemia. *N Engl J Med* **287:**341–342, 1972.

94. Saulsbury FT, Bernstein MT, Winkelstein JA. Pneumocystis carinii pneumonia as the presenting infection in congenital hypogammaglobulinemia *J Pediatr* **95:**559–561, 1979.

95. Wright PF, Hatch MH, Kasselberg AG, et al: Vaccine associated poliomyelitis in a child with sex-linked agammaglobulinemia. *J Pediatr* **91:**408–412, 1977.

96. Wilfert CM, Buckley RH, Mohanakumar T, et al. Persistent and fatal central-nervous-system echovirus infections in patients with agammaglobulinemia. *N Engl J Med* **296:**1485-1489, 1977.

97. Erlendsson K, Schwarz T, Dwyer JM: Successful reversal of echovirus encephalitis in X-linked hypogammaglobulinemia by intraventricular administration of immunoglobulin. *N Engl J Med* **312:**351–353, 1985.

98 Saulsbury FT, Winkelstein JA, Yolken RH: Chronic rotavirus infection in immunodeficiency. *J Pediatr* **97:**61-65, 1980.

99. So AK, Furr PM, Taylor-Robinson D, et al: Arthritis caused by Mycoplasma salivarium in hypogammaglobulinaemia *Br Med J* **286:**762–763, 1983.

100 Amman AJ, Hong R: Selective IgA deficiency. Presentation of 30 cases and a review of the literature, *Medicine (Baltimore)* **50:**223–236, 1971.

101 DeGraeff PA, The TH, van Munster PJ, et al: The primary immune response in patients with selective IgA deficiency. *Clin Exp Immunol* **54:**778–785, 1983.

102. Oxelius VA, Laurell AB, Lindquist B, et al: IgG subclasses in selective IgA deficiency: Importance of IgG2–IgG4 deficiency. *N. Engl J Med* **304:**1476–1477, 1981.

103. Hobbs JR, Milner RDG, Watt PJ. Gamma-M deficiency predisposing to meningococcal septicaemia. *Br Med J* **4:**583–586, 1967.

104. Lefranc MP, Lefranc G, de Lange G, et al. Instability of the human immunoglobulin heavy chain constant region locus indicated by different inherited chromosomal deletions *Mol Biol Med* **1:**207–217, 1983

105 Reinherz EL, Geha R, Wohl ME, et al. Immunodeficiency associated with loss of T4 + inducer T cell function. *N Engl J Med* **304:**811–816, 1981

106 Eibl MM, Mannhalter JW, Zlabinger G, et al Defective macrophage function in a patient with common variable immunodeficiency. *N Engl J Med* **307:**803–806, 1982.

107. Cronkite EP, Fliedner TM: Granulocytopoiesis *N Engl J Med* **270:**1347–1352, 1964

108 Joyce RA, Boggs DR, Hasiba U, et al: Marginal neutrophil pool size in normal subjects and neutropenic patients as measured by epinephrine infusion. *J Lab Clin Med* **88:**614–620, 1976

109. Craddock PRE, Hammerschmidt D, White JG, et al. Complement (C5a)-induced granulocyte aggregation in vitro. a possible mechanism of complement-mediated leukostasis and leukopenia. *J Clin Invest* **60:**260–264, 1977.

110. Craddock PRE, Fehr J, Bringham KL, et al Complement and leucocyte-mediated pulmonary dysfunction in hemodialysis. *N Engl J Med* **296:**769–774, 1977.

111. Gallin JI (moderator): Disorders of phagocyte chemotaxis *Ann Intern Med* **92:**520–538, 1980.

112 Klempner MS, Gallin JI, Balow JE, et al: The effect of hemodialysis on neutrophil subpopulations *Blood* **55:**777–783, 1980.

113. Arnaout MA, Hakim RM, Todd RF III, et al. Increased expression of an adhesion promoting surface glycoprotein in the granulocytopenia of hemodialysis *N Engl J Med* **312:**457–462, 1985.

114. Metcalf D, Parker J, Chester RHM, et al. Formation of eosinophilic granulocytic colonies by mouse bone marrow in vitro. *J Cell Physiol* **84:**275–289, 1974.

115. Bass DA: Eosinophil behavior during host defense reactions. In Gallin JE, Fauci AS (eds). *Advances in Host Defense Mechanisms. Vol. 1* Raven, New York, 1982, pp 211–241.

116. van Furth R, Cohn ZA: The origin and kinetics of mononuclear phagocytes. *J Exp Med* **128:**415–435, 1968.

117. Goud ThJLM, Schotte C, van Furth R: Identification and characterization of the monoblast in mononuclear phagocyte colonies grown in vitro. *J Exp Med* **142:**1180–1199, 1975.

118. van der Meer JWM, van de Gevel JS, Beelen RHJ, et al: Culture of human bone marrow in the Teflon culture bag. Identification of the human monoblast. *J Reticuloendothel Soc* **32:**355–369, 1982.

119. van Furth R, Raeburn JR, van Zwet TL. Characteristics of human mononuclear phagocytes *Blood* **54:**485–500, 1979

120. van Furth R, Diesselhoff-den Dulk MMC, Sluiter W, et al: New perspectives on the kinetics of mononuclear phagocytes. In van Furth (ed): *Mononuclear Phagocytes. Characteristics, Physiology, and Function* Martinus Nijhoff, Boston, 1983, pp. 201–208.

121. van Furth R, Cohn ZA, Hirsch JG, et al. The mononuclear phagocyte system. A new classification of macrophages, monocytes and their precursor cells. *Bull WHO* **46:**845–852, 1972.

122. van Furth R: Cells of the mononuclear phagocyte system. Nomenclature in terms of sites and conditions. In van Furth R (ed): *Mononuclear Phagocytes*. Martinus Nijhoff, Boston, 1980, pp. 1–30.

123. Burger EH, van der Meer JWM, van de Gevel JS, et al: In vitro formation of osteoclasts from long-term cultures of bone marrow mononuclear phagocytes. *J Exp Med* 156:1604–1614, 1982.

124. Snyderman R, Goetzl EJ: Molecular and cellular mechanisms of leucocyte chemotaxis. *Science* 213:830–837, 1981.

125. Walker RI, Willemze R: Neutrophil kinetics and the regulation of granulocytopoiesis. *Rev Infect Dis* 2:282–292, 1980.

126. Dinarello CLA: Interleukin-1. *Rev Infect Dis* 6:52-95, 1984.

127. Sluiter W, van Waarde D, Hulsing-Hesselink E, et al: Humoral control of monocyte production during inflammation. In van Furth R (ed): *Mononuclear Phagocytes. Functional Aspects*. Martinus Nijhoff, Boston, 1980, pp. 325–339.

128. Griffin FM, Griffin JA, Leider JE, et al: Studies on the mechanisms of phagocytosis. I. Requirement for circumferential attachment of particle bound to specific receptors on the macrophage plasma membrane. *J Exp Med* 142:1263–1282, 1975.

129. Leijh PCJ, van den Barselaar MT, van Furth R: Kinetics of phagocytosis and intracellular killing of Staphylococcus aureus and Escherichia coli by human monocytes. *Scand J Immunol* 13:159–174, 1981.

130. Roos D: The metabolic response to phagocytosis. In Weissmann G (ed): *Handbook of Inflammation*. vol. II: The Cell Biology of Inflammation. Elsevier/North-Holland, Amsterdam, 1985, pp. 337–385.

131. Klebanoff SJ: Oxygen dependent cytotoxic mechanisms of phagocytes. In Gallin JI, Fauci AS (eds): *Advances in Host Defense Mechanisms*. Vol. I, Raven, New York, 1982, pp. 111–162.

132. Wright DG: The neutrophil as a secretous organ of host defense. In Gallin JI, Fauci AS (eds): *Advances in Host Defense Mechanism*. Vol. I. Raven, New York, 1982, pp. 75–110.

133. Leijh PCJ, van den Barselaar MT, van Zwet TL, et al: Requirement of extracellular complement and immunoglobulin for intracellular killing of microorganisms by human monocytes. *J Clin Invest* 63:772–784, 1979.

134. Gleich GM, Loegering DA: Immunobiology of eosinophils. *Annu Rev Immunol* 2:429–459, 1984.

135. Arend WP, Mannik M: Studies on antigen–antibody complexes. II. Quantitation of tissue uptake of soluble complexes in normal and complement depleted rabbits. *J Immunol* 107:63-75, 1971.

136. van Es LA, Daha MR, Kijlstra A: Clearance of soluble immune complexes and aggregates. In Peeters H (ed): *Protides of the Biological Fluids*. Pergamon, New York, 1979, pp. 159–162.

137. Haakenstadt AO, Mannik M: Saturation of the reticuloendothelial system with soluble immune complexes. *J Immunol* 112:1939–1948, 1974.

138. Atkinson JP, Frank MM: Studies on the in vivo effects of antibody, interaction of IgM antibody and complement in the immune clearance and destruction of erythrocytes in man. *J Clin Invest* 54:339–348, 1974.

138a. Beutler B, Cerami A: Cachectin: more than a tumor necrosis factor. *New Engl J Med* 316:379–385, 1987.

139. Gordon S: Lysozyme and plasminogen activator: constitutive and induced secretory products of mononuclear phagocytes. In van Furth R (ed): *Mononuclear phagocytes. Functional Aspects*. Martinus Nijhoff, Boston, 1980, pp. 1273–1294.

140. Unanue ER: Antigen presenting function of the macrophage. *Annu Rev Immunol* 2:395–428, 1984.

141. Bodey GP, Buckley M, Sathe YS, et al: Quantitative relationships between circulating leucocytes and infection in patients with acute leukemia. *Ann Intern Med* 64:328–340, 1966.

142. van der Meer JWM, Alleman M, Boekhout M: Infections episodes in severely granulocytopenic patients. *Infection* 7:171–175, 1979.

143. Dale DC, Dupont G, Wewerka JR, et al: Chronic neutropenia. *Medicine (Baltimore)* 58:128–144, 1979.

144. van Furth R, van Zwet TL, Leijh PCJ: In vitro determination of phagocytosis and intracellular killing by polymorphonuclear and mononuclear phagocytes. In Weir DM, Herzenberg LA, Blackwell C (eds): *Handbook of Experimental Immunology Vol 2*, Blackwell, Oxford, 1985, pp. 46.1–46.21.

145. Miles AA, Miles EM, Burke J: The value and duration of defense reactions of the skin to the primary lodgment of bacteria. *Br J Exp Pathol* 38:79–96, 1957.

146. Frank MM, Hamburger MI, Lawley TJ, et al: Defective reticuloendothelial system Fc-receptor function in systemic lupus erythematosus. *N Engl J Med* 300:518–523, 1979.

147. Hamburger MI, Moutsopoulos HM, Lawley TJ, et al: Sjögren syndrome: A defect in reticuloendothelial system Fc receptor specific clearance. *Ann Intern Med* 91:534–538, 1979.

148. Hamburger MI, Gerardi EH, Fields TR, et al: Lymphoplasmapheresis and reticuloendothelial system Fc receptor function in rheumathoid arthritis. *Arthritis Rheum* 24 (suppl. 399):4, 1981.

149. Kimberly RP, Imman RD, Bussel JB, et al: Modulation of mononuclear phagocyte system function and circulating immune complexes by lyophilized concentrates in patients with classic hemophilia. *Clin Immunol Immunopathol* 31:321–330, 1984.

150. Lawley TJ, Hall RP, Fauci AS, et al: Defective Fc receptor functions associated with the HLA B8 DRW3 haplotype. *N Engl J Med* 304:185–192, 1981.

151. Kimberly RP, Gibofsky J, Salmon JE, et al: Impaired Fc receptor mediated mononuclear phagocyte system clearance in HLA DR2 and MT1 positive healthy young adults. *J Exp Med* 157:1698–1703, 1983.

152. Jaffe CJ, Vierling JM, Jones EA, et al: Receptor specific clearance by the reticuloendothelial system in chronic liver diseases: Demonstration of defective C3b-specific clearance in primary biliary cirrhosis. *J Clin Invest* 62:1069–1077, 1978.

153. Biozzi G, Benacerraf B, Halpern BN, et al: Exploration of the phagocyte function of the reticuloendothelial system

with heat denatured human serum albumin labeled with
I-131 and applications to the measurement of liver blood
flow in normal man and in some pathological conditions. *J
Lab Clin Med* **51**:230–238, 1958.

154. Lahnborg G, Friman L, Berghem L: Reticuloendothelial
function in patients with alcoholic liver cirrhosis. *Scand J
Gastroenterol* **16**:481–489, 1981.

155. Rimola A, Soto R: Reticuloendothelial system phagocytic
activity in cirrhosis and its relation to bacterial infection and
prognosis. *Hepatology* **4**:53–58, 1984.

156. Fischer GW, Hunter KW, Wilson SR, et al: Diminished
bacterial defences with intralipid. *Lancet* **2**:819–820, 1980.

157. Fraser I, Pearson H, Bowly V, et al. The intravenous intralipid tolerance test. *J Leukocyte Biol* **36**:647–649, 1984.

158. Editorial: Block the phagocytes. *Lancet* **2**:199, 1983.

159. Ortaldo JR, Herberman RB: Heterogeneity of natural killer
cells. *Annu Rev Immunol* **2**:359–394, 1984.

159a. Herberman RB: Natural killer cells, *Ann Rev Med* **37**:347–
352, 1986.

160. Timonen T, Saksela E: Isolation of human NK cells by density gradient centrifugation. *J Immunol Methods* **36**:285–
291, 1980.

161. Podack ER: The molecular mechanism of lymphocyte mediated tumor cell lysis. *Immunol Today* **6**:21–27, 1985.

162. Ching C, Lopez C: Natural killing of herpes simplex virus
type 1-infected target cells: Normal human responses and
influence of antiviral antibody. *Infect Immun* **26**:49–56,
1979.

163. Quinnan GV, Kirmani N, Rook AH: Cytotoxic T cells in
cytomegalovirus infection HLA-restricted T lymphocyte
and non-T lymphocyte cytotoxic responses correlate with
recovery from cytomegalovirus infection in bone marrow
transplant recipients. *N Engl J Med* **307**:7–13, 1982.

164. Seligmann M, Chess L, Fahey JL, et al: AIDS—An immunologic reevaluation. *N Engl J Med* **311**:1286–1292, 1984.

165. Van Voorhis WE, Valinsky J, Hoffman E, et al: The relative
efficacy of human monocytes and dendritic cells as accessory cells for T cell replication. *J Exp Med* **158**:174–191,
1983.

166. Stingl G, Katz SI, Clement L, et al: Immunological functions of Ia-bearing epidermal Langerhans cells. *J Immunol*
121:2005–2013, 1978.

167. Mizel SB: Interleukin 1 and T cell activation. *Immunol Rev*
63:51–72, 1982.

168. Dinarello CA: Interleukin-1 and the pathogenesis of the
acute phase response. *N Engl J Med* **311**:1413–1418, 1984.

169. Smith KA: Interleukin 2. *Annu Rev Immunol* **2**:319–323,
1984.

170. Cantor H, Gershon RK: Immunological circuits: Cellular
composition. *Fed Proc* **38**:2058–2064, 1979.

171. Ballieux RE, Heynen CJ: Functional T cell subsets defined
by monoclonal antibodies. *Immunol Rev* **74**:5–28, 1983.

172. Meuer SC, Schlossmann SF, Reinherz EL: Clonal analysis
of human cytotoxic T lymphocytes: T4⁺ and T8⁺ recognize
products of different major histocompatibility complex regions. *Proc Natl Acad Sci USA* **128**:463–468, 1982

173. Thomas Y, Rogozinski L, Irigoyen OH, et al: Functional
analysis of human T cell subsets defined by monoclonal

antibodies. IV. Induction of suppressor cells within the
OKT4⁺ population. *J Exp Med* **154**:459–467, 1981.

173a. Young M, Geha RF: Human regulatory T cell subsets, *Ann
Rev Med* **37**:165–172, 1986.

174. Hahn H, Kaufmann SHE: The role of cell-mediated immunity in bacterial infections. *Rev Infect Dis* **3**:1221–1250,
1981.

175. Murray HW: How protozoa evade intracellular killing. *Ann
Intern Med* **98**:1016–1018, 1983.

176. Cohn ZA: The activation of mononuclear phagocytes. Fact,
fancy and future. *J Immunol* **121**:813–816, 1978.

177. Adams DO, Hamilton TA: The cell biology of macrophage
activation. *Annu Rev Immunol* **2**:283–318, 1984.

178. Siegel RL, Issekutz T, Schwaber J: Deficiency of T helper
cells in transient hypogammaglobulinemia of infancy. *N
Engl J Med* **305**:1307–1313, 1981.

179. Hunninghake GW, Crystal RG: Pulmonary sarcoidosis. A
disorder mediated by excess helper-T lymphocyte activity at
sites of disease activity. *N Engl J Med* **305**:429–434, 1981.

180. Weinberg ED: Pregnancy-associated depression of cell-mediated immunity. *Rev Infect Dis* **6**:814–831, 1984.

181. Skamene E, Stevenson MM: Genetic control of macrophage
response to infection. In van Furth R (ed): *Mononuclear
Phagocytes. Characteristics, Physiology, and Function.*
Martinus Nijhoff, Boston, 1985, pp. 647–653.

182. De Vries RRP, van Rood JJ: Immunogenetics and disease. In
King RA, Rotter JI, Motulsky AC (eds): *Genetic Basis of
Common Disease.* Oxford University Press, New York (in
press).

183. Legrand L, Rivat-Perrau L, Huttin C, et al: HLA and Gm
affecting the degradation rate of antigens (sheep red blood
cells) endocytized by macrophages. *Hum Immunol* **4**:1–13,
1982.

184. De Vries RRP, Meera Khan P, Bernini LF, et al: Genetic
control of survival in epidemics *J Immunogenet* **6**:271–287,
1979.

185. van Eeden W, Gonzalez NM, de Vries RRP, et al. HLA
linked control of predisposition to lepromatous leprosy. *J
Infect Dis* **151**:9–14, 1985

186. Svejgaard A, Platz P, Rijder LP: HLA and disease 1982. A
survey. *Immunol Rev* **70**:193–218, 1983.

187. Pollack MS, Rich RR: the HLA complex and the pathogenesis of infectious diseases. *J Infect Dis* **151**:1–8, 1985.

188. Chandra RK. Nutrition, Immunity and Infection: Present
knowledge and future directions. *Lancet* **1**:688–691, 1983.

189. Keusch GT: Host defense mechanisms in protein energy
malnutrition. *Adv Exp Med Biol* **135**:183–209, 1981.

190. Salimonu LS, Ojo-Amaize E, Williams AIO, et al: Depressed natural killer cell activity in children with protein
calorie malnutrition. *Clin Immunol Immunopathol* **24**:1–7,
1982.

191. Sugarman B. Zinc and infection. *Rev Infect Dis* **5**:137–147,
1983.

192. Tucker SB, Schroeter AL, Brown PW Jr, et al: Acquired
zinc deficiency: Cutaneous manifestations typical of acro-
dermatitis enteropathica. *JAMA* **235**:2399–2402, 1976.

193. Chandra RK, Au B, Woodford G, et al: Iron status, immunocompetence and susceptibility to infection. In *Iron Metab-*

olism. Ciba Foundation Symposium, No. 51. Elsevier, Amsterdam, 1977, pp. 249–268.

194. Bullen JJ: The significance of iron in infection: *Rev Infect Dis* 3:1127–1138, 1981.

195. Murray MJ, Murray AB, Murray MB, et al: The adverse effect of iron repletion on the course of certain infections. *Br Med J* 2:113–115, 1978.

196. van Asbeck BS, Verbrugh HA, van Oost BA, et al: Listeria monocytogenes meningitis and decreased phagocytosis associated with iron overload, *Br Med J* 284:542–544, 1982

197. Melby K, Slørdahl S, Gutteberg TJ: Septicaemia due to Yersinia enterocolitica after oral overdoses of iron. *Br Med J* 285:467–468, 1982.

198. Craddock PR, Yawata Y, van Santen L: Acquired phagocyte dysfunction. A complication of the hypophosphatemia of parenteral hyperalimentation. *N Engl J Med* 290:1403–1407, 1974.

199. Smith D, Peter G; Ingram DL, et al: Responses of children immunized with the capsular polysaccharide of Hemophilus influenzae type B. *Pediatrics* 52:637–640, 1973.

200. Adamkin D, Stitzel A, Urmson J, et al: Activity of the alternative pathway of complement in the newborn infant. *J Pediatr* 93:604–608, 1978.

201. Maródi L. Leijh PCJ, Braat A, et al.: Opsonic activity of cord blood sera against various species of micro-organisms. *Pediatr Res* 19:433–436, 1985.

202. Park BH, Holmes B, Good RA: Metabolic activities in leucocytes of newborn infants. *J Pediatr* 76:237–241, 1970.

203. McCracken GH, Eichenwald HF: Leucocyte function and the development of opsonic and complement activity in the neonate. *Am J Dis Child* 121:120–126, 1971.

204. Schuit KE, Powall DA: Phagocyte dysfunction in monocytes of normal newborn infants. *Pediatrics* 65:501–504, 1980.

205. Maródi L. Leijh PCJ, van Furth R: Characterization and functional capacities of human cord blood granulocytes and monocytes. *Pediatr Res* 18:1127–1131, 1984

206. Maródi L, Jzerniczky J, Csorba S, et al: Chemotactic and random movement of cord blood granulocytes. *Experientia* 40:1407–1410, 1984.

207. Maródi L, Csorba S, Nagy B: Chemotactic and random movement of human newborn monocytes. *Eur J Pediatr* 135:73–85, 1980.

208. van Tol MJD, Zijlstra J, Thomas CMG, et al: Distinct role of neonatal and adult monocytes in the regulation of the in vitro antigen-induced plaque-forming cell response in man. *J Immunol* 133:1902–1908, 1984.

209. Kohl S, Frazier JJ, Greenberg SB, et al: Interferon induction of natural killer cytotoxicity in human neonates. *J Pediatr* 98:379–384, 1981.

210. Wakasugi N, Virelizier JL: Defective IFN γ production in the human neonate. Dysregulation rather than intrinsic abnormality *J Immunol* 134:167–171, 1985.

211. Phair J, Kauffman CA, Bjornson A: Failure to respond to influenza vaccine in the aged: correlation with B cell number of function. *J Lab Clin Med* 92:822–828, 1978.

212. Roberts-Thomson IC, Whittingham S, Youngchaiyud U, et al: Aging, immune response and mortality. *Lancet* 2:368–370, 1974.

213. Gardner ID: The effect of aging on susceptibility to infection. *Rev Infect Dis* 2:801–810, 1980.

214. Mackowiak PA: Direct effects of hyperthermia on pathogenic microorganisms: Teleologic implications with regard to fever. *Rev Infect Dis* 3:508–520, 1981.

215. Jampel HD, Duff GW, Gershon RK, et al: Fever and immunoregulation. III. Hyperthermia augments the primary in vitro humoral response. *J Exp Med* 157:1229–1238, 1983.

216. Hanson DF, Murphy PA, Silicano R, et al: The effect of temperature on the activation of thymocytes by interleukins I and II. *J Immunol* 130:216–221, 1983.

217. Giard DJ, Fleischaker RJ, Sinskey AT, et al: Kinetics of human beta inferferon production under different temperature conditions. *J Interferon Res* 2:471–477, 1982.

218. Dinarello CA, Dempsey RA, Allegretta M, et al: Inhibitory effects of elevated temperature on human cytokine production and natural killer activity. *Cancer Res* 46:6236–6241, 1986.

219. van der Meer JWM, Guiot HFL, van den Broek PJ, et al: Infections in bone marrow transplant recipients. *Semin Hematol* 21:123–140, 1984.

220. Witherspoon RP, Lum LG, Storb R: Immunological reconstitution after human marrow grafting. *Semin Hematol* 21:2–10, 1984.

221. Engleman EJ, Benike CJ, Hoppe RT, et al: Autologous mixed lymphocyte reaction in patients with Hodgkin's disease. *J Clin Invest* 66:149–158, 1980.

222. Ward PA, Berenberg JC: Defective regulation of inflammatory mediators in Hodgkin's disease. *N Engl J Med* 290:76–80, 1974.

223. Weitzman SA, Aisenberg AC, Siber GR, et al: Immunity in treated Hodgkin's disease. *N Engl J Med* 297:245–248, 1977.

224. Chilcote RR, Baehner RL, Hammond D: Septicemia and meningitis in children splenectomized for Hodgkin's disease. *N Engl J Med* 295:798–800, 1976.

225. Weitzman S, Aisenberg AC: Fulminant sepsis after the successful treatment of Hodgkin's disease. *Am J Med* 62:47–50, 1977.

226. Schwartz PE, Sterioff S, Mucha P, et al: Post splenectomy sepsis and mortality in adults. *JAMA* 284:2279–2283, 1982.

227. Fibbe W, Ligthart G, van der Broek PF, et al: Septicaemia with a dysgonic fermenten (DF-2) bacterium in a compromised host, *Infection* 6:286–287, 1985.

228. Hosea SW, Brown EJ, Hamburger MI, et al: Opsonic requirements for intravascular clearance after splenectomy. *N Engl J Med* 304:245–250, 1981.

229. Benner R, Hijmans W, Haayman JJ: The bone marrow: The major source of serum immunoglobulins but still a neglected site of antibody formation. *Clin Exp Immunol* 46:1–8, 1981.

230. Schumacher MJ: Serum immunoglobulin and transferrin levels after childhood splenectomy. *Arch Dis Child* 45:114–117, 1970.

231. Di Padova F, Düng M, Harder F, et al: Impaired antipneumococcal antibody production in patients without spleens. *Br Med J* 290:14–16, 1985.

231a. Amlot PL, Hayes AE: Impaired human antibody response to the thymus independent antigen DNP-Ficoll after splenectomy, *Lancet* **1**:1000–1011, 1985.

232. Carlisle HN, Saslaw S: Properdin levels in splenectomized persons. *Proc Soc Exp Biol* **102**:150–155, 1959.

233. Broome CV, Facklam RR, Fraser DW: Pneumococcal disease after pneumococcal vaccination. An alternative method to estimate the efficacy of pneumococcal vaccine. *N Engl J Med* **303**:549–552, 1980.

234. Barret-Connor E: Infection and sickle cell anemia. In Allen JC (ed): *Infection in the Compromised Host. Clinical Correlations and Therapeutic Approaches.* 2nd ed. Williams & Wilkins, Baltimore, 1981, pp. 107–120.

235. Ballester OF, Prasad AS: Anergy, zinc deficiency and decreased nucleoside phosphorylase activity in patients with sickle cell anemia.. *Ann Intern Med* **98**:180–182, 1983.

236. Amman AJ, Addiego J, Wara DW, et al: Polyvalent pneumococcal-polysaccharide immunization of patients with sickle cell anemia and patients with splenectomy. *N Engl J Med* **297**:897–900, 1977.

237. Allen JC: The diabetic as a compromised host. In Allen JC (ed): *Infection and the Compromised Host. Clinical Correlations and Therapeutic Approaches.* 2nd ed., Williams & Wilkins, Baltimore, 1981, pp. 229–270.

238. Meyers BR, Wormser G, Hirschman SZ, et al: Rhinocerebral mucormycosis Premortem diagnosis and therapy. *Arch Intern Med* **139**:557–563, 1979.

239. Doroghazi RM, Nadol JB Jr, Hyslop NE Jr, et al: Invasive external otitis, report of 21 cases and review of the literature. *Am J Med* **71**:603–614, 1981.

240. Brayton RG, Stokes PE, Schwartz MS, et al: Effect of alcohol and various diseases on leukocyte mobilization phagocytosis and intracellular bacterial killing. *N Engl J Med* **282**:123–128, 1970.

241. Mowat AG, Baum J: Chemotaxis of polymorphonuclear leucocytes from patients with diabetes mellitus. *N Engl J Med* **284**:621–627, 1971.

242. Miller ME, Baker L: Leukocyte functions in juvenile diabetes mellitus: Humoral and cellular aspects. *J Pediatr* **81**:979–982, 1972.

243. Hill HR, Augustine NH, Rallison ML, et al: Defective monocyte chemotactic responses in diabetes mellitus. *J Clin Immunol* **3**:70–77, 1983.

244. Sheldon WH, Bauer H: The development of the acute inflammatory response to experimental cutaneous mucormycosis in normal and diabetic rabbits. *J Exp Med* **110**:845–859, 1959.

245. Bagdade JD, Root RK, Bulger RJ: Impaired leukocyte function in patients with poorly controlled diabetes. *Diabetes* **23**:9–15, 1974.

246. Chernew I, Braude AI: Depression of phagocytosis by solutes in concentrations found in the kidney and urine. *J Clin Invest* **41**:1945–1951, 1962.

247. Nolan CM, Beaty HN, Bagdade JD: Further characterization of the impaired bactericidal function of granulocytes in patients with poorly controlled diabetes. *Diabetes* **27**:889–894, 1978.

248. Tan JS, Anderson JL, Watanakunakorn C, et al. Neutrophil dysfunction in diabetes mellitus *J Lab Clin Med* **85**:26–33, 1975.

249. Berken A, Sherman AA: Reticuloendothelial system phagocytosis in diabetes mellitus. *Diabetes* **23**:218–220, 1974.

250. Maccuish AC, Urbaniak SJ, Cambell CJ, et al: Phytohemagglutinin ·transformation and circulating lymphocyte subpopulations in insulin-dependent diabetic patients. *Diabetes* **23**:708–712, 1974.

251. Eliashiv A, Olumide F, Norton L, et al: Depression of cell-mediated immunity in diabetes *Arch Surg* **113**:1180–1183, 1978.

252. Mahmoud AAF, Rodman HM, Mandel MA, et al: Induced and spontaneous diabetes mellitus and suppression of cell-mediated immunologic responses. *J Clin Invest* **57**:362–367, 1976.

253. Parry MF, Root RK, Metcalf JA, et al: Myeloperoxidase deficiency, prevalence and clinical significance. *Ann Intern Med* **95**:293–301, 1981.

254. Cech P, Stalder H. Widmann JJ, et al: Leucocyte myeloperoxidase deficiency and diabetes mellitus associated with Candida albicans liver abscess. *Am J Med* **66**:149–153, 1979.

255. Montgomerie JZ, Kalmanson GM, Guze LB: Renal failure and infection, *Medicine (Baltimore)* **47**:1–32, 1968.

256. Clarke IA, Ormond DJ, Miller TE: Host immune status in uremia. V. Effect of uremia on resistance to bacterial infection. *Kidney Int* **24**:66–73, 1983.

257. Perescenschi G, Zakouth V, Spirer Z, et al: Leucocyte mobilization by epinephrine and hydrocortisone in patients with chronic renal failure. *Experientia* **33**:1529–1530, 1977.

258. Perillie PE, Nolan JP, Finch SC: Studies of the resistance to infection in diabetes mellitus: Local exudative cellular response. *Lab Clin Med* **59**:1008–1015, 1962

259. Salant DF, Glover AM, Anderson R, et al: Depressed neutrophil chemotaxis in patients with chronic renal failure and after renal transplantation. *J Lab Clin Med* **88**:536–545, 1976.

260. Abrutyn E, Solomons NW, St Clair L, et al: Granulocyte function in patients with chronic renal failure: Surface adherence, phagocytosis, and bactericidal activity in vitro. *J Infect Dis* **135**:1–8, 1977.

261. Urbanitz D, Sieberth HG: Impaired phagocytic activity of human monocytes in respect to reduced antibacterial resistance in uremia. *Clin Nephrol* **4**:13–17, 1975.

262 Nelson J, Ormrod DJ, Muller TE: Host immune status in uremia. IV. Phagocytosis and the inflammatory response in vivo. *Kidney Int* **23**:312–319, 1983.

263. Kirkpatrick CH, Wilson WEC, Talmage DW: Immunologic studies in human organ transplantation. I. Observation and characterization of suppressed cutaneous reactivity in uremia. *J Exp Med* **119**:727–742, 1964.

264. Newsberry WM, Sanford JP: Defective cellular immunity in renal failure: depression of reactivity of lymphocytes to phytohemagglutinin by renal failure serum. *J Clin Invest* **50**:1262–1271, 1971.

265. Daniels JC, Sakae H, Remmers AR, et al: In-vitro reactivity of human lymphocytes in chronic uraemia. Analysis and interpretation. *Clin Exp Immunol* **8**:213–227, 1971.

266. Miller TE, Stewart E: Host immune status in uraemia. I. cell-mediated immune mechanisms. *Clin Exp Immunol* **41**:115–122, 1980.

267. Stevens CE, Alter HJ, Taylor PE, et al: Hepatitis B vaccine in patients receiving hemodialysis. Immunogenicity and efficacy. *N Engl J Med* 311:496–511, 1984.
268. Crosnier J, Jungers P, Couroucé AM, et al: Randomized placebo-controlled trial of hepatitis B surface antigens vaccine in French haemodialysis units. *Lancet* 1:797–800, 1981.
269. Desmyter J, Colaert J, de Groote G, et al: Efficacy of heat-inactivated hepatitis B vaccine in haemodialysis patients and staff: Double-blind placebo-controlled trial. *Lancet* 2:1323–1328, 1983.
270. Lelie PN, Reesink HW, De Jong-van Manen STh, et al: Immune response to a heat-inactivated hepatitis B vaccine in patients undergoing hemodialysis. Enhancement of the response by increasing the dose of hepatitis B surface antigen from 3 to 27 µg. *Arch Intern Med* 145:305–309, 1985.
271. Ruddy MC, Rubin AL, Novogrodsky A, et al: Decreased macrophage-mediated suppression of lymphocyte activation in chronic renal failure. *Am J Med* 75:571–579, 1983.
272. Sengar DPS, Rashid A, Harris JE: In-vitro reactivity of lymphocytes obtained from uraemic patients maintained by haemodialysis. *Clin Exp Immunol* 21:298–305, 1975.
273. Langhoff E, Ladefoged J: Cellular immunity in renal failure: Depression of lymphocyte transformation by uraemia and methylprednisolone. *Int Arch Allergy Appl Immunol* 74:241–245, 1984.
274. Gloor HJ, Nichols WK, Sorkin MI, et al: Peritoneal acces and related complications in continuous ambulatory peritoneal dialysis. *Am J Med* 74:593–598, 1983.
275. Verbrugh HA, Keane WF, Hoidal JR, et al: Peritoneal macrophages and opsonins: Antibacterial defense in patients on chronic peritoneal dialysis. *J Infect Dis* 147:1018–1029, 1983.
276. Keane WF, Peterson PK: Host defense mechanisms of the peritoneal cavity and continuous ambulatory peritoneal dialysis. *Peritoneal Dialysis Bull* 4:122–127, 1984.
277. Amair P, Khanna R, Leibel B, et al: Continuous ambulatory peritoneal dialysis in diabetics with endstage renal disease. *N Engl J Med* 306:625–630, 1982.
278. MacGregor RR, Spagnuolo PJ, Lentnek AE: Inhibition of granulocyte adherence by ethanol, prednisone, and aspirin measured with an assay system. *N Engl J Med* 291:642–646, 1974.
279. Gluckman SJ, Dvorak VC, MacCregor RR: Host defenses during prolonged alcohol consumption in a controlled environment. *Arch Intern Med* 137:1539–1543, 1977.
280. Berenyi MR, Straus B, Cruz D: In vitro and in vivo studies of cellular immunity in alcoholic cirrhosis. *Am J Dig Dis* 19:199–205, 1974.
281. Lundy J, Raaf JH, Deakins S, et al: The acute and chronic effects of alcohol in the human immune system. *Surg Gynecol Obstet* 141:212–218, 1975.
282. Tisman G, Herbert V: In vitro myelosuppression and immunosuppression by ethanol. *J Clin Invest* 52:1410–1414, 1973.
283. DeMeo AN, Andersen BR: Defective chemotaxis associated with a serum inhibitor in cirrhotic patients. *N Engl J Med* 286:735–740, 1972.
284. Blussé van Oud Alblas A, Janssens AR, Leijh PCJ, et al: Functions of granulocytes and monocytes in primary biliary and alcoholic cirrhosis. *Clin Exp Immunol* 62:724–731, 1985.
285. Wijke RJ, Rajkovic IA, Williams R: Impaired opsonization by serum from patients with chronic liver disease. *Clin Exp Immunol* 51:91–98, 1983.
286. Sorrell MF, Leavy CM: Lymphocyte transformation and alcoholic liver injury. *Gastroenterology* 63:1020–1028, 1972.
287. Staples PJ, Gerding DN, Decker JL, et al: Incidence of infection in systemic lupus erythematosus. *Arthritis Rheum* 17:1–10, 1974.
288. Abeles M: The reumatic patient as a compromised host. In Allen JC (ed): *Infection and the Compromised Host. Clinical Correlations and Therapeutic Approaches.* 2nd ed. Williams & Wilkins, Baltimore, 1981, pp. 197–227.
289. Ginzler E, Diamond H, Kaplan D, et al: Computer analysis of factors influencing frequency of infection in systemic lupus erythematosus. *Arthritis Rheum* 21:37–47, 1978.
290. Moutsopoulos HM, Gallagher JD, Decker JL, et al: Herpes zoster in patients with systemic lupus erythematosus. *Arthritis Rheum* 21:798–802, 1978.
291. Clark RA, Kimball HR, Decker JL: Neutrophil chemotaxis in systemic lupus erythematosus. *Ann Rheum Dis* 33:167–172, 1984.
292. Perez HD, Lipton M, Goldstein IM: A specific inhibitor of complement (C5) derived chemotactic activity in serum from patients with systemic lupus erythematosus. *Clin Res* 26:519A, 1978.
293. Jasin HE, Orozco JH, Ziff M: Serum heat labile opsonins in systemic lupus erythematosus. *J Clin Invest* 53:343–353, 1974.
294. Zurier RB: Reduction of phagocytosis and lysosomal enzyme release from human leucocytes by serum from patients with lupus erythematosus. *Arthritis Rheum* 19:73–78, 1976.
295. Kimball HR, Wolff SM, Talal N, et al: Marrow granulocyte reserves in the rheumatic disease. *Arthritis Rheum* 16:345–352, 1973.
296. Rosenthal CJ, Franklin EC: Depression of cellular mediated immunity in systemic lupus erythematosus. *Arthritis Rheum* 18:207–217, 1975.
297. Mowat AG, Baum J: Chemotaxis of polymorphonuclear leucocytes from patients with rheumatoid arthritis. *J Clin Invest* 59:2541–2549, 1971.
298. BarEli M, Ehrenfeld M. Litvin Y, et al: Monocyte function in rheumatoid arthritis. *Scand J Rheumatol* 9:17–23, 1980.
299. Turner RA, Schumacher HR, Myers AR: Neutrophil chemotaxis in rheumatic diseases. *J Clin Invest* 52:1632–1635, 1974.
300. Barnes CG, Turnbull AL, Vernon-Roberts B. Felty's syndrome: A clinical and pathological survey of 21 patients and their response to treatment. *Ann Rheum Dis* 30:359–374, 1971.
301. Ruderman M, Miller LM, Pinals RS: Clinical and serological observations on 27 patients with the Felty syndrome. *Arthritis Rheum* 11:377–384, 1968.
301a. Breedveld FC, Fibbe WE, Hermans J, et al: Factors influencing the incidence of infections in Felty's syndrome. *Arch Intern Med* 147:915–920, 1987.

302. Mackowiak PA: Microbial synergism in human infections. *N Engl J Med* **298**:21–87, 1978.

303. O'Grady F, Smith H (eds): *Microbial Perturbation of Host Defences.* Academic, London, 1981, pp. 1–254.

304. Solberg CO, Hellum KB: Neutrophil granulocyte function in bacterial infection. *Lancet* **2**:727–730, 1972.

305. Barbour AG, Allred CD, Solberg CO, et al: Chemiluminescence by polymorphonuclear leukocytes from patients with active bacterial infection. *J Infect Dis* **141**:14–20, 1980.

306. Parenti DM, Snydman DR: Capnocytophaga species: infections in nonimmunocompromised and immunocompromised hosts. *J Infect Dis* **151**:140–147, 1985.

307. Shurin SB, Socransky SS, Sweeney E, et al: A neutrophil disorder induced by capnocytophaga, a dental micro-organism. *N Engl J Med* **301**:849–854, 1979.

308. Rubin RH, Cosimi AB, Tolkoff-Rubin NE, et al: Infectious disease syndromes attributable to cytomegalovirus and their significance among renal transplant recipients. *Transplantation* **24**:458–464, 1977.

309. Chatterjee SN, Fiala M, Weiner J, et al: Primary cytomegalovirus infection and opportunistic infections. Incidence in renal transplant recipients. *JAMA* **240**:2446–2449, 1978.

310. Rand KH, Pollard RB, Merigan TC: Increased pulmonary superinfections in cardiac transplant patients undergoing primary cytomegalovirus infection. *N Engl J Med* **298**:951–953, 1978.

311. Carney WP, Rubin RH, Hoffman RA, et al: Analysis of T lymphocyte subsets in cytomegalovirus mononucleosis. *J Immunol* **126**:2114, 1981.

312. van Es A, van Gemert GW, Baldwin WK, et al: Viral infection and T-lymphocyte subpopulations in renal transplant recipients. *N Engl J Med* **309**:110–111, 1983.

313. La Quaglia MP, Tolkoff-Rubin NE, Dienstag J, et al: Impact of hepatitis on renal transplantation. *Transplant* **32**:504–507, 1981.

314. Fauci AS, Dale DC, Balow JE: Glucocorticosteroid therapy. Mechanisms of action and clinical considerations. *Ann Intern Med* **84**:304–315, 1976.

315. Schneiderman CA, Wilson JW: Effects of corticosteroids on complement and the neutrophilic polymorphonuclear leucocyte. *Transplant Proc* **7**:41–48, 1979.

316. Butler WT, Rossen RD: Effects of corticosteroids on immunity in man. *J Clin Invest* **52**:2629–2640, 1973.

317. Suda T, Miura Y, Ijima H: The effect of hydrocortisone on human granulopoiesis in vitro. *Exp Hematol* **11**:114–121, 1983.

318. Dale DC, Fauci AS, Guerry D, et al: Comparison of agents producing a neutrophilic leukocytosis in man: Hydrocortisone, prednisone, endotoxin and etiocholanolone. *J Clin Invest* **56**:808–813, 1975.

319. Dale DC, Fauci AS, Wolff SM: Alternate-day prednisone: Leukocyte kinetics and susceptibility to infections. *N Engl J Med* **291**:1154–1158, 1974.

320. Wiener SL, Wiener R, Urivetzky M, et al: The mechanism of action of a single dose of methylprednisolone on acute inflammation in vivo. *J Clin Invest* **56**:679–689, 1975.

321. Thompson J, van Furth R: The effect of glucocorticosteroids on the kinetics of mononuclear phagocytes *J Exp Med* **131**:429–442, 1970.

322. Rinehart JJ, Sagone AL, Balcerzak SP, et al: Effects of corticosteroid therapy on human monocyte function. *N Engl J Med* **292**:236–241, 1975.

323. Rinehart JJ, Balcerzak SP, Sagone AL. Effects of corticosteroid on monocyte function *J Clin Invest* **53**:1327–1343, 1974.

324. van Zwet TL, Thompson J, van Furth R: Effect of glucocorticosteroids on the phagocytosis and intracellular killing by peritoneal macrophages *Infect Immun* **12**:699–705, 1975.

325. van Furth R, Jones TC: Effect of glucocorticosteroids on phagosome–lysosome interaction. *Infect Immun* **12**:888–890, 1975.

326. Atkinson JP, Frank MM: Cortisone inhibition of complement independent erythrocyte clearance *Blood* **44**:629–637, 1974.

327. Werb ZA: Hormone receptors and hormonal regulation of macrophage physiological functions. In van Furth R (ed): *Mononuclear Phagocytes Functional Aspects.* Martinus Nijhoff, Boston, 1980, pp. 809–829.

328. Bondy PK, Bodel PT: Mechanisms of pyrogenic and antipyretic steroids. In Wolstenholme GEW, Birch J (eds): *Pyrogens and Fever.* Churchill Livingstone, Edinburgh, 1971, pp. 101–113.

329. Dannenberg AM Jr: The anti-inflammatory effects of glucocorticosteroids. A brief review of the literature. *Inflammation* **3**:329–343, 1979.

330. Cupps TR, Fauci AS: Corticosteroid-mediated immunoregulation in man. *Immunol Rev* **65**:134–155, 1982

331. Gershwin ME, Goetzl EJ, Steinberg AD: Cyclophosphamide: Use in practice. *Ann Intern Med* **80**:531–540, 1974.

332. Balow JE: Cyclophosphamide suppression of established cell-mediated immunity. *J Clin Invest* **56**:65–70, 1975.

333. Fauci AS, Wolff SM, Johnson JS: Effect of cyclophosphamide upon the immune response in Wegener's granulomatosis. *N Engl J Med* **285**:1493–1496, 1971.

334. Skinner MD, Schwartz RS: Immunosuppressive therapy. *N Engl J Med* **287**:221–286, 1972.

335. Gassmann AE, van Furth R: The effect of azathioprine on the kinetics of monocytes and macrophages during the normal steady state and an acute inflammatory reaction. *Blood* **46**:51–64, 1975.

336. TenBerge RJM, Schellekens PTA: A critical analysis of the use of azathioprine in clinical medicine. *Neth J Med* **26**:164–171, 1983.

337. Hyams JS, Donaldson MH, Metcalf JA, et al. Inhibition of human granulocyte function by methotrexate. *Cancer Res* **38**:650–655, 1978.

338. Rubin RH, Cosimi AB, Hirsch MD, et al: Effects of antithymocyte globulin on cytomegalovirus infection in renal transplant recipients. *Transplantation* **31**:143–145, 1981.

339. van Hooff JP, van Es, A, Koolen MI, et al: Less aggressive rejection therapy and low-dose corticosteroids leading to satisfactory cadaveric kidney graft survival and low morbidity rate. *Proc Eur Dial Transplant Assoc* **17**:435–439, 1980.

340. Cohen DJ, Loertscher R, Rubin MF, et al. Cyclosporine: A

new immunosuppressive agent for organ transplantation. *Ann Intern Med* **101**:667–682, 1984.

341. Granelli-Piperno A, Inaba K, Steinman RM: Stimulation of lymphokine release from T lymphoblasts, requirements for mRNA synthesis and inhibition by cyclosporin A. *J Exp Med* **160**:1792–1802, 1984.

342. Hauser WE, Remington JS: The effect of antibiotics on the humoral and cell-mediated immune responses. In Sabath LD (ed): *Action of Antibiotics in Patients*. H Huber, Berne, 1982, pp. 127–147.

343. Heyworth MF: Clinical experience with antilymphocyte serum. *Immunol Rev* **65**:79–97, 1982.

344. Cosimi AB: Clinical usefulness of antilymphocyte antibodies. *Transplant Proc* **15**:583–589, 1983.

345. Lederman MM, Ratnoff OD, Scillian JJ, et al: Impaired cell-mediated immunity in patients with classic hemophilia. *N Engl J Med* **308**:79–82, 1983.

346. Editorial: Blood transfusion haemophilia and AIDS. *Lancet* **2**:1433–1435, 1984.

347. Gascón P. Zoumbos NC, Young NS, et al: Immunological abnormalities in patients receiving multiple blood transfusions. *Ann Intern Med* **100**:173–177, 1984.

348. Doria G, Agarossi G, Adorini L: Selective effects of ionizing radiations on the immunoregulatory cells. *Immunol Rev* **65**:23–54, 1982.

349. Baehner RL, Neiburger RG, Johnson DE, et al: Transient bactericidal defect of peripheral blood phagocytes from children with acute lymphoblastic leukemia receiving craniospinal irradiation. *N Engl J Med* **289**:1209–1213, 1973.

350. Slater JM, Ngo E, Lau BHS: Effect of therapeutic irradiation on the immune responses. *AJR* **126**:313–320, 1976.

351. Strober S, Slavin S, Gottlieb M, et al: Allograft tolerance after total lymphoid irradiation (TLI). *Immunol Rev* **46**:87–112, 1979.

352. Gallico III GG, O'Connor NE, Compton CC, et al: Permanent coverage of large burn wounds with autologous cultured human epithelium. *N Engl J Med* **311**:448–451, 1984.

353. Hirsch MS, Schooley RT, Cosimi AB, et al: Effects of interferon-alpha on cytomegalovirus reactivation syndromes renal transplant recipients. *N Engl J Med* **308**:1489–1493, 1983.

354. Schwartmann WB, Tillotson JR, Taft EG, et al: Plasmapheresis for meningococcemia with disseminated intravascular coagulation. *N Engl J Med* **300**:1277, 1979.

355. Bjorvatn B, Bjertnals L, Fadnes HO, et al: Meningococcal septicaemia treated with combined plasmapheresis and leu-

copheresis or with blood exchange. *Br Med J* **288**:439–441, 1984.

356. Roord JJ, van der Meer JWM, Kuis W, et al: Treatment of antibody deficiency syndromes with subcutaneous infusion of gammaglobulin. *Birth Defects* **19**:217–271, 1983.

357. Nydegger UE (ed): *Immunohemotherapy. A Guide to Immunoglobulin Prophylaxis and Treatment*. Academic, London, 1981.

358. Winston DJ, Young LS: Immunization of the compromised host against infectious complications. In Allen JC (ed): *Infection and the Compromised Host. Clinical Correlations and Therapeutic Approaches*. Williams & Wilkins, Baltimore, 1981, pp. 37–89.

359. Ziegler EJ, McCutchan JA, Fierer J, et al: Treatment of Gram-negative bacteremia and shock with human antiserum to a mutant Escherichia coli. *N Engl J Med* **307**:1225–1230, 1982.

360. Stein RS, Beamon C, Ali MY, et al: Lithium carbonate attenuation of chemotherapy-induced neutropenia. *N Engl J Med* **297**:427–428, 1977.

361. Winston DJ, Ho WG, Gale RP: Therapeutic granulocyte transfusions in documented infections. A controlled trial in ninety five infectious granulocytopenic episodes. *Ann Intern Med* **97**:509–515, 1982.

362. Keusch GT, Ambinder EP, Kovacs I, et al: Role of opsonins in clinical response to granulocyte transfusion in granulocytopenic patients. *Am J Med* **73**:552–563, 1982.

363. van der Meer JWM, van den Broek PJ: Present status of the management of patients with defective phagocyte function. *Rev Infect Dis* **6**:107–121, 1984.

364. Buescher ES, Gallin JI: Leukocyte transfusions in chronic granulomatous disease. *N Engl J Med* **307**:800–803, 1982.

365. Hong R: Thymus transplants: A look to the future. *Birth Defects* **11**:357–360, 1975.

366. Editorial: Which thymic hormone? *Lancet* **1**:1309-1311, 1983.

367. Massicot JG, Goldstein RA: Transfer factor. *Ann Allerg* **49**:326–329, 1982.

368. Zegers BJM, Stoop JW: Therapy in adenosine deaminase and purine nucleoside phosphorylase deficient patients. *Clin Biochem* **16**:43–47, 1983.

369. Sparks FC: Hazards and complications of BCG immunotherapy. *Med Clin North Am* **60**:499–509, 1976.

370. Bakker W, Nijhuis-Heddes JM, Brutel de la Revière A, et al: Complications of post-operative intrapleural BCG in lung cancer. *Ann Thorac Surg* **33**:267–272, 1982.

4

Fever and Septicemia

LOWELL S. YOUNG

1. Introduction

Fever is the hallmark of infection but is not specific for it. Infection can begin and progress in the absence of fever. When fever occurs in the immunocompromised host, the single major challenge in clinical decision making is to ascertain whether the onset of temperature elevation is a reliable indication of the onset of infection rather than a manifestation of the underlying disease, a hypersensitivity reaction, or a factitious development. Another major issue that frequently stirs acrimonious bedside debate involves the clinical wisdom of suppressing fever with or without evidence of documented infection. Despite many decades of controversy, it has not been conclusively established whether fever is "good" for the patient or just adds to patient discomfort without benefitting host defenses against infection or the underlying disease.

Whatever the cause and however major the temperature elevation, the appearance of fever in the immunocompromised host is an urgent signal to initiate a comprehensive search for its etiology. If the clinical situation warrants, a presumptive diagnosis of systemic infection is made, and empirical drug therapy may be initiated in the absence of microbiologic confirmation. "Unstable" patients will require constant observation in a well-staffed setting. Although the decision to initiate therapy may be precipitous, the clinician who cares for immunocompromised patients must be flexible, per-

LOWELL S. YOUNG • Kuzell Institute for Arthritis and Infectious Disease, Division of Infectious Diseases, Pacific Presbyterian Medical Center, San Francisco, California 94115.

sistently inquisitive, and willing to change course as more clinical and laboratory information becomes available.

2. Criteria for Fever, Fever of Undetermined Origin, and Septicemia

A widely read textbook of infectious disease defines fever as a body temperature in excess of 100.2°F (37.8°C) orally or above 101.2°F (38.4°C) rectally.[1] These are practical criteria for distinguishing febrile from normal states. Nonetheless, it must be recognized that a single definition of fever is quite arbitrary, and there is a considerable range in temperatures even in normal individuals. For instance, 42% of subjects in one study had temperatures exceeding 98.6°F (37°C) and reaching 100°F (37.8°C) in some instances.[2] A wide variety of factors, including ovulation, smoking, exercise, and psychoneural factors, may affect body temperature.

Fever of undetermined origin (FUO) is a well-known term used by various investigators to describe persistence of fever over a period of several (2–5) weeks during which conventional diagnostic measures are unfruitful.[3] Several "thresholds" for FUO have been proposed, such as temperature elevations above 100.5°F (38°C) or 101°F (38.3°C). Regardless of definitions, we believe that the experience reported in several classic studies of FUO[4,5] has limited applicability to the immunocompromised host for several reasons. First, the classic studies have summarized the clinical experience obtained from evaluating febrile patients who present without a known underlying disease. In the immunocompromised host, the nature of the basic disorder is usually identified, and when fever appears, the challenge is to determine whether something else, i.e., of infectious etiology, is also present. Second, the classic definitions of FUO require a period of weeks of febrility. When fever develops in an immunocompromised subject, an immediate therapeutic decision is often required. The clinician does not enjoy the luxury of a diagnostic evaluation that may span 1 or 2 weeks. Conversely, a diagnosis of FUO after a single initial evaluation by a physician is inappropriate because the results of initial diagnostic studies will not be available for 12–72 hr, and the patient could have a readily identifiable bacterial infection.

We believe that a practical working definition of FUO in the immunocompromised subject can be made after initial diagnostic measures to rule out an acute bacterial or fungal infection. Since 90% of positive blood cultures for bacteria are identified within 72 hr of incubation,[6] and candidal growth takes perhaps a day longer, this working definition sets a boundary of perhaps 100 hr. Beyond that point, more aggressive and invasive diagnostic measures may be required. Obviously, if indicated by clinical developments such as progressive diffuse pulmonary infiltrates, such procedures should be undertaken even earlier than that.

In clinical parlance, the terms septicemia and bacteremia are used interchangeably, usually with little chance for misunderstanding. Bacteremia can be transient (as following mastication), whereas septicemia implies systemic spread of infection. For reasons that are poorly understood, some bacterial (nocardiosis and tuberculosis) and fungal infections (Candida and Aspergillus) may spread systemically in the face of negative blood cultures. Therefore, in addition to positive blood cultures or blood smears, we would accept as evidence of septicemia or disseminated infection histologic evidence of the presence of an organism in muscle, soft tissue, bone marrow, organ sections, or skin lesions. In the impaired host, we would accept as evidence of septicemia positive cultures of peripheral venous blood, even though the bacteremia or fungemia might result from contaminated intravascular lines. Foreign bodies may serve as an iatrogenic source of infection that nonetheless results in systemic spread. By contrast, we cannot accept the recovery of an organism from mucosal surfaces, expectorated respiratory secretions, stool, or skin surfaces as prima facie evidence of systemic infection with organ involvement because of the well-known bacterial and fungal overgrowth that can take place when the host has a debilitating illness and is treated with a variety of antimicrobial agents.

3. Pathogenesis of Fever

A scientific understanding of the pathogenesis of fever in animal models dates back to the pioneering discovery of Beeson,[7] who reported in 1948 that a pyrogen distinct from bacterial endotoxin could be recovered from rabbit leukocytes. More recent work has indicated that at least one protein moiety, so-called "endogenous pyrogen," is elaborated by a variety of cell types, including blood monocytes, alveolar and peritoneal macrophages, and the phagocytic cells of the reticuloendothelial system present in liver (Kupffer cells), spleen, and lymph nodes.[8,9] By contrast, lymphocytes are apparently incapable of pyrogen production.

Important work has also demonstrated the identity between endogenous pyrogen and interleukin-1 (IL-1), an important lymphokine elaborated by macrophages.[8,9] IL-1 appears to be responsible for muscle wasting and protein catabolism during severe infection.[9,10]

The basic mechanism underlying the production of fever in rabbits involves a period during which certain exogenous agents (activators) stimulate protein synthesis, because normal phagocytic cells from rabbits neither contain nor produce endogenous pyrogen when incubated in vitro. These activators include both gram-positive and gram-negative bacteria, endotoxins derived from gram-negative cell walls, viruses, phagocytizable particles such as Latex, and certain pyrogenic steroids. Incubation of activating agents with phagocytic cells results in phagocytosis within minutes and the elaboration of endogenous pyrogen, which continues for many hours in vitro. In the rabbit, endogenous pyrogen appears in the blood at the same time that the fever develops. Following removal of the provocative agent, injection of supernatant fluids from cells activated in vitro into blood or brain at sites in or near the anterior hypothalamus results in prompt elevation of

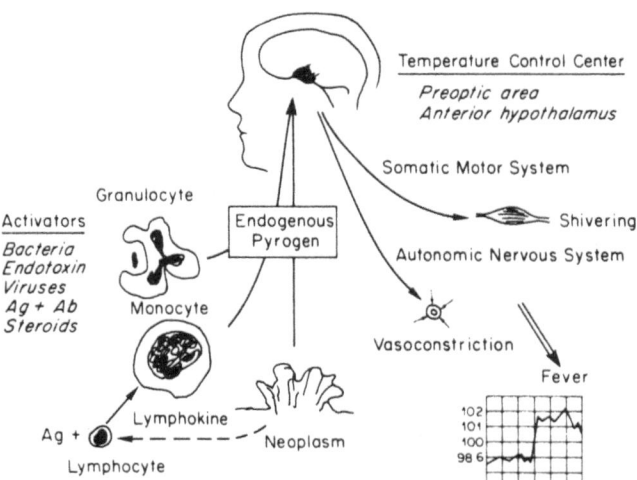

FIGURE 1. Pathogenesis of fever This schematic diagram summarizes the mechanisms by which fever is induced in man. Activating substances consist of microorganisms or drugs such as steroids. Phagocytosis by granulocytes or antigen interaction with lymphocytes followed by lymphocyte–monocyte collaboration can lead to release of endogenous pyrogen. The latter acts directly on the hypothalamic temperature control center by initiating events like shivering and vasoconstriction that lead to temperature elevation

animal body temperature. Thus, as shown in Fig. 1, the pathway to temperature elevation includes (1) elaboration of endogenous pyrogen by activated cells after an exposure to the proper stimulus, (2) the release of endogenous pyrogen into the circulation, (3) interaction of pyrogen with neurons of the temperature control center of the anterior hypothalamus, and (4) a change in the set point of the body temperature resulting in initiation of processes involving heat conservation (e.g., vasoconstriction through the autonomic nervous system) and increased heat production (e.g., the muscular action of shivering).

Purification of endogenous pyrogen has been accomplished. It has been made immunogenic, and a radioimmunoassay (RIA) for its detection has been reported.[8] Further application of this approach would be a great boon to the understanding of fever and for the evaluation of patients with the syndrome of FUO. Less sensitive methods for pyrogen detection, e.g., bioassay, have led to reports of the finding of pyrogen in the urine of febrile patients with neoplastic disorders, but demonstration of circulating human endogenous pyrogen has been accomplished only infrequently in a rabbit bioassay system.[11]

Much interest has been focused on the mechanism of fever production in hypersensitivity reactions and in neoplastic diseases. There appear to be two separate pathways for the development of hypersensitivity fevers in experimental animals. One mechanism, as shown in Fig. 1, involves the reaction of antigen with antibody. Immune complexes can function as activators and are probably phagocytized by

monocytes with the subsequent release of endogenous pyrogen. The other mechanism appears to involve cell-mediated immune recognition. When lymphocytes harvested from lymph nodes of rabbits sensitized with an antigen are incubated with the antigen in vitro, the lymphocytes fail to produce pyrogen but are able to stimulate normal blood leukocytes to release pyrogen when these two types of cells are incubated together.[12] Thus, it appears that antigen recognition by lymphocytes results in release of a nonpyrogenic intermediate substance, such as a lymphokine, which then activates mononuclear cells, resulting in release of endogenous pyrogen.

Recurrent fever is a common manifestation of many neoplastic disorders such as leukemias, lymphomas (Hodgkin disease in particular), hypernephromas, sarcomas of bone, and atrial myxomas (see Tables 6 and 7). There are many reports of fever associated with a wide variety of tumor types. A common observation is that fever can coincide with tumor growth, disappears with appropriate treatment or extirpation of malignant disease, but reappears upon return or recrudescence of the neoplasm. Several major hypotheses have been advanced to explain tumor-associated fever including elaboration of a toxin by the tumor, tissue necrosis with leukocyte infiltration and release of tissue pyrogen, obstruction of secretary functions (as in the case of solid tumor metastatic to liver), abnormal liver function with altered conjugation of pyrogenic steroids, or excessive heat production by tumor cells. There is a surprising paucity of evidence that really supports these hypotheses. The popular concept of tumor necrosis being associated with fever has been supported by one study but refuted by others.[13]

Since normal human leukocytes neither contain pyrogen nor produce it in vitro unless stimulated by some agent, the focus of investigations into tumor-associated fever has been on the possible elaboration of pyrogens by malignant cells. Bodel[13] presented evidence that certain tissues, including hypernephromas and spleens and lymph nodes from patients with Hodgkin disease, contain cells that spontaneously release pyrogen when incubated in vitro. Mononuclear cells and probably malignant cells appear to be the most likely source of pyrogen, and they differ from phagocytes, which require an activating stimulus. Fever characteristic of endogenous pyrogen resulted when spleen cells from 11 of 20 patients with Hodgkin disease were incubated in vitro and their supernatant fluids were injected into rabbits. By contrast, febrile responses were observed with only two of 70 supernatants following incubations of spleen cells from patients with nonmalignant diseases. Pyrogenic responses were similarly observed with supernatant fluids prepared after incubation of cells from lymph nodes of patients with Hodgkin disease. Because such cell preparations contain few if any granulocytes, mononuclear cells are apparently responsible for pyrogen production. Recent studies have shown that cultured Hodgkin disease cell lines produce endogenous pyrogen spontaneously.[8]

The work on tumor-associated fever indicates that malignant cells per se can be the source of a pyrogenic material, but it is also possible that tissue inflammatory cells that respond to tumor growth might be activated by products released from the tumor to release endogenous pyrogen. Such products could include tumor antigens, and they may vary with different neoplastic diseases, thus accounting for differences in incidence of tumor-associated fever. Furthermore, tumor-associated fever might well result from a hypersensitivity reaction. As Bodel[13] postulated, it is possible that the early release of pyrogen that is characteristic of spleen cells from patients with Hodgkin disease is also mediated by lymphocytes in tissue that are reacting with a tumor-associated antigen. These lymphocytes may then activate other tissue cells (i.e., phagocytes) to release pyrogen.

4. Syndrome-Oriented Approach to Fever and Suspected Infection: Differential Diagnosis

The onset of fever should immediately trigger an exhaustive evaluation to determine what clues can be found to its etiology. Tables 1–5 summarize infectious etiologies suggested by certain clinical findings. In adopting this syndrome-oriented approach, we make no claims to completeness and refer the reader to other chapters for more detailed coverage of pneumonia (Chapter 5) and central nervous system (CNS) infection (Chapter 6). What is desirable, however, is to formulate an orderly approach to differential diagnosis whereby the most likely causes of symptoms referable to an organ system or a physical finding are most expeditiously considered and then ruled in or out. Unfortunately, too many reviews of opportunistic infection stress the organism rather than the presenting manifestations, whereas in actuality the reverse is what is encountered. The problems posed by specific opportunistic pathogens are highlighted in Chapters 7–14.

Evidence of disseminated disease with skin lesions—abscesses, vesicles, macules, vasculitis, infarcts, ulcers, maculopapular lesions—should suggest certain groups of bacterial, fungal, and viral pathogens (Table 1). *Staphylococcus aureus* classically has been associated with hematogenously spread abscesses that can involve any skin or subcutaneous area.

Of all the gram-negative rods causing sepsis in the compromised host, *Pseudomonas aeruginosa* has been most associated with vasculitic skin lesions. Ecthyma gangrenosum is the term applied to the clas-

TABLE 1. Infectious Disease Syndromes and Etiologic Agents in the Compromised Host: Disseminated Disease with Skin Lesions

Bacteria	Fungi
S. aureus	*Aspergillus*
Gram-negative bacilli	*Zygomycetes*
P. aeruginosa	*Candida* species
Aeromonas hydrophila	*Cryptococcus neoformans*
Marine *Vibrios* (halophilic)	*Trichosporin* species
Nocardia species	
	Viruses
	Herpes simplex
	Varicella–zoster

TABLE 2. Infectious Disease Syndromes and Etiologic Agents in the Compromised Host: Central Nervous System Infection[a]

Bacteria	Fungi
Listeria monocytogenes	*Cryptococcus neoformans*
Nocardia spp.	*Aspergillus fumigatus*
S. aureus	*Zygomycetes* (*Mucor* and
P. aeruginosa	*Rhizopus*)
M. tuberculosis	*Candida* species
	Viruses[b]
	Varicella–zoster
	Herpes simplex

[a]Meningoencephalitis, possibly brain abscess
[b]In patients with AIDS, the possibility of retrovirus encephalopathy or infection with papovavirus should be considered

TABLE 4. Infection Mimicking Neoplasm: Diagnostic Considerations

Finding	Causative organism
Brain metastases	*Nocardia asteroides*
	Toxoplasma gondii
Budd–Chiari syndrome	*Mucor* spp., *Aspergillus*
Intestinal obstruction	*Strongyloides*
	Entamoeba histolytica
Nephrotic syndrome	*Mucor* spp., *Aspergillus*
Renal vein thrombosis	Gram-negative bacilli
Obstructive nephropathy	*Candida*
Oculomotor palsy	Zygomycosis
Pulmonary nodules	Histoplasmosis, pneumocystosis
Superior vena cava syndrome	Histoplasmosis

sic cutaneous lesions of *P. aeruginosa*.[14] These lesions are striking in appearance. They may begin as small macules enlarging into an oval or round halo of erythema. Within this halo of erythema (which becomes indurated and slightly raised), a vesicular lesion may develop which may enlarge and become frankly bullous. Palpation of the skin and detection of a round or oval area of induration are valuable means of detecting early ecthyma lesions. It is not unusual to see multiple crops of ecthyma gangrenosum lesions evolve over a matter of hours. The centers of these lesions may become frankly necrotic and ulcerate while the surrounding areas become ecchymotic. One of the major problems in the differential diagnosis of these lesions is that they often tend to occur in thrombocytopenic patients and may be misinterpreted as ecchymoses. Two areas that must be searched assiduously for ecthyma lesions are the per-

TABLE 3. Infectious Disease Syndromes and Etiologic Agents in the Compromised Host: Pathogens in the Head and Neck

Bacteria	Viruses
Anaerobes	Herpes simplex
Aerobes: Streptococci and	Cytomegalovirus
gram-negative rods,	
particularly *P. aeruginosa*	
Fungi	
Candida	
Aspergillus	
Zygomycetes	
Histoplasma capsulatum	

irectal area and groin. A perirectal abscess may be the first of a series of disseminated pseudomonal skin lesions. In a strict sense, a perirectal abscess is not an ecthyma gangrenosum lesion. (For that matter, in a granulocytopenic patient, a perirectal lesion is more likely to be cellulitis rather than an abscess because of the lack of a neutrophil response.) However, *Pseudomonas* vasculitis may spread from a perirectal cellulitis, and ecthyma lesions may be present in the perirectal area. Perirectal lesions (including thrombosed hemorrhoids) in the neutropenic patient should be regarded as caused by *P. aeruginosa* until proved otherwise.

Some observers have believed that ecthyma gangrenosum lesions might represent a hypersensitivity reaction in the skin analogous to a local Shwartzman reaction. However, in most cases in which antimicrobial therapy has not been initiated, either biopsy or culture will reveal the causative organism. Histopathologic studies carried out on ecthyma gangrenosum lesions indicate that the initial mechanism is a venous thrombosis triggered by invasion of small vessels by microorganisms.[15] Furthermore, it is likely that microbial products such as enzymes and exotoxins are responsible for the evolution of the progressive gross and microscopic changes. Nonetheless, the initial event appears to be localized intravascular thrombosis caused by direct invasion of small and medium-sized blood vessels by viable bacilli.

It has become increasingly apparent that other gram-negative organisms besides *P. aeruginosa*

TABLE 5. Some Emerging Pathogens in the Immunocompromised Host[a]

Organism	Reference	Host	Clinical patterns
Aeromonas hydrophila	Ketover et al.[16]	Neutropenic patients	Necrotizing vasculitis or myositis
Bacillus species	Ihde and Armstrong[41]	Cancer patients	Sepsis and pneumonia
Candida tropicalis	Wingard et al.[42]	Neutropenic patients	Skin lesions, myositis, polyarthralgias
Corynebacterium species	Kressel and Szewczyk[43]		Lung abscess and sepsis
Equi	Berg et al.[44]	Lymphoma patients	Sepsis and pneumonia linked to hyper-
Other	Stamm et al.[45]	Marrow transplants	alimentation lines, organism sensitive
			only to vancomycin
Eiknella corrodens	Brooks et al.[46]	Cancer and rheumatology patients	Infections of bites around head and neck
Hemophilus influenza	Nixon and Aisenberg[47]	Lymphoma patients	Overwhelming septicemia
Petriellidium boydii	Winston et al.[48]	Neutropenic patients	Vascular thrombosis and infarction
Pseudomonas cepacia	Bottone et al.[49]	Chronic granulomatous disease	Sepsis, multiple abscesses
Staphylococcus epidermidis	Winston et al.[40]	Patients with intra-vascular devices	Catheter-associated sepsis, often highly antibiotic resistant
Torulopsis glabrata[b]	Aisner et al.[50]	Cancer patients	Sepsis and pneumonia
Trichosporin sp.[51]	Haupt et al.[51]	Neutropenic patients	Pneumonia, necrotizing skin lesions
Vibrio (halophilic sp.)	Blake[17]	Hepatic disease	Wound infection, sepsis with necrotizing vasculitis

[a]See also Chapters 5–8 for pulmonary and central nervous system pathogens
[b]Taxonomically renamed *Candida glabrata*

have the capacity to produce ecthyma–gangrenosum-like lesions. Septicemic infections caused by the gram-negative bacillus *Aeromonas hydrophila* are uncommon compared to *P. aeruginosa,* but in one series of *Aeromonas* bacteremias, some 40% of neutropenic patients had either cutaneous lesions that were indistinguishable from *Pseudomonas aeruginosa* or a gangrenous type of cellulitis accompanied by myonecrosis.[16] *Aeromonas* species are taxonomically distinct from pseudomonads and the enteric bacilli. Like *Pseudomonas,* such organisms can be quite antibiotic resistant. In addition, there are several reports of marine vibrios (parahemolyticus, alginolyticus, and vulnificus) causing septicemia characterized by necrotizing skin lesions.[17–19]

Over the past 15 years, we have had the opportunity to study a number of neutropenic patients who developed colorful cutaneous lesions in association with gram-negative rod bacteremia. Some lesions have been ecthyma-like, whereas others have been violaceous blisters, orange-yellow vesicles tensely filled with fluid, or a rapidly progressing angry cellulitis. The causative organisms have included *Escherichia coli, Klebsiella, Enterobacter, Proteus,* and *Serratia* species. The appearance of these cutaneous lesions has been an indication for both immediate culturing of the blood and other potentially infected sites and initiating systemic antimicrobial therapy. If possible, these lesions should be biopsied as well as aspirated or cultured. Some organisms may not be grown (particularly if antimicrobial therapy has already been given), but biopsy followed by appropriate stains will reveal the infecting pathogen.

Nocardia species are higher bacteria previously classified among the fungi. *Nocardia* initially infect the lung, but the next most common sites of involvement are subcutaneous tissues and brain. If *P. aeruginosa* and *S. aureus* have been reasonably excluded in a patient with pulmonary abscesses, subcutaneous abscesses, or brain abscesses, *Nocardia* infection is one of the leading diagnostic possibilities. The species *N. asteroides* is the most commonly encountered organism, but *N. brasiliensis* can cause an indistinguishable clinical syndrome. Nocardial organisms are gram-positive, beaded in appearance, acid-fast, and branch at 90° angles (see Chapter 9). Although a fair number of cases of *Nocardia* infection have been described in immunosuppressed hosts, particularly those receiving corticoids or with underlying lymphoma, the isolation of this organism in our recent experience has been on the decline. A possible explanation for this trend is the widespread empirical use of broad-spectrum agents that display activity against *Nocardia asteroides* such as carbenicillin, trimethoprim–sulfamethoxazole, and some cephalosporins. If patients suspected of having nocardiosis are already receiving antimicrobial therapy, diagnostic efforts must concentrate on microscopic identification of the organism in respiratory secretions or metastatic lesions.

As pointed out in Chapters 8 (fungal infections) and 18 (infections complicating leukemia and lymphoma), one area of major concern in the management of the immunocompromised hosts is the rising incidence of disseminated fungal infection. Deep infections are notoriously difficult to diagnose, but cutaneous involvement is an important clue that may spare the patient an invasive diagnostic procedure. There have been well-described examples of cutaneous involvement by *Candida*,[20] *Cryptococcus*,[21] zygomycetes (*Mucor* and *rhizopus* species),[22] and *Aspergillus*.[23] The candidal skin lesions may have an indwelling vascular catheter as the source, and patients may have other evidence of metastatic candidal disease in, for example, the eye (although in our experience, we have never seen *Candida* endophthalmitis in a markedly neutropenic patient). Cutaneous lesions with *Candida* are maculopapular in appearance and may be frankly purulent providing that the patient has an adequate cellular inflammatory response. The lesions of *Aspergillus* and *Phycomycetes* can be oval, raised, and easily mistaken for ecthyma gangrenosum as in one interesting case published by Meyer et al.[22] Although most of the lesions reflect blood-borne dissemination, one recent report has associated cutaneous *Rhizopus* infection with contaminated adhesive dressing.[24] Cutaneous lesions of herpes simplex and varicella–zoster virus (VZV) infection are so familiar that they need not be commented on further. Any doubt about the underlying nature of the viral infection can be resolved by aspiration of these lesions and inoculation into tissue culture (see Chapter 13). A preliminary diagnosis can be made with the Tzank stain, which will reveal multinucleated giant cells in the case of both herpes simplex and varicella–zoster infection; usually (but not always), the two infections can be distinguished on clinical grounds alone.

The pneumonitic processes covered in Chapter 6 may logically be assessed by systematically considering bacterial, fungal, viral, and parasitic etiologies. Diffuse pulmonary infiltrates call for vigorous diagnostic efforts to rule out such life-threatening yet treatable complications as *Pneumocystis* pneumonia. As a result of extensive coverage in the current medical literature, the role of organisms such as *P. carinii* and *Legionella pneumophila* has probably been emphasized out of proportion to their true incidence. No physician who cares for the immunocompromised patient can ignore these possibilities in a patient with pneumonitis, but the initial diagnostic emphasis should be placed on detecting infection caused by the more common gram-negative and gram-positive bacteria. As studies using the transtracheal aspiration technique have documented, gram-negative bacilli are the most common cause of nosocomial aspiration pneumonia,[25] and aspiration is the probable mechanism for the development of most pneumonias. Patients who develop fever and have pneumonitis secondary to inhospital treatment are likely candidates for infection by the more antibiotic-resistant bacilli such as *P. aeruginosa*, *Proteus* species, *Enterobacter* species, and *S. marcescens*.[25]

Many reviews cite the lung as the most common locus for infection in the immunocompromised host.[26,27] This conclusion must be accepted with some caution, however, because a chest radiograph is a readily obtainable noninvasive procedure associated with negligible inconvenience and risk. Thus, pulmonary disease may be documented more frequently than other types of organ involvement. Appearance of pulmonary infiltrates, however, may often reflect a noninfectious pulmonary process. The pitfalls of diagnosing pulmonary infiltrates by examination of expectorated sputum have been emphasized by many investigators, but there are obvious hazards to obtaining samples of intrapulmonary secretions or lung tissue. To compound the problem of defining the nature of infection, it has been claimed that a number of neutropenic patients lack early radiographic evidence of pneumonia, and evidence for pneumonitis has cited such findings as rôles in the absence of pulmonary infiltrates.[28] However, reliance on auscultatory or radiologic findings alone may be misleading, since congestive heart failure (CHF) may be difficult to rule out in such subjects. There is little doubt that one of the major current problems in evaluating fever and pulmonary changes in the immunocompromised host is the multitude of noninfectious etiologies of lung infiltrates, including radiation pneumonitis, a number of drug reactions (due to busulfan, bleomycin, and methotrexate), intrapulmonary hemorrhage, neoplasm, or a combination of these factors.

There are a limited number of tools for determining the etiology of CNS infection. Much of the information published on opportunistic fungal infection involving the nervous system has been based on autopsy studies. The bacteria, fungi, and viruses that should be considered are listed on Table 3. In the initial diagnostic evaluation, emphasis should be placed on those possibilities that are not only common but are treatable. Two CNS pathogens, *Listeria monocytogenes* and *Cryptococcus neoformans,* are so readily treatable even in markedly immunosuppressed patients that it would be most unfortunate to overlook them. In most cases, therapy directed against these two pathogens is curative in spite of marked impairment of host defenses.

In our experience, *L. monocytogenes* is the most common cause of bacterial meningitis in the immunocompromised host and has a special predilection for patients on corticosteroid therapy or with impaired T-cell function, as in Hodgkin disease. Interestingly, *Listeria* infections have been rare in patients with acquired immunodeficiency syndrome (AIDS), when everything we know about the latter would have led to the prediction of fairly frequent *Listeria* infections. *Listeria monocytogenes* involvement in the CNS is primarily a meningocephalitis, although a few cases of brain abscess have been described.[29] By contrast, involvement of the brain by *Nocardia* species or *Toxoplasma gondii* usually is a more focal infectious process, with the patient presenting with a seizure disorder or a mass lesion with neurologic impairment. *Pseudomonas aeruginosa* can cause meningitis, but this process usually reflects overwhelming septicemia. Thus, the prognosis is particularly poor because spread of *P. aeruginosa* to the brain or meninges clearly reflects an inability to contain bloodstream infection. *Mycobacterium tuberculosis* can cause meningitis, and the well-known difficulty of diagnosing tuberculous meningitis in even a normal host is further compounded in the immunosuppressed subject in whom cerebrospinal fluid (CSF) pleocytosis may not be as striking because of drug-induced immunosuppression. Howev-

er, it is our impression that CNS tuberculosis in immunosuppressed hosts has become a relatively rare event because of the tendency to use isoniazid (INH) prophylaxis in patients with exposure history and/or positive tuberculin tests.

Of the fungal pathogens, *Cryptococcus neoformans* ranks highest on the list of organisms that must be considered if there are signs of CNS infection. The availability of a highly accurate diagnostic test, the cryptococcal antigen test, and improved antimicrobial therapy of proven disease make it imperative to rule out cryptococcal disease in patients having any sign of a meningeal inflammation. However, we have encountered a case in a febrile renal transplant recipient in whom the initial lumbar puncture (performed for fever and headache) showed entirely normal values for CSF protein, cell count, and sugar. After many days' incubation, the CSF from this patient grew out a yeastlike organism. On recognition of the possibility of cryptococcal infection, we performed the Latex agglutination antigen detection test and found it to be positive on both CSF and serum. Only in retrospect was it appreciated that the patient had a solitary lung abscess consistent with cryptococcal involvement that predated CNS infection.

The outlook for the therapy of other types of mycotic involvement of the CNS is less sanguine. *Candida* infection of the CNS (like *Aspergillus,* zygomycosis, and cryptococcosis) is on a metastatic basis and is frequently associated with infection of lung, liver, and other deep organs. The prognosis in *Aspergillus* and zygomycotic involvement in the CNS has been extremely poor, but this is probably a reflection of late or terminal recognition of the problem. Some investigators have questioned whether *Aspergillus* or zygomycoses involving the brain is a curable condition.[30] Isolated instances of recovery from zygomycotic infection (*Mucor* or *Rhizopus* species) when the internal carotid artery has been occluded have been reported.[31,32] It appears that the chance of recovery, with or without therapy with agents such as amphotericin B, is critically related to improvement in underlying disease and/or amelioration of predisposing factors such as immunosuppressive treatment. Using a new serodiagnostic test,[33] we have followed several leukemic patients who developed focal CNS signs during the nadir of their white blood cell (WBC) counts and then were found to have elevated levels of serum *Aspergillus* antibodies. They fortunately achieved remission, and neurologic findings resolved. However, these examples can only be considered presumed cases of fungal involvement of the brain in the absence of histopathologic documentation.

With the introduction of drugs that can be used to treat herpes virus meningoencephalitis, adenine arabinoside and acylovir, measures to diagnose this infection have become more justified. In varicella–zoster, another DNA virus infection, involvement of the CNS may be observed. Lumbar puncture performed on patients with localized zoster may show a CSF pleocytosis. In most cases, this pleocytosis will resolve as the disease resolves. Unfortunately, we have seen situations in which patients have concurrently had *Pneumocystis carinii* pneumonia, disseminated herpes zoster infection, and cryptococcal infection of the CNS. Thus, documentation of CNS pleocytosis in the patient with varicella–zoster pneumonia should not lead to the assumption that this is a reactive process occurring in the CSF, but an assiduous search should be initiated for another concomitant treatable infection.

A fourth major category of signs and symptoms relates to the head and neck region: the oral cavity, the nasal passages, and the esophagus. Although the hemolytic *Streptococcus* is the most commonly occurring bacterial organism causing acute pharyngitis, hemolytic streptococci belonging to many serogroups besides group A can cause pharyngitis and infection around the tonsillar crypts.[34] *Staphylococcus* has not been convincingly shown to cause pharyngitis but may be the primary pathogen in a number of soft tissue infections of the head and neck. Anaerobic organisms are a major part of the normal flora of the mouth but can cause serious soft tissue infections of the floor of the mouth, of the retropharyngeal area, and of the sinuses. Generally speaking, gram-negative rods and *P. aeruginosa* in particular cannot be considered causes of bacterial pharyngitis. However, with the aggressive use of certain antineoplastic agents such as daunorubicin, pharyngeal ulceration can occur followed by colonization and infection by gram-negative bacteria. Indeed, we have observed a number of cases in which *P. aeruginosa* was isolated from the pharynx in association with bacteremia caused by a *Pseudomonas* serotype of identical nature and antimicrobial susceptibility. Furthermore, in such cases, *P. aeruginosa*

was not isolated from stool, suggesting that the origin of the bacteremia was actually the oropharynx.

By far the most common type of fungal involvement of the oropharynx is candidal colonization of the mouth, tongue, and mucosal surfaces. Initially, this can be a mild mucositis, but the inflammation may progress to a state wherein the patient virtually becomes unwilling to eat or swallow. Candidal involvement of the esophagus can be a prelude to systemic invasion. A characteristic symptom in candidal esophagitis is pain on swallowing accompanied by postglutition substernal burning. However, caution should be exercised in assuming that all substernal burning pain is the result of *Candida* esophagitis. Herpes simplex can involve the esophagus and be associated with a radiologic picture indistinguishable from the feathery or ulcerative pattern observed when barium is swallowed by a patient with advanced *Candida* esophagitis. Occasionally, cytomegalovuris (CMV) has been recovered from similar esophageal lesions, but the virus may have originated from a higher (pharyngeal) source. Definitive diagnosis of esophageal involvement will require some endoscopic procedure with biopsy rather than reliance solely on the barium-swallow procedure.

Both *Aspergillus* and the zygomycetes can cause infection of the esophagus and nasal tissues, as well as the paranasal sinuses. Histoplasmosis has been associated with oral ulcerations.[35] Although progressive clouding of the sinuses is suggestive of aerobic and anaerobic bacterial infection, fungal invasion of the sinuses can occur in the absence of glucose intolerance. Pain over the sinuses or dysesthesias of the face can also be important early manifestations of fungal involvement. Pain and clouding of the sinuses should not be attributed to bleeding per se, but an exhaustive evaluation should be initiated to determine the etiology of sinus inflammation in the neutropenic, thrombocytopenic patient. Aspiration or biopsy of this sinus involvement is clearly necessary to distinguish a fungal e.g., *Aspergillus*, from an anaerobic bacterial process (as in chronic sinusitis).

A large proportion of immunosuppressed patients in any hospital have underlying neoplasms, and an important aspect of any diagnostic evaluation is to distinguish spread of tumor from an infectious complication. In addition, it is now well recognized that patients with one neoplasm may develop second primary tumors and that recipients of organ transplants are at increased risk of developing cancers of a variety of cell types. The finding of a space-occupying lesion of the brain or a nodular (coin type) mass in the lung could obviously represent spread of tumor. In the febrile patient, however, the possibility that such a finding can be caused by an infectious process such as toxoplasmosis or histoplasmosis must be evaluated in a comprehensive manner.

Table 4 summarizes some of the infectious agents that might be responsible for a laboratory, radiologic, or physical finding mimicking tumor. Mass lesions in the CNS are particularly suggestive of nocardial brain abscess or toxoplasmosis. The ability of the zygomycoses and *Aspergillus* species to invade blood vessels and precipitate thrombosis can result in a Budd–Chiari syndrome, nephrotic syndrome, and oculomotor palsy.[23,31,35] Fungal involvement need not be direct, however; in the case of histoplasmosis, fibrosing mediastinitis can lead to a superior vena cava syndrome.[36] In some instances, the growth of organisms rather than the reactive inflammation can be so dense as to cause or enhance an obstructive clinical picture. One example is heavy candidal growth in both ureters, which leads to a clinical picture of postrenal obstructive uropathy characterized by oliguria and rising serum creatinine. Intestinal overgrowth of *Strongyloides* may exacerbate a clinical picture of paralytic ileus, although the role of the parasite may not be primary. One form of intestinal amebiasis is a dense localized area of inflammation, the ameboma, containing viable trophozoites, that mimics colon carcinoma clinically, radiologically, and even in gross appearance. Solitary or multiple pulmonary nodules can be caused by a variety of infectious processes. Those caused by histoplasmosis can "grow" like a tumor.[37] Even *P. carinii*, whose pattern of pulmonary involvement is usually diffuse, can present as a solitary nodule.[38]

Finally, one of the more annoying symptoms in immunosuppressed patients is onset of diarrhea. While typical causes of gastroenteritis (e.g., *Salmonella, Campylobacter,* and *Shigella*) need to be considered, a common cause of diarrhea is use of antibiotics. Antibiotic-associated diarrhea is not synonymous with pseudomembraneous colitis, and the clinical evaluation of patients with diarrhea often results in negative cultures for *C. difficile* and negative tests for enterotoxin. Nonetheless, a patient with severe diarrhea may have high fever solely on the basis of colitis; sigmoidoscopy that reveals typical pseudomembranes can be diagnostic. Viral causes of diarrhea include adenoviruses, coxsackie viruses, and rotaviruses. The parasitic causes of diarrhea are being much more commonly recognized, especially cryptosporidia and isospora. These parasitic entities, as well as *Giardia lamblia,* are reviewed in Chapter 10.

5. Some Emerging Pathogens in the Immunocompromised Host

The major categories of opportunistic pathogens afflicting the immunocompromised host have not changed significantly during the past decade. On the other hand, some specific pathogens within a group—a previously uncommon species or a more antibiotic-resistant organism belonging to a generally susceptible group—may become more common or have attracted attention because of their role in well-defined nosocomial outbreaks. Perhaps the most important trend among hospitalized patients is the increase in bacteremias due to gram-positive organisms—coagulase-positive and coagulase-negative *Staphylococcus* (*S. epidermidis*) and *Corynebacterium* (commonly referred to as diphtheroids).[39,40] Changes in the types of opportunistic pathogens can be a real challenge to the clinician who should be prepared for unusual microorganisms even though his basic diagnostic thinking is oriented along the lines outlined in the previous sections.

Table 5[41–51] lists some of the more unusual emerging pathogens and their major clinical manifestations. No claim is made that the clinical patterns listed are comprehensive or that these disease-producing agents are really new. Indeed, *H. influenzae* is a well-known pathogen in young children, but its appearance in adult septicemias has been uncommon. The isolation of these organisms should lead to careful consideration of their disease-causing potential, and they should not be dismissed as nonpathogenic organisms or as saprophytes. Conversely, the findings of vasculitis, myositis, or necrotizing pneumonia in immunosuppressed subjects should raise suspicion that some of these more unusual pathogens might be involved.

6. Clinical Approach to Fever: History and Physical Examination

The initial evaluation of the patient must always begin with a carefully taken history. Recognition that the patient is immunocompromised by virtue of his (her) underlying disease (e.g., a neoplasm) or some form of treatment (e.g., cyclophosphamide and steroids for pemphigus) should be followed by a careful review and analysis of the following factors:

1. *Time of initial disease diagnosis or procedure:* The date of organ transplant or date of surgery should be noted.

2. *History of treatment for underlying disorder:* Factors such as radiation, drug treatment, or transfusion of blood products will be extremely important in interpreting new findings such as a pulmonary infiltrate or an allergic reaction. The nature of drug therapy, corticosteroids in particular, can be important in considering or excluding such important infectious etiologies as listeriosis, nocardiosis, and pneumocystosis. The time of administration and dose of medication may be crucial in diagnosing drug-induced fevers. Perhaps more important, such information is useful in assessing the magnitude of risk to the patient from drug-induced neutropenia following use of cytotoxic or myelosuppressive agents. Patients whose circulating neutrophil counts are rapidly plummeting are those in maximum danger from gram-negative bacillary and opportunistic fungal diseases.

Records of transfusions of all blood products should be carefully scrutinized. Prior use of analgesic/antipyretic medications and their effect on masking previous symptomatology may alert the clinician to the fact that illness has actually been of longer duration than suspected or that important manifestations such as fever had been masked. Often, as with use of steroids, an apparent flareup of symptoms and fever is related to reduction in dosage (see Chapter 10, Section 2). Recent (e.g., abdominal) exploration or antecedent surgery (splenectomy in a patient with Hodgkin disease) are obviously crucial in pointing to possible infectious complications. Even "minor" surgical procedures should be noted, such as the date of insertion of an intravenous cutdown or the date of a tracheostomy.

3. *Stage of the underlying disease:* This information is sometimes helpful in predicting some opportunistic infections. Freshly diagnosed leukemics and patients with plasma cell dyscrasias are more likely to have pyogenic infections (streptococcal and staphylococcal) than disseminated mycotic infections and pneumocystosis. Similarly, the more drug-resistant systemic or pulmonary gram-negative bacillary infections are more likely to follow repeated courses of chemotherapy or long-term immunosuppression and thus are complications of advanced stages of disease (or, in the case of transplants, multiple episodes of rejection). The clinician should, however, be alerted to possible exceptions to the latter rule if there has been a delay in diagnosis of the underlying disease and the patient has received courses of broad-spectrum antibiotics for fever. Thus, we have seen patients with marrow aplasia, lymphoma, or leukemia who were treated with ampicillin or oral cephalosporins prior to accurate diagnosis of the underlying disease and who, in the interim, became heavily colonized by antibiotic-resistant gram-negative rods. Septicemia caused by organisms such as *P. aeruginosa* occurred early during attempts to treat the underlying disease.

4. *History of previous infections and antibiotic treatment:* This information can be both helpful and misleading to the clinician. Infections can certainly recur in immunosuppressed individuals even after appropriate therapy and often in the setting of an underlying disease that fails to improve. Persistently positive cultures of a local site (e.g., wound drainage, deep cough sputum) can be a helpful but not infallible clue to the possibility of recurrence. On the other hand, if the patient has experienced a microbiologic and clinical cure of a documented infection, our experience has been that the reappearance of fever and signs of infection, more often than not, signals the onset of a new process rather than a recrudescence of an old one. Thus, our working rule has always been "the cause of the first successfully treated infection is not the same as a new infection," and a vigorous search for the etiology of fever is renewed without any preconceptions. The clinician should also be aware of the possibility of the presence of multiple infections, each involving the same area, such as lung. Knowledge of previous antibiotic treatment can also be applied with the same principle, since the more antibiotic-susceptible infections tend to occur earlier. *Pseudomonas aeruginosa* infections usually follow staphylococcal disease, but we have

almost never seen staphylococcal superinfection after treatment of *P. aeruginosa.*

5. *Presence of symptoms other than fever:* This factor is often crucial to localizing the source of infection and extent of involvement. Particular attention should be focused on the symptom of pain as one of the major clues to the presence of infection. In a recent review of infection in neutropenic patients, only local pain or tenderness and erythema were present in all patients irrespective of site of infection and level of granulocyte count.[52] Headache has always been an important finding pointing to the possibility of CNS infection.

6. *Travel history, dietary history, and exposure history:* Often components of a routine history, these factors should be broadened to include whether fever and evidence of infection developed in the community or in the hospital setting. A history of illness in the patient's family or community may occasionally be a helpful clue. By contrast, the development of infection in a nosocomial setting alerts the clinician to the severity of infection (tending to be more antibiotic resistant) and of suggested underlying disease/pathogen associations: the intensive care unit (ICU) with gram-negative pneumonia, the burn unit with *Pseudomonas* infections, and so forth. Salmonellosis may be a nosocomial problem related to specific dietary exposure. An avocational or pet history is like a travel history in usually being of little value. Rarely, knowledge that a patient is a pigeon fancier, raises cats, or has a pet turtle will lead to the diagnosis of cryptococcosis, toxoplasmosis, or salmonellosis, but the vast majority of owners of such pets suffer no ill consequences even if they become immunocompromised.

7. *Complications of previous therapy:* Knowledge of side effects, including drug reactions, may be helpful in evaluating the possibility of hypersensitivity reactions mimicking infection.

8. *History of recurrent temperature elevations and their pattern:* This is usually of very limited value in diagnosis. Rare instances of morning fever pointing to tuberculosis or periodic fever suggesting malaria are often cited, but it is unusual for classic fever patterns to occur and actually be of major importance in establishing a specific diagnosis. The evidence for this conclusion is well presented in a study by Musher et al.[53]

A complete physical examination should be car-ried out as expeditiously as possible in a period of no more than 45 min. It always must be borne in mind that patients who are immunosuppressed and/or granulocytopenic suffer the consequences of an impaired inflammatory response. Many typical physical signs of infection such as induration, fluctuance, local heat, reactive regional lymphadenopathy, and exudation of pus tend to be less frequent than in normal subjects who are infected. In pneumonia there may be decreased cough and little sputum production; in pharyngitis there may be an absence of a prominent exudate, and with urinary tract infection, patients may not have significant symptoms nor may they develop pyuria. The classic sign of nuchal rigidity may be absent in meningitis; thus, two very important clues are headache and poor performance on the mental status component of the neurologic examination. Of the physical findings in neutropenic subjects, erythema is the most reliable clue to the presence of infection irrespective of the absolute level of the WBC count.[52]

Within the context of a complete physical examination, emphasis should be placed on the following:

1. Neurologic examination covering both mental status and cranial nerves, including examination of optic fundi
2. Skin: major flat and intertriginous surfaces, perirectal area in particular
3. Oropharynx
4. Chest: careful auscultation of lungs and heart
5. Abdomen: liver and spleen enlargement
6. Lymph nodes: careful examination of all node-bearing areas
7. Pelvic examination in female if any symptoms are referable to this area
8. Site of insertion of any catheter site or drain
9. Site of a diagnostic procedure (e.g., thoracentesis, lumbar puncture)

Special examinations have some risk but should be done if symptoms are present:

1. *Rectal examination in patient with perirectal pain:* The latter may be the major clue to a perirectal (and often pseudomonal) abscess in a neutropenic patient. If the patient has neither obvious induration from external examination nor infected, thrombosed hemorrhoids, gentle rectal examination is indicated despite the danger of triggering bacteremia.

2. *Lumbar puncture:* This subject is covered

with CNS infections in Chapter 7. The examination of spinal fluid should be an initial diagnostic study for anyone with suspected CNS infection. On the other hand, caution must be observed in two specific situations: (a) if there is any suggestion of increased intracranial pressure, computed tomography (CT) should be performed to rule out a mass lesion that might result in brain herniation if lumbar puncture is performed; and (b) if the patient is markedly thrombocytopenic, platelet transfusions should be given as soon as possible. Lumbar puncture in the presence of a low platelet count has a small but definite hazard, and there should be clear-cut indication for the procedure if the patient is thrombocytopenic (<40,000 platelets/mm^3). We do not routinely recommend a lumbar puncture as part of the fever workup in the patient who does not have neurological signs or a change in mental status.

7. Interaction between the Clinician and the Microbiology Laboratory

If a group of clinicians and the hospital where they practice is to become involved in the care of immunocompromised patients, the clinical microbiology laboratory must assume a major role in the total effort. Such a laboratory must provide work of high quality and accuracy and, in important situations, be willing to perform special studies irrespective of when specimens become available. By the same token, microbiologists cannot be expected to be mind readers in anticipating what the clinician wants or considers desirable. Improved communication between the wards and the laboratory will help microbiologists select the most appropriate isolation techniques for any special problem that a clinician may have in mind. On our clinical service, we expect that house officers and fellows spend some time in the microbiology laboratory each day, not only collating laboratory results but discussing challenging problems of clinical and laboratory diagnosis.

8. Specific Laboratory Studies

A fundamental approach involves cultures taken of blood and any site or body fluid suspected of being infected. For the more rapid and accurate detection of

bacteremia, one major advance in recent years has been the so-called blind subculture technique for processing blood cultures. The conventional procedure for detecting positive growth in blood cultures involves daily (or twice-daily) observation of broth cultures for visible turbidity. However, it has been well documented that as many as 10^6 organisms can be present in broth without rendering these suspensions turbid. The blind subculture or blind passage technique involves subculturing apparently clear broth culture bottles to both aerobic and anaerobic plate media. Pseudomonads are obligate aerobes, and the blind subculture technique is a useful method for decreasing the time to isolation of these important organisms from blood cultures. Not surprisingly, anaerobic organisms may be detected by blind subculture even from the aerobe bottle, particularly if the specimen is removed from the bottom of the culture bottle with a long pipette and immediately incubated in an anaerobic atmosphere.

In addition to the relatively simple technique of blind subculture, a whole variety of laboratory equipment has become available for the more rapid identification of disease-causing bacteria. Some offer real improvements, whereas others have major technologic drawbacks. This emphasizes the need for the clinician to become familiar with the basic methods (and potential pitfalls) employed where one practices.

With the trend toward greater laboratory automation, an obviously desirable goal is the development of approaches that might either speed recovery of fastidious pathogens or increase test sensitivity. Two such approaches have been widely introduced into laboratory medicine. The first consists of devices containing resins or materials that remove antibiotics, thus improving detection rates if patients have been inadvertently treated. Some studies support the latter claim, but many of the isolates are gram-positive saprophytic organisms of dubious clinical importance.[54] Our own clinical experience with such devices suggest that they help diagnose bacterial endocarditis occurring in nonimmunosuppressed hosts, a situation in which a patient may have received oral antimicrobial agents prior to hospitalization and definitive diagnostic studies. On the other hand, in immunosuppressed patients who are persistently febrile and neutropenic while on broad-spectrum antimicrobial agents, the routine use of such antibiotic removing devices has infrequently yielded reliable information, over and above what could be obtained with carefully collected specimens (of adequate blood volume) for routine aerobic and anerobic blood cultures.

The other relatively new development is the introduction into blood culture systems of devices that lyse phagocytic cells (usually a compound such as saponin is incorporated into the test system) after differential centrifugation of blood has concentrated the leukocyte-rich fraction.[55] The rationale for such approaches is that some organisms such as fungi and microbes may remain viable within phagocytes. Centrifugation concentrates white cells and lysis releases viable organisms that may then be detected by a variety of routine or radiometric methods. The earliest studies have been highly encouraging in selected situations, particularly those in which an underlying fungal (candidal) or gram-negative infection is a good possibility.[56] In addition, the use of lysis centrifugation methods has now made it possible to detect bloodstream infections caused by mycobacteria routinely, particularly isolates of *M. avium* complex from patients with AIDS.[56,57] These techniques are costly and should probably be used in selected situations rather than on a routine basis. Furthermore, the usage of the lysis centrifugation methods for detection of fungi or acid-fast organisms should be probably incorporated with a method for rapid detection of microbial growth, such as commercially available devices, that measures the respiration or metabolism of slow-growing bacteria or fungi.

Several studies of blood cultures have indicated that for patients not previously receiving antimicrobial therapy most pyogenic organisms show detectable growth after 72 hr or 3 days of incubation.[6] If, however, the patient has received antimicrobial therapy, the growth of organisms may be suppressed for longer periods (although modern blood culture media contain antibiotic inhibitors and "dilute out" the blood sample by virtue of a large volume of broth so the suppressive effects of antimicrobials are often obviated). Another important observation is that three sets of blood cultures are adequate to diagnose bacteremia, and any more than this number is likely to be a waste of effort and expense.[57] Thus, we have evolved the rule of three: if three sets of blood cultures (three separate venipunctures) have been drawn, and 3 days of incubation have elapsed, the probability of documenting aerobic bacteremia is less than 10%. We advise that the interval between obtaining such blood cultures be determined by clinical circumstances: certainly no more than a total of 30 min should elapse in the critically ill patient, during which blood cultures are obtained from several sites.

Any patient who develops skin lesions should have them promptly aspirated, cultured, and biopsied. Occasionally, bacterial, fungal, and viral pathogens may not grow even when obviously present in histological sections, but morphology alone can establish the diagnosis. If antimicrobial therapy has already been initiated, ecthyma gangrenosum lesions may still reveal bacterial growth. In addition, immunofluorescence may be a way to identify pathogens in skin lesions, CSF, or other body fluids (e.g., tubercle bacilli in pleural biopsies, *L. pneumophila* in respiratory secretions after antimicrobial therapy has been initiated).

Fungal cultures may require long periods of incubation, so the above guidelines for judging the likelihood of bacterial blood cultures becoming positive are not applicable. Well-documented cases of *Cryptococcus neoformans* have taken several months' incubation of spinal fluid before growth became detectable. Although the problem of diagnosing cryptococcosis has been significantly reduced by methods for detection of capsular polysaccharide antigen, other fungal organisms such as *Rhizopus* and more unusual fungi may grow very slowly. No mycology laboratory should discard culture plates before at least a minimum of 1 month of incubation.

One of the most frustrating areas in laboratory medicine is the failure to detect fungal growth in blood cultures taken from patients who are eventually found to have widespread disseminated mycotic disease. The reasons for this are not clear, but some fungi, like *Candida* species, may spread through the lymphatics rather than through the bloodstream. On the other hand, hematogenous spread of organisms such as the zygomycetes and *Aspergillus* has been documented on a few occasions, but this is still rare. Fungal endocarditis, such as caused by *Aspergillus* species, may occasionally present with embolic phenomena, and removal of the blood clot may reveal fungal elements contained therein.

Anaerobic cultures of blood, of transtracheal aspirates, and of any abscess are clearly indicated. Anaerobes can cause CNS and urinary tract infection, but routine anaerobic cultures of CSF and urine are probably not indicated. Viral cultures of blood are probably not indicated except for CMV infection, and these may require a long duration of incubation to become positive.

Occasionally the clinician encounters a situation in which an isolate from blood, sputum, or wounds may be a contaminant. The therapeutic decision must be based on the gravity of the underlying disease and the relationship of an isolate to an objective clinical finding. We have occasionally observed isolation of cryptococci and *Nocardia* from sputum in the absence of pulmonary lesions.[58] Such patients can probably be followed carefully without treatment, but we would unhesitatingly initiate therapy if the patient were to develop fever or any pneumonic process.

Interpreting the significance of blood cultures drawn through a catheter is often difficult. Multiple positive cultures may reflect infection in and around the catheter rather than a true sustained bacteremia or fungemia. We do not recommend that cultures be obtained in this manner, but simple expediency is the best explanation for this practice surviving. A positive culture obtained on blood drawn through a catheter should be validated by samples drawn by conventional venipuncture, but unfortunately, the patient may have been started on antibiotics in the interim, and not all bacteremias are constant. Therefore, it seems prudent to eschew catheter-drawn blood cultures whenever possible.

9. Diagnosis of Infection: Antibody Measurements and Skin Tests

A variety of serologic tests for diagnosis of infection are available in most clinical laboratories, but some are probably overused and others significantly underused. In our experience, obtaining febrile agglutinins rarely has been helpful in establishing the diagnosis of an opportunistic infection in the immunocompromised host. Serologic tests for diagnosis of infection are most helpful when positive, and a negative test in an immunosuppressed subject cannot serve as the basis for excluding a diagnostic possibility. Measuring complement-fixing antibodies against *Coccidioides immitis*, Sabin–Feldman dye titers against *Toxoplasma gondii*, and detection of

cryptococcal antigen are usually quite reliable tests with few false-positive or false-negative results. On the other hand, fewer than half of all cases of opportunistic histoplasmosis are associated with elevated complement-fixing antibody titer,[35] and the status of diagnostic tests for systemic candidiasis and aspergillosis remain in dispute (see Chapter 8). Reliance on antibody measurements to diagnose infection in immunosuppressed subjects is obviously perilous, and the information obtained must be carefully integrated with other clinical and laboratory findings. Similarly, skin tests for diagnosis of infection are of very limited usefulness and are helpful, if positive, in validating prior exposure to a potential pathogen. A negative skin test is of no value in excluding a diagnostic possibility.

10. Noninvasive Diagnostic Procedures

Radioactive scans of liver and spleen have been available for some years and are very helpful in delineating both organ enlargement and filling defects that could be caused by infectious or neoplastic processes. Liver scanning, in particular, may be useful if coupled with such studies as diagnostic ultrasound, because the latter can be useful in distinguishing solid from fluid-containing lesions. The localization of lesions can be important in selecting the most appropriate approaches to diagnosis and treatment.

Considerable experience has evolved in the use of ^{67}Ga scintography for the detection of abscesses. This radionuclide is taken up by some tumors and by inflammatory masses as well, probably because it is concentrated by phagocytes. Late uptake of gallium (>24 hr) is more suggestive of tumor, whereas early uptake (4–8 hr) is suggestive of an abscess. Gallium scans have been most useful in detecting intraabdominal and subphrenic abscesses, but significant problems remain because of (1) confusion of areas of uptake with tumor, (2) uptake of radionuclide by reticuloendothelial cells and large bowel, and (3) inability to distinguish pus from an inflammatory reaction. Thus, a high incidence of false-positive results should lead clinicians to be wary about relying on this procedure alone to detect a localized or deep-seated abscess. Improved accuracy of diagnosis may be achieved by combining gallium scanning with diagnostic ultrasound or using it in conjunction with

[^{99}Tc]sulfur colloid scanning of liver and spleen. The latter compound defines the limits of the liver and spleen, making gallium uptake in other areas more helpful for localization of infection. An alternative to gallium scans is the use of radiolabeled leukocyte scans, which can target an area of inflammation. These scans may take several days to yield positive results, however.

Bone scans employing ^{99}Tc-labeled phosphate compounds have been used to establish an early diagnosis of osteomyelitis before significant bone destruction occurs. It has long been recognized that approximately 30–50% of mineral content of bone must be lost before a lytic lesion is detectable by radiography, and this process may take several weeks. Bone scans are particularly valuable in detecting multiple areas of involvement and identifying sites for biopsy, although it has been argued that documented bacteremia occurring concomitantly with scintiscan evidence of osteomyelitis obviates the need for biopsy. It should be remembered, however, that scintiscan cannot be used as a method for following treatment or assessing cure, because bone remodeling continues after eradication of infection.

Computed tomography was initially applied to diagnosis of CNS lesions and more recently has been extended to evaluation of intrathoracic and intraabdominal disease. More information is likely to be forthcoming on the value of this method in comparison with, or as a supplement to, ultrasound and radionuclide scanning.

11. Invasive Diagnostic Procedures

Invasive procedures may be divided into two categories: (1) those of brief duration, limited risk, and not requiring general anesthesia (e.g., arteriography, lymphangiography, and liver biopsy) and (2) those carried out in an operating suite with all the hazards associated with a major surgical undertaking.

Bone marrow biopsy probably carries little more risk than venipuncture and is a routine approach to the diagnosis of neoplasm. It has been helpful in evaluating granulomatous involvement of marrow. In two series of disseminated histoplasmosis in immunocompromised subjects, the diagnosis was established in approximately one-half of the patients by careful histologic examination and culture[35,59]; the

diagnostic yield increased to 61% if liver biopsy was also performed.[35] In our recent experience, culture of marrow for acid-fast organisms has been relatively unfruitful except in patients with AIDS. Any patient with the latter condition who is severely debilitated and who has persistent unexplained fever should have several blood and bone marrow aspirates cultured for mycobacteria, preferably by the lysis centrifugation technique.

Lymphangiography has been available for almost two decades and has been valuable for delineating the extent of involvement of retroperitoneal lymphomas. Patterns suggesting tumor have also been observed in some infectious granulomatous processes. It is clear, therefore, that lymphangiography is not a means for making an etiologic diagnosis but rather for determining if an abnormal lymph node architecture is present. If the latter is confirmed, attempts to make a tissue diagnosis are obviously indicated.

Angiography has been particularly useful in detecting anatomical structures with abnormal vasculature, particularly neoplastic processes. An abscess or occult purulent collection is suggested in filling defects or localized areas of hypoperfusion. Angiography should follow ultrasound and radioactive scintiscanning to delineate the nature of any abnormalities detected.

Ultimately, if conventional approaches to the diagnosis of infection are unrewarding, and noninvasive techniques also yield negative results, consideration should be given to a more invasive approach such as percutaneous biopsy of liver, lung biopsy, and/or exploratory laparotomy. The closed-needle approach to liver biopsy is widely employed. Unfortunately, the specimens obtained are often inadequate for comprehensive microbiological studies, but the histopathologic examination is often quite useful. Even though a relatively small core of tissue is removed by needle biopsy, washing of the needle with broth media and incubating the washings may improve the yield from culture. When liver biopsy in a patient with AIDS or suspected AIDS shows the presence of granulomas, blood, and bone marrow aspirates should be cultured for fungi and mycobacteria.

Exploratory laparotomy has been considered the definitive diagnostic approach to prolonged fever of unexplained origin.[4] With the introduction of newer noninvasive diagnostic techniques, abdominal exploration is performed less often, and two conditions should be met before deciding to undertake this approach: (1) clinical signs, symptoms, and laboratory findings that suggest intraabdominal pathology; and (2) ultrasound, scans, and liver biopsy that are uninformative, equivocal, or give conflicting interpretations. Although laparatomy has been considered a last resort in the diagnostic approach, we have no hesitation to recommend this procedure if the indications are present. The choice is often between laparotomy and a long course of empirical and potentially toxic antimicrobial treatment, following which laparotomy may still be required.

12. Diagnostic Tests of Limited Usefulness

The limited value of standard laboratory tests such as WBC count, urinalysis, and the erythrocyte sedimentation rate (ESR) in immunosuppressed patients must be recognized. Neutropenic patients may register no neutrophilic response in the presence of overwhelming sepsis and may become even more neutropenic through a "consumption" type of mechanism. The ESR is occasionally useful as a marker for inflammation. However, the ESR is a crude reflection of serum fibrinogen, and in hepatic disease states or during consumption coagulopathy triggered by sepsis, the ESR may actually drop secondary to a decline in serum fibrinogen. We believe that the ESR has some value if there is reason to doubt the presence of an inflammatory or infectious process such as in suspected factitious fever. On the other hand, if the patient is both febrile and immunocompromised, there appears to be little value in measuring the ESR because it should be elevated. If it were not elevated, we would suspect that a depressed level of fibrinogen is the cause.

There have been many efforts aimed at developing rapid, simple "bedside tests" that could aid in the diagnosis of infection and thereby serve as a guide to initiation of antimicrobial therapy. The goal is laudible, but the proposed approaches have not been validated in a number of prospective studies. Two such tests are the nitroblue tetrazolium (NBT) dye test[60] and the limulus lysate gelation test.[61] Nitroblue tetrazolium in its unreduced form is an orange material that can be taken up by phagocytizing leukocytes and converted to blue/black formazan. Neutrophils stimulated by whole bacteria, bacterial products, or endotoxins will demonstrate enhanced uptake and reduction of NBT corresponding to their intraleukocytic microbicidal mechanism. On the other hand, it has been shown that reduction of NBT is no more useful than detecting other morphologic indices of leukocyte reactivity in the presence of infection, and the claims that a certain percentage of NBT-positive cells in peripheral blood correlates with bacterial infection have not been borne out in other studies.[62] Thus, although the NBT dye-reduction test is very useful in ruling out intrinsic defects of granulocyte killing (see Chapter 16), it is not a reliable procedure for making a presumptive diagnosis of bacterial infection or for excluding that possibility.

The limulus lysate test is based on the observation that minute quantities of bacterial lipopolysaccharide (endotoxin) can trigger coagulation of extract prepared from the amebocyte cell of *Limulus polyphemus*, the Eastern horseshoe crab.[61] The horseshoe crab, like man, has a complex clotting system which can be activated by endotoxin or endotoxin-like products. This is a very sensitive in vitro technique for quantitating lipopolysaccharides, but in the study of human gram-negative bacterial infection, particularly bacteremia, only one-half to two-thirds of patients have had positive tests, and there have been studies reporting a significant number of false positive tests.[63,64] Perhaps one of the major reasons for false negativity is the presence in serum of inhibitors or antibodies which block the effects of endotoxin in triggering the coagulation sequence.[64] In examining CSF, the limulus assay appears to be a very reliable method for ruling out gram-negative meningitis,[65] but the test is not reliable for detecting hematogenously circulating gram-negative bacterial endotoxin. A modification of the *Limulus* test, using spectrophotometry for precisely measuring gelation is now available but still yields a significant number of false-negative results in specimens from patients with gram-negative bacteremia.

13. Persistent or Recurrent Fever in the Patient with Negative Cultures: Diagnostic Considerations

One of the most frustrating clinical situations to deal with in the management of immunocompromised patients is persistent or recurrent fever despite negative bacterial and fungal cultures. The major clinical choices are to pursue the search for a cryptic infectious process or to attribute fever to underlying disease (or in the case of organ transplants, graft rejection). We would strongly argue that the latter should be a diagnosis of exclusion, and the failure to detect an infectious cause of fever after an initial evaluation mandates a comprehensive reappraisal of diagnostic strategies with emphasis still being placed on finding an infectious cause.

Table 6 summarizes the major causes of fever that should be considered after an initial "negative" evaluation. Some, such as CHF or pulmonary emboli, call for diagnostic and therapeutic approaches outside of the infectious disease sphere. The possibility of drug fever calls for careful review of all medications (including topical ones). If a medication is suspected of triggering fever, it should be discontinued, but one must bear in mind that convincing proof of drug fever will depend on provoking fever on rechallenge. An indwelling vascular catheter may have a cutaneous site of insertion that looks benign, but removal of this foreign body may reveal distal infection. Adrenal insufficiency must always be borne in mind for patients who have received long-term steroids and have then had their dose reduced. Fever of adrenal insufficiency tends to be low grade and may be accompanied by feelings of marked general weakness and hyperkalemia.

If initial cultures for bacterial and fungal patho-

TABLE 6. Causes of Recurrent or Persistent Fever in Patients with Negative Bacterial and Fungal Cultures

Adrenal insufficiency
Anicteric viral hepatitis
  Hepatitis A, B, non-A–non-B
Catheter-associated infection (including candidiasis)
Congestive heart failure
Cryptic abscess
Cytomegalovirus infection (with or without hepatitis)
Drug fever
Epstein–Barr virus infection
Graft-vs.-host disease (bone marrow transplants, recipients of nonirradiated leukocytes)
Hematomas, infected or uninfected
Other viral infections
Pulmonary emboli
Splenic infarct
Tuberculous or other granulomatous infection
Underlying disease even though all other evidence is negative

gens are negative, the thrust of further diagnostic efforts aimed at uncovering an infectious cause should be directed towards granulomatous and chronic viral infections or a cryptic abscess. Extrapulmonary tuberculosis should always be considered in the febrile immunocompromised patient irrespective of what initial studies show, i.e., in the face of negative tuberculin tests, negative chest radiographs, and absence of cough. It is well known that miliary or disseminated TB can progress without radiologic involvement of the chest.[3] One helpful clue is the tendency for the alkaline phosphatase of the hepatic type or other liver enzymes that are elevated in "obstructive" liver disease to be mildly to moderately elevated in disseminated tuberculosis. Tuberculous involvement of the fundi, bone marrow, and urine are other helpful clues to this diagnosis, but the yield is quite low in culturing bone marrow or in culturing urine in every patient with suspected tuberculosis.

Anicteric viral hepatitis is another possibility of which there are several causes. Hepatitis of the A, B, or non-A, non-B type as well as that caused by the CMV can produce fever and liver function test abnormalities in the absence of clinical jaundice. Hepatitis serology and measurement of complement-fixing or other types of antibodies against CMV may be important in establishing this diagnosis.

Unfortunately, the category of other viral infection must now include the retrovirus, which is identified as the cause of AIDS [human immunodeficiency virus (HIV) or lymphadenopathy-associated virus]. The possibility of transfusion-acquired AIDS must be considered in any immunocompromised patient who has received fresh blood products since the late 1970s. While it is hoped that routine screening for antibodies in blood donors, begun in 1985, will reduce this infection risk, the long incubation period for AIDS should remind clinicians of the potential hazard of AIDS superimposed on another disorder (like cancer) or following organ transplantation. Furthermore, one cannot be confident that antibody screening in a previously immunosuppressed patient (non-AIDS) will reveal prior exposure to the virus.

A cryptic abscess has classically been one of the major entities to consider in any patient with an unexplained fever. Traditionally, the search for cryptic abscesses has focused on the abdomen. However, consideration should also be given to soft tissue lesions in the extremities, flanks, and perirectal areas.

In many reviews, CHF has been listed as one of the causes of fever of undetermined origin. It would be unusual, however, for CHF to cause high temperature, in excess of 102.1°F (39°C), accompanied by rigors and chills. The evidence for CHF may be subtle and may consist of only mild pulmonary congestion. Fever associated with cardiac failure may quickly respond to a diuretic such as intravenous furosemide.

Pulmonary emboli have long been recognized as causes of high recurrent fever, and these may be accompanied by chills and rigors. It is also well known that many patients with pulmonary emboli and fever may not have clear-cut clinical signs or the classic radiologic findings. Further, patients with pulmonary emboli may not have readily identifiable sources of these emboli. We have observed pulmonary emboli in patients who were markedly thrombocytopenic or who had prolonged prothrombin times (PPT) secondary to far advanced hepatic disease. Most patients with angiographically documented pulmonary emboli have fever, and in some 80% of febrile patients with pulmonary emboli, it has been attributed solely to pulmonary thromboembolism and not to a concomitant process.[66] In these studies high fever, i.e., temperature greater than 102.2°F (39°C), caused by pulmonary embolism may occur early, and low-grade fever may continue for a week or more, but fever persisting beyond 6 days, especially with temperatures in excess of 101.3°F (38.5°C), should not be ascribed to pulmonary thromboembolism unless other causes have been carefully excluded. An interesting report details superinfection of pulmonary emboli in neutropenic patients or patients receiving steroids.[67] This should be a consideration in patients who have fever more than a week after the acute episode.

Hematomas located in a wide variety of body sites, and particularly in the central nervous system, can be the cause of recurrent fever. An assiduous search for hematomas, particularly in the central nervous system if there is any evidence of altered mentation, is an important part of the diagnostic reevaluation of the patient with persistent fever. Hematomas outside of the nervous system may become easily infected, but even bland hematomas are associated with fever.

Infarcts of the spleen are usually observed in conditions where there is splenomegaly such as chronic myelocytic leukemia or lymphoma. These infarcts may be bland or secondary to a bacteremia, and the mortality associated with splenic abscess that follows septic infarcts may be quite high. Patients who have septic infarcts usually have easily documented bacteremia, but bland infarcts may still be accompanied by high hectic fevers and prominent symptoms of pain in the left upper abdominal quadrant.

In recipients of bone marrow transplants, one of the major causes of fever, particularly that which occurs more than 2 weeks after engraftment of new marrow, is onset of graft-vs.-host (GVH) disease. The manifestations of GVH include pruritis, arthralgias, liver function abnormalities, hepatomegaly, and a diarrhea of varying severity which may not respond to conventional antidiarrheal medications. GVH disease may require a histopathologic diagnosis. Our experience with allogeneic bone marrow transplantation indicates that in the face of a rising white count (representing engraftment), the onset of fever suggests early GVH disease. On the other hand, a demonstration of abnormal liver function studies, diarrhea, and other typical findings of GVH should not exclude a persistent search for infectious causes or coexistent infection caused by an organism such as CMV.

The two major categories of underlying diseases that have been recognized as causes of fever per se are connective tissue disorders and neoplasms. Prior to the availability of effective antiinflammatory agents for systemic lupus erythematosus, fever was a prominent disease manifestation that could not be attributed to infection.[68,69] In neoplastic diseases, fever unassociated with infection may be a presenting symptom of leukemia or lymphoma. In patients who achieve a hematological remission, the subsequent reappearance of fever may be an ominous sign heralding an intramedullary relapse. In patients with hematologic malignancies who have a bone marrow that still shows remission, the recurrence of fever may signal a relapse in an extramedullary site such as meninges or testicles.

The problem of fever in lymphoma and leukemia will be considered in more detail in Chapter 18. Table 7 is an attempted summary of the association between neoplastic processes and fever. Fever is most common with unremitting hematologic malignancies and is relatively uncommon in the chronic

Table 7. Fever and Neoplasia

Neoplasia	Often	Occasional	Rare
Hematologic malignancies			
Acute myelogenous leukemia	+		
Acute monocytic leukemia		+	
Chronic myelocytic leukemia (blast crises)		+	
Acute lymphatic leukemia	+		
Chronic lymphatic leukemia			+
Hodgkin disease	+		
Multiple myeloma		+	
Non-Hodgkin lymphoma		+	
Solid tumors (without obstruction or metastatic tumor)			
Adrenal carcinoma and pheochromocytoma	+		
Hepatoma	+		
Hypernephroma	+		
Hypothalamic tumor		+	
Ovary		+	
Pancreas		+	
Testicular		+	
Thyroid		+	
Bowel		+	
Breast			+
Colon			+
Lung			+

leukemias and common solid tumors of breast, lung, and gastrointestinal origin. Classically, hypernephroma, hepatoma, adrenal carcinoma, pheochromocytoma, and malignant tumors of the pancreas, thyroid, and hypothalamic areas have been associated with fever. However, it seems clear that all tumors can be associated with fever if they are the cause of obstruction, and metastatic tumor in the liver is an accepted cause of fever even without gross obstruction or infection.

14. Findings Suggestive of Microbial Infection Rather Than Fever Secondary to Underlying Disease

There are no hard and fast rules for distinguishing between fever of infection and underlying disease, but Table 8 is an attempt to summarize some of the important findings that would point toward an infectious etiology in the seriously ill patient. None of these findings is specific for infection. For instance, neoplastic processes such as acute promyelocytic leukemia can trigger consumption coag-

ulopathy, and hemolysis may be a prominent feature of a connective tissue disorder complicated by an autoimmune anemia. Nonetheless, the factors listed in Table 8 have been extremely helpful in certain situations. Change in mental status is often seen during the onset of septicemia, as is hyperventilation with ensuing respiratory alkalosis. Hypotension may be a terminal event in patients with far advanced malignancy, but an acute hypotensive episode (although also possibly caused by noninfectious causes

TABLE 8. Findings Suggestive of Microbial Infection Rather Than Fever Secondary to Underlying Disease

Appearance of skin lesions
Change in mental status
Consumption coagulopathy, particularly thrombocytopenia
Hemolysis
Hyperventilation and/or respiratory alkalosis
Hypotension
Increased fluid volume requirements
Localized pain
Metabolic acidosis
Oliguria

such as pulmonary emboli) should be strongly considered an indication for initiation of empirical antimicrobial therapy. Similarly, oliguria is a frequent sequel of systemic hypotension, and a sudden fall in urine output may be a clue to an underlying gram-positive or gram-negative septicemia. Both hypotension and oliguria may be associated with impaired tissue perfusion and metabolic acidosis.

15. Initial or Empirical Antimicrobial Therapy: Indications for Treatment

For any immunocompromised patient, the sudden appearance of fever should trigger both an intensive diagnostic evaluation and consideration of presumptive or empirical antimicrobial therapy. The concept of giving antimicrobial agents without definite microbiological proof of infection is disturbing to some physicians who are schooled with the principle of knowing what they treat. However, information obtained from cultures may take days (and sometimes weeks) to become available, and a delay in treating a rapidly progressing infection may be disastrous. A more pragmatic approach is to give treatment based on the best available information and subsequently make adjustments in therapy or discontinue it altogether as the results of specific laboratory tests return. Previously available microbiological studies, however recent in relation to a febrile episode, should be interpreted with some caution, as new events (e.g., superinfection) can be fast developing.

Any finding on physical or laboratory examination that establishes the presence of infection in lungs, soft tissues, gastrointestinal (GI) tract, or urine should prompt a decision to treat. In the absence of pain, inflammation, and exudate, any of the findings listed in Table 8 may tip the balance toward giving antimicrobial therapy. If neither objective findings of infection are present nor any of the changes cited in Table 8 are present, we would still treat the febrile patient if (1) underlying disease is worsening and/or (2) the neutrophil count is falling. It is hard to cite a defininte cutoff point for the neutrophil count, but infection risk is definitely increased at levels below 500/mm^3.[70] We would still give empirical broad-spectrum antibacterial therapy

if the neutrophil count is rapidly plummeting, even though the absolute value of the WBC count is above the 1000/mm^3 mark. For instance, in acute leukemia, it is not unusual for the white count to successively halve as the result of intensive cytotoxic treatment. Even though the number of normal neutrophils exceeds 1000/mm^3, the precipitous fall in the WBC count will virtually ensure that the patient will become functionally aplastic within a matter of days. Thus, the sudden appearance of fever and findings suggestive of septicemia such as hyperventilation, acidosis, and hypovolemia would be decisive factors in opting for antimicrobial treatment. On the other hand, if the patient's peripheral WBC count is quite low, but a marrow examination reveals repopulation of the marrow with normal morphological elements, and the peripheral WBC is slowly rising, we would be less inclined to be aggressive about antibacterial treatment with onset of low-grade fever.

If patients suddenly become febrile despite treatment with very high doses of antiinflammatory agents such as corticosteroids, we would be extremely concerned about the possibiility of a bacterial or fungal septicemia. We are not proposing that corticosteroids can be used as a diagnostic test for an infectious etiology of fever but feel that the fever in the face of antipyretic medications is a stronger indication for considering therapy.

Among the principles that must be exercised in the clinical management of the immunocompromised host who has fever and suspected septicemia is the speed with which the diagnostic evaluation should be undertaken and empirical therapy initiated. Any significant delay could be dangerous, particularly in the presence of hemodynamic instability. Our clinical rule is to make a decision about giving treatment within an hour of being notified that the patient has signs of fever and/or infection. The necessary diagnostic steps for culturing of blood, secretions, and other infected sites can usually be performed within 60 min. During this interval, the clinician should assure himself or herself of at least one reliable route for giving intravenous therapy. This may require the insertion of an intravenous plastic cannula or intravenous cutdown. Appropriate monitoring devices should be set in place and, if necessary, the patient moved to an area where vital signs can be carefully monitored.

16. Relationship of Antimicrobial Therapy and Underlying Disease to Outcome of Infection

The importance of effective antimicrobial therapy in the management of the immunocompromised host cannot be overemphasized, but it would be difficult to establish unequivocally that antibacterial agents alone have improved survival in certain disease states. More than a decade ago, several major reviews of gram-negative rod septicemias pointed out the extremely poor prognosis for patients with so-called rapidly fatal diseases.[71-73] Such diseases were defined as bone marrow failure (aplastic anemia) or hematologic malignancies in which the outlook for survival was a matter of months. In a combined series of gram-negative rod bacteremias reviewed in 1971 (which reflected the clinical experience prior to the introduction of antipseudomonal penicillins and modern aminoglycosides), the mortality was 84% among patients with rapidly fatal diseases irrespective of whether appropriate or inappropriate antimicrobial treatment was given (appropriate therapy was defined as use of at least one antibiotic that inhibited the infecting organism). In other underlying disease categories, i.e., so-called nonfatal or ultimately fatal diseases, the use of appropriate antimicrobial agents could be correlated with lower mortality.[73]

In contrast, there appears to be a definite improvement in survival rates, particularly in those patients who would be classified as having rapidly fatal diseases, since the introduction of antipseudomonal penicillins and aminoglycosides beginning with gentamicin.[74] Our recent experience is that as many as 80% of patients with leukemias, lymphomas, and bone marrow transplants have survived gram-negative bacillary infections, although the mortality is still higher from bacteremic infections caused by *P. aeruginosa*.[75] A widely accepted concept is that recovery from a septic episode is directly related to the status of host defenses and that ultimate survival is closely linked to improvement in underlying disease. Although we have always subscribed to this, it must be acknowledged that it represents a circular pattern of reasoning that leaves the relationship between cause and effect unresolved. In the management of the cancer patient, it has been argued that antibiotics keep patients alive while allowing antineoplastic

drugs to work. On the other hand, the belief that ultimate recovery from infection is not possible without improvement in the basic disorder implies that effective treatment of the basic disease is crucial to the success of antimicrobial therapy. In the final analysis, these concepts need not be mutually exclusive. In many instances, it is possible to sterilize the blood of patients in the absence of marrow recovery with aggressive use of modern antimicrobial agents even though the basic disease has not improved.[76] This is usually a temporary gain, however, because patients whose underlying condition fails to improve often develop new episodes of gram-negative bacillary, fungal, and viral infections within a short period of time. Nonetheless, antimicrobial therapy "buys time"—an interval during which additional attempts can be undertaken to control the underlying disease. If the latter is successful, the improved treatment of underlying disease (leading to remission or control of cancer, collagen vascular disorder, etc.) leads to better control or cure of infectious complications.

17. Factors Underlying Recommendation of Initial or Empirical Antimicrobial Therapy Regimens

The major factors influencing selection of antimicrobial agents for use in serious bacterial infections include spectrum, potency, pharmacokinetics, stability, and resistance to inactivation by enzymes of bacteria or inactivation secondary to use of other pharmacologic agents. We consider safety a highly desirable feature as well, but in the acute stages of a life-threatening infection, we are more concerned with efficacy rather than avoiding complications of treatment. In order to enhance the potency of therapy, we believe substantial evidence exists for the use of multiple antimicrobial agents as initial therapy. In addition, there is need to ensure that these agents are given in sufficient dosage so as to achieve adequate therapeutic levels.

Despite the extremely large number of clinical trials of antimicrobial agents reported in the medical, surgical, or pediatric literature, a limited number have included a comparison or control group, and there is a paucity of studies demonstrating the superiority of one regimen over another. Clearly, it is not ethical to have untreated control groups when sepsis is the clinical diagnosis, but comparison of different regimens in large numbers of treated patients is vastly preferable to anecdotal reports or ''open,'' i.e., non-comparative evaluations. Studies that use historical controls cannot easily be condoned because of the multiplicity of factors that have changed in the management of different underlying disease conditions.

It has been our policy for more than a decade and a half to initiate antimicrobial therapy in the immunocompromised host with no less than two agents and to consider adding a third, depending on the history, laboratory findings, and clinical findings. For the neutropenic patient with an absolute granulocyte count of <500 cells/mm³ (and particularly the markedly neutropenic patient with <100 neutrophils/mm³) we still believe that an essential component of empirical therapy should be an aminoglycoside paired with a β-lactam agent. There is persistent debate about (1) the relative merits of agents within the aminoglycoside class and (2) whether the β-lactam agent should be either a cephalosporin, an antipseudomonal penicillin, or one of the newer compounds, such as a monobactam (e.g., aztreonam), carbapenem (e.g., imipenem), or β-lactamase inhibitor paired with a penicillin (clavulanate plus ticarcillin). Many new compounds belonging to the β-lactam class have been introduced into clinical use during the past 5 years; many of these agents are considerably augmented in their gram-negative coverage. Nonetheless, a consistent finding has been a relative decrease in antistaphylococcal activity, against both coagulase-positive and coagulase-negative organisms (*Staphylococcus epidermidis*). Some classes of new compounds, such as the monobactams (e.g., aztreonam), completely lack gram-positive activity and cannot be used alone in empirical therapy.

By employing two agents, we achieve not only a broadening of antibacterial spectrum but take advantage of possibly synergistic interactions between agents. Antimicrobial synergism between aminoglycosides and β-lactam agents has been documented in in vitro experiments and experimental infections.[75,77,78] Although laboratory criteria have differed, synergism implies an antibacterial effect greater than the sum of the individual activities of the components of a regimen. In the treatment of human infection—whether the infection is enterococcal endocarditis or gram-negative rod bacteremia—it has not been possible to conduct a rigorous clinical trial

that proves the superiority of synergistic combinations of antimicrobial agents. Such a definitive study would have to involve randomization of patients to receive synergistic versus nonsynergistic combinations of agents. On the other hand, Klastersky et al.[79,80] and our group[81,82] have shown that the use of synergistic combinations in human gram-negative infections is associated with significantly better results than nonsynergistic combinations. In actuality, whether two agents interact additively or synergistically is probably moot. The net result is greater activity than with the use of a single agent, and antagonism is rarely seen. (In fact, we have not documented antagonism in the study of more than 200 episodes of gram-negative rod bacteremia treated with aminoglycoside/β-lactam agent combinations.)

The greater in vitro antibacterial activity against gram-negative rods obtained with combinations seems to translate into better clinical results. Table 9 pools results from two studies in which fairly similar treatment protocols were used empirically in febrile neutropenic patients suspected of having systemic gram-negative bacillary infections.[76,83] The aminoglycoside was either amikacin, gentamicin, or netilmicin, while the antipseudomonal penicillin was either carbenicillin or ticarcillin. Each study shows the same trend, and the combined results demonstrate that responses, as measured by defervescence and clearing of bacteremia, were significantly better in patients treated with two agents active against the infecting strain than when only one of the assigned agents in a combination inhibited the bacteremic

TABLE 9. Combination Therapy of Gram-Negative Rod Bacteremia in Neutropenic Patients[a,b]

	UCLA +	UCLA −	BCRC +	BCRC −	Percent response
Pathogen susceptibility					
Both antibiotics	31	8	28	5	82
One agent	2	5	18	9	59
Neither agent	0	3	2	5	20
Total	33	16	48	19	70

[a]Pooled results of UCLA[83] and Baltimore Cancer Research Center[76] Experience
[b]+, survived, improved, or temporarily improved, −, died or failed therapy, BCRC, Baltimore Center Cancer Research Center, UCLA, University of California, Los Angeles

pathogen in vitro. Such results argue for the use of the most broadly active agents in an initial empirical regimen. The 82% response rate for combination therapy of gram-negative bacteremia when both agents inhibit the infecting strain is a standard against which other studies may be compared. Indeed, variations on the themes expressed above showed similar response rates when piperacillin–amikacin[84,85] moxalactam/amikacin,[86] and ceftazidime–tobramycin[87] were used as empirical therapy in cancer patients. While studies of some newer β-lactam agents used as monotherapy claim results equivalent to combination with an aminoglycoside,[87] the numbers of severely neutropenic patients with documented bacteremia in such series have been much smaller than the numbers of cases represented in Table 9.

With regard to specific recommendations, our initial choices would therefore involve selection of the most broadly active compounds of the aminoglycoside and β-lactam classes. Admittedly, there will be a number of alternative choices and no clearcut regimen that most investigators and clinicians would consider ideal. As implied in subsequent chapters and as summarized in Table 10, the following combinations would appear to be the reasonable therapeutic equivalents: either amikacin, netilmicin, or tobramycin plus either piperacillin, azlocillin, ceftazidime, or cefoperazone. A recent study of empiric antimicrobial therapy organized by the European Organization for the Research and Treatment of Cancer (EORTC) involved more than 800 patients and compared regimens in which either azlocillin, ticarcillin, or cefotaxime were combined with amikacin.[88] For *P. aeruginosa* bacteremia, the results with antipseudomonal penicillins were significantly better than when cefotaxime was paired with amikacin. In addition, the overall results in the treatment of all gram-negative rod bacteremias with azlocillin plus amikacin were superior to results with either of the other two-comparison regimen. There is no evidence that addition of a first-generation cephalosporin such as cefazolin improves results over that obtained with an aminoglycoside and an antipseudomonal penicillin.[89]

Cefotaxime, the first of the third-generation cephalosporins, has markedly augmented activity against many important gram-negative rods such as *E. coli* and *Klebsiella* species. There are some excellent well-conducted studies, such as that reported by

TABLE 10. Summary of Recommendations for Empirical Therapy

I. Neutropenia (neutrophils <500 mm³) or rapidly falling WBC.
   Aminoglycoside (tobramycin or amikacin) + β-Lactam (piperacillin, azlocillin, ceftazidime or cefoperazone)
   (cephalosporin or imipenem can be used in penicillin allergy)
II. Neutropenia plus (one or more):
   Creatinine 1 2 mg% or greater
   Age ≥60 years
   Eighth nerve damage
   Potential nephrotoxic medication (ceftazidime + piperacillin)
III. Neutrophil count >1000 (stable):
   Aminoglycoside + first generation cephalosporin (oxacillin or nafcillin)
                     or
   Third-generation cephalosporin (alone)
                     or
   Imipenem (alone)
IV. Add therapy in specific situations:
   Diffuse lung infiltrates: trimethoprim/sulfamethoxazole
   Multiple areas of lung consolidation: erythromycin
   Catheter site inflammation/pain: vancomycin
   Severe diarrhea or abdominal symptoms: metronidazole

Smith et al.,[95] indicating that cefotaxime used alone as a monotherapeutic agent was superior to and less toxic than the combination of nafcillin plus tobramycin. It must be noted, however, that this study did not include immunocompromised neutropenic patients, nor were there large numbers of patients who had bacteremic infections due to organisms like *P. aeruginosa*, *Enterbacter* species, and *Klebsiella* species. The relatively poor results observed in the cefotaxime-containing arm in the EORTC studies seems related, in part, to deficiencies in activity against *Pseudomonas*.[88] Klastersky and colleagues[91] demonstrated that cefoperazone plus amikacin is a highly effective combination in a small study of gram-negative rod infections. Cefoperazone would appear to be superior to cefotaxime in antipseudomonal coverage but is probably not as active as ceftazidime, which has been successfully used in immunosuppressed neutropenic patients as monotherapy for *P. aeruginosa* bacteremia with a better than 80% clinical response rate.[87] Either one of these antipseudomonal cephalosporins (cefoperazone, ceftazidime) usually can be used safely in patients with history of penicillin allergy. Further comments on the newer cephalosporin and related β-lactam agents are presented in Section 18.3. It should be noted that even use of cetazidime alone as empirical therapy may still offer problems, as it is relatively less active (compared with first-generation cephalosporins) against staphylococcal species. Both grampositive and anerobic superinfections have been observed secondary to ceftazidime usage.[92] Experiences of this nature still argue for the prudent use of combinations as initial therapy in patients who are severely neutropenic.

An alternative to conventional aminoglycoside plus β-lactam agents has been a resurrection of a therapeutic strategy employed earlier in the 1970s, in which two so-called double β-lactam trials in neutropenic hosts were disappointing, particularly with regard to the response in the treatment of *Klebsiella* infection.[94,95] Admittedly, compounds used in earlier studies, such as carbenicillin as the penicillin and cefazolin as the cephalosporin, were relatively less active than newer agents belonging to the same respective drug classes. More recently, double β-lactam therapy has been reevaluated with the pairing of third-generation cephalosporins with more potent antipseudomonal penicillins. Several large studies of moxalactam–piperacillin[96] and moxalactam–ticarcillin[97] indicate that overall response rates are quite similar to those obtained using comparison regimens of broad-spectrum penicillin with an aminoglycoside. In one of these studies, there was less nephrotoxicity in the double β-lactam regimen as contrasted with the aminoglycoside-containing regimen,[97] but in the other study[96] no difference in ototoxicity or nephrotoxicity was observed. Interestingly, one of these reports shows poorer responses in patients with *P. aeruginosa* infections given a double β-lactam combination of piperacillin and moxalactam[96] compared with the aminoglycoside-containing arm. Furthermore, in that study several patients treated with two β-lactam agents experienced relapse of *P. aeruginosa* bacteremia with emergence of multiple β-lactam-resistant organisms, suggesting a selection for strains elaborating inducible β-lactamases by one of the mechanisms suggested by Sanders and Sanders.[98] A review of these recent studies[93] has suggested that these types of double β-lactam regimens may be associated with significantly more fungal superinfection[97] and significantly prolonged neutropenia.[96] It

is well known (perhaps related to prolonged duration of therapy) that some patients may develop neutropenia secondary to β-lactam antibiotic therapy. Use of two such agents in large doses for prolonged periods of time may impede marrow recovery, creating a paradoxical situation in which an attempt is made to treat infection in neutropenic patients, but the net result is actually prolongation of neutropenia (and therefore infection risk).

Nonetheless, despite the problems encountered thus far, modern double beta lactam therapy has some attractive features. An increasing proportion of patients being treated with cytotoxic and immunosuppressive therapy have either borderline or impaired eighth nerve and renal function. Many immunocompromised patients are receiving nephrotoxic agents such as cis-platinum, amphotericin B, and organ transplant recipients may be receiving cyclosporine. For these reasons, the initiation of double β-lactam therapy in patients above the age of 60 or in patients with impaired or borderline renal and eighth nerve function appears prudent, particularly when infection due to the more problematic gramnegative rods seems less likely (*P. aeruginosa, Enterobacter* sp. and *Serratia* sp.). Probably the most active double β-lactam regimen widely available is the combination of piperacillin and ceftazidime, as suggested in Table 10. With known or likely *Pseudomonas* infection of the lungs or the bloodstream, it would still seem prudent to use an aminoglycoside coupled with either a potent antipseudomonal penicillin or cephalosporin.

There are still gaps in empiric therapy coverage if one focuses on combining a traditional aminoglycoside with a β-lactam agent. The choice of one of the newer cephalosporins risks enterococcal superinfection, particularly when moxalactam is used.[96] With widespread use of indwelling vascular catheters, *S. epidermidis* bacteremia is one of the leading causes of bloodstream infection; many physicians have added vancomycin as an initial component of the early treatment regimen. Such a decision should probably be related to physical findings. If physical examination reveals an obviously infected indwelling catheter, such a finding would favor empirical vancomycin. It is interesting to note, however, that there has never been a convincing therapeutic trial in which three initial antimicrobial agents given as empiric therapy have proved superior to a two-drug regimen. The second major multicenter EORTC study found that amikacin plus carbenicillin was no less effective than amikacin–carbenicillin–cefazolin.[89] However, the addition of vancomycin to an aminoglycoside and β-lactam agent combination would be justifiable when staphylococcal or enterococcal infections are frequently encountered or appear likely on clinical grounds.

Finally, an alternative non-nephrotoxic empirical therapy regimen that might be used with considerable success would include vancomycin plus cetazidime, or ceftazidime plus trimethoprim–sulfamethoxazole given parenterally.

Table 10 summarizes currently recommended regimens for empirical antibacterial therapy of immunocompromised patients. These recommendations must be interpreted only as general guidelines that need to be modified if more specific clinical and laboratory information (e.g., history of recent documented infection, results of surveillance cultures) is available.

18. Antimicrobial Agents

18.1. Aminoglycosides

The primary indication for aminoglycoside agents is in the therapy of documented or presumed gram-negative rod infections, since these antibiotics inhibit most clinically significant bacilli.

The greatest clinical experience has been with gentamicin, which has been available for more than a decade. Tobramycin is identical to gentamicin in pharmacokinetics and is resistant to one enzyme that can inactivate gentamicin. Amikacin is a semisynthetic derivative of kanamycin, and both of these agents achieve blood levels about four times higher than gentamicin. Kanamycin, like streptomycin, lacks anti-*Pseudomonas* activity and has no real indications in the immunocompromised patient. Amikacin is susceptible to inactivation by only one of the plasmid-mediated enzymes that can modify gentamicin and tobramycin. Netilmicin is also a semisynthetic aminoglycoside. It is more stable to enzymic inactivation than tobramycin but less stable than amikacin.

If infecting agents are equally susceptible to any of these aminoglycoside agents, and therapeutic levels of each are achieved, there is no evidence that one compound is clinically superior to the other. Differences in in vitro susceptibility (taking into account potency by weight and achievable blood levels) do exist, including: (1) increased activity of tobramycin against *P. aeruginosa* and (2) increased activity of amikacin against *Klebsiella, Enterobacter, Serratia,* and *Providencia*. It has not been demonstrated, however, in randomized, prospective human studies that such in vitro superiority results in enhanced clinical efficacy if patients are carefully monitored and have drug doses adjusted so that peak blood levels fall within therapeutic ranges.[82,99] Table 10 summarizes current dosage recommendations for these aminoglycosides and emphasizes the desired therapeutic ranges.

Many authorities have emphasized the need to monitor blood levels to ensure adequate dosage.[100-102] There is a wide range of dose–blood level relationships for gentamicin (the best-studied agent), and this observation is probably true for the other aminoglycosides as well. Adequate blood levels are crucial for the successful treatment of septicemia and pulmonary infections in the impaired host, and many treatment failures and breakthroughs on gentamicin therapy have occurred in association with subtherapeutic levels.[103] Monitoring of blood levels may also alert clinicians to the potentially toxic accumulation of these agents so that dosage can be adjusted.[104] We recommend twice- to three-times-weekly measurements in septicemic patients. In urinary tract infection, urine levels of drug correlate best with outcome, and all aminoglycosides achieve very high concentrations in urine so that blood level monitoring is not critical. Some authors have recommended continuous infusions of aminoglycosides but have not demonstrated convincingly superior results.[105] In addition, infusions given in this manner usually require special equipment and additional intravenous lines. From a purely pragmatic view, we recommend pulsed infusions of approximately 30-min duration and prefer IV to IM treatment in seriously ill patients.

Information on the clinical prevalence of resistance to gentamicin and tobramycin shows considerable interinstitutional differences. Clearly, knowledge of local patterns of antimicrobial susceptibility as well as the bacterial species most prevalent in immunocompromised hosts should have the most important bearing on initial antimicrobial selection. While we prefer to use amikacin for empirical therapy before the results of cultures are known, a justifiable concern is the emergence of broad aminoglycoside resistance. Fortunately, this appears to have occurred rather infrequently in the face of widespread usage.[106,107] Organisms that are resistant to all aminoglycosides are not rare, however, and such multiresistant strains have developed permeability barriers to drug penetration. The selection of such resistant strains may occur secondary to the use of any aminoglycoside.

Although aminoglycosides are routinely given with penicillins, clinicians should be aware that under certain circumstances agents such as gentamicin and tobramycin can be inactivated by carbenicillin. The basis for the inactivation is the formation of a biologically inactive amide between penicillin and aminoglycoside.[108] This phenomenon is dose, time, and temperature related, and inactivation is probably most significant in patients with renal failure in whom both agents circulate and have adequate time for the inactivation to occur. Closed space infections or urinary tract infection may be other situations when inactivation occurs.[109] A report indicates that even in patients without renal failure, some inactivation of gentamicin will occur when a penicillin (ticarcillin) is given.[110] We believe that documented renal failure is an indication for amikacin because it is least subject to inactivation, perhaps 10% in 24 hr.[111] If gentamicin or tobramycin are used with a penicillin in renal failure, even more care should be paid to following blood levels because it will probably be necessary to augment the dosage.

18.2. Antipseudomonal Pencillins

Following the introduction of ticarcillin, three other agents in this category have become clinically available: mezlocillin, pipercillin, and azlocillin. It is important to remember that all antipseudomonal penicillins are not reliably effective against staphylococcal infection, with all these agents being readily hydrolyzed by staphylococcal β-lactamase.

Mezlocillin and pipercillin exhibit modest but variable activity against *Klebsiella* species. In both cases, this activity is not predictably reliable against klebsiella organisms. Mezlocillin is relatively less potent than azlocillin and pipercillin against *P.*

aeruginosa. The primary advantage of ticarcillin, mezlocillin, azlocillin, and piperacillin compared with carbenicillin is greater potency by weight, permitting lower dosages. The net result tends to be less hypokalemia and less sodium overloading. These differences may be clinically significant.[85] When used in appropriate dosage, all the antipseudomonal penicillins combined with appropriate aminoglycoside appear to give comparable results. Pipercillin and azlocillin are most potent against *Pseudomonas* and for this reason are to be favored in severe infection caused by this pathogen.

18.3. Cephalosporins

Within the past half-decade, the most rapidly changing area in systemic antimicrobial therapy has been the field of parenteral cephalosporins. Traditionally, the activity of the cephalosporins, as exemplified by cephalothin and cefazolin (so-called first-generation compounds) included reliable activity against coagulase-positive staphylococci compared with penicillins such as ampicillin or carbenicillin. In addition, they were usually active against *E. coli* and *Klebsiella*. First- and second-generation (e.g., cefoxitin) cephalosporins lacked activity against the more resistant gram-negative rods, such as *Pseudomonas* and *Serratia*. First-generation cephalosporins have been traditionally favored in surgical prophylaxis. The major development in the cephalosporin field, as commonly acknowledged by many investigators, has been the rapid introduction of compounds belonging to the so-called third generation. Some of these compounds and recommended dosage regimens are summarized in Table 12. For completeness, related compounds such as aztreonam and imipenem are included as well with recommended dosing intervals.

The third-generation cephalosporins are exceedingly potent against pathogens such as *E. coli* and *Klebsiella* species, pathogens traditionally susceptible to cephalosporins. They are some one hundred times more active than predecessor compounds of their class if one considers gravimetric potency. Furthermore, the coverage against enteric organisms is comprehensive, with very low minimum inhibitory concentrations (MIC) for *Proteus* species and related organisms. The activity against *P. aeruginosa* has been variable. Agents such as ceftazidime exhibit

TABLE 11. Calculation of Aminoglycoside Therapy for Systemic Therapy

Agent	Dose		Interval (hr)	Anticipated	
	mg/kg	mg/body surface area (m²)		Peak (μg/ml)	Valley (μg/ml)
Gentamicin	1.5[a]	60	8	>4	<2
Tobramicin	1.5[a]	60	8	>4	<2
Amikacin	7.5[b]	280	12	>20	<10
	5[b]	200	8	>14	<10

[a]For seriously ill patients, an initial loading dose of 2 mg/kg or 105 mg/m² is recommended
[b]The total daily dose of amikacin should be 15 mg/kg or less In seriously ill patients, dosage every 8 hr (5 mg/kg) is preferred

considerably more activity than cefotaxime, ceftizoxime, and ceftriaxone. Caution must still be expressed about the activity of these agents against Pseudomonas species, *Enterobacter* species, *Serratia,* and *Citobacter* species, in which there is potential for inducible β-lactamase resistance.[98] It seems prudent, therefore, to employ these potent agents in combinations at least until the nature of infecting bloodstream pathogens is known. Furthermore, it should be pointed out that many of these compounds may have adverse effects, which undermine the traditional concept that cephalosporins are extremely safe compounds for antimicrobial therapy. Coagulopathy and disulfiram-like reactions are associated with cefoperazone and moxalactam.[110] The potential bleeding complications are a genuine concern for the clinician who must manage thrombocytopenic patients. Minor disulfiram-like reactions may, in fact, occur in patients receiving medications that contain small amounts of alcohol (e.g., cough medications).

Aztreonam is very much like ceftazidime in its anti-gram-negative spectrum, and the two compounds do exhibit major structural similarities. The major deficiency of aztreonam, however, is lack of activity against all gram-positive pathogens, thereby mandating its use in combination when empiric therapy is given.

Imipenem, a compound marketed with an inhibitor of its metabolism, cilastatin, is a very potent, novel β-lactam agent with broad gram-positive and gram-negative activity. There may still, however, be

TABLE 12. Recommended Dosage and Selected Pharmacokinetic Properties of Third-Generation Cephalosporins and Other New β-Lactam Agents

Agent	Peak serum level (μg/ml)[a]	Half-life (hr)	Protein binding (%)	Daily IV dose[b] interval (g)
Aztreonam	50	1.7	60	2 q8h
Cefotaxime[c]	40	1.1	40	1–2 q6–8h
Ceftizoxime	75	1.4	30	2 q8–12h
Ceftriaxone	150	8.0	90	1–2 q24h
Ceftazidime	80	1.8	20	2 q8h
Cefoperazone	125	2.0	90	2 q8–12h
Imipenem	50	1.0	50	0.5–1 q6h
Moxalactam	75	2.3	50	1 5 q8h

[a]After administration of 1 g IV
[b]Doses recommended are for an average-size adult with moderately severe infection who has normal renal function
[c]Cefotaxime is metabolized to an active derivative with a longer half-life (1 6 hr)

problems with the emergence of resistance among problematic organisms such as *Pseudomonas*[111] and its effect against *Enterococcus* is not bactericidal. Nevertheless, its use has occasionally been life-saving in pseudomonal and other gram-negative infections that have been resistant to other forms of antimicrobial chemotherapy.

18.4. Antistaphylococcal Semisynthetic Penicillins

Methicillin, oxacillin, and nafcillin are equally effective antistaphylococcal agents when used in appropriate dosage. Methicillin is preferred for CNS infections because of superior penetration into spinal fluid; however, there may be more hypersensitivity nephritis and neutropenia associated with its use.

19. Is Specific Antistaphylococcal Therapy Necessary?

One of the most frequently asked questions regards the advisability of including an antistaphylococcal agent such as oxacillin, a cephalosporin, or vancomycin with the initial combination of an antipseudomonal penicillin and an aminoglycoside. The experience of several centers including our own is that empirical use of an aminoglycoside and an antipseudomonal penicillin will prevent serious progression of staphylococcal infection (including bacteremia) and that no ground is lost by not giving specific antistaphylococcal coverage.[82] In some countries where methicillin-resistant organisms are prevalent, the use of an aminoglycoside for staphylococcal infections has been associated with satisfactory clinical response rates. Nevertheless, we do not advocate continued use of aminoglycosides when it is known that the patients have methicillin- and cephalosporin-susceptible staphylococcal infections (based on in vitro susceptibility tests). specifically, we will add an antistaphylococcal agent and probably alter the initial antibiotic coverage (by stopping the aminoglycoside).

One potential detraction from our assumption that aminoglycosides constitute adequate initial coverage for staphylococci is the recognition that some hospitals, particularly those treating patients with thermal injury, have observed infections caused by

both gentamicin- and amikacin-resistant staphylococci.[113] These organisms appear to be resistant by virtue of their elaboration of enzymes that inactivate gentamicin and amikacin, respectively. If infections caused by such organisms are documented, alternative therapy must include vancomycin inasmuch as such strains can also be methicillin resistant. The problem of dealing with catheter-associated *S. epidermidis* infection is covered in Section 23.

20. Alteration of Empirical Therapy after Documentation of Bacterial Infection

After documentation of bacterial infection, therapy can justifiably be altered according to the results of in vitro susceptibility tests. Such instances include the following:

1. Resistance to one or more components of the empirical regimen. If azlocillin or ticarcillin was initially used, and infection proves to be caused by *Klebsiella* species, substitution of a cephalosporin or trimethoprim/sulfamethoxazole (if supported by in vitro tests) is indicated.
2. A less expensive, better tolerated alternative is available. If the infection proves to be *E. coli*, ampicillin can be substituted for carbenicillin or a cephalosporin (providing the patient is not penicillin allergic). Trimethoprim–sulfamethoxazole appears to be a reasonable alternative to β-lactam agents for enterobacterial infection (but not gram-positive infection where we would recommend vancomycin).
3. Quantitative in vitro susceptibility tests (MIC or equivalent) showing that one agent is at least fourfold more potent than another. For instance, it is generally recognized that aminoglycosides have a narrow ratio of therapeutic/toxic levels. If the MIC of gentamicin is 4 μg/ml and that of tobramycin is 1 μg/ml against an infecting strain, we would switch to the latter agent.

Although we believe there is evidence that synergistic interactions have a favorable impact on clinical outcome, routinely performing synergy tests is time consuming and expensive. Results are available usually after 2–3 days, which is often a week or so after the initial culture was taken. The late availability of these results is likely to have little impact on therapeutic decision making.

Should the infecting pathogen be susceptible in vitro to both agents that were initially used, an important question is whether to continue their use or discontinue the more potentially toxic component, i.e., the aminoglycoside. Our studies[83] suggest the benefit of continuing multiple agents in the more severe underlying diseases (rapidly fatal) and certainly in patients whose neutrophil counts are less than 500/mm³. For the remainder we would wait until defervescence occurs and the patient has been afebrile for 72 hr. Even with patients who present less severe underlying disease, we tend to continue double-agent therapy if the infection proves to be *P. aeruginosa*, *Serratia*, *Enterobacter*, or indole-positive *Proteus* species.

21. Role of Other Antibacterial Agents in Therapy

Chloramphenicol, the polymyxins (colistin and polymyxin B), clindamycin, trimethoprim–sulfamethoxazole, rifampin, and tetracycline may have certain indications, but we would not use them as initial compounds of empirical therapy. The polymyxins have impressive in vitro activity against *P. aeruginosa*, *E. coli*, and *Klebsiella* but are inactive against *Serratia* and *Proteus* species. A principal virtue is that R-factor (plasmid)-mediated resistance to these compounds has not been documented. However, there are persistent doubts about their efficacy, and their role is primarily in the treatment of aminoglycoside-resistant organisms.[74] Occasionally, it can be demonstrated that sulfonamides will potentiate the action of a polymyxin against the highly resistant strains of *Serratia* or *Proteus*, and in such situations such combination therapy may be considered.[114]

Clindamycin and chloramphenicol have occasionally been added to empirical therapy regimens, particularly for patients with possible anaerobic infection. Although their activity against anaerobes is unquestioned, our experience has been that anaerobic organisms are infrequently a major component of infections in immunocompromised patients unless there has been some violation of the integrity of the mucosal surfaces of the GI tract. Furthermore, our experience has been that antipseudomonal penicillins are probably satisfactory antianaerobic agents. Occasionally, we have observed a patient to defervesce following addition of carbenicillin even though bacteremic infection remains undocumented. An unanswered question is whether the effect of carbenicillin against anaerobic microorganisms is responsible for this improvement. No substantial data have been presented to support this hypothesis. By the same token, clindamycin or chloramphenicol added to an initial combination of carbenicillin or ticarcillin and aminoglycoside adds little in terms of antibacterial coverage, poses some risk of toxicity, and has not been shown in any comparative or randomized study to improve significantly the clinical response rate.

Trimethoprim–sulfamethoxazole, on the other hand, is an agent with interesting pharmacologic properties and impressive antimicrobial activity. The excellent tissue penetration of the trimethoprim and sulfonamide components is an advantage over aminoglycosides. There are some strains of Enterobacteriaceae, particularly *Serratia*, that are resistant to all other agents including the aminoglycosides, and it is in the treatment of infections caused by these organisms that trimethoprim–sulfamethoxazole may be distinctly beneficial. In vitro this agent inhibits most clinically significant gram-positive and gram-negative organisms except for *Enterococcus*, anaerobes, and *P. aeruginosa*. We do not believe that the problem of pneumocystosis or toxoplasmosis is sufficiently great to justify empirical use of this compound or its therapeutic trial in persistently febrile patients. On the other hand, this agent might make an effective partner in combination with an aminoglycoside or an antipseudomonal penicillin; such therapeutic approaches require further clinical study.

The dose of trimethoprim–sulfamethoxazole for certain infections will vary depending on severity of infection, presence of bacteremia, and source of infection. We have extensive experience with the intravenous preparation. Although there are some technical problems with this preparation (including the necessity for administration of large volumes of fluid to maintain solubility of the product), it would clearly be advantageous to use a parenteral preparation in seriously ill patients. We recommend the intravenous trimethoprim–sulfamethoxazole in a dosage of 240 mg or 3 mg/kg every 8 hr IV with the intravenous infusion proceeding over approximately 1 hr duration. In more serious infections (and including *Pneumocystis carinii* pneumonia), that dose may be doubled with little risk of major acute toxicity.

Tetracyclines are bacteriostatic agents that are infrequently used to treat bacterial infection in immunocompromised subjects. Infections caused by non-*aeruginosa* pseudomonads, some anaerobic pathogens, and mycoplasmas are some indications. Some tetracyclines such as minocycline are an effective component of multidrug therapy of *Nocardia* infection.

Rifampin is a highly effective antituberculous agent and one of the two drugs of choice (along with isoniazid) for the treatment of rapidly progressing tuberculosis. It will inhibit a number of other bacteria as well, but clinical experience with this agent when used alone was that emergence of resistance developed fairly rapidly. Rifampin is a highly effective antistaphylococcal agent, possibly because of its penetration into leukocytes. Consequently, its use has been in combination with agents such as vancomycin against staphylococci resistant to semisynthetic penicillins or against which the effect of vancomycin is bacteriostatic and not bactericidal. There are a number of strains of *Staphylococcus epidermidis* that are inhibited by vancomycin but are not killed until fairly high concentrations are used. Against these strains, the addition of rifampin results in bactericidal activity at clinically achievable levels. *Staphylococcus epidermidis* infections are occasionally encountered in infected shunts and catheters, and there could be major problems associated with removal of the infected prosthetic device.

22. Therapeutic Drug Monitoring

It is clearly desirable to monitor aminoglycoside blood levels during severe infections. The problem of breakthrough bacteremias[103] and the demonstration of better clinical results when targeted levels are achieved[115] support this policy. Other tests have been proposed, such as the monitoring of serum bactericidal activity in a manner akin to measurements obtained during the treatment of endocarditis.[116–118]

Some impressive correlations have been demonstrated between high cidal levels and clinical success in treating cancer patients[119] and patients with endocarditis.[118] The test, however, is cumbersome, poorly standardized, and takes days to execute. Equally useful information (in terms of identifying patients whose dosing regimen requires modification) may be derived by using some of the rapid antibiotic assays that yield results within minutes.

23. Management of Catheter-Associated Infection

During the past half decade, a remarkable trend has gone unchecked in major centers dealing with immunocompromised hosts: the tendency to use large indwelling vascular catheters for delivery of parenteral fluids, blood transfuions, hyperalimentation, and so forth. The advantages of this approach are obvious because such indwelling catheters facilitate infusion of large quantities of medications and nutritional support.[120] In addition, it may be possible with multiple-lumen catheter to also draw blood from a central site, thereby reducing the number of venipunctures that a patient may require. The almost universal acceptance of indwelling central catheters in patients undergoing organ transplantation or intensive chemotherapy underscores their current popularity.

Much of the risk of long-term indwelling catheters is related to infection hazards. Clearly, the technique and experience of physicians inserting such catheters and those who manage such catheters (nursing personnel or the patient him or herself should the individual choose or want to elect to manage the catheter) will affect the subsequent incidence of infectious complications. When highly experienced personnel are involved in surgical insertion of these catheters and their daily maintenance, cleaning, and care, the infection rate may decline to almost negligible levels. With less experienced catheter care, more than half of such catheters can be infected in spite of the use of parenteral antimicrobial agents.

Major clinical dilemmas arise when neutropenic patients have fever and no readily identified source. The catheter becomes suspect as the source of sepsis by a "process of elimination." Nonetheless, because of the impaired inflammatory response of immunosuppressed patients, there may be slight or even no evidence of inflammation of the cutaneous entry site of even an infected catheter. Thus, the catheter is always a suspected candidate for the source of the fever in a patient with FUO, yet clinicians are reluctant to remove such catheters because they are so convenient to use and the removal of one catheter in a patient who has a venous access problem may merely mean that another one will have to be reinserted within a fairly short interval.

Another area of controversy relates to the fact that patients who have indwelling catheters will clearly have bacteremias from multiple sources and the source obviously may not be the catheter. If there is clinical evidence of localized infection around the catheter, such a finding is fairly incriminating. If the organism cultured from blood has the same morphologic and antimicrobial susceptibility pattern as an organism in urine or wound, the catheter is far less suspect. However, the possibility exists that the catheter may become secondarily infected (seeded) if the bacteremia was sustained. What seems clear is that routine removal of a catheter in any patient with fever is to be discouraged. When a patient has documented bacteremia due to a gram-negative organism one should not automatically incriminate the vascular catheter as the predisposing factor. By contrast, bloodstream recovery of *S. epidermidis*, *Corynebacterium*, and *Candida* species should lead to the catheter being the prime suspect, unless there is another more readily identifiable focus of infection.

Once a catheter is identified as the source of infection (by multiple positive peripheral blood cultures and culture of blood drawn through the catheter), controversy exists about the alternatives of treating the infection in situ or removing the catheter. Infectious disease dogma maintains that foreign bodies that are the focus of infection should be removed, and this remains a generally sound principle. Nonetheless, Pizzo and others have reported that more than half of such catheters can be maintained in place with appropriate antibiotic therapy.[121] This allows a patient to complete a course of cancer chemotherapy or to be supported during the immediate posttransplantation period (if the patient has undergone such a transplant) and obviate the need for yet another catheter insertion procedure in a very sick patient. From the careful studies of catheters infected by *S.*

epidermidis, antibiotic therapy such as with vancomycin either alone or in combination with rifampin or gentamicin can lead to eradication or suppression of *S. epidermidis* infection. Often, defervescence of the patient is but a reflection of the suppression of infection caused by a relatively less virulent organism. Still, suppression may be an acceptable goal providing that only a few additional weeks of treatment of the underlying disease is necessary.

We believe that there are rational guidelines to catheter management. Our own experience is that it is possible to suppress *S. epidermidis* or corynebacterial bacteremia that is associated with a catheter in more than half of cases, using vancomycin with or without rifampin or gentamicin (but sometimes requiring all three agents). On the other hand, we have never been able to sterilize the blood of patients who have had bloodstream infections due to *Candida* species, more resistant gram-negative organisms such as *P. aeruginosa*, *Serratia*, or *Enterobacter*. With the latter bacteria, the catheter should be removed at the earliest possible opportunity and specific antimicrobial therapy given for 7–10 days (or longer, if there are metastatic foci of infection). Most *S. aureus* and *E. coli* bacteremias that are clearly linked to catheters are not easily suppressed even with very potent antibacterial chemotherapy and catheter removal is usually necessary. For the more sensitive organisms (*S. epidermidis*, *Corynebacterium*), a trial of 3–5 days of therapy may be justified if the overall clinical condition is stable. If the patient has not defervesced and improved by the end of such a trial period, then the catheter must be removed. If the patient does respond to suppressive therapy, such treatment should be continued for a total of 10–14 days, with the recognition that the infection may well recrudesce (the value of longer treatment is unclear).

24. Should Fever Be Suppressed?

Despite much controversy there has been no satisfactory resolution to this much-debated issue. Substantial evidence exists that fever is beneficial to the host in experimental infections.[3] On the other hand, there is no convincing evidence that, providing adequate antimicrobial therapy is given for a documented infection, the concomitant suppression of fever is detrimental to the clinical outcome. Proponents of suppressing fever argue that patients are more comfortable, have less metabolic demand, and elderly patients in particular benefit from reduced stress on cardiovascular function.

A prudent clinical approach argues that it would be misleading to routinely administer antipyretics while searching for a cause of fever or while assessing the response to treatment. On the other hand, if patients become markedly febrile (temperature 102.2°F, or >39°C), the use of antipyretics can be justified particularly in the elderly or anemic patient. We would recommend initiating a 24–48-hr trial of acetoamiphen, 600 mg every 4–6 hr or naproxen, 250 mg every 12 hr, and then stopping the antipyretic and observing for a "rebound" in temperature. This seems preferable to intermittent use of antipyretics for single temperature elevations, a practice that leads to "seesaw" temperature changes, drenching sweats, and much patient discomfort. Younger patients tolerate fever much better, and suppression of temperature is not strongly advocated in this group.

25. Therapy of Underlying Disease during Documented Infection

Whenever an immunosuppressed patient develops documented infection, it is entirely appropriate to consider the possibility of decreasing, perhaps temporarily, the intensity of treatment of the basic disease to aid in combating the infection. However, in some diseases such as acute leukemia where there is rapid cell proliferation, this concept is unrealistic because the malignancy is likely to progress during the hiatus. In bone marrow transplantation, the nature of the conditioning is such that, once begun, a point of no return is quickly reached. Similarly in collagen vascular disease or acute graft rejection, the principal aim of therapy is control of the inflammatory or rejection process, and reducing immunosuppression jeopardizes the basic therapeutic approach. In selected situations, decreasing immunosuppression is feasible such as with an infection that occurs during remission consolidation of leukemia. Although every attempt is usually made to save a renal graft, the ultimate consideration in a life-threatening infection is whether to allow the patient to reject it. The renal

transplant recipient enjoys one advantage over the recipient of cardiac or bone marrow transplant: the patient can be supported by dialysis while the complicating infection is being treated.

26. Duration of Antimicrobial Therapy in Documented Infection

The immunocompromised patient who develops infection should be treated for no shorter duration than for the same type of infection in the normal host, but some patients may require a longer course of therapy. There is no substitute for clinical judgment in this decision-making process, with the critical variable being the status of the underlying disease. For neutropenic patients who develop bacteremia, pneumonia, or extensive cellulitis, we would treat for at least 14 days total until the patient became afebrile. If the patient remains febrile and still has signs of infection, we would continue until the neutrophil count exceeds 500/mm^3. This might require many more weeks of treatment. We have given one leukemic patient with extensive necrotizing cellulitis of an extremity because of *P. aeruginosa* 4 months of aminoglycosides and carbenicillin until satisfactory healing had been achieved. If there is persistent evidence of a localized or systemic infection, it would be foolish to terminate effective therapy "by the calendar."

On the other hand, there are situations where shorter courses of treatment may be as beneficial as longer courses. In uncomplicated lower urinary tract infection, a day of treatment may be adequate.[122] In vascular and catheter-associated infections, a week of therapy following their removal is usually satisfactory if a rapid defervescence and clinical response are observed.

27. Undocumented Infection and the Decision to Continue or Withhold Antimicrobial Agents

Perhaps one of the greatest clinical dilemmas facing the physician who treats immunocompromised subjects is how long to wait to assess the clinical effect after empirical therapy is started and what to do if no infection has been documented. Thus, the crucial question is: should therapy be stopped, modified, or intensified? It is clear that many patients given empirical treatment may take more than 4 days to become afebrile; Rodriguez et al.[123] isolated bacteria after an initial 4 days of fever in 21% of treated patients. Thus, empirical coverage should likely extend beyond 4 days and probably up to a week. In another study,[124] the incidence of superinfection increased after 7 days of empirical therapy, and if infection was not documented by 4–7 days of fever, no patient deteriorated when antibiotics were stopped. Pennington[26] goes on to advocate that a reasonable approach would be that for patients who defervesce within 3 to 4 days, a total of 5 afebrile days of therapy should be given if cultures are negative, and at least 7 if positive. If patients fail to respond to empirical treatment, alteration in therapy is indicated. The clinically stable but continuously febrile patient who turns out to have negative cultures should receive empirical antibiotics for more than 4 but not more than 7 days. If these patients continue to deteriorate for more than a week, consideration of empirical antifungal therapy is indicated, especially if a fungus is isolated from other body sites.

Unfortunately, there is no uniformity of opinion as to each step in the decision-making process. Although there have been many trials of empirical therapy, particularly in the neutropenic patient, relatively few details have been provided about the factors that influence decisions to continue or discontinue antimicrobial agents. Unquestionably, a large number of patients have fever with undocumented infection (see Chapter 18). In our recent experience with neutropenic patients more than 70% of patients fall into this category. On the other hand, the clinical response rate to initiation of empirical antimicrobial therapy now exceeds 70% and is no different from the patient population with documented bacterial infection.[82] This raises the tantalizing question about what processes may be responsible for febrility that are yet responsive to empirical antimicrobials.

An interesting study was described by Pizzo et al.[125] at the National Cancer Institute (NCI). It acknowledges that the complications of broad-spectrum antibacterial therapy argue for brief treatment, whereas the risk of inadequately treated infection in the granulocytopenic patient favors longer therapy. Of more than 300 patients at the NCI initially treated

with cephalothin, gentamicin, and carbenicillin, an infectious etiology of fever was not identified in 142 of 306 (46%) of episodes. Of those patients with persistent granulocytopenia, 33 defervesced, and their granulocytes remained at less than 500/mm^3. These were randomized after 7 days of the empirical regimen to continue or to discontinue treatment. There was no problem with patients whose WBC counts exceeded 500/mm^3 because they had no infectious sequelae. However, seven of the 17 (41%) of those patients randomly selected to discontinue agents experienced infectious sequelae a median of 2 days after discontinuing antibiotics. This result was statistically significant. No patient continuing on therapy had a resistant superinfection or developed resistant microbial flora. Analysis of the seven patients who had their therapy discontinued and then experienced a rebound fever or infection showed that two had fever alone, but five experienced documented infections, of which two were ultimately fatal. If the two groups are compared by numbers of documented infections, the significance of the difference is marginal. Nonetheless, this study argues for continued therapy during the duration of granulocytopenia.

The conclusions of Pennington[26] and Pizzo et al.[121] are essentially contradictory. The former sees no problem discontinuing antimicrobials in febrile patients (and danger in continuing them without proven infection), whereas the latter group suggests that empirical therapy be continued even if the patient is afebrile. Certainly, the risk of a rebound fever or infection should, if anything, be greater in febrile patients with undocumented infection. The lack of a consensus is even more apparent in the clinically more challenging situation of persistent fever, granulocytopenia, and undocumented infection. Some investigators cite examples of catastrophic developments if antimicrobial agents are stopped.[125,126] Another alternative is suggested by Rodriguez et al.[123] who, based on a relatively small number of cases studied, recommend adding a third antibacterial agent. If an aminoglycoside and a cephalosporin formed the initial combination, addition of an antipseudomonal (and better antianaerobic) penicillin may occasionally lead to defervescence, but we have rarely seen improvement if the third agent is chloramphenicol or clindamycin. Usually, little is to be gained by adding a cephalosporin to the initial regimen of an aminoglycoside and penicillin unless the patient has a *Klebsiella* or *S. aureus* infection.

A more recent follow-up to the initial study by Pizzo and collaborators has been published, and offers substantial guidelines for the management of the febrile neutropenic patient who fails to respond to an empiric antibacterial regimen.[127] The initial treatment regimen employed at the NCI has been the combination of cephalothin, gentamicin, and carbenicillin. Satisfactory response rates at that institution have been observed with relatively few problems with drug resistance. Patients who had persistent fever and neutropenia for 1 week were randomized as follows. Group I was randomized to stop all three antibacterial agents. Three of these patients developed rebound bacterial infections and six experienced shock. Group II was randomized to continue the empirical three-drug antimicrobial regimen in the absence of documented infection. Subsequently, five patients were found to have a systemic fungal infection, an incidence of almost one-third (consistent with some projections and estimates by other investigators). Group III was randomized to continue parenteral antibacterial therapy with the addition of empirical amphotericin B. In this group, only one opportunistic fungal infection was documented, due to *Petriellidium boydii,* an organism resistant to amphotericin B. An important observation was that patients randomized to receive empirical antifungal defervesced more rapidly than patients in the other two groups.

This study clearly gives support to empirical addition of amphotericin B to empirical antibacterial therapy, but it would be dangerous, and certainly wasteful of a valuable drug, if every patient who did not respond within a finite number of days to antibacterial treatment were blindly started on amphotericin B. A number of factors might enter into clinical decision making; these are reviewed in the next section.

28. Recommendations for Continuing or Discontinuing Antimicrobial Therapy and Initiating Empirical Antifungal Therapy

We believe that a rational decision can be made based on the clinical and laboratory factors summarized in Table 13. We agree with many investigators

TABLE 13. Factors Affecting the Decision to Stop or Continue Antibiotics in the Face of Fever and Negative Blood Cultures

Factor	Suggested course
Magnitude of WBC	Stop if $\geq 500/\text{mm}^3$ for 2 days
Condition of bone marrow	Stop if normocellular and rising by 50% daily increase in peripheral white count even if total $<500/\text{mm}^3$
Continuation of treatment for underlying disease	Continue antibiotics
Surveillance cultures	Continue antibiotics if *P. aeruginosa* or *K. pneumoniae* recovered until white count reaches $500/\text{mm}^3$
Recovery of *Candida* or other fungus from blood or urine	Start amphotericin B
Radiography	
Diffuse infiltration consolidation, cavity	Invasive procedure, consider trimethoprim–sulfa or amphotericin B
Severe esophagitis	Start amphotericin B

that the magnitude of the circulating white count is of crucial importance in determining susceptibility to infection. Thus, if patients have persistent fever, we recommend discontinuing antibiotics after a 7-day trial providing that the granulocyte count exceeds $500/\text{mm}^3$ for 2 or more days and all cultures are negative. Perhaps as important as circulating neutrophil count, however, is the condition of the bone marrow. If afebrile patients have evidence of normocellularity of the marrow after a course of cytotoxic treatment, and the peripheral white count is rising by 50% per day, we recommend discontinuing antibacterial therapy even if the peripheral WBC count is low. An even more important factor in decision making is the anticipated effect of further treatment. In the face of plans to augment the dose of adrenocorticosteroids, give a cytotoxic agent to prevent graft rejection, or resume another cycle of antileukemic treatment, we believe it would be perilous to discontinue antibiotic therapy if the patient has persistent fever. We place considerable reliance on the results of the surveillance cultures in adult patients being treated for acute leukemia and in patients of all ages who are subject to the bone marrow transplant procedure. The rationale for surveillance cultures is that colonization precedes infection in a vast majority of immunosuppressed hosts and that a substantial interval exists between acquisition of colonization and the development of infection (see Chapter 2). Thus, we can have an early warning system about potential infecting organisms. It is an expensive procedure that should not take the place of the clinical acumen and careful examination. Of the sites that are sampled, the three most important areas for surveillance cultures are the oropharynx, stool, and nares. The first two sites are important for detecting gram-negative rod colonization, and the nose culture for staphylococcal carriage.

The manner in which surveillance culture results influence our management of antibiotic therapy is as follows. For the neutropenic patient who has responded to empirical antibacterial treatment, we would treat for the interval to defervescence plus 3 afebrile days or a total of 7 days, whichever is greater, unless surveillance cultures reveal *P. aeruginosa, Klebsiella pneumoniae, Enterobacter* species, or *Aeromonas* species. In both afebrile, colonized (by the latter organisms) neutropenic patients and febrile neutropenic patients irrespective of colonization status, we treat with systemic agents until the white count reaches 500/mm³. The only exception to this working principle is the patient with severe aplastic anemia or myelofibrosis in whom it is unlikely that a circulating level of neutrophils approximating 500/mm³ will ever be reached. In these patients, we continue treatment until they are clinically stable and afebrile and discontinue antibiotics under close observation.

One of the most dramatic findings in an immunocompromised patient is the rapid development of new pulmonary infiltrates accompanied by hypoxia and hemoptysis. This may be the first evidence of a fungal or parasitic superinfection because of the difficulty of making the diagnosis of systemic or pulmonary disease based on cultures of blood or expectorated sputum. Of those patients who have received more than a week of broad-spectrum antibiotic therapy directed against gram-negative pathogens such as *Pseudomonas aeruginosa* and *Klebsiella pneumoniae* and then develop pulmonary infiltrates, the etiology—if proven to be infectious—will be fungal in perhaps 90% of instances. The remainder of infectious etiologies include *Pneumocystis,* tuberculosis,

and toxoplasmosis, but fungal superinfection is by far the most likely infectious possibility.

Clearly, we are in favor at this point of obtaining a histologic diagnosis of intrapulmonary pathology but would favor use of empirical amphotericin B if the chest radiograph shows consolidation mimicking a pulmonary infarct, a cavity, or lobar consolidation.[127] If pneumonitis is more diffuse, *P. carinii* infection is a major possibility, but we cannot exclude many other etiologies including fungal infection. In the diffuse pneumonias occurring in neutropenic patients in whom no invasive diagnostic procedure can be undertaken, we feel fungal infection is more likely than pneumocystosis. Thus, we would also use amphotericin B empirically in this setting.

In view of the mounting evidence for fungal superinfections following a prolonged course of antibacterial treatment, several realistic guidelines have evolved that form the basis for a rational approach to empirical therapy if histopathologic evidence or blood culture confirmation is not available. Such evidence would be as follows:

1. The development of new pulmonary infiltrates while the patient is receiving an aminoglycoside and a β-lactam agent.
2. Refractory oropharyngeal *Candida* lesions with symptoms of esophagitis.
3. Onset of candiduria with hyphal forms detected in the urine in the absence of a Foley catheter or an anatomical urinary tract abnormality.
4. Evidence of peripheral embolic phenomena such as large arterial or vein occlusion in the extremities and occasionally the central nervous system. In the young person who develops sudden cerebral infarction unaccompanied by CNS hemorrhage, a supratentorial fungal process should be strongly suspected. Additionally, the arterial vasculature should not be the only site suspected of involvement by disseminated opportunistic fungal organisms. Some fungi, like *Mucor* species and *Aspergillus,* can invade the vena cava and cause thrombosis of the hepatic vein and a resultant Budd–Chiari syndrome or cause thrombosis of the renal veins with development of nephrotic syndrome.[128]

If a persistently neutropenic patient remains febrile on broad-spectrum antibacterial agents after a period of 7 days but has no objective findings as suggested above (points 1–4), empirical amphotericin B should still be strongly considered if bone marrow examination shows a hypoplastic marrow or a marrow filled with malignant cells. In this circumstance, marrow recovery will take a week and usually longer. The dose should be escalated to a goal of 0.7 mg/kg per day and duration of empirical amphotericin B keyed to the clinical response. If no fungal pathogen is subsequently documented but the patient defervesces, treatment should be given for at least a week after temperature normalizes.

For recommended doses of antifungal agents and techniques for administration, see Chapter 8.

References

1. Hoeprich PD, Boggs DR: Manifestations of infectious diseases. In Hoeprich PD (ed): *Infectious Diseases*. ed. 3. Harper & Row, Philadelphia, 1983, pp. 85–107.
2. Weinstein L, Fields BN: Fever of obscure origin. In Weinstein L, Fields BN (eds): *Seminars in Infectious Diseases*. Vol. 1. Stratton Intercontinental, New York, 1978, pp. 1–33.
3. Murray HW: *FUO—Fever of Undetermined Origin*. Futura, Mt. Kisco, New York, 1983.
4. Petersdorf RG, Beeson PB: Fever of unexplained origin: Report on 100 cases. *Medicine (Baltimore)* **40**:1–30, 1961.
5. Baker RR, Tumulty PA, Shelly WM: The value of exploratory laparatomy in fever of undetermined etiology. *Johns Hopkins Med J* **125**:159–170, 1969.
6. Young LS, Martin WJ, Meyer RD, et al: Gram negative rod bacteremia: Microbiologic, immunologic and therapeutic considerations. *Ann Intern Med* **86**:456–471, 1977.
7. Beeson PB: Temperature elevating effect of a substance obtained from polymorphonuclear leukocytes *J. Clin Invest* **27**:527–534, 1948.
8. Dinarello CA, Wolff SM: Molecular basis of fever in humans. *Am J Med* **72**:799–819, 1982.
9. Baracos V, Rodemann HP, Dinarello CA, Goldberg AL: Stimulation of muscle protein degradation and prostaglandin E_2 release by leukocytic pyrogen (Interleukin-1). *N Engl J Med* **308**:553–558, 1983.
10. Beisel WR: Mediators of fever and muscle proteolysis. *N Engl J Med* **308**:585–587, 1983.
11. Snell ES: An examination of the blood of febrile subjects for pyrogenic properties. *Clin Sci* **21**:115–124, 1961.
12. Atkins E, Feldman JD, Francis L, et al: Studies on the mechanism of fever accompanying delayed hypersensitivity: The role of the sensitized lymphocyte. *J Exp Med* **135**:1113–1132, 1972.
13. Bodel P: Tumors and fever. *Ann NY Acad Sci* **230**:6–13, 1974.
14. Young LS, Armstrong D: Pseudomonas aeruginosa infections. *CRC Crit Rev Clin Lab Sci* **3**:291–347, 1972.
15. Dorff BJ, Geimer NF, Rosenthal DR, et al: Pseudomonas septicemia. *Arch Intern Med* **128**:591–595, 1971.
16. Ketover BP, Young LS, Armstrong D: Septicemia due to *Aeromonas hydrophila:* Clinical and immunologic aspects. *J Infect Dis* **127**:284–290, 1973
17. Blake PA, Merson MH, Weaver RE, et al: Disease caused by a marine vibrio. *N Engl J Med* **300**:1–5, 1979.
18. Schmidt U, Chmel H, Cobbs C: *Vibrio alginolyticus* infections in humans. *J Clin Microbiol* **10**:666–668, 1979.
19. Tacket CO, Brenner F, Blake PA: Clinical features and an epidemiologic study of vibrio vulnificus infection. *J Infect Dis* **149**:558–561, 1984.
20. Edwards JE, Lehrer RI, Stiehm ER, et al: Severe candidal infections. *Ann Intern Med* **89**:91–106 1978.
21. Gander JP: Cryptococcal cellulitis. *JAMA* **237**:672–673, 1977.
22. Meyer RD, Kaplan MH, Ong M, et al: Cutaneous lesions in disseminated mucormycosis. *JAMA* **225**:737–738, 1973.
23. Young LS: Aspergillosis. In Warren KS, Mahmoud AAF (eds): *Tropical Geographic Medicine*. McGraw-Hill, New York, 1984, pp. 890–897.
24. Gartenberg G, Bottone EJ, Keusch GT, et al: Hospital acquired mucormycosis (*Rhizopus rhizopodiformis*) of skin and subcutaneous tissue: Epidemiology, mycology, and treatment. *N Engl J Med* **299**:1115–1118, 1978.
25. Lorber B, Swenson RM: Bacteriology of aspiration pneumonia: A prospective study of community- and hospital-acquired cases. *Ann Intern Med* **81**:329–331, 1974.
26. Pennington JE: Infection in the compromised host: Recent advances and future directions. In Weinstein L, Fields BN (eds): *Seminars in Infectious Diseases*. Vol. 1. Stratton Intercontinental, New York, 1978, pp. 142–168.
27. Chang H-Y, Rodriguez V, Narboni G, et al: Causes of death in adults with acute leukemia. *Medicine (Baltimore)* **55**:259–268, 1976.
28. Valdivieso M, Gil-Extremera B, Zornoza J, et al: Gram-negative bacillary pneumonia in the compromised host. *Medicine (Baltimore)* **56**:241–254, 1977.
29. Louria DB, Hensle T, Armstrong D, et al. Listeriosis complicating malignant disease. *Ann Intern Med* **67**:261–281, 1967.
30. Krick JA, Remington JS: Opportunistic invasive fungal infections in patients with leukemia and lymphoma *Clin Haematol* **5**:249–309, 1976.
31. Meyer RD, Rosen P, Armstrong D: Phycomycosis complicating leukemia and lymphoma. *Ann Intern Med* **77**:871–879, 1972.
32. Meyers BR, Wormser G, Hirschman SZ, et al: Rhinocerebral mucormyosis. *Arch Intern Med* **139**:557–560, 1979.
33. Holmberg K, Berdischewsky M, Young LS. Serodiagnosis of aspergillosis. *J Infect Dis* **141**:656–664, 1980.
34. Armstrong D, Blevins A, Louria DB, et al: Groups B, C, and G streptococcal infections in a cancer hospital. *Ann NY Acad Sci* **174**:511–522, 1970.

35. Kauffman CA, Israel KS, Smith JW, et al: Histoplasmosis in immunosuppressed patients. *Am J Med* **64**:923–932, 1978.

36. Strimlan CV, Dines DE, Payne WS: Mediastinal granuloma. *Mayo Clin Proc* **50**:702–705, 1975.

37. Goodwin RA, Nickell JA, DesPrez RM: Mediastinal fibrosis complicating healed primary histoplasmosis and tuberculosis. *Medicine (Baltimore)* **51**:227–246, 1972.

38. Cross AS, Steigbigel RT: *Pneumocystis carinii* pneumonia presenting as localized nodular desities. *N Engl J Med* **291**:831–832, 1974.

39. Wade JC, Schimpff SC, Newman KA, Wiernik PA: *Staphylococcus epidermidis:* An increasing cause of infection in patients with granulocytopenia. *Ann Intern Med* **97**:503–508, 1982.

40. Winston DJ, Dudnik DV, Chapin M, et al: Coagulase negative staphyloccal bactermia in patients receiving immunosuppressive therapy. *Arch Intern Med* **143**:32–36, 1983.

41. Ihde DC, Armstrong D: Clinical spectrum of infection due to *Bacillus* species. *Ann J Med* **55**:839–845, 1973.

42. Wingard JR, Merz WG, Saral R: *Candida tropicalis.* A major pathogen in immunocompromised patients. *Ann Intern Med* **91**:539–543, 1979.

43. Kressel B, Szewczyk C, Tuazon C: Early clinical recognition of disseminated candidiasis by muscle and skin biopsy. *Arch Intern Med* **138**:429–433, 1978.

44. Berg R, Chmel H, Mayo J, et al: *Corynebacterium equi* infection complicating neoplastic disease. *Am J Clin Pathol* **68**:73–77, 1977.

45. Stamm WE, Tompkins LS, Wagner KF, et al: Infection due to *Corynebacterium* species in marrow transplant patients. *Ann Intern Med* **91**:167–173, 1979.

46. Brooks GF, O'Donoghue J, Morgan R, et al: *Eikenella corrodens,* a recently recognized pathogen: Infections in medical–surgical patients and in association with methylphenidate abuse. *Medicine* **53**:325–342, 1974.

47. Nixon DW, Aisenberg AC: Fatal *Hemophilus influenzae* sepsis in an asymptomatic splenectomized Hodgkin's disease patient. *Ann Intern Med* **77**:69–73, 1972.

48. Winston DJ, Jordan MC, Rhodes J: *Alleschena (Petriellidium boydii)* infections in the immunosuppressed host. *Am J Med* **63**:830–835, 1977.

49. Bottone EJ, Douglas SD, Rausen AR, et al: Association of *Pseudomonas cepacia* with chronic granulomatous disease, *J Clin Microbiol* **1**:425–428, 1975.

50. Aisner J, Schimpff SC, Sutherland JC, et al: *Torulopsis glabrata* infections in patients with cancer. *Am J Med* **61**:23–28, 1976.

51. Haupt HM, Merz WG, Beschorner WE, et al: Colonization and infection with trichosporon species in the immunosuppressed host. *J Infect Dis* **147**:199–203, 1983.

52. Sickles EA, Greene WH, Wiernik PH: Clinical presentation of infection in granulocytopenic patients. *Arch Intern Med* **135**:715–719, 1975.

53. Musher DM, Fainstein V, Young EJ, et al: Fever patterns—their lack of clinical significance. *Arch Intern Med* **139**:1225–1228, 1979.

54. Washington JA II: Role of the microbiology laboratory in the diagnosis and antimicrobial treatment of infective endocarditis. *Mayo Clin Proc* **57**:22–32, 1982.

55. Henry NK, McLimans CA, Wright AJ, et al: Microbiological and clinical evaluation of an isolator-lysis centrifugation blood culture tube. *J Clin Microbiol* **17**:864–869, 1983.

56. Kiehn TE: Quantitative blood cultures: A review of 52 years. In Brown AE, Armstrong E (eds): *Infectious Complications of Neoplastic Disease* Yorke, New York, 1985, pp. 87–103.

57. Washington JA II: Blood cultures—principles and techniques. *Mayo Clin Proc* **59**:91–98, 1975.

58. Young LS, Armstrong D, Blevins A, et al: *Nocardia asteroides* infection complicating neoplastic disease. *Am J Med* **50**:356–367, 1971.

59. Dismukes WE, Royal SA, Tynes BS: Disseminated histoplasmosis in corticosteroid-treated patients. *JAMA* **240**:1495–1498, 1978.

60. Matula G, Paterson PY: Reduction of nitroblue tetrazolium by neutrophils of adults with infection. *N Engl J Med* **285**:311–314, 1971.

61. Levin J, Poore TE, Zauber NP, et al: Detection of endotoxin in the blood of patients with sepsis due to gram-negative bacteria. *N Engl J Med* **283**:1313–1316, 1970.

62. Steigbigel RT, Johnson PK, Remington JS: The nitroblue tetrazolium reduction test versus conventional hematology in the diagnosis of bacterial infections. *N Engl J Med* **290**:235–243, 1974.

63. Elin R, Robinson RA, Levine AS, et al: Lack of clinical usefulness of the limulus test in the diagnosis of endotoxemia. *N Engl J led* **293**:521–524, 1975.

64. Young LS: Opsonizing antibodies, host factors, and the limulus assay for endotoxin. *Infect Immunol* **12**:88–92, 1975.

65. Nachum R, Lipsey A, Siegel SE: Rapid detection of gram-negative bacterial meningitis by the limulus lysate test. *N Engl J Med* **289**:931–933, 1973.

66. Murray HW, Ellis GC, Blumenthal DS, et al: Fever and pulmonary thromboembolism. *Am J Med* **67**:232–235, 1979.

67. Ramsey PG, Rubin RH, Tolkoff-Rubin NE, et al: The renal transplant patient with fever and pulmonary infiltrates: Etiology, clinical manifestations, and management. *Medicine (Baltimore)* **59**:206–222, 1980.

68. Ropes MW: Natural course of disseminated lupus erythematosus. *Medicine (Baltimore)* **43**:387–391, 1964.

69. Harvey AM, Shulman LE, Tumulty PA, et al: Systemic lupus erythematosus: Review of the literature and clinical analysis of 138 cases. *Medicine (Baltimore)* **33**:291–437, 1954.

70. Bodey GP, Buckley M, Sathe YS, et al: Quantitative relationships between circulating leukocytes and infection in patients with acute leukemia. *Ann Intern Med* **64**:328–340, 1966.

71. McCabe WR, Jackson GG: Gram-negative bacteremia. II. Clinical, laboratory, and therapeutic observations. *Arch Intern Med* **110**:856–864, 1962.

72. Freid MA, Vosti KL. Importance of underlying disease in patients with gram-negative bacteremia. *Arch Intern Med* **121**:418–423, 1968.

73. Bryant RE, Hood AF, Hood CE, et al: Factors affecting

mortality of gram-negative rod bacteremia. *Arch Intern Med* **127:**120–128, 1971.

74. Young LS: Gram-negative sepsis. In Mandell G, Doublas JG, Bennett JV et al (eds): *Hospital Infections* Little, Brown, Boston, 1979, pp. 489–506.

75. Young LS: Combination or single drug therapy for gram-negative sepsis. In Remington JS, Swarts MN (eds): *Current Clinical Topics in Infectious Diseases,* Vol. 3. McGraw-Hill, New York, 1982, pp. 177–205.

76. Love LJ, Schimpff SC, Schiffer CA, et al: Improved prognosis for granulocytopenic patients with gram-negative rod bacteremia. *Am J Med* **68:**643–648, 1980.

77. Winston DJ, Sidell J, Hairston J, et al: Antimicrobial therapy of *Klebsiella pneumoniae* septicemia in neutropenic rats. *J Infect Dis* **139:**377–388, 1979.

78. Lumish RM, Norden CW: Therapy of neutropenic rats infected with *Pseudomonas aeruginosa. J Infect Dis* **133:**538–547, 1976.

79. Klastersky J, Hensgens C, Meunier-Carpentier F: Comparative effectiveness of combinations of amikacin with penicillin G and amikacin with carbenicillin in gram-negative septicemia: Double-blind clinical trial. *J Infect Dis (Suppl.)* **134:**S433–S440, 1976.

80. Klastersky J, Meunier-Carpentier F, Prevost J-M: Significance of antimicrobial synergism for the outcome of gram-negative sepsis. *Am J Med Sci* **273:**157–167, 1977.

81. Anderson ET, Young LS, Hewitt WL: Antimicrobial synergism in the therapy of gram-negative bacteremia. *Chemotherapy* **24:**45–54, 1978.

82. Lau WK, Young LS, Black RE, et al: Comparative efficacy and toxicity of amikacin/carbenicillin versus gentamicin/carbenicillin in leukopenic patients. *Am J Med* **62:**212–219, 1977.

83. Young LS: Amikacin: Experience in a comparative clinical trial with gentamicin in leukopenic subjects. In Luthy R, Siegenthaler W (eds): *Current Chemotherapy.* American Society for Microbiology, Washington, D.C., 1978, pp. 246–248.

84. Wade, JC, Schimpff SC, Newman KA, et al: Piperacillin or ticarcillin plus amikacin. *Am J Med* **71:**983–990, 1981.

85. Winston DJ, Ho WG, Young LS, et al: Piperacillin plus amikacin therapy in febrile neutropenic patients. *Arch Intern Med* **142:**1663–1667, 1982.

86. DeJongh CA, Wade JC, Schimpff SC, et al: Empiric antibiotic therapy for suspected infection in granulocytopenic cancer patients. A comparison between the combination of moxalactam plus amikacin and ticarcillin plus amikacin. *Am J Med* **73:**89–96, 1982.

87. Fainstein V, Bodey GP, Elting L, et al: A randomized study of ceftazidime compared to ceftazidime and tobramycin for the treatment of infections in the cancer patient. *J Antimicrob Chemother* (Suppl. A) **12:**101–110, 1983.

88. Klastersky J, Glauser MP, Schimpff SC, et al: Prospective randomized comparison of three antibiotic regimens for empirical therapy of suspected bacteremic infection in febrile granulocytopenic patients. *Antimicrob Ag Chemother* **29:**263–270, 1986.

89. EORTC Antimicrobial Therapy Project Group: Combination of amikacin and carbenicillin with or without cefazolin as empirical treatment of febrile neutropenic patients. *J Clin Oncol* **1:**597–603, 1983.

90. Smith CR, Ambinder R, Lipsky JJ, et al: Cefotaxime compared with nafcillin plus tobramycin for serious bacterial infections: A randomized prospective trial. *Ann Intern Med* **101:**469–477, 1984.

91. VanLaethem Y, Lagast H, Klastersky J: Serum bactericidal activity of ceftazidime and cefoperazone alone and in combination with amikacin against *P. aeruginosa* and *K. pneumoniae. Antimicrob Ag Chemother* **23:**435–439, 1983.

92. Ramphal R, Kramer BS, Rand KH, et al: Early results in a comparative trial of ceftazidime versus cephalothin, carbenicillin, and gentamicin in the treatment of febrile granulocytopenic patients. *J Antimicrob Chemother* (Suppl A) **12:**81–88, 1983.

93. Young LS: Double beta-lactam therapy in the immunocompromised host. *J Antimicrob Chemother* **16:**4–6, 1985.

94. Bodey GP, Valdivieso M, Feld R, et al: Carbenicillin plus cephalothin or cefazolin as therapy for infections in neutropenic patients. *Am J Med Sci* **273:**309–318, 1977.

95. EORTC Antimicrobial Therapy Project Group. Three antibiotic regimens in the treatment of infection in febrile granulocytopenic patients with cancer. *J Infect Dis* **137:**14–29, 1978.

96. Winston DJ, Barnes RC, Ho WG, et al: Moxalactam plus piperacillin versus moxalactam plus amikacin in febrile granulocytopenic patients. *Am J Med* **77:**442–450, 1984.

97. Fainstein V, Bodey GP, Bolivar R, et al: Moxalactam plus ticarcillin or tobramycin for treatment of febrile episodes in neutropenic cancer patients. *Arch Intern Med* **144:**1766–1770, 1984.

98. Sanders CC, Sanders WE Jr: Microbial resistance to newer generation beta-lactam antibiotics: Clinical and laboratory implications. *J Infect Dis* **151:**399–406, 1985.

99. Smith CR, Baughman KL, Edwards CQ, et al: Controlled comparison of amikacin and gentamicin. *N Engl J Med* **296:**349–355, 1977.

100. Dahlgren JG, Anderson ET, Hewitt WL: Gentamicin blood levels: A guide to nephrotoxicity. *Antimicrob Agents Chemother* **8:**58–62, 1975.

101. Barza M, Brown RB, Shen D, et al: Predictability of blood levels of gentamicin in man. *J Infect Dis* **132:**165–174, 1975.

102. Kaye D, Levison ME, Labovitz ED: The unpredictability of serum concentrations of gentamicin. Pharmacokinetics of gentamicin in patients with normal and abnormal renal function. *J Infect Dis* **130:**150–154, 1974.

103. Anderson ET, Young LS, Hewitt WL: Simultaneous antibiotic levels in "breakthrough" gram negative rod bacteremia. *Am J Med* **61:**493–497, 1976.

104. Smith CR, Maxwell RR, Edwards CQ, et al: Nephrotoxicity induced by gentamicin and amikacin. *Johns Hopkins Med J* **142:**85–90, 1978.

105. Feld R, Valdivieso M, Bodey GP, et al: A comparative trial of sisomicin therapy of intermittent versus continuous infusion. *Am J Med Sci* **274:**179–184, 1977

106. Gerding DN, Larson TA: Aminoglycoside resistance in gram-negative bacilli during increased amikacin use. *Am J Med* (Suppl. 1a) **79:**1–7, 1985.

107. Young LS: The use of aminoglycosides in immunocompromised patients. *Am J Med* (Suppl. 1A) **79**:21–27, 1985.

108. Waitz JA, Drube CG, Moss EL, et al: Biological aspects of the interaction between gentamicin and carbenicillin. *J Antibiot* **25**:219–225, 1972

109. Young LS, Decker G, Hewitt WL: Inactivation of gentamicin by carbenicillin in the urinary tract. *Chemotherapy* **20**:212–220, 1974.

110. Murillo J, Standiford HC, Schimpff SC, et al: Gentamicin and ticarcillin serum levels. *JAMA* **241**:2401–2403, 1979

111. Holt HA, Broughall JM, McCarthy M, et al: Interactions between aminoglycoside antibiotics and carbenicillin or ticarcillin. *Infection* **4**:107–109, 1976.

112. Schimpff SC, Aisner J: Empiric antibiotic therapy. *Cancer Treatm Rep* **62**:673–680, 1978.

113. Crossley K, Loesch D, Landesman B, et al: An outbreak of infections caused by strains of *Staphylococcus aureus* resistant to methicillin and aminoglycosides. I. Clinical studies. *J Infect Dis* **139**:273–279, 1979.

114. Rosenblatt JE, Stewart PR: Combined activity of sulfamethoxazole, trimethoprim, and polymyxin B against gram-negative bacilli. *Antimicrob Agents Chemother* **6**:84–92, 1974.

115. Moore RD, Smith CR, Lietman PS: Association of aminoglycoside plasma levels with therapeutic outcome in gram-negative pneumonia. *Am J Med* **77**:657–662, 1984.

116. Schlichter JG, Maclean H: A method of determining the effective therapeutic level in the treatment of subacute bacterial endocarditis with penicillin. *Am Heart J* **34**:209–211, 1947.

117. Wolfson JS, Swartz MN: Serum bactericidal activity as a monitor of antibiotic therapy. *N Engl J Med* **312**:968–973, 1985.

118. Weinsten MP, Stratton CW, Ackley A, et al: Multicenter collaborative evaluation of a standardized serum bactericidal test as a prognostic indicator in infective endocarditis *Am J Med* **78**:262–269, 1985.

119. Sculier JP, Klastersky J: Significance of serum bactericidal activity in gram-negative bacillary bacteremia in patients with and without granulocytopenia *Am J Med* **76**:429–435, 1984.

120. Hickman RO, Buckner CP, Clift RA: Modified right atrial catheter for access to the venous system in marrow transplant recipients *Surg Gynecol Obstet* **148**:871–875, 1979.

121. Pizzo PA, Commers J, Cotton D, et al: Approaching the controversies in the antibacterial management of cancer patients *Am J Med* **76**:436–439, 1981.

122. Fang LST, Tolkoff-Rubin NE, Rubin RH: Efficacy of single dose and conventional amoxicillin therapy in urinary tract infection localized by the antibody coated bacteria technic *N Engl J Med* **298**:413–416, 1978.

123. Rodriguez V, Burgess M, Bodey GP: Management of fever of unknown origin in patients with neoplasms and neutropenia. *Cancer* **32**:1007–1012, 1973.

124. Pennington JE. Fever, neutropenia, and malignancy. A clinical syndrome in evolution. *Cancer* **39**:1345–1349, 1977.

125. Pizzo PA, Robichand KJ, Gill FA, et al: Duration of empiric antibiotic therapy. *Am J Med* **67**:194–205, 1979.

126. Burke PJ, Braine HG, Rathbun HK, et al: The clinical significance and management of fever in acute myelocytic leukemia. *Johns Hopkins Med J* **139**:1–12, 1976.

127. Pizzo PA, Robichand KJ, Gill FA, et al: Empiric antibiotic and antifungal therapy for cancer patients with prolonged fever and granulocytopenia. *Am J Med* **72**:101–106, 1982.

128. Meyer RD, Young LS, Armstrong D, et al. Aspergillosis complicating neoplastic disease. *Am J Med* **54**:6–15, 1973.

5

Dermatologic Manifestations of Infection in the Compromised Host

JOHN S. WOLFSON and ARTHUR J. SOBER

1. Introduction

Among the most formidable challenges to the clinician is the care of the patient with an impaired immune system—the compromised host.[1-4] Two characteristics in particular contribute to the complexity of management of infection in these patients: the exceptionally broad variety of potential microbial pathogens, and the wide spectrum of clinical manifestations of disease resulting from the abnormal immune response.[5-7]

In the compromised patient, cutaneous and subcutaneous tissues may be expected to be an important aspect of infection, for three reasons.[8-13] First, the skin together with the mucosal surfaces represents the first line of defense of the body against the external environment. These barriers assume an even greater importance when secondary defenses, such as phagocytosis, cell-mediated immunity, and antibody production, are impaired. Second, the rich blood supply of the skin provides a route of spread of infection both from the skin to other bodily locations and also to the skin from other infected sites[14] (Fig. 1). In the latter case, a skin lesion may serve as an early warning system to alert the patient and the clinician to the existence of a systemic infection.[14] Importantly, these lesions may be benign in appearance, presum-

ably because of the impaired host-immune response, and therefore be easily missed or dismissed as not significant. And third, skin infections are common, occurring in up to one-third of significantly compromised hosts.[9-17]

It is the purpose of this chapter to give an overview of infection of the cutaneous and subcutaneous tissues in compromised hosts. Topics of discussion are the skin as a barrier to infection, a four part classification of skin infection in compromised patients,[12,13] dermatologic lesions associated with the acquired immunodeficiency syndrome (AIDS), and diagnostic considerations. Three illustrative cases are presented.

2. Skin as a Barrier to Infection

The skin is usually quite resistant to infection. The mechanisms by which this resistance occurs are not well understood. Three important components contributing to microbial resistance are nonspecific: (1) intact keratinized layers of the skin, which prevent penetration of microorganisms; (2) dryness of the skin, which retards the growth of certain organisms such as the aerobic gram-negative bacilli and *Candida* sp., and (3) the suppressant effect of the normal skin flora, which appears to reduce colonization of pathogens, a phenomenon known as bacterial interference.[18] Within this framework, then, one might expect potentially serious skin infection to develop under the following three circumstances: (1) destruction by trauma or bypass by introduction of intravascular catheters of the previously intact ker-

JOHN S. WOLFSON • Infectious Disease Unit, Medical Services, Massachusetts General Hospital; and Department of Medicine, Harvard Medical School, Boston, Massachusetts 02114   ARTHUR J. SOBER • Dermatology Service, Massachusetts General Hospital; and Department of Dermatology, Harvard Medical School, Boston, Massachusetts 02114.

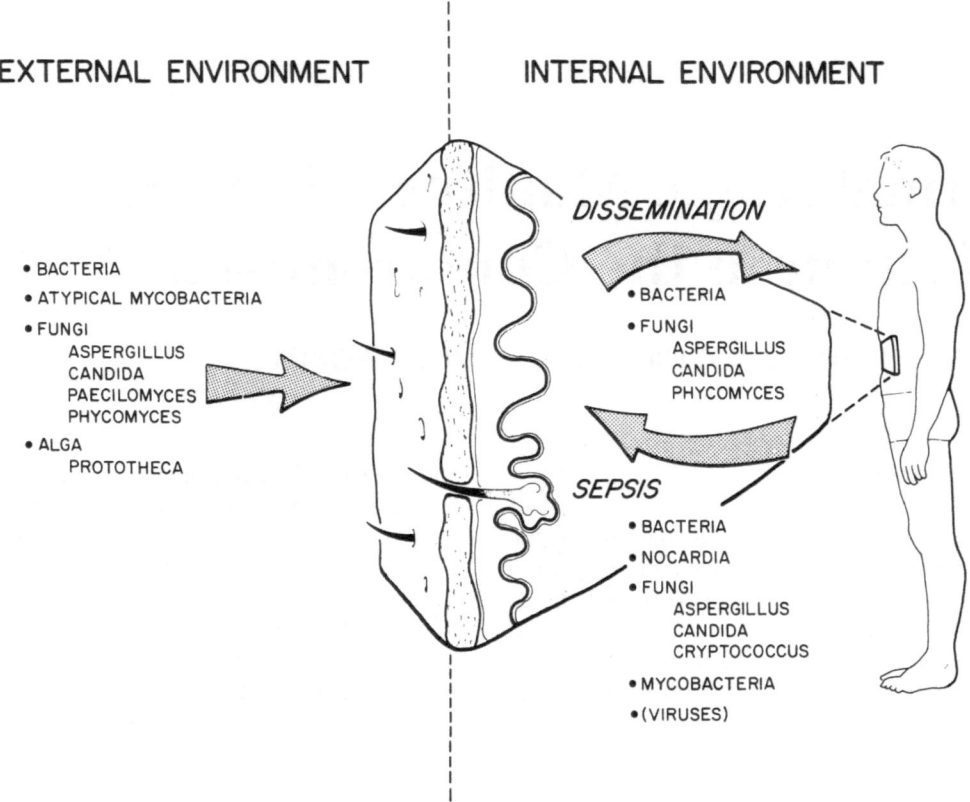

FIGURE 1. Schematic representation of the role of the skin in the occurrence of localized and disseminated infection in the compromised patient. (From Wolfson et al [12])

atinized layer of skin; (2) moistening of the skin, such as under occlusive dressings; and (3) alteration of the normal colonizing flora, such as after administration of antimicrobial agents. These types of events would represent risk to the normal patient but are considerably more threatening to the compromised patient with impaired immunologic defenses that are likely to be more readily overwhelmed when the primary cutaneous barrier breaks down.

An example of these phenomena is the development of invasive fungal infection in compromised patients whose skin has been traumatized by tape holding intravascular lines in place.[19-27] Infection with *Rhizopus* sp. has been associated with use of Elastoplast tape to secure intravascular catheters.[21-24] Skin infection with *Rhizopus* and *Aspergillus* sp. has occurred with the use of adhesive tape and boards to stabilize arms to protect intravenous lines. Because of the occurrence of these types of infections, the

following approach would seem warranted. Occlusive dressings in immunocompromised patients should be avoided when possible and skin covered by such dressings should be routinely inspected. Paper tape should be used in preference to cloth tape, and surgical dressings might be secured with girdles of elasticized netting rather than tape whenever possible.[11]

The effect of chronic administration of corticosteroids on the skin is another factor that may contribute to increased susceptibility to infection of compromised patients.[28] Steroid therapy appears to inhibit proliferation of fibroblasts, synthesis of mucopolysaccharides, and deposition of collagen. The net effect is thin and atrophic skin that heals poorly.[9,28] Minor trauma generates lesions that tend to persist, providing potential portals of entry for pathogens. An example of this phenomenon that has been observed is recurrent staphylococcal cellulitis about the elbow in patients receiving chronic immunosuppressive therapy after renal transplantation.[12,13] These patients exhibited two adverse effects of chronic corticosteroid administration: thinning of the skin leading to enhanced susceptibility of the tissue to trauma, and steroid-induced proximal myopathy. Because of the myopathy, the patients tended to rise from the sitting position by pushing off with their elbows and thus traumatizing them. Cellulitis about the elbows recurred in these patients until protection was provided to their elbows and the steroid dose was decreased.

3. Types of Skin Infection

Infection of the cutaneous and subcutaneous tissues in compromised patients can be classified in a variety of ways: by pathogen, by underlying immunologic defect, or by pace of illness. An additional categorization considers pathophysiologic events and consists of four groups[11-13]: (1) infection taking origin in skin and being typical of that which occurs in immunocompetent persons, albeit with the potential for more serious illness; (2) extensive cutaneous involvement with pathogens that normally produce trivial or well-localized disease in immunocompetent patients; (3) infection originating from a cutaneous source and caused by opportunistic pathogens that rarely cause disease in immunocompetent patients but that may cause either localized or widespread disease in compromised persons; and (4) cutaneous or subcutaneous infection which represents metastatic spread from a noncutaneous site. Cutaneous and subcutaneous infections in compromised patients will be discussed in Section 3.1 within the framework of these four groups.

3.1. Primary Skin Infection with Common Pathogens

There appears to be an increased incidence and severity of conventional forms of infections originating in the skin. Gram-positive organisms, such as group A streptococci and *Staphylococcus aureus*, commonly cause these infections. In addition, granulocytopenic patients are also susceptible to cellulitis caused by less usual bacterial pathogens, such as the *Enterobacteriaceae* and *Pseudomonas* sp., and by

anaerobic bacteria. Also, patients with leukemia or diseases altering cell-mediated immunity may have cellulitis caused by opportunistic pathogens such as *Cryptococcus neoformans* or *Candida* sp. identical in appearance to cellulitis caused by gram-positive bacteria. When evaluating routine-appearing cellulitis in a compromised patient, clinicians therefore need to include in their differential diagnoses the unusual as well as the usual etiologic agents. Importantly, if a patient does not respond to conventional antimicrobial therapy, an aggressive approach to diagnosis, with biopsy of lesions for Gram and other stains, cultures, and histopathologic evaluation is warranted to identify correctly the offending pathogen.

3.2. Unusually Widespread Cutaneous Infection

Viruses and a variety of nonvirulent skin fungi constitute the two major causes of infection in this category. These pathogens typically cause minor infections in immunocompetent persons but in compromised patients tend to generate more extensive disease that may lead to more serious systemic illness.

3.2.1. Viral Infections

Viral exanthems (e.g., those caused by rubella, rubeola, or enterovirus) may occur in compromised patients, but the more problematic pathogens include the papillomaviruses and the family of herpes viruses.

DNA papillomaviruses cause human warts. In immunocompetent persons, the virus tends to generate single verrucous lesions, but in the chronically immunosuppressed patient warts either may be extremely numerous or may form large confluent lesions.[9,10,29,30] Approximately 40% of renal transplant recipients develop warts following transplantation,[9,31] and up to 1% have extensive disease.[9,30] The incidence and severity of warts seem to be related to immunosuppression, with previously acquired latent virus reactivating with institution of immunosuppressive therapy.[9,31,32]

In compromised patients, warts represent a potential danger because malignant transformation, particularly in the sun-exposed areas of the body,[9,30,33] occurs not infrequently.[9,30] Recently in skin cancers of a renal transplant recipient human papillomavirus DNA has been detected.[34] Therefore, management of patients with extensive warts should include avoidance of sun exposure, use of strong sun blockers (SPF 15), reduction in immunosuppressive therapy when possible, and careful observation of the patient for the development of malignant lesions that require local destructive therapy.[9]

Illustrative Case 1: Papillomavirus Infection

A 35-year-old man with confluent warts on both feet had systemic lupus erythematosus (SLE) with renal involvement, for which he had been receiving corticosteroid therapy for 3 years, most recently prednisone 25 mg/day PO. On physical examination, warts were found to be confluent on both feet in pressure-bearing areas of his toes, balls, and heels (Fig. 2A). Treatment by multiple courses of therapy with podophyllin over several years had failed. Finally, when prednisone was tapered to 3 mg/day PO, the lesions on both feet completely resolved within 2 months (Fig. 2B).

Comment. This patient illustrates that extensive confluent warts may occur in an immunosuppressed patient and that the lesions may dramatically improve when the extent of immunosuppression is reduced.

Skin infections with members of the herpesvirus family, particularly herpes simplex virus (HSV) and varicella zoster virus (VZV), are very common in compromised patients.[9,35,36] Thorough reviews of infections with these two viruses in compromised patients have been written[34,36] (see Chapter 13, for a detailed discussion). Within the context of cutaneous infection, however, some aspects are worthy of emphasis.

Nasolabial or anogenital infections due to HSV occur in as many as one-half of renal transplant patients, patients with malignancy, patients receiving chemotherapy, and persons with the acquired immunodeficiency syndrome (AIDS).[9,35–38] In addition, compromised patients may have more serious forms of HSV infection[36]:

1. *Herpes phagenda:* This large ulcerated lesion, which persists for periods of months, may occur in patients immunosuppressed because of renal transplantation, hematologic malignancy, or AIDS. The cutaneous lesion may cause severe pain or bladder or rectal dysfunction and may also be the site of bacterial superinfection. It is noteworthy that the lesion is often without vesicles and that Tsanck preparations are usually negative; thus, viral cultures are needed for diagnosis.

2. *Dissemination:* Although uncommon, spread of HSV infection from the skin to other sites may occur in patients with hematologic malignancy (especially lymphoma) or bone marrow transplant recipients and in neonates. Dissemination rarely also occurs in renal, cardiac, or liver transplant recipients.

3. *Esophageal or respiratory tract infection:* HSV infection at these sites may develop in patients with orolabial infection. Particularly prone to esophageal or respiratory tract infection are those patients with orolabial infection and mucosa traumatized by a nasogastric tube or an endotracheal tube.

Management of such HSV infections includes treatment with acyclovir[39–45] and reduction of immunosuppressive therapy when possible. This latter maneuver remains important despite the availability of acyclovir therapy because there is a high recurrence rate when acyclovir is discontinued unless the level of immunosuppression has been reduced.

In compromised patients, reactivation of VZV is not uncommon, occurring in about 14% of Hodgkin disease patients, 8% of non-Hodgkin lymphoma and renal transplant patients, and 2% of patients with solid tumors.[36] Visceral dissemination occurs in 15–30% of Hodgkin disease patients with zoster, but such spread is uncommon in renal transplant recipients.[35,36] VZV infection is particularly problematic for bone marrow transplant recipients, of whom one-half will develop VZV infection. In one-third of these infections, viral infection will disseminate and in one-fourth a generalized atypical recurrent chickenpox illness will develop.[46,47] For the treatment of disseminated infection, such agents as systemic acyclovir, interferon, and adenine arabinoside appear promising.[36,45] For the treatment of localized infection, acyclovir has proved efficacious in halting progression of disease.[48]

3.2.2. Nonvirulent Fungi

This group of organisms includes the dermatophytes (*Epidermophyton, Microsporum* sp.,

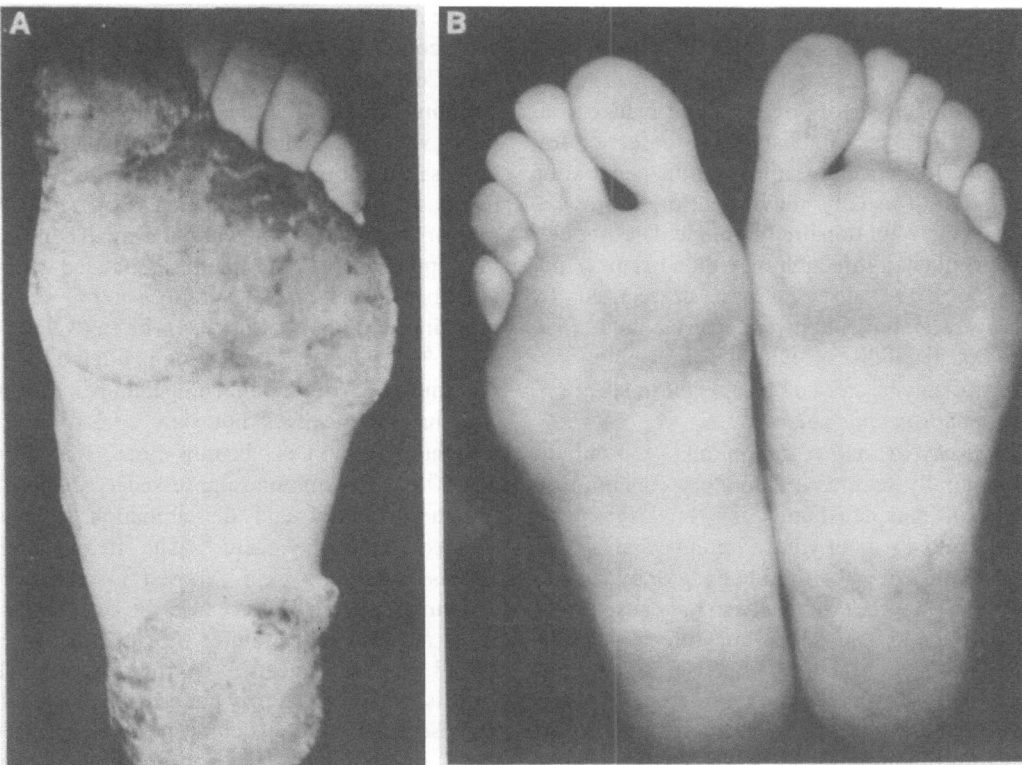

FIGURE 2. Papillomavirus infection in a man with systemic lupus erythematosus (SLE) receiving corticosteroid therapy. Confluent warts on the plantar surfaces of the feet (A) cleared 1 month after reduction of the dose of corticosteroid therapy (B). (From Wolfson et al.[13])

and *Trichophyton* sp.), *Candida* sp., *Pityrosporium* sp., *Fusarium solani*, and *Alternaria alternata*. Like the papillomavirus, HSV, and VZV, these microbes may cause unusually widespread cutaneous infection in compromised patients. These fungal species are ubiquitous in the environment and intermittently colonize and may establish localized, superficial skin infection in immunocompetent persons, particularly when skin has been traumatized. For compromised patients, there appears to be both an increased incidence[8,49,50] and an increased severity of infection.[49] Local infection, particularly on the extremities, may be extensive, being both disfiguring and also providing a site of entry for bacterial superinfection. Nail involvement may be extensive and life long. Studies of grossly normal skin of renal transplant recipients and patients with malignancy have demonstrated an increased frequency of colonization with these fungi (in comparison with immunocompetent persons) and colonization of bodily sites normally free of these organisms, such as the back, chest, and abdomen.[49] Small breaks in the skin presumably permit these colonizers to invade deeper, and suppressed cell-mediated immunity impairs eradication of the infection.

Treatment of these infections in compromised patients with topical therapy or with griseofulvin usually fails. In anecdotal experiences, treatment with systemic ketoconazole resulted in marked clearing of infections of the skin and nails in renal transplant recipients. Within a few months of cessation of therapy, however, infection recurred, a response similar to that seen in treatment of candidal infection with ketoconazole in another disease related to an immune defect, chronic mucocutaneous candidiasis.[51] If in the future ketoconazole is approved for the therapy of compromised patients with extensive infection with these nonvirulent fungi, the clinician will need to weigh the problems of the infection against the risk of drug toxicity in deciding whether to recommend treatment with chronic or intermittent ketoconazole.[52]

3.3. Opportunistic Primary Cutaneous Infection

The pathogenesis of disease in this category almost always involves establishment of infection following some form of injury that permits penetration or inoculation of usually nonvirulent organisms beneath the skin. With impaired immune defenses, local or disseminated infection may then occur. Troublesome localized disease may be caused by *Paecilomyces*, atypical mycobacteria, and *Prototheca*. Localized disease with life-threatening systemic spread may be caused by *Aspergillus* sp., *Candida* sp., and *Rhizopus* sp.

Paecilomyces is a ubiquitous saprophytic fungus generally seen as a laboratory contaminant. The organism may cause infection, however, when introduced into a patient whose immune status is altered by the presence of a foreign body or by chemotherapy. For instance, *Paecilomyces* has caused prosthetic valve endocarditis[53–56] or infection of an implanted intraocular lens.[57,58] Also, three renal transplant recipients have been reported in whom an ulcerating cellulitis following lacerating trauma to their anterial tibial region.[13,59] For renal transplant recipients, therapy included local excision with or without skin grafting and treatment of bacterial superinfection. Systemic miconazole therapy may also be of value.[59]

Both typical and atypical mycobacteria may cause infection of the cutaneous and subcutaneous tissues in compromised patients.[60–67] Beyt and associates[63] categorized cutaneous mycobacterial infection as resulting from (1) inoculation from an exogenous source, (2) hematogenous spread, and (3) nonhematogenous spread from an endogenous source. In the last circumstance, contiguous spread usually occurred from a site of osteomyelitis. *Mycobacterium tuberculosis* was the offending species for most cases resulting from contiguous or hematogenous spread. By contrast, atypical mycobacteria, such as *Mycobacterium marinum*, *Mycobacterium chelonei*, *Mycobacterium kansasii*, and *Mycobacterium haemophilium*,[68] were responsible for cases resulting from direct inoculation from an exogenous source, particularly among immunosuppressed patients. Wallace and associates[67] described 125 patients with infection caused by *M. fortuitum*, *M. chelonei*, and other rapidly growing mycobacteria.

Of the nine patients with disseminated disease, eight were compromised and had skin lesions.

Cutaneous and subcutaneous lesions associated with mycobacterial infection in compromised patients vary and include panniculitis, cellulitis, and abscess formation. A common lesion is a papule or nodule that may ulcerate.[63] For *M. marinum*, a papule or a nodule with or without a small central ulcer may appear weeks after trauma associated with water immersion (such as exposure to water of aquariums or swimming pools or at fresh- or saltwater beaches).[13,63,69] The site of infection is often over a bony prominence.[63] In immunocompetent persons, the lesion usually resolves but may spread in a sporotrichoid fashion or, in rare cases, may disseminate.[63,69] In immunosuppressed patients, sporotrichoid spread and dissemination to multiple cutaneous sites may occur.[63] The site of dissemination is usually to skin exposed to ambient temperatures, presumably because the organisms grow better at lower temperatures (30°–32°C), but rarely spread may be to deeper, warmer viscera.[69] Diagnosis is by biopsy but may not be established initially because of difficulty in demonstrating acid-fast organisms in tissue and because granuloma formation may be retarded in the setting of immunosuppression. In addition, with ulceration, superinfection may occur, further altering the histologic pattern. Therefore, repeated biopsies and culturing of tissue at 30°C may be needed for diagnosis. Therapy with multiple drug regimens, including rifampin, ethambutol, minocycline, and trimethoprim is usually effective, even for disseminated disease.[67] If diagnosis and therapy are delayed, superinfection may extend to bone and joints, leading to a need for surgery (such as amputation of a finger) to effect cure.[13]

Prototheca species are unicellular, achlorophyllic algalike organisms that are ubiquitous in nature and that may rarely cause disease in humans.[13,70–81] *P. wickerhamii* is the usual offending species, but infections with *P. zopfi* occasionally occur.[70] Infection appears to develop after inoculation of the organism under the skin during trauma or surgery. The lesion that results is usually a localized papule or nodule which may ulcerate and intermittently drain. Wound infection with local spread to lymph nodes and an olecranon bursa have also been reported. Prototheca has been described in five compromised patients, including three renal transplant recipients,[13,75,76] one patient receiving chemotherapy for carcinoma of the breast,[81] and one patient with a defect in phagocytic function.[77,78] Diagnosis was by biopsy. Treatment included therapy with amphotericin B with local debridement, including amputation of fingers in one renal transplant recipient.[13]

In marked contrast to infections with *Paecilomyces* sp., atypical mycobacteria, and *Prototheca* sp., primary cutaneous infections caused by the opportunistic organisms of *Aspergillus*,[19,20,26,27,82] *Rhizopus*[21,24,83–85] or *Candida* sp.[13] are more dangerous to the compromised patient because of the potential for disseminated disease. Cutaneous primary infection with these fungi has been associated with the use of adhesive tape, Elastoplast tape, or extravasation of intravenous fluids. The histopathology of tissue involvement for *Aspergillus* and *Rhizopus* sp. includes invasion of blood vessels,[86,87] which may lead to gangrene, hemorrhage, and dissemination. Because of hematogenous spread, therapy with the systemic antifungal agent amphotericin B is indicated. Blood supply to infected tissue is impaired, however, so amphotericin B alone may be inadequate, and excision of infected tissues may be required.[85]

Illustrative Case 2: Aspergillosis

The patient was a 4-year-old boy with fever and an erythematous chest lesion in the setting of acute myelogenous leukemia and neutropenia. The diagnosis of leukemia had been made 3 weeks earlier, at which time therapy with daunarubicin, cytosine arabinoside, vincristine, and prednisone had been initiated with favorable response. The patient became neutropenic and then developed fever, for which nafcillin, ticarcillin, and tobramycin were administered. The fever persisted, and a source was not identified. An episode of upper gastrointestinal (GI) bleeding necessitated transfer to an intensive care unit (ICU), where cardiac rhythm was continuously monitored. His bleeding resolved; several days later, an area of skin on his right anterior chest appeared abraded where a cardiac electrode lead had been attached. Two days later, the minor skin lesion persisted but was considered by some observers not to be infected. Fever persisted, with the patient neutropenic, despite continuing therapy with broad-spectrum antibacterial agents.

Physical examination showed the patient to be a pale, quiet child in no acute distress. Temperature was 101°F (axillary), and respirations were 24 per min and unlabored. An ophthalmologic examination revealed no signs of fungal infection. The lungs were clear to percussion and auscultation. The right anterior chest lesion was 5 mm in diameter, erythematous, slightly raised, and non-tender. Minimal diffuse lymphadenopathy was present. The white blood count (WBC) was 200 per mm^3. Chest radiographs showed no infiltrates.

A punch biopsy of the chest lesion was taken. Stains and a potassium hydroxide (KOH) fungal wet preparation showed no pathogens. Intravenous amphotericin B therapy was initiated because of the possibility of fungal infection of the chest wall or elsewhere.

One day later, histopathologic studies of the skin biopsy material revealed branching, septate fungal forms consistent with aspergillosis (Fig. 3). Cultures subsequently grew *Aspergillus fumigatus.* Blood cultures remained negative. The chest lesion was excised. The patient defervesced 4 days after institution of amphotericin B therapy, except during periods of infusion of the drug. One week later, his neutropenia resolved, and systemic antibacterial agents were discontinued. The patient received a total of 500 mg amphotericin B IV over a 50-day period. One year later, he was in remission on maintenance chemotherapy for leukemia, without recurrence of *Aspergillus* infection.

Comment. This patient's infection with *Aspergillus* illustrates several of the previously discussed points. The setting of invasive infection with this opportunistic organism was that of a neutropenic patient with acute leukemia. The patient presumably had markedly altered skin flora because of his residence in a hospital and therapy with antibacterial agents. His skin was traumatized with a cardiac electrode lead. After removal of the lead, a persisting abraded lesion appeared so benign that some observers doubted infection. The benignity of the lesion likely reflected the inability of a patient with impaired host defenses to respond to the pathogen. Biopsy was necessary to establish the diagnosis. Therapy was successful and included local excision of the lesion and administration of systemic amphotericin B for presumed undetected fungal infection metastatic from the skin.

3.4. Systemic Infection Metastatic to Cutaneous and Subcutaneous Sites

In a recent retrospective study of dermatologic manifestations of infection in compromised patients, eight of 31 patients (26%) had apparent spread of systemic infection to cutaneous and subcutaneous tissues.[13] Importantly, in six of these eight patients, cutaneous or subcutaneous lesions were the first clinical sign of disseminated infection.

In compromised patients, cutaneous lesions resulting from hematogenous spread of infection are caused in general by three classes of pathogens: (1) *Pseudomonas aeruginosa* and other bacteria; (2) the endemic systemic mycoses *Histoplasma capsulatum, Coccidioides immitis,* and *Blastomyces dermatitidis;* and (3) the opportunistic organisms *Aspergillus* sp., *Cryptococcus neoformans, Candida* sp., *Rhizopus* sp., and *Nocardia* sp.

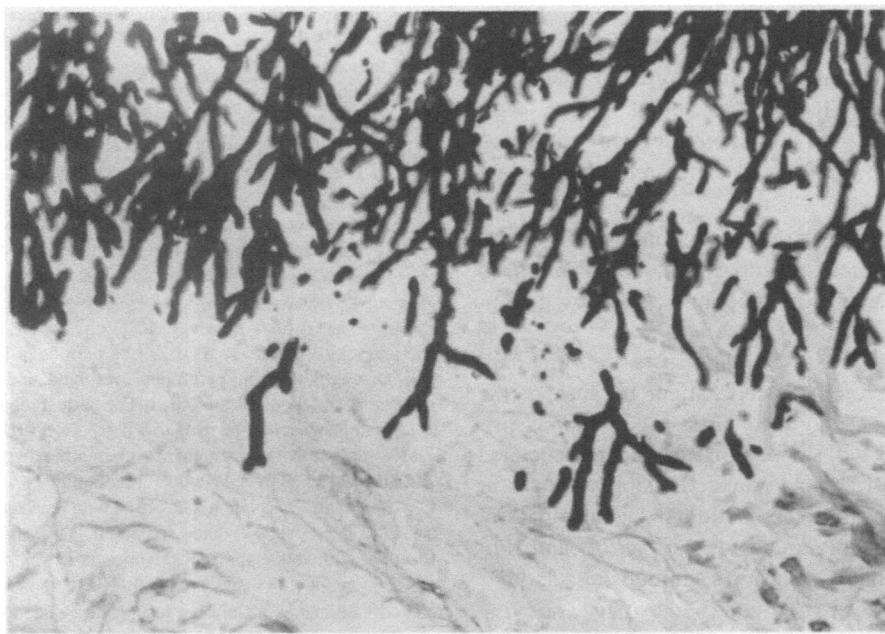

FIGURE 3. Histologic section of a skin biopsy showing *Aspergillus* (dark branching forms) in a patient with acute myelogenous leukemia and neutropenia. The tissue was stained with methenamine-silver. (×500)

3.4.1. Infection with *Pseudomonas aeruginosa*

In the setting of compromised patients undergoing chemotherapy for acute leukemia, the causes of bacterial infection metastatic to the skin are often gram-negative bacilli, particularly *Pseudomonas aeruginosa*.[88,89]

For tissue infection with *P. aeruginosa,* necrotizing vasculitis is an important pathologic lesion. In the skin, the result may be a variety of gross lesions,[88] including bullae or vesicles, which may be hemorrhagic; gangranous cellulitis, which with sharp margins and superficial and necrotic appearance is similar to a decubitus ulcer, except for location in a nonpressure area; nodular cellulitis, which is erythematous, warm, and often fluctuant; macules or papules that may ulcerate; erysipelas-like lesions; and ecthyma gangrenosum. This last lesion, which is often associated with bacteremia, is a round, indurated ulcer with a black area of central necrosis and surrounding erythema. Ecthyma gangrenosum is often located in the perineal or axillary region and may evolve from a vesicle. Aspiration of material from each of these various lesions may yield gram-

negative rods on Gram stain and *P. aeruginosa* on culture. Less commonly, ecthyma gangrenosum may be caused by other bacterial species, including *Escherichia coli,* or rarely by fungi such as *Candida* sp. or Mucoraceae.[13,89]

The clinical setting in which these life-threatening infections occur is often the patient with acute leukemia or profound granulocytopenia or both. Clinical management of such patients in whom these lesions develop[89] should include prompt aspiration or biopsy, or both, of the lesions, blood culturing, and initiation of therapy with an antipseudomonal penicillin and an aminoglycoside.

3.4.2. Systemic Mycotic Infection

Fungi causing systemic infection may also manifest metastatic skin lesions. The three major systemic fungal infections endemic in the United States—histoplasmosis, coccidioidomycosis, and blastomycosis—have several pathogenetic characteristics in common. Infections with these three organisms occur in immunocompetent persons living in, or traveling through, defined geographic areas where the pathogens are in the soil, are aerosolized, and penetrate through the respiratory tract. Immunocompetent persons with primary pulmonary infection usually are either asymptomatic or have minimal self-limited disease, after which the organisms may lie dormant. In patients with deficiencies in cell-mediated immunity at the time of infection, progressive primary infection with dissemination may occur. In addition, an immunosuppressed patient who acquired the organism asymptomatically many years earlier while living in an endemic area may have reactivation years later in a nonendemic region following the development of an immunosuppressive condition.[11] Thus obtaining a detailed epidemiologic history from a compromised patient may be important in excluding these three fungal infections from the differential diagnosis of a skin lesion.

Of these three fungal pathogens, *Histoplasma capsulatum*, appears to be the most likely to cause cutaneous lesions.[90–98] For renal transplant recipients with histoplasmosis, up to one-third have skin involvement, often early during the course of infection and often as the presenting manifestation of illness.[96] *H. capsulatum* commonly causes cellulitis, but papules, nodules, pustules, and hemorrhagic lesions may occur as well (Table 1).

3.4.3. Opportunistic Fungal and Nocardial Infections

Skin and subcutaneous infection that represents metastatic spread from noncutaneous sites in compromised patients may also occur with opportunistic fungi such as *Aspergillus* sp., *Candida* sp., *Cryptococcus neoformans,* and *Rhizopus* sp. and with species of the bacterium *Nocardia.*[14,86,99–107] The portal of infection for these pathogens (except for *Candida* sp.) is usually the respiratory tract, although primary cutaneous infection may also occur. Initial respiratory infection may be asymptomatic, with the first signs of systemic disease in the skin or in other organs following blood vessel invasion and hematogenous dissemination.[14,86,98,105,108–114]

For infection with *C. neoformans,* central nervous system (CNS) disease is the major life-threatening complication.[104,106] In one series, cryptococcal skin lesions that antedated CNS disease by weeks to months occurred in up to 20% of patients with cryptococcal meningitis.[104] In another series, four renal

TABLE 1. Cutaneous and Subcutaneous Lesions Caused by Opportunistic Organisms that Infect Compromised Patients

Type of lesion	Organism that may cause lesion
Abscess	*Aspergillus* sp ,[9,82] *Chaetoconidium,*[144] *Cryptococcus neoformans,*[112,145] *Fusarium solani,*[146] Mucoraceae,[22] *Mycobacterium avium-intracellulare,*[142] *M. fortuitum,*[62], *M. kansasii,*[62,147] *M. tuberculosis,*[63] *Nocardia* sp.[100]
Cellulitis	*Aspergillus* sp.,[20,82] *Candida* sp.,[116] *C. neoformans,*[110,112] *Histoplasma capsulatum,*[90,93,96,98] Mucoraceae,[24,84,85,143] *M. kansasii,*[147] *Nocardia* sp ,[113] *Paecilomyces*[59]
Ecthyma gangrenosum	*Candida* sp.,[89,148] Mucoraceae,[83,109] *Pseudomonas aeruginosa,*[88,89] other gram-negative bacteria
Erythematous macules	*Alternaria alternata,*[149] *Aspergillus* sp.,[20] Mucoraceae[109]
Hemorrhagic lesions	*A alternata,*[149] *Aspergillus* sp.,[26] *Candida* sp.,[126] *C. neoformans,*[112] *H. capsulatum,*[93] *Trichosporon beigelii*[50]
Papules, nodules	*Aspergillus* sp.,[20] *Candida* sp.,[115,116,123,124,126,127,128,148] *C. neoformans,*[112,150] *H. capsulatum,*[95,96] Mucoraceae,[21,83,109] *M. chelonei,*[151] *M. fortuitum,*[9] *M. kansasii,*[147] *M. marinum,*[69] *M. szulgai,*[152] *Prototheca* sp.,[72,76,78] *T. beigelii*[50,153]
Plaques	*A alternata,*[154,155] *Aspergillus* sp ,[20] *Candida* sp.,[148] *C. neoformans,*[150] *M kansasii,*[64] *M tuberculosis,*[63] *Prototheca* sp.[71,73]
Pustules	*Aspergillus* sp.,[9,82] *C neoformans,*[112,150] *H capsulatum,*[94] Mucoraceae,[22] *M. kansasii,*[147] *Prototheca* sp.[71]
Subcutaneous nodules, panniculitis	*Candida* sp ,[116] Chaetoconidium,[144] *H. capsulatum,*[93,96] Mucoraceae,[105] *M fortuitum,*[63] *M. intracellulare,*[156] *M kansasii,*[64] *M. marinum,*[69] *M. tuberculosis,*[63] *Nocardia* sp ,[100] *Scytalidium hyalinum*[157]
Vesicles, bullae	*Aspergillus* sp.,[26] *Candida* sp.,[8] *C neoformans,*[110] Herpes simplex, Herpes zoster, Mucoraceae,[23,158] *Prototheca* sp ,[75] *P. aeruginosa*

transplant recipients with cutaneous cryptococcosis had skin lesions as the initial sign of systemic infection.[13] The gross appearance of cutaneous lesions varies and includes papules, nodules, pustules, ulcers, and cellulitis (Table 1). Biopsy of a cryptococcal skin lesion may lead to curative therapy prior to development of the more difficult to treat CNS disease.

Illustrative Case 3: Cryptococcosis

A 45-year-old man was a renal transplant recipient who presented with a macular lesion on his scalp. The patient had insulin-requiring diabetes mellitus with blindness caused by diabetic reti-

nopathy Diabetic nephropathy had produced renal failure, for which the patient had received a cadaveric renal transplant 1 year earlier. Since transplantation, he had been treated with prednisone and-azathioprine. One month prior to admission, he had noticed a small, rough lesion on his scalp He denied fevers, headache, stiff neck, dyspnea, and cough.

On physical examination, the patient was in no distress. He was afebrile. His neck was supple. A 0.5×1.0-cm non-erythematous, dry, rough, and nontender scalp lesion was present. Lungs were clear to percussion and auscultation. Neurologic examination was remarkable for changes of diabetic retinopathy and blindness. WBC count was 4900 per mm³ with a normal differential count. Blood urea nitrogen (BUN) was 40 mg/dl, and serum creatinine was 2.4 mg/dl. Chest radiographs showed no infiltrates. Cerebrospinal fluid (CSF) was clear and contained no cells and had a glucose level of 233 mg/dl and a protein level of 99 mg/dl. Gram stain and India ink preparation of CSF revealed no organisms.

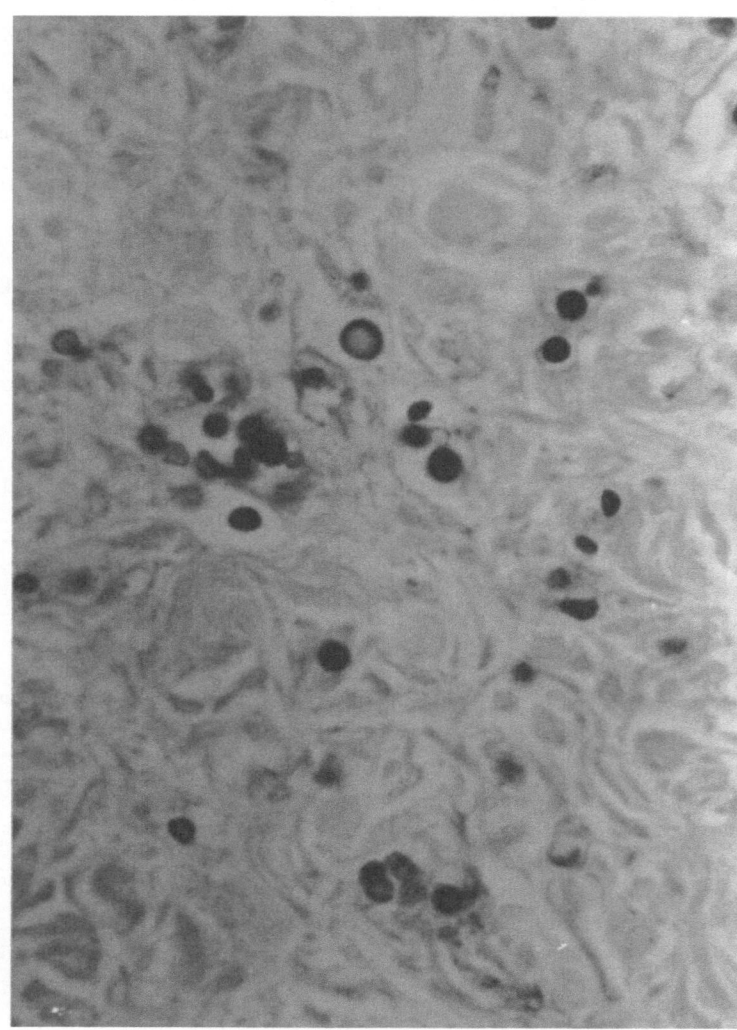

FIGURE 4. Histologic section of a skin biopsy showing *Cryptococcus* (dark spheres) in a renal transplant recipient receiving therapy with prednisone and azathioprine. The tissue was stained with methenamine-silver. (×400)

Cryptococcal antigen was not detected in the CSF or in the serum. Cultures of CSF and blood were negative.

The skin lesion was removed by excisional biopsy. Evaluation of the tissue in the microbiology laboratory revealed no pathogens, but histologic studies showed cryptococcal organisms (Fig. 4). The patient received systemic amphotericin B for a period of 6 weeks (total dose 1.2 gm). Five years later, the patient was free of cryptococcal disease, even with continuation of immunosuppressive therapy.

Comment. This case illustrates the presentation of a potentially life-threatening systemic infection as a benign-appearing skin lesion in a compromised patient. Treatment included not only local excisional biopsy but also systemic antifungal chemotherapy, because the skin lesion almost certainly represented metastatic spread from an undetected pulmonary site. This patient and the patient presented in case 2 emphasize that patients with disseminated fungal infections appear to respond more readily to therapy prior to the development of CNS disease.

Candidal infections, which represent the most common of all disseminated opportunistic fungal infections,[14] have cutaneous lesions in 10–13% of cases.[14,115,116] The portal of entry is usually the GI tract or an infected intravascular line rather than the respiratory tract.[116–121] An important clinical syndrome seen in leukemic or neutropenic patients is that of a nonspecific erythematous eruption composed of macular and papular skin lesions, fever, myalgias (due to candidal myositis), and positive blood cultures.[115,116,122–128] The rash may be similar to that seen in a drug reaction. The most common species that causes this syndrome is *C. tropicalis.*[14,115,116,126]

For systemic infection with *Candida* and other fungal species, early diagnosis by skin biopsy may be a life-saving maneuver, as blood cultures may not become positive for many days or may remain negative despite disseminated disease.

In compromised patients, *Nocardia asteroides*[99–101,113] and, less commonly, *Nocardia brasiliensis*[129] typically cause pulmonary infections but also not uncommonly cause nodules and abscesses in the subcutaneous tissues. The portal of entry for these bacteria is occasionally the skin but is usually the lungs with subsequent spread not only to subcutaneous tissues but to the CNS and other sites as well. In a series of 16 patients with *N. asteroides,*[100] seven patients were compromised, and five of these seven had subcutaneous lesions. In a series of 21 cardiac transplant recipients with *N. asteroides,*[113] involvement of subcutaneous tissues occurred in four patients, in two of whom it was the presenting manifestation of infection. For *N. brasiliensis* infection,[129] seven of 12 compromised patients had cutaneous or subcutaneous infection. Diagnosis of nocardial skin or subcutaneous infection requires aspiration or biopsy of the lesion.

4. Dermatologic Lesions Associated with AIDS

The cutaneous and subcutaneous lesions associated with AIDS may be conveniently categorized as noninfectious and infectious. The noninfectious associations include prominently the diffuse lymphadenopathy of AIDS,[38,130] Kaposi sarcoma,[38,130] and adverse reactions to drugs such as sulfamethoxazole and trimethoprim.[131–133] Less common noninfectious dermatologic lesions include those of lymphoma,[134,135] autoimmune thrombocytopenic purpura,[136] seborrheic dermatitis,[137] and hyperalgesiac pseudothrombophlebitis.[138]

The cutaneous infectious associations with AIDS include lesions caused by HSV[37] and herpes zoster infection,[38,139] bacterial skin flora (cellulitis),[140,141] *Nocardia* sp.,[141] and atypical mycobacteria.[142] In particular, herpes phagenda is a not uncommon problem in this patient population.[37] Chronic cutaneous infection with *Candida* sp., papillomavirus, and molluscum contagiosum have also been seen (A. J. Sober, unpublished observations). Other pathogens that cause systemic disease in AIDS patients that might produce cutaneous or subcutaneous lesions include *M. tuberculosis, Cryptococcus neoformans, Candida* sp., *Aspergillus* sp., *H. capsulatum,* and hepatitis B.

5. Diagnostic Aspects of Skin Infections in the Compromised Patient

In the immunocompetent patient, the gross appearance of a skin lesion is an important aspect of diagnosis. By contrast, the clinical value of the gross appearance of a cutaneous lesion in a compromised person is likely for two reasons to be limited.[10–14,19,90,93,126,143,144] First, in compromised patients, the variety of organisms that may cause infection is substantially greater than in immunocompetent persons.[3,4] Second, in compromised patients, the inflammatory response to infection may be altered.[5-7] It is noteworthy that a cutaneous lesion results not only from the invading pathogen itself but from the inflammatory response of the body to the microbe as well. Thus, with an impaired inflammatory response, the prediction is that the diagnostic usefulness of gross appearance would be suboptimal. For these two reasons, it is key to realize that the differential diagnosis of a particular skin lesion in a compromised patient is extensive. This point is emphasized in Table 1, which indicates that no gross morphology of a skin lesion in a compromised person is pathognomonic for a single etiologic agent. All these considerations stress the value of skin biopsy in establishing a diagnosis.

The approach to biopsy of a cutaneous lesion suspected to be infectious should include two considerations: the most rapid and most sensitive methods for detecting microbes both histologically and immunologically should be used, and appropriate cultures and stains should be obtained to optimize the chance of identifying the pathogen. Biopsy, if possible, should be a generous wedge excision. Half the tissue then is sent for histopathologic evaluation by routine methods and also by special stains for fungi, mycobacteria, and bacteria. The other half is sent to the microbiology laboratory for culture for aerobic and anaerobic bacteria, mycobacteria, and fungi (at 25°C and 37°C) and also for Gram, acid-fast, modified acid-fast, and direct fungal stains of touch preparations or ground material.

In conclusion, to take advantage of the skin as an early warning system of serious infection in compromised patients, both the physician and the patient should routinely search for cutaneous and subcutaneous lesions. Unexplained skin lesions then should be evaluated by biopsy for culture and histologic examination. Otherwise an undesirable outcome might result if one waits and allows an infectious process to declare itself at additional sites.

ACKNOWLEDGMENTS. We thank Robert H. Rubin for many interesting discussions and critical reading of the manuscript. We are grateful to Ben R. Bronstein for preparation of Figure 3. We thank Ms. Judy Feiner for valuable assistance with preparation of the manuscript.

References

1. Hill RB, Dahrling BE, Starzl TE, et al: Editorial: Death after transplantation. *Am J Med* **42**:327–334, 1967.
2. Anderson RJ, Schafer LA, Olin DB, et al: Infectious risk factors in the immunosuppressed host. *Am J Med* **54**:453–460, 1973.
3. Rubin RH, Young LS (eds). *Clinical Approach to Infection in the Compromised Host.* Plenum, New York, 1981.
4. Klastersky J (ed): *Infections in Cancer Patients.* European Organization for Research on Treatment of Cancer Monograph Series. Vol 10. Raven, New York, 1982.
5. Dale DC, Petersdorf RG: Corticosteroids and infectious diseases. *Med Clin. North Am.* **57**:1277–1287, 1973.
6. Dale DC. Defects in host defense mechanisms in compromised patients. In Rubin RH, Young LS (eds): *Clinical Approach to Infection in the Compromised Host.* Plenum, New York, 1981, pp. 35–74.
7. Wiernik PH. The management of infection in the cancer patient. *JAMA* **244**:185–192, 1980.
8. Haim S, Freidman-Birnbaum R, Better O, et al: Skin complications in immunosuppressed patients: Follow-up of kidney recipients. *Br J Dermatol* **89**:169–173, 1973.
9. Koranda F, Dehmel E, Kahn G, Penn I: Cutaneous complications in immunosuppressed renal homograft recipients. *JAMA* **229**:419–424, 1974.
10. Savin JA, Nobel WC: Immunosuppression and skin infection. *Br J Dermatol* **93**:115–120, 1975.
11. Rubin RH: Infection in the renal transplant patient. In Rubin RH, Young LS (eds): *Clinical Approach to Infection in the Compromised Host.* Plenum, New York, 1981, pp. 553–606.
12. Wolfson JS, Sober AJ, Rubin RH: Dermatologic manifestations of infection in the compromised host. *Annu. Rev. Med.* **34**:205–217, 1983.
13. Wolfson JS, Sober AJ, Rubin RH: Dermatologic manifestations of infections in immunocompromised patients. *Medicine (Baltimore)* **64**:115–133, 1985.
14. Ray TL: Cutaneous signs of systemic disease: Fungal infections in the immunocompromised host. *Med Clin North Am* **64**:955–968, 1980.
15. Eickhoff T, Olin B, Anderson R, et al: Current problems and approaches to diagnosis of infection in renal transplant recipients. *Transplant Proc* **4**:613–697, 1972.
16. Notter D, Grossman P, Rosenberg S, et al: Infections in patients with Hodgkin's disease: A clinical study of 300 consecutive adult patients. *Rev Infect Dis* **2**:761–800, 1980.
17. Bishop T, Schimpff S, Diggs C, et al: Infections during intensive chemotherapy for non-Hodgkins lymphoma. *Ann Intern Med* **95**:549–555, 1981.
18. Weinberg AN, Swartz MN. General considerations of bacterial diseases. Fitzpatrick TB, Eisen AZ, Wolff K, et al (eds): In *Dermatology in General Medicine.* McGraw-Hill, New York, 1979, pp. 1415–1426.
19. Prystowsky S, Vogelstein B, Ettinger D, et al: Invasive aspergillosis. *N Engl J Med* **295**:655–658, 1976.
20. Carlile JR, Millet RE, Cho CT, et al: Primary cutaneous

aspergillosis in a leukemic child. *Arch Dermatol* **114**:78–80, 1978.

21. Gartenberg G, Bottone E, Keusch G, et al: Hospital-acquired mucormycosis (*Rhizopus rhizopodiformis*) of skin and subcutaneous tissue. *N Engl J Med* **299**:1115–1118, 1978.

22. Keys T, Haldorson A, Rhodes K, et al: Nosocomial outbreak of *Rhizopus* infections associated with Elastoplast wound dressings—Minnesota. *MMWR* **27**:33–34, 1978.

23. Sheldon DL, Johnson WC: Cutaneous mucormycosis: Two documented cases of suspected nosocomial cause. *JAMA* **241**:1032–1034, 1979.

24. Dennis JE, Rhodes KH, Cooney DR, et al: Nosocomial *Rhizopus* infection (zygomycosis) in children. *J Pediatr* **96**:824–828, 1980.

25. Biro L, Gibbs RC, Leider M: Staphylococcal infections. A study of incidence on a dermatologic ward. *Arch Dermatol* **82**:205–211, 1960

26. Grossman ME, Fithian EC, Behrens C, et al: Primary cutaneous aspergillosis in six leukemic children. *J Am Acad Dermatol* **12**:313–318, 1985.

27. Granstein RD, First LR, Sober AJ: Primary cutaneous aspergillosis in a premature neonate. *Br J Dermatol* **103**:681–684, 1980.

28. Lorenzen I: The effects of glucocorticoids on connective tissue. *Acta Med Scand (Suppl.)* **50**:17–21, 1969.

29. Smithers DW: Hodgkin's disease. II. *Br Med J* **2**:337–340, 1967.

30. Mullen DL, Silverberg SG, Penn I, et al: Squamous cell carcinoma of the skin and lip in renal homograft recipients. *Cancer* **37**:729–734, 1976.

31. Hersh EM, Freireich EJ: Focus on cutaneous host–defense failure in transplant recipients. *JAMA* **229**:457–458, 1974.

32. Spencer ES, Anderson HK: Clinically evident, non-terminal infections with herpes viruses and the wart virus in immunosuppressed renal allograft recipients. *Br Med J* **3**:251–254, 1970.

33. Hardie IR, Strong RW, Hartley CJ, et al: Skin cancer in Caucasian renal allograft recipients living in a subtropical climate. *Surgery* **87**:177–183, 1980.

34. Lutzner MA, Orth G, Dutronquay V, et al: Detection of human papillomavirus type 5 DNA in skin cancers of an immunosuppressed renal allograft recipient. *Lancet* **2**:422–424, 1983.

35. Dolin R, Reichman RC, Mazur MH. et al: NIH Conference: Herpes zoster-varicella infections in immunosuppressed patients. *Ann Intern Med* **89**:375–388, 1978.

36. Hirsch MS: Herpes group virus infections in the compromised host. In Rubin RH, Young LS (eds): *Clinical Approach to Infection in the Compromised Host*. Plenum, New York, 1981, pp. 389–415.

37. Siegel FP, Lopez C, Hammer GS, et al: Severe acquired immunodeficiency in male homosexuals, manifested by chronic perianal ulcerative herpes simplex lesions. *N Engl J Med* **305**:1439–1444, 1981.

38. Gottlieb MS, Groopman JE, Weinstein WM, et al: UCLA Conference: The acquired immunodeficiency syndrome *Ann Intern Med* **99**:208–220, 1983.

39. Chou S, Gallagher JG, Merigan TC: Controlled clinical trial of intravenous acyclovir in heart-transplant patients with mucocutaneous herpes simplex infection. *Lancet* **1**:1392–1394, 1981.

40. Mitchell CD, Bean B, Gentry SR, et al: Acyclovir therapy for mucocutaneous herpes simplex infections in immunocompromised patients. *Lancet* **1**:1389–1392, 1981.

41. Straus SE, Smith HA, Brickman C, et al: Acyclovir for chronic mucocutaneous herpes simplex virus infection in immunosuppressed patients. *Ann Intern Med* **96**:270–277, 1982.

42. Wade JC, Newton B, McLaren C, et al: Intravenous acyclovir to treat mucocutaneous herpes simplex virus infection after marrow transplantation: A double-blind trial. *Ann Intern Med* **96**:265–269, 1982.

43. Hirsch MS, Schooley RT: Treatment of herpesvirus infections. *N Engl J Med* **309**:963–970, 1034–1039, 1983.

44. Whitley RJ, Levin M, Barton N, et al: Infections caused by herpes simplex virus in the immunocompromised host: Natural history and topical acyclovir therapy. *J Infect Dis* **150**:323–329, 1984.

45. Wong KK, Hirsch MS: Herpes virus infections in patients with neoplastic disease. Diagnosis and therapy. *Am J Med* **76**:464–478, 1984.

46. Schimpff S, Serpick A, Stoler B, et al: Varicella-zoster infection in patients with cancer. *Ann Intern Med* **76**:241–254, 1972.

47. Meyers JD, Thomas ED: Infection complicating bone marrow transplantation. In Rubin RH, Young LS (eds): *Clinical Approach to Infection in the Compromised Host*. Plenum, New York, 1981, pp. 507–551.

48. Balfour HH, Bean B, Laskin OL, et al: Acyclovir halts progression of herpes zoster in immunocompromised patients. *N Engl J Med* **308**:1448–1453, 1983.

49. Alteras I, Aryeli G, Feuerman EJ: The prevalence of pathogenic and potentially pathogenic fungi on the apparently healthy skin of patients with neoplastic diseases. *Mycopathologia* **71**:85–87, 1980.

50. Manzella JP, Berman IJ, Kukrilca MD: *Trichosporon beigelii* fungemia and cutaneous dissemination. *Arch Dermatol* **118**:343–345, 1982.

51. Horsburgh CR, Kirkpatrick CH: Long-term therapy of chronic mucocutaneous candidiasis with ketoconazole: Experience with 21 patients. *Am J Med* **74**:23–29, 1983.

52. Dismukes WE, Stamm AM, Graybill JR, et al: Treatment of systemic mycoses with ketaconazole: Emphasis on toxicity and clinical response in 52 patients. *Ann Intern Med* **98**:13–20, 1983.

53. Uys CT, Don PA, Schire V, et al: Endocarditis following cardiac surgery due to the fungus Paecilomyces. *S Afr Med J* **37**:1276–1280, 1963.

54. Silver MD, Tuffnell PG, Bigelow WG: Endocarditis caused by *Paecilomyces varioti* affecting an aortic valve allograft. *J Thorac Cardiovasc Surg* **61**:278–281, 1971.

55. Haldane EV, MacDonald JL, Gittens WO, et al: Prosthetic valvular endocarditis due to the fungus Paecilomyces. *Can Med Assoc J* **111**:963–968, 1974.

56. McClellan JR, Hamilton JD, Alexander JA, et al:

Paecilomyces varioti endocarditis on a prosthetic valve. *J Thorac Cardiovasc Surg* **71:**472–475, 1976.

57. Mosier MA, Lusk B, Pettit TH, et al: Fungal endophthalmitis following intraocular lens implantation. *Am J Ophthalmol* **83:**1–8, 1977.

58. O'Day DM: Fungal endophthalmitis caused by *Paecilomyces lilacinus* after intraocular lens implantation. *Am J Ophthalmol* **83:**130–131, 1977.

59. Harris LF, Dan BM, Lefkowitz LB, et al: *Paecilomyces* cellulitis in a renal transplant patient: Successful treatment with intravenous miconazole. *South Med J* **72:**897–898, 1979.

60. Fogan L: Atypical mycobacteria. *Medicine (Baltimore)* **49:**243–255, 1970.

61. Kaplan MH, Armstrong D, Rosen P: Tuberculosis complicating neoplastic disease. *Cancer* **33:**850–858, 1974.

62. Wolinsky E: Nontuberculous mycobacteria and associated diseases. *Am Rev Respir Dis* **119:**107–158, 1979.

63. Beyt BE, Ortbals DW, Santa Cruz DJ, et al: Cutaneous mycobacteriosis: Analysis of 34 cases with a new classification of the disease. *Medicine (Baltimore)* **60:**95–109, 1981.

64. Lloveras J, Peterson PK, Simmons RL, et al: Mycobacterial infections in renal transplant recipients: Seven cases and a review of the literature. *Arch Intern Med* **142:**888–892, 1982.

65. Lichtenstein IH, MacGregor RR: Mycobacterial infections in renal transplant recipients: Report of five cases and review of the literature. *Rev Infect Dis* **5:**216–226, 1983.

66. Grice, K: Sarcoidosis and *Mycobacterium avium-intracellulare* cutaneous abscesses. *Clin Exp Dermatol* **8:**323–327, 1983.

67. Wallace RJ, Swenson JM, Silcox VA, et al: Spectrum of disease due to rapidly growing mycobacteria. *Rev Infect Dis* **5:**657–679, 1983.

68. Davis BR, Brumback J, Sanders WJ, et al: Skin lesions caused by *Mycobacterium haemophilum*. *Ann Intern Med* **97:**723–724, 1982.

69. Gombert ME, Goldstein EJC, Corrado ML, et al: Disseminated *Mycobacterium marinum* infection after renal transplantation. *Ann Intern Med* **94:**486–487, 1981.

70. Davies RR, Wilkinson JL: Human protothecosis: Supplementary studies. *Ann Trop Med Parasitol* **61:**112–115, 1967.

71. Tindall JP, Fetter BF: Infections caused by achloric algae (protothecosis). *Arch Dermatol* **104:**490–500, 1971.

72. Cox GE, Wilson JD, Brown P: Protothecosis: A case of disseminated algal infection. *Lancet* **2:**379–382, 1974.

73. Sudman MS: Protothecosis: A critical review. *Am J Clin Pathol* **61:**10–19, 1974.

74. Mayhall CG, Miller CW, Eisen AZ, et al: Cutaneous protothecosis: Successful treatment with amphotericin B. *Arch Dermatol* **112:**1749–1752, 1976.

75. Wolfe ID, Sacks HG, Samorodin CS, et al: Cutaneous protothecosis in a patient receiving immunosuppressive therapy. *Arch Dermatol* **112:**829–832, 1976.

76. Dagher FJ, Smith AG, Pankoski D, et al: Skin protothecosis in a patient with renal allograft. *South Med J* **71:**222–224, 1978.

77. Phair JP, Williams JE, Bassaris HP, et al: Phagocytosis and algicidal activity of human polymorphonuclear neutrophils against *Prototheca wickerhamii* *J Infect Dis* **144:**72–76, 1981.

78. Venezio FR, Lavoo E, Williams JE, et al: Progressive cutaneous protothecosis. *Am J Clin Pathol* **77:**485–493, 1982.

79. Pegram PS, Kerns FT, Wasilauskas BL, et al: Successful ketoconazole treatment of protothecosis with ketoconazole-associated hepatotoxicity. *Arch Intern Med* **143:**1802–1805, 1983.

80. Vernon SE, Goldman LS: Protothecosis in the Southeastern United States. *South Med J* **76:**949–950, 1983.

81. Klintworth GK, Fetter BF, Nielsen HS: Protothecosis: An algal infection: Report of a case in man. *J Med Microbiol* **1:**211–216, 1968

82. Langlois RP, Flegel KM, Meakins JL, et al: Cutaneous aspergillosis with fatal dissemination in a renal transplant recipient. *Can Med J* **22:**673–676, 1980.

83. Lehrer RI, Howard DH, Sypherd PS, et al: UCLA conference: Mucormycosis. *Ann Intern Med* **93:**93–108, 1980.

84. Fisher J, Tuazon CU, Geelhoed GW: Mucormycosis in transplant patients. *Am Sur* **46:**315–322, 1980.

85. Bateman CP, Umland ET, Becker LE: Cutaneous zygomycosis in a patient with lymphoma *J Am Acad Dermatol* **8:**890–894, 1983.

86. Young RC, Bennett JE, Vogel CL, et al: Aspergillosis: The spectrum of the disease in 98 patients. *Medicine (Baltimore)* **49:**147–173, 1970.

87. Meyer RD, Rosen P, Armstrong D: Phycomycosis complicating leukemia and lymphoma. *Ann Intern Med* **77:**871–879, 1972.

88. Forkner CE, Frei E, Edgecomb JH, et al: Pseudomonas septicemia: Observations on twenty-three cases. *Am J Med* **25:**877–889, 1968.

89. Greene SL, Su WP, Muller SA: Ecthyma gangranosum: Report of clinical, histopathologic, and bacteriologic aspects of eight cases. *J Am Acad Dermatol* **11:**781–787. 1984.

90. Park RK, Goltz RW, Carey TB: Unusual cutaneous infections associated with immunosuppressive therapy. *Arch Dermatol* **95:**345–350, 1967.

91. O'Dorisio TM, Jasper DA, Sullivan J: A cutaneous manifestation of untreated disseminated histoplasmosis. *Chest* **67:**616–617, 1975.

92. Studdard J, Sneed WF, Taylor MR, et al: Cutaneous histoplasmosis. *Am Rev Respir Dis* **113:**689–693, 1976.

93. Daman LA, Hashimoto K, Kaplan RJ, et al: Disseminated histoplasmosis in an immunosuppressed patient. *South Med J* **70:**355–356, 1977.

94. Cott GR, Smith TW, Hinthorn DR, et al: Primary cutaneous histoplasmosis in immunosuppressed patients. *JAMA* **242:**456–457, 1979.

95. Johnston CA, Tang CK, Jiji R: Histoplasmosis of skin and lymph nodes and chronic lymphocytic leukemia. *Arch Dermatol* **115:**336–337, 1979.

96. Davies SR, Sarosi GA, Peterson PK, et al: Disseminated histoplasmosis in renal transplant recipients. *Am J Surg* **137:**686–691, 1979.

97. Goodwin RA, Shapiro JL, Thurman GH, et al: Disseminated histoplasmosis: Clinical and pathologic correlations. *Medicine (Baltimore)* **59:**1–33, 1980.

98. Farr B, Beacham BE, Atuk NO: Cutaneous histoplasmosis after renal transplantation. *South Med J* **74**:635–637, 1981.

99 Palmer DL, Harvey RL, Wheeler JK: Diagnostic and therapeutic considerations in *Nocardia asteroides* infection. *Medicine (Baltimore)* **53**:391–401, 1974.

100. Frazier AR, Rosenow EC, Roberts GD: Nocardiosis: A review of 25 cases occurring during 24 months. *Mayo Clin Proc* **50**:657–663, 1975.

101. Beaman BL, Burnside J, Edwards B, et al: Nocardial infections in the United States, 1972–1974. *J Infect Dis* **134**:286–289, 1976.

102. Brown E, Freedman S, Arbeit R, et al: Invasive pulmonary aspergillosis in an apparently non-immunocompromised host. *Am J Med* **69**:624–627, 1980.

103. Fisher BD, Armstrong D, Yu B, et al: Invasive aspergillosis: Prognosis in early diagnosis and treatment. *Am J Med* **71**:571–577, 1981.

104. Kerkering TM, Duma RJ, Shadomy S: The evolution of pulmonary cryptococcosis. *Ann Intern Med* **94**:611–616, 1981.

105. Myskowski PL, Brown AE, Dinsmore R, et al: Mucormycosis following bone marrow transplantation. *J Am Acad Dermatol* **9**:111–115, 1983.

106. Perfect JR, Durack DT, Gallis HA: Cryptococcemia. *Medicine (Baltimore)* **62**:98–109, 1983.

107. Rinaldi MG: Invasive aspergillosis. *Rev Infect Dis* **5**:1061–1077, 1983.

108. Sarosi GA, Silberfarb PM, Tosh FE: Cutaneous cryptococcosis: A sentinel of disseminated disease. *Arch Dermatol* **104**:1–3, 1971.

109. Meyer RD, Kaplan MH, Ong M, et al: Cutaneous lesions in disseminated mucormycosis. *JAMA* **225**:737–738, 1973.

110. Schupbach CW, Wheeler CE, Briggaman RA, et al: Cutaneous manifestations of disseminated cryptococcosis. *Arch Dermatol* **112**:1734–1740, 1976.

111. Kramer BS, Hernandez AD, Reddick RL, et al: Cutaneous infarction: Manifestation of disseminated mucormycosis. *Arch Dermatol* **113**:1075–1076, 1977.

112. Greene MH, Macher AM, Hernandez AD, et al: Disseminated cryptococcosis presenting as palpable purpura. *Arch Intern Med* **138**:1412–1413, 1978.

113. Simpson GL, Stinson EB, Egger MJ, et al: Nocardial infections in the immunocompromised host: A detailed study in a defined population. *Rev Infect Dis* **3**:492–507, 1981.

114. Bernhardt MJ, Ward WQ, Sams WM: Cryptococcal cellulitis. *Cutis* **34**:359–361, 1984.

115. Bodey GP, Luna M: Skin lesions associated with disseminated candidiasis. *JAMA* **229**:1466–1468, 1974.

116. Wingard JR, Merz WG, Saral R: *Candida tropicalis.* A major pathogen in immunocompromised patients. *Ann Intern Med* **91**:539–543, 1979.

117 Louria DB, Stiff DP, Bennett B: Disseminated moniliasis in the adult. *Medicine (Baltimore)* **41**:307–337, 1962.

118. De Vita VT, Utz JP, Williams T, et al: Candida meningitis. *Arch Intern Med* **117**:527–535, 1966.

119. Curry CR, Quie PG: Fungal septicemia in patients receiving parenteral hyperalimentation. *N Engl J Med* **285**:1221–1225, 1971.

120. Bayer AS, Edwards JE, Seidel JS, et al: Candida meningitis.

Report of seven cases and review of the English literature. *Medicine (Baltimore)* **55**:477–486, 1976.

121. Myerowitz RL, Pazin GJ, Allen CM: Disseminated candidiasis. Changes in incidence, underlying diseases, and pathology. *Am J Clin Pathol* **68**:29–38, 1977.

122. Balandran L, Rothschild H, Pugh N, et al: A cutaneous manifestation of systemic candidiasis. *Ann Intern Med* **78**:400–403, 1973.

123. Edwards JE, Lehrer RI, Stiehm ER, et al: UCLA Conference: Severe candidal infections: Clinical perspective, immune defense mechanisms, and current concepts of therapy. *Ann Intern Med* **89**:91–106, 1978.

124. Jarowski CI, Fialk MA, Murray HW, et al: Fever, rash, and muscle tenderness: A distinctive clinical presentation of disseminated candidiasis. *Arch Intern Med* **138**:544–546, 1978.

125. Kressel B, Szewczyk C, Tuazon CU: Early clinical recognition of disseminated candidiasis by muscle and skin biopsy. *Arch Intern Med* **138**:429–433, 1978.

126. Grossman ME, Silvers DN, Walther RR: Cutaneous manifestations of disseminated candidiasis. *J Am Acad Dermatol* **2**:111–116, 1980.

127. Jacobs MI, Magid MS, Jarowski CI: Disseminated candidiasis: Newer approaches to early recognition and treatment. *Arch Dermatol* **116**:1277–1279, 1980.

128. Arena FP, Perlin M, Brahman H, et al: Fever, rash, and myalgias of disseminated candidiasis during antifungal therapy. *Arch Intern Med* **141**:1233, 1981.

129. Smego RA, Gallis HA: The clinical spectrum of *Nocardia brasiliensis* infection in the United States. *Rev Infect Dis* **6**:164–180, 1984.

130. Fauci AS, Macher AM, Longo DL, et al: NIH conference. Acquired immunodeficiency syndrome: Epidemiologic, clinical, immunologic, and therapeutic considerations. *Ann Intern Med* **100**:92–106, 1984.

131. Jaffe HS, Abrams DI, Ammann AJ, et al: Complications of co-trimoxazole in treatment of AIDS-associated *Pneumocystis carinii* pneumonia in homosexual men. *Lancet* **2**:1109–1111, 1983.

132. Mitsuyasu R, Groopman J, Volberding P: Cutaneous reaction to trimethoprim-sulfamethoxazole in patients with AIDS and Kaposi's sarcoma. *N Engl J Med* **308**:1535–1536, 1983.

133. Gordin FM, Simon GL, Wofsy CB, et al: Adverse reactions to trimethoprim-sulfamethoxazole in patients with the acquired immunodeficiency syndrome. *Ann Intern Med* **100**:495–499, 1984.

134. Ziegler JL, Beckstead JA, Volberding PA, et al: Non-Hodgkin's lymphoma in 90 homosexual men. Relation to generalized lymphadenopathy and the acquired immunodeficiency syndrome. *N Engl J Med* **311**:565–570, 1984.

135. Lind SE, Gross PL, Andiman WA, et al: Malignant lymphoma presenting as Kaposi's sarcoma in a homosexual man with the acquired immunodeficiency syndrome. *Ann Intern Med* **102**:338–340, 1985.

136. Morris L, Distenfeld A, Amorosi E, et al: Autoimmune thrombocytopenic purpura in homosexual men. *Ann Intern Med* **96**:714–717, 1982.

137. Eisenstat BA, Wormser GP: Seborrheic dermatitis and butterfly rash in AIDS. *N Engl J Med* **311**:189, 1984.

138. Abramson SB, Odajnyk CM, Grieco AJ, et al: Hyperalgesic pseudothrombophlebitis. New syndrome in male homosexuals. *Am J Med* **78**:317–320, 1985.

139. Sandor E, Croxson TS, Millman A, et al: Herpes zoster ophthalmicus in patients at risk for AIDS. *N Engl J Med* **310**:1118–1119, 1984.

140. Ho DD, Murata GH: Streptococcal lymphadenitis in homosexual men with chronic lymphadenopathy. *Am J Med* **77**:151-153, 1984.

141. Holtz HA, Lavery DP, Kapila R: Actinomycetales infection in the acquired immunodeficiency syndrome. *Ann Intern Med* **102**:203–205, 1985.

142. Macher AM, Kovars JA, Gill V, et al: Bacteremia due to *Mycobacterium avium-intracellulare* in the acquired immunodeficiency syndrome. *Ann Intern Med* **99**:782–785, 1983.

143. Wilson CB, Siber GR, O'Brien TF, et al: Phycomycotic gangrenous cellulitis. *Arch Surg* **111**:532–538, 1976.

144. Lomvardias S, Madge GE: *Chaetoconidium* and atypical acid-fast bacilli in skin ulcers. *Arch Dermatol* **106**:875–876, 1972.

145. Lewis JL, Rabinovich S: The wide spectrum of cryptococcal infections. *Am J Med* **53**:315–322, 1972

146. Cho CT, Vats TS, Lowman JT, et al: *Fusarium solani* infection during treatment for acute leukemia. *J Pediatr* **83**:1028–1031, 1973.

147. Bolivar R, Salterwhite TK, Floyd M: Cutaneous lesions due to *Mycobacterium kansasii. Arch Dermatol* **116**:207–208, 1980.

148. Fine JD, Miller JA, Harrist TJ, et al: Cutaneous lesions in disseminated candidiasis mimicking ecthyma gangrenosum. *Am J Med* **70**:1133–1135, 1981

149. Farmer SG, Komorowski RA: Cutaneous microabscess formation from *Alternaria alternata. Am J Clin Pathol* **66**:565–569, 1976.

150. Moore M: Cryptococcus with cutaneous manifestations. *J Invest Dermatol* **28**:159–182, 1957.

151. Heironimus JD, Winn RE, Collins CB: Cutaneous nonpulmonary *Mycobacterium chelonei* infection. *Arch Dermatol* **120**:1061–1063, 1984.

152. Cross GM, Guill MA, Aton JK: Cutaneous *Mycobacterium szulgai* infection. *Arch Dermatol* **121**:247–249, 1985.

153. Apaliski SJ, Moore MD, Reiner BJ, et al: Disseminated *Trichosporon beigelii* in an immunocompromised child. *Pediatr Infect Dis* **3**:451–454, 1984.

154. Hernanz AD, Conde-Zurita JM, Pecharroman SR, et al: A case of *Alternaria alternata* (Fr.) Keissler infection of the knee. *Clin Exp Dermatol* **8**:641–646, 1983.

155. Bourlond A, Alexandre G: Dermal alternariasis in a kidney transplant recipient. *Dermatologica* **168**:152–156, 1984.

156. Sanderson TL, Moskowitz L, Hensley GT, et al. Disseminated *Mycobacterium avium-intracellulare* infection appearing as a panniculitis. *Arch Pathol Lab Med* **106**:112–114, 1982.

157 Zaatari GS, Reed R, Morewessel R: Subcutaneous hyphomycosis caused by *Scytalidium hyalinum. Am J Clin Pathol* **82**:252–256, 1984.

158. Baker RD, Seabury JH, Schneidau JD: Subcutaneous and cutaneous mucormycosis and subcutaneous phycomycosis. *Lab Invest* **11**:1091–1102, 1962.

6

Etiology and Management of the Compromised Patient with Fever and Pulmonary Infiltrates

ROBERT H. RUBIN and REGINALD GREENE

1. Febrile Pneumonitis Syndrome and Its Importance

The immunocompromised patient in whom fever and pneumonitis develop presents a formidable challenge to the clinician. A legion of microbial invaders ranging from common viral and bacterial pathogens to exotic fungal and protozoan agents have been reported to cause pulmonary infection in these patients. Given the array of infectious etiologies, it is little wonder that pneumonia is the most frequent cause of fatal infection in the compromised host.[1-8] For example, in one large series of 227 renal transplant patients, inflammatory disease of the lung occurred in 20% of patients and was associated with 50% of fatalities.[6] Patients with acute leukemia in relapse develop an episode of pneumonia approximately once every 60 days at risk.[9] In patients with hematologic malignancy who developed fever and pulmonary infiltrates, the mortality rate (45%) was five times that for such patients with fever alone.[10] In a similar study of pneumonia in patients with cancer, the mortality rate (76%) for patients with pulmonary

infection was many time greater than the mortality associated with infection at other sites.[11] In most patients with acquired immunodeficiency syndrome (AIDS) pneumonia develops, and in virtually all these patients pneumonia is an important factor in their demise.

A variety of factors account for these observations. Perhaps most important are the abnormal local and systemic host defenses that are present. Damage to the mucocutaneous surfaces of the respiratory tract, impaired drainage of secretions from the tracheobronchial tree, deficiencies in T and B lymphocytes, decreases in the number and function of circulating granulocytes, and alveolar macrophage dysfunction may all result from the underlying disease and its treatment.[1,6] Studies in animal models suggest that immunosuppressed patients receiving either corticosteroids or cyclophosphamide, or both, and probably other cytotoxic agents and radiation as well, do not mount a normal local inflammatory response to challenge with microorganisms. Thus, initial infection will be poorly contained, and extensive pulmonary infection will rapidly ensue.[12]

Exposure to the hospital environment can play an important role in the pathogenesis of infectious pneumonia in the compromised patient. We had observed a very high rate of *Pseudomonas aeruginosa* pulmonary infection among renal transplant patients temporarily housed on the same isolation floor, although in different rooms with separate nursing and

ROBERT H. RUBIN • Infectious Disease and Transplantation Units, Massachusetts General Hospital; and Department of Medicine, Harvard Medical School, Boston, Massachusetts 02114   REGINALD GREENE • Chest Division, Radiology Service, Massachusetts General Hospital; and Department of Radiology, Harvard Medical School, Boston, Massachusetts 02114.

physician staffs, as burn patients. Since the transplant patients have been moved to a different hospital site, apart from the burn patients who are heavily contaminated with *P. aeruginosa,* there has not been a single instance of *Pseudomonas* pulmonary infection in 500 consecutive transplants. However, colonization and superinfection with other relatively antibiotic-resistant gram-negative bacilli in the hospital environment such as *Klebsiella, Serratia, Enterobacter,* and *Acinetobacter* remain significant problems for us as they are for all other centers dealing with patients with compromised host defenses.[6]

The pathogenesis of nosocomial gram-negative pneumonias appears to involve the colonization of the upper respiratory tract with these organisms, followed by aspiration of these virulent bacteria into the lower respiratory tract. In normal persons, the upper respiratory tract is primarily gram positive, nonvirulent, and penicillin sensitive. This normal flora is maintained in large measure because of a selective advantage provided by the specific interaction of bacterial surface adhesins with specialized receptors on the surfaces of upper respiratory epithelial cells. The selective advantage that this adhesive mechanism provides is normally sufficient to prevent colonization of the respiratory tract with gram-negative organisms.[13-15]

In seriously ill patients, such as hospitalized immunocompromised patients undergoing acute immunosuppressive therapy, the ecology of the normal flora is disturbed, making possible a high rate of upper respiratory tract gram-negative colonization. In large part, the increased rates of gram-negative colonization are due to alterations in the epithelial cell surface, which now favors the adherence of gram negative bacteria at the expense of the normal flora. The tendency toward gram-negative carriage is greatly accentuated within the hospital setting when there is excess nosocomial exposure to these organisms. Once gram-negative colonization occurs, aspiration can result in the delivery of virulent, relatively antibiotic-resistant bacteria to the lungs. The severity of the patient's underlying illness and the intensity of the immunosuppressing therapy, then, influence the type of bacterial adherence that develops, the nature of the colonizing flora, and the subsequent rate of gram-negative pneumonia.[13-15] Miniaspiration of the upper respiratory flora probably occurs more frequently in this population as well, particularly in patients with oral, pharyngeal, and esophageal ulcerations re-

sulting from chemotherapy or herpetic or candidal infections. Many of these patients have difficulty handling their pharyngeal secretions because of these painful lesions, and aspiration and subsequent pneumonia develop.[1]

Other, more opportunistic, pathogens have caused epidemics of nosocomial pneumonia in the immunosuppressed patient. The most important of these are the epidemics due to *Legionella* sp. (Chapter 11) and *Aspergillus* sp. (Chapter 8). Epidemic disease due to *Legionella pneumophila* infection has occurred on several occasions among immunosuppressed patients being cared for within the hospital.[16-21] The great majority of *L. micdadei* cases occur in hospitalized patients being treated with intensive immunosuppressive therapy—the setting in which it was first discovered.[22-26]

Of all the opportunistic infections apt to invade the respiratory tract of the compromised host from a nosocomial source, *Aspergillus* species have been the most virulent problem. The presence of excessive numbers of *Aspergillus fumigatus* and/or *A. flavus* spores in hospital environments may be associated with highly lethal epidemic disease. Epidemic invasive aspergillosis has been documented to have occurred in the following circumstances: *A. fumigatus* spores were contaminating the air ducts leading to the rooms of immunosuppressed patients; *A. fumigatus* was growing in pigeon excreta that was being sucked into the intake duct of ventilating systems leading to an operating room; and there have now been several documented outbreaks involving transplant patients and cancer patients, caused by *Aspergillus* spores present in fireproofing and/or insulating materials that were disturbed during renovation or used in the building of a new hospital facility.[3,6,27-34]

The majority of recognized nosocomial *Aspergillus* epidemics have been due to contamination of the air in the patients' rooms, so-called domiciliary epidemics. Recently, we noted a second form of epidemic: an outbreak of invasive *Aspergillus fumigatus* infection among immunosuppressed patients being cared for in widely separated portions of the hospital with very different air supplies. In this instance, the epidemic was due to construction in the central radiology suite these patients all visited for radiologic studies—a nondomiciliary, common source epidemic. Such epidemics are probably not uncommon but are more difficult to detect.[34]

Less commonly, other organisms may also

cause nosocomial outbreaks of pulmonary infection among immunosuppressed persons. For example, Singer et al.[35] reported on apparent outbreak of *Pneumocystis carinii* infection involving patients and staff on an oncology ward.

The implications of these observations are that constant surveillance of the immunosuppressed patient is essential to identify the existence of an important infectious disease hazard before a major epidemic occurs. In a very real sense, the compromised patient is much like the oldfashioned "sentinel chicken" staked out in swamps to monitor the circulation of arboviruses between mosquitoes and birds. In this instance, the immunosuppressed patient is placed out into the hospital environment, and if there is much microbial activity, he will quickly reflect it, with the respiratory tract being particularly at risk. This increased hazard may encompass both conventional bacterial and unusual fungal or even protozoan infection. Although nosocomial pulmonary infection is an important problem for all hospitalized patients, it is of critical importance in this population that has little reserve to withstand the effects of microbial invasion.

Compounding the problem further for the clinician is the fact that noninfectious causes of pulmonary inflammation—radiation lung injury, drug reactions, the underlying neoplasm, pulmonary embolic disease, leukoagglutinin transfusion reactions, pulmonary hemorrhage, and atypical pulmonary edema—may present a clinical picture similar to that produced by infection.[1,4,6,8,10] The clinical problem in this patient population is not just the differential diagnosis of pulmonary infection in the compromised host but rather the differential diagnosis of fever and pulmonary infiltrates in this patient population. At the Massachusetts General Hospital, approximately one-fourth of renal transplant patients and patients with malignant disease who present with the febrile pneumonitis syndrome have a noninfectious process. In renal transplant patients, pulmonary emboli and atypical pulmonary edema are the major etiologies of this process; in cancer patients, recurrent tumor, radiation pneumonitis, drug-induced pneumonitis, and pulmonary emboli are the major causes (Table 1).[1,6]

The clinician dealing with fever and pneumonitis in the compromised patient, then, must contend with an impressive array of diagnostic possibilities. In addition, particularly with the infections, the clinical presentation, course, and impact of the pulmonary process may be greatly modi-

TABLE 1. Etiology of Febrile Pneumonitis Syndrome in 100 Cancer Patients and 51 Renal Transplant Patients at Massachusetts General Hospital[a]

Etiology	Number of cancer patients	Number of renal transplant patients	Total	Percent
Infectious causes				
Conventional bacterial infection	26	10	36	23 8
Viral infection	11	9	20	13 2
Fungal infection	10	6	16	10.6
Nocardia asteroides	5	8	13	8 6
Pneumocystis carinii	6	2	8	5 3
Mycobacterium tuberculosis	1	0	1	0.7
Mixed infections	14	1[b]	15	9.9
Total	73	36	109	72.2
Noninfectious causes				
Pulmonary emboli	3	9	12	7 9
Recurrent tumor	8	0	8	5 3
Radiation pneumonitis	7	0	7	4.6
Pulmonary edema	1	6	7	4 6
Drug-induced pneumonitis	5	0	5	3.3
Leukoagglutinin reaction	2	0	2	1.3
Pulmonary hemorrhage	1	0	1	0.7
Total	27	15	42	27.8

[a]Data taken and modified from Rubin[1] and Ramsey et al[6]
[b]This one case was that of an aspiration pneumonia from whom mixed oropharyngeal flora were grown from a transtracheal aspirate In addition, 23 renal transplant patients with a primary pulmonary process developed superinfection

fied by the underlying disease and its treatment. Severe granulocytopenia will have the most profound effect. The incidence of cough and purulent sputum production, rate of development and progression of radiologic findings, the occurrence of cavitation, and pleural space involvement are all markedly diminished in patients with profound granulocytopenia.[1,2,5,36,37] In addition, the consequences of the pulmonary process in such granulocytopenic patients may also be modified. For example, in children with acute leukemia and pneumonia who have absolute granulocyte counts of less than 1000/mm[3], the incidence of positive blood cultures has been reported to be 64%, with the incidence of positive cultures falling to 0% in children with leukemia, pneumonia, and absolute granulocyte counts greater than 1000/mm[3].[38] Similarly, although septic shock is a rare occurrence in a normal patient with pneumonia, it is not that unusual in a severely granulocytopenic patient.[1] It is not surprising, then, that as many as 58% of patients with cancer and profound granulocytopenia who die have been shown to have clinically unrecognized and, hence, inadequately treated pneumonia at autopsy.[38]

Despite the obvious difficulties, a variety of clues are available to the clinician in approaching this clinical problem: (1) the clinical and epidemiologic setting in which the pulmonary process is occurring, (2) the rate of progression of the illness, (3) the pattern of radiologic abnormality produced on chest radiography, and (4) the effect of the pneumonitis on pulmonary function tests and arterial blood gas (ABG) measurements.[1,6] A logical approach using these clues and a graduated sequence of diagnostic procedures will enable the clinician to arrive rapidly at the appropriate diagnosis. Such rapid diagnosis and appropriate institution of therapy can, even in this population, result in a gratifying rate of clinical response and meaningful patient survival.

2. Epidemiologic Clues to the Diagnosis of Pulmonary Infection

Three aspects of the epidemiologic history are of importance in evaluating the immunocompromised patient with possible pulmonary infection: the remote epidemiologic history (even dating back to the period prior to the development of the illness that

has resulted in compromised host defenses); the epidemiologic history referable to community and household contacts; and the epidemiologic history related to hospital contacts.[1]

There are three important questions to be asked when the clinician considers the remote epidemiologic history: First, has the patient been exposed to or had evidence of dormant infection with one of the endemic systemic mycotic infections (blastomycosis, coccidioidomycosis, or histoplasmosis) or tuberculosis? Rapidly progressive primary pulmonary infection in compromised hosts has been well documented to occur.[39,40] Far more common is reactivation of dormant infection with one of these agents years after first exposure. Reactivation fungal or mycobacterial infection is of particular concern in patients receiving prolonged corticosteroids and/or cyclophosphamide or azathioprine therapy (i.e., organ transplant recipients and patients with collagen disease receiving such therapy), patients with lymphoma, those with cancer of the lung (especially after the initiation of chemotherapy), and those with AIDS. A controversial issue, in the case of both mycotic infection and tuberculosis, is whether exogenous reinfection occurs in immunocompromised patients with long-dormant tuberculosis or fungal infection.[39-46]

Illustrative Case 1

A 46-year-old man with known lymphoblastic lymphoma previously treated with radiotherapy and chemotherapy, but for the past 6 months on prednisone and weekly vincristine, entered with a 2-week history of a "cold." He had been relatively well until the gradual onset of fever, night sweats, anorexia, 10-lb weight loss, increased fatiguability, and mild dyspnea on exertion. He did not complain of chest pain but had noted some dyspnea on exertion There was no history of past tuberculosis or tuberculous exposure. Although a resident of New England for the past 10 years, for more than 30 years of his life, he had lived and worked on a farm in the San Joaquin Valley Physical examination revealed a chronically ill man with a respiratory rate of 18, temperature of 101°F (38.3°C) coarse rhonchi over the right upper lung field, and an enlarged spleen. Laboratory data revealed a hematocrit (Hct) of 32%, white blood cell (WBC) count of 11,000/mm[3] with 85% polys, 3% bands, and 12% lymphs Both second-strength PPD and *Candida albicans* skin tests were negative, as was a skin test with coccidioidin. Sputum examination revealed abundant polymorphonuclear leukocytes and normal throat flora. Chest radiography revealed a cavitary lesion in the right upper lobe. Room air arterial blood gases (ABGs) revealed Pao_2 88 mm Hg, $Paco_2$ 36 mm Hg, and pH 7.45. Complement-fixing antibody to *Coc-*

cidioides immitis drawn prior to skin testing was positive at a titer of 1 : 64, rising to a titer of 1 : 128 over a 3-week period.

Comment. This is an example of pulmonary coccidioidomycosis reactivating in a patient immunosuppressed by both malignant disease and its treatment. The important clue to the diagnosis lay in the patient's epidemiologic history, with the diagnosis established by serologic testing. A negative coccidioidin skin test and a positive serologic test is the characteristic pattern observed in this circumstance. The combination of well-preserved room air ABGs, focal cavitary lung lesion, and a subacute presentation is quite characteristic of fungal, nocardial, and tuberculous infection (see Section 3). The patient was treated with amphoterocin B (at a total of 3 g) and discontinuation of his prednisone therapy with an excellent clinical response.

The second question to be asked is: Has the patient been exposed to *Strongyloides stercoralis* infection in the past? *S. stercoralis* is unique among the intestinal nematodes affecting humans in that it has an autoinfection cycle that can take place entirely within a person's gastrointestinal (GI) tract. As a result, chronic asymptomatic GI infestation can be maintained for decades after the person has been exposed in an endemic area. With the onset of depressed cell-mediated immune function, either due to disease or its therapy, overwhelming systemic invasion by this organism can occur. Hemorrhagic pulmonary consolidations or diffuse, bilateral alveolar infiltrates, often with accompanying gastrointestinal complaints, may develop. Alternatively, systemic strongyloidiasis may be accompanied by the adult respiratory distress syndrome[47,48] (Chapter 10).

Illustrative Case 2

An 18-year-old Cambodian-born male resident of the United States for 3 years developed end-stage renal disease due to rapidly progressive glomerulonephritis. During a 3-month period of hemodialysis, multiple stool specimens were found free of ova and parasites. The patient then underwent cadaveric renal transplantation, with immunosuppression provided by antithymocyte globulin, azathioprine, and prednisone therapy. Six months posttransplant, at a time when his serum creatinine was 1.2 mg/dl and his immunosuppressive therapy had reached a maintenance level of 100 mg azathioprine and 15 mg prednisone per day, the patient presented to the hospital with a 3-day illness of fever, abdominal cramps, bloody diarrhea, dyspnea, and hemoptysis. Chest radiography revealed a diffuse alveolar infiltrate involving both lungs consistent with that observed with *Pneumocystis carinii*, viral infection, or *Mycoplasma pneumoniae* infection Sputum was bloody and revealed no pathogens. Fiberoptic bronchoscopy with transbronchial biopsy revealed motile *Strongyloides* larvae Despite therapy with Thiabendazole, the patient succumbed on the third hospital day. At postmortem examination, disseminated

strongyloidiasis was found involving the lungs, GI tract, peritoneal cavity, and brain.

Comment. A patient with an otherwise successful renal transplant was tragically lost due to disseminated *S stercoralis* infection predominantly involving his lungs. Such problems have been particularly common in recent years among immigrants from Southeast Asia, such as this patient, and from Central America, who become immunosuppressed. It is noteworthy that repeated examinations for ova and parasites in the stool of this patient pretransplant were unavailing. This is quite common, with purged specimens or some sort of duodenal intubation often being necessary to rule out asymptomatic infestation with this nematode. Unfortunately, although treatment pretransplant is simple, after the onset of immunosuppression and the occurrence of disseminated disease, treatment is quite difficult.

The third question to be asked is: Has the patient received blood transfusions? Post-transfusion leukoagglutinin reactions or transmission of such viruses as cytomegalovirus (CMV) have long been recognized. What is new is the occurrence of post-transfusion AIDS. We have seen, as has every other center caring for AIDS patients, patients without any other risk factor for AIDS presenting from the community with *Pneumocystis* or some other opportunistic pneumonia as the first manifestation of AIDS acquired from a blood transfusion years before.

Illustrative Case 3

A 56-year-old heterosexual business executive presented with a 3-day history of fever, nonproductive cough, and increasing shortness of breath He had no history of drug abuse or homosexual experiences. However, 2½ years previously he had been transfused with 4 units of blood because of an episode of upper GI bleeding from a duodenal ulcer. Since that episode, he had remained completely well, with antacids and cimetidine being his only medication. There was no other significant epidemiologic history. Physical examination revealed a middle-aged man in acute respiratory distress with a respiratory rate of 45. Otherwise, the physical examination was negative. Room air ABGs drawn on admission revealed Pao_2 38 mm Hg, $Paco_2$ 29 mm Hg, and pH 7.56. Chest radiography revealed a bilateral lower lobe peribronchovascular infiltrate. He was immediately intubated and placed on 100% oxygen. Bronchoalveolar lavage yielded both CMV and *Pneumocystis carinii*. Despite therapy with high-dose intravenous trimethoprim–sulfamethoxazole, the patient died on his third hospital day. Serum drawn on admission was positive for antibody to the human immunodeficiency virus (previously known variously as human T-cell Leukemia virus III, lymphadenopathy-associated virus, and AIDS-associated retrovirus). Retrospective tracing of his blood donors revealed that one of his donors, although asymptomatic at the time of blood donation, had subsequently died of AIDS.

Comment The possibility of transfusion-associated AIDS

and the presence of opportunistic infection must now be considered in every patient who presents from the community with pneumonia. Such cases have been observed in persons who have received their transfusions as part of treatment for another illness. This problem is likely to increase.

Most published series devoted to pulmonary infections in immunocompromised patients have emphasized the importance of opportunistic gram-negative, fungal, protozoan, nocardial, and herpes group viral infections.[3-5,10-12] Such series have been primarily concerned with infections in patients with acute leukemia or other illnesses undergoing intensive immunosuppressive therapy within the hospital environment. In our experience, *Streptococcus pneumoniae* is the single most common bacterial infection in the cancer patient and renal transplant patient population, as it is in the normal host, and influenza is the most common viral infection, other than CMV, in the renal transplant patient (see Section 3). These patients with pneumococcal and influenzal infection differ from those with more opportunistic infection in several respects: they acquired their pneumonia in the community when their primary disease was either in remission or relatively quiescent; immunosuppressive therapy was at a minimum; there was a predominance of patients with stable renal transplants, solid tumors, or collagen disease, and a dearth of patients with acute allograft rejection, acute leukemia, etc.; and there was a relatively high level of influenza activity in the community and within their family units. Therefore, for the clinician it is essential to define the status of the patient's primary illness and to differentiate between community-acquired and nosocomially acquired pulmonary infection. If community acquired, then information regarding infectious disease present in the patient's household and community is of great help in diagnosis.[1,68]

Illustrative Case 4

A 32-year-old renal transplant patient was admitted with a 4-hr history of fever, rigors, pleurisy, purulent sputum production, and shortness of breath. The patient had received an HLA-identical kidney from his brother 18 months previously. Since then he had had no episodes of rejection and was maintained on alternate-day prednisone (30 mg every other day) and azathioprine 100 mg/day, with a stable serum creatinine of 1.2 mg/dl. One week prior to admission, he developed an upper respiratory infection characterized by low-grade fever, malaise, anorexia, myalgias, and nonproductive cough. Both his wife and one of his children had similar

illnesses. He appeared to be getting somewhat better, when he was awakened early on the morning of admission with a shaking chill, pleuritic chest pain, an increased cough now productive of purulent blood-tinged sputum, and shortness of breath. Physical examination revealed a toxic, tachypneic gentleman with a temperature of 103.4°F (39.7°C) and a respiratory rate of 35. Herpes labialis was evident to the right of his mouth. Signs of consolidation were present at the left lung base. The renal transplant was of normal size and nontender. Laboratory data revealed Hct of 43%, WBC count of 14,000/mm^3, with 80% polys, 14% bands, 3% lymphs, 3% monocytes, BUN 26 mg/dl, creatinine 1.1 mg/dl. Sputum examination revealed sheets of polymorphonuclear leukocytes and gram-positive diplococci. Sputum and two-blood cultures grew *Streptococcus pneumoniae*. Chest radiography (Fig 1) revealed a focal air space consolidation in the left lower lobe. Room air ABGs indicated Pao$_2$ 44 mm Hg, Paco$_2$ 28 mm Hg, and pH 7.54.

Comment. This is the classic presentation of pneumococcal pneumonia following a viral upper respiratory infection. In this stable renal transplant patient receiving minimal immunosuppressive therapy, the community-acquired pulmonary infection is identical and presents in identical fashion to that seen in the normal host. Physical findings, chest radiography, and ABG pattern are typical for this type of infection. The patient made a complete recovery on conventional penicillin therapy.

The impact of nosocomial pulmonary infection on the compromised host has already been commented on but cannot be overemphasized. The clustering in time and space of two or more cases of pneumonia caused by a particular gram-negative bacillus, fungus, etc., suggests an important environmental hazard worthy of investigation. In dealing with the individual patient, it is useful to know the most common causes of nosocomial infection at a given institution.[1,3-9,16-35,49]

Illustrative Case 5

A 37-year-old woman with acute myelogenous leukemia was undergoing intensive chemotherapy in an attempt to induce remission with cytosine arabinoside, thioguanine, and daunorubicin. She had been severely granulocytopenic for 1 week (absolute granulocyte count of less than 100/mm^3). Chemotherapy had been complicated by frequent nausea and vomiting and by painful ulcerations within her mouth. She had been afebrile until the day in question when she complained of a shaking chill and spiked a temperature of 104°F (40°C). A dry cough and mild shortness of breath were noted. Physical examination revealed an acutely ill woman with a temperature of 103.6°F (39.8°C), a respiratory rate of 30, and a pulse rate of 110. Her skin was remarkable for multiple petechiae and ecchymoses, particularly at blood-drawing sites. Faint rales were heard at the right lung base. Laboratory data included Hct 29%, WBC count of 400 (100% lymphocytes), platelet count of 10,000. Chest radiography revealed atelectasis

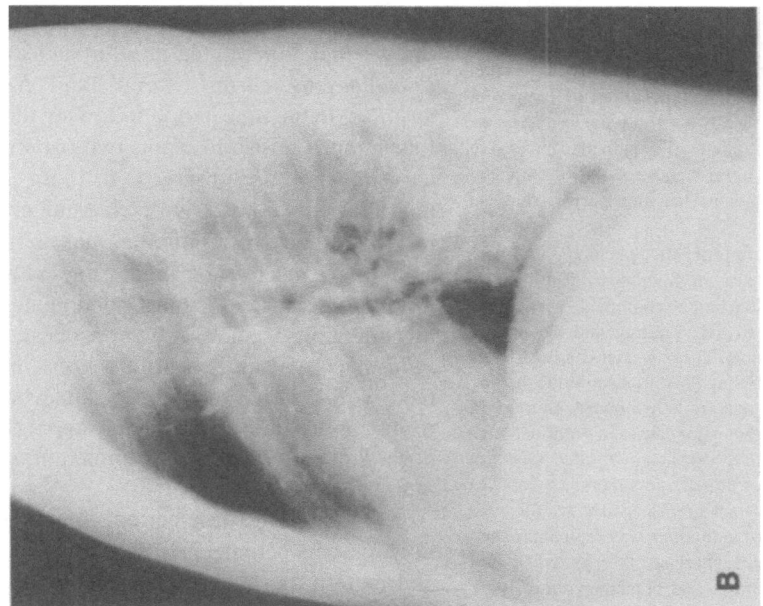

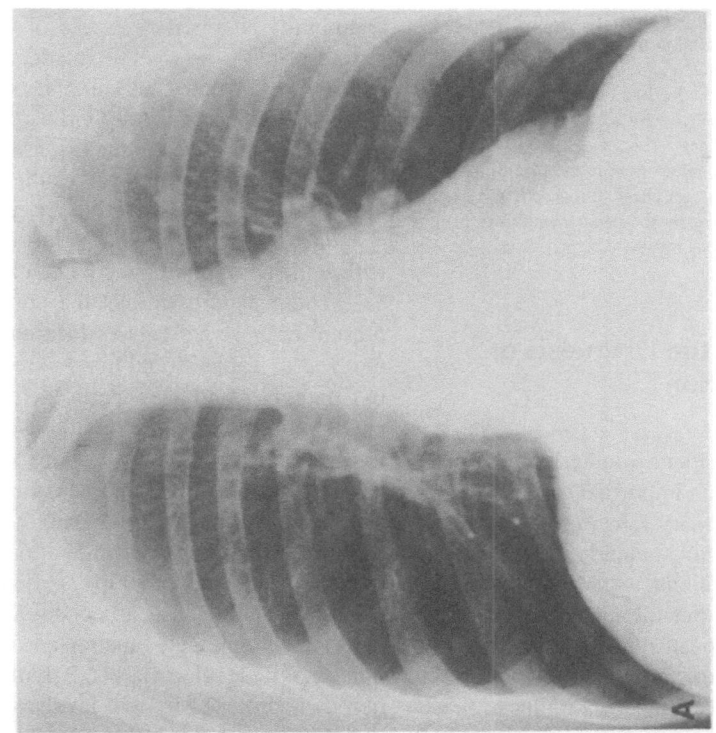

FIGURE 1. Left lower lobe pneumococcal pneumonia. (A) A left lower lobe consolidation is hidden behind the heart. (B) The lateral view, however, clearly shows a large, posterior basal density. This appearance is typical of the peripheral, nonsegmental consolidation associated with pneumonococcal pneumonia.

with or without a small infiltrate at the right base. After platelet transfusion brought the platelet count to 60,000, transtracheal aspiration was carried out and yielded a small amount of sputum, which on Gram stain revealed gram-negative rods. She was begun on therapy with cephalothin and gentamicin. Culture of the sputum and three blood cultures subsequently grew out *Klebsiella pneumoniae* sensitive to these two antibiotics. The patient responded to her antimicrobial therapy and ultimately went into a complete remission of her acute myelogenous leukemia, with complete clearing of her chest radiograph.

Comment. In this setting, gram-negative pneumonia is by far the most likely diagnosis, as it was in this patient. Presumably, gram-negative pharyngeal colonization combined with mini-aspiration episodes secondary to the vomiting and the painful mouth lesions led to this pneumonia. The physicians caring for this patient were greatly helped in chosing the initial antibiotic therapy by being aware of the following data from their own institution. In this population at this hospital, the major causes of gram-negative pneumonia were *Klebsiella* and *Escherichia coli*, with *Pseudomonas* being an uncommon cause of primary pneumonia. Second, at this institution, gentamicin-resistant gram-negative bacilli were rare. Hence, the initial choice of antibiotics was cephalothin and gentamicin in an attempt to obtain synergistic therapy, whereas at other institutions where *Pseudomonas* and/or gentamicin-resistant gram-negative bacilli occur in appreciable numbers, initial therapy would require the substitution of amikacin for gentamicin and the use of ticarcillin, carbenicillin, pipercillin, or mezlocillin in place of, or in addition to, the cephalothin to provide potentially synergistic therapy against possible *Pseudomonas* infection. In other circumstances, imipenem or a third-generation cephalosporin might be employed, although usually not alone or as initial therapy. The other point to be emphasized here is the occurrence of bacteremia in this granulocytopenic patient in the face of a rather unimpressive infiltrate visible on her chest radiograph. The extent of the infiltrate is clearly limited by the decreased ability of the patient to mount an inflammatory response.

3. Clinical Clues to the Diagnosis of Pulmonary Infection

The status of the patient's underlying disease and its therapy will have an important effect in determining the type of pulmonary infection that will develop. This may be seen most clearly in renal transplant patients and in patients with lymphoma. In renal transplant patients, pneumonias occurring during the first 3–4 weeks post-transplant are virtually never caused by opportunistic pathogens but rather are the result of bacterial pathogens similar to those causing postoperative pneumonia in other surgical patients—aspiration pneumonia resulting from mouth flora or gram-negative bacilli. In the period 1–4 months post-transplant, the most important factor is CMV infection (see Chapters 3 and 21), with CMV

being the most important single cause of pulmonary infection at this time and also predisposing to potentially lethal superinfection with such organisms as *Pneumocystis carinii*, fungi, and *Nocardia asteroides*. In the time period following this, more than four months post-transplant, two patterns of pulmonary infection are observed. In those patients with normally functioning grafts (serum creatinine ≤ 2 mg/dl) who are receiving minimal immunosuppression (<20 mg/day of prednisone plus ≤ 100 mg azathioprine per day), most pneumonias are caused by community-acquired pneumococcal, *Hemophilus influenzae*, and influenzal infections. For those patients with poorly functioning grafts who continue to receive more intensive immunosuppression, fungal, nocardial, and *Pneumocystis* infection are most common.[6,50–53]

Although the time period–infection correlation in lymphoma patients is less clear cut, a similar general pattern may be observed. Patients with newly diagnosed lymphoma have a low incidence of pneumonia, and, when present, the pneumonias are of the community-acquired type. As disease and therapy progress, both the overall incidence of pneumonia and the occurrence of fungal, nocardial, *Pneumocystis*, and herpes group virus infections increase. In the terminal stages of the disease or at times when intensive chemotherapy has resulted in severe granulocytopenia, gram-negative pneumonia and *Aspergillus* infections similar to those seen in patients with acute nonlymphocytic leukemia predominate.[51]

These patterns reflect the host defense defects present in these patients at different times. As summarized in Table 2 (and more extensively discussed in Chapters 2 and 3), specific defects predispose to pneumonia with specific microbial agents. Of special importance are the net effect of the underlying disease, the therapy employed, and the modifying effect of other infections in decreasing host defenses. For example, following a combination of splenectomy, radiation, and chemotherapy, patients with Hodgkin disease, which itself is associated with profound defects in T-lymphocyte function and cell-mediated immunity, will develop marked B-lymphocyte dysfunction as manifested by low levels of serum IgM and specific antibody against *Hemophilus influenzae* type B, poor response to pneumococcal vaccine, and an increased risk of life-threatening systemic and pulmonary infection with these two organisms.[54,55] Although the incidence of *Pneumocystis carinii* infec-

TABLE 2. Pulmonary Infections to which Patients with Specific Host-Defense Defects Are Predisposed[a]

Host-defense defect	Pulmonary infections to which patient is predisposed
Oral and tracheobronchial ulceration and/or obstruction	Oral bacteria flora Enterobacteriaceae
Decrease in the number of fully functional granulocytes	Oral bacterial flora Enterobacteriaceae Aspergillus sp Pseudomonas aeruginosa
Hypogammaglobulinemia	Streptococcus pneumoniae Hemophilus influenzae type B (Pneumocystis carinii)
Depressed cell-mediated immunity	Typical and atypical mycobacteria Fungi Viruses (cytomegalovirus, varicella–zoster virus, herpes simplex, measles virus) Pneumocystis carinii Toxoplasma gondii Strongyloides stercoralis
Complement defects	Streptococcus pneumoniae H. influenzae type B

[a]Modified from Rubin [1] Infections uncommonly associated with a particular defect are listed in parentheses

tion is somewhat increased in patients with defects in cell-mediated immunity and antibody synthesis, the occurrence rate is markedly increased when corticosteroid therapy and/or CMV infection are added to the underlying illness.[3,6,56,57] Thus, it is best to think in terms of the net state of immunosuppression, which is contributed to by the underlying disease, its therapy, the presence of such immune-modulating viruses as the AIDS virus, CMV, Epstein-Barr virus (EBV), and non-A, non-B hepatitis, and certain metabolic factors. Of the metabolic factors so far defined that have adverse effects on host defenses, the most important appear to be uremia, hyperglycemia, and protein-calorie malnutrition.[51]

Perhaps the most useful clue to the correct diagnosis in patients with the febrile pneumonitis syndrome comes from an assessment of the mode of onset and rate of progression of the pulmonary process. Thus, an acute onset over less than 24 hr of symptoms severe enough to bring the patient to medical attention would suggest conventional bacterial infection (and, of the noninfectious causes, pulmonary embolic disease, pulmonary edema, a leukoagglutinin reaction, or pulmonary hemorrhage). A subacute onset over a few days to a week would suggest viral or *Mycoplasma* infection, *Pneumocystis*, or, in some instances, *Aspergillus* or *Nocardia*. A more chronic course over 1 or more weeks would suggest fungal, nocardial, or tuberculous infection (as well as tumor, radiation- or drug-induced pneumonitis). When the mode of clinical presentation is combined with the radiologic finding, the range of etiologic possibilities becomes considerably smaller and much more manageable for the clinician (Table 3).

Additional useful information may also be obtained by measuring the arterial partial pressure of oxygen (Pao_2) while the patient is breathing room air. Most of the disease processes causing the febrile

TABLE 3. Differential Diagnosis of Fever and Pulmonary Infiltrates in the Compromised Host According to Roentgenographic Abnormality and the Rate of Progression of the Symptoms[a]

Chest radiographic abnormality	Etiology according to the rate of progression of the illness	
	Acute	Subacute–chronic
Consolidation	Bacterial (including Legionnaires' disease) Thromboembolic Hemorrhage (pulmonary edema)	Fungal Nocardial Tuberculous Tumor (Viral, *Pneumocystis,* radiation, drug-induced)
Peribronchovascular ("interstitial") infiltrate	Pulmonary edema Leukoagglutinin reaction (bacterial)	Viral *Pneumocystis* Radiation Drug-induced (fungal, nocardial, tuberculous, tumor)
Nodular infiltrate[b]	(Bacterial, pulmonary edema)	Tumor Fungal Nocardial Tuberculous (*Pneumocystis*)

[a]Modified from Rubin [1] An acute illness is one developing and requiring medical attention in a matter of a relatively few hours (less than 24) A subacute–chronic process develops over several days to weeks Note that unusual causes of a process are placed in parentheses

[b]A nodular infiltrate is defined as one or more large (>1 cm² on chest radiography) focal defects with well-defined, more-or-less-rounded edges, surrounded by aerated lung Multiple tiny nodules of smaller size, as sometimes caused by such an agent as varicella–zoster virus or cytomegalovirus, are not included here

pneumonitis syndrome in the compromised host are associated with significant impairment in oxygenation early in the clinical course (room air Pao_2 <65 mm Hg). By contrast, most patients with pulmonary disease caused by fungi, tuberculosis, *Nocardia*, and tumor will have relatively well-maintained oxygenation (room air Pao_2 >70 mm Hg) despite massive consolidation on chest radiography until very late in the clinical course. Although a rare patient with these three forms of infection will have an acute overwhelming pneumonia resembling acute bacterial infection both in clinical presentation and ABG findings, the great majority will have subacute or chronic presentations associated with well-preserved oxygenation. For example, among 14 renal transplant patients with primary fungal or nocardial pulmonary infections, 12 had a Pao_2 value of >70 mm Hg. The two exceptions had concomitant congestive heart failure (CHF) and chronic obstructive pulmonary disease (COPD) to explain their low Pao_2 values. The hypoxemia in patients with acute bacterial and viral infection and the noninfectious causes of the febrile pneumonitis syndrome results from a large shunt combined with regions of low ventilation–perfusion (V/Q) ratios in the involved lung tissues. Maintenance of the Pao_2 in the fungal, nocardial, tuberculous, and, presumably, tumor patients appears to be because of diversion of blood flow away from the involved lung, thus minimizing V/Q mismatch. The pathogenetic mechanism for this may be either direct invasion of the blood vessels or a strong, unopposed reflex arteriolar vasoconstriction in response to regional alveolar hypoxia. This is best shown by the inadequate rise in Pao_2 when 100% oxygen is inhaled in those patients with a large shunt (the patients with viral, bacterial, and other causes of pneumonia), whereas there is a relatively normal Pao_2 (>450 mm Hg) when perfusion and ventilation have both been interrupted (as in the fungal, nocardial, and tuberculous cases). It may also be possible to show this feature by particulate radioisotope scanning.[1,6,51]

4. Clinical Clues to the Diagnosis of Noninfectious Causes of Febrile Pneumonitis Syndrome

The occurrence of noninfectious causes of the febrile pneumonitis syndrome in the compromised host is related to the underlying disease and how it is treated. Thus, in the patient with malignant disease, the major causes of this syndrome are radiation pneumonitis, drug-induced pulmonary injury, and parenchymal tumor invasion. In the renal transplant patient, in the patient receiving corticosteroids, and in other groups of patients immunocompromised by nonmalignant disease, the major considerations are pulmonary emboli and pulmonary edema. Less commonly, any patient with a major clotting or platelet disorder can develop pulmonary hemorrhage, and any transfused patient is at risk for the development of a leukoagglutinin reaction (Table 1).[1,6,8,59]

4.1. Radiation Pneumonitis

Radiation lung injury is of two types: an acute type, radiation pneumonitis, which begins 1–6 months after completion of a course of radiation therapy; and a chronic type, radiation fibrosis, which may follow acute disease or begin without previous symptoms 6 or more months following the completion of therapy. Pathologically, radiation pneumonitis is characterized by the desquamation of bronchiolar and alveolar cells and by the formation of protein-rich hyaline membranes as a result of the exudation of plasma into the alveolar spaces through injured pulmonary capillaries. Engorgement and thrombosis of capillaries and arterioles are evident, and the alveolar septa are thickened by lymphocytic infiltrates and immature collagen deposition. Radiation fibrosis is characterized by the replacement of normal pulmonary parenchyma and architecture by dense connective tissue. Clinically, radiation pneumonitis begins insidiously with fever without rigors, nonproductive cough, progressive dyspnea, and a characteristic pattern of pulmonary infiltrates on chest radiography (see Illustrative Case 6). Radiation fibrosis, as its name suggests, is not associated with symptoms of inflammation: it is usually asymptomatic, and, when symptoms are present, these are related to the progressive pulmonary fibrosis: dyspnea, orthopnea, cyanosis, clubbing, and cor pulmonale.[60–64]

Because of the nature of the radiation therapy administered, symptomatic radiation injury of the lung is most common in patients receiving radiotherapy for breast cancer, lung cancer, and lymphoma, patients in whom symptomatic disease develops in approximately 5–15% of those at risk.[60] The incidence and severity of radiation lung injury are largely determined by the characteristics of the radiation administered: the volume of lung exposed, the total dose, and the rate at which the radiation is delivered. The greater the volume of lung exposed, the higher the dose (radiation pneumonitis rarely occurs at doses of less than 2000 rad but is almost invariable with doses of greater than 6000 rad), and the shorter the period of time over which the therapy is administered (fractionation of therapy permits repair of sublethal damage between doses), the higher is the incidence of radiation lung disease. In addition, certain modifying factors greatly enhance the risk of radiation damage, the most important of these being previous radiotherapy to the lung, abrupt withdrawal of corticosteroid treatment, and the concomitant administration of cytotoxic cancer chemotherapy. Surprisingly, preexisting chronic obstructive pulmonary disease (COPD) appears not to play an important role. Finally, there appears to be individual variability in susceptibility to radiation injury, as there are several reports of severe pneumonitis developing after relatively small doses of radiation.[49,60,65-73]

Thus, the clinician should be highly suspicious of the possibility of radiation pneumonitis in a patient with one of the tumor types noted who has a subacute–chronic onset of respiratory symptoms following the completion of a course of radiotherapy and from whom a history of one or more of the adjunctive factors can be obtained. Early diagnosis by biopsy can lead to effective therapy with corticosteroids, although such therapy will be ineffective if significant delay occurs.[60,74]

Illustrative Case 6

A 41-year-old woman with known Hodgkin disease presented with a 3-week history of increasing dyspnea, nonproductive cough, fever, night sweats, and malaise. Stage IIIB Hodgkin disease was diagnosed 6 months previously and was treated with 5000 rad to the mediastinum and paraaortic lymph nodes followed by cyclic MOPP chemotherapy (nitrogen mustard, vincristine, prednisone, and procarbazine), the most recent cycle having been completed 2 weeks previously. The patient noted the insidious onset of fever, nonproductive cough, malaise, and dyspnea on exertion. Although she was quite dyspneic by the time she sought medical attention, the patient could not designate any one time when a major change in her clinical status occurred. No significant travel exposures had occurred, and there were no illnesses in her family. Physical examination revealed a dyspneic woman with a temperature of 101°F (38.3°C) and a respiratory rate of 35. General physical examination was unrevealing. Laboratory data included Hct 34%, WBC count 5400/mm³ with 82% polys, 11% lymphs, 7% monocytes. ABGs on Room air revealed a Pao_2 value of 42 mm Hg, $Paco_2$ 28

mm Hg, $Paco_2$ 28 mm Hg, and pH 7.52. Chest radiography revealed a diffuse peribronchovascular infiltrate predominantly central in distribution (Fig. 2). Transtracheal aspiration was nonrevealing. The diagnosis of radiation pneumonitis was made by transbronchial biopsy taken through the fiberoptic bronchoscope. The patient was treated with corticosteroids with marked improvement. Two weeks after the initiation of steroids, room air ABGs revealed a Pao_2 value of 90 mm Hg, $Paco_2$ 36 mm Hg, and pH 7 45.

Comment. This is a classic case of radiation pneumonitis—insidious onset of febrile pneumonitis syndrome in the appropriate clinical setting with a typical chest radiograph. However, the clinicians dealing with this patient could not rule out *Pneumocystis carinii* infection, and since the therapy for *Pneumocystis* (trimethoprim–sulfamethoxazole) is so different from the therapy for radiation pneumonitis (corticosteroids), an invasive diagnostic procedure was necessary to establish the diagnosis. In this situation, with this type of radiographic abnormality, transbronchial biopsy is the initial diagnostic procedure of choice.

4.2. Drug-Induced Pneumonitis

Several chemotherapeutic agents, most notably bleomycin, busulfan, cyclophosphamide, and chlorambucil produce pulmonary injury akin to that caused by radiation (Table 4). It should be assumed that all alkylating agents have this ability because of their radiomimetic and mutagenic capabilities. In the lung, these effects cause injury, particularly to the lining epithelium of the alveoli and to the alveolar capillary endothelium, resulting, as in radiation lung injury, in two clinical syndromes: a progressive interstitial pneumonitis characterized by fever without chills, as well as dyspnea, nonproductive cough, and progressive hypoxia beginning weeks to months after significant amounts of the drug have been administered, and a chronic interstitial fibrosis that may follow symptomatic inflammatory lung disease or occur insidiously without previous warning. Some patients may have symptoms due to drug-induced lung injury but negative chest radiographs. In these instances, a decrease in CO diffusing capacity or a positive ^{67}Ga scan can be helpful.[8]

The inflammatory manifestations, like early radiation pneumonitis, may be responsive to the cessation of the provoking drug and the initiation of steroid therapy, whereas the chronic fibrotic process often is not. Again, as with radiation pneumonitis, both the dose of the agent administered (and the time course over which it is administered) and individual susceptibility to lung injury appear to be important in the pathogenesis of this process. Given the similarities among the presumed pathogenesis, radiographic and

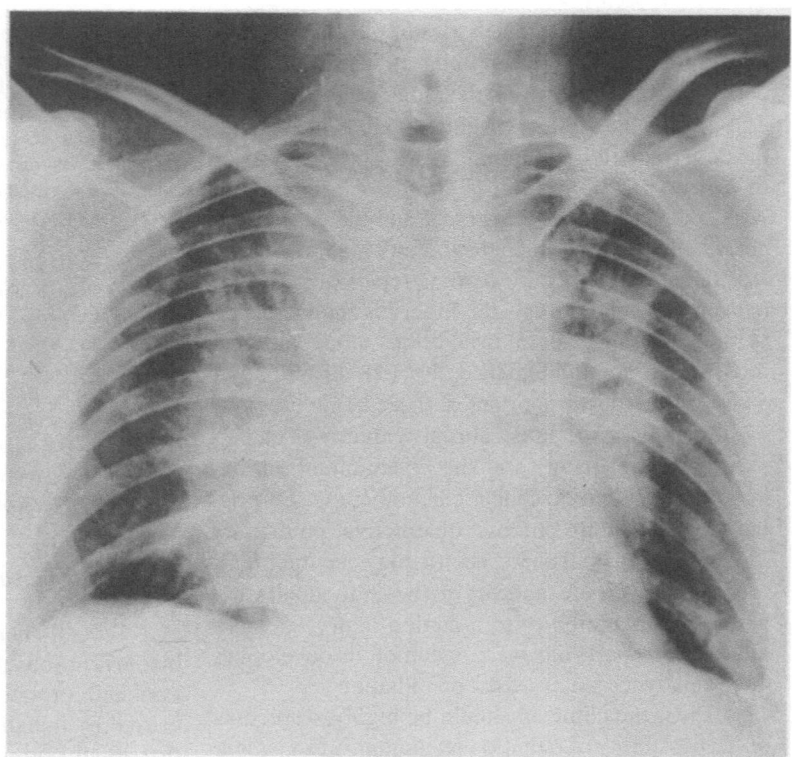

FIGURE 2. Radiation pneumonitis. The bilateral paramediastinal opacification of the lungs corresponding to radiation portals is typical of radiation pneumonitis 2 months after completion of treatment.

histologic appearances, and clinical presentation of drug-induced and radiation lung injury, it is not surprising that the combination of these treatment modalities is associated with a greater risk of pulmonary disease than is either type of agent used alone.[75–77] It has been suggested that both the drug and radiation induce local production of oxygen radicals such as hydrogen peroxide and superoxide anions, which then produce lung injury. Consistent with this hypothesis is the observation that oxygen administration to a patient receiving bleomycin will accelerate drug-induced pulmonary toxicity.[78–80] Both types of lung injury are associated with restrictive defects and lowered diffusing capacities on pulmonary function testing.[81–83] Given the subacute onset of symptoms, the interstitial pulmonary infiltrate, and the clinical setting, the major differential diagnostic considerations are *Pneumocystis carinii* infection and viral pneumonitis. Usually, these can only be distinguished by lung biopsy.[84–91]

Of all the cancer chemotherapeuic agents, busulfan and bleomycin are the drugs most commonly implicated as causes of pulmonary injury. In the case of busulfan, pulmonary injury is usually observed in patients placed on maintenance long-term therapy with this agent in the treatment of chronic myelogenous leukemia or, less commonly, polycythemia vera. In these patients, pulmonary disease may develop as early as 1 year after the initiation of such therapy but more commonly requires up to 4 years.[92,93] The incidence of busulfan lung injury is not well established but appears to be less than 5%. For example, in one series of 23 well-studied patients followed for an average period of approximately 2 years, only one patient developed clinical pulmonary disease, and this patient received a smaller dose of busulfan than did several of the other patients. Pathologically, intraalveolar fibrosis and large atypical alveolar mononuclear cells may be seen in a much higher percentage of patients receiving chronic busulfan therapy.[94–97]

Bleomycin is the single most common cause of drug-induced pulmonary injury; in an estimated 2.5–10% of patients receiving this agent, symptomatic pulmonary disease develops, and the reported mortality approaches 50%.[86–102] Clinically manifest lung injury will occur in most patients receiving a cumulative bleomycin dose greater than 500 mg.[99] In

TABLE 4. Cytotoxic and Noncytotoxic Chemotherapeautic Agents Known to Induce Pulmonary Disease[a,b]

Cytotoxic	Noncytotoxic
Azathioprine	Bleomycin sulfate
Bleomycin sulfate	Cytosine arabinoside
Busulfan	Methotrexate sodium
Chlorambucil	Procarbazine hydrochloride
Cyclophosphamide	
Hydroxyurea	
Melphalan	
Mitomycin	
Nitrosourea (BCNU, CCNU, methyl-CCNU)	
Procarbazine hydrochloride	

[a]Modified from Rosenow et al [8]

[b]Not that although both bleomycin and procarbazine are mainly associated with cytotoxic reactions, noncytotoxic reactions have also been observed, albeit uncommonly

addition, there have now been several reports[102–104] of life-threatening pulmonary disease when as little as 50–180 mg has been administered. Early pulmonary injury may be detected by the demonstration of a decrease in diffusing capacity and vital capacity at a time when the chest radiograph is still normal.[100,103] An important clue for the clinician is the relatively high rate of bleomycin toxicity in patients who have received prior radiotherapy. For example, in one study of 101 patients receiving bleomycin therapy, 5 of 12 who had received previous radiotherapy showed the development of pulmonary disease, whereas only 4 of 89 not receiving radiotherapy showed the development of comparable pulmonary injury.[101,102]

The nitrosourea compounds (BCNU, CCNU, and methyl-CCNU) have also emerged as important causes of cytotoxic drug-associated pulmonary injury.[105,106] The pulmonary injury appears to be identical to that caused by busulfan and bleomycin. Less commonly, cyclophosphamide[75,107–109] and chlorambucil[110–112] appear to be associated with the same process.

Illustrative Case 7

A 51-year-old man with Hodgkin disease was admitted with a 2-week history of fever, night sweats, and increasing shortness of breath. Two years earlier, Hodgkin disease was diagnosed and was treated with splenectomy, total nodal irradiation, and several cycles of MOPP therapy after it had been staged as IIIA. Eight months previously, recurrent disease involving the lung, liver, and bone was diagnosed, and bleomycin was begun with a total dose of 340 mg given by the time of admission. Over the 2 weeks prior to admission, fever, night sweats, nonproductive cough, and slowly increasing dyspnea were noted. No travel exposures were reported, and all family members were well. On physical examination his temperature was 100.6°F (38.1°C), respiratory rate was 30, and pulse rate was 90. He was a chronically ill appearing man in mild respiratory distress. Fine rales were heard over both lung bases. Laboratory evaluation revealed Hct 34%, WBC count of 3200 with 83% polys, 4% lymphs, 13% monocytes. Room air ABGs revealed a Pao_2 of 54 mm Hg, $Paco_2$ 32 mm Hg, and pH 7.50. Chest radiography revealed a diffuse peribronchovascular infiltrate in both lung fields, most prominent at the bases (Fig. 3). Transtracheal aspiration was negative, but transbronchial biopsy via the fiberoptic bronchoscope yielded characteristic changes of bleomycin-induced lung disease, with no evidence of infection. Therapy with corticosteroids was associated with symptomatic improvement and an increase in room air Pao_2 to approximately 60–65 mm Hg. Over the next 3 months, he remained stable with respect to respiration and showed no major change in the chest radiograph. However, he succumbed to progressive Hodgkin disease at this point. At postmortem examination, a mixed pulmonary picture consisting of extensive intraalveolar fibrosis, interstitial pneumonitis with frequent large atypical alveolar mononuclear cells were observed—the typical picture of bleomycin (and busulfan) lung injury.

Comment. This was a typical presentation of bleomycin-induced lung disease in a patient predisposed to its development by the previous radiotherapy he had received. The dose of bleomycin he received, although not excessive, was clearly in the range associated with at least a 5–10% risk of pulmonary toxicity. Again, the treatable differential diagnostic possibilities based on the chest radiograph and clinical course lay chiefly between bleomycin lung disease and *Pneumocystis*. Transbronchial biopsy provided an easy, well-tolerated means of diagnosis. Only a moderate response to corticosteroid therapy was observed in this case.

Methotrexate, an antimetabolite widely used in the chemotherapy of leukemia and other neoplastic conditions, in bone marrow transplantation, and in the treatment of certain skin diseases such as psoriasis may also be associated with subacute and chronic pulmonary injury syndromes. However, there are important differences from the pulmonary injury syndromes produced by radiation and the alkylating agents: methotrexate appears to cause an acute allergic granulomatous reaction that may subside despite the continuation of therapy, although progressive chronic interstitial fibrosis may also develop. The duration of methotrexate therapy before the onset of symptoms can range from less than 1 month to more than 5 years with an average weekly dose during this period of 25–50 mg. Clinical disease and radiographic findings resemble those seen with

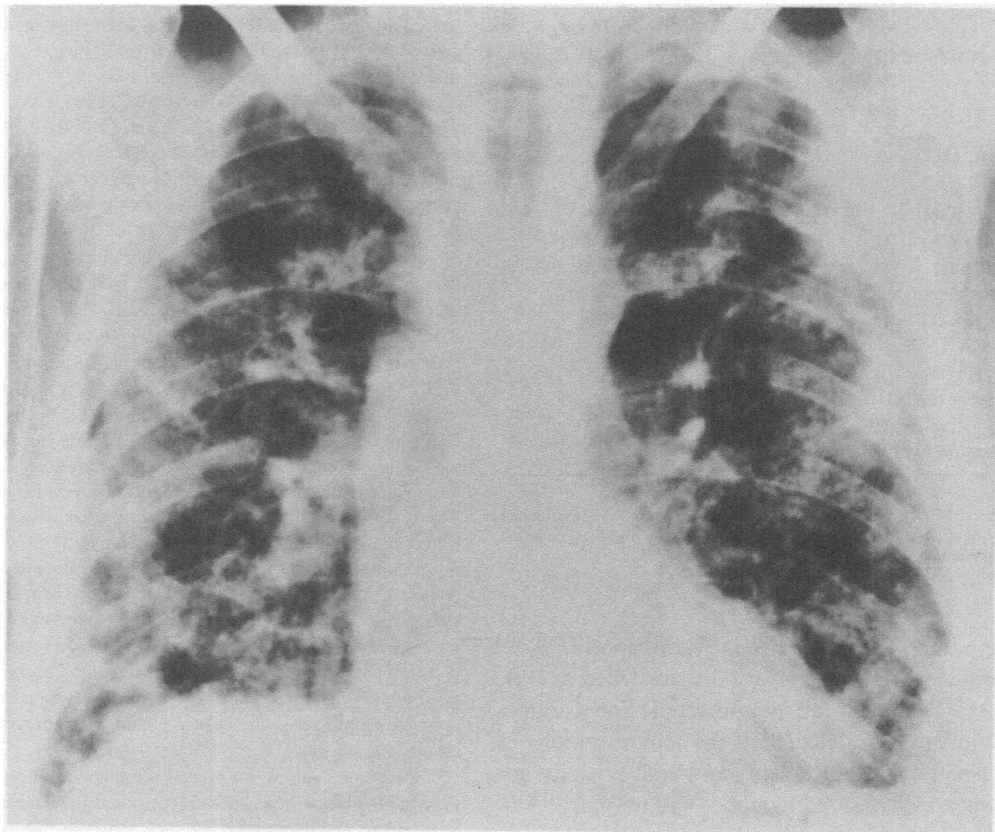

FIGURE 3. Bleomycin lung. Multiple irregular opacities are present throughout the periphery of the lungs. This is the most characteristic appearance of bleomycin lung

the other agents but, reflecting the probable allergic nature of the process, eosinophilia is the rule rather than the exception.[75,113–121] The incidence of at least transient methotrexate-induced pulmonary injury can be exceedingly high, with 41% of children receiving maintenance methotrexate therapy in one report manifesting pulmonary symptoms.[122] Not surprisingly, preceding radiation therapy appears to play no role in predisposing patients to this form of pulmonary injury. Rarely, bleomycin, cytosine arabinoside, and procarbazine can produce lung injury with a methotrexate-like pathologic picture—presumably due to a similar allergic rather than cytotoxic mechanism.[8,121]

Other agents to which compromised patients may be exposed that may be associated with the production of either or both the febrile pneumonitis syndrome and chronic interstitial fibrosis include melphalan,[123] azathioprine,[124] diphenylhydantoin,[125] amitriptyline,[126] and parenteral gold therapy.[127] It is likely that other agents will also be recognized in the future.

4.3. Neoplastic Pulmonary Invasion

Fever and a clinical presentation suggesting pneumonia caused by neoplastic invasion of the lung may sometimes occur, particularly in patients with lymphoma. In patients with Hodgkin disease, pulmonary involvement occurs in 20–30% of patients, with most of these having the nodular sclerosis type of tumor. Almost invariably, Hodgkin disease of the lung is associated with mediastinal lymph node involvement (or at least a history of previously treated mediastinal disease). In the rare Hodgkin disease patient with pulmonary invasion in the absence of mediastinal adenopathy, there is almost always evidence of extrathoracic disease.[128-131]

Primary intrathoracic disease is uncommon in patients with non-Hodgkin lymphoma (4% in one series of 1269 patients,[132] but in approximately half of these, thoracic disease will eventually develop). Primary pulmonary disease accounts for only 10% of these thoracic cases, with lymphocytic lymphoma being the histologic type most frequently encountered.[132,133] Unlike the situation in Hodgkin disease, a significant proportion of these patients may have pulmonary involvement in the absence of mediastinal nodal disease.[131-134]

Leukemia patients may occasionally have leukemic infiltrates in their lungs with associated fever, especially in patients with acute monocytic and chronic lymphatic leukemia. Necropsy studies would suggest that as many as 25% of such patients will have leukemic pulmonary invasion. Occasionally, particularly in leukemic patients with WBC counts greater than 200,000/mm^3, and a high percentage of blast cells, leukostasis and occlusion of pulmonary vessels may produce pulmonary symptoms and even infiltrates on chest radiographs. Superinfection of such areas is quite common. Because of decreased compliance within small blood vessels, leukemic blast cells may be particularly important in the pathogenesis of the intravascular leukostasis.[8,135-137] A variation of this process is what has been termed *leukemic cell lysis pneumonopathy*, in which persons with large numbers of circulating leukemic blasts develop fever, respiratory distress, and patchy lung infiltrates within a few days of rapid chemotherapy-induced destruction of blasts. It has been suggested that this represents either diffuse alveolar or pulmonary capillary damage due to enzymes released locally by the destroyed blast cells.[8,138] However, infiltrates in such patients sufficient to cause radiographic abnormalities are much more frequently the result of infection, hemorrhage, or heart failure, and the clinician should proceed on this basis rather than passing off such infiltrates as being caused by the leukemia.[139,140]

Perhaps the most common association between neoplastic pulmonary invasion and the febrile pneumonitis syndrome is related to endobronchial lesions from primary or metastatic cancer that may cause bronchial obstruction, distal atelectasis, and bacterial infection. Bronchoscopic demonstration of such lesions can be quite useful and lead to effective surgical or radiation therapy.[131]

Illustrative Case 8

A 58-year-old man with a long history of cigarette smoking (at least 50 pack-years) presented with a 2-day history of fever, rigors, an increasing cough productive of blood-tinged, greenish sputum, and progressive shortness of breath. The patient had had a long history of COPD, with a history of several hospitalizations for acute bronchitis/bronchopneumonia over the past 5 years. Over the 3 months prior to admission, he had an increased morning cough, occasionally productive of blood-tinged sputum. During this period, he was more easily fatigued than usual and was somewhat anorectic. Two days prior to admission, he developed a fever, felt chilly, and began coughing an increasingly purulent sputum that was occasionally blood tinged. Over the 12 hr prior to admission, he had noted increasing shortness of breath.

Physical examination on admission revealed a temperature of 100.6°F (38.1°C), respiratory rate of 36, BP 130/60, pulse rate of 110. Examination of his fingers revealed definite clubbing of the nails. Chest examination showed an increased anterior–posterior diameter, low-lying diaphragm, and signs of consolidation over his left upper lung field. There were diffuse rhonchi on both sides of the chest, more prominent on the left than on the right.

Laboratory evaluation revealed Hct 34%, WBC count of 14,000 with 81% polys, 7% bands, 6% lymphs, 6% monocytes. Room air ABGs revealed a Pao$_2$ of 58 mm Hg, Paco$_2$ 34 mm Hg, and pH 7.46. Chest radiography demonstrated a left upper lobe consolidation with air bronchograms (Fig. 4). Gram stain of the expectorated sputum revealed abundant polymorphonuclear leukocytes and a mixed flora of gram-positive cocci and gram-negative rods. Cultures grew normal throat flora and *E. coli*. Therapy was begun with clindamycin and gentamicin, with no clinical response over the first 48 hr. Initial sputum cytologies were negative, but on the third hospital day bronchoscopy revealed a partially obstructing bronchogenic carcinoma. Drainage of the involved lung was initially accomplished via bronchoscopic biopsy. With this, aggressive chest physical therapy, and continued antibiotics, the pneumonia responded to therapy. A course of palliative radiation therapy was given to further improve pulmonary drainage.

Comment. The radiographic pattern in which the pulmonary infiltrate was contained within particular bronchopulmonary segments was highly suggestive of a pneumonia in association with a partially obstructing mass lesion—in this case, a bronchogenic carcinoma. The index of suspicion for lung cancer was particularly high in this chronic smoker with evidence of clubbing of his fingernails. The failure of response to initial therapy led rapidly to bronchoscopy and appropriate diagnosis and therapy.

4.4. Other Noninfectious Causes of Febrile Pneumonitis Syndrome

Even in immunosuppressed patients without neoplastic disease, noninfectious causes of the feb-

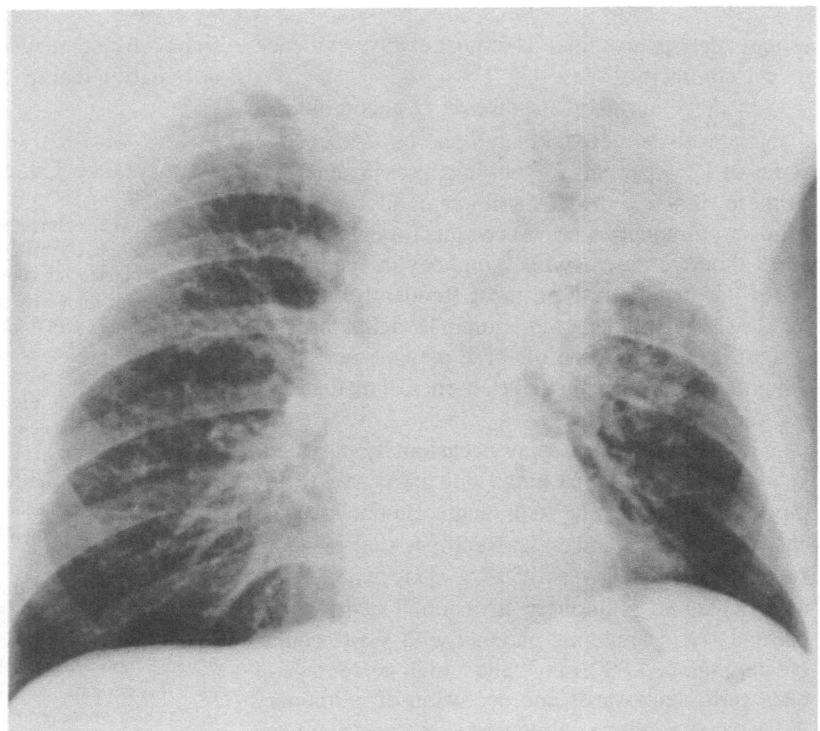

FIGURE 4. Pneumonia distal to left upper lobe carcinoma. The left upper lobe consolidation demonstrates multiple air bronchograms. The partially obstructing left upper lobe carcinoma is not visible, but the pneumonia distal to the tumor is apparent.

rile pneumonitis syndrome account for approximately 25% of such cases. Here, pulmonary emboli and atypical pulmonary edema are the major causes. Such difficulties are particularly prominent in renal transplant patients.[6,141,142] In these patients, surgical manipulation of pelvic or lower extremity venous structures are especially associated with pulmonary emboli, acute allograft failure, oliguria, and fluid overload (rather than primary cardiac disease) in patients with pulmonary edema. In particular, Freidman et al.[142] reported two renal transplant patients in whom the radiographic findings of pulmonary edema were almost entirely unilateral, thus closely mimicking an infectious process. A major difference between immunosuppressed patients and normal patients with these forms of primary pulmonary disease is the high rate of superinfection in the immunosuppressed patient. For example, in one series of renal transplant patients, eight of nine patients with pulmonary embolic disease developed life-threatening superinfection,[6] with rates of superinfection nearly as high being noted in patients on high-dose corticosteroids, those with lymphoma, and

those with other causes of significant immunosuppression.

An unusual cause of fever and pulmonary infiltrate in the compromised host is a leukoagglutinin reaction. Leukoagglutinin reactions result in a syndrome of febrile pulmonary edema of noncardiac origin characterized by the abrupt onset of fever, chills, tachypnea, nonproductive cough, and respiratory distress in the first 24 hr following blood transfusion (and most commonly during the transfusion or in the first few hours following it). Such reactions are initiated by the interaction of preformed agglutinating antibodies with antigens on leukocyte surfaces, probably both of HLA and non-HLA type. The antibodies may be present in the patient's serum because of sensitization by past transfusions or pregnancies and are directed against leukocytes transfused with the unit of blood; conversely, the antibodies may be present in the plasma of the blood being transfused and be acting against the patient's leukocytes. Clearly, such reactions can best be avoided by using red cell preparations for transfusion such as frozen red blood cells (RBCs) or washed, packed RBCs relatively free of both exogenous leukocytes and plasma that could contain preformed leukoagglutinins.[143–146]

Illustrative Case 9

A 22-year-old woman with a relapse of her acute myelogenous leukemia developed fever and acute respiratory distress 4 hr after a blood transfusion. The patient had been well until 7 months previously when she presented with fever and ecchymoses, and a diagnosis of acute myelogenous leukemia was made. Full remission was induced with cytosine arabonoside, daunorubicin, and thioguanine therapy after a stormy course requiring multiple RBC, WBC, and platelet transfusions for bleeding and gram-negative sepsis. Once in remission, she remained well until a few days prior to admission when a bone marrow aspiration revealed recurrent disease, and she was found to be anemic and thrombocytopenic with a guaiac-positive stool. She was admitted to the hospital and given two units of packed RBCs and 15 units of platelets. Approximately 4 hr after the initiation of the transfusion therapy, she complained of a shaking chill, spiked a fever, and developed progressive respiratory distress. Physical examination revealed an acutely dyspneic young woman with a temperature of 103°F, respiratory rate of 40, and diffuse rales over both lung fields. Cardiac examination revealed a regular tachycardia, no gallops, and a grade 2/6 pulmonic-flow murmur. Room air ABGs revealed a Pao_2 value of 39 mm Hg, $Paco_2$ 28 mm Hg, and pH 7.52. Chest radiography revealed a normal-size heart with a diffuse patchy infiltrate consistent with pulmonary edema (Fig. 5A). Sputum examination revealed no polymorphonuclear leukocytes or organisms. The patient was treated with intubation, positive end-expiratory pressure (PEEP), and oxygen supplementation as needed. Twelve hours after intubation, she was extubated, and by 24 hr, her chest radiography had returned to normal (Fig. 5B).

Comment. Noncardiogenic pulmonary edema secondary to a leukoagglutinin reaction is evident in this case. The therapy here does not include digitalization or more than mild diuresis but rather is centered on adequate respiratory support with oxygen, PEEP, and intubation as needed. As in any immunosuppressed host, extubation should be carried out as soon as possible.

5. Radiologic Clues to the Diagnosis of Febrile Pneumonitis Syndrome

It is well recognized that no particular chest radiographic pattern is specific for a given pathologic process or microbial invader, particularly in the immunosuppressed patient.[3] It is also true, however, that certain patterns on radiography are more characteristic of some processes than of others, and the recognition of such patterns can aid greatly in narrowing down the differential diagnostic possibilities.

In describing such patterns, we find the following radiographic characteristics useful when making clinical–radiologic–pathologic correlations.[6]

1. The time of appearance, progression, or resolution of new pulmonary abnormalities as correlated with clinical findings.

2. The distribution and location of radiographic abnormalities. Opacities confined to one anatomic area (e.g., segment or lobe) are considered focal, whereas widespread or innumerable lesions are considered diffuse. Abnormalities that are distributed in more than one area but are not so numerous as to be uncountable are termed multifocal.

3. Lung abnormalities are divided into three groups: consolidations, peribronchovascular (interstitial) opacities, and nodules. Consolidations are defined as lung opacities in which there is substantial replacement of alveolar air by tissue density material. Anatomic regions of the lung that are more or less homogeneously opacified are included in this group. The presence of air bronchograms is considered confirmatory but is not a necessary finding for inclusion in this group. Opacities that are predominantly oriented along the peribronchial or perivascular bundles are termed peribronchovascular (or interstitial) opacities. Multiple tiny nodules with diameters of ≤3 mm are termed miliary. Interstitial pneumonitis is occasionally manifested as miliary nodules. In those instances in which this type of lesion progresses to total air replacement by tissue-density material, it is then considered a consolidation. Nodules greater than 1 cm^2 are defined as space-occupying nonanatomic lesions with well-defined, more or less rounded edges surrounded by aerated lung. Occasionally, it is difficult to differentiate small well-defined peripheral consolidations from macronodules. In such cases, well-defined lesions that abut the pleura are called consolidations, and those that are totally surrounded by aerated lung are called nodules.

4. Other characteristics that should be looked for include pleural fluid, atelectasis, cavitation, lymphadenopathy, and cardiac enlargement.

The value of such an approach is illustrated by the following findings in a renal transplant population[6]: of 12 patients with proven bacterial pneumonia, the distribution of lesions in 10 was focal and in two multifocal; the type of lesion was a consol-

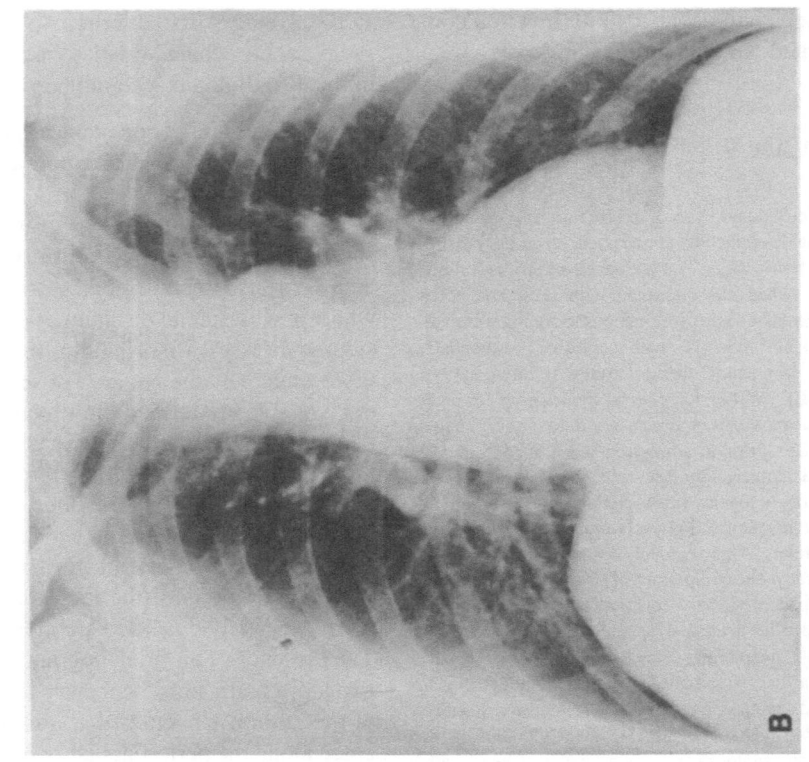

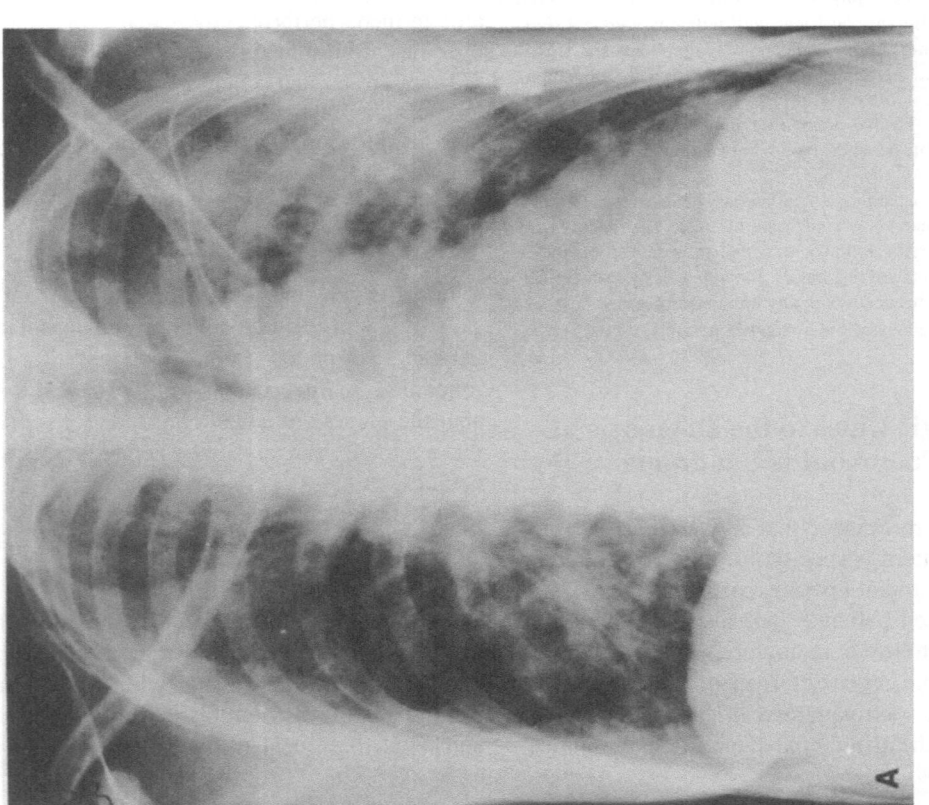

FIGURE 5. Leukoagglutinin reaction. Several hours after an intravenous transfusion, a patchy but widespread consolidation characteristic of leukoagglutinin reaction (A); 24 hr after therapy, the lungs became clear (B).

idation in 10, peribronchovascular in one, and nodular in one. Of 14 patients with fungal or nocardial infection, six were focal in distribution, seven multifocal, and one diffuse; five were consolidations, and nine nodular in type. By contrast, of nine patients with viral or *Pneumocystis* infection, six were diffuse, two were focal, and one multifocal; one was a consolidation, six were peribronchovascular in type, and two manifested miliary micronodules. When such data are combined with information concerning the rate of progression of the illness (acute vs. subacute or chronic) as outlined in Table 3, this information becomes even more useful. Focal or multifocal consolidation of acute onset will quite likely be caused by bacterial infection; similar lesions with subacute–chronic histories are most likely secondary to fungal or nocardial infection (or tuberculosis). Nodules are usually a sign of fungal or nocardial disease, particularly if they are subacute in onset; and subacute disease with diffuse abnormalities, either of peribronchovascular type or miliary micronodules, are caused by viruses or *Pneumocystis*. Noninfectious causes are added to the differential diagnosis, as noted in Table 3, when the history is appropriate, the radiographic findings are consistent, and ancillary radiographic signs (such as hilar adenopathy in patients with Hodgkin disease) are present.

Additional clues can be found by examining the pulmonary lesion for the development of cavitation or by carefully delineating the location of the infiltrate. Cavitation suggests necrotizing infection such as that caused by fungi, *Nocardia*, certain gram-negative bacilli (most commonly *Klebsiella* and *Pseudomonas*), and *Staphylococcus aureus*, or necrotic tumor.

The best clues to the radiographic diagnosis of radiation pneumonitis are the timing of onset with respect to radiation treatment and the location of the infiltrate, which is almost always confined to the outlines of the radiation portals. Thus, the diagnosis of radiation pneumonitis should be suspected when an infiltrate (particularly a peribronchovascular one) with relatively sharp margins that do not correspond to bronchopulmonary anatomy but adjoin the edges of the radiation field is present on radiography (Fig. 2). Changes occurring outside this area should be minor and are presumably related to stray or oblique irradiation. Since many cases of radiation pneumonitis follow mediastinal irradiation, the infiltrates are often central in location in contrast to the usual peripheral location of most other processes affecting this population. A rare case demonstrating extensive changes outside the field of radiation has been reported, as have a few cases of bilateral pneumonitis following unilateral irradiation. It has been suggested that such occurrences are caused by a delayed hypersensitivity reaction to an antigen resulting from radiation injury. The long latent period, the involvement of unirradiated tissue, the idiosyncratic occurrence of the process, and the clinical response to corticosteroid therapy that is seen are all consistent with this hypothesis.[1,60–68,73,74,147]

The depressed inflammatory response of the immunocompromised host may greatly modify or delay the appearance of a pulmonary infiltrate on radiography. This is most frequently seen in patients with severe neutropenia (absolute granulocyte count <500/mm^3, especially <100/mm^3). When such severe neutropenia is present, atelectasis may be the only radiologic clue to the presence of clinically important pulmonary infection. In particular, radiographic evidence of fungal invasion, which normally excites a less exuberant inflammatory response than does bacterial invasion, will often be very slow to appear. This may result, for example, in the first evidence of invasive *Aspergillosis* emanating from a pulmonary focus being metastatic lesions of the brain or other organs. By contrast, in patients recovering from neutropenia, there may be paradoxical increase in the radiologic findings (and sputum production) as the granulocyte count recovers despite a good clinical response to treatment.[2,9,36]

Despite these confounding factors, the chest radiograph is the major clue to the presence of pneumonitis. When patterns of radiographic abnormality are combined with a determination of the rate of progression of the illness (acute vs. subacute–chronic), the differential diagnosis is greatly simplified (Table 3).

6. Definitive Diagnosis

The effective therapy of the febrile pneumonitis syndrome in immunocompromised patients requires rapid and precise diagnosis. Although the diagnostic clues discussed thus far may greatly limit the differential diagnostic possibilities, the definitive answer should be sought whenever possible. Such an approach will limit drug toxicity and the risk of potentially lethal superinfection without exposing the patient to potentially inadequate therapy. Not surprisingly, several studies have shown that the rapidity with which the diagnosis is made has a major impact on determining the results of therapy, whether one is dealing with a noninfectious disease, a conventional bacterial infection, or invasive fungal or nocardial disease.[1,3,5,6,73,75,104,148] For example, in renal transplant patients diagnosed appropriately in the first 5 days of illness, a 79% survival rate was achieved; by contrast, if diagnosis and therapy were delayed for greater than 5 days, only a 35% survival rate was observed.[6] Therefore, great emphasis must now be placed on the techniques available for making a precise diagnosis: immunologic studies, conventional examination of expectorated sputum, and a variety of invasive procedures designed to sample either lower respiratory tract secretions or lung tissue, or both.[1]

6.1. Immunologic Techniques

Measurement of antibody and delayed hypersensitivity skin test responsiveness to microbial antigens are time-honored techniques for diagnosing invasive infection. However, such methods have limited applicability when caring for immunosuppressed patients with febrile pneumonitis syndrome for several reasons:

1. Even under the best of circumstances in the normal host there is a delay between the onset of infection and the development of a measurable immune response. In the compromised patient, such responses may be further delayed or totally abrogated. Thus, to wait for the development of such a response will greatly interfere with the need and desire to arrive at a rapid diagnosis.

2. Since many of the opportunistic infections causing life-threatening disease in the compromised host cause asymptomatic subclinical infection in the normal population, the presence of a positive result may have little meaning. The classic examples of this phenomenon are the many attempts to make the diagnosis of invasive candidiasis or aspergillosis on the basis of the presence of precipitating or agglutinating antibodies directed against these organisms. It is now clear that because of the failure of development of such antibodies in many compromised patients and

because of their presence in many normals, these tests are of limited diagnostic value.[149–151]

3. Appropriate serologic or skin tests are not available for many of the disease processes under consideration.

Therefore, the effectiveness of such traditional immunologic techniques has been disappointing. Even in patients with possible AIDS, the demonstration of HIV only connotes infection with the virus and does not correlate with the presence or absence of full-blown AIDS. The major exception has been in patients with histories of exposure to *Coccidioides immitis* or *Histoplasma capsulatum,* in whom the demonstration of elevated or rising titers of complement-fixing antibody is an excellent clue to the presence of active infection with these agents (see Illustrative Case 1).[1,39]

Far more promising are techniques that are currently being developed to demonstrate the presence of microbial antigens or products of microbial metabolism in body fluids and tissues. Immunofluorescent staining for antigens of *Legionella pneumophila* can lead to immediate diagnosis of Legionnaire disease from biopsy specimens as can the demonstration of *Legionella pneumophila* antigen in the urine by immunoassay (see Chapter 11). Similarly, CMV infection can be diagnosed rapidly in pulmonary specimens using either immunofluorescent techniques with highly specific monoclonal antibodies or in situ DNA hybridization with a labeled DNA probe homologous for a portion of the virus genome. The finding of cryptococcal antigen in the serum of patients with cryptococcal pulmonary infection (interstitial disease)[152,153] is an important specific diagnostic technique. Reports of the demonstration of circulating *Aspergillus* antigens in both animal models and humans with invasive aspergillosis[154,155] and of fungal metabolites in patients with invasive candidiasis[156] suggest that such approaches will be of great use in the future. What one is looking for are the "fingerprints" of the invading organism, be they circulating antigens or circulating unique products of metabolism.

6.2. Conventional Sputum Examination

The usual clinical approach to the diagnosis of pneumonia is based on the Gram stain and cultural examination of expectorated sputum specimens. It should be emphasized that strict criteria should be employed when viewing the Gram stain of an expectorated sputum specimen before trusting the validity of the specimen: few squamous epithelial cells (<10 per low-power field) and many polymorphonuclear leukocytes (>25 per low-power field). If such criteria are not met, the validity of the specimen is in question. For a variety of reasons, such an approach is often of little diagnostic value in the compromised patient. First, many of these patients, particularly those with significant leukopenia, fail to produce sputum, and usual methods of inducing sputum are frequently unsuccessful.[5,36,37,158-160] Second, the upper respiratory tract of many of these patients is frequently colonized with a large number of potential pathogens, particularly gram-negative bacilli and fungi. Expectorated sputum specimens will therefore be contaminated by these potential pathogens, and differentiation between organisms truly invading the lung and those that colonize the pharynx may be quite difficult.[13-15] This is particularly true in the granulocytopenic patient who is unable to mount a polymorphonuclear leukocyte response to invasive infection; review of Gram-stained specimens will lose a major clue—the presence of polymorphs on smear in proximity to the invading pathogens. Third, certain organisms that commonly cause pneumonia in this population, such as *Aspergillus* and *Pneumocystis*, rarely shed sufficient organisms into the sputum to permit diagnosis by cultural or microscopic examination.[1,3,6,161] Finally, the noninfectious causes of pulmonary infiltrates will not be diagnosed by examination of expectorated sputum specimens. For all these reasons, then, the invasive diagnostic techniques, which include transtracheal aspiration, bronchial brushing, percutaneous lung aspiration, cutting needle biopsy, fiberoptic bronchoscopy with bronchial brushing and/or transbronchial biopsy, and open lung biopsy, have been developed in order to permit specific diagnosis.[1] The proper deployment of these techniques is the major diagnostic responsibility of the clinician dealing with immunocompromised patients presenting with febrile pneumonitis syndrome.

6.3. Transtracheal Aspiration

The first invasive diagnostic technique to be considered is transtracheal aspiration. Transtracheal aspiration is most useful in diagnosing conventional bacterial infection, where we have had a 92% diagnostic yield with essentially no false positives when the procedure is performed correctly.[1] Similar success may be obtained in diagnosing viral or mycoplasmal infection. Even in such difficult-to-diagnosis infections as those caused by *Pneumocystis* and *Aspergillus*, the diagnosis may be made 15–20% of the time on transtracheal aspiration, provided the specimens are processed appropriately.[1,6,162] Any specimens obtained by this procedure or by any other invasive technique should ideally be cultured aerobically and anaerobically for bacterial pathogens, mycobacteria, fungi, viruses, mycoplasma, and on special media for *L. pneumophila* (see Chapter 11). In addition, materials should be processed for methenamine silver staining for *Pneumocystis*, immunofluorescent staining for *L. pneumophila*, routine staining by the Ziehl–Neelsen and Gram methods, and be examined on fungal wet mounts for the appropriate organisms. When, as if so often the case, limited diagnostic material is available, those staining and cultural techniques should be employed that are most likely to point to a diagnosis on the basis of the clues previously discussed.

The proper deployment of transtracheal aspiration in the diagnosis of pneumonia in the immunocompromised host is at present controversial. In expert hands, there is clearly considerably less oropharyngeal contamination of the specimen than is seen with expectorated sputum specimens, thus making Gram stain and cultural results more believable.[163-167] It is also clear that this technique is particularly useful in the diagnosis of anaerobic pleuropulmonary infection, although such infections are relatively uncommon in this population of patients.[8,163] Considerable concern has been expressed regarding the occurrence of hemorrhage or cervical cellulitis with this procedure, and some centers have abandoned its use, particularly in thrombocytopenic patients.[8,59] Other centers view this procedure with considerable enthusiasm.[1,6,163,167]

We ourselves have carried out more than 500 such procedures on immunocompromised patients (primarily organ transplant patients and patients with leukemia) with a complication rate of less than 1% and no deaths, using the following precautions:

1. There are three absolute contraindications to transtracheal aspiration: an uncooperative patient; a

patient (such as an obese person, a child, or one who has undergone surgery or radiation therapy in this area) with anatomic characteristics that make the procedure technically difficult; and those with uncorrectable bleeding diatheses.

2. In the process of anesthetizing the area over the cricothyroid membrane where the lavage needle and catheter will be inserted, a small 25-gauge needle is employed both to deliver the local anesthesia and to delineate the track that the larger needle will follow.

3. In neutropenic patients, broad-spectrum antibacterial therapy is initiated immediately after the procedure and continued for a minimum of 48 hr postprocedure.

4. In patients, such as those with leukemia, who are subject to bleeding difficulties, appropriate clotting studies and platelet counts are carried out, with abnormalities corrected, for 48 hr post-transtracheal aspiration. Even in patients with acute leukemia or other causes of severe thrombocytopenia, this procedure can be safely carried out if platelet transfusions are available, if they can sustain a platelet count of greater than 50,000 mm^3 for more than 24 hr after the procedure, and if other causes of bleeding are not present. We carry out this procedure routinely in immunocompromised patients who have pneumonia with an acute clinical course suggesting a bacterial process, who fulfill these criteria, and whose condition are not diagnosed on the basis of the expectorated sputum examination.

6.4. Invasive Diagnostic Techniques

If the diagnosis has not been made by transtracheal aspiration, a more invasive procedure in which direct sampling of pulmonary tissue is carried out is then required. Choice of procedure is dependent on several factors: the degree of illness of the patient, the rate of progression of the disease, type of pulmonary infiltrate present on radiography, and the expertise and experience of personnel at a given institution. If the pneumonitis and the degree of hypoxia are progressing rapidly, the definitive diagnostic procedure—the open lung biopsy—should be carried out immediately. This is particularly true when the radiographic pattern of infiltrate is diffuse or multifocal. Despite the need for general anesthesia, thoracotomy, and a postoperative chest tube, it is remarkable how well this procedure is tolerated, especially if a treatable process is identified.[1,8,59]

If the pulmonary process is progressing at a more desultory pace, progressive hypoxia is not an immediate problem, and the clinical problem is more of a diagnostic dilemma than a therapeutic emergency, then less invasive techniques can be attempted, with the open lung biopsy held in reserve if these techniques fail. Which of these procedures should be employed in the individual patient can be decided on the basis of the following data. Bronchial brushing with special catheters introduced into the lower respiratory tract via the nose or mouth is well tolerated, with the incidence of major pneumothorax requiring chest tube placement or major hemorrhage being less than 1%. This procedure will result in the correct diagnosis of more than 90% of viral infections of *Pneumocystis* infection in approximately 75% of patients, and of fungal or nocardial disease in 50–75% of cases. Because of upper airway contamination, this technique is less useful in diagnosing bacterial infection and appears to be quite insensitive for diagnosing tumor invasion, radiation, or drug-induced disease.

In performing both this procedure and fiberoptic bronchoscopy, great care must be taken in the use of topical anesthetic agents for two reasons. Particularly in the elderly debilitated patient, too much local anesthesia for the procedure will leave the patient with an impaired gag reflex, inadequate airway protection after the procedure, and a resulting significant risk of aspiration pneumonia. Second, contamination of diagnostic material obtained with the bactericidal anesthetic agents can lower the diagnostic yield.[1,3,160,169—171]

An attempt has been made to combine the advantages of transtracheal aspiration with those of bronchial brushing by introducing the bronchial brushes transtracheally through the cricoid membrane, thereby avoiding oral contamination and allowing meaningful evaluation of bacterial cultures.[160] Of 17 patients not receiving broad-spectrum antibiotics at the time of the procedure, the correct diagnosis was made in 14; the false-negative results were obtained in three patients with fungal infection. In this study as in similar studies evaluating the diagnostic usefulness of needle aspiration of the lung and transbronchial biopsy in association with fiberoptic bronchoscopy, the use of broad-spectrum antibiotics at the time of the procedure may result in negative cultures despite the presence of active bacterial infection. Despite the high rate of diagnostic accuracy with transtracheal bronchial biopsy, this procedure has not received widespread use because of an apparently high rate of complications (approximately 15%): cellulitis of the neck, major pneumothorax, and significant hemorrhage.[160]

A variety of techniques has been employed to obtain diagnostic specimens directly from the involved lung percutaneously. The turbine-powered trephine biopsy technique yielded excellent specimens for diagnosis but was associated with an unacceptably high rate of major complications, including death, from hemorrhage or air embolism and has now been largely abandoned. Similar difficulties were encountered when percutaneous lung biopsies were carried out with a modified Vim–Silverman cutting needle.[1,3,172,173] By contrast, needle aspiration under fluoroscopic control, employing a thin-walled 18-gauge noncutting needle, has yielded excellent results, particularly in patients with focal, peripherally located pulmonary lesions—especially when cavitation has been present. Accordingly, this technique has had its highest yield in patients most likely to have this type of lung lesion, i.e., those with focal bacterial, fungal, nocardial, or tuberculous lesions. At our institution, we have successfully diagnosed more than 90% of fungal or nocardial infections occurring in immunosuppressed patients approached in this manner and regard this procedure as the one of choice for such peripherally placed, focal pulmonary lesions not diagnosed by the initial transtracheal aspiration. Major complications such as significant hemorrhage or the need for chest tube placement are most unusual, occurring in fewer than 3% of patients. This technique appears to be less useful in diagnosing diffuse lung disease.[1,3,6,171-178]

The diagnostic procedure of choice in immunocompromised patients with diffuse lung disease not requiring immediate open lung biopsy is fiberoptic bronchoscopy combined with transbronchial biopsy, bronchial brushing, and bronchoalveolar lavage via the bronchoscope. With this technique, the most common treatable causes of diffuse interstitial lung disease in the immunosuppressed host, *Pneumocystis carinii*, appears to be diagnosable in approximately 90% of patients. In addition, biopsy material adequate for the diagnosis of radiation- and drug-induced disease appears to be obtainable in a comparable percentage of patients with these conditions (see Illustrative Cases 6 and 7). Tumor invasion may be missed, however, as the biopsy forceps tends to slide off the tumor. Although the most important application of this technique is for the diagnosis of diffuse lung disease, focal fungal and nocardial infections may also be diagnosed, particularly when bronchial brushings as well as transbronchial biopsy are carried out through the fiberoptic bronchoscope.

The range of diagnostic effectiveness of this procedure may be considerably increased by a modification described by Wimberley and colleagues.[179] By employing a telescoping cannula distally occluded with a plug of ethylene glycol through a conventional fiberoptic bronchoscope, contamination of lower respiratory samples by upper airway resident flora may be effectively bypassed, thus making possible the reliable diagnosis of bacterial pneumonias and expanding the utility of the procedure.[179] Winterbauer et al.[180] suggested that the diagnostic yield for bacterial pneumonias could be considerably increased by doing quantitative bacteriology and staining for antibody coating of bacteria on a slide smeared with material obtained at bronchoscopy. More than 4000 colony-forming units on quantitative culture and the presence of immunoglobulin on the bacteria were both highly associated with the presence of invasive bacterial infection. The complication rates associated with fiberoptic bronchoscopy with biopsy and brushing are as follows: an approximately 5% risk for pneumothorax, 1–2% for significant hemorrhage, and a mortality rate of approximately 0.2%.[1,4,10,181-185]

In recent years, particularly in patients with AIDS but also in patients with a borderline coagulation status, there has been increasing enthusiasm for carrying out bronchoalveolar lavage alone without the biopsy procedures. This involves the positioning of the bronchoscope into an area of pulmonary infiltrate, and then lavaging this area with approximately 200 ml sterile isotonic saline. The lavage fluid is then aspirated and submitted for appropriate cytologic and microbiologic studies.[8] Stover et al.[186] reported in non-AIDS immunocompromised patients that 83% of opportunistic infections, but only 46% of malignancies and 40% of drug toxicities, were diagnosed by this technique. The fact that biopsies via the bronchoscope add to the diagnostic yield is illustrated by studies of *Pneumocystis carinii* pneumonia in patients with AIDS. It should be emphasized that this group of patients carries the largest parasite burden of any immunocompromised patient with *Pneumocystis* infection and that there is the greatest spillover from the alveolar spaces into the bronchial tree. Thus, it is fair to say that bronchoalveolar lavage will be most successful in the AIDS patient. Approximately 90% of *P. carinii* pneumonias were diagnosed by transbronchoscopic fixed-tissue and touch-imprint biopsies, 40–50% by brush biopsies and 80% for bronchoalveolar lavage.[187–189] Thus, biopsies still have a higher yield than lavage. It should be emphasized, however, that transbronchial biopsy carries a complication rate for bleeding and significant pneumothorax that is considerably higher than lavage alone or open biopsy under direct vision.

The severely neutropenic patient is at particular risk for the development of serious complications of fiberoptic bronchoscopy, with life-threatening bacteremia and postbronchoscopy pneumonia well-described risks of this procedure in this population.[190,191] In order to avoid these problems, we routinely begin broad-spectrum intravenous antimicrobial therapy with ticarcillin and tobramycin (or a cephalosporin–aminoglycoside combination) as soon as adequate specimens are obtained in the neutropenic patient. Such antibiotics are continued for 48 hr after the procedure unless some untoward event has occurred that requires further antibiotic therapy. With this precaution, we have not encountered this problem during the last 48 months.

At many centers, including our own, there has been increasing concern regarding the quality of the biopsy obtained, particularly in non-AIDS patients. Because of this, there has been a revival of interest in an older procedure—transpleural lung biopsy by the thoracoscopic route. This appears to be particularly useful in the diagnosis of patients with diffuse interstitial pulmonary disease. Although an artificial pneumothorax is induced to carry out the procedure and a chest tube is needed for 1–3 days postprocedure, it may be carried out under local anesthesia and appears to be well tolerated, even in bone marrow transplant patients.[192–195] Thus Dijkman et al.[192] reported 100% success in the diagnosis of acute pulmonary disease in 26 immunocompromised patients with acute diffuse pulmonary disease and 90% success among 63 nonimmunocompromised patients. They report that in their hands better diagnostic material was obtained and that the procedure was better tolerated than fiberoptic bronchoscopy, especially in hypoxic patients. We have had a similar experience in 10 non-AIDS immunocompromised patients.

The definitive diagnostic procedure remains open lung biopsy which should be carried out as expeditiously as possible if arterial hypoxemia is intensifying, the pulmonary infiltrates are spreading rapidly, and the patient has a hopeful prognosis from his underlying disease. Despite the need for general anesthesia, thoracotomy, and a postoperative chest tube, the procedure is remarkably well tolerated, especially in those patients in whom a treatable disorder is identified. A specific diagnosis is made in approximately 80% of immunosuppressed patients who come to open lung biopsy. The undiagnosed cases probably represent instances of unrecognized pulmonary drug toxicity, the effects of antecedent antimicrobial therapy in modifying the disease process, or even some new pulmonary infection. Recent experiences with *Legionella pneumophila* and *L. micdadei* suggest that there are as yet undiagnosed pathogens causing human disease and that immunocompromised persons are those most likely to be infected with such agents. There is a false-negative rate with open lung biopsy of <4%—those instances presumably related to sampling error or inappropriate handling of specimens.[196–201]

A more important question is how frequently the knowledge obtained results in meaningful therapy. The answer to this question is clearly different for different patient populations. In a transplant patient or an AIDS patient, for example, there is a high likelihood of useful information being obtained. By contrast, in a leukemic patient, for example, that may not be true. Tenholder and Hooper,[145] as well as others[202,203] have pointed out that the timing of the process and its radiographic appearance were important determinants of open-biopsy yield in leukemic patients. In untreated leukemic patients presenting with pneumonitis, localized disease was almost invariably due to conventional bacterial pathogens, whereas diffuse disease was usually due to such noninfectious causes as hemorrhage, pulmonary edema or leukemic infiltrates. Localized disease after treatment was instituted was due to infection three-fourths of the time, but in only 10% of cases was it opportunistic (the search for which is a major indication for open lung biopsy). In those patients in whom diffuse disease developed on therapy, there was a high rate of opportunistic infection. Therefore, a graded diagnostic approach is indicated at different stages of the disease.

The final issue here is the question of the circumstances in which empirical therapy without invasive diagnostic procedures is indicated. The following circumstances should be included: (1) far-advanced AIDS or relapsing acute myelogenous leukemia, with a limited life expectancy because of the severity of the underlying illness; (2) leukemia prior to therapy, with a low probability of opportunistic infection; (3) either an uncorrectable bleeding diathesis or such impaired pulmonary function that invasive diagnostic techniques would not be tolerated; and (4) refusal of invasive diagnostic studies. In such patients, the choice of empirical therapy is made on the basis of the indirect clues outlined previously: the epidemiologic and clinical setting, the nature of the immune defect(s) present, the pace of the pulmonary process, and the radiographic pattern.

Although it is clear that one or another of these techniques is particularly well adapted for certain types of pulmonary lesion and is less useful for others, this information must be tempered by an assessment of the experience and expertise that can be called on at a particular institution. Such information should supersede published statistics obtained elsewhere when the diagnostic approach to be followed is determined. For example, in the case of fiberoptic bronchoscopic procedures, probably the most versatile single technique short of open lung biopsy that can be brought to bear on this problem, success is directly dependent on effective communication between an expert bronchoscopist, a pathologist experienced in the evaluation of biopsy material obtained in this manner, and the utilization of appropriate diagnostic stains and culture media.[1]

7. Pulmonary Infiltrates in the Patient with AIDS

The epidemic of AIDS has had a major impact on the practice of medicine in general and on the specialties of infectious disease and pulmonary medicine in particular. The possibility of any patient presenting with a community-acquired pneumonia having AIDS and an opportunistic infection must be considered, particularly if the individual had received transfusions in the past. By contrast, because of the wide variety of pathogens and processes, pulmonary disease is a major manifestation of AIDS, with virtually every patient with AIDS having at least one major episode of pulmonary infection or neo-

plasm during his clinical course, and pulmonary infection usually playing a major role in the patient's demise. Although this subject is covered more completely in Chapter 15, several points bear emphasis:

1. *Pneumocystis carinii* accounts for more than one-half of the episodes of pneumonia in this patient population. It is frequently a presenting manifestation of AIDS. Unlike other immunosuppressed patients, recurrent episodes are the rule rather than the exception. *P. carinii* pneumonia should be particularly suspected in the absence of rigors, persistent sputum production, and a radiographic picture of lobar consolidation, adenopathy, or pleural effusion. It should be suspected in the presence of a subacute presentation with a dry cough, repeated fevers, and a radiographic picture of interstitial pneumonitis, particularly if bilateral.[204–208] A significant minority of AIDS patients with early *P. carinii* pneumonia present with nonproductive cough and fever, who belong to one of the population groups at high risk for AIDS (or are known to have AIDS or to have antibody to the human immunodeficiency virus) and have clear chest radiographs. In this situation, gallium scanning and pulmonary function testing are often very helpful in terms of suggesting the possibility of *P. carinii* infection. Gallium scanning is quite sensitive but is not specific; it reveals early inflammation but does not tell the physician the cause. Similarly, the pulmonary function abnormalities of arterial hypoxemia, decreased lung volumes, and reduced single-breath CO_2 diffusing capacity are sensitive but nonspecific abnormalities.[206,208–210]

2. Other opportunistic infections, particularly fungal and mycobacterial (typical and atypical) infections, and viral processes (especially CMV) are commonly present, reflecting the profound defect in cell-mediated immunity that is the major defect in these patients.[204–208]

3. It is important to recognize that there is also a profound defect in other elements of the host defense in the AIDS patient, particularly a defect in B-cell function and antibody formation. Not surprisingly then, bacterial infection, especially with such encapsulated organisms as *Pneumococcus* and *Hemophilus influenzae* type B must be considered. Bacterial pneumonia is suggested by an acute onset, purulent sputum production, rigors, and a consolidation on chest radiography.[211]

4. Tumor, especially Kaposi sarcoma, may have significant pulmonary effects in these patients, and must be considered in the differential diagnosis.[204-208]

5. Sequential or simultaneous involvement of the lungs with a variety of processes is the rule and not the exception.[204-208]

6. Although there is a temptation to just treat these patients empirically with trimethoprim-sulfamethoxazole for *Pneumocystis,* every effort should be made to establish a diagnosis. Relatively noninvasive procedures such as bronchoalveolar lavage have a high yield; by contrast, untoward reactions to therapy are common and other treatable conditions may be present.[208]

8. Superinfection

Implicit in this review and in most published reports concerning the febrile pneumonitis syndrome in the immunocompromised patient is that a single etiology is responsible for the disease syndrome. That this is not always the case is shown in Table 1 in which 10% of the subjects, particularly the cancer patients, were shown to have mixed infections. Particular combinations of agents that are likely to be present together are CMV with *Pneumocystis carinii,* gram-negative, or fungal infection; *Nocardia* and *Aspergillus; Cryptococcus* and *Nocardia; Cryptoccus* and *P. carinii;* and radiation pneumonitis with gram-negative bacillary infection.[1,8]

Even more important is the occurrence of superinfection. For example, in one series of renal transplant patients,[6] it was noted that pulmonary superinfection developed in 43% of the patients and accounted for 81% of the fatalities, with all but one of the 23 patients who developed superinfection dying. Superinfection appears to be most common in three groups of patients, those with pulmonary embolic disease, those with preceding CMV infection, and those with severe leukopenia or who are receiving high-dose corticosteroid therapy. Unlike the situation in normal hosts, in whom secondary infection of a sterile pulmonary infarct is quite uncommon, over 50% of such immunocompromised patients will develop superinfections (89% of renal transplant patients in this series[6]).

The important role of primary CMV infection in predisposing to potentially lethal superinfection cannot be overemphasized, particularly in organ transplant recipients, be they kidney, heart, or bone marrow.[6,50,212-216] The explanation for this association appears to lie in the adverse effects of this agent on the already compromised host defenses of the patient infected. In important experiments carried out by Hamilton and colleagues,[217] sublethal CMV infection of mice led to a striking increase in mortality following subsequent challenge with sublethal doses of *Staphylococcus aureus, Pseudomonas aeruginosa,* or *Candida albicans.* It is likely that a similar effect is operative in humans.

The pathogens responsible for superinfection are somewhat different from those responsible for primary infection. Virtually all the instances of bacterial superinfection are by gram-negative bacilli, particularly *Pseudomonas aeruginosa* and relatively antibiotic-resistant *Enterobacteriaceae.* Two organisms that rarely produce primary pulmonary infection, Herpes simplex and *Candida albicans,* are not uncommon causes of superinfection, as are *Aspergillus fumigatus* and *Torulopsis glabrata.*[1,6,51]

The clinician should be particularly alert to the possibility of superinfection in the following circumstances: in the patient who has shown an initial clinical response to therapy in terms of temperature curve, ABGs, well-being, WBC count, and sputum production, but who now shows deterioration in one or more of these parameters; in any patient with significant leukopenia or who continues to receive high-dose (>20 mg prednisone per day) corticosteroid therapy; and the patient with progressive deterioration despite apparently effective treatment. In any of these instances, aggressive diagnostic techniques should be again undertaken. At postmortem examination in too many patients, the primary cause of fever and pneumonitis is no longer present, but instead, multiple superinfecting microorganisms can be demonstrated. Both earlier recognition and better prevention are necessary in dealing with this unsolved problem complicating the febrile pneumonitis syndrome in the compromised host.[1-3,5,6]

Illustrative Case 10

A 36-year-old patient with stage IVB Hodgkin disease entered with a week's history of increased fever, cough, and shortness of breath. The patient had had IVB Hodgkin for a total of 5 years and had received multiple courses of radiation, MOPP therapy, and, most recently, bleomycin (total dose 160 mg) and daily prednisone, 20 mg/day. Approximately 1 week prior to admission he, along with other members of his family, developed a nonproductive cough, a low-grade fever, malaise, and fatiguability. On the day of admission, he noted the onset of shaking chills, fever to 104°F (40°C), increasing dyspnea, right-sided pleurisy, and an increased cough. Physical examination on admission revealed a cachectic white male who was acutely ill with a temperature of 103°F (39.4°C) and a respiratory rate of 40. Signs of consolidation were evident at his right base. Laboratory evaluation disclosed Hct 32%, WBC count 1600/mm^3 with 45% polys, 12% bands, 9% lymphs, 29% monocytes, 5% eosinophils. Room air ABGs revealed a Pao$_2$ of 48 mm Hg, Paco$_2$ 29 mm Hg, and pH 7.53. Chest radiography revealed a focal air space consolidation in the right lower lobe. Transtracheal aspirate yielded a specimen containing a few polymorphonuclear leukocytes and numerous gram-positive diplococci. Culture of this material and blood cultures yielded *Streptococcus pneumoniae*. Therapy was started with 2.4 million units of penicillin G per day, with improvement over the first 4–5 days of hospitalization. On the fifth hospital day his room air ABGs were Pao$_2$ 65 mm Hg, Paco$_2$ 30 mm Hg, and pH 7.48. There was a marked improvement in his well-being. On the seventh hospital day, increased fevers were noted, and the patient appeared and felt less well. Over the next 3 days there was clear-cut clinical deterioration in terms of temperature curve, appetite, well-being, and so forth. There were no significant changes in his ABGs or the chest radiograph. A transtracheal aspiration was repeated, and *Aspergillus* was seen on fungal wet mount, and *A. fumigatus* was grown on culture. Despite the institution of amphotericin B therapy, the patient steadily deteriorated and succumbed on the twenty-first hospital day. At autopsy there was no evidence of pneumococcal infection, but there was considerable evidence for widespread invasive aspergillosis.

Comment. This patient was at high risk for the development of superinfection because of his severely immunosuppressed state from his far-advanced Hodgkin disease, leukopenia, and corticosteroid therapy. The clue to the onset of superinfection was the change in fever curve and well-being. In this circumstance, the chest radiograph is usually an insensitive measure of the onset of superinfection, as shown by the failure of the development of significant new lesions until very late in his course. A significant degree of fungal infection is often present without major changes in the ABGs, so this is a rather insensitive test for the diagnosis of superinfection by fungi as well. Earlier diagnosis of superinfection such as this is needed, but even more important is the development of ways to prevent this form of lethal infection. As witnessed by the absence of pneumococci at autopsy in this patient, the treatment of primary pulmonary infection in the compromised host has become quite good; unfortunately, the prevention and treatment of secondary infection is not nearly so efficacious, particularly in the high-risk patient.

References

1. Rubin RH: The cancer patient with fever and pulmonary infiltrates; Etiology and diagnostic approach. In Remington JS, Swartz MN (eds): *Current Clinical Topics in Infectious Disease.* Vol. I. McGraw-Hill, New York, 1980, pp. 288–303.

2. Levine AS, Schimpff SC, Graw RG, et al: Hematologic malignancies and other marrow failure states: Progress in the management of complicating infections. *Semin Hematol* 11:141–202, 1974.

3. Williams DM, Krick JA, Remington JS: Pulmonary infection in the compromised host. *Am Rev Respir Dis* 114:359–394, 593–627, 1976.

4. Schimpff SC: Diagnosis of infection in patients with cancer. *Eur J Cancer (Suppl.)* 11:29–38, 1975.

5. Pennington JE, Feldman NT: Pulmonary infiltrates and fever in patients with hematologic malignancy: Assessment of transbronchial biopsy. *Am J Med* 62:581–587, 1977.

6. Ramsey PG, Rubin RH, Tolkoff-Rubin NE, et al: The renal transplant patient with fever and pulmonary infiltrates: Etiology, clinical manifestations, and management. *Medicine (Baltimore)* 59:206–222, 1980.

7. Bishop JF, Schimpff SC, Diggs CH, *et al:* Infections during intensive chemotherapy for non-Hodgkin's lymphoma. *Ann Intern Med* 95:549–555, 1981.

8. Rosenow EC III, Wilson WR, Cockerill FR III: Pulmonary disease in the immunocompromised host. *Mayo Clin Proc* 60:473–487, 610–631, 1985.

9. Sickles EA, Young VM, Greene WH, *et al:* Pneumonia in acute leukemia. *Ann Intern Med* 79:528–534, 1973.

10. Singer C, Armstrong D, Rosen PP, et al: Diffuse pulmonary infiltrates in immunosuppressed patients: Prospective study of 80 cases. *Am J Med* 66:115–120, 1979.

11. Singer C, Kaplan MH, Armstrong D: Bacteremia and fungemia complicating neoplastic disease. *Am J Med* 62:731–742, 1977.

12. Pennington JE: Infection in the compromised host; recent advances and future directions. In Weinstein L, Fields BN (eds): *Seminars in Infectious Disease.* Vol. 1. Stratton Intercontinental, New York, 1978, pp. 142–168.

13. Johanson WG Jr, Pierce AK, Sanford JP: Changing pharyngeal bacterial flora of hospitalized patients. *N Engl J Med* 281:1137–1140 1969.

14. Johanson WG Jr, Higuchi JJ, Chadhuri TR, Woods DE: Bacterial adherence to epithelial cells in bacterial colonization of the respiratory tract. *Am Rev Respir Dis* 121:55–63, 1980.

15. Woods DE: Bacterial colonization of the respiratory tract: Clinical significance. In Pennington JE (ed): *Respiratory Infections: Diagnosis and Management.* Raven, New York, 1983, pp. 25–29.

16. Beatty HN, Miller AA, Broome CV, et al: Legionnaires' disease in Vermont, May to October 1978, *JAMA* 240:127–131, 1978.

17. Bock BV, Kirby BD, Edelstein PH, et al: Legionnaires' disease in renal transplant recipients, *Lancet* 1:410–413, 1978.

18. Gump DW, Frank RO, Winn WC Jr, et al. Legionnaires' disease in patients with associated serious disease. *Ann Intern Med* 90:538–542, 1979.

19. Haley CE, Cohen ML, Halter J, et al: Nosocomial Legionnaires' disease: A continuing common-source epidemic at

Wadsworth Medical Center. *Ann Intern Med* **90:**583–586, 1979

20. England AC III, Fraser DW, Plikaytis BD, et al. Sporadic legionellosis in the United States: The first thousand cases *Ann Intern Med* **94:**164–170, 1981

21. Arnow PM, Chou T, Weil D, et al. Nosocomial Legionnaires' disease caused by aerosolized tap water from respiratory devices. *J Infect Dis* **146:**460–467, 1982.

22. Pasculle AW, Myerowitz RL, Rinaldo CR: New bacterial agent of pneumonia isolated from renal transplant recipients *Lancet* **2:**58–61, 1979

23. Myerowitz RL, Pasculle AW, Dowling JN, et al. Opportunistic lung infection due to "Pittsburgh pneumonia agent." *N Engl J Med* **301:**953–958, 1979.

24. Rogers BH, Donowitz GR, Walker GK, et al: Opportunistic pneumonia. A clinicopathogenic study of five cases caused by an unidentified acid-fast bacterium. *N Engl J Med* **301:**495–961, 1979.

25. Muder RR, Yu VL, Zuravleff JJ. Pneumonia due to the Pittsburgh Pneumonia Agent: New clinical perspective with a review of the literature. *Medicine (Baltimore)* **62:**120–128, 1983.

26. Rudin JE, Wing EJ: A comparative study of *Legionella micdadei* and other nosocomial acquired pneumonias *Chest* **86:**675–680, 1984.

27. Aisner J, Schimpff SC, Benett JE, et al: Aspergillus infections in cancer patients. Association with fireproofing materials in a new hospital. *JAMA* **235:**411–413, 1976

28. Arnow PM, Andersen P, Mainous PD, et al Pulmonary aspergillosis during hospital renovation. *Am Rev Respir Dis* **118:**49–53, 1978.

29. Burton JR, Sachery JB, Bessin R, et al: Aspergillosis in four renal transplant patients; diagnosis and effective treatment with Amphoterocin B. *Ann Intern Med* **77:**383–388, 1972

30. Rose HD: Mechanical control of hospital ventilation and aspergillus infections. *Am Rev Respir Dis* **105:**306–307, 1972.

31. Sarubbi FA Jr, Kopf HB, Wilson MB, et al: Increased recovery of *Aspergillus flavus* from respiratory specimens during hospital construction. *Am Rev Respir Dis* **125:**33–38, 1982

32. Rhame FS, Streifel AJ, Kersey JH Jr, et al. Extrinsic risk factors for pneumonia in the patient at high risk of infection. *Am J Med* **75(5A):**42–52, 1984.

33. Opal SM, Asp AA, Cannady PB Jr, et al: Efficacy of infection control measures during a nosocomial outbreak of disseminated aspergillosis associated with hospital construction. *J Infect Dis* **153:**634–637, 1986

34. Hopkins CC, Weber D, Rubin RH. Non-domiciliary, nosocomial epidemic of invasive aspergillosis: A common source epidemic due to construction in a radiology suite *Amer Rev Resp Dis* (in press), 1986.

35. Singer C, Armstrong D, Rosen PP, et al: *Pneumocystis carinii* pneumonia: A cluster of 11 cases *Am J Med* **82:**772–777, 1975.

36. Sickles EA, Greene WH, Wiernik PH: Unusual presentation of infection in granulocytopenic patients. *Arch Intern Med* **135:**715–719, 1975

37. Zornoza J, Goldman AM, Wallace S, et al. Radiologic features of gram-negative pneumonias in the neutropenic patient **127:**989–996, 1976.

38. Bodey GP, Buckley M, Sathe YS, et al: Quantitative relationships between circulating leukocytes and infection in patients with acute leukemia. *AJR* **64:**328–340, 1966.

39. Rubin RH: Systemic mycotic infections. In Rubenstein E, Federman DD (eds): *Scientific American's Medicine*. Section 7, Subsection IX. Scientific American, New York, 1987, pp. 1–20.

40. Millar JW, Horne NW. Tuberculosis in immunosuppressed patients *Lancet* **1:**1176–1180, 1979

41. Kaplan MH, Armstrong D, Rosen P: Tuberculosis complicating neoplastic disease. *Cancer* **33:**850–858, 1974

42 Feld R, Bodey GP, Groschel D. Mycobacteriosis in patients with malignant disease. *Arch Intern Med* **136:**67–78, 1976.

43. Roberts CJ: Coccidioidomycosis in acquired immune deficiency syndrome. Depressed humoral as well as cellular immunity *Am J Med* **76:**734–736, 1984.

44. Bonner JR, Alexander WJ, Dismukes WE, et al: Disseminated histoplasmosis in patients with the acquired immune deficiency syndrome *Arch Intern Med* **144:**2178–2181, 1984

45. Taylor MN, Baddour LM, Alexander JR· Disseminated histoplasmosis associated with the acquired immune deficiency syndrome. *Am J Med* **77:**579–580, 1984

46 Wheat LJ, Slama TG, Zeckel ML. Histoplasmosis in the acquired immune deficiency syndrome. *Am J Med* **78:**203–210, 1985.

47. Scowden EB, Schaffner W, Stone WJ. Overwhelming strongyloidiasis: An unappreciated opportunistic infection. *Medicine (Baltimore)* **57:**527–544, 1978

48. Morgan JS, Schaffner W, Stone WJ. Opportunistic strongyloidiasis in renal transplant recipients. *Transplantation* (in press), 1986.

49. Meyer RD, Young LS, Armstrong D, et al· Aspergillosis complicating neoplastic disease *Am J Med* **54:**6–15, 1973.

50. Rubin RH, Cosimi AB, Tolkoff-Rubin NE, et al. Infectious disease syndromes attributable to cytomegalovirus and their significance among renal transplant recipients, *Transplantation* **24:**458–464, 1977

51 Rubin RH, Cosimi AB. Infection in the immunocompromised host 2nd ed In Simmons RL, Howard R (eds): *Surgical Infectious Disease*, Appleton-Century Crofts, E. Norwalk, Connecticut, 1987, (in press)

52. Masur H, Cheigh JS, Stubanbord WT. Infection following kidney transplantation: A changing pattern. *Rev Infect Dis* **6:**1208–1219, 1982.

53. Rubin RH, Wolfson JS, Cosimi AB, et al. Infection in the renal transplant patient. *Am J Med* **70:**405–411, 1981

54. Weitzman SA, Aisenberg AC Fulminant sepsis after the successful treatment of Hodgkin's disease *Am J Med* **62:**47–50, 1977

55. Weitzman SA, Aisenberg AC, Siber GR, et al. Impaired humoral immunity in treated Hodgkin's disease. *N Engl J Med* **297:**245–248, 1977.

56 Siber GR, Weitzman SA, Aisenberg AC, et al Impaired antibody response to pneumococcal vaccines after treatment for Hodgkin's disease *N Engl J Med* **299:**442–446, 1978.

57. Burke BA, Good RA: *Pneumocystis carinii* infection. *Medicine (Baltimore)* 52:23–49, 1973.

58. Rand KH, Pollard RB, Merigan TC. Increased pulmonary superinfections in cardiac-transplant patients undergoing primary cytomegalovirus infection. *N Engl J Med* 298:951–953, 1978

59. Masur H, Shelhamer J, Parrillo JE: The management of pneumonias in immunocompromised patients *JAMA* 253:1769–1773, 1985

60. Gross NJ: Pulmonary effects of radiation therapy *Ann Intern Med* 86:81–92, 1977.

61. Jennings FL, Arden A. Development of radiation pneumonitis Time and dose factors *Arch Pathol Lab Med* 74:351–360, 1962.

62. Teates, CD The effects of unilateral thoracic irradiation on pulmonary blood flow. *AJR* 102:875–882, 1968

63. Margolis LW, Phillips TL: Whole-lung irradiation for metastatic tumor. *Radiology* 93:1173–1179, 1969.

64. Deeley TJ: The effects of radiation on the lungs in the treatment of carcinoma of the bronchus. *Clin Radiol* 11:33–39, 1960

65. Fleming JAC, Filbee JF, Wiernik G· Sequelae to radical irradiation in carcinoma of the breast. An inquiry into the incidence of certain radiation injuries. *Br J Radiol* 34:713–719, 1961

66. Lougheed MN, Maguire GH: Irradiation pneumonitis in the treatment of carcinoma of the breast. *J Can Assoc Radiol* 11:1–9, 1960.

67. Whitfield AGW, Bond WH, Kunkler PB: Radiation damage to thoracic tissues *Thorax* 18:371–380, 1963.

68. Boushy SF, Helgason AH, North LB: The effect of radiation on the lung and bronchial tree. *AJR* 108:284–292, 1970.

69. Phillips TL, Wharam MD, Margolis LW. Modification of radiation injury to normal tissues by chemotherapeutic agents. *Cancer* 35:1678–1684, 1975

70. Castellino RA, Glatstein E, Turbow MM, et al: Latent radiation injury of lung or heart activated by steroid withdrawal. *Ann Intern Med* 80:593–599, 1974

71. Kun LE, DeVita VT, Young RC, et al. Treatment of Hodgkin's disease using intensive chemotherapy followed by irradiation *Int J Radiat Oncol Biol Phys* 1:619–626, 1976.

72. Poussin-Rosillo H, Nisce LZ, et al. Complications of total nodal irradiation of Hodgkin's disease stages III and IV *Cancer* 42:437–441, 1978.

73. Goldman AL, Enquist R: Hyperacute radiation pneumonitis *Chest* 67:613–615, 1975.

74. Roswit B, White DC· Severe radiation injuries of the lung. *AJR* 129:127–136, 1977.

75. Rosenow EC III. The spectrum of drug-induced pulmonary disease. *Ann Intern Med* 77:977–991, 1972.

76. Brettner A, Heitzman ER, Woodin WG: Pulmonary complications of drug therapy *Radiology* 96:31–38, 1970

77. Whitcomb ME· Drug-induced lung disease. *Chest* 63:418–422, 1973

78. Goldiner PL, Schweizer O· The hazards of anesthesia and surgery in bleomycin-treated patients *Semin Oncol* 6:121–124, 1979

79. Tryka AF, Skornik WA, Godleski JJ, et al. Potentiation of bleomycin-induced lung injury by exposure to 70% oxygen. Morphologic assessment. *Am Rev Respir Dis* 126:1074–1079, 1982.

80. Einhorn L, Krause M, Hornback N, et al: Enhanced pulmonary toxicity with bleomycin and radiotherapy in oat cell lung cancer. *Cancer* 37:2414–2416, 1976

81. Littler WA, Ogilvie C: Lung function in patients receiving busulphan. *Br Med J* 4:530–532, 1970.

82. Rodman T, Karr S, Close HP: Radiation reaction in the lung. Report of a fatal case in a patient with carcinoma of the lung, with studies of pulmonary function before and during prednisone therapy. *N Engl J Med* 262:431–434, 1960.

83. Brady LW, Germon PA, Cander L: The effects of radiation therapy on pulmonary function in carcinoma of the lung. *Radiology* 85:130–134, 1965.

84. Sostman HD, Matthay RA, Putman CE: Cytotoxic drug-induced lung disease. *Am J Med* 62:608–615, 1977.

85. Willson JVK: Pulmonary toxicity of antineoplastic drugs. *Cancer Treatm Rep* 62:2003–2008, 1978.

86. Holoye PY, Luna MA, MacKay B, et al. Bleomycin hypersensitivity pneumonitis *Ann Intern Med* 88:47–49, 1978.

87. Rosenow EC III: Chemotherapeutic drug-induced pulmonary disease. *Semin Respir Med* 2:89–96, 1980.

88. Collis CH: Lung damage from cytotoxic drugs. *Cancer Chemother Pharmacol* 4:17–27, 1980.

89. Weiss RB, Muggia FM: Cytotoxic drug-induced pulmonary disease *Am J Med* 68:259–266, 1980.

90. Batist G, Andrews JL Jr: Pulmonary toxicity of antineoplastic drugs. *JAMA* 246:1449–1453, 1981

91. Ginsberg SJ, Comis RL: The pulmonary toxicity of antineoplastic agents. *Semin Oncol* 9:34–51, 1982

92. Oliner H, Schwartz R, Rubio F Jr, et al: Interstitial pulmonary fibrosis following busulfan therapy. *Am J Med* 31:134–139, 1961.

93. Leake E, Smith WG, Woodliff HJ. Diffuse interstitial pulmonary fibrosis after busulphan therapy. *Lancet* 2:432–434, 1963.

94. Heard BE, Cooke RA: Busulphan lung. *Thorax* 23:187–193, 1968

95. Kirschner RH, Esterly JR. Pulmonary lesions associated with busulfan therapy of chronic myelogenous leukemia *Cancer* 27:1074–1080, 1971.

96. Manning DM, Strimlan CV, Turbiner EH: Early detection of busulfan lung: Report of a case. *Clin Nucl Med* 5:412–414, 1980.

97. Hankins DG, Sanders S, MacDonald FM, et al: Pulmonary toxicity recurring after a six week course of busulfan therapy and after subsequent therapy with uracil mustard. *Chest* 73:415–416, 1978.

98. Horowitz AL, Friedman M, Smith J, et al: The pulmonary changes of bleomycin toxicity, *Radiology* 106:65–68, 1973.

99. Blum RH, Carter SK, Agre K A clinical review of bleomycin—A new antineoplastic agent, *Cancer* 31:903–914, 1973.

100. Pascual RS, Mosher MB, Sikand RS, et al. Effects of bleomycin on pulmonary function in man, *Am Rev Respir Dis* 108:211–217, 1973

101. Samuels ML, Johnson DE, Itoloye PY, et al: Large-dose bleomycin therapy and pulmonary toxicity: A possible role of prior radiotherapy. *JAMA* **235**:1117–1120, 1976.

102. Iacovino JR, Leitner J, Abbas AK, et al: Fatal pulmonary reaction from low doses of bleomycin. An idiosyncratic tissue response. *JAMA* **235**:1253–1255, 1976.

103. Perez-Guerra F, Harkleroad LE, Walsh RE, et al: Acute bleomycin lung. *AM Rev Respir Dis* **106**:909–913, 1972.

104. Brown WG, Hasan FM, Barbee RA: Reversibility of severe bleomycin-induced pneumonitis. *JAMA* **239**:2012–2014, 1978.

105. Aronin PA, Mahaley MS Jr, Rudnick SA, et al: Prediction of BCNU pulmonary toxicity in patients with malignant gliomas: An assessment of risk factors. *N Engl J Med* **303**:183–188, 1980.

106. Durant JR, Norgard MJ, Murad TM, et al: Pulmonary toxicity associated with bischloroethyl nitrosourea (BCNU). *Ann Intern Med* **90**:191–194, 1979.

107. Rodin AE, Haggard ME, Travis LB: Lung changes and chemotherapeutic agents in childhood: Report of a case associated with cyclophosphamide therapy. *Am J Dis Child* **120**:337–340, 1970.

108. Dohner VA, Ward HP, Standard RE: Alveolitis during procarbazine, vincristine and cyclophosphamide therapy. *Chest* **62**:636–639, 1972.

109. Patel AR, Shah PC, Rhee HL, Sassoon H, Rao KP: Cyclophosphamide therapy and interstitial pulmonary fibrosis. *Cancer* **38**:1542–1549, 1976.

110. Rubio FA: Possible pulmonary effects of alkylating agents. *N Engl J Med* **287**:1150–1151, 1972.

111. Rose MS: Busulphan toxicity syndrome caused by chlorambucil. *Br Med J* **2**:123–127, 1975.

112. Godard P, Marty JP, Michel FB: Interstitial pneumonia and chlorambucil. *Chest* **76**:471–473, 1979.

113. Clarysse AM, Cathey WJ, Cartwright GE, et al: Pulmonary disease complicating intermittent therapy with methotrexate. *JAMA* **209**:1861–1864, 1969.

114. Whitcomb ME, Schwarz MI, Tormey DC: Methotrexate pneumonitis: Case report and review of the literature. *Thorax* **27**:636–639, 1972.

115. Goldman GC, Moschella SL: Severe pneumonitis occurring during methotrexate therapy. Report of two cases. *Arch Dermatol* **103**:194–197, 1971.

116. Everts CS, Westcott JL, Bragg DG: Methotrexate therapy and pulmonary disease. *Radiology* **107**:539–543, 1973.

117. Lisbona A, Schwartz J, Lachance C, et al: Methotrexate-induced pulmonary disease. *J Can Assoc Radiol* **24**:215–220, 1973.

118. Sostman HD, Matthay RA, Putman CE, et al: Methotrexate-induced pneumonitis. *Medicine (Baltimore)* **55**:371–388, 1976.

119. Gutin PH, Green MR, Bleyer WA, et al: Methotrexate pneumonitis induced by intrathecal methotrexate therapy: A case report with pharmacokinetic data. *Cancer* **38**:1529–1534, 1976.

120. Lascari AD, Strano AJ, Johnson WW, et al: Methotrexate-induced sudden fatal pulmonary reaction. *Cancer* **40**:1393–1397, 1977.

121. Rosenow EC III, Unni KK: Drug-induced pulmonary granulomas. *Lung Biol Health Dis* **20**:469–484, 1983.

122. Cooperative study: Acute lymphocytic leukemia in children. Maintenance therapy with methotrexate administered intermittently. Acute leukemia group B. *JAMA* **207**:923–928, 1969.

123. Codling BW, Chakera TM: Pulmonary fibrosis following therapy with melphalan for multiple myeloma. *J Clin Pathol* **25**:668–673, 1972.

124. Rubin G, Baume P, Vandenberg R: Azathioprine and acute restrictive lung disease. *Aust NZ J Med* **2**:272–274, 1972.

125. Hazlett DR, Ward GW, Madison DS: Pulmonary function loss in diphenylhydantoin therapy. *Chest* **66**:660–664, 1974.

126. Marshall A, Moore K: Pulmonary disease after amitriptyline overdosage. *Br Med J* **1**:716–717, 1973.

127. Winterbauer RH, Wilske KR, Wheelis RF: Diffuse pulmonary injury associated with gold treatment. *N Engl J Med* **294**:919–921, 1976.

128. Whitcomb ME, Schwarz MI, Keller AR, et al: Hodgkin's disease of the lung. *Am Rev Respir Dis* **106**:79–85, 1972.

129. Martin JJ: The Nisbet Symposium: Hodgkin's disease. Radiological aspects of the disease. *Australas Radiol* **11**:206–218, 1967.

130. Strickland B: Intra-thoracic Hodgkin's disease. Part II. Peripheral manifestations of Hodgkin's disease in the chest. *Br J Radiol* **40**:930–938, 1967.

131. Fraser RG, Paré JAP (eds): Neoplastic diseases of the lungs. In *Diagnosis of Diseases of the Chest*. Vol. II. 2nd ed. WB Saunders, Philadelphia, 1978, pp. 981–1134.

132. Rosenberg SA, Diamond HD, Jaslowitz B, et al: Lymphosarcoma: A review of 1269 cases. *Medicine (Baltimore)* **40**:31–84, 1961.

133. Rose HA: Primary lymphosarcoma of the lung. *J Thorac Cardiovasc Surg* **33**:254–263, 1957.

134. Baron MG, Whitehouse WM: Primary lymphosarcoma of the lung. *AJR* **85**:294–308, 1961.

135. Vernant JP, Brun B, Mannoni P, et al: Respiratory distress of hyperleukocytic granulocytic leukemias. *Cancer* **44**:264–268, 1979.

136. McKee LC Jr, Collins RD: Intravascular leukocyte thrombi and aggregates as a cause of morbidity and mortality in leukemia. *Medicine (Baltimore)* **53**:463–478, 1974.

137. Myers TJ, Cole SR, Klatsky AU, et al: Respiratory failure due to pulmonary leukostasis following chemotherapy of acute non-lymphocytic leukemia. *Cancer* **51**:1808–1813, 1983.

138. Tryka AF, Godleski JJ, Fanta CH: Leukemic cell lysis pneumonopathy: A complication of treated myeloblastic leukemia. *Cancer* **50**:2763–2770, 1982.

139. Green RA, Nichlos NJ: Pulmonary involvement in leukemia. *Am Rev Respir Dis* **80**:833–844, 1959.

140. Blank N, Castellino RA, Shah V: Radiographic aspects of pulmonary infection in patients with altered immunity. *Radiol Clin North Am* **11**:175–190, 1973.

141. Simmons RL, Uranga VM, LaPlante ES, et al: Pulmonary complications in transplant recipients. *Arch Surg* **105**:260–268, 1972.

142. Friedman M, Libert R, Michaelson ED: Unilateral pulmonary edema after renal transplantation. *N Engl J Med* **293**:343–344, 1975.

143. Ward HN: Pulmonary infiltrates associated with leukoagglutinin transfusion reactions. *Ann Intern Med* **73**:689–694, 1970.

144. Thompson JS, Severson CD, Parmely MJ, et al: Pulmonary "hypersensitivity" reactions induced by transfusion of non-HL-A leukoagglutinins. *N Engl J Med* **284**:1120–1125, 1971.

145. Tenholder MF, Hooper RG: Pulmonary infiltrates in leukemia. *Chest* **78**:468–473, 1980.

146. Popovsky MA, Abel MD, Moore SB: Transfusion-related acute lung injury associated with passive transfer of anti-leukocyte antibodies. *Am Rev Respir Dis* **128**:185–189, 1983.

147. Roswit B, White DC: Severe radiation injuries of the lung. *AJR* **129**:127–136, 1977.

148. Aisner J, Schimpff SC, Wiernik PH: Treatment of invasive aspergillosis: Relation of early diagnosis and treatment to response. *Ann Intern Med* **86**:539–543, 1977.

149. Schaefer JC, Yu B, Armstrong D: An aspergillus immunodiffusion test in the early diagnosis of aspergillosis in adult leukemia patients. *Am Rev Respir Dis* **113**:325–329, 1976.

150. Filice G, Yu B, Armstrong D: Immunodiffusion and agglutination tests for candida in patients with neoplastic disease: Inconsistent correlation of results with invasive disease. *J Infect Dis* **135**:349–357, 1977.

151. Edwards JE Jr, Lehrer RI, Stiehm ER, et al: Severe candidal infections: Clinical perspective, immune defense mechanisms, and current concepts of therapy. *Ann Intern Med* **89**:91–106, 1978.

152. Fisher BD, Armstrong D: Cryptococcal interstitial pneumonia: Value of antigen determination. *N Engl J Med* **297**:1440–1441, 1977.

153. Jensen WA, Rose RM, Hammer SM, et al: Serologic diagnosis of focal pneumonia caused by *Cryptococcus neoformans*. *Am Rev Respir Dis* **132**:198–200, 1985.

154. Shaffer PJ, Medoff G, Kobayashi GS: Demonstration of antigenemia by radioimmunoassay in rabbits experimentally infected with *Aspergillus*. *J Infect Dis* **139**:313–319, 1979.

155. Weiner MH, Talbot GH, Gerson SL, et al: Antigen detection in the diagnosis of invasive aspergillosis; utility in controlled blinded trials. *Ann Intern Med* **99**:777–784, 1983.

156. Kiehn TE, Bernard EM, Gold JWM, et al: Candidiasis: Detection by gas–liquid chromatography of D-arabinitol, a fungal metabolite, in human serum. *Science* **206**:577–580, 1979.

157. Murray PR, Washington JA II: Microscopic and bacteriologic analysis of expectorated sputum. *Mayo Clin Proc* **50**:339–344, 1975.

158. Bodey GP, Powell RD, Hersh EM, et al: Pulmonary complications of acute leukemia. *Cancer* **19**:781–793, 1966.

159. Sickles EA, Young VM, Greene WH, et al: Pneumonia in acute leukemia. *Ann Intern Med* **79**:528–534, 1973.

160. Aisner J, Kuols LK, Sickles EA, et al: Transtracheal selective bronchial brushing for pulmonary infiltrates in patients with cancer. *Chest* **69**:367–371, 1976.

161. Walzer PD, Perl DP, Krogstad DJ, et al: *Pneumocystis carinii* pneumonia in the United States: Epidemiologic, diagnostic, and clinical features. *Ann Intern Med* **80**:83–93, 1974.

162. Lau WK, Young LS, Remington JS: *Pneumocystis carinii* pneumonia: Diagnosis by examination of pulmonary secretions. *JAMA* **236**:2399–2402, 1976.

163. Bartlett JG: Diagnostic accuracy of transtracheal aspiration: Bacteriologic studies. *Am Rev Respir Dis* **115**:777–782, 1977.

164. Hahn HH, Beaty HN: Transtracheal aspiration in the evaluation of patients with pneumonia. *Ann Intern Med* **72**:183–187, 1970.

165. Ries K, Levison ME, Kaye D: Transtracheal aspiration in pulmonary infection. *Arch Intern Med* **133**:453–458, 1973.

166. Davidson M, Tempest B, Palmer DL: Bacteriologic diagnosis of acute pneumonia: Comparison of sputum, transtracheal aspirates, and lung aspirates. *JAMA* **235**:158–163, 1976.

167. Matthay RA, Moritz ED: Invasive procedures for diagnosing pulmonary infection: A critical review. *Clin Chest Med* **2**:3–19, 1981.

168. Bartlett JG, Alexander J, Mayhew J, et al: Should fiberoptic bronchoscopy aspirates be cultured? *Am Rev Respir Dis* **114**:73–78, 1976.

169. Thiede WH, Banaszak GF: Selective bronchial catheterization. *N Engl J Med* **286**:525–528, 1972.

170. Repsher LH, Schroter G, Hammon WS: Diagnosis of *Pneumocystis carinii*. *N Engl J Med* **287**:340–341, 1972.

171. Finley R, Kieff E, Thompson S, et al: Bronchial brushing in the diagnosis of pulmonary disease in patients at risk for opportunistic infection. *Am Rev Respir Dis* **109**:379–386, 1974.

172. Zavala DC, Bedell GN, Rossi NP: Trephine Lung biopsy with a high-speed air drill. *J Thorac Cardiovasc Surg* **64**:220–228, 1972.

173. McCartney RL: Hemorrhage following percutaneous lung biopsy. *Radiology* **112**:305–307, 1974.

174. Bandt PD, Blank N, Castellino RA: Needle diagnosis of pneumonitis. Value in high-risk patients, *JAMA* **220**:1578–1583, 1972.

175. Greenman RL, Goodall PT, King D: Lung biopsy in immunocompromised hosts. *Am J Med* **59**:488–497, 1975.

176. Krick JA, Stinson EB, Remington JS: Nocardia infection in heart transplant patients. *Ann Intern Med* **82**:18–26, 1975.

177. Zavala DC, Schoell JE: Ultrathin needle aspiration of the lung in infectious and malignant disease. *Am Rev Respir Dis* **123**:125–131, 1981.

178. Bandt PD, Blank N, Castellino RA: Needle diagnosis of pneumonitis; value in high-risk patients. *JAMA* **220**:1578–1580, 1972.

179. Wimberley N, Faling LJ, Bartlett JG: A fiberoptic bronchoscopy technique to obtain uncontaminated lower airway secretions for bacterial culture. *Am Rev Respir Dis* **119**:337–343, 1979.

180. Winterbauer RH, Hutchinson JF, Reinhardt GN, et al: The use of quantitative cultures and antibody coating of bacteria to diagnose bacterial pneumonia by fiberoptic bronchoscopy. *Am Rev Respir Dis* **128**:98–103, 1983.

181. Ellis JH Jr.: Transbronchial lung biopsy via the fiberoptic bronchoscope: Experience with 107 consecutive cases and comparison with bronchial brushing. *Chest* **68:**524–532, 1975.

182. Cunningham JH, Zarala DC, Corry RJ, et al: Trephine air drill, bronchial brush, and fiberoptic transbronchial lung biopsies in immunosuppressed patients. *Am Rev Respir Dis* **115:**213–220, 1977.

183. Ellis JH Jr: Diagnosis of opportunistic infections using the flexible fiberoptic bronchoscope. *Chest (Suppl)* **73:**713–715, 1978.

184. Matthay RA, Farmer WC, Odero D: Diagnostic fiberoptic bronchoscopy in the immunocrompromised host with pulmonary infiltrates. *Thorax* **32:**539–545, 1977.

185. George RB, Jenkinson SG, Light RW: Fiberoptic bronchoscopy in the diagnosis of pulmonary fungal and nocardial infections. *Chest* **73:**33–36, 1978.

186. Stover DE, Zaman MB, Hajdu SI, et al: Bronchoalveolar lavage in the diagnosis of diffuse pulmonary infiltrates in the immunosuppressed host. *Ann Intern Med* **101:**1–7, 1984.

187. Coleman DL, Dodek PM, Luce JM, et al: Diagnostic utility of fiberoptic bronchoscopy in patients with *Pneumocystis carinii* pneumonia and the acquired immune deficiency syndrome. *Am Rev Respir Dis* **128:**795–799, 1983.

188. Murray JF, Felton CP, Garay SM, et al: Pulmonary complications of the acquired immunodeficiency syndrome. *N Engl J Med* **310:**1682–1688, 1984.

189. Young JA, Hopkin JM, Cuthbertson WP: Pulmonary infiltrates in immunocompromised patients: Diagnosis by cytological examination of bronchoalveolar lavage fluid *J Clin Pathol* **37:**390–397, 1984.

190. Beyt BE Jr, King DK, Glew RH: Fatal pneumonitis and septicemia after fiberoptic bronchoscopy. *Chest* **72:**105–107, 1977.

191. Robbins H, Goldman AL: Failure of a "prophylactic" antimicrobial drug to prevent sepsis after fiberoptic bronchoscopy. *Am Rev Respir Dis* **116:**325–326, 1977.

192. Dijkman JH, van der Meer JWM, Bakker W, et al: Transpleural lung biopsy by the thoracoscopic route in patients with diffuse interstitial pulmonary disease. *Chest* **82:**76–83, 1982.

193. Lloyd MS: Thoracoscopy and biopsy in the diagnosis of pleurisy with effusion. *Q Bull Sea View Hosp* **14:**128–133, 1953.

194. DeCamp PT, Mosley PW, Scott ML, et al: Diagnostic thoracoscopy. *Ann Thorac Surg* **16:**79–84, 1973.

195. Oldenburg FA, Newhouse MT: Thoracoscopy. A safe, accurate diagnostic procedure using the rigid thoracoscope and local anesthesia. *Chest* **75:**45–50, 1979.

196. Toledo-Pereyra LH, DeMeester TR, Kinealey A, et al: The benefit of open lung biopsy in patients with previous nondiagnostic transbronchial lung biopsy; a guide to appropriate therapy. *Chest* **77:**647–650, 1980.

197. Jaffe JP, Maki DG: Lung biopsy in immunocompromised patients: One institution's experience and an approach to management of pulmonary disease in the compromised host. *Cancer* **48:**1144–1153, 1981.

198. Haverkos HW, Dowling JN, Pasculle AW, et al. Diagnosis

199. McKenna RJ Jr, Mountain CF, McMurtrey MJ: Open lung biopsy in immunocompromised patients. *Chest* **86:**671–674, 1984.

200. Cockerill FR III, Wilson WR, Carpenter HA, et al: Open lung biopsy in immunocompromised patients. *Arch Intern Med* **145:**1398–1404, 1985.

201. Cheson BD, Samlowski WE, Tang TT, et al: Value of open-lung biopsy in 87 immunocompromised patients with pulmonary infiltrates. *Cancer* **55:**453–459, 1985.

202. Maile CW, Moore AV, Ulreich S, et al: Chest radiographic-pathologic correlation in adult leukemia patients. *Invest Radiol* **18:**495–499, 1983.

203. McCabe RE, Brooks RG, Mark JBD, et al: Open lung biopsy in patients with leukemia. *Am J Med* **78:**609–616, 1985.

204. Murray JF, Felton CP, Gonay SM, et al: Pulmonary complications of the acquired immunodeficiency syndrome: Report of a National Heart, Lung, and Blood Institute Workshop. *N Engl J Med* **310:**1682–1688, 1984.

205. Hopewell PC, Luce JM: Pulmonary involvement in the acquired immune deficiency syndrome. *Chest* **87:**104–112, 1985.

206. Stover DE, White DA, Romano PA, et al: Spectrum of pulmonary disease associated with the acquired immunodeficiency syndrome. *Am J Med* **78:**429–437, 1985.

207. Catterall JR, Potasman I, Remington JS: Pneumocystis carinii pneumonia in the patient with AIDS *Chest* **88:**758–762, 1985.

208. Talaverda W, Mildvan D. Pulmonary infections in the acquired immunodeficiency syndrome. *Semin Respir Infect* **1:**202–211, 1986.

209. Coleman DL, Hattner RS, Luce JM, et al· Correlation between gallium lung scan and fiberoptic bronchoscopy in patients with suspected *Pneumocystis carinii* pneumonia and the acquired immune deficiency syndrome. *Am Rev Respir Dis* **130:**1166–1169, 1984.

210. Tuazon CU, Delaney MD, Simon GL, et al. Utility of gallium 67 scintigraphy and bronchial washings in the diagnosis and treatment of *Pneumocystis carinii* pneumonia in patients with the acquired immune deficiency syndrome. *Am Rev Respir Dis* **132:**1087–1092, 1985.

211. Polsky B, Gold JWM, Whimby E, et al. Bacterial pneumonia in patients with acquired immune deficiency syndrome. *Ann Intern Med* **104:**38–41, 1986.

212 Betts RF, Freeman RB, Douglas RG, et al: Clinical manifestations of renal allograft derived primary cytomegalovirus infection *Am J Dis Child* **131:**759–763, 1977.

213. Chatterjee SN, Fiala M, Weiner J, et al: Primary cytomegalovirus and opportunistic infections: Incidence in renal transplant recipients. *JAMA* **240:**2446–2449, 1978.

214. Rand KH, Pollard RB, Merigan TC: Increased pulmonary superinfections in cardiac transplant patients undergoing primary cytomegalovirus infection *N Engl J Med* **298:**951–953, 1978.

215. Neiman PE, Reeves W, Ray G, et al: A prospective analysis of interstitial pneumonia and opportunistic viral infection

among recipients of allogenic bone marrow grafts. *J Infect Dis* **136:**754–767, 1977.

216. Rubin RH, Russell PS, Levin M, et al: Summary of a workshop on cytomegalovirus infections during organ transplantation. *J Infect Dis* **134:**728–734, 1979.

217. Hamilton JR, Overall JC, Glasgow LA: Synergistic effect on mortality in mice with murine cytomegalovirus and *Pseudomonas aeruginosa, Staphylococcus aureus* or *Candida albicans* infection. *Infect Immun* **14:**982–989, 1976.

7

Central Nervous System Infections in the Compromised Host

DONALD ARMSTRONG and BRUCE POLSKY

1. Introduction

Meningitis and other types of central nervous system (CNS) infection in the immunocompromised patient are usually caused by different organisms than in the general population.[1-3] For instance, *Streptococcus pneumoniae* or *Neisseria meningitidis* may produce meningitis in an immunocompromised patient, but it is more common to find *Listeria monocytogenes* or *Pseudomonas aeruginosa* as the cause. The latter organisms may cause meningitis in the general population, but much less commonly as compared with the *Pneumococcus* or the *Meningococcus*.[4-6] Similarly, the most common type of brain abscess seen in the general population is caused by mixed aerobic and anaerobic bacterial flora[7,8] by a process that generally extends from the nasopharynx. In contrast, *Aspergillus fumigatus*[9,10] or *Nocardia asteroides*[11,12] more frequently cause brain abscess in the immunocompromised patient,[1,2] and the apparent route of access is hematogenous.

Our past experience suggests that we may be able to predict, with some degree of accuracy, the organisms that will be responsible for a particular type of CNS infection depending on the nature of the underlying disease and associated defects in host-defense mechanisms.[1-3,13] These observations have

been substantiated in a series of patients from a general hospital.[14] For instance, the patient with Hodgkin disease is more likely to develop an infection caused by an organism that exploits a defect in the thymus-derived (or T-lymphocyte) mononuclear phagocyte system. A patient with leukemia who is neutropenic, either because of his basic disease or from chemotherapy, is more likely to develop CNS infection with an organism against which the neutrophil is a critical component of host defense. Various chemotherapeutic regimens tend to alter one immune system more than another. Adrenocorticosteroids affect predominantly the T-lymphocyte, mononuclear phagocyte system, although at the same time, these agents may alter (to a lesser degree) the ability of neutrophils to phagocytose and kill.[15]

Cytotoxic agents, such as the nitrogen mustards, the antimetabolites, or antitumor antibiotics may also alter the T-lymphocyte, mononuclear phagocyte immune response. Azathioprine, commonly used following renal transplantation, predominantly affects T-cell and bursa-derived (B)-cell function. However, it occasionally leads to significant neutropenia which places the host at great risk to infection with pyogenic microorganisms. Even before the neutrophil count declines, the function of these cells can be altered by antineoplastic chemotherapy.[15] It has also been noted that after prolonged treatment with cytotoxic chemotherapeutic agents for a disease such as Hodgkin disease, immunoglobulin levels may fall.[16] This can be reflected in a decline of specific levels of opsonizing and bactericidal antibodies. Splenectomy may be associated with decreased IgM

DONALD ARMSTRONG and BRUCE POLSKY • Department of Medicine, Infectious Disease Service and Microbiology Laboratory, Memorial Sloan-Kettering Cancer Center, Cornell University Medical College, New York, New York 10021.

levels in the setting of additional antineoplastic treatment.

Thus, in CNS infection, when the predominant immune defect is known, the list of likely opportunistic organisms can be narrowed down to a relative few[1-3,13] (Tables 1-4). In general, the underlying condition, such as a lymphoma or organ transplantation plus adrenocorticosteroid therapy, tends to make the patient more susceptible to organisms that take advantage of the depression of the T-lymphocyte, mononuclear phagocyte system. These organisms are obligate or facultative intracellular parasites and are listed in Table 1. The total neutrophil count can be helpful in diagnosing the microbial etiology of a CNS infection. Certain organisms are much more likely to be responsible for meningitis or brain abscess when the total peripheral white blood cell (WBC) count is less than 1000/mm^3 (Table 2). With the knowledge of the underlying disease and the peripheral WBC, the responsible organisms can be predicted with considerable accuracy in a patient with either meningitis, encephalitis, or clinical brain abscess.

For the purpose of a complete presentation of the problem of meningitis and CNS infections in the immunocompromised host, infections are discussed first according to microorganisms, followed by a review of clinical syndromes and the differential diagnosis. There is thus some repetition, but we believe it worthwhile. Since definite patterns have been recognized in CNS disease in patients with the acquired immune deficiency syndrome (AIDS), this subject is discussed separately.

2. Microorganisms

2.1. Bacteria

The most common microorganisms causing CNS infections according to the immune defect in the immunocompromised host are listed in Tables 1-4.

2.1.1. Gram-Positive Rods

2.1.1a. *Listeria monocytogenes.* *Listeria monocytogenes* is a gram-positive rod that is motile and hemolytic. On Gram stain of cerebrospinal fluid (CSF), the rods can readily appear as coccobacillary forms or be mistaken for the *Pneumococcus*. They can also be overdecolorized and appear as small, delicate, gram-negative rods. The characteristic tumbling motility is best seen at room temperature. Hemolysis may not be appreciable on initial isolation but usually becomes quite apparent on first subculture. This can cause some confusion with groups A and B streptococci, which commonly cause meningitis in the neonate.[17] The organism appears to be widespread in nature, having been isolated from tap water and sewage and a number of different animal species including mammals and birds. It can be isolated from the stool of asymptomatic individuals and appears to be more commonly isolated from individuals who work in abattoirs.

A cold enrichment technique appears to yield a higher incidence of isolation, at least from stools, but this has not been true with CSF specimens in many laboratories.[18-20] In some instances of *Listeria monocytogenes* septic syndrome, diarrhea has preceded the bacteremia, but this has not been consistent. The organism may reside in the gastrointestinal (GI) tract, and when the host becomes immunocompromised, it may disseminate from there. Recently, there have been three epidemics due to cole slaw,[21] pasteurized milk,[22] and Mexican-style cheese[23] containing *Listeria monocytogenes*. In each of these outbreaks pregnant women were the immunocompromised hosts most affected.

The two syndromes usually seen in the immunocompromised host other than the neonate are a pattern of sepsis with bacteremia and a meningitis or a meningoencephalitis with or without cerebritis. Clinically, the patient may have no CNS signs, although the organism can be recovered from the CSF. For example, a patient who has a septic syndrome caused by *Listeria monocytogenes* and no clinical evidence of meningitis can still have a pleocytosis and *Listeria monocytogenes* isolated from the spinal fluid. Other patients may show minimal signs, such as personality changes, mild headaches, and/or low-grade fever, although more rarely a rather fulminant syndrome with a cerebritis may be observed.[20] In the patient with the subtle meningitis syndrome, a stiff neck may be absent both by history and physical examination.

With *Listeria monocytogenes* meningitis high on the list of possible etiologies, lumbar puncture should be performed at the earliest clinical suspicion in an immunocompromised patient. The procedure is

TABLE 1. Thymus-Derived (T) Lymphocyte, Mononuclear Phagocyte Defect

	Bacteria	Fungi	Parasites	Viruses
Meningitis	Listeria monocyto-genes	Cryptococcus neoformans	Toxoplasma gondii Strongyloides ster-coralis	Varicella–zoster Herpes simplex
Meningoencephalitis	Listeria monocyto-genes Legionella sp.	Cryptococcus neoformans	Toxoplasma gondii Strongyloides ster-coralis	Varcella–zoster Papovavirus
Abscess	Nocardia asteroides	Cryptococcus neoformans	Toxoplasma gondii	Papovavirus

indicated in the presence of fever and/or headache in a patient with impaired T-lymphocyte, mononuclear phagocyte function. In addition, the slightest CNS signs such as increased irritability, personality change, or forgetfulness should alone suggest the diagnosis and prompt a diagnostic lumbar puncture. Patients may present with focal signs such as facial nerve palsy or even hemiplegia. Although we have frequently noted RBCs in the CSF of patients with Listeria monocytogenes, this does not appear to be any more common than in any other type of meningitis. The pleocytosis may be either predominantly mononuclear or polymorphonuclear; however, in most cases, the predominant cell type is the neutrophil.[6,20] Cell counts have ranged from null to 1200/mm^3, protein concentrations have ranged from within normal limits to 735 mg/dl, and sugars from normal to undetectable. The diagnosis is frequently not made by Gram stain of the CSF, since the organisms are often not present in large numbers. The typical gram-positive diphtheroid-like rods have been seen on smear in approximately 10% of our cases where the organism has been isolated.[24] In the appropriate clinical setting, a prolonged search for Listeria on Gram stain of the spinal fluid should be made using the centrifuged sediment from a minimum of 10 ml CSF.

Antibiotic sensitivity studies have shown that all isolates of Listeria monocytogenes are susceptible to ampicillin but that some strains are resistant to penicillin.[6] The organism is usually also sensitive to the cephalosporins, erythromycin, chloramphenicol, tetracycline, and the aminoglycosides. There are both in vitro evidence and animal studies to document that a combination of ampicillin plus an aminoglycoside such as gentamicin acts synergistically against Listeria monocytogenes.[6] The treatment of choice, in our opinion, is ampicillin in doses of 200 mg/kg per day, although we cannot argue strongly against penicillin in doses of 125 mg/kg per day[25] (Table 5). Whether the addition of an aminoglycoside such as gentamicin will appreciably affect the outcome is uncertain. If aminoglycosides are to be used for meningitis, they should be given both systemically and intrathecally (gentamicin doses of 2–10 mg/ml once or twice a day) because of poor blood–brain barrier penetration with systemic administration. If the patient is penicillin allergic, the choice is either to desensitize the patient to ampicillin or penicillin or to use an alternate therapeutic regimen. The combination of erythromycin and tetracycline or chloramphenicol has been used successfully in a number of cases.[20] Trimethoprim–sulfamethoxazole has been used successfully in cases of

TABLE 2. Neutrophil Defect

	Bacteria	Fungi	Parasites	Viruses
Meningitis	Enteric bacilli	Candida sp.	—	—
Meningoencephalitis	Enteric bacilli	Aspergillus sp. Mucoraceae	—	—
Abscess	Enteric bacilli	Aspergillus sp.	—	—

TABLE 3. Surgery

	Bacteria	Fungi	Parasites	Viruses
Meningitis	Enteric bacilli *Staphylococcus aureus* *Staphylococcus epidermidis* *Corynebacterium* sp.	*Candida* sp.	Trichomonads	—
Meningoencephalitis	Enteric bacilli *Staphylococcus aureus* *Staphylococcus epidermidis* *Corynebacterium* sp.	*Candida* sp.	Trichomonads	—
Abscess	Enteric bacilli *Staphylococcus aureus* *Staphylococcus epidermidis* *Corynebacterium* sp.	*Candida* sp.	—	—

penicillin allergy or when initial therapy has failed.[26,27]

Duration of therapy should be at least 2 weeks, with 3–4 weeks considered if response to antimicrobials is not prompt (defervescence in 72 hr). Cases of *Listeria* bacteremia should always be treated with meningeal doses of drug, and any relapse taken as evidence of deep-seated CNS involvement, i.e., brain abscess.

2.1.1b. *Bacillus* **Species.** Two gram-positive organisms that have infected immunocompromised patients with leukemia and neutropenia are *Bacillus subtilis* and *Bacillus cereus*.[28] These have a tendency to cause brain abscess, but meningitis can coexist. They appear as large, plump gram-positive rods with spores. They can be readily identified, and sensitivities are important because they may vary considerably. Not all are susceptible to penicillin, and therapy may necessitate use of an aminoglycoside or chloramphenicol.

2.1.2c. *Nocardia asteroides.* *Nocardia asteroides* is a gram-positive, beaded, branching rod that is one of the Actinomycetales. Contrary to popular impression, it is a higher bacterium rather than a fungus. It belongs to the same family as *Actinomyces* and *Mycobacterium*. Like the latter, it is sometimes

TABLE 4. Miscellaneous Defects

	Bacteria	Fungi	Parasites	Viruses
Splenectomy meningitis	*Streptococcus pneumoniae* *Hemophilus influenzae* *Neisseria meningitidis*	—	—	—
Hypogammaglobulinemia meningitis	*Streptococcus pneumoniae* *Hemophilus influenzae* *Neisseria meningitidis*	—	—	Coxsackie B

TABLE 5. Treatment of Common Causes of CNS Infection in the Immunocompromised Host

Organism	Recommended therapy	Alternate therapy[a]
Listeria monocytogenes	Ampicillin IV, 35 mg/kg q4h	Erythromycin IV, 10 mg/kg q6h plus tetracycline IV, 5 mg/kg q6h
Streptococcus pneumoniae	Penicillin IV, 5000 units/kg q4h	Chloramphenicol IV, 15 mg/kg q6h
Cryptococcus neoformans	Amphotericin B IV, 1–2 mg/kg q48h plus 5-flucytosine PO, 40 mg/kg q6h, +/− intraventricular amphotericin B	Miconazole IV, 8 to 15 mg/kg q6–8h
Escherichia coli	A third-generation cephalosporin plus gentamicin, 1.25 mg IV q6h and gentamicin IT,[b] 0.1 mg/kg q12–24h	Chloramphenicol IV plus gentamicin IV and IT[b] Cotrimoxazole IV 2.5 mg/kg q6h trimethoprim plus gentamicin IV and IT[b]
Klebsiella pneumoniae	A third generation cephalosporin plus gentamicin IV, 1.25 mg/kg q6h plus gentamicin IT,[b] 0.1 mg/kg q12–24h	Chloramphenicol IV 50–100 mg/kg q6h plus gentamicin IV and IT[b] Cotrimoxazole IV 2.5 mg/kg q6h trimethoprim plus gentamicin IV and IT[b]
Pseudomonas aeruginosa	Piperacillin 50 mg/kg q4h plus tobramycin IV, 1.25 mg/kg q6h plus tobramycin IT,[b] 0.1 mg/kg q12–24h	Cefotaxime 35 mg/kg[c] q4h, cefoperazone 70 mg/kg[c] q8h or ceftazidime 70 mg/kg[c] q8h plus tobramycin IV and IT[b]
Nocardia asteroides	Sulfadiazine IV, 30 mg/kg q6h	Cotrimoxazole as above
Toxoplasma gondii	Sulfadiazine IV, 30 mg/kg plus pyrimethamine PO, 1 mg/kg PO × 1, then 0.3 mg/kg PO qd	Cotrimoxazole as above
Strongyloides stercoralis	Thiabendazole PO, 25 mg/kg q12h × 10 days	None
Staphylococcus aureus	Oxacillin IV, 35 mg/kg q4h	Vancomycin IV 10 mg/kg q6h; rifampin 5 mg/kg q12h
Staphylococcus epidermidis	Oxacillin IV, 35 mg/kg q4h[d]	Vancomycin IV 10 mg/kg q6h; rifampin 5 mg/kg q12h
Corynebacterium sp.	Penicillin IV, 5000 mg/kg q4h	Vancomycin Oxacillin

[a]Other semisynthetic penicillins such as methicillin or nafcillin may be substituted for oxacillin, aminoglycosides such as amikacin or tobramycin may be substituted for gentamicin; cotrimoxazole is the same preparation as trimethoprim–sulfamethoxazole
[b]IT, intrathecal administration
[c]Maximum dose of 12 g/day
[d]Vancomycin should be used initially, change to oxacillin if organism sensitive

acid-fast with either the regular or a modified Ziehl–Nielsen stain.[11,12] The organism has been isolated from soil and occasionally in respiratory secretions of normal individuals and patients with chronic bronchitis or chronic obstructive pulmonary disease. Some of the latter have not had obvious invasive nocardiosis. We have occasionally isolated it when it appeared not to be causing invasive disease in immunocompromised patients,[11] but nevertheless, we should take its isolation very seriously in any secretion of an immunocompromised individual.

If Nocardia asteroides is clinically suspected,

the laboratory should be alerted to that fact because the organism grows slowly. Sometimes 4–5 days may elapse before typical colonies appear. In mixed cultures, such as sputum, it may be obscured by rapidly growing organisms, or the cultures may be discarded before the colonies appear. In addition, specimens should be delivered to the laboratory as quickly as possible, because the gram-positive beaded, branching rods of Nocardia asteroides can fragment and take on the appearance of chains of gram-positive cocci.

Nocardia asteroides enters the host by the respiratory route and most frequently causes a pneumonia. It spreads from the lung to the brain and meninges via the hematogenous route. The usual CNS manifestation is that of brain abscess or as one or more space-occupying lesions that may cause focal signs and symptoms and defy diagnosis except by brain biopsy. On occasion, if the abscess is close to the meninges, there may be a meningeal spillover and inflammation. Either a polymorphonuclear leukocyte response or mononuclear cell response can be observed, but unfortunately, the organisms are infrequently detected by stains of the CSF. There is no reported experience with counterimmunoelectrophoresis to detect antigen in the CSF, and the experience with serologic tests for antibody has not been encouraging in that many patients with *Nocardia asteroides* infections do not develop antibody responses.[29] Those affected with CNS infections are usually patients with a T-lymphocyte, mononuclear phagocyte defect. The organism may be isolated from sputum or subcutaneous abscesses, and the presumptive diagnosis of central nervous system nocardiosis made if the patient also has CNS signs or symptoms. Brain biopsy should still be considered for two reasons: (1) concomitant infection with another organism such as toxoplasmosis may be present, and (2) drainage appears to be important in the treatment of *Nocardia* abscesses in the brain as well as elsewhere in the body. In addition to the lung, subcutaneous tissues, and brain, other organs such as the liver and kidneys are frequently involved.

The organism is variably susceptible to a number of antimicrobial agents. Sulfonamides, including sulfisoxazole and sulfadiazine, are generally regarded as the most effective agents for treatment. Trimethoprim–sulfamethoxazole has also been used, but there is insufficient evidence that trimethoprim adds significantly to the therapeutic effects of the sulfonamide.[30] Isolates have been found susceptible to cycloserine, minocycline, erythromycin, rifampin, and penicillins like ampicillin or carbenicillin. The treatment of choice remains a sulfonamide, presumably sulfadiazine because of its good distribution in extracellular fluid, including the CSF. In severely ill patients, a second agent such as ampicillin or erythromycin is often added, but it is not clear whether this really improves therapy. It may be wise to perform in vitro testing with sulfonamides and several other agents because some strains have been

found to be sulfonamide resistant. The recommended dose of sulfadiazine is 100 mg/kg per day, at first intravenously and subsequently by mouth. We have treated patients successfully with sulfisoxazole in similar doses. After the first week or so, according to the severity of the illness, 60 mg/kg may be better tolerated. Attention to adequate hydration is an important aspect of sulfonamide therapy.

2.1.1d. *Mycobacterium* Species. *Mycobacterium tuberculosis* might be expected to be a more common cause of meningitis or brain abscess in the immunocompromised host because mycobacterial species tend to disseminate in the T-lymphocyte-, mononuclear phagocyte-deficient patients. However, there is no convincing evidence of an increased incidence of CNS infection by *Mycobacterium tuberculosis* or other mycobacterial species, such as *Mycobacterium avium-intracellulare, Mycobacterium kansasii*, or *Mycobacterium scrofulatium*, although infections in other anatomical sites (non-CNS) caused by these organisms have been reported.[31,32]

2.1.2. Gram-Positive Cocci

2.1.2a. *Streptococcus pneumoniae*. This well-known organism is carried in the nasopharynx of up to 10% of asymptomatic people and is best known for its ability to cause pneumonia in man. It can, however, cause a fulminant bacteremia, otitis media, and, rarely, a pharyngitis. It is frequently isolated from patients with sinusitis or chronic purulent bronchitis. Pneumococci can infect almost any organ or tissue, and they are one of the most common causes of meningitis in the general adult population.[4] The susceptibility of splenectomized patients to develop severe septic syndromes and meningitis because of pneumococci is particularly well known.[33–35] The route of entry to the CNS may be via the nasopharynx or via an otitis media or bacteremia.

Other than in splenectomized and hypogammaglobulinemic patients, pneumococcal meningitis is not definitely more common in patients with any other type of immune defect. Nonetheless, any patient (immunocompromised or not) who has had head and neck surgery resulting in damage to anatomic barriers between the nasopharynx and the meninges is more at risk of developing meningitis caused by *Streptococcus pneumoniae* as well as by other constituents of the nasopharyngeal flora.[12] Gram stain of the CSF usually reveals a predominance of neutrophils and gram-positive diplococci both within and outside the phagocytes. These gram-positive diplococci can sometimes be confused with *Listeria monocytogenes,* particularly if the capsule is small and not readily apparent on Gram stain.

It is important to remember that very early in a pneumococcal meningitis, only a few to no neutrophils and no organisms may be present in the CSF. If the patient has been partially treated, lymphocytes in the 100–200 cell/mm³ range may predominate, and no organisms may be detectable. In either case, a large volume of CSF, such as 10 ml or more, would be helpful for diagnostic studies. Omniserum, a potent pooled antiserum directed against most of the common serotypes that infect man (available through the State Serum Laboratories, Copenhagen, Denmark), can be used to detect antigen present in the CSF by counterimmunoelectrophoresis. This technique has been very useful in a number of cases of pneumococcal meningitis characterized by an absence of visible or culturable organisms. The treatment of choice is still penicillin G in doses of 125 mg/kg per day (for adults, 20 million units/day). There is no good evidence that intrathecal penicillin offers any advantage over systemic treatment, and intrathecal administration may cause seizures. Alternate therapy is chloramphenicol, 50 mg/kg per day, or erythromycin at 50 mg/kg per day.

A pneumococcal vaccine[36] containing multiple serotypes has been licensed in the United States. Although considerable doubts have been raised about its ability to engender protective antibody in immunosuppressed or immunodeficient patients[37,38] (see Chapter 16), it can be argued that the vaccine is safe: no harm and possibly some good will result from its immunoprophylactic use. At one cancer hospital, pneumococci responsible for bacteremias were of the serotypes contained in the vaccine in only 62% of cases[39]; poorly immunogenic (even in normal volunteers) type VI organisms were the most common pneumococcal isolates from blood. A follow-up study has shown similar results, and many experts would use prophylactic penicillin in patients at high risk of pneumococcal meningitis.[40] The important lesson to the clinician is not to exclude the possibility of fulminant systemic and CNS infection in patients who have been previously immunized.

2.1.2b. *Staphylococcus aureus.* *Staphylococcus aureus* meningitis is usually the result of an artificial access of the bacteria into the CNS, for instance, as a result of head or spine surgery. These organisms can also reach the brain or the meninges via the hematogenous route. Meningitis has occurred following extensive nasopharyngeal surgery in areas directly adjacent to the CNS after penicillin has been used as a prophylactic antibiotic. *Staphylococcus aureus* also appears in shunt infections or in Ommaya reservoirs. The organism is usually sensitive to a semisynthetic penicillin such as methicillin, oxacillin, or nafcillin. Although methicillin binds less readily to the plasma proteins and therefore, theoretically, would reach higher levels in the CSF, there is no evidence that it is more effective against *Staphylococcus aureus* meningitis or brain abscess than the other semisynthetic penicillins. Resistance to a semisynthetic penicillin has usually been associated with equal resistance to the cephalosporins. Vancomycin appears to be a reasonable alternative because virtually all of the isolates that are methicillin resistant are sensitive to vancomycin. However, CNS penetration of this agent may be variable, and measurement of CSF levels are strongly recommended for any patient being treated with vancomycin for meningitis. Clindamycin, which does not penetrate the blood–brain barrier is not a reasonable alternative.

2.1.2c. *Staphylococcus epidermidis.* *Staphylococcus epidermidis* was an unusual complication of head and spine surgery prior to development of surgical procedures that involved implantation of foreign-body devices in the CNS. The typical example is the Ommaya reservoir. With such devices, the most common superinfecting organism is *Staphylococcus epidermidis.* It is a gram-positive coccus which occurs in clusters and can be seen in tetrads just as *Staphylococcus aureus.* It cannot be differentiated from the latter organism on Gram stain but can be tentatively identified by colonial morphology and ultimately by its negative coagulase or DNase reaction. It is frequently resistant to the semisynthetic penicillins and the cephalosporins and can elaborate β-lactamases. When vancomycin is used for central nervous system infections with this organism, intraventricular therapy may be necessary. This has been successfully employed for susceptible organisms with doses of vancomycin of 10–50 mg once daily or bacitracin, 1000–5000 units twice daily.

2.1.3. Gram-Negative Rods

2.1.3a. *Pseudomonas aeruginosa.* This, in a 20-year review of CNS bacterial infections at our hospital, was the most common cause of bacterial meningitis in the neutropenic patient. It is a gram-negative, aerobic bacillus commonly isolated from the GI tract of the immunocompromised host as are the Enterobacteriaceae. *Pseudomonas aeruginosa* is also commonly isolated from environmental sources such as sinks, humidifiers, bathtubs, and water. It has been isolated from food and plant vegetable matter. It can be isolated from the GI tract of normal individuals in 23% of instances but has been found to colonize patients admitted to cancer hospitals at an increased incidence.[41] It is also found on the skin, especially in moist areas. It is one of the most common causes of life-threatening infection in the neutropenic patient, and the portal of entry usually appears to be the GI tract. This may be via invasion in a rectal fissure or abscess, or it may be along the GI tract in inapparent ulcers associated with chemotherapy and thrombocytopenia in patients with leukemias and lymphomas. It usually reaches the CNS through hematogenous spread. It also may colonize the nasopharynx of patients who are hospitalized and treated with broad-spectrum antibiotics and may reach the CNS via anatomic defects between the nasopharynx and the meninges. In neutropenic or diabetic patients, a source of CNS infection has occasionally been an otitis media or even a purulent sinusitis.

Like *Enterobacteriaceae, Pseudomonas aeruginosa* can superinfect wounds or surgical sites of the head and neck or spine, leading directly to CNS infection.[42] There have been reports of *Pseudomonas* meningitis following lumbar punctures.

When *Pseudomonas aeruginosa* causes meningitis, the CSF is usually purulent. However, in the profoundly neutropenic host, there may be few WBCs and little in the way of pleocytosis. Organisms are usually seen in large numbers in the cerebrospinal fluid in the neutropenic patient and grow rapidly, yielding the definitive diagnosis. *Pseudomonas aeruginosa* is usually sensitive to one of the three commonly used aminoglycosides: gentamicin, to-

bramycin, or amikacin. Choice of a particular aminoglycoside should depend on the predominant sensitivity among the isolates in the particular hospital. Most isolates are sensitive to relatively high levels of ticarcillin, piperacillin, and the third-generation cephalosporins (moxalactam, cefoperazone, cefotaxime, and ceftazidime), all of which have been used successfully.[42] These agents penetrate the blood–brain barrier,[43–45] but the aminoglycosides do so unreliably. In addition to combination therapy with parenteral aminoglycoside and an antipseudomonal penicillin, or third-generation cephalosporin, aminoglycosides should be administered intrathecally: gentamicin or tobramycin 6–10 mg or amikacin 30–50 mg. Twice-daily dosage may be preferable, and measurement of CSF levels just prior to the next injection is highly recommended as a guide to adequacy of therapy. Care should be taken in using an aminoglycoside preparation that does not contain preservatives, otherwise a severe arachnoiditis may ensue. It is also evident that better levels in ventricular fluid and in cerebrospinal fluid after repeated inoculations are obtained by using an Ommaya reservoir.[46] In an infection with as high a mortality rate as *Pseudomonas aeruginosa* meningitis, it is reasonable to consider the use of an Ommaya reservoir if the patient does not respond immediately to systemic therapy plus intrathecal therapy or if the patient at the outset is very ill. Duration of therapy is variable, but since the infection tends to persist, particularly in the face of neutropenia, 4–6 weeks of therapy should be considered.

Illustrative Case 1

The patient was an 11-year-old white girl who was admitted to the hospital because of a relapse of acute lymphoblastic leukemia. She had on previous occasions been successfully induced into a remission with the combination of vincristine and prednisone. It was decided to attempt reinduction with a rotating protocol of vincristine, high-dose prednisone, adriamycin, and L-asparaginase. When the WBC count plummeted below 200 normal neutrophils/mm^3, high fevers in the range of 102.2–105 8°F (39°–41°C) occurred as often as 3–4 times daily. The patient subsequently developed right lower quadrant pain and a number of cutaneous vasculitic lesions on the abdomen and forearm, which had the classic appearance of ecthyma gangrenosum. Aspirates of one of these lesions grew abundant *Pseudomonas aeruginosa* as well as five out of seven blood cultures for a type 3 (Fisher Serotyping System) *Pseudomonas aeruginosa*. Because of persistent right lower quadrant pain and classic findings of appendicitis on physical examination, the patient was taken to the operating room after gentamicin–carbenicillin therapy was initiated, and a gangrenous appendix was removed. *Pseudomonas aeruginosa* of the same serotype present in blood was isolated from the appendix. Approximately 11–12 hr postoperatively, the patient developed severe headache, nuchal rigidity, and chest radiographic evidence of fluffy infiltrates in both lung fields. A lumbar puncture revealed only 23 neutrophils, all of which were mature forms, protein 171 mg/dl, and a CSF glucose 11 mg/dl. A few gram-negative rods were seen on a spun sediment from 10 ml CSF. In addition to carbenicillin, 80 mg/kg IV every 4 hr, and gentamicin, 2 mg/kg IV every 8 hr, the patient was begun on intrathecal gentamicin (without preservative), 5 mg intrathecally every 12 hr. Daily granulocyte transfusions were also begun. CSF cultures became negative after 72 hr of treatment. The patient gradually defervesced over a period of 8 days coincidental with evidence of an early hematologic remission in her bone marrow. Of interest is that the appendiceal drain continued to grow *Pseudomonas aeruginosa* for an additional 4 weeks until healing occurred. The patient had no neurologic sequelae.

Comment. This case illustrates a relatively uncommon phenomenon, bacteremic *Pseudomonas aeruginosa* meningitis associated with clinical recovery. Prior to the availability of antipseudomonal penicillins that penetrate the CSF when the meninges are inflamed, the mortality with this complication approached 100%. Even the introduction of aminoglycosides, such as gentamicin, has been associated with low recovery rates because of unreliable diffusion into the CSF. Intrathecal aminoglycosides are one method of overcoming the problem of poor CSF penetration, but patients who develop *Pseudomonas* meningitis, and particularly those who have a ventricular catheter for hydrocephalus, may require intraventricular therapy because the administration of aminoglycoside into the CSF at the lumbar level may not result in therapeutic aminoglycoside levels at the level of the basal cisterns and above. The patient's focus of infection was, curiously, a gangrenous appendix, which on histologic section revealed necrotizing vasculitis characteristic of *Pseudomonas* infection. Disease spread via the bloodstream to the lungs, and seeded the meninges. Unquestionably, the patient's clinical recovery was related not only to aggressive antimicrobial treatment but achievement of hematologic remission. The decline in the incidence of bacteremic meningitis caused by gram-negative rods like *Pseudomonas* over the last 15 years is most likely related to the prompt initiation of empirical systemic agents that cover not only *S aureus,* pneumococci, and meningococci, but gram-negative bacilli as well.

2.1.3b. *Escherichia coli.* *Escherichia coli* is the most common aerobic gram-negative rod in the GI tract and is one of the most common causes of meningitis in the neutropenic patient. Its access to the meninges appears to be similar to that of *Pseudomonas aeruginosa,* and the identification is made similarly, usually within 8–12 hr of the time the CSF is cultured. Some strains with the K-1 capsular antigen will agglutinate with group B meningococcal antiserum because of immunochemical similarity of the capsular antigen.[47] Optimal therapy is unknown, and

many strains of *Escherichia coli* are now resistant to ampicillin. Therefore, the safest treatment is to combine ticarcillin, piperacillin, and the third-generation cephalosporin, since the latter penetrates the blood–brain barrier well and because more than 90% of hospital-isolated *E. coli* are susceptible. Most strains of *E. coli* are susceptible to aminoglycosides, but intrathecal plus systemic therapy is warranted in the critically ill patient. Alternatives to a third-generation cephalosporin include chloramphenicol or trimethoprim–sulfamethoxazole.

2.1.3c. *Klebsiella pneumoniae.* *Klebsiella pneumoniae* is a gram-negative aerobic bacillus that cannot be reliably differentiated on gram stain from *Pseudomonas aeruginosa* or *E. coli.* *Klebsiella pneumoniae* may have a large capsule and occur in pairs, giving a rather characteristic appearance. One should not base the diagnosis, however, on Gram stain. *Klebsiellae* sometimes do not decolorize well and can then appear as gram-positive rods or even cocci. Growth in culture is usually rapid, and within a matter of hours it will be possible to distinguish *K. pneumoniae* from the other two common gram-negative causes of meningitis in the neutropenic patient.

Klebsiella pneumoniae differs importantly from *Escherichia coli* as far as in vitro antimicrobial susceptibility. *Klebsiellae* are almost always resistant to ampicillin, carbenicillin, and ticarcillin but are usually sensitive to cephalosporins, piperacillin, chloramphenicol, trimethoprim–sulfamethoxazole, and aminoglycosides. First- and second-generation cephalosporins do not reliably penetrate the blood–brain barrier, and chloramphenicol alone may not be effective. As with *E. coli* meningitis, combination systemic therapy with a third-generation cephalosporin and an aminoglycoside is advisable, and intrathecal aminoglycosides may be indicated in the very ill patient.

2.1.3d. *Proteus* **Species.** *Proteus* species rarely cause meningitis in the neutropenic patient, but when CNS infections caused by this group do occur, *Proteus mirabilis* is the most commonly isolated species. These organisms are usually susceptible to ampicillin and large doses of penicillin G. We recommend a similar approach to *Proteus* CNS infections as with *Klebsiella.* However, since most *Proteus* species (both indole-positive and -negative) are ticarcillin susceptible, this agent may substitute for a third-generation cephalosporin. Most of the isolates of *E. coli, Klebsiella,* or *Proteus* species remain sensitive to chloramphenicol, an antibiotic that readily penetrates the CSF. It should be substituted for a β-lactam in a penicillin-allergic patient.

2.1.3e. Other Enteric Bacilli. Among the Enterobacteriaceae that appear to be increasing as a cause of sepsis in the neutropenic patient and therefore are occasionally encountered as causes of meningitis are *Enterobacter* species, especially *Enterobacter aerogenes* and *Enterobacter cloacae.* These organisms are more drug resistant than *Escherichia coli* and *Proteus mirabilis,* however, a combination of piperacillin or a third-generation cephalosporin with an aminoglycoside may be effective. Trimethoprim–sulfamethoxazole may be effective against most of the Enterobacteriaceae and this combination of antimicrobial agents may be paired with parenteral aminoglycosides in the initial treatment of gram-negative meningitis in the immunocompromised host, especially in the setting of penicillin allergy.[26]

2.1.3f. *Hemophilus influenzae.* *Hemophilus influenzae* is a small pleomorphic gram-negative coccobacillus that commonly causes meningitis in young children. Immunocompromised patients with hypogammaglobulinemia or who have been splenectomized are probably also more at risk of *H. influenzae* meningitis. There is nothing diagnostic about the appearance of these delicate gram-negative organisms on smear, and they frequently are found within neutrophils. Specific *H. influenzae* capsular antigen (polyribose phosphate) can be detected in the CSF in most cases using counterimmunoelectrophoresis or Latex particle agglutination. Commercially available kits for these tests are available. Resistance to ampicillin has increased, and recent reports suggest that chloramphenicol-resistant organisms are emerging.[48] Some experts advocate the use of newer cephalosporins such as cefuroxime, ceftriaxone, and cefotaxime when *H. influenzae* meningitis is anticipated.

A polysaccharide vaccine against disease caused by *H. influenzae* type b has recently been licensed in the United States. A large randomized, controlled trial in Finland demonstrated a 90% protective efficacy among children 18 months of age or older.[49] Although only limited data on immu-

nogenicity and clinical efficacy are available in children at increased risk for invasive *H. influenzae* infection, the vaccine appears to be safe; consequently, the Advisory Committee on Immunization Practices has recommended that such children be immunized at 18 months of age.[50]

2.1.4. Gram-Negative Cocci

2.1.4a. *Neisseria meningitidis.* *Neisseria meningitidis* is a gram-negative coccus that causes meningitis sporadically or in epidemic form. In the immunocompromised host it causes severe disease in the same patients as *Streptococcus pneumoniae* and *Hemophilus influenzae,* namely, those with splenectomies or hypogammaglobulinemia. On Gram stain it may be confused with *H. influenzae* if only a rare organism is present. Specific group A and C polysaccharide antigens may be detectable by counterimmunoelectrophoresis. *Neisseria meningitidis* is still highly sensitive to penicillin, and an alternate therapeutic choice is chloramphenicol.

2.1.4b. *Acinetobacter* Species. *Acinetobacter* species, formerly identifed as *Mima polymorpha,* or *Herellea vaginicola,* are small gram-negative coccobacillary organisms that may rarely cause meningitis in an immunocompromised host. There are no clear-cut predisposing factors except head and spine surgery. On Gram stain they may appear as gram-negative cocci or bacilli. The diagnosis of *Acinetobacter* meningitis should be considered if coccobacillary organisms are present on Gram stain but counterimmunoelectrophoresis tests for neisserial and *H. influenzae* type b antigens are negative. Since these organisms are consistently resistant to penicillins, and chloramphenicol susceptibility is variable, both systemic and intrathecal aminoglycoside therapy will be necessary. Ticarcillin, piperacillin, a third-generation cephalosporin, or trimethoprim–sulfamethoxazole may also be used parenterally.

2.2. Fungi

Fungi are among the most common organisms causing CNS infection in the immunocompromised host. In most instances the patient has a T-lymphocyte, mononuclear phagocyte defect. Thus, susceptible patients include those with lymphoma, leukemia, transplant patients, and individuals with collagen vascular disease who receive treatment aimed at suppressing delayed hypersensitivity. In a large series of patients with neoplastic disease, one fungus, *Cryptococcus neoformans*, was the second most common cause of CNS infection, surpassed only by *Listeria monocytogenes*.[2]

2.2.1. *Cryptococcus neoformans*

This organism appears to be ubiquitous in soil and is found on fresh vegetables. Thus, human contact with *Cryptococcus* is common, but only a few individuals develop systemic infection. In about one-half of all cases there is a clear underlying disorder such as a lymphoma or immunosuppression.[51] In the other half, there are no obvious immune defects, but subtle defects could be detected. The organism is isolated in abundant numbers from pigeon feces, but most patients who develop cryptococcal CNS infection have had no special contact with pigeons.

Cryptococcus neoformans can be well visualized by an India ink preparation where the capsule excludes the India ink particles, thereby projecting a halo around the organism. This, however, can be imitated by WBCs, RBCs, and even talcum powder granules. A positive India ink preparation should contain a budding yeast. On Gram stain, the organisms show a gram-negative capsule and a dense blue center; however, the center of the yeast occasionally may be stippled in blue (Fig. 1). Rather pale oval forms with a central line or lines forming a Y can sometimes appear on Gram stain. The organisms become more and more pale pink as patients respond to therapy. The capsule contains a polysaccharide antigen that is characteristic of *Cryptococcus neoformans*. Capsular detection may be of great help diagnostically, and serial measurements of antigen titers are a useful guide to treatment. In many instances, the organism is not apparent on India ink preparation or Gram stain even when more than 10 ml CSF is obtained for study; however, we have found that when both the Gram stain and India ink preparation are used more than 50% of CSF specimens from which *C. neoformans* is isolated will be smear positive.[52] Less frequently, the organism is not isolated on culture, particularly on the first few lumbar punctures. These spinal fluids, even in the absence of

visible or culturable *Cryptococcus,* usually contain cryptococcal antigen. On a rare occasion, small-capsule *Cryptococcus* will not produce detectable amounts of antigen.

Various serologic methods have been used to detect cryptococcal antigen, but the most common is particle agglutination. Latex agglutination is a relatively simple, rapid, and commercially available method. A hyperimmune rabbit globulin against cryptococcal antigen is incubated with and adheres to the Latex particles; these in turn combine with antigen in body fluid and cause visible clumping. The more antigen present, the more the CSF or serum can be diluted and still clump the antibody-coated Latex particles. The presence of clumping of the Latex particles by the CSF in titer of 1 : 4 or higher has in almost every instance been associated with a cryptococcal infection of the CNS. Nonetheless, appropriate controls are needed to rule out the presence of rheumatoid factor, which nonspecifically agglutinates Latex particles coated with globulin. In this case, another serologic test such as complement fixation or counterimmunoelectrophoresis will be needed for serodiagnosis. Small-capsule variants may not produce much antigen, and cryptococcomas may not be associated with detectable levels of antigen in the CSF.

Serologic tests can also be used to guide duration of therapy. As patients respond to therapy, antigen levels in the CSF decrease, and usually once sufficient therapy has been administered the antigen is no longer detectable. On a rare occasion, we and others have found low levels of antigen to persist in the absence of active cryptococcal disease or in the absence of recurrent cryptococcosis in that particular patient. In one instance, we have found at autopsy granulomatous lesions within the brain containing what appeared to be cryptococci. They did not grow in culture, and their viability was questionable.[53] Whether the cryptococci can persist in the brain in the nonviable state and slowly leak antigen into the CSF is still unclear.

Cryptococci are almost uniformly sensitive to amphotericin B. Most isolates are also initially sensitive to 5-fluorocytosine, although resistance may develop during exposure to that antimicrobial agent by itself. Recommended treatment includes amphotericin B and 5-flucytosine.[54] *Cryptococcus neoformans* is usually sensitive in vitro to micona-

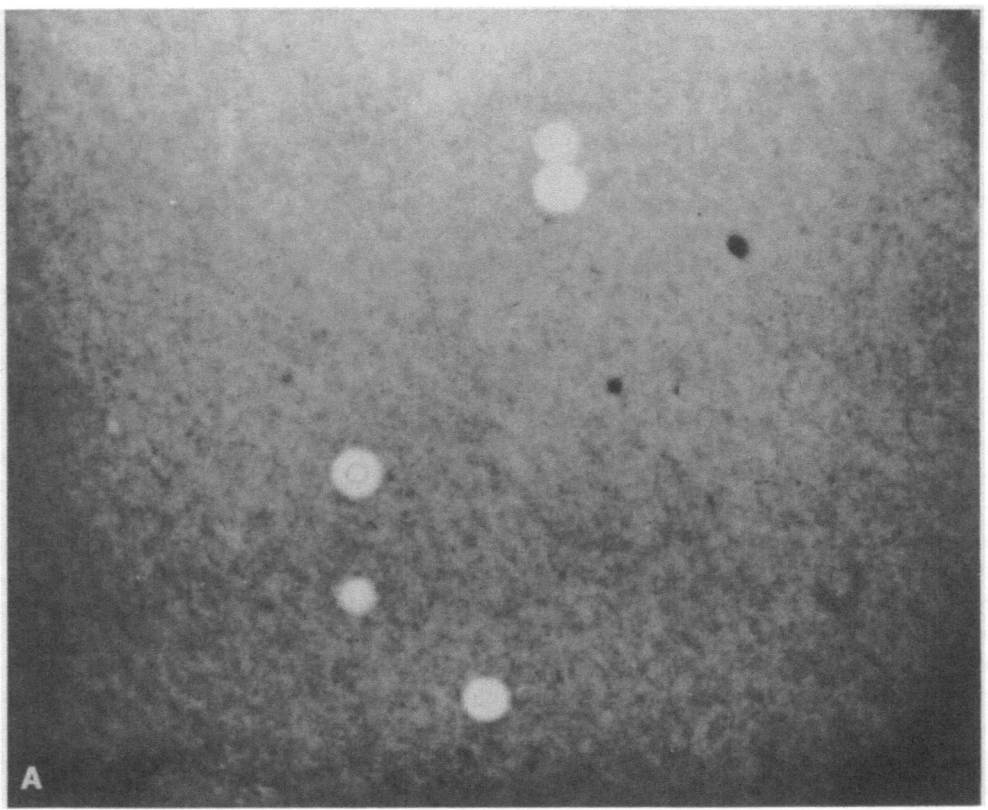

FIGURE 1. (A) *Cryptococcus neoformans* identified by the classic India ink preparation involving the mixture of equal amounts of CSF and India ink. Note that a defined halo is an absolute prerequisite for identification (budding also is helpful) because red blood cells and starch granules can be confusing artifacts. (B) *Cryptococcus* identified by Gram stain. Wherever possible, Gram staining should also be carried out. The body of the yeast contains gram-positive stippled structures, and the yeast cell wall is also gram positive. There is a suggestion of a capsule because of the halo effect against the inflammatory cell response. The halo is an amorphous gram-negative staining material.

zole, but clinical experience in the treatment of meningitis is limited.[55] There have been individual case reports where patients failing to respond to initial courses of amphotericin B have responded to miconazole. In severe or recurrent cases, systemic amphotericin B and 5-flucytosine in combination with intraventricular amphotericin B administered via an Ommaya reservoir may be effective.[52]

2.2.2. Coccidioides immitis

Systemic coccidioidomycosis has often been associated with defects in cell-mediated immunity. *Coccidioides immitis*, the causative agent, is found in the soil and sands of the southwestern United States,

Central America, and northern and central South America. Infections in normal individuals living in those areas are frequent and usually asymptomatic; occasional flulike syndromes or an infectious-mononucleosis-like syndrome may occur. In the immunocompromised host as well as those relatively few apparently normal individuals with extrapulmonary involvement, the disease usually disseminates from the lungs and then spreads to the CNS. The organisms cannot be readily isolated from the CSF and are only infrequently seen as a budding yeast. In the immunocompetent individual, the diagnosis is almost always supported by a serologic response. Usually a rise in complement-fixation titer can readily be demonstrated. In the immunocompromised indi-

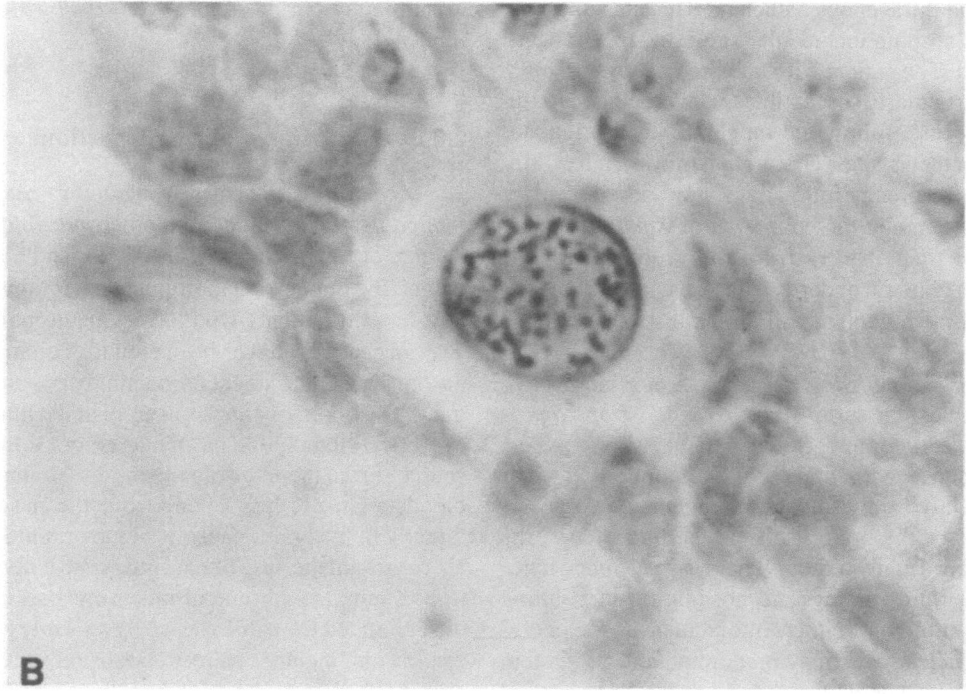

FIGURE 1. (*Continued*)

vidual, there may be no detectable serologic response.[56]

The organism is sensitive to amphotericin B and miconazole, but the former remains the agent of choice. Coccidioidal meningitis should always be initially treated with intrathecal amphotericin B 0.3–0.7 mg, 2–4 times weekly, along with systemic amphotericin B. Duration of treatment usually exceeds 1 year (particularly for the intrathecal component) and may extend for several years. Nonetheless, treatment failures often occur or recur after an initial response. Intraventricular reservoirs have been used with limited success, and the rate of secondary infection is high. In addition to amphotericin B, miconazole has been used to treat pulmonary coccidioidomycosis,[55] but this drug is not reliably effective in meningitis. The latter conclusion also applies to ketoconazole.

2.2.3. *Histoplasma capsulatum*

Disseminated infections from this organism are now recognized as an opportunistic infection occur-ring in the immunocompromised host.[57] Disseminated histoplasmosis has also been reported occurring in nonendemic areas.[58] It does not usually involve the CNS; however, meningitis and brain abscesses have been reported, usually following relapse of inadequately treated disseminated disease.[59] The diagnosis is usually made on the basis of bone marrow, liver, lung, or skin biopsy or even by positive blood cultures. Serologic responses usually do not occur in immunocompromised patients with histoplasmosis.[57] The organism is susceptible to amphotericin B and some imidazoles.

2.2.4. *Candida* Species

Candida species are ubiquitous. They are found in the GI tract of normal humans and are readily isolated after initiation of antimicrobial therapy. They are also found in other animal species. The species usually infecting humans are *Candida albicans, tropicalis, parapsilosis, krusii,* and *pseudotropicalis.*[60]

Candida species frequently enter the bloodstream via intravenous catheters. The sites of hematogenous seeding include the kidneys, spleen, heart, and lungs. The patient with impaired neutrophil function is particularly susceptible to developing disseminated disease following fungemia that originates from a catheter site. The organism may infect kidneys via the ureters following Foley catheterization. Another source of dissemination of Candida species is the GI tract. Ulcers from the esophagus to the rectum may be secondarily infected by Candida species, and the organism will disseminate from such a source.

Candida albicans is the most commonly isolated species. In some series Candida tropicalis is encountered far more often in patients with leukemia than in those with other types of underlying disease.[61] Only rarely does dissemination involve the meninges or the brain itself. When this occurs, the infection is usually a relatively low-grade one. Cerebrospinal fluid findings are not helpful in pointing toward etiology: either mononuclear or polymorphonuclear cells may predominate, CSF protein may be normal or elevated, and sugar may be normal or depressed.[60] For reasons that are poorly understood, Candida species are hard to isolate from the CSF.

In addition to patients with hematological malignancy, those susceptible to CNS Candida species infections include neonates.[60] Candida meningitis in the neonate may be acute or subacute. In these patients the organism usually can be isolated from the CSF.

Candida serology has not been very helpful in those patients who are at high risk of becoming colonized, because colonization alone may result in a rise in antibody titer.[62]

There are preliminary results suggesting that antigen can be detected in the serum of patients with disseminated candidiasis.[63,64] This should be applied to the cerebrospinal fluids of patients with suspected CNS Candida infections. Gas–liquid chromatography and other biochemical methods have also been used to demonstrate either cell-wall constituents such as mannan[65] or metabolites of Candida such as arabinatol[66-68] in the sera and CSF of patients with invasive disease.

The basis of treatment of invasive candidiasis is amphotericin B, however, combined amphotericin B and flucytosine therapy may be superior to amphotericin B alone in C. tropicalis fungemia.[69]

2.2.5. Aspergillus Species Infections

Aspergillus species, including Aspergillus fumigatus, flavus, niger, and others are ubiquitous in nature, occurring in dust, in plants, and sometimes colonizing humans. Opportunistic infections are usually seen in patients who have a neutrophil defect. The organisms have been found colonizing the nasopharynx, the tracheobronchial tree, and the GI tract. The portal of entry is usually in the lungs; however, occasionally the nasopharynx or GI tract is the source. From there the organisms disseminate via the bloodstream or, less often, from the nasopharnyx directly to the brain, causing single or multiple brain abscesses. In the case of nasopharyngeal invasion the rhinocerebral syndrome of mucormycosis cannot be differentiated from that caused by an Aspergillus species. This includes direct extension through the cribriform plate or the orbit from the sinus. The organisms show acutely branching septate hyphae and are seen better on wet mount than on Gram stain. The CSF ranges from normal to purulent, but usually there is only a moderate (100–300) pleocytosis, slightly elevated protein, and slightly depressed glucose levels.[10] On fixed tissue section, Gomori's methenamine silver stain is especially effective in delineating morphology. In the rhinocerebral syndrome (which is rare with aspergillosis), a nasal scraping may reveal the organism, but if not, a biopsy usually will. A brain biopsy is usually necessary to show aspergillosis as a cause of CNS involvement. If the patient has documented pulmonary disease caused by Aspergillus, the presence of a brain abscess can be assumed to be caused by Aspergillus and therapy started on that basis. Extirpation of an Aspergillus abscess may be important therapeutically because the organism invades blood vessels, causing clotting and then infarction beyond the clot. Tissue levels of antifungal agents will not be high in such an area that becomes secondarily invaded by the fungus.

Aspergillus species are variably sensitive to amphotericin B. In vitro sensitivity studies are very hard to interpret because the fungus grows primarily as a mold. There have been enough clinical cures of Aspergillus lung disease and a rare cure of As-

pergillus brain abscess with amphotericin B, so that the use of this drug is justified. Most improvement, however, has occurred concurrent with improvement in the underlying disease. There are no well-documented responses to other antifungal agents.

Illustrative Case 2

The patient was a 23-year-old Hispanic woman who was readmitted to the hospital because of a relapse in her acute myelocytic leukemia. Nine months previously, a full hematologic remission had been induced with the combination therapy of cytosine arabinoside, thioguanine, and daunorubicin. On admission, the patient had mild posterior pharyngeal pain and erythema, a clear chest radiograph, and a slightly enlarged spleen. Her temperature was 102.2°F (39.0°C) and all diagnostic studies failed to identify an infectious cause of her temperature elevations. During the ensuing 3 weeks, the patient received another course of her initial induction regimen but without evidence of a bone marrow response. A sustained (17-day) period of neutropenia with normal granulocyte count less than 500/mm³ was managed with a prolonged course of gentamicin and carbenicillin. These medications were stopped after a total of 19 days with a rise in neutrophil counts to >1000/mm³. After a week's pause, a second cycle of treatment was initiated that included cytosine arabinoside, vincristine, cyclophosphamide, and 5-azacytidine. Following a 4-day pulse of this treatment, the white counts inexorably declined to negligible levels (<100/mm³), and fevers returned. Gentamicin and carbenicillin were again reinstituted, but on this occasion, *Klebsiella pneumoniae*, susceptible to gentamicin but resistant to carbenicillin, was isolated from four of four blood cultures. Cefazolin 4 g IV per day was then added to the regimen, but on this treatment, two additional blood cultures were positive. The putative source of the bacteremia was never identified but was presumed to be the GI tract. After 5 days on IV cefazolin, carbenicillin, and gentamicin, the patient's temperature persisted, and oral trimethoprim–sulfamethoxazole (240 mg trimethoprim every 8 hr) was given with erratic patient compliance because of severe nausea and pain. Five days after the trimethoprim was initiated, the patient's temperature declined to near normal. However, a routine follow-up chest radiograph revealed consolidation in the left lower lung field and retrocardiac areas as well as the right lower lung field. The lesions on both sides during the following week progressed to dense consolidation, with the area on the left containing a central area of cavitation. Multiple sputum cultures were negative for any bacteria or fungi except for a few colonies of *Candida albicans*. It was felt that the progression of radiologic changes most likely represented *Aspergillus* pneumonia, and the patient was begun on a rising dosage schedule of amphotericin B (see Chapter 8). Despite the aggressive use of amphotericin B, the areas of consolidation in the lung increased, occupying the lower two-thirds of both lung fields with the development of an effusion on the left. Ten days after development of the pulmonary infiltrates, a thoracentesis was performed and *A. fumigatus* isolated from the pleural fluid after 5 days of incubation. At this point, the patient's clinical course was critical

with return of high fevers. Some of these temperature elevations seemed related to concomitant amphotericin B administration. On the 45th hospital day, the patient developed severe headache, obtundation, and a left central facial nerve paresis. Lumbar puncture revealed an elevated pressure of 270 mm H₂O, a protein of 113 mg/dl, a normal CSF glucose, and a WBC cell count of 12/mm³, most of which were lymphocytes (peripheral white count remained less than 100 cells/mm³). The following day the patient developed a right hemiparesis. Efforts were initiated to perform a radionuclide brain scan, but at the start of the procedure the patient had a cardiac arrest and could not be resuscitated.

At autopsy the patient had diffuse *Aspergillus* pneumonia with consolidation and infarction in two distinct areas. Subsequent sectioning of the brain revealed a left cerebral cortical infarct with extension of this infarct into the thalamus. There were also infarcts in the brain stem. Interestingly, *Aspergillus fumigatus* was not isolated from the tissue at autopsy, presumably because the patient had received approximately 12 days of intravenous amphotericin B. Nonetheless, abundant branching septate hyphae were apparent in sections of the lung and brain.

Comment. This patient had achieved a brief hematologic remission in her acute myelocytic leukemia but relapsed and was readmitted to the hospital for a course of treatment on an experimental protocol. Failure to achieve remission, the prolonged courses of broad-spectrum antibacterial treatment, and the attendant fungal superinfection are now commonly recognized events in neutropenic patients. The appearance of a cavitary lesion on chest radiograph could have been the result of anaerobic infection, but in the neutropenic host it is much more likely to reflect fungal pneumonia caused by filamentous fungi such as *Aspergillus* and *Mucor* species. It is of interest that *Aspergillus fumigatus* was cultured from the pleural effusion. Diagnostic thoracentesis should be undertaken in any patient who has evidence of pleural effusion. Aggressive diagnostic measures should include both thoracentesis and pleural biopsy if the platelet count permits. The sudden appearance of CNS disease and impaired neurologic function, particularly in a patient who has lung lesions, is most suggestive of a fungal process, although gram-negative rods can sometimes cause CNS vasculitis and infarcts. No single anatomic lesion could explain the constellation of cranial nerve palsies, headache, and pyramidal track signs. Diffuse involvement of the CNS because of fungi invading the vascular structures and the ensuing infarction were the terminal clinical events.

This patient was seen and evaluated at a time when computed tomography (CT) was not available for the localization of mass lesions. Nonetheless, the entire clinical picture is so striking and so typical of CNS involvement by filamentous fungi in a patient with neutropenia that empirical antifungal therapy was justified. Had CT been available, it would have added relatively little to the management of the patient. The primary reasons this type of infectious complication fails to respond include: (1) failure to control underlying disease, and (2) poor CNS penetration of amphotericin B and/or other antifungal agents. It is not clear whether or not amphotericin alone or in combination with other agents such as rifampin or flucytosine might have enhanced activity against organisms such as *Aspergillus* species. Nonetheless, it is unrealistic to expect that a patient will recover from CNS fungal infection if an underlying hematologic malignancy is unremitting.

2.2.6. *Mucoraceae (Zygomycetes)*

There are four different genera among the *Mucoraceae* that cause clinical disease in immunocompromised patients. The genera found to cause invasive disease in immunocompromised hosts have been *Mucor, Absidia, Rhizopus,* and *Cunninghamella.*[70–72]

Mucor, Rhizopus, and *Absidia* have been responsible for reported CNS disease. In many instances, the organism has been seen in histological material but not isolated and identified in the microbiology laboratory. Classically, a rhinocerebral syndrome characterized by invasion of the CNS from the sinuses occurs in diabetic patients in acidosis. In contrast, in patients with leukemia and lymphoma, the mold usually invades the lungs and then disseminates to the brain. In about one-third of cases, there may be the classic rhinocerebral syndrome, with the classic triad of coma, ophthalmoplegia, and proptosis. Perhaps just as commonly, the patient may present merely with proptosis and cellulitis around the eye that progresses to ophthalmoplegia. Direct extension to the brain usually occurs in the latter cases. This classic rhinocerebral syndrome is most often associated with diabetics in ketoacidosis, although a number of cases have been observed in nonacidotic diabetics. Rhinocerebral cases have also occurred in children who are acidotic following severe diarrhea. The common denominator between the neutrophil defect seen in patients with leukemia and lymphoma who develop disseminated mucormycosis and those with diabetes, particularly in acidosis, has not as yet been elucidated.

The diagnosis is most difficult unless the patient with the rhinocerebral syndrome has a nasal or sinus scraping and/or a biopsy that reveals typical organisms. Some patients may have pulmonary infection along with one or more CNS lesions, a situation requiring a brain biopsy to establish the diagnosis of intracerebral mucormycosis. Computed tomography of both the brain and orbit of the involved eye can be helpful in establishing the extent of disease. Sometimes a proptotic eye (usually with intact vision) is displaced forward by the fungal mass and accompanying inflammation, which is valuable information for the head and neck surgeon. The CSF is not diagnostic and is much like that seen in CNS aspergillosis with mild pleocytosis and a few erythrocytes, usually elevated protein, and diminished glucose.[70] In patients with pulmonary infection, the organism is infrequently recovered from sputum. Since occasional sputum isolates are made in the absence of invasive pulmonary disease, biopsies are necessary to establish the diagnosis. There is no reliable serological test for this fungal infection. Amphotericin B is the only proven antimicrobial therapy for the rhinocerebral syndrome, but it must be coupled with aggressive surgery to debride the sinuses and paraorbital areas (including bone) of involvement. Enucleation of the eye, particularly if vision is lost, is often necessary. When diabetic acidosis has been controlled, either surgery or amphotericin B alone has been effective[70] although combined therapy is preferable.[72]

Illustrative Case 3

A 47-year-old woman was transferred from another hospital with a 17-day history of progressive monocular blindness and proptosis, headache, fevers, and diabetes. The patient had undergone renal transplantation 4 months previously and had received high-dose immunosuppressive therapy for ongoing rejection. Her underlying renal disease had been diabetic nephropathy, and she had been an insulin-dependent diabetic for 34 years. One month previously, while receiving high-dose steroids for allograft rejection, she developed diabetic ketoacidosis and fever and complained of right-sided orbital headaches. Over the next week, despite control of the diabetes, her headaches became more severe, and she began noting numbness over areas of the right side of the face. Subsequently, a black necrotic eschar was noted on her hard palate. Biopsy revealed invasive mucormycosis. Therapy was started with high-dose amphotericin B. However, up until the time of transfer, there was a progressive loss of vision, development of severe proptosis and total ophthalmoplegia, and gradual obtundation.

Physical examination was remarkable for a temperature of 101°F (38.3°C) and a respiratory rate of 34 in a cushingoid, obtunded woman. Her right eye was proptotic, paralyzed, and the pupil did not respond to light. Anesthesia was noted over the distribution of the second division of the right trigeminal nerve. A mild left hemisparesis was present, with a Babinski response present on the left.

Laboratory data revealed a hematocrit (Hct) of 29% and WBC count of 2900 with 78% polys, 6% bands, 11% lymphs, 5% monos. The BUN was 95 mg/dl, creatinine 8.6 mg/dl, blood sugar of 387 mg/dl, and an arterial pH of 7.27. A CT scan revealed direct invasion of the orbit, right-sided nasal sinuses, and multiple mass lesions in the right hemisphere.

The patient's infection was felt to be too far advanced to be surgically approachable, and although amphotericin therapy was continued, she succumbed on the third hospital day. At postmortem examination, *Mucor* species were found to be invading contiguously into the eye, orbit, and sinuses with involvement of cranial nerves II–VI. In addition, metastatic abscesses were present in the brain.

Comment. This is a classical case of rhinocerebral mucormycosis occurring in a diabetic, acidotic, immunosuppressed host. As in most such cases, the infection began in the nasal sinuses and palate and then spread contiguously to neighboring structures. In addition, noncontiguous spread via hematogenous metastasis occurred, in this case to the brain. The pathologic hallmarks of mucormycosis are the invasion of blood vessels producing extensive tissue infarction and the typical blackish inflammatory exudate. Because of the extent of the blood vessel involvement, it is exceedingly difficult to deliver effective antifungal therapy to the site of involvement. Therefore, radical surgery akin to that performed for head and neck cancers, is a cornerstone of therapy. The error that was made in this case was to delay surgery and treat just medically until the patient had become inoperable.

2.3. Parasites

The parasites that infect the CNS of immunocompromised patients are usually those that exploit a T-lymphocyte mononuclear phagocyte host defect. The two most common examples are *Toxoplasma gondii* and *Strongyloides stercoralis*. There have been a few cases of amebiasis with dissemination to the brain seen in immunocompromised patients as well as in normals, but these have not been sufficient to establish a syndrome such as one sees with *Toxoplasma gondii* and *Strongyloides stercoralis*.

2.3.1. *Toxoplasma gondii*

This organism is a protozoan parasite whose definitive host is the cat. However, it can infect most other mammals. It is excreted as an oocyst in the feces of the cat, whereupon it is ingested by other mammals. The oocysts yield trophozoites that penetrate the GI tract and then pass usually to muscle, lymph nodes, and sometimes to heart, lung, and brain as well as liver and spleen. The infection is usually asymptomatic but with some encystment in organs or various tissues, which in the human includes muscle just as it does in cows and other animals.[73] Cysts have also been found in human brain. It can be transmitted from mother to a fetus in utero by the transplacental route and has also been transmitted by blood cell transfusions, particularly WBCs. There is some question whether it has been transmitted via heart transplantation. One of the most common

modes of transmission is by eating undercooked or raw meat such as beef, mutton, or lamb.

It is probable that many cases of toxoplasmosis in the immunocompromised host are a result of the encysted organism reactivating and releasing trophozoites. When the organism infects the brain of the immunocompromised host, it causes an encephalitis or a picture of brain abscess. Even the immunocompromised host, however, may recover from a symptomatic febrile infection with *Toxoplasma gondii*, so the effectiveness of a treatment is difficult to judge. There are no controlled studies and probably will not be, since once toxoplasmosis becomes apparent in the immunosuppressed patient, it may be a rapidly life-threatening infection. (See Chapter 10 for additional information on clinical presentation and diagnosis.) The diagnosis is made most often by serology where titers by indirect immunofluorescence, complement fixation, or Sabin–Feldman dye test are the usual assays. An indirect test for IgM antibody has been successful in some laboratories where titers above 1 : 40 suggest an ongoing infection.[73] Since asymptomatic infections occur even in immunocompromised patients, serologic changes do not prove that CNS disease is caused by toxoplasmosis. Cerebrospinal fluid findings are not very helpful and usually consist of a mild to moderate pleocytosis with mostly mononuclear cells, normal to elevated protein content, and normal to decreased glucose concentration.[74] In the neonate, by the time the disease is treated, brain damage may have already occurred, but treatment will probably alter the course, preventing further brain damage, and control, to some extent, hepatic disease. A combination of a sulfonamide and pyrimethamine is the treatment of choice, especially since both achieve effective CNS levels.

2.3.2. *Strongyloides stercoralis*

This organism is found in the soil of subtropical and tropical countries and the southeastern and south-central United States. It penetrates the skin of individuals who have contact with infected soil. It makes its way via the venous system to the lungs where the larvae are coughed up and swallowed, and then the parasite lodges and resides in the upper intestine. This is usually a relatively benign infestation and may merely cause some upper abdominal discomfort and fullness. This is the only common worm with which endogenous reinfection often occurs. The patient may carry the organism for up to or more than 20 years, and then, during immunosuppression, the hyperinfection syndrome may develop (see Chapter 10). This consists of invasion of the gut wall by the larvae and dissemination in the bloodstream. Bacteremia, normally caused by gram-negative rods, frequently accompanies the parasitemia. One of the areas of the body to which the larvae may disseminate and invade is the CNS. Both the meninges and the brain may be involved, producing the picture of a meningoencephalitis. Just as in the blood, the CNS may also be invaded by bacteria transported there by the *Strongyloides,* causing a bacterial meningitis as well.[75]

The diagnosis should be suspected from the clinical picture and confirmed by visualization of the organisms in the stool, duodenal aspirates, or sputum. On a rare occasion, organisms may be seen in the CSF. The CSF findings are not significantly different from other causes of aseptic meningitis, and the presence of the bacteria may confuse the picture. Serologic tests are not always positive and must be obtained through reference laboratories. There is seldom time, when the clinician suspects the hyperinfection syndrome in a patient, to wait for serological results.

The organisms are sensitive to thiabendazole, and there have been clinical cures of the hyperinfection syndrome using this antiparasitic agent. Dose and duration of therapy in this syndrome are uncertain, but the latter should probably exceed the 2 days recommended for intestinal disease. In one case report, 8 days of therapy did not eradicate the organisms.[76] Decreasing the magnitude of immunosuppressive therapy may aid clinical recovery. If the infestation can be documented before immunosuppressive therapy is given, thiabendazole, 25 mg/kg PO, bid for 2 days should be administered. Consideration should be given to treating high-risk patients from an endemic area (who are about to be immunosuppressed) who have indications of possible infection such as unexplained eosinophilia. It can be difficult to prove infection by stool examination, and duodenal aspiration may be necessary.

2.4. Viral Infections

The viruses that may involve the CNS in the immunocompromised patient belong to two major classes[1,2]: (1) the herpes group of viruses, which have long been recognized to infect normal as well as immunocompromised patients, and (2) a papovavirus, the virus of multifocal leukoencephalopathy, which more recently has been identified as a cause of CNS disease in the immunocompromised host.

2.4.1. Herpes Group of Viruses

Herpes simplex types 1 or 2 (HSV-1, HSV-2) can cause encephalitis in the immunocompromised host, but there is no known increased incidence of herpes simplex encephalitis in immunocompromised individuals over the general population.[77] Some severe, disseminated cases of herpes simplex involving the liver and lungs have been reported in immunocompromised patients and in neonates. These do not usually also involve the CNS. It appears that impairment of the T-lymphocyte, mononuclear phagocyte system is associated with increased susceptibility to dissemination with herpes simplex, but not necessarily in the CNS.

HSV-1 is carried in the pharnyx of many normal individuals. It causes no symptoms, or in some instances, recurrent herpes labialis. HSV-2 is carried in the genitourinary tract of some individuals and occasionally cause herpes progenitalis. On first exposure, HSV-2 may produce a vaginitis just as HSV-1 can cause a stomatopharyngitis after initial exposure. There has been no evidence that individuals developing vaginitis or stomatopharyngitis are immunocompromised in the sense that we usually think of that term. One case of HSV-2 encephalitis seen in a patient with Hodgkin disease was reported because the course seemed so indolent. It was speculated that this was due to decreased delayed hypersensitivity, which, when intact, may be responsible for severe symptoms in nonimmunocompromised patients with herpes encephalitis.[78]

Diagnosis of herpes meningoencephalitis is usually made by brain biopsy since the virus is seldom isolated from the CSF. HSV-2 is more likely to cause meningitis, but isolation even of this type from CSF is rare. Serology is not particularly helpful, since rises in titer may occur with asymptomatic infections. The CSF findings usually include erythrocytes but are not sufficiently different to be diagnostic.

A compound that inhibits DNA synthesis, adenine arabinoside (ara-A), has been used to treat herpes simplex encephalitis with effectiveness according to some studies[79] (see Chapter 13). Acyclovir, a purine nucleoside analogue, is also effective in herpes simplex encephalitis and in two controlled studies was shown to be superior to ara-A.[80,81] Acyclovir is now considered the preferred treatment for herpes simplex encephalitis.

Varicella–zoster virus (VZV) causes chickenpox after first exposure and then remains latent. Inexplicably, it may recur along the dermatome of a sensory nerve root in some patients. The later condition, herpes zoster, occurs in normal, healthy individuals, and it also occasionally occurs in a dermatome that contains a tumor or that has received radiation. The incidence is much higher among patients with lymphomas, particularly Hodgkin disease, than in the general population. Not only is the incidence higher, but once the dermatomal disease occurs, it is more likely to disseminate from there in contrast to the limited infection seen in normal individuals. The dissemination usually involves the skin and occasionally internal organs such as the lungs, liver, or more rarely, the brain.

Once herpes zoster occurs in the dermatome of a cranial nerve, involvement of the CNS is more likely to occur, sometimes with a fatal encephalitis. Like herpes simplex, VZV is a highly cell-associated virus. It is rarely isolated from the CSF but may be isolated from a brain biopsy.

The diagnosis is usually obvious because of the dermatomal distribution of the original lesion. Wright-stained smears of the fluid from a vesicle should reveal multinuclear giant cells and intranuclear and intracytoplasmic inclusions. A biopsy with a hematoxylin and eosin stain (H & E) should show similar cells, although appearance alone does not distinguish VZV effect from herpes simplex. Culture of vesicular fluid, particularly if the base of the lesion is scraped and cells obtained, will usually afford a specific diagnosis. In immunocompromised patients with clinical herpes zoster, there appears to be some amelioration with the use of ara-A[81] or interferon[82] if the disease is treated within 72 hr of the first symptom. Acyclovir, when compared with placebo, halted the progression of herpes zoster and reduced the period of viral shedding as well as preventing visceral dissemination and is now the treatment of choice for herpes zoster in the immunocompromised host.[84]

Cytomegalovirus (CMV) can cause a febrile syndrome, pneumonia, or bleeding from the gastrointestinal tract in the immunocompromised host.[85] There have been a few cases of encephalitis reported, but they are extremely rare. The organism is very common; it spreads from human to human by intimate contact and may be found in throat or saliva cultures of individuals who are asymptomatic carriers despite intense immunosuppression. It is also found in the gynecologic tract of the female and the genital tract of the male. It is excreted in the urine of either sex from days to months following an initial infection. Most severe CMV infections observed following renal transplantation have been caused by initial exposures to the virus, whereas recrudescent infections subsequent to the immunosuppression used for renal transplantation do not as frequently result in such severe disease.

The diagnosis is usually made by rises in antibody titers or biopsy of tissues that show the classic "owl's eye" inclusion and giant cells. A rise in antibody titer may result from an asymptomatic infection, and indeed, viremia may be accompanied by no symptoms whatever, so that the isolation of the virus from the blood or even from an organ may not implicate it in a disease. Most authorities accept only histopathologic proof.

There is no known effective treatment for CMV infection, although interferon may have some prophylactic benefit (see Chapter 13). Although the nucleoside analogue DHPG and the DNA polymerase inhibitor phosphonoformate appear to be active against CMV in vitro,[86,87] studies of their efficacy in vivo are just under way.

2.4.2. Papovaviruses

Progressive multifocal leukoencephalopathy is caused by a papovavirus that appears to be similar to the Simian virus 40 (SV40) virus. In some instances, isolates have cross-reacted serologically with that virus, but other studies show them to be separate entities. The papovavirus is a small DNA virus resembling the human wart virus as well as the monkey SV40 virus. It has been grown in vitro only in human brain cells, although more recently isolates from the urine have been grown in monkey kidney cell cultures.

The organism was originally found at autopsy, usually in patients with far advanced carcinoma of the lung or lymphoma. It is rarely found in patients without an underlying disease. It has occasionally been isolated from patients with conditions other than neoplasia or post-transplant immunosuppression. The virus has sometimes been found in the urine of asymptomatic renal transplant patients. Its origin is not known; that it could be the wart virus is a possibility. The clinical syndrome is that of a waxing and waning multifocal cerebral disease with a CSF that is not diagnostic. There is no known treatment for this virus.

3. Clinical Presentation: The Approach to the Patient

Central nervous system infection in the immunocompromised host is often accompanied by subtle signs and symptoms because immunosuppression usually decreases the inflammatory response. However subtle the presentation, detection of headache, localizing neurologic signs, or an altered mental state is an immediate indication for a comprehensive physical examination and initiation of diagnostic tests. The most important tests are sampling of CSF by the conventional lumbar route (but if necessary by cisternal tap) and noninvasive, but increasingly important procedures, such as CT or magnetic resonance imaging (MRI). Fever per se is probably not an indication for these procedures, but fever accompanied by subtle neurologic signs, obtundation, disorientation, or agitation is adequate justification.

Although it is absolutely essential that CSF be sampled for a suspected case of CNS infection, the major contraindication to immediate lumbar puncture is the presence of focal neurologic findings with or without a decreased state of consciousness. If the patient presents with the syndrome of fever and headache, careful fundoscopic examination is clearly mandatory. Any evidence of papilledema, unilateral or bilateral, constitutes a focal neurologic finding. If these are present—focal findings, papilledema, decreased consciousness—a CT study, preferably with injection of contrast material, should be performed without hesitation prior to carrying out the lumbar puncture. Lumbar puncture in the presence of focal findings or with a suggestion of increased intracranial pressure assumes an unacceptable risk of brain stem herniation.

Provided that the examining physician can be assured that no papilledema is present, he may pro-

ceed at once to perform a lumbar puncture. If for technical reasons CT cannot be performed, other tests such as brain scan or arteriography (the latter posing significant risks in thrombocytopenic hosts), might be considered. Magnetic resonance imaging, a new technique, may supplement or replace some of the older imaging methods. The other alternative if such test procedures are not available, albeit far less satisfactory, is to initiate empirical therapy based on the severity of the patient's condition and the likely infecting pathogens.

Examination of CSF should be undertaken by both physicians and technologists experienced in the handling of these materials. If the flow of the CSF is brisk, there is probably not much danger in taking a large volume, e.g., 10 ml as opposed to a small volume, 2 ml. The larger volume may increase the chance of detecting microorganisms. Diagnostic yield may also be increased by examination of the centrifuged sediment of the CSF. Sugar and protein concentrations of the CSF will be the same whether they are measured on the whole spinal fluid or on the supernatant after centrifugation. Because examination of the cellular content and detection of any microorganisms are of crucial importance, the most expeditious procedure involves obtaining a fairly large volume of fluid, in the neighborhood of 8–12 ml, in a series of at least four tubes.

The first tube can be a small sample to compare with the last tube in case clearing of the fluid to assess the significance of a traumatic tap is necessary (0.5 ml). The last (fourth) tube is probably most valuable for assessment of the total cell count (0.5–1.0 ml). The second tube can be used for cytology (1 ml), and the third tube for the large volume that will be centrifuged. The centrifuged sediment is obviously valuable for microscopic examination and appropriate staining for bacteria, mycobacteria, and fungi. A differential cell count may also be easier to perform on the centrifuged sediment if a cytocentrifuge device is available. The supernatant can be used for the glucose and protein determinations without any significant error in comparison with an uncentrifuged sample. Cryptococcal antigen determination can also be accurately carried out on the supernatant after centrifugation. Other studies that can be performed on the supernatant are counterimmunoelectrophoresis for the presence of antigens of the *Pneumococcus*, *Neisseria meningitidis*, *Hemophilus influenzae*, and for the limulus lysate assessment of bacterial endotoxin.[47,88] With the electrophoretic technique, it should be remembered that the test result is most useful when positive. Because of variations in the quality and potency of some of the test antisera, false-negative clinical results have been well documented, and this often occurs in the case of meningococcal infection where the antiserum may not be of adequate potency.

Demonstration of lactic acid in the CSF[89] has been regularly associated with infectious meningitis and should add weight to the decision to treat such a patient. In addition, gas–liquid chromatography is a new experimental technique whereby certain patterns have been associated with CSF infections caused by tuberculosis, viruses, and bacteria.[90–92] This type of work is promising but needs corroboration. From the clinical viewpoint, if the spinal fluid is grossly turbid and a quick examination by Wright or Giemsa stain documents the presence of granulocytes or inflammatory cells, a decision should be made to initiate empirical treatment within minutes of perceiving the abnormality.

Occasionally, some conditions may mimic CNS infection and need to be considered according to underlying disease. Patients with acute leukemia may develop leukemic meningitis accompanied by fever, stiff neck, and blastic cells in the CSF. Although in the past this has been more commonly seen in lymphatic rather tham myelocytic leukemia, CNS involvement may be partly related to duration of disease. With increasing survival of patients with acute myelocytic leukemia, CNS involvement may become more common. High peripheral blast counts may correlate with likelihood of organ (including CSF) infiltration, but many patients (particularly with childhood leukemia) have had a CNS relapse while their bone marrow appeared to be in a remission state. The important laboratory test for diagnosing leukemic meningitis is some type of cytologic study. Chemical examination of the CSF may not be helpful because a low sugar content and elevated protein concentration may be present in leukemic meningitis. It is also important to remember that if a patient's leukemia is in relapse, detection of blast cells in the CSF does not exclude an infectious etiology of meningitis.

In addition to leukemia, CNS infiltration by lymphoma, Hodgkin disease, or breast cancer, in particular, may imitate chronic meningitis. A brain abscess can be mimicked by almost any type of solid tumor.

3.1. Meningitis

When an organism is readily detected by Gram stain, India ink preparation or serology, then selection of treatment is straightforward (Tables 5 and 6). Often this is not the case, and empirical therapy must be started without the help of a presumptive or definitive microbial diagnosis. This may be because the patient was already receiving antibiotics or because the organisms are present in only small numbers. In such instances empirical therapy may be necessary because the meningitis can be life-threatening and requires prompt treatment. Table 6 suggests an approach to common types of problem patients that considers the nature of the primary immune defect, the blood leukocyte count, and the CSF findings.

A syndrome of persistent neutrophilic meningitis has been described and is characterized by a persistence of neutrophils in the CSF lasting more than 1 week and ongoing signs of meningeal irritation.[93] Smears and cultures of CSF are regularly negative. In the immunocompromised host, the zygomycetes and actinomycetes are the predominant infectious etiologies, and some would consider empirical use of amphotericin B and a sulfonamide in undiagnosed cases where there is clinical deterioration.

3.2. CNS Infections Complicating AIDS

CNS disease in patients with AIDS can be caused by (1) the human immunodeficiency virus (HIV), (2) the organisms that cause opportunistic infections, and (3) the tumors that complicate AIDS (Table 7).

The most common CNS disease is due to HIV and the manifestations are those of a subacute encephalitis that was described early in the epidemic,[94] but at that time it was not known that HIV was responsible. Patients developed loss of short-term memory as well as slowness of thought and motor responses. Periods of lethargy were followed by withdrawal and semicoma. Death occurred due to either an opportunistic infection or a complication of

TABLE 6. Empirical Therapy According to Clinical Presentation of CNS Infection
in Immunocompromised Patients

Primary immune defect	Blood leukocyte count	CSF findings	Recommended therapy	Alternate therapy[a]
T-lymphocyte, mono-nuclear phagocyte defect	Normal	No organisms, pleocytosis, negative cryptococcal antigen	Ampicillin for *Listeria monocytogenes* or *Streptococcus pneumoniae*	Erythromycin, tetracycline, or chloramphenicol
	Normal	No organisms ± pleocytosis positive cryptococcal antigen	Obtain more CSF Consider amphotericin B + 5-fluorocytosine for *Cryptococcus neoformans*	Start amphotericin B + 5-FC, miconazole
	Low	No organisms ± pleocytosis	A third-generation cephalosporin, gentamicin IV, IT[b] for gram-negative meningitis	None[c]
Neutrophil defect	Low	No organisms ± pleocytosis	A third-generation cephalosporin, gentamicin IV, IT[b]	None
	Normal	No organisms ± pleocytosis	A third-generation cephalosporin; gentamicin IV, IT[b]	None
Splenectomy	Normal	No organisms, pleocytosis	Penicillin and chloramphenicol	Ampicillin, cotrimoxazole, or a third-generation cephalosporin
Surgery	Normal	No organisms, pleocytosis	A third-generation cephalosporin; gentamicin IV, IT,[b] and oxacillin	Vancomycin can be substituted for oxacillin

[a]Other semisynthetic penicillins such as methicillin or nafcillin may be substituted for oxacillin, aminoglycosides such as amikacin or tobramycin may be substituted for gentamicin, cotrimoxazole is the same preparation as trimethoprim–sulfamethoxazole
[b]IT, intrathecal administration
[c]For the penicillin-allergic patient, desensitize to the cephalosporin chosen

the semicomatose state or a hospital-associated infection. The diagnosis is made from the signs and symptoms and laboratory studies. A brain biopsy is unnecessary, since the other CNS diseases seen with AIDS are sufficiently different in that they are more focal, or acute, and show more evidence of disease on CT scan. Examination of the CSF is usually negative. HIV has been isolated from the CSF and neural tissue in several cases,[95] and HIV specific nucleic acid sequences have been detected in others.[96] Acute aseptic meningitis has also been described[95] with isolation of HIV from the CSF. Once the diagnosis is clinically established, therapy is still not available. Of the experimental antiviral agents, trisodium phosphonoformate (foscarnet) does cross the blood–brain barrier. There is no available prevention except for prevention of the HIV infection itself. Vacuolar degeneration of the spinal cord resulting in paraparesis, ataxia, and incontinence occurs in approximately 20% of patients with AIDS,[97] and may also be due to HIV infection of the CNS.

Toxoplasma gondii encephalitis is the second most common opportunistic infection involving the CNS in patients with AIDS. Almost all cases are due to recrudescent disease as evidenced by preexisting antibody. In 30% of our patients with preexisting antibody, CNS toxoplasmosis has developed. Patients regularly have headache and fever and also recognize localizing evidence of focal disease by focal weakness or even seizures. Rarely, impaired vision occurs due to retinal involvement. Physical examination usually reveals localizing signs and rarely exudative retinal lesions typical of toxoplasmosis. The CSF is not diagnostic and the

TABLE 7. CNS Infections Complicating AIDS

Organism	Syndrome	Comment
Viruses		
HIV	Dementia, aseptic meningitis, ?vacuolar myelopathy	Isolated from CSF and/or nucleic acid sequences detected in CNS tissues in some cases; no treatment currently available
Cytomegalovirus	Chorioretinitis, ?encephalitis	Some cases of chorioretinitis respond to DHPG
Papovavirus–JC	Progressive multifocal leuko-encephalopathy	Brain biopsy required to confirm the diagnosis; no proven treatment available
Epstein–Barr virus	Lymphoma	Aggressvie B-cell lymphomas of CNS may be related to EBV infection
Parasites		
Toxoplasma gondii	Encephalitis, brain abscess	After HTLV-III/LAV, the most common CNS infection seen in AIDS; antibody response usually poor, especially IgM; prolonged therapy necessary
Fungi		
Cryptococcus neoformans	Meningitis, brain abscess	Concomitant pulmonary involvement and disseminated disease common, with high antigen titers in CSF and serum; relapse after usual courses of therapy the rule; consider chronic suppression with amphotericin B on outpatient basis
Bacteria		
Nocardia asteroides	Brain abscess	Seen in association with *Salmonella* in one case

serology that has been so helpful in other patients is usually not helpful in AIDS. The rule is absent or low IgM titers and no rise (or a prolonged rise) in IgG antibody titers. CSF titers have shown a significant rise in titer in the absence of a serum rise in one patient in one report.[98] Computed tomography scans of the brain usually, but not always, show ring-enhancing lesions; lymphomas may cause similar lesions. If the serology is not diagnostic, the definitive test is a brain biopsy. In the presence of considerable necrosis on biopsy, organisms may not be seen, but an immunoperoxidase stain for antigen may be diagnostic.[99] Definitive diagnosis in many cases requires brain biopsy.

One method of management, when the clinical diagnosis strongly suggests toxoplasmosis with a nondiagnostic serology, is for treatment empirically with pyrimethamine and sulfadiazine.[100] If there is no response after 4–7 days, a brain biopsy can be done. If it is a CNS neoplasm, the few days lost in such a therapeutic trial for toxoplasmosis are not crucial in the subsequent management of the neoplasm. If the patient responds to empirical therapy, it should be continued indefinitely. We have no criteria for knowing when to stop therapy. We do know that the usual courses of 6–8 weeks may be inadequate. Because of this uncertainty and the experience that so

many infections in AIDS patients recur regularly, recommendations for indefinite therapy have been made. It is worthwhile to continue following with serologic tests for rises in antibody titer, which may be delayed in these patients. Reactions to the sulfadiazine may occur in the form of rash, fever, neutropenia, or thrombocytopenia. In the presence of neutropenia, lowering the dose of sulfadiazine was effective in one case in our experience. When reactions to sulfadiazine have been severe, we have continued therapy with pyrimethamine alone and found that it controlled the CNS toxoplasmosis.

Cryptococcus neoformans is the most common cause of meningitis in patients with AIDS. Symptoms and signs are the same as those of other immunocompromised hosts with one remarkable exception. Extensive pulmonary involvement has been present at the same time as the presenting meningitis in patients with AIDS but has occurred rarely in others. Another unusual feature of the disease in patients with AIDS is that the CSF shows many yeasts, but few host cells. Cryptococcal antigen titers in the CSF and serum are extraordinarily high, regularly above a titer of 1 : 1024. The patients' symptoms and signs usually respond promptly to therapy but organisms in the CSF and high antigen titers in the CSF and serum persist.[101] As relapses after a 6-week course of therapy are the rule,[101] we believe that an initial 6-week course of amphotericin B and flucytosine (5-FC) should be followed by continuation of amphotericin B indefinitely. This can usually be managed in an outpatient clinic with the patient coming in for therapy 1–2 days per week at doses of 0.75–1 mg/kg. Tissue levels[102] should be maintained for prolonged periods on this schedule. Some patients, with appropriate supervision, can have amphotericin B administered at home. Small capsule cryptococci have been reported as common in patients with AIDS at one hospital,[103] and this interesting finding remains to be confirmed.

Cytomegalovirus is among the microorganisms most frequently causing disease in patients with AIDS; however, the precise incidence of infection and disease due to this virus is unknown. Although some neurologic manifestations of AIDS have been thought to be due to CNS infection with CMV, it has only rarely been found on histopathology or culture of CNS tissues at postmortem examination. Many of the CNS syndromes previously attributed to CMV[94] are most likely due to HIV infection of the CNS.

A severe, progressive chorioretinitis characterized by hemorrhages, exudates, and vascular sheathing due to CMV occurs commonly in patients with AIDS and usually results in blindness. The experimental antiviral agent 9-[2-hydroxy-l-(hydroxymethyl)ethoxymethyl]guanine (DHPG) has halted progression or improved the retinitis in some patients.[104–106] As with other infections in patients with AIDS, relapse is common and therefore, some have recommended prolonged outpatient therapy with DHPG if there has been an initial response.

Papovavirus–JC infections manifested by progressive multifocal leukoencephalopathy have been documented in several patients.[94] The clinical syndrome of slowly progressive, multifocal, neurologic disease suggests the diagnosis, but brain biopsy is necessary for confirmation. No proven effective treatment is available.

Primary CNS B-cell lymphomas have been seen in patients with AIDS and are usually refractory to therapy.[107] It has been suggested that Epstein–Barr virus (EBV) may be responsible for this progressive neoplastic disease. If this can be documented, antiviral therapy could be an important component in the treatment of such lymphomas.

Bacterial infections of the CNS occur rarely in patients with AIDS. A mixed brain abscess with *Nocardia asteroides* and *Salmonella enteriditis* group B has been reported.[108] Although we would have anticipated seeing listeriosis in patients with AIDS due to their severe T-cell defect, only two cases of *Listeria monocytogenes* bacteremia have been reported.[109] There have been no reports of *Listeria* meningitis in patients with AIDS.

References

1. Chernik NL, Armstrong D, Posner JB: Central nervous system infections in patients with cancer. *Medicine (Baltimore)* **52:**563–581, 1973.
2. Chernik NL, Armstrong D, Posner JB: Central nervous system infections in patients with cancer: Changing patterns. *Cancer* **40:**268–274, 1977.
3. Lukes SA, Posner JB, Nielsen S, et al: Bacterial infections of the CNS in neutropenic patients. *Neurology (NY)* **34:**269–275, 1984.
4. Swartz MN, Dodge PR: Bacterial meningitis: A review of selected aspects. *N Engl J Med* **272:**725–731, 1965.
5. Mangi RJ, Quintiliani R, Andriole VT: Gram negative meningitis. *Am J Med* **59:**829–836, 1975.
6. Armstrong D: Listeria monocytogenes. In Mandell GL, Douglas RG, Bennett JE (eds): *Principles and Practice of Infectious Diseases.* 2nd Ed. Wiley, New York, 1985, pp. 1177–1182.
7. Scheld WM, Winn HR: Brain abscess. In Mandell GL, Douglas RG, Bennett JE (eds): *Principles and Practice of Infectious Diseases.* 2nd Ed. Wiley, New York, 1985, pp. 585–592.
8. Samson DS, Clark K: A current review of brain abscess. *Am J Med* **54:**201–210, 1973.
9. Young RC, Bennett JE, Vogel CL, et al: Aspergillosis: The spectrum of disease in 98 patients. *Medicine (Baltimore)* **49:**147–173, 1970.
10. Meyer RD, Young LS, Armstrong D, et al: Aspergillosis complicating neoplastic disease. *Am J Med* **54:**6–15, 1973
11. Young LS, Armstrong D, Blevins A, et al: Nocardia asteroides infection complicating neoplastic disease. *Am J Med* **50:**356–367, 1971.
12. Palmer DL, Harvey RL, Wheeler JK: Diagnostic and therapeutic considerations in *Nocardia asteroides* infection. *Medicine (Baltimore)* **53:**391–401, 1974
13. Polsky B, Armstrong D: Infectious complications of neoplastic disease. *Am J Infect Control* **13:**199–209, 1985.
14. Hooper DC, Pruitt AA, Rubin RH: Central nervous system infection in the chronically immunocompromised. *Medicine (Baltimore)* **61:**166–188, 1982.
15. Hersh EM, Freireich EJ: Host defense mechanisms and their modification by cancer chemotherapy. *Methods Cancer Res* **4:**355–451, 1968.
16. Walzer PD, Armstrong D, Weisman P, et al: Serum immunoglobulin levels in childhood Hodgkin's disease: Effect of

splenectomy and long-term follow-up. *Cancer* **45**:2084–2089, 1980.

17. Moffet, HL: *Pediatric Infectious Disease: A Problem Oriented Approach. Acute Neurologic Syndromes.* JB Lippincott, Philadelphia, 1975.

18. Killenger AH: *Listeria monocytogenes.* In Lenette EH, Spaulding EH, Travet JP (eds): *Manual of Clinical Microbiology.* American Society for Microbiology, Washington, DC, 1974, pp. 135–139.

19. Gray ML (ed): *Second Symposium on Listeria Infections.* Artcraft Printers, Bozeman, Montana, 1962.

20. Louria DB, Hensle T, Armstrong D, et al: Listeriosis complicating malignant disease: A new association. *Ann Intern Med* **67**:261–281, 1967.

21. Schlech WF III, Lavigue PM, Bortolussi RA, et al: Epidemic listeriosis—Evidence for transmission by food. *N Engl J Med* **308**:203–206, 1983.

22. Fleming DW, Cochi SL, MacDonald KL, et al: Pasteurized milk as a vehicle of infection in an outbreak of listeriosis. *N Engl J Med* **312**:404–407, 1985.

23. Centers for Disease Control: Listeriosis outbreak associated with Mexican-style cheese—California. *MMWR* **34**:357–359, 1985.

24. Gersten MJ, Ognibene F, Blevins A, et al: Listeria infections and neoplastic disease: An old association, recent observations. (In preparation.)

25. Medoff G, Knuz LJ, Weinberg AN: Listeriosis in humans: An evaluation. *J Infect Dis* **123**:247–250, 1971.

26. Levitz R, Quintiliani R: Trimethoprim–sulfamethoxazole for bacterial meningitis. *Ann Intern Med* **100**:881–890, 1984.

27. Jacquette G, Dennehy PH: Trimethoprim–sulfamethoxazole in *Listeria monocytogenes meningitis. (Letter.) Ann Intern Med* **102**:866–867, 1985.

28. Ihde DC, Armstrong D: Clinical spectrum of infection due to *Bacillus* species. *Am J Med* **55**:839–845, 1973.

29. Humphreys DW, Crowder JG, White A: Serological reactions to nocardia antigens. *Am J Med Sci* **269**:323–326, 1975.

30. Present CA, Wiernik PH, Serpick AA: Factors affecting survival in nocardiosis. *Am Rev Respir Dis* **108**:1444–1448, 1973.

31. Kaplan MH, Armstrong D, Rosen PP: Tuberculosis complicating neoplastic disease: A review of 201 cases. *Cancer* **33**:850–858, 1974.

32. Ortballs DW, Marr JJ: A comparative study of tuberculosis and other mycobacterial infections and their associations with malignancy. *Am Rev Respir Dis* **117**:39–45 1978.

33. Bisno AL: Hyposplenism and overwhelming pneumococcal infection: A reappraisal. *Am J Med Sci* **262**:101–107, 1971.

34. Chilcote RR, Baehner RL, Hammond D, et al: Septicemia and meningitis in children splenectomized for Hodgkin's disease. *N Engl J Med* **295**:798–800, 1976.

35. Ravry M, Maldonado N, Vélez-Gárcia E, et al: Serious infection after splenectomy for the staging of Hodgkin's disease. *Ann Intern Med* **77**:11–14, 1972.

36. Austrian R, Douglas RM, Schiffman G, et al: Prevention of pneumococcal pneumonia by vaccination. *Trans Assoc Am Physicians* **89**:184–194, 1976.

37. Hosea SW, Burch C, Brown EJ, et al: Impaired immune response of splenectomized patients to polyvalent pneumococcal vaccine. *Lancet* **1**:804–807, 1981.

38. Siber GR, Weitzman SA, Aisenberg CA, et al: Impaired antibody response to pneumococcal vaccine after treatment for Hodgkin's disease. *N Engl J Med* **299**:442–448, 1978.

39. Folland D, Armstrong D, Seides S, et al: Pneumococcal bacteremia in patients with neoplastic disease. *Cancer* **33**:845–849, 1974.

40. Chou MY, Brown AE, Blevins A, et al: Severe pneumococcal infection in patients with neoplastic disease. *Cancer* **51**:1546–1550, 1983.

41. Schimpff SC, Young VM, Greene WH, et al: Origin of infection in acute non-lymphocytic leukemia: Significance of hospital acquisition of potential pathogens. *Ann Intern Med* **77**:707–714, 1972.

42. Fong IW, Tomkins KB: Review of *Pseudomonas aeruginosa* meningitis with special emphasis on treatment with ceftazidime. *Rev Infect Dis* **7**:604–612, 1985.

43. Kaplan SL, Mason EQ, Garcia H, et al: Pharmacokinetics and cerebrospinal fluid penetration of moxalactam in children with bacterial meningitis. *J Pediatr* **98**:152–157, 1981.

44. Neu HC: The new beta-lactamase stable cephalosporins. *Ann Intern Med* **97**:408–419, 1982.

45. Landesman SH, Corrado ML, Cherubin CE, et al: Diffusion of a new beta-lactam (LY 127935) into cerebrospinal fluid. *Am J Med* **69**:92–98, 1980.

46. Kaiser AB, McGee ZA: Aminoglycoside therapy of gram negative bacillary meningitis. *N Engl J Med* **293**:1215–1220, 1975.

47. McCracken GH, Saiff LD: Endotoxin in cerebrospinal fluid: Detection in neonates with bacterial meningitis. *JAMA* **235**:617–620, 1976.

48. Campos J, Garcia-Tornel G, Sanfeliu I: Susceptibility studies of multiply-resistant *Haemophilus influenzae* isolated from pediatric patients and contacts. *Antimicrob Agents Chemother* **25**:706–709, 1984.

49. Peltola H, Käyhty H, Virtanen M, et al: Prevention of *Hemophilus influenzae* Type B bacteremia infections with the capsular polysaccharide vaccine. *N Engl J Med* **310**:1561–1566, 1984.

50. Centers for Disease Control: Polysaccharide vaccine for prevention of *Haemophilus influenzae* Type b disease. *MMWR* **34**:201–205, 1985.

51. Diamond RD, Bennett JE: Prognostic factors in cryptococcal meningitis: A study in 111 cases. *Ann Intern Med* **80**:176–181, 1974.

52. Polsky B, Depman MR, Gold JWM, et al: Intraventricular therapy of cryptococcal meningitis via a subcutaneous reservoir. *Am J Med* **81**:25–28, 1986.

53. Kaplan MH, Rosen PP, Armstrong D: Cryptococcosis in a cancer hospital: Clinical and pathological correlates in forty-six patients. *Cancer* **39**:2265–2274, 1977.

54. Bennett JE, Dismukes WE, Duma RJ, et al: Amphotericin B–flucytosine in cryptococcal meningitis. *N Engl J Med* **301**:126–131, 1979.

55. Medoff G, Kobayoishi GS: Strategies in the treatment of systemic fungal infections. *N Engl J Med* **302**:145, 1980.

56. Deresinski SC, Stevens DA: Coccidioidomycosis in com-

promised hosts. Experience at Stamford University. *Hosp Med* **54:**377–386, 1974.

57. Kaufman CA, Israel KS, Smith JW, et al: Histoplasmosis in immunocompromised patients. *Am J Med* **64:**923–932, 1978.

58. Davies SF, Khan M, Sarosi GA. Disseminated histoplasmosis in immunologically suppressed patients. *Am J Med* **64:**94–100, 1978.

59. Sathapatayavongs B, Batteiger BE, Wheat J, et al: Clinical and laboratory features of disseminated histoplasmosis during two large urban outbreaks. *Medicine (Baltimore)* **62:**263–270, 1983.

60. Odds FC: *Candida and Candidosis.* University Park Press, Baltimore, 1979.

61. Meunier-Carpentier F, Kiehn TE, Armstrong D: Fungemia in the immunocompromised host: Changing patterns, antigenemia, high mortality. *Am J Med* **71:**363–70, 1981.

62. Filice G, Yu B, Armstrong D: Immunodiffusion and agglutination tests for candida in patients with neoplastic disease: Inconsistent correlation of results with invasive infection. *J Infect Dis* **135:**349–357, 1977

63. Weiner MH, Yong WJ: Mannan antigenemia in the diagnosis of invasive candidiasis. *J Clin Invest* **58:**1045–1053, 1976.

64. Segal E, Berg RA, Pizzo PA, et al: Detection of candida antigen in sera of patients with candidiosis by an enzyme-linked immunosorbent assay-inhibition technique. *J Clin Microbiol* **10:**116–118, 1979.

65. Miller GG, Witwer MW, Braude AL, et al: Rapid identification of *Candida albicans* septicemia in man by gas–liquid chromatography. *J Clin Invest* **54:**1235–1240, 1974.

66. Kiehn TE, Bernard EM, Gold JWM, et al: Candidiosis: Detection by gas–liquid chromatography of D-arabinatol, a fungal metabolite, in human sera. *Science* **206:**577–580, 1979.

67. Gold JWM, Wong B, Bernard EM, et al: Serum arabinitol concentrations and arabinitol/creatinine ratios in invasive candidiasis. *J Infect Dis* **147:**504–514, 1983.

68. Scheld WM, Lee D, Bernard EM, et al: CSF arabinitol in experimental *Candida albicans* meningitis. Abstract #1168. In *Twenty-fourth Interscience Conference of Antimicrobial Agents and Chemotherapy, Washington, D C., October 8–10, 1984.*

69. Horn R, Wong B, Kiehn TE, et al: Fungemia in a cancer hospital: Changing frequency, earlier onset, and results of therapy. *Rev Infect Dis* **7:**646–655, 1985.

70. Meyer RD, Armstrong D: Mucomycosis: Changing status. *CRC Crit Rev Clin Lab Sci* **4:**421–451, 1073.

71. Kiehn TE, Edwards F, Armstrong D, et al: Pneumonia caused by *Cunninghamella bertholletiae* complicating chronic lymphatic leukemia. *J Clin Microbiol* **10:**374–379, 1979.

72. Lehner RI, Howard OH, Sypherd PS, et al: Mucormycosis. *Ann Intern Med* **93:**93–108, 1980.

73. Ruslein J, Remmington JS: Toxoplasmosis in the compromised host. *Ann Intern Med* **84:**193–199, 1976.

74. Hakes TB, Armstrong D: Toxoplasmosis complicating neoplastic disease. *Cancer* **52:**1535–40, 1983.

75. Purtilo DT, Meyers AM, Connor DH: Fatal strongyloidiasis in immunosuppressed patients. *Am J Med* **56:**488–493, 1974.

76. Meltzer RS, Singer C, Armstrong D, et al: Antemortem diagnosis of central nervous system strongyloidiasis. *Am J Med Sci* **277:**91–98, 1979.

77. Nahmias AJ, Roizman B: Infection with herpes simplex viruses 1 and 2. *N Engl J Med* **289:**667–674, 1973.

78. Price RW, Chernik NL, Horta-Barbosa, L, et al: Herpes simplex encephalitis in an anergic patient. *Am J Med* **54:**222–228, 1973.

79. Natural Institute of Allergy and Infectious Diseases Collaborative Antiviral Study: Adenine arabinoside therapy of biopsy proved herpes simplex encephalitis. *N Engl J Med* **297:**289–294, 1977.

80. Skoldenberg B, Alestig K, Burman L, et al: Acyclovir versus vidarabine in herpes simplex encephalitis. *Lancet* **2:**707–711, 1984.

81. Whitley RJ, Alford CA, Hirsch MS, et al: Vidarabine versus acyclovir therapy in herpes simplex encephalitis. *N Engl J Med* **314:**144–149, 1986

82. Whitely RJ, Chien LT, Dolin R, et al: Adenine arabinoside therapy of herpes zoster in the immunosuppressed; Natural Institute of Allergy and Infectious Diseases Collaborative Antiviral Study. *N Engl J Med* **294:**1193–1199, 1976.

83. Merigan R, Rand KH, Pillard RB, et al: Human leucocyte interferon for the treatment of herpes zoster in patients with cancer. *N Engl J Med* **298:**981–987, 1978.

84. Balfour HH, Bean B, Laskin OL, et al: Acyclovir halts progression of herpes zoster in immunocompromised patients. *N Engl J Med* **308:**1448–1453, 1983.

85. Weller TH: The cytomegaloviruses: Ubiquitous agents with protean clinical manifestations. *N Engl J Med* **285:**203–214, 1971.

86. Mar E-C, Cheng Y-C, Huang E-S: Effect of 9-(1,3-dihydroxy-2-propoxymethyl)guanine on human cytomegalovirus replication in vitro. *Antimicrob Agents Chemother* **24:**518–521, 1983.

87. Oberg B: Antiviral effects of phosphonoformate (PFA, forscarnet sodium). *Pharmacol Ther* **19:**387–415, 1983

88. Berman NS, Siegel SE, Nachim R, et al: Cerebrospinal fluid endotoxin concentrations in gram negative bacterial meningitis. *J Pediatr* **88:**553–556, 1976.

89. Bland RD, Lister RL, Ries JP: Cerebrospinal fluid lactic acid levels and pH in meningitis. *Am J Dis Child* **128:**151–156, 1974.

90. Craven RB, Brooks JB, Edman DC, et al: Rapid diagnosis of lymphocytic meningitis by frequency-pulsed electron capture gas–liquid chromatography: Differentiation of tuberculosis, cryptococcal and viral meningitis. *J Clin Microbiol* **6:**27–32, 1977.

91. Brice JL, Tornabene TG, LaForce FM: Diagnosis of bacterial meningitis by gas–liquid chromatography I. Chemotyping studies of *Streptococcus pneumoniae, Haemophilus influenzae, Neisseria meningitidis, Staphylococcus aureus* and *Escherichia coli. J Infect Dis* **140:**443–452, 1979.

92. LaForce FM, Brice JL, Tornabene TG: Diagnosis of bacterial meningitis by gas–liquid chromatography. II. Analysis of spinal fluid. *J Infect Dis* **140:**453–464, 1979.

93. Peacock JE, McGinnis MR, Cohen MS: Persistent neu-

trophilic meningitis. *Medicine (Baltimore)* **63**:379–395, 1984.

94 Snider WD, Simpson DM, Nielsen S, et al: Neurological complications of acquired immune deficiency syndrome: analysis of 50 patients. *Ann Neurol* **14**:403–418, 1983.

95 Ho DD, Rota TR, Schooley RT, et al: Isolation of HTLV-III from cerebrospinal fluid and neural tissues of patients with neurologic syndromes related to the acquired immunodeficiency syndrome. *N Engl J Med* **313**:1493–1497, 1985.

96. Shaw GM, Harper ME, Hahn BH, et al: HTLV-III infection in brains of children and adults with AIDS encephalopathy. *Science* **227**:177–82, 1985.

97. Petito CK, Navia BA, Cho E-S, et al: Vacuolar myelopathy pathologically resembling subacute combined degeneration in patients with the acquired immunodeficiency syndrome. *N Engl J Med* **312**:874–879, 1985.

98 Wong B, Gold JWM, Brown AE, et al: Central nervous system toxoplasmosis in homosexual men and parenteral drug abusers. *Ann Intern Med* **100**:36–42, 1984.

99. Luft BJ, Brooks RG, Conley FR, et al: Toxoplasmic encephalitis in patients with acquired immune deficiency syndrome. *JAMA* **252**:913–917, 1984.

100. Navia BA, Petito CK, Gold JWM, et al: Cerebral toxoplasmosis complicating the acquired immune deficiency syndrome (AIDS): Clinical and neuropathological findings in 27 patients. *Ann Neurol* **19**:224–238, 1986.

101. Kovacs JA, Kovacs AA, Polis M, et al: Cryptococcosis in the acquired immunodeficiency syndrome. *Ann Intern Med* **103**:533–538, 1985.

102. Christiansen KJ, Bernard EM, Gold JWM, et al: Distribution and activity of amphotericin B in humans. *J Infect Dis* **5**:1037–1043, 1985.

103. Bottone EJ, Toma M, Johansson BE, et al: Capsule-deficient *Cryptococcus neoformans* in AIDS patients *Lancet* **1**:400, 1985.

104. Felsenstein D, D'Amico DJ, Hirsch MS, et al: Treatment of cytomegalovirus retinitis with 9-[2-hydroxy-1-(hydroxymethyl)ethoxymethyl]guanine. *Ann Intern Med* **103**:377–380, 1985

105. Bach MC, Bagwell SP, Knapp NP, et al. 9-(1,3-dihydroxy-2-propoxymethyl)guanine for cytomegalovirus infections in patients with the acquired immunodeficiency syndrome. *Ann Intern Med* **103**:381–382, 1985.

106. Masur H, Lane HC, Palestine A, et al: Effect of 9-(1,3-dihydroxy-2-propoxymethyl)guanine on serious cytomegalovirus disease in eight immunosuppressed homosexual men. *Ann Intern Med* **104**:41–44, 1986.

107. Gill PS, Levine AM, Meyer PR, et al. Primary central nervous system lymphoma in homosexual men. Clinical, immunologic, and pathologic features. *Am J Med* **78**:742–748, 1985.

108. Holtz HA, Lavery DP, Kapila R: Actinomycetales infection in the acquired immunodeficiency syndrome. *Ann Intern Med* **102**:203–205, 1985

109. Real FX, Gold JWM, Krown SE, et al: *Listeria monocytogenes* bacteremia in the acquired immunodeficiency syndrome. (Letter.) *Ann Intern Med* **101**:883–884, 1984

8

Fungal Infections in the Compromised Host

FRANÇOISE MEUNIER

1. Introduction

As the numbers of patients with host defenses compromised by disease and/or therapy have increased, so has the importance of invasive fungal infection as a cause of significant morbidity and mortality in this patient population.[1-6] The most important fungal infections in the compromised host are those caused by *Candida* and *Aspergillus* species, Mucoraceae, and *Cryptococcus neoformans*—organisms rightfully considered opportunistic invaders. The difference between fungal infection in the impaired host as opposed to the normal individual is strikingly demonstrated by a study from California that compared the types of fungal infection observed in different patient populations.[2] Of 72 fungal infections occurring in immunocompromised people, 80% were caused by *Candida, Aspergillus,* and Mucoraceae, with an additional 12% caused by *Cryptococcus;* of 62 fungal infections occurring in normal hosts, 71% were caused by *Coccidioides* and *Histoplasma,* 5% by *Cryptococcus,* and none by *Candida, Aspergillus,* or Mucoraceae.

This is not to say that histoplasmosis and coccidioidomycosis do not occur on occasion in the immunocompromised host who has been exposed to these organisms within geographically well-defined areas of the world. Indeed, infection with these

agents and such other fungi as *Trichosporon cutaneum, Blastomyces dermatitidis* (another geographically restricted mycotic infection), *Sporothrix schenckii,* and others have been noted in immunocompromised patients. Rather, the point to be emphasized is that *Candida, Aspergillus,* Mucoraceae, and *Cryptococcus* are ubiquitous in the environment and have a particular virulence for the compromised host.[2,5,6]

The challenge to the clinician in dealing with the fungal infections is that noninvasive diagnostic techniques are insensitive, clinical presentation is often occult, and therapy is prolonged and often hazardous. Despite these inherent problems, fungal infection can be prevented and treated in this patient population. This chapter presents an approach that will enable the clinician to accomplish these tasks.

2. Diagnostic Approach: A General Overview

Although invasive fungal infection is frequently suspected, accurate diagnosis remains extremely difficult in the immunocompromised patient.[7] On the one hand, such noninvasive tests as blood culturing and testing for antibodies to these organisms is quite insensitive, with a high rate of false-positive and false-negative results; on the other hand, definitive biopsy procedures may be impossible because of bleeding disorders or severe respiratory failure.

The definitive diagnostic test for invasive fungal infection is histologic demonstration of the fungal

FRANÇOISE MEUNIER • Department of Internal Medicine and Henri Tagnon Laboratory of Clinical Investigation, Section of Microbiology and Infectious Diseases Unit, Jules Bordet Institute, 1000 Brussels, Belgium.

pathogen invading tissue, followed by the identification of the organism by cultures of the same specimen. Because of the difficulty in fulfilling these rather stringent diagnostic criteria in many immunocompromised patients with potentially life-threatening invasive fungal infection, increased emphasis is being placed on newer techniques of diagnosis, such as antigen detection (e.g., the demonstration of cryptococcal antigen in the cerebrospinal fluid (CSF) of a patient with cryptococcal meningitis) and detection of unique fungal metabolites. In evaluating these new techniques, however, they must always be compared with the gold standard of histopathology.

2.1. Histology

This approach is mandatory to confirm a presumptive diagnosis of opportunistic fungal infection. The demonstration of fungal elements in tissue establishes the diagnosis of invasive infection and eliminates the possibility of colonization. However, numerous factors may interfere with the value of the biopsy, including the size and site of the biopsy, the staining procedures employed, as well as the expertise of the pathologist. Some fungal pathogens are easily identified in tissue sections, but others do not always show typical forms that permit an accurate diagnosis. Complicating the interpretation of biopsy specimens is the fact that the range of inflammatory response incited by fungal pathogens may be very great—from frank caseation to a granuloma, to an acute polymorphonuclear leukocyte response, to no response. This wide range of response is in large part determined by the nature and extent of the host-defense defects present in the patient. In addition, particularly in compromised patients, multiple pathogens, including nonfungal pathogens, must be considered. The most useful specific stains for fungal organisms are the Gomori methenamine silver (GMS), Gridley fungus (GF), and periodic acid–Schiff (PAS) stains. The characteristic histopathologic features of most fungal infection have been illustrated extensively by Chandler et al.[8] The diagnostic value of biopsy and demonstration of fungus in tissues is essential in patients with suspected invasive candidiasis or aspergillosis, as the responsible pathogens frequently colonize the compromised patient without concomitant deep-seated invasion. Thus, cultures alone will not necessarily yield the definitive diagnosis. The optimal approach in these situations seems to rely on specimens obtained from suspected sites such as pulmonary or hepatic tissue, cutaneous emboli, or splenic lesions. Unfortunately, cutaneous manifestations that represent easily accessible sites for biopsy are not frequent early in the evolution of most opportunistic fungal diseases.

2.2. Cultures

Only cultures permit correct identification of the causative fungal pathogen. Isolation of the organism permits determination of the infectious species, which is impossible on a histologic basis for most fungi, particularly *Candida* species. In addition, antimicrobial sensitivity testing is only possible following cultural isolation of the organism. The combination of cultures and histology is therefore crucial in establishing a specific diagnosis of fungal disease. It must be emphasized, however, that the significance of a positive culture is usually determined by the origin of the specimen: the isolation of pathogenic fungi in several blood cultures or in any sample obtained from a sterile closed space (e.g., CSF) represents valid diagnostic information. By contrast, the isolation of *Aspergillus* or *Candida* species from the sputum is usually of unclear significance. It should be stressed that false-negative cultures are common even in cases of extensive fungal opportunistic infections. Routine autopsy studies performed in compromised patients have established a high rate of invasive mycoses that are clinically unsuspected and only discovered postmortem.

2.3. Serology

2.3.1. Detection of Antibodies

Various approaches have been used in an effort at making a specific diagnosis of fungal infection by measuring the level of circulating antibodies against fungi.[5,9,10] Numerous methods have recently been developed with the aim of increasing the sensitivity and specificity of such tests. Moreover, the purification of antigens has somewhat improved the yield of this approach. However, a great lack of standardization of reagents still exists and precludes the comparison of data obtained from various laboratories.[11]

Overall, specific antibody detection has been useful in the diagnosis of coccidioidomycosis[12] and histoplasmosis.[13] The value of detection of antibodies against *Aspergillus* species or *Candida* species still remains controversial but does not appear to be a satisfactory diagnostic tool, particularly in immunocompromised hosts who are often unable to produce specific antibodies in response to fungal invasion.[5,7,14–17]

In addition, many persons have preexisting antibodies to these organisms that are ubiquitous in the environment. The testing for antibodies against *Cryptococcus neoformans* appears to be of little diagnostic use but may have prognostic significance; that is, patients with cryptococcal invasion who produce antibody appear to have a better chance of responding to therapy.[18,19] Antibody measurements in the diagnosis of invasive infection due to such other less common pathogens such as *Blastomyces* species.[20] *Sporothrix* species, *Trichosporon* species, and *Petriellidium boydii* have not proven to be of diagnostic value.

2.3.2. Detection of Antigen or Fungal Metabolites

Since the ability of compromised patients to produce specific antibodies is well known to be impaired, numerous studies have been performed to detect fungal antigens or metabolites in the blood of patients suspected of having invasive fungal infections. The value of detection of fungal antigen is best illustrated for cryptococcosis and particularly for the diagnosis of cryptococcal meningitis. The detection of capsular antigen appears to be a useful test, with a high sensitivity (greater than 95%) and excellent specificity (99%) provided adequate controls are performed to rule out the possibility of false-positive reactions, such as those produced by the presence of rheumatoid factor.[18] By analogy with this successful approach, many investigations have been undertaken to apply this concept to other opportunistic fungal infections. Most studies have been performed in patients with suspected disseminated candidiasis. Circulating antigens of various composition (mannan, mannose)[21–30] and metabolites (e.g., arabinitol) have been detected in the blood of these patients.[31–35] However, the optimal approach remains to be defined, since false-positive and false-negative reactions have been reported. Fewer studies have been realized in aspergillosis, but promising data are already available.[36,37,38,39] Improvement of the available techniques may be useful in establising a rapid diagnosis earlier in the evolution of opportunistic infections, but these techniques remain investigational and do not yet provide a rapid diagnostic tool at the bedside that is routinely applicable in all community hospitals.

3. Candidiasis

3.1. *Candida* Species

Infections caused by *Candida* species are the commonest fungal disease in immunocompromised patients.[3,5,6] Numerous species of yeasts have been recognized as offending pathogens and careful identification is mandatory.[30,40–53] *C. albicans, C. tropicalis, C. krusei,* and *C. parapsilosis* are frequently isolated, but *C. guillermondii, C. pseudotropicalis,* and other species may also be responsible for a similar clinical picture. In addition, the closely related yeast, *Torulopsis glabrata,* is a not uncommon cause of infection in this patient population. In general, *C. albicans* and *C. tropicalis* are the species most associated with invasive candidiasis following fungemia. By contrast, fungemia with the other species of yeast are infrequently associated with invasive disease.[5,30]

In the normal host, neutrophils, monocytes, and eosinophils phagocytize and kill *Candida* blastospores, and neutrophils and monocytes kill hyphal forms. Not surprisingly, then, the prime candidates for life-threatening invasive candidal infection are those with defects in white blood cell (WBC) number and function, the prime example being the severely neutropenic leukemic patient. The second host defense of importance against yeast infection is cell-mediated immunity. Therefore, persons with profound defects in cell-mediated immunity, such as transplant recipients, patients with acquired immunodeficiency syndrome (AIDS), and patients receiving chronic steroid therapy are at significant risk of invasive candidal infection. Finally, therapeutic maneuvers that compromise normal mucocutaneous barriers to infection, such as indwelling intravenous catheters, and medications such as antibiotics and steroids that enhance *Candida* colonization, predispose to candidemia and systemic candidiasis.[5,54–58]

3.2. Clinical Presentation

3.2.1. Disseminated Candidiasis

The characteristic clinical setting is most commonly the neutropenic patient (e.g., with an hematologic malignancy) or the patient with a solid tumor at a terminal stage. The prognosis of such opportunistic infections is extremely poor, and disseminated candidiasis represents an increasing cause of mortality in cancer patients.[3,5,30,43,59,60] This infection usually occurs in patients hospitalized for a prolonged period, treated with numerous agents, including antibiotics, antineoplastic chemotherapy, and steroids. The diagnosis should be suspected for each debilitated patient (neutropenic or not) who remains febrile without a documented source of fever. Disseminated candidiasis usually involves many organs, such as the kidneys, the liver, the spleen, the myocardium, the skin, the gastrointestinal (GI) tract, the central nervous system (CNS), the eyes, and the lungs. Occasionally, other organs such as the thyroid, the ovaries, the adrenals, the joints, or the lymph nodes may also be invaded by the yeasts.[60] Numerous syndromes have been associated with hematogenous dissemination.[59] Unfortunately, there is no characteristic finding allowing the clinician to ascertain the diagnosis since the clinical manifestations are generally nonspecific; except for fever, which is almost always present, other signs and symptoms such as shaking chills, hypotension, tachycardia, dyspnea, hepatomegaly, or splenomegaly are noted in only 10–30% of cases. Typical skin rash, endophthalmitis, and myalgia occur in fewer than 5% of the patients with disseminated candidiasis. Hypercalcemia has also been occasionally reported in leukemic patients with disseminated candidiasis.[61] The duration of the evolution varies: symptoms may progress rapidly, indicating an acute and rapidly fatal infection; for other patients, however, the onset of clinical manifestations is more insidious.

Illustrative Case 1

A 70-year-old man with multiple myeloma was hospitalized for fever and neutropenia, which developed after a course of antineoplastic chemotherapy, including melphalan (2 mg/kg) The clinical site of infection on admission was a dental abscess. The patient was treated intravenously with broad-spectrum antibiotics (ticarcillin and amikacin) resulting in improvement of signs and symptoms of infection as well as eradication of fever. As neutropenia persisted, antibiotics were continued and the patient became febrile again 19 days after initiation of the antibacterial therapy without any clinical site of infection evident. Ticarcillin and amikacin were discontinued after 21 days of therapy; reevaluation of the fever was carried out, including multiple blood cultures, which were all positive for *Escherichia coli*. The clinical status of the patient deteriorated rapidly and death occurred within 48 hr despite resumption of ticarcillin and amikacin. Autopsy revealed an unsuspected disseminated candidiasis (digestive tract, liver, spleen and lungs) and persistence of neoplastic cells in the bone marrow.

Comment Disseminated candidiasis remains often a postmortem discovery. No fungemia was documented in this patient despite multiple blood cultures. Surveillance cultures revealed a few colonies of *C. tropicalis* in the mouth and more than 100,000 CFU/ml in the urine (yeast forms were noted in the urinary sediment) 3 weeks before death. Two subsequent urine cultures were negative. Throat swabs obtained during the last 3 days of life also revealed *C. tropicalis* without clinical signs or symptoms of oral thrush. Postmortem cultures from the lungs and spleen were also positive for *C. tropicalis*. This case also demonstrates the potential risks of prolonged administration of broad-spectrum antibiotics, with emergence of resistant organisms such as *E. coli* in blood cultures as well as superinfection and bloodstream invasion with *C. tropicalis*. The precise pathogenic role of the latter in the fulminant evolution of this patient is unclear and controversial. Nevertheless, it should be stressed that disseminated candidiasis should be considered in febrile patients with extensive neoplastic disease even when another pathogen has already been isolated.

3.2.2. Fungemia

The clinical presentation of fungemia is nonspecific and may be similar to bacterial sepsis. Fever, chills, hypotension, and even shock (observed in 30% of cases) are the major clinical manifestations of fungemia. Various sources of fungemia have to be taken into consideration: fungemia may occur as a result of an intravenous catheter-related infection or a deep-seated candidiasis. Transient candidemia may also occur without obvious source; however, colonization of the gastrointestinal (GI) tract constitutes the major endogenous source of candidiasis. Occasionally, exogenous sources such as contamination of intravenous solutions[47] have also been recognized. The significance of candidemia may be difficult to ascertain in some circumstances. Only 30–50% of patients with disseminated candidiasis have a positive blood culture. Although candidemia may not indicate a deep-seated infection, particularly in normal hosts, a positive blood culture in immunocompromised patients should always suggest the existence of deep tissue invasion; specific therapy should be initiated pending further investigations. Major complications such as vision loss, endocarditis, fungal arthritis, or osteomyelitis[62-71] have been recognized following an episode of fungemia that has been considered transient and that has remained untreated. The clinical significance of fungemia in cancer patients has been evaluated in the United States in a series of 70 patients and indicated that only 8 (11%) episodes were transient. Our own data obtained at the Institut Jules Bordet, the Cancer Center of the University of Brussels, also indicated the poor outcome of patients with fungemia.[41] It should be stressed that the precise pathogenic role of fungemia is often difficult to determine in cancer patients with a progressive underlying disease. Nevertheless, fungemia appears to be the immediate cause of death in 10–30% of the cases. Weinstein et al.[66] also demonstrated that the mortality rate during an episode of fungemia was 68%, although only one-half of these patients succumbed to infection. Documented fungemia should therefore initiate a careful evaluation of each patient, consisting of complete culturing, biopsy of any skin or muscle lesions, and then serious consideration of initiating empiric therapy if the patient remains immunocompromised, particularly if the species of yeast isolated is *C. albicans* or *C. tropicalis*.

Illustrative Case 2

A 13-year-old boy with acute lymphocytic leukemia in first relapse, unresponsive to treatment despite numerous chemotherapeutic trials, was hospitalized for allogeneic bone marrow transplantation Two days after receiving cyclophosphamide (60 mg/kg), he became febrile without evidence of infection, and broad-spectrum antibiotics (azlocillin and amikacin) were initiated. Within 48 hr, severe myalgias developed in the lower legs, and he became febrile again without a documented site of infection. At that time, the patient underwent total body irradiation and was randomized not to receive empiric amphotericin B. The patient continued to remain febrile, particularly after transfusions. Bone marrow transplatation was performed and antifungal prophylaxis (nystatin) was discontinued because of GI intolerance and poor compliance. The patient complained again of pain in the lower legs, 4 days after the transplantation and oral thrush was first noted.

In addition, a few skin lesions appeared on the face, the trunk, and the lower legs. Cutaneous lesions were erythematous nodules compatible with septic emboli. The nodules were biopsied and

amphotericin B was initiated. The patient was febrile and had shaking chills and bilateral calf pain. The cultures of the cutaneous lesions as well as the urine cultures revealed *C. tropicalis*. The clinical status deteriorated rapidly, and the patient expired 48 hr after the skin lesions had developed. All blood cultures drawn after the appearance of the septic nodules were reported to be positive for *C. tropicalis*, but only after the patient expired. Autopsy revealed disseminated candidiasis involving the myocardium, the lungs, lymph nodes, and kidneys.

Comment. Fungemia in patients with severe neutropenia (less than 100 polymorphonuclear leukocytes/mm³) is rapidly fatal. Moreover, blood cultures are usually inadequate for providing a specific early diagnosis. Myalgias and skin nodules seem particularly characteristic of disseminated candidiasis due to *C. tropicalis*. This case illustrates the potential role of empiric initiation of amphotericin B in severely neutropenic patients who remain febrile despite antibiotics. The potential benefit of this approach relies on treatment of occult fungal diseases which are too often diagnosed too late and when the situation is irreversible. In addition, the need for better effective prophylactic measures with good compliance is also obvious.

3.2.3. Cardiac Candidiasis

The incidence of fungal endocarditis is increasing in cancer patients as well as in other diseases. *Candida* sp. endocarditis is also a complication observed in drug abusers or in patients who have undergone cardiac surgery. Pathogenic mechanisms are similar to those described for bacterial endocarditis. The clinical presentation varies and may consist of an abrupt onset of fever with emboli to the major vessels or may be insidious with protean signs and symptoms. Antemortem diagnosis is established in 60% of cases. Approximately 80% of patients with endocarditis due to *Candida* species have a positive blood culture. However, it has been recommended that a large volume of blood be cultured, since fungemia may be transient, and the level of fungemia is usually low. Occasionally, emboli in the coronary arteries may cause either ischemia or cardiac failure, or both. Pericardial involvement is rare. Cardiac candidiasis has also been demonstrated in the setting of disseminated infection with multiple emboli to deep tissue. Numerous microabscesses in the myocardium as well as the conducting system have also been described and may be responsible for dysrhythmias.[73]

3.2.4. Gastrointestinal Candidiasis

The proliferation of yeasts within the GI tract constitutes the major source of deep-seated candidiasis in the immunocompromised host. Fungal colonization of the digestive tract has been recognized in 20–30% of normal persons, but in debilitated patients such as cancer patients, yeasts are identified in the GI tract in as many as 85% of patients.[44,74–76]

Severe oral thrush is frequently observed in debilitated patients, particularly those hospitalized for a prolonged period of time. This infection is painful and may result in impaired nutritional intake. Diagnosis should rely on signs and symptoms as well as the presence of yeasts with pseudomycelia on smears, associated with a positive culture. Invasion of the mucosal membranes may be localized, such as in the esophagus, or may extend to the entire GI tract. Dissemination usually occurs from these sites of infection in persons with fungemia. However, the intensity of colonization in the GI tract does not permit the establishment of a diagnosis of invasive infection. Autopsies performed in cancer patients have shown that 11–27% of patients with acute leukemia, lymphoma, or Hodgkin disease show evidence of GI candidiasis.[77] Candidal esophagitis usually results from the progression of oral thrush. Up to 25% of patients with autopsy-proven severe esophagitis are asymptomatic. The specific diagnosis of *Candida* esophagitis may be difficult to ascertain, as viral lesions due to herpes simplex virus (HSV) or cytomegalovirus (CMV) can mimic candidiasis. Endoscopy is necessary to determine the correct etiology as well as to establish progression or cure with therapy.[78] Gastrointestinal candidiasis has also been associated with severe bleeding.[77]

Other not infrequent sites of GI candidiasis include the hepatobiliary tree and the peritoneum. Hepatic microabscesses are generally observed in the setting of disseminated candidiasis; however, recently, another entity has been described and consists of focal hepatic candidiasis associated with abdominal pain, elevated alkaline phosphatase, and serum bilirubin.[79–81]

Respiratory alkalosis and negative hepatic cultures may also be a common feature of this syndrome. Fungus balls within the biliary tract and obstruction of the common bile duct have also been reported occasionally.[82,83]

Fungal peritonitis is a rare infection in cancer patients that usually results from perforation[84] in the abdomen after multiple GI resections for extensive tumor[85,86] or as a complication of peritoneal dialysis.[87,88]

3.2.5. Urinary Tract Candidiasis

The recovery of yeasts from the urine is frequent, particularly in patients with an indwelling bladder catheter, since colonization of the bladder via the catheter is common. The significance of candiduria in the individual patient is often difficult to ascertain. Bladder candidiasis, renal candidiasis, and obstructive uropathy should be considered different entities. Colonization from the GI tract and the perineal area constitutes a major reservoir responsible for the contamination of the urinary tract. In immunocompromised patients, renal invasion should always be suspected in the presence of candiduria, particularly if renal function is deteriorating. Pseudohyphae do invade the renal tubules and proliferate easily, probably due to an impaired phagocytosis and intracellular killing by polymorphonuclear leukocytes in that tissue. As opposed to bacteriuria, the quantitative evaluation of funguria is not reliable in ascertaining the severity of infection.[89] Several studies have demonstrated renal candidiasis in patients with 5,000–10,000 colonies of yeast per ml urine. Therefore, the cutoff point between contamination and infection remains controversial.[90,91] The presence of fungal casts in the urinary sediments may be useful.[92–94] Various species of yeasts, including *T. glabrata*, may produce severe renal infections.[95] Fungus balls have been mainly observed in diabetic patients[96–98] but may also occur in patients with neoplastic disease[99] or following renal transplantation, causing anuria. Bladder candidiasis as well as obstructive uropathy usually result from an ascending process. Renal candidiasis appears more generally as a consequence of hematogenous dissemination and is characteristic of disseminated infection. In the absence of fungal lesions in the bladder, the vagina or the urethra, the finding of yeast in the urine should suggest the diagnosis of deep-seated disseminated infection.[89,100,101] Similarly, candiduria in the absence of bladder dysfunction or a bladder catheter can be a clue to disseminated infection with renal seeding. Unfortunately, not uncommonly, urine cultures are negative despite the existence of disseminated infection.

3.2.6. Pulmonary Candidiasis

Yeasts are frequently isolated from respiratory secretions, but the clinical relevance of those cultures is limited. Colonization of the mouth and upper airway may produce contamination of the sputum. Moreover, pulmonary infection with *Candida* species usually results from hematogenous dissemination, and in many instances patients do not produce sputum or the cultures obtained remain negative. Primary pulmonary infection with *Candida* is quite unusual, and definitive diagnosis usually requires histologic demonstration of yeasts invading the pulmonary parenchyma. Secondary pulmonary candidiasis, either due to dissemination via the bloodstream from another site (most common) or superinfection of lung tissue previously damaged by other microbial pathogens is not uncommon. Pulmonary candidiasis by itself is rarely a cause of death.[102,103] The closely related yeast, *Torulopsis glabrata,* produces a similar array of clinical syndromes.[44,45]

3.2.7. Cerebromeningeal Candidiasis

This localization was relatively uncommon among cancer patients but occurred mainly in debilitated children.[104-107] However, recent autopsy reports seem to indicate an increased incidence of meningitis caused by *Candida* species.[108,109] In fact, cerebromeningeal candidiasis seems to be the commonest fungal infection discovered in the CNS at autopsy. Antemortem diagnosis is rare. The mortality rate is extremely high. The clinical presentation is nonspecific (e.g., fever and headache) as well as variable findings in the CSF.[110,111] Recommendations have been made to culture large volumes of CSF in order to avoid false-negative cultures. Occasionally, *Candida* meningitis occurs as a complication of extensive neurosurgical procedures. In addition, CNS infection with *Candida albicans* has been reported following a lumbar puncture.[112] Cerebral abscesses may cause focal deficits related to their localization, but in immunosuppressed patients lesions are usually numerous and small, resulting from hematogenous dissemination and are more often associated with no neurologic findings on examination or depressed level of consciousness than with focal deficits.

3.2.8. Osteoarticular Candidiasis

This localization is also infrequent in cancer patients and results mainly from hematogenous dissemination.[113,114] Large joints such as the knee and hip are principally involved. This complication may present several weeks after an episode of fungemia which had been considered as transient and self-limited.[115] These lesions may also persist and develop over prolonged periods of time, even in immunocompromised hosts.[116] Other localizations such as vertebral osteomyelitis have been reported in leukemic patients[117] but also in patients receiving total parenteral nutrition[118] or in drug addicts.[119] Aspiration of the infected joint is useful for diagnostic as well as therapeutic purposes.

3.2.9. Other Forms of Candidiasis

Every organ may be involved in cases of disseminated candidiasis. However, occasionally isolated lesions in cervical nodes, without other localization, have been described in leukemic patients.[120] Classic ocular manifestations have been well characterized, particularly endophthalmitis occurring in the setting of fungemia or disseminated infections.[121] Other ocular lesions such as keratitis are rare, but extensive *Candida* corneal ulcers have been reported in a burn patient.[122] Superficial candidiasis such as nail infections, vaginal candidiasis, as well as chronic mucocutaneous candidiasis represent separate entities and do not have a specific pattern in immunocompromised hosts and are not discussed in this chapter.

4. Aspergillosis

4.1. *Aspergillus* Species

The genus *Aspergillus* includes numerous species. *Aspergillus fumigatus* and *Aspergillus flavus* are the commonest pathogens identified in immunocompromised hosts, but other species may cause severe disease as well. These molds are common contaminants found in decaying organic debris; their distribution is widespread in the environment.[123] Aspergillosis results from inhalation of spores and this occurs both inside or outside hospitals. Airborne spore counts vary with seasons, construction work, or air-filtration systems.[124] Several nosocomial epidemics of invasive aspergillosis have been reported in immunocompromised patients hospitalized in units undergoing construction or renovation, with aerosolization of large numbers of spores resulting from manipulation of contaminated walls, fireproofing, or weatherproofing materials. Alternatively, ventilation systems may become contaminated and serve as sources of infection.[123–128] One other potential source of *Aspergillus* infection is the smoking of marijuana. *Aspergillus* can be cultured from most marijuana samples, antibodies to *Aspergillus* can be found in one-half of immunologically normal marijuana smokers, and invasive aspergillosis has developed in immunosuppressed marijuana smokers who had no other exposure.[5,123]

4.1.1. Pulmonary Aspergillosis

The lungs are the classic site of invasive infection caused by *Aspergillus* species. *Aspergillus* species are responsible for a variety of pulmonary manifestations, including allergic bronchopulmonary aspergillosis, aspergilloma, and invasive aspergillosis. Only the last entity is considered in this chapter, as this is the disease that occurs in compromised patients, the other two conditions occurring in persons with normal immune function. Invasive aspergillosis occurs almost exclusively in immunocompromised patients.[123–131] However, invasive infections have been described on rare occasions in apparently normal hosts or in patients with either liver disease or chronic lung disease, or both.[132,132a] These infections are air-borne and occur particularly in patients who remain neutropenic for a prolonged period of time. The duration of granulocytopenia seems to be crucial.[133] In addition, patients such as transplant recipients, receiving high-dose steroids are at significant risk of invasive aspergillosis.[134–136] Also, patients with WBC functional defects such as chronic granulomatous disease are at increased risk of *Aspergillus* invasion.[137] These three important risk factors—granulocytopenia, WBC dysfunction, and steroid administration—correlate well with the two major host defenses against the initiation of invasive infection in the lungs: alveolar macrophages, which are inhibited by steroids, block spore germination and eradicate inhaled spores; and neutrophils eradicate the hyphae that escape the alveolar macrophages.[138–141] *Aspergillus* spores are ubiquitous, and epidemiologic data must be taken into consideration, since clusters of invasive aspergillosis may develop, particularly in hematologic units.[124–128,142,143] The patient isolated within laminar airflow rooms or whose air supply is passed through a high-efficiency particulate air (HEPA) filter appears to be protected from acquisition of invasive aspergillosis.

The clinical presentation is usually fever unresponsive to broad-spectrum antibiotics in patients without an identified pathogen. Usually, a new pulmonary infiltrate develops, and the evolution of the lesion may result in consolidation and subsequent cavitation. The most common site of primary invasion is within the upper lobes, but multiple lesions also occur. The typical chest radiographic picture is that of a triangular infiltrate resulting from lung infarction due to blood vessel invasion, but various other abnormalities on the chest radiograph have been reported. However, there are no pathognomonic findings on chest radiography, and the absence of lesions does not rule out invasive aspergillosis in neutropenic patients. Massive hemoptysis is relatively rare. Sputum production is an inconsistent finding. The diagnostic value of isolation of *Aspergillus* species from bronchial secretions remains controversial; contamination of the specimen may occur, colonization of the bronchial tree or of the nasopharynx may also exist without evidence of invasive aspergillosis. In addition, numerous patients have autopsy-proven pulmonary aspergillosis without a positive premortem culture for *Aspergillus* species.[130] Routine surveillance cultures from the nose have been helpful in predicting infection in compromised hosts.[144] The optimal approach for obtaining an early diagnosis has not yet been defined: some authorities favor fiberoptic bronchoscopy[145] and bronchoalveolar lavage[146] but in some circumstances, the open lung biopsy may be useful.[147] Both techniques have advantages and disadvantages. Even such aggressive and invasive diagnostic approaches may be misleading[148]; therefore, the final decision should rest with the physician in charge of the patient according to individual clinical considerations, hospital facilities, and the skills of the available team. However, the prognosis also relies on the status of the underlying disease and recovery of an adequate granulocyte count. Residual lesions may be surgically removed in patients who achieve remission. Serodiagnosis remains difficult. Precipitins may be absent, since patients have impaired humoral immunity. The demonstration of *Aspergillus* antigens in serum or in bronchoalveolar fluid appears promising. Early diagnosis of invasive aspergillosis is imperative, as the chance of recovery is directly related to rapid initiation of adequate therapy.[149]

4.1.2. Other Forms of Aspergillosis

Invasive aspergillosis has also been described in sites other than the lungs. It usually results from hematogenous dissemination. Occasionally, however, a primary focus occurs without pulmonary aspergillosis.

Secondary sites classically observed in compromised hosts with pulmonary lesions are localized in the CNS.[3,4,123,129,130,150] Vascular invasion of *Aspergillus* species produces infarction and necrosis of tissue. Cerebral aspergillosis is not a rare complication, and its correct diagnosis should rely on brain biopsy. Recent data seem to indicate that aggressive diagnostic and therapeutic approaches may change the outcome of the patients. Prompt adequate therapy is occasionally life saving.

Occasionally, heroin abusers may develop cerebral aspergillosis or endophthalmitis without other manifestation of systemic infection.[151,152] Besides the localization into the CNS, the major complication of pulmonary aspergillosis, other metastatic sites include the bones, kidneys, liver, spleen, and thyroid.[3,4,123–133] Occasionally, primary foci of aspergillosis occur in the accessory nasal sinuses, the external auditory canal, the eyes, or the cardiac valves. The GI tract may also be invaded primarily without clinical evidence of lung infection. Bleeding and perforation are major complications of this entity. Recently, involvement of sinuses by *Aspergillus* species has been more frequently observed in immunocompromised patients[153] and mimics mucormycosis. Invasive external otitis has also been described, associated with documented fungemia.[154]

Aspergillus endocarditis occurs mainly after valve replacement.[72,155] Epidural abscesses have also been reported in renal transplant patients without pulmonary aspergillosis,[156,157] but direct extension to the spinal cord from pulmonary aspergillosis may also develop in leukemia patients.

Illustrative Case 3

A 23-year-old man was admitted for therapy of an acute lymphocytic leukemia. Induction chemotherapy included prednisone, vincristine, adriamycin, methotrexate, and cytosine arabinoside; complete remission of leukemia was achieved within 30 days. During the first episode of neutropenia, fever developed necessitating initiation of broad-spectrum antibiotics. No bacteria were isolated, but numerous infectious complications were documented. Oropharyngeal candidiasis developed that was successfully treated with ketoconazole (600 mg/day) for 18 days; herpes labialis was treated with acyclovir. In addition, three sputum cultures obtained on 3 consecutive days (immediately after discontinuation of ketoconazole) were positive for *Aspergillus fumigatus* without clinical signs throughout the course. Neurologic disorders, including behavioral changes and headaches, developed within 3 days after positive cultures for *Aspergillus fumigatus* and cerebral CT scan showed two lesions (one frontal and one parietal) suggestive of abscesses (Fig. 1). Cerebral aspiration was performed and showed filamentous fungi on smears; the culture of the specimen was positive for *Aspergillus fumigatus*. Amphotericin B treatment was immediately initiated, but within 13 days generalized seizures and hemiparesis developed. At that time, the patient had received 450 mg amphotericin B. Surgical excision of the parietal lesion was performed and at histologic examination, filamentous fungi were still identified, but the culture remained negative. Neurologic status improved and the patient underwent brain irradiation as prophylactic therapy for his leukemia. Amphotericin B was administered continuously and surgical excision of the frontal lesion was performed 2 months after its appearance. At that time, the patient had received 2.5 g amphotericin B. The histology was still positive for filamentous fungi, but the culture remained negative. Amphotericin B was, however, continued until a total dose of 4 g was achieved, after a duration of 3.5 months. Thirty-two months after discontinuation of amphotericin B (3 years after induction of therapy) the patient is still in remission from his leukemia and without any evidence of aspergillosis nor neurologic defect.

Comment. This case is particularly noteworthy for several reasons. Despite the administration of ketoconazole for 3 weeks for oropharyngeal candidiasis, positive sputum cultures and cerebral aspergillosis developed. Indeed, the ketoconazole could have played a role in selecting for the *Aspergillus*.[158] The definite source of this fungal infection remains unclear, since sinus and pulmonary investigations did not show evidence of invasive aspergillosis. However, it should be stressed that this patient had three positive sputum cultures prior to the neurologic symptoms. Such findings in debilitated patients should be taken into consideration and aspergillosis should be suspected in these settings. Positive surveillance cultures obtained from the nose have also shown to be of significant predictive value of invasive aspergillosis by other investigators.[144] In addition, the final favorable outcome seems to rely exclusively on aggressiveness in diagnostic pro-

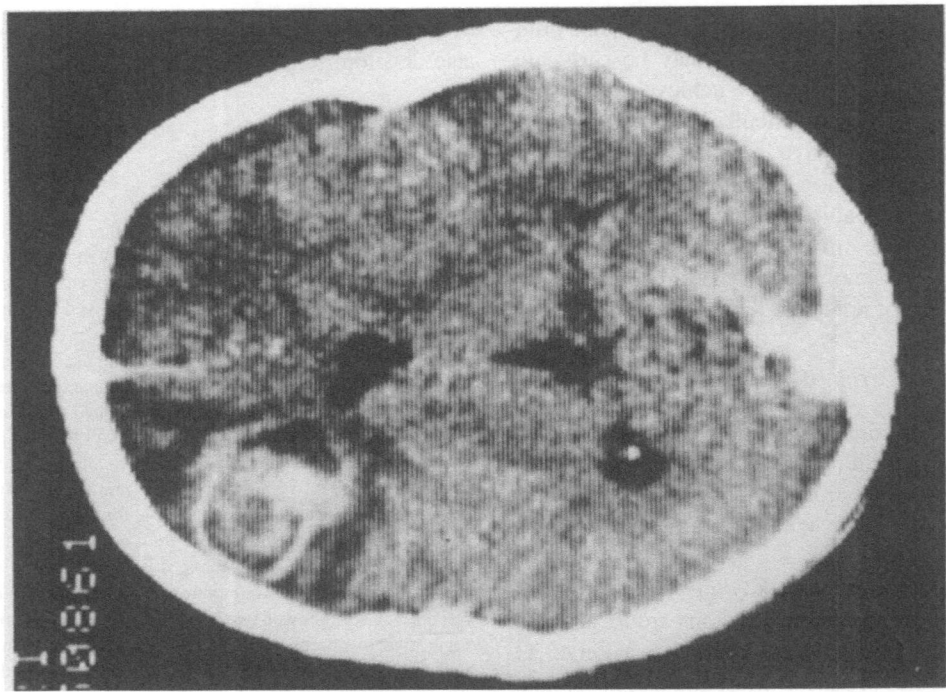

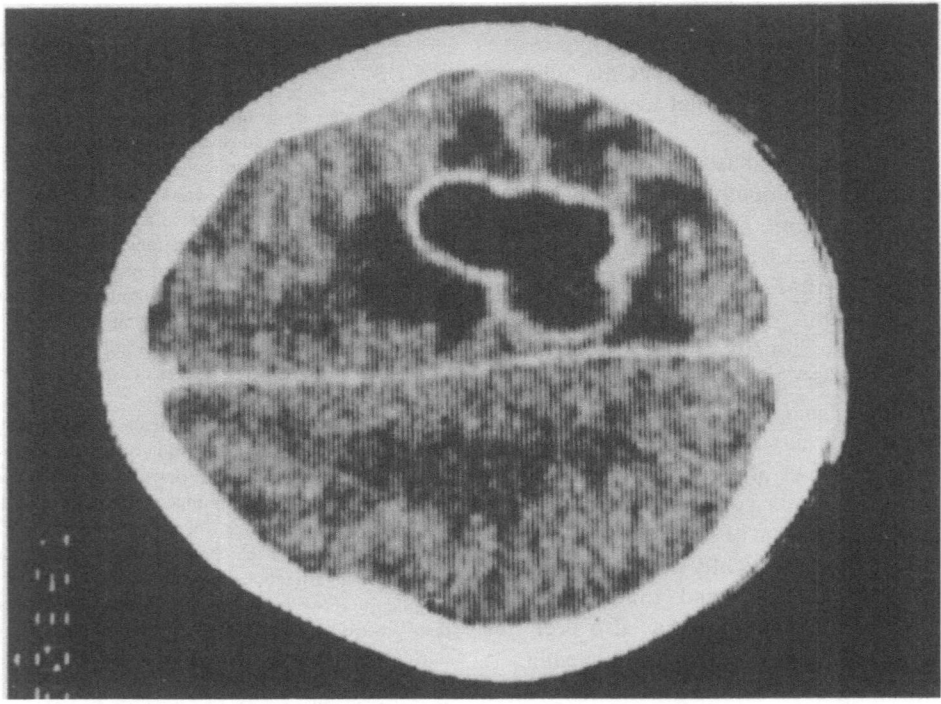

FIGURE 1. Cerebral lesions caused by *Aspergillus fumigatus* visualized by computed tomography (CT) scan in a leukemic patient.

cedures and treatment. Brain biopsies or aspiration should be done early to obtain a specific diagnosis. Although this patient had two extensive cerebral lesions, surgical management was possible without causing a permanent neurologic deficit The combination of intravenous amphotericin B therapy and surgery allowed the control of a disease usually considered uniformly fatal.[4] However, the decision to perform the neurosurgical excision depends on the hematologic status as well as neurologic findings. In this case, despite the fact that surgery had to be somewhat delayed, the outcome of the patient was excellent. Whether a total dose of 4 g amphotericin is necessary remains controversial. However, prolonged therapy may be mandatory for patients receiving antineoplastic chemotherapy and therefore developing prolonged episodes of neutropenia. Finally, invasive aspergillosis appears generally as an opportunistic infection in patients with end-stage underlying disease, but this case also illustrates that a patient in first induction of chemotherapy may develop life-threatening complications caused by *Aspergillus fumigatus*.

5. Mucormycosis

5.1. Mucoraceae

This family includes several genuses, such as *Absidia, Mucor,* and *Rhizopus,* which are classic pathogens in immunocompromised hosts. These molds are ubiquitous and may cause diseases similar to those caused by *Aspergillus* species.[5] The mode of infection in humans is the inhalation of airborne spores. These spores are relatively resistant to host defenses, but germination of these spores, the critical first step in the initiation of invasive infection is normally inhibited by bronchoalveolar macrophages. These macrophages become ineffective in diabetes or following the administration of steroids. (This is in contrast to *Aspergillus* infection, in which steroids but not diabetes will inhibit the effectiveness of the macrophages.) Normal host serum, but not serum from diabetic patients with ketoacidosis, will inhibit hyphal growth of the Mucoraceae. Finally, normally functioning granulocytes in adequate numbers destroy germinating spores that escape the macrophages and develop into the tissue invading hyphal forms. Thus, invasive mucormycosis is not uncommonly seen in the setting of uncontrolled diabetes, neutropenia, and/or high-dose steroid therapy.[5,140,159] Histopathologic findings allow one to distinguish *Aspergillus* species from Mucoraceae, since *Aspergillus* filaments are narrow and septate and branch at acute angles, while Mucor hyphae are wide and nonseptate and branch at right angles.[8]

5.2. Clinical Presentation

5.2.1. Rhinocerebral Mucormycosis

This infection is particularly severe and the evolution is usually fulminant. After inhalation, the spores proliferate within the nasal mucosa, and invasion occurs in susceptible hosts. Patients with uncontrolled diabetes mellitus (such as those in acidosis) are susceptible to this classic syndrome as well as neutropenic cancer patients.[160] However, the exact role of ketoacidosis remains to be ascertained. Nasal lesions and facial cellulitis may progress and extend to the sinuses as well as the orbit, with involvement of cranial nerves and then the brain, resulting in meningoencephalitis.[160] Direct examination and culture from nasal swabs or scrapings may be negative despite the demonstration of filamentous fungi on histologic examination of a biopsy, which should be performed for all suspected cases. Cerebral lesions may occur without nasal or facial signs, particularly in cancer patients and heroin addicts, as a result of hematogenous dissemination from a primary focus in the lungs.[161] Therefore, computed tomography (CT) should be obtained in predisposed patients according to the clinical setting.

The classic presentation of rhinocerebral mucormycosis consists of coma, proptosis, and ophthalmoplegia. Initially, a black nasal ulcer may be observed, but the evolution is usually fulminant after a few days of unilateral headache and nasal congestion. Rapid extension results from vascular invasion and thrombosis with infarction and necrosis. Cerebrospinal fluid findings are not specific, and culture is almost always negative. Serodiagnosis is not yet available. Occasionally, the patients have a concomitant positive sputum culture. Rapid therapeutic effects are mandatory in attempts to control these usually fatal infections.[162] Only extensive surgical resection associated with high doses of intravenous amphotericin B offer the possibility of success, but the morbidity and mortality remain high.

5.2.2. Pulmonary Mucormycosis

Foci of infection due to Mucoraceae may develop in the lungs of debilitated patients, producing lesions identical to those observed in pulmonary aspergillosis.[160] However, this clinical entity is less common. Specific diagnosis should be established by histopathologic examination and positive cultures. Occasionally, the air crescent sign on chest radiographs due to cavitation and the development of a necrotic area of lung within the cavity has also been observed.[163] The management and outcome of this opportunistic infection is similar to that for aspergillosis, except that surgical resection is almost always required for invasive pulmonary mucormycosis, while medical therapy alone with amphotericin B is often sufficient for invasive pulmonary aspergillosis.

5.2.3. Other Forms of Mucormycosis

Disseminated infections occur mainly in patients with hematologic malignancies.[160] If cutaneous lesions exist, the biopsy of metastatic skin lesions in this setting allows a specific diagnosis to be obtained without other invasive procedures.[5] However, cutaneous aspiration may be negative. Other involved organs can include the brain, the kidneys, the liver, the heart and the GI tract. Cutaneous infections due to Mucoraceae may also be primary and may result from various sources, including contamination of extensive burns.[164] Occasionally, diabetic patients may also develop cellulitis or mucormycotic ulcers secondary to minor trauma to the skin. Localized cutaneous lesions have also been described in a lymphoma patient.[165] In addition, contamination of bandages (Elastoplast) used to cover surgical wounds has also been responsible for necrotizing cutaneous mucormycosis.[166] Gastrointestinal mucormycosis, endocarditis, infection from a vascular graft, and renal invasion are rare.[5]

6. Cryptococcosis

6.1. *Cryptococcus neoformans*

The distribution of this yeast is worldwide. The organism is commonly found in vegetable matter, in the soil, as well as in avian feces.[167] However, there is a lack of epidemiologic data demonstrating a correlation between contact with pigeon droppings and cryptococcosis. *Cryptococcus neoformans* is not considered a contaminant from the air in clinical laboratories. Most strains have a polysaccharide capsule

which inhibits the phagocytosis of the yeast by macrophages. Various serotypes (A–D) have been identified, according to the capsular composition. There is a variation in the geographic distribution. In addition, serotypes B and C correspond to the *gattii* variety and have never been isolated from the environment.[18,168] The polysaccharide capsule excludes India ink and therefore is responsible for the halo visualized on smears stained with India ink. However, caution is mandatory, since erythrocytes, leukocytes, and some artifacts such as starch particles occasionally show similar halos. Therefore, a presumptive diagnosis of cryptococcal meningitis should only be considered if budding yeasts are demonstrated on the India ink preparation.

6.2 Clinical Presentation

6.2.1. Central Nervous System Infection

Cryptococcus neoformans is a common cause of fungal meningitis in immunocompromised patients but the syndrome may occur without underlying disease. Patients with defects of cell-mediated immunity, such as after renal transplantation, or patients with lymphomas or AIDS are highly predisposed.

The onset of infection may be insidious without dramatic neurologic findings.[18,167] Cerebrospinal fluid is usually clear and typically reveals a lymphocytic pleocytosis, hypoglycorrachia, and an elevated protein level. A poor prognosis has been related to low glucose level, high opening pressure, and fewer than 20 leukocytes/mm^3, as well as the observation of numerous cryptococci on smears.[19] A definitive diagnosis should rely on a positive culture. However, cryptococcal meningitis may be suspected earlier in the evolution on direct examination of the CSF if the India ink preparation is positive or if capsular antigen has been detected. The most common technique used to detect cryptococcal antigen is a commercially available latex agglutination test. This last test appears to have a higher sensitivity (95%) as compared with the India ink preparation (50%), but adequate controls should be performed routinely to rule out false positive reactions.[169–174] Persistent high posttreatment titers of cryptococcal antigen in CSF or in serum, as well as isolation of cryptococci from extraneuronal sites have been correlated with relapse.[19] Occasionally, antigen has been detected in lumbar

CSF with *Cryptococcus neoformans* grown only from ventricular fluid.[175]

In addition to meningitis, *Cryptococcus neoformans* also can cause intracerebral lesions[176] or lesions confined to the spinal cord.[4] Most patients with CNS cryptococcosis complain of headache, but fever is not constant. However, despite the chronicity of the symptoms, prompt therapy should be considered, since the mortality, particularly in cancer patients, remains high.[177] Meningitis caused by cryptococcosis is currently the major indication for a combined treatment regimen of amphotericin B and 5-fluorocytosine (5-FC).[178] The definitive role of intrathecal or intraventricular administration of amphotericin B remains controversial and should probably be considered for patients with poor prognostic signs, or with relapse.[179] In patients without apparent underlying disease, an indolent course has occasionally been described even without therapy.[180]

6.2.2. Other Forms of Cryptococcosis

Cryptococcus neoformans may also cause pulmonary and cutaneous infections or occasionally dissemination.[181—183] These entities are relatively uncommon in cancer patients but frequent in patients with the AIDS syndrome.[184,185] Pulmonary cryptococcosis may present as a localized nodule, or as a lobar or interstitial pneumonia. Patients with CNS cryptococcosis usually fail to show evidence of concomitant lung infection.[18] Although the portal of entry seems to be the bronchial tree, most pulmonary lesions remain asymptomatic.

Cutaneous cryptococcosis presents as small nonspecific lesions which are generally underestimated. Biopsy of skin lesions permits the establishment of a diagnosis of dissemination without more aggressive diagnostic procedures. Involvement of other organs such as bone, prostate, liver, and heart is rare.[5,18]

7. Coccidioidomycosis

7.1. *Coccidioides immitis*

This fungus is dimorphic and exists in the soil in a mycelial phase, while in tissue the characteristic appearance is a spherule with endospores.[12] The optimal temperature for incubation is 30°C but recovery of *Coccidioides immitis* is also possible at 37°C. Areas of endemicity are located in North, Central, and South America. Acquisition of this airborne infection has been demonstrated after exposure in the desert in endemic areas as well as secondary to archeologic digging. In addition, inanimate objects such as packages contaminated in endemic locales can, when sent to individuals outside these areas, carry the infection to those handling such objects.

7.2. Clinical Presentation

7.2.1. Pneumonia

Most infections in immunocompetent hosts are asymptomatic or present as a transient upper respiratory infection. About 40% of the hosts will develop symptomatic pulmonary infections and only a small proportion will evolve and present a thin-walled cavity or a pulmonary nodule that may mimic cancer. Patients with impaired cell mediated immunity are predisposed to severe infections due to *Coccidioides immitis,* as well as to reactivation. However, the prognosis of lesions localized to the lungs remains comparable to that of normal hosts.

The diagnosis should be considered in patients living (or who have been living) in endemic areas. A history of a positive skin test can be helpful. It is interesting to stress that serology may be of great help to detect specific antibody even in debilitated patients. This is the one fungal infection in the immunocompromised host where antibody measurement is an essential part of diagnosis and clinical management. Demonstration of the organism in the sputum may be difficult and requires experienced personnel due to potential problems of contamination. Silver stains have proved useful to visualize spherules in such tissues as lung biopsies.[169]

7.2.2. Other Forms of Coccidioidomycosis

Dissemination from pulmonary lesions occurs rarely in normal hosts but more commonly in debilitated patients such as cancer patients or in pregnant women or in certain racial groups such as blacks and Filipinos. The various factors affecting the host–parasite interactions and predisposing to dissemination were extensively reviewed recently.[186]

The prognosis of extrapulmonary lesions in compromised hosts is poor.[186] Skin tests may be negative in this setting. The main areas of localization are skin, soft tissue, liver, bone, joints, and especially the meninges.[5]

Central nervous system infections are particularly difficult to diagnose and treat.[188] The presence of specific antibody (by complement-fixation test) in CSF should be accepted as evidence of coccidioidal meningitis requiring intrathecal therapy. Occasionally, liver biopsy may also be helpful in a setting of disseminated coccidioidomycosis.[189] Routine serologic determination may provide antemortem diagnosis. The pathologic findings are comparable to those of tuberculous lesions with granulomatous reaction and occasionally caseation. The outcome is dependent on the initiation of appropriate therapy, which relies mostly on amphotericin B.[190,191] However, imidazoles such as miconazole and ketoconazole have been promising in some studies, but their definite role remains controversial and relapses have already been reported.[5,191−193]

8. Histoplasmosis

8.1. *Histoplasma capsulatum*

This dimorphic fungus is endemic in the central United States but may also be encountered in some tropical, subtropical, or temperate zones.[13] Two types of histoplasmosis must be distinguished. *Histoplasma capsulatum* var. *capsulatum* is responsible for classic histoplasmosis with a global distribution and is characterized by a small size (2–4 μm) yeast in tissues. *Histoplasma capsulatum* var. *duboisii* produces a larger yeast (8–15 μm) and causes the African histoplasmosis probably strictly confined to the African continent.[8] In endemic areas, cultures of soil reveal the mycelial phase, which reverts to the pathogenic phase (yeast phase) after inhalation of spores. A correlation has been established between heavy contamination of the soil with avian or bat excrement and the recovery of *Histoplasma capsulatum* in soil samples.[13]

8.2. Clinical Presentation

8.2.1. Primary Infection

In endemic areas, most people have been contaminated, as shown by a positive skin reaction to histoplasmin. The primary infection may mimic tuberculosis. These organisms normally demonstrate low virulence. However, dissemination may occur in cases of depressed host immunity, particularly if cell-mediated immunity is affected. Patients undergoing organ transplantation or cancer chemotherapy and AIDS patients are highly predisposed to reactivate primary foci of infection[194] or to develop progressive primary infection. The primary focus of infection caused by *Histoplasma capsulatum* var. *capsulatum* is located in the lung and may be heralded by a flulike illness characterized by fever, myalgia, and cough. Asymptomatic infection is even more common but is difficult to document.

Occasionally, infection is severe and disseminates to the spleen and liver, even in normal hosts. In tissue, yeasts are mainly localized within the macrophages. Primary infection caused by *Histoplasma capsulatum* var. *duboisii* is also mainly localized to the lungs but also with a particular tropism for the bones and skin.[8]

8.2.2. Disseminated Infection

This entity is typical in immunocompromised hosts and results from dissemination of the yeasts by way of hilar lymph nodes.[5,195,196] Most often, symptomatic infections are reactivation in these patients. However, occasionally, dissemination has also been described in apparently normal individuals.[197] Fever, hepatosplenomegaly, anemia, leukopenia, and thrombocytopenia are common in the severe form.[13] Dissemination to other organs such as adrenals, GI tract, and skin may also occur. Central nervous system infection is rare.

The correct diagnosis relies on the isolation of *Histoplasma capsulatum* from clinical specimens and identification in tissue sections. Silver stains are helpful in these situations as well as bone marrow biopsy.[5] Occasionally, blood cultures may be positive.[169]

Serologic tests are usually not effective to permit an early diagnosis in debilitated patients, and false-negative tests have been reported. As documented for other disseminated fungal infections,[61] hypercalcemia may also occur.[198] Amphotericin B is the treatment of choice but failures are numerous and the role of imidazoles such as ketoconazole remains to be further investigated. Meanwhile, the use of this agent should be restricted to mild cases.[13]

9. Other Fungal Infections

Other fungal pathogens have also been identified in immunocompromised hosts.[5] Disseminated infection caused by *Trichosporon* species has been well documented in leukemia patients.[51,53] The clinical presentation of this entity may mimic invasive candidiasis. Blastomycosis and sporotrichosis may occasionally cause opportunistic infection.[5,20,199,200]

Pseudoallescheria boydii is also a saprophytic fungus commonly isolated in soil or decaying vegetable matter and can be responsible for invasive disseminated infections, particularly in immunocompromised hosts.[5,201–205] The characteristic features of this infection are compatible with invasive aspergillosis and differential diagnosis may be impossible on a clinical basis. However, the correct etiology may be important to obtain by isolation of the pathogen, as this organism may be resistant to amphotericin B and sensitive to imidazoles, while the presently available imidazoles are ineffective in the treatment of invasive aspergillosis.

Recently, invasive infections caused by *Fusarium* species were documented in bone marrow transplant recipients.[206] This pathogen is generally responsible for superficial infections such as those localized to the eyes. However, dissemination has previously been described in burn patients[207] as well as in a patient with lymphoma.[208]

10. Prevention of Opportunistic Fungal Infection

10.1. General Considerations

The sources of fungal complications are numerous in debilitated hosts. Epidemiologic data have to be taken into consideration. Unnecessary exposure to dust or soil such as camping or digging in heavily contaminated areas are not recommended for susceptible hosts, and such advice appears to be the only measure suitable to prevent infections such as invasive histoplasmosis or coccidioidomycosis. There are no effective prophylactic means to prevent exposure to the causative agents of cryptococcosis or mucormycosis. Most studies have been performed with the aim of preventing candidiasis or aspergillosis in neutropenic cancer patients. Nonspecific means, including patient education (as well as family and personnel), excellent hygiene, restricted cooked-food diet, dental care, avoidance of invasive procedures (e.g., indwelling catheters), are mandatory to reduce colonization and infection caused by fungal pathogens.[209–211] Adequate control of the underlying disease and reduction of immunosuppressive therapy also play a major role in the pathogenesis of opportunistic fungal infections.

Prophylactic granulocyte transfusions have been disappointing. They are currently not recommended to prevent infection and, in particular, invasive mycoses.[212]

10.2. Chemoprophylaxis

10.2.1. Prevention of Candidiasis

Numerous studies have been carried out evaluating various antifungal agents in neutropenic patients. However, only a few controlled trials have been published and this prophylactic approach remains controversial.[213] Nystatin has been administered at various dosages, but the compliance of neutropenic patients to high doses of this antifungal agent is generally poor. There is no proof of the efficacy of nystatin at low doses.[214–216] Persistence of fungal colonization has been documented at high doses.[217–219] In addition, fungemia has been described in patients receiving nystatin prophylactically.[30]

Another polyene, amphotericin B, has also been widely investigated, with conflicting results. In patients receiving up to 6 g of amphotericin B orally each day, stool cultures revealed in 30% the persistence of fungal pathogens.[220] Nevertheless, amphotericin B used at low dose (200 mg/day) has been shown to be effective in reducing the incidence of autopsy-proven candidiasis in one placebo-controlled study.[221] Our own data in neutropenic patients comparing a placebo with the administration of 1.5 g amphotericin B show a significant reduction in fungal colonization for the patients receiving amphotericin B. Disappointingly, there was no decreased incidence of candidiasis.

Imidazoles, another class of antifungal agents, have also been extensively investigated. Miconazole was not proved to be effective, when administered orally or even intravenously.[222] Ketoconazole is better absorbed after oral administration than miconazole. Contradictory data have been observed by several investigators, but the dosage of ketoconazole varied from 200–600 mg/day.[215,223–225] The individual variation in absorption may also be responsible for conflicting results and ketoconazole levels should be monitored routinely. In addition, reduction of serum levels of ketoconazole has been noted after bone marrow transplantation.[226] Our own data evaluating the potential value of a daily dose of 600 mg ketoconazole show a reduction of fungal colonization, comparable to the effect of oral amphotericin B, as opposed to the high rate of colonization by yeasts in the patients receiving a placebo but again fail to show a significant decrease in candidiasis. It should be stressed, however, that only oropharyngeal candidiasis occurred in patients receiving ketoconazole, while disseminated candidiasis was described for the patients in the placebo or in the amphotericin B group.

The selection of *Torulopsis glabrata* in the surveillance cultures obtained from the patients receiving ketoconazole has been definitely demonstrated in our studies as well as by other investigators.[227–230] Therefore, pending further studies, there is no uniformly accepted prophylactic means to prevent candidiasis in neutropenic patients. Further evaluation should establish the potential benefit of topical administration of antifungal agents, such as oral troches of clotrimoxazole, which appears to reduce oropharyngeal colonization by yeasts.[231] Considerable efforts have been made to eradicate yeasts from the stools and subsequent studies should probably also concentrate the investigations on oropharyngeal colonization. A new triazole (fluconazole), which is active on yeasts, has recently been developed and studies evaluating its potential role as a chemoprophylactic agent have been initiated.

10.2.2. Prevention of Aspergillosis

Invasive aspergillosis occurs mainly in neutropenic patients or in individuals such as transplant patients who are receiving prolonged courses of corticosteroids. Prophylactic modalities were recently reviewed.[232] This infection is airborne. Currently no antifungal agent (e.g., nystatin, amphotericin B, miconazole, or ketoconazole) is administered orally that is effective in preventing aspergillosis. Nystatin and amphotericin B are not absorbed from the GI tract and are mainly active on digestive fungal flora. Aspergillosis has been demonstrated despite the administration of these agents.[233] Similarly, ketoconazole has been shown to be ineffective in preventing aspergillosis. In our placebo-controlled study, overall 10% of the neutropenic patients developed aspergillosis whether they received amphotericin B, ketoconazole, or the placebo. Recently, another imidazole, itraconazole which is more active on *Aspergillus* species has been developed and should be further investigated.

Topical chemoprophylaxis is probably more promising, as acquisition of *Aspergillus* spores occurs via the nasopharynx. We are currently evaluating the potential prophylactic value of nasal sprays of amphotericin B in neutropenic patients and preliminary data are encouraging.[234]

10.3. Isolation

Colonization with *Aspergillus* species may occur in hospitals, with neutropenic patients being particularly predisposed. Airborne contamination has been well documented and represents a major epidemiological problem in units located within areas of hospital renovation or construction work.[142–144,235] Surveillance cultures from the environment in which susceptible patients are hospitalized seem mandatory.[124] In addition, ornamental plants or flowers should not be permitted within the units in which neutropenic patients are hospitalized.[236] However, *Aspergillus* spores are ubiquitous and may be difficult to eradicate from the environment. Therefore, sophisticated units such as laminar airflow rooms equipped with HEPA filters have been recommended and several studies have shown them to decrease the incidence of infections. In fact, these units are particularly effective in reducing hospital acquired aspergillosis.[209,237] Nevertheless, this type of isolation is expensive and unavailable for all neutropenic patients. The use of laminar airflow rooms should probably be restricted to patients undergoing intensive chemotherapy and who remain neutropenic for a prolonged period of time, such as bone marrow transplant patients. HEPA filters by themselves do provide significant degrees of protection. Particularly during periods of hospital construction, every effort should be made to provide HEPA-filtered air to hospitalized immunosuppressed patients.[124–128]

11. Antifungal Therapy

11.1. Antifungal Agents

This section will only deal with systemic antifungal chemotherapy for invasive or deep-seated fungal infections in compromised hosts, excluding the treatment of cutaneous infections such as those caused by dermatophytes.

11.1.1. Polyenes

Nystatin and amphotericin B belong to this class of agent. Nystatin is only administered topically or orally. The potential role of nystatin in preventing candidiasis has been discussed in Section 10.2.1. The classic indication for this nonabsorbable agent remains oropharyngeal candidiasis[238] or topical administration. Nystatin is too toxic to be administered intravenously.

Amphotericin B is a substance insoluble in water and is administered intravenously as a complex to desoxycholate (Fungizone). This agent may be administered orally, but its absorption should be considered as negligible.[239–241] The oral mode of administration is therefore only used as a prophylactic approach. Intravenous administration of amphotericin B remains the treatment of choice for invasive fungal infections in immunocompromised hosts. Amphotericin B is active on most commonly encountered fungi, except some *Pseudoallescheria* strains.

Schedules of the various modalities of administration have been reviewed.[169,242–245] The total daily dose should be administered within 24 hr after initiation of the first injection to rapidly achieve therapeutic levels. Meperidine has been shown to decrease side effects.[246] Some patients tolerate rapid infusions.[245] However, the duration of administration should not be less than 1 hr to avoid dysrhythmias or cardiac arrest.[247–249]

Correlation between serum or tissue levels and efficacy has not been extensively evaluated. Daily administration or infusion on alternate days seems to be as effective. The daily dose ranges between 0.5–1.3 mg/kg according to the severity of the disease. Elimination in the urine accounts only for 15–20% of drug metabolism, but nephrotoxicity is the major complication. Hypokalemia is also common, and an acquired renal tubular acidosis may develop. Pro-

longed administration of amphotericin B may produce anemia. Pulmonary toxicity has been described in patients receiving concomitant WBC transfusions. This syndrome remains controversial; pending further studies, the administration of amphotericin B and WBC should probably be on alternate day regimens.[250–252] Pregnancy may produce immunosuppression and predispose to disseminated mycosis. Amphotericin B has been administered safely to pregnant women.[253] Because of high-protein binding, penetration in the CSF is low; thus, intrathecal administration of amphotericin B has been useful in some circumstances and may occasionally be advocated for severe cryptococcal meningitis.[38,169,175,254] Intraarticular injections have also been administered[255] as well as intravesical irrigations for cystitis[256] and intraperitoneal irrigations for peritonitis.[257,258] Despite the administration of amphotericin B, the prognosis of invasive fungal infections in the immunocompromised hosts is still poor. Failures as well as relapses are numerous. The final outcome of these opportunistic infections relies mainly on the recovery of an adequate neutrophil count, the cessation of exogenous immunosuppressive therapy (when possible), the remission of a leukemia or the control of the underlying disease. A new therapeutic modality, i.e., the administration of amphotericin B encapsulated in liposomes, is presently under investigation to establish the value of this approach.

11.1.2. 5-Fluorocytosine

5-Fluorocytosine is commercially available only for oral administration. Intravenous preparations can be obtained under special circumstances from Roche. Oral absorption is generally excellent. The recommended daily dose is 150 mg/kg in three or four divided doses per day.[245,259] The rapid emergence of resistant strains precludes the administration of 5-FC alone, except for some specific indications such as urinary tract infection caused by *Candida* species. 5-Fluorocytosine is mainly active on yeasts and has no significant antifungal effect on filamentous fungi. 5-Fluorocytosine has been extensively investigated as a combined therapy with amphotericin B in cryptococcal meningitis and has been shown useful.[178,179] In addition, such combined therapy is probably the best available treatment for serious invasive candidal infection.[5,6]

Toxicity related to 5-FC is mainly gastrointestinal,[260-262] including nausea and vomiting, but also occasionally bowel perforation and hepatitis, and hematologic (due to bone marrow aplasia).[243,263,264] Monitoring of blood levels of 5-FC should be routinely performed to avoid serum concentrations higher than 100 µg/ml.[36,243,245] 5-Fluorocytosine should not be used as a prophylactic agent.

11.1.3. The Imidazoles

This new class of agents has been extensively investigated in the last decade.[245] Miconazole had been initially evaluated, but the absorption after oral administration is poor; only the intravenous form is currently available. The daily dose range is 30–50 mg/kg. Cardiorespiratory toxicity has been reported after rapid infusion.[265] The protein binding of this agent is high and metabolism occurs mainly in the liver. Side effects are numerous[245] but tend to be more manageable than those observed with amphotericin B. Intrathecal administration of miconazole has also been advocated.[266,267] The definite indication for this agent remains to be determined, particularly in immunocompromised hosts, except for infections caused by *Pseudoallescheria boydii*, where it appears to be the drug of choice.[268]

More recently, ketoconazole has been evaluated. This agent may be administered orally, but monitoring of serum levels is mandatory because of individual variations in absorption. Cimetidine and antacids have been reported to interfere with the absorption of ketoconazole, as absorption requires the presence of an acid pH in the stomach. The recommended dose of ketoconazole ranges between 200 and 1200 mg/day. Reported side effects include minor GI disturbances,[245] nausea, vomiting, but also occasionally severe hepatitis.[269-273] Monitoring of liver function tests is mandatory. Endocrine side effects have also been reported and include gynecomastia,[274] inhibition of testosterone synthesis,[275-277] as well as adrenal steroid synthesis.[278] Those effects seem reversible.[279] Interactions with other medications may also occur. We have observed in human volunteers, a significant reduction of serum levels of ketoconazole when administered concomitantly with rifampin,[279a] and this observation has been confirmed in patients.[280] Interaction of ket-

oconazole with cyclosporine has also been reported, and this is of particular importance for patients receiving organ transplants.[281-283] Hepatic oxidative metabolism may be altered by ketoconazole and other drug interactions may also occur.[284] Ketoconazole, like miconazole, has poor activity on filamentous fungi such as *Aspergillus* species or Mucoraceae. Promising data have been observed in chronic mucocutaneous candidiasis[285] as well as coccidioidomycosis[118] or histoplasmosis.[13] However, failures have been described. Therefore, the definitive role of this agent remains to be proven in the treatment of fungal infections in debilitated hosts.[286] The potential prophylactic value of ketoconazole has been reviewed in detail[286a] and is discussed in Section 10.2. Other imidazoles such as clotrimazole only have a role as topical agents. Itraconazole is being investigated currently and may be more effective in the treatment of infection due to *Aspergillus* species. Preliminary studies done with fluconazole, particularly in oropharyngeal candidiasis, have also provided encouraging data. There is also suggestion that this agent could be effective in treating cryptococcal meningitis, but further investigations are mandatory.

11.2. Current Controversies in the Management of Fungal Infections in the Immunocompromised Host

11.2.1. Empiric Therapy

The aim of this approach is primarily to improve the prognosis of invasive mycoses in neutropenic patients. It has been suggested that early administration of intravenous amphotericin B may prevent dissemination of an occult fungal infection.[75,287] Since early diagnosis is difficult, empiric administration of antifungal therapy seems rational. However, in a large collaborative randomized trial within the EORTC, evaluating the role of administration of amphotericin B to neutropenic patients who remain febrile despite broad-spectrum antibiotics, we observed a benefit from such an approach in a selected group of patients, i.e., those with severe and persistent neutropenia, who did not previously receive an antifungal prophylaxis. We failed to demonstrate a significant improvement in the survival of these patients despite the reduction of fever in the patients receiving amphotericin B compared with patients without antifungal treatment. However, no fungal deaths occurred among the 68 patients receiving empiric amphotericin B, while 4 deaths were described in the 64 patients not receiving empiric amphotericin B. Whether febrile patients who are colonized with fungi would benefit from early administration of amphotericin B is still unclear. Positive surveillance cultures for *Aspergillus* species have been useful to predict infection[144] and to improve the outcome,[149] but the clinical implication of positive surveillance cultures for other fungi remains controversial. The optimal empiric antifungal therapy should also be investigated; in particular, the potential value of ketoconazole or fluconazole in this situation has not yet been reported.

11.2.2. Optimal Dose and Duration of Therapy

There is no consensus to recommend the total dose of amphotericin B that needs to be administered for most fungal infections occurring in compromised hosts. In addition, the optimal duration of therapy has not been studied either. As an example, oropharyngeal candidiasis or esophagitis usually respond favorably and require a small dose of amphotericin B (250 mg) over a short period of time (a few days). Transient fungemia is usually treated with a total dose of 500 mg amphotericin B. Disseminated candidiasis is a rapidly fatal disease when not treated. Total doses of ≥2 g amphotericin B may be necessary. However, therapy seems only beneficial if the neutrophil count becomes normal.

Aspergillosis, mucormycosis, and other disseminated fungal infections usually also require more than 2 g amphotericin B, but no study is available to establish this statement. In addition, invasive fungal infections have been demonstrated at autopsy in patients who had received more than 2 g amphotericin B prior to death. Resection of persistent foci of infection is mandatory, particularly for cerebral abscesses or pulmonary lesions caused by *Aspergillus* species. Distribution of amphotericin B in tissues, has been recently studied in humans[287a] and, despite detection of high levels of drug, fungal growth as well as histologic invasion could be demonstrated from the same tissues. The lack of bioavailability of amphotericin B probably constitutes a contributing factor to the numerous failures observed in patients.

11.2.3. Combined Regimens

Since failures of therapy are numerous despite the use of amphotericin B, various combinations have been investigated *in vitro* and *in vivo* to enhance the activity of amphotericin B as well as decrease its toxicity. This subject has been recently reviewed.[244] Except for cryptococcal meningitis,[178,179,245,288] there is no indication that a combined regimen (amphotericin B + 5-FC) is more effective than amphotericin B alone although there is preliminary evidence that it is also true in invasive candidal infection.[5,6,288a] A few isolated case reports have described beneficial therapy with amphotericin B plus rifampin or other combinations but these observations remain anecdotal. In addition, antagonistic reactions may occur, particularly between amphotericin B and ketoconazole and this combination should not be used pending further information.[289]

11.2.4. Emergence of Resistant Strains

Most fungi were long considered uniformly sensitive to amphotericin B. However, emergence of resistant strains of yeasts has been observed, particularly in previously treated patients or in patients hospitalized in hematological units where polyenes are commonly used.[290-293] Fatal fungal infection due to organisms resistant to amphotericin B has been reported[294] and represents a major complication for the future. Emergence of resistant strains of yeasts during therapy with 5-FC alone has been well documented[295,296] and precludes the administration of 5-FC alone.

Whether the emergence of resistant strains of yeasts, initially sensitive to ketoconazole, represents a clinical problem, is difficult to ascertain and remains controversial. In addition, the prolonged administration of ketoconazole results in selection of *T. glabrata* and, possibly, *Aspergillus*.

11.2.5. Role of Granulocyte Transfusions

The potential role of granulocyte transfusions has only been investigated in an animal model with candidiasis in leukopenic dogs. Until now, there is no clinical data to support the therapeutic value of WBC transfusions, except for anecdotal reports.[297,298] The potential pulmonary toxicity related to concomitant administration of amphotericin B and WBC has been previously discussed.

12. Perspectives for the Future

This review demonstrates the need for several areas of investigation to improve the outcome of invasive fungal infections in immunocompromised patients in the future. The optimal approaches to these complications should rely on better diagnostic, prophylactic, and therapeutic techniques.

The detection of circulating fungal antigens or metabolites appears to be a particularly promising means of effecting early diagnosis. Monoclonal antibodies to fungal antigens may improve the value of these techniques.

Pharmacologic and clinical studies evaluating in humans various modalities of administration of amphotericin B (such as encapsulated into liposomes) are under way. We have observed in vitro an enhanced antifungal activity using amphotericin B entrapped into unilamellar liposomes.[299] Preliminary data obtained in patients from our unit,[300,300a] as well as by other investigators[301] have already shown encouraging data, and may represent a significant improvement for the management of deep-seated mycoses.

Finally, the development of new antifungal agents is clearly needed. Itraconazole and fluconazole both hold great promise as agents that may improve prophylaxis and treatment of invasive fungal infections in immunocompromised hosts.[302–305]

References

1. Bodey G: Fungal infections complicating acute leukemia. *J Chron Dis* **19**:667–687, 1966.
2. Hart PO, Russel E, Remington JS: The compromised host and infection. Deep fungal infection. *J Infect Dis* **120**:169–191, 1969.
3. DeGregorio M, Lee W, Linker C, et al: Fungal infections in patients with acute leukemia. *Am J Med* **73**:543–548, 1982.
4. Salaki JS, Louria DB, Chmel H: Fungal and yeast infections of the central nervous system. *Medicine (Baltimore)* **63**:108–132, 1984.
5. Hawkins C, Armstrong D: Fungal infections in the immunocompromised host. *Clin Haematol* **13**:599–630, 1984.
6. Gold JWM: Opportunistic fungal infections in patients with neoplastic disease. *Am J Med* **76**:458–463, 1984.
7. Evans EG: Diagnosis of systemic fungal infections In Reeves D, Geddes A (eds): *Recent Advances in Infection.* Churchill Livingstone, Edinburgh, 1979, pp. 55–75.
8. Chandler F, Kaplan W, Ajello L (eds): *Histopathology of Mycotic Diseases.* Wolfe Medical, London, 1980.
9. Louria D: The usefulness of antibody tests in systemic fungal, yeasts and higher bacterial infections: A limited overview. In Baxter M (ed): *Proceedings of the International Society for Human and Animal Mycology* Palmerston North (New Zealand), Massey University, 1982, pp. 174–177.
10 Penn R, Lambert R, George R: Invasive fungal infections. The use of serologic tests in diagnosis and management. *Arch Intern Med* **143**:1215–1220, 1983.
11. Gordon MA, Gwinn DD: Summary of a workshop on serodiagnosis of systemic mycoses, *J Infect Dis* **146**:570–574, 1982.
12. Stevens DA. Coccidioides immitis. In Mandell GC, Douglas GR, Bennett JE (eds): *Principles and Practice of Infectious Diseases.* Wiley, New York, 1985, pp. 1485–1493.
13. Goodwin RA, Des Prez RM: Histoplasma capsulatum. In Mandell GC, Douglas GR, Bennett JE (eds): *Principles and Practice of Infectious Diseases.* Wiley, New York, 1985, pp. 1468–1477.
14. Bennett JE: Aspergillus species. In Mandell GC, Douglas GR, Bennett JE (eds): *Principles and Practice of Infectious Diseases.* Wiley, New York, 1985, pp. 1447–1451.
15. Guinan M, Portas M, Hill H: The candida precipitation test in an immunosuppressed population. *Cancer* **43**:299–302, 1979.
16. Jones S, Bremman M, Kundsin R. Candida serology: An aid in diagnosis of deep-organ candidiasis. *J Surg Res* **14**:235–237, 1973
17. Taschdjian C, Kozinn P, Finck H, et al: Post mortem studies of systemic candidiasis. I. Diagnosis validity of precipitation reaction and probable origin of sensitization to cytoplasmic candidal antigens. *Sabouraudia* **7**:110–117, 1969.
18. Diamond RD: Cryptococcus neoformans. In Mandell GC, Douglas GR, Bennett JE (eds): *Principles and Practice of Infectious Diseases.* Wiley, New York, 1985, pp. 1460–1468.
19. Diamond RD, Bennett JE: Prognostic factors in cryptococcal meningitis. A study of 111 cases. *Ann Intern Med* **80**:176–181, 1974.
20. Chapman SW: Blastomyces dermatidis. In Mandell GC, Douglas GR, Bennett JE (eds): *Principles and Practice of Infectious Diseases.* Wiley, New York, 1985, pp. 1477–1485.
21. Araj G, Hopfer R, Chesnut S, et al: Diagnostic value of the enzyme-linked immunosorbent assay for detection of Candida albicans cytoplasmic antigen in sera of cancer patients. *J Clin Microbiol* **16**:46–52, 1982.
22. Kerkering T, Espinell-Ingroff A, Shadomy S: Detection of Candida antigenemia by counterimmunoelectrophoresis in patients with invasive candidiasis. *J Infect Dis* **140**:659–664, 1979.
23. Lew M, Siber G, Donahue D, et al: Enhanced detection with

an enzyme linked immunosorbent assay of Candida mannan in antibody containing serum after heat extraction. *J Infect Dis* **145**:45–56, 1982.

24. Meckstroth K, Reiss E, Keller J, et al: Detection of antibodies and antigenemia in leukemia patients with candidiasis by enzyme linked immunosorbent assay. *J Infect Dis* **144**:24–32, 1981.

25. Segal E, Berg R, Pizzo P, et al: Detection of Candida antigen in sera of patients with candidiasis by an enzyme-linked immunosorbent assay-inhibition technique. *J Clin Microbiol* **10**:116–118, 1979.

26. Weiner M, Coats-Stephen M: Immunodiagnosis of systemic candidiasis: Mannan antigenemia detected by radioimmunoassay in experimental and human infections. *J Infect Dis* **140**:989–993, 1979.

27. Weiner M, Yount W: Mannan antigenemia in the diagnosis of invasive candida infections. *J Clin Invest* **58**:1045–1053, 1976.

28. Meunier-Carpentier F: Rapid diagnosis of fungal infections: Serology for antigen. In Baxter M (ed): *Proceedings of the International Society for Human and Animal Mycology.* Palmerston North (New Zealand), Massey University, 1982, pp. 178–183.

29. Meunier-Carpentier F, Armstrong D. Candida antigenemia as detected by passive hemagglutination in patients with disseminated candidiasis or candida colonization. *J Clin Microbiol* **13**:10–14, 1981.

30. Meunier-Carpentier F, Kiehn T, Armstrong D: Fungemia in the immunocompromised host: Changing patterns, antigenemia high mortality. *Am J Med* **1**:363–370, 1981.

31. Miller G, Witwer M, Braude A, et al: Rapid identification of C. albicans septicemia in man by gas liquid chromatography. *J Clin Invest* **54**:1235–1240, 1974.

32. Kiehn T, Bernard E, Gold J, et al: Candidiasis: Detection by gas liquid chromatography of D-arabinitol, a fungal metabolite in human sera. *Science* **206**:577–580, 1979.

33. Wong B, Bernard E, Gold J, et al: The arabinitol appearance rate in laboratory animals and humans: Estimation from the arabinitol/creatinine ratio and relevance to the diagnosis of candidiasis. *J Infect Dis* **146**:353–359, 1982.

34. Wong B, Bernard E, Gold J, et al: Increased arabinitol levels in experimental candidiasis in rats: Arabinitol appearance rates, arabinitol/creatinine ratios and severity of infection *J Infect Dis* **146**:346–352, 1982.

35. Gold J, Wong B, Bernard E, et al: Serum arabinitol concentrations and arabinitol/creatinine ratios in invasive candidiasis. *J Infect Dis* **147**:504–513, 1983.

36. Andrews CP, Weiner MH: Aspergillus antigen detection in bronchoalveolar lavage fluid from patients with invasive aspergillosis and aspergillomas. *Am J Med* **73**:372–380, 1982.

37. Weiner MH, Talbot GH, Gerson SL, et al: Antigen detection in the diagnosis of invasive aspergillosis. *Ann Intern Med* **99**:777–782, 1983.

38. DeRepentigny L, Reiss E: Current trends in immunodiagnosis of candidiasis and aspergillosis. *Rev Infect Dis* **6**:301–312, 1984.

39. Sabetta JR, Miniter P, Andriole VT: The diagnosis of invasive aspergillosis by an enzyme-linked immunoabsorbent assay for circulating antigen. *J Infect Dis* **152**:946–953, 1985

40. Ahearn D: Medically important yeasts. *Annu Rev Microbiol* **32**:59–68, 1978.

41. Gerain J, Snoeck R, Muller C, et al: Fongemie chez des malades immunocompromis. *Med Mal Infect* **14**:605–606, 1984

42. Louria D, Blevins A, Armstrong D, et al: Fungemia caused by "nonpathogenic" yeasts. *Arch Intern Med* **119**:247–252, 1967.

43. Wingard J, Merz W, Saral R: Candida tropicalis: A major pathogen in immunocompromised patients. *Ann Intern Med* **91**:539–543, 1979.

44. Aisner J, Schimpff S, Sutherland J, et al: Torulopsis glabrata infections in patients with cancer; increasing incidence and relationship to colonization. *Am J Med* **61**:23–28, 1976.

45. Aisner J, Sickles E, Schimpff S, et al: Torulopsis glabrata pneumonitis in patients with cancer. *JAMA* **230**:584–585, 1974.

46. Kiehn T, Edwards F, Armstrong D: The prevalence of yeasts in clinical specimens from cancer patients. *Am J Clin Pathol* **73**:518–521, 1980.

47. Plouffe J, Brown D, Silua J, et al: Nosocomial outbreak of Candida parapsilosis fungemia related to intravenous infusions. *Arch Intern Med* **137**:1686–1689, 1977.

48. Baker J, Salkin I, Pincus D, et al: Pathogenicity of C. paratropicalis. *Arch Pathol Lab Med* **107**:577–579, 1983.

49. Hurley R, Winner H: The pathogenicity of C. tropicalis *J Pathol* **84**:33–38, 1962.

50. Louria D, Stiff D, Bennett B: Disseminated moniliasis in the adult. *Medicine (Baltimore)* **41**:307–337, 1962.

51. Gold J, Poston W, Mertelsmann R, et al: Systemic infection with Trichosporon cutaneum in a patient with acute leukemia *Cancer* **48**:2163–2167, 1981.

52. Jameson B, Carter R, Watson J, et al: An unexpected fungal infection in a patient with leukemia. *J Clin Pathol* **34**:267–270, 1981.

53. Winston D, Balsley G, Rhodes J, et al: Disseminated Trichosporon capitatum infection in an immunosuppressed host. *Arch Intern Med* **137**:1192–1195, 1977.

54. Lehrer RI: The fungicidal mechanisms of human monocytes. I. Evidence for myeloperoxidase-linked and myeloperoxidase-independent candidacidal mechanisms. *J Clin Invest* **55**:338–346, 1975.

55. Diamond RD, Krzesicki R, Jao W: Damage to pseudohyphal forms of *Candida albicans* by neutrophils in the absence of serum in vitro, *J Clin Invest* **61**:349–359, 1978.

56. Diamond RD, Krzesicki R: Mechanisms of attachment of neutrophils to *Candida albicans* pseudohyphae in the absence of serum, and of subsequent damage to pseudohyphae by microbicidal process of neutrophils in vitro. *J Clin Invest* **61**:360–369, 1978.

57. Diamond RD, Haudenschild CC: Monocyte-mediated serum-independent damage to hyphal and pseudohyphal forms of *Candida albicans* in vitro. *J Clin Invest* **67**:173–182, 1981.

58. Rogers TJ, Balish E: Immunity to *Candida albicans*. *Microbiol Rev* **44**:660–682, 1980.

59. Bodey G: Candidiasis in cancer patients. *Am J Med* **77**(4D):13–19, 1984.

60. Maksymiuk A, Thongprasert S, Hopfer R, et al. Systemic

candidiasis in cancer patients. *Am J Med* **77**(4D):20–27, 1984.

61. Kantarjian H, Saad M, Estey E, et al: Hypercalcemia in disseminated candidiasis. *Am J Med* **77**:721–724, 1983.

62. Fishman D, Griffin J, Sapico F, et al: Hematogenous Candida endophtalmitis. A complication of candidemia. *N Engl J Med* **286**:675–681, 1972.

63. Klein J, Watanakunakorn C: Hospital acquired fungemia Its natural course and clinical significance. *Am J Med* **67**:51–58, 1979.

64. Montgomerie J, Edwards J: Association of infection due to Candida albicans with intravenous hyperalimentation. *J Infect Dis* **137**:197–201, 1978.

65. Sixbey J, Caplan E: Candida parapsilosis endophthalmitis. *Ann Intern Med* **89**:1010–1011, 1978

66. Weinstein A, Reller B, Murphy J, et al: The clinical significance of positive blood cultures: A comprehensive analysis of 500 episodes of bacteremia and fungemia in adults. *Rev Infect Dis* **5**:35–70, 1983.

67. Murray H, Fialk M, Roberts R: Candida arthritis: A manifestation of disseminated candidiasis. *Am J Med* **60**:587–595, 1976.

68. Noble M, Lyne E: Candida osteomyelitis and arthritis from hyperalimentation therapy. *J Bone Joint Surg* **56B**:825–829, 1974.

69. Gazzaniga A, Mir-Sepasi M, Jefferies M, et al: Candida endocarditis complicating glucose total intravenous nutrition. *Ann Surg* **179**:902–905, 1974

70. Rubinstein E, Noriega E, Simberkoff M, et al: Fungal endocarditis: Characterization of the disease and response of the disease and response to therapy. *Infect Immun* **17**:140–147, 1977.

71. Edwards JE: Candida endophthalmitis. In Remington JS, Swartz MN (eds): *Current Clinical Topics in Infectious Disease.* Vol. 3. McGraw-Hill, New York, 1982, pp. 381–397.

72. MacLeod R, Remington J: Fungal endocarditis. In Rahimtoola S (ed): *Infective Endocarditis.* Grune & Stratton, New York, 1978, pp. 211–290.

73. Van Kirk J, Simon A, Armstrong W: Candida myocarditis causing complete atrioventricular block. *JAMA* **227**:931–933, 1974.

74. Pizzo P, Robichaud K, Edwards B, et al. Oral antibiotic prophylaxis in patients with cancer. *J Pediatr* **102**:125–133, 1983.

75. Pizzo P, Robichaud K, Gill F, et al: Empiric antibiotic and antifungal therapy for cancer patients with prolonged fever and granulocytopenia. *Am J Med* **72**:101–111, 1982.

76. Smits F, Prior A, Arblaster P. Incidence of Candida in hospitals in patients and the effects of antibiotic therapy. *Br Med J* **1**:208–210, 1966.

77 Eras P, Goldstein M, Sherlock P: Candida infection of the gastrointestinal tract. *Medicine (Baltimore)* **51**:367–379, 1972.

78. Jones J: Necrotizing Candida oesophagitis. Failure of symptoms and roentgenographic findings to reflect severity. *JAMA* **244**:2190–2191, 1980.

79. Jones J: Granulomatous hepatitis due to Candida albicans in patients with acute leukemia. *Ann Intern Med* **94**:475–477, 1981

80. Moseley R, Kris M, Einzig A, et al: Respiratory alkalosis and abdominal pain heralding Candida hepatitis *Arch Intern Med* **142**:1495–1497, 1982

81. Tashjian L, Abramson J, Peacock J: Focal hepatic candidiasis: A distinct clinical variant of candidiasis in immunocompromised patients *Rev Infect Dis* **6**:689–703, 1984.

82 Marcucci R, Whitelly H, Armstrong D: Common bile duct obstruction secondary to infection with Candida. *J Clin Microbiol* **7**:490–492, 1978.

83. Schreiber M, Black L, Noah Z, et al: Gallbladder candidiasis in a leukemic child. *Am J Dis Child* **136**:462–463, 1982

84. Gordon R, Simmons B, Applebaum P, et al: Intraabdominal abscess and fungemia caused by Candida krusei. *Arch Intern Med* **140**:1239–1240, 1980.

85. Solomkin J, Flohr A, Quie P, et al: The role of Candida in intraperitoneal infections. *Surgery* **88**:524–530, 1980.

86. Solomkin J, Simmons R. Candida infection in surgical patients *World J Surg* **4**:381–394, 1980.

87 Eisenberg E, Alpert B, Weiss R, et al: Rhodotorula rubra peritonitis in patients undergoing continuous ambulatory peritoneal dialysis. *Am J Med* **75**:349–352, 1983.

88. Kerr C, Perfect J, Craven P, et al. Fungal peritonitis in patients on continuous ambulatory peritoneal dialysis. *Ann Intern Med* **99**:334–337, 1983.

89. Michigan S: Genitourinary fungal infections. *J Urol* **116**:390–397, 1976.

90. Goldberg P, Kozinn P, Wise G, et al: Incidence and significance of candiduria. *JAMA* **241**:582–584, 1979.

91. Kozinn P, Taschdjian C, Goldberg F, et al: Advances in the diagnosis of renal candidiasis. *J Urol* **119**:184–187, 1978.

92. Argyle C, Schumann GB, Genack L, et al: Identification of fungal casts in a patient with renal candidiasis. *Hum Pathol* **15**:480–481, 1984.

93. Gregory MC, Schumann GB: Antemortem diagnosis of disseminated fungal infection. *N Engl J Med* **312**:124, 1985.

94. Gregory MC, Schumann GB, Schumann JL, Argyle JC: The clinical significance of candidal casts *Am J Kidney Dis* **4**:179–184, 1984

95. Kauffman C, Tan J: Torulopsis glabrata renal infection. *Am J Med* **57**:217–224, 1974.

96. Boldus R, Brown R, Culp D: Fungus balls in the renal pelvis. *Radiology* **102**:555–557, 1972.

97. Dembner A, Pfister R: Fungal infection of the urinary tract: Demonstration by antegrade pyelography and drainage by percutaneous nephrostomy. *AJR* **129**:415–418, 1977.

98. McDonald D, Fagan C: Fungus balls in the urinary bladder. *AJR* **114**:753–757, 1972.

99. Armstrong D, Chmel H, Singer C, et al: Non-bacterial infections associated with neoplastic diseases. *Eur J Cancer* **11**:79–94, 1975.

100. Ellis C, Spivack M: The significance of candidemia. *Ann Intern Med* **67**:511–522, 1967.

101. Krick J, Remington J: Opportunistic invasive fungal infection in patients with leukemia and lymphoma. *Clin Haematol* **5**:249–310, 1976.

102. Masur H, Rosen P, Armstrong D. Pulmonary disease caused by Candida species. *Am J Med* **63**:914–925, 1977.

103. Rose H, Sheth N: Pulmonary candidiasis. A clinical and

pathological correlation. *Arch Intern Med* **138**:964–965, 1978.

104. Bennett JE. Treatment of cryptococcal, candidal and coccidioidal meningitis. In Remington J, Swartz M (eds): *Current Clinical Topics in Infectious Diseases*. Vol. 2. McGraw-Hill, New York, 1981, pp. 54–67.

105. Chesney PJ, Teets KC, Mulvihill JJ, et al: Successful treatment of Candida meningitis with amphotericin B and 5-fluorocytosine in combination. *J Pediatr* **89**:1017–1019, 1976.

106. Chesney PJ, Justman RA, Bogdanowicz WM: Candida meningitis in new-born infants: A review and report of combined amphotericin B-fluocytosine therapy. *Johns Hopkins Med J* **142**:155–160, 1978.

107 Lilien LD, Ramamurthy RS, Pildes RS: Candida albicans meningitis in a premature neonate successfully treated with 5-fluorocytosine and amphotericin B A case report and review of the literature *Pediatrics* **61**:57–61, 1978.

108. Lipton S, Hickey W, Morris J, et al: Candidal infection in the central nervous system. *Am J Med* **76**:101–108, 1984

109. Parker JC, McCloskey JJ, Lee RS: The emergence of candidiasis. The dominant post mortem cerebral mycosis. *Am J Clin Pathol* **70**:31–36, 1978.

110. DeVita V, Utz J, Carbone P: Candida meningitis. *Arch Intern Med* **117**:527–535, 1966.

111. Odds F: Candidosis of the central nervous system In Odds (ed): *Candida and Candidosis*. University Park Press, Baltimore, 1979, pp. 166–170.

112. Cheml H: Candida albicans meningitis following lumbar puncture. *Am J Med Sci* **266**:465–467, 1973.

113 Fainstein V, Hopfer R, Trier P, et al: Bone marrow cultures: their value in diagnosing fungal and fecal flora in patients with acute leukemia. *J Infect Dis* **144**:79, 1981.

114. Bayer A, Guze L: Fungal arthritis. Candida arthritis: Diagnostic and prognostic implications and therapeutic considerations. *Semin Arthritis Rheum* **8**:142–150, 1978.

115 Murray H, Fialk M, Roberts R: Candida arthritis: A manifestation of disseminated candidiasis. *Am J Med* **60**:587–595, 1976.

116. Gerster J, Glauser M, Delacretaz F, et al. Erosive Candida arthritis in a patient with disseminated candidasis. *J Rheumatol* **7**:911–914, 1980.

117. Shaikh BS, Applebaum PC, Aber RC: Vertebral disc space infection and osteomyelitis due to candida albicans in a patient with acute myelomonocytic leukemia *Cancer* **45**:1025–1028, 1980.

118. Nobel M, Lyne E: Candida osteomyelitis and arthritis from hyperalimentation therapy. *J Bone Joint Surg* **56B**:825–829, 1984.

119. Dupont B, Drouhet E: Cutaneous, occular and osteoarticular candidiasis in heroin addict *J Infect Dis* **152**:577–591, 1985.

120. Epstein J, Tuazon C: Isolated lymphadenitis caused by Candida albicans in a patient with acute leukemia. *Arch Intern Med* **141**:1697–1698, 1981

121. Edwards J (moderator): Severe candidal infections: Clinical perspective, immune defense mechanisms and current concepts of therapy *Ann Intern Med* **89**:91–106, 1978.

122 Brownstein S, Mahoney-Kinsner J, Harris R Ocular candida with pale-centered hemorrhages. *Arch Ophthalmol* **101**:1745–1748, 1983.

123. Rinaldi MG: Invasive aspergillosis *Rev Infect Dis* **5**:1061–1077, 1983

124. Rhame ES, Streifel AJ, Kersey JH, et al: Extrinsic risk factors for pneumonia in the patient at high risk of infection. *Am J Med (Suppl)* **15**:42–52, 1984.

125. Arnow PM, Anderson RL, Mainous PD, et al. Pulmonary aspergillosis during hospital renovation *Am Rev Respir Dis* **118**:49–53, 1978.

126. Sarubbi FA Jr, Kopf HB, Wilson MB, et al: Increased recovery of *Aspergillus flavus* from respiratory specimens during hospital construction. *Am Rev Respir Dis* **125**:33–38, 1982.

127. Streifel AJ, Lauer JL, Vesley D, et al: *Aspergillus fumigatus* and other thermotolerant fungi generated by hospital building demolition. *Appl Environ Microbiol* **46**:375–378, 1983.

128. Opal SM, Asp AA, Cannady PB Jr, et al: Efficacy of infection control measures during a nosocomial outbreak of disseminated aspergillosis associated with hospital construction. *J Infect Dis* **153**:634–637, 1986.

129. Young RC, Bennett JE, Vogel CL, et al. Aspergillosis: The spectrum of the disease in 98 patients *Medicine (Baltimore)* **49**:143–147, 1970.

130 Fischer BS, Armstrong D, Yu B, et al. Invasive aspergillosis. Progress in early diagnosis and treatment *Am J Med* **71**:571–577, 1981.

131. Meyer D, Young LS, Armstrong D, et al: Aspergillosis complicating neoplastic disease. *Am J Med* **54**:6–15, 1973.

132. Pennington JE: Aspergillus lung disease. *Med Clin North Am* **64**:475–627, 1980.

132a. Brown E, Freedman S, Arbeit R, Come S: Invasive pulmonary aspergillosis in an apparently nonimmunocompromised host. *Am J Med* **69**:624–627, 1980.

133. Gerson SL, Talbot GH, Hurwitz S, et al: Prolonged granulocytopenia: The major risk factor for invasive pulmonary aspergillosis in patients with acute leukemia. *Ann Intern Med* **100**:345–351, 1984.

134. Ramsey PG, Rubin RH, Tolkoff-Rubin NE, et al: The renal transplant patient with fever and pulmonary infiltrates Etiology, clinical manifestations and management *Medicine (Baltimore)* **59**:206–222, 1978.

135. Weiland D, Ferguson RM, Peterson PK, et al: Aspergillosis in 25 renal transplant patients; epidemiology, clinical presentation, diagnosis and management. *Ann Surg* **198**:622–629, 1983

136. Gustafson TL, Schaffner W, Lavely GB, et al. Invasive aspergillosis in renal transplant recipient: Correlations with corticosteroid therapy *J Infect Dis* **148**:230–238, 1983

137. Cohen MS, Isturiz RE, Malech HL, et al: Fungal infection in chronic granulomatous disease, the importance of the phagocyte in defense against fungi. *Am J Med* **71**:59–66, 1981

138. Schaffner A, Herndon D, Brande A Selective protection against candida by mononuclear and against mycelia by polymorphonuclear phagocytes in resistance to *Aspergillus J Clin Invest* **69**:617–631, 1982

139. Levitz SM, Diamond RD: Changing patterns of aspergillosis infections, *Adv. Intern Med* **30**:153–174, 1984

140. Waldorf AR, Levitz SM, Diamond RD. In vivo bron-

choalveolar macrophage defense against *Rhizopus oryzae* and *Aspergillus fumigatis*. *J Infect Dis* 150:752–760, 1984.

141 Levitz SM, Diamond RD: Mechanisms of resistance of *Aspergillus fumigatus Candida* to killing by neutrophils *in vitro*. *J Infect Dis* 152:33–41, 1985

142. Aisner J, Schimpf SC, Bennett JE, et al: Aspergillus infection in cancer patients. Association with fire proofing material in a new hospital. *JAMA* 235:411–412, 1976.

143. Cairns MR, Durack DT: Fungal pneumonia in the immunocompromised host. *Semin Respir Infect* 1:166–185, 1986.

144 Aisner J, Murrillo J, Schimpf SC, et al: Invasive aspergillosis in acute leukemia: Correlation with nose culture and antibiotic use. *Ann Intern Med* 90:4–9, 1979

145 Albelda SM, Talbot GH, Gerson SL, et al: Role of fiberoptic bronchoscopy in the diagnosis of invasive pulmonary aspergillosis in patients with acute leukemia *Am J Med* 76:1027–1034, 1984.

146 Stover DE, Zamman MB, Hajdu SI, et al: Bronchoalveolar lavage in the diagnosis of diffuse pulmonary infiltrates in the immunosuppressed host. *Ann Intern Med* 101:1–7, 1984

147. Young LS: Diagnosis and treatment of diffuse pneumonias In Grieco MH (ed): *Infections in the Abnormal Host*. Yorke, New York, 1980, pp. 601–622.

148. McCabe RE, Brooks RG, Mark JB, et al: Open lung biopsy in patients with acute leukemia. *Am J Med* 78:609–616, 1985

149 Aisner J, Schimpff SC, Wiernik PH: Treatment of invasive aspergillosis: Relation of early diagnosis and treatment to response. *Ann Intern Med* 86:539–543, 1977

150. Beal MF, O'Carroll CP, Kleinman GM, et al: Aspergillosis of the nervous system *Neurology (NY)* 32:473–479, 1982

151. Morrow R, Wong B, Finkelstein WE, et al. Asgillosis of the cerebral ventricles in a heroin abuser. *Arch Intern Med* 143:161–164, 1983

152. Doft BH, Clarkson JF, Rebell G, et al. Endogenous aspergillus endophthalmitis in drug abusers. *Arch Ophthalmol* 98:859–862, 1980.

153. Morgan MA, Wilson WR, Meel HB, et al. Fungal sinusitis in healthy and immunocompromised individuals *Am J Pathol* 82:597–601, 1984

154. Petrak RM, Pottage JC, Levin S. Invasive external otitis caused by Aspergillus fumigatus in an immunocompromised patient. *J Infect Dis* 151:196, 1985.

155. Kammer RB, Utz JP: Aspergillus species endocarditis *Am J Med* 56:506–521, 1974

156. Byrd BF, Weiher MH, McGee ZA: Aspergillus spinal epidural abscess. *JAMA* 248:3138–3139, 1982.

157. Ingwer I, McLeish KR, Tight RD, et al: Aspergillus fumigatus epidural abscess in a renal transplant recipient *Arch Intern Med* 138:153–154, 1978

158 Schaffner A, Frick PG. The effect of ketoconazole on amphotericin B in a model of disseminated aspergillosis *J Infect Dis* 151:902–910, 1985.

159. Waldorf AR, Ruderman N, Diamond RD: Specific susceptibility to mucormycosis in murine diabetes and bronchoalveolar macrophage defense against *Rhizopus*. *J Clin Invest* 74:150–160, 1984

160 Meyer RD, Rosen P, Armstrong D Phycomycosis complicating leukemia and lymphoma *Ann Intern Med* 77:871–879, 1972

161 Masucci EF, Fabara JA, Saini M, et al. Cerebral mucormycosis in a heroin addict *Arch Neurol* 139:304–306, 1982

162. Abedi E, Sismanis A, Choi K, et al. Twenty-five years's experience treating cerebro-rhino-orbital mucormycosis *Laryngoscope* 94:1060–1062, 1984

163 Funada H, Misawa T, Nakao S, et al The air crescent sign of invasive pulmonary mucomycosis in acute leukemia *Cancer* 53:2721–2723, 1984

164 Bruck HM, Nash G, Foley FD, et al: Opportunistic fungal infection of the burn wound with phycomycetes and aspergillus *Arch Surg* 102:476–482, 1971

165. Bateman CP, Umland ET, Becker LE. Cutaneous zygomycosis in a patient with lymphoma *J Am Acad Dermatol* 8:890–894, 1983.

165 Gartenberg G, Bottone EJ, Keusch GT, et al. Hospital-acquired mucormycosis (Rhizopus rhizopodiformis) of skin and subcutaneous tissue Epidemiology, mycology and treatment. *N Engl J Med* 299:1115–1118, 1978

167 Hoeprich PD. Cryptococcosis In Hoeprich PD (ed): *Infectious Diseases* Harper & Row, New York, 1977, pp 902–910.

168 Bhattacharjee AK, Bennett JE, Glaudemans CPJ Capsular polysaccharides of *Cryptococcus neoformans* *Ref Infect Dis* 6:619–624, 1984.

169 Goodman JS, Kaufman L, Keonig MG. Diagnosis of cryptococcal meningitis· Value of immunologic detection of cryptococcal antigen *N Engl J Med* 285:434–436, 1971.

170. Wu TC, Koo SY. Comparison of 3 commercial cryptococcal latex kits for detection of cryptococcal antigen *J Clin Microbiol* 18:1127–1130, 1983.

171 Bloomfield N, Gordon MA, Elmendorf DF. Detection of *Cryptococcus neoformans* antigen in body fluids by latex particle agglutination. *Proc Soc Exp Biol Med* 114:64–67, 1963

172 Bennett JE, Bailey JW: Control for rheumatoid factor in the latex test for cryptococcosis *Am J Clin Pathol* 56:360–365, 1971

173 Snow RM, Dismukes WE: Cryptococcal meningitis Diagnostic value of cryptococcal antigen in cerebrospinal fluid. *Arch Intern Med* 135:1155–1157, 1975.

174. Mackinnon S, Kane JG, Parker RH: False-positive cryptococcal antigen test and cervical prevertebral abscess. *JAMA* 240:1982–1983, 1978

175. Meunier-Carpentier F Cryptococcal meningitis. A case report and review of diagnostic procedures and therapy *Acta Clin Belg* 36:300–302, 1981

176. Fujita NK, Reynard M, Sapico FL, et al: Cryptococcal intercerebral mass lesions *Ann Intern Med* 94:382–388, 1981.

177 Kaplan MH, Rosen PP, Armstrong D· Cryptococcosis in a cancer hospital: Clinical and pathological correlates in 46 patients. *Cancer* 39:2265–2274, 1977

178. Bennett JE, Dismukes WE, Duma RJ, et al A comparison of amphotericin B alone and combined with flucytosine in the treatment of cryptococcal meningitis *N Engl J Med* 301:126–131, 1979

179 Bennett JE Treatment of cryptococcal, candidal and coc-

cidiodal meningitis In Remington JS, Swartz M (eds) *Current Clinical Topics in Infectious Diseases.* Vol. 2. McGraw-Hill, New York, 1981, pp. 54–67

180 Campbell GD, Currier RD, Busey JF: Survival in untreated cryptococcal meningitis *Neurology (NY)* 31:1154–1157, 1981

181. Fisher BD, Armstrong D: Cryptococcal interstitial pneumonia *N Engl J Med* 297:1440–1441, 1977.

182. Jensen WA, Rose RM, Hammer SM, et al Serologic diagnosis of focal pneumonia caused by *Cryptococcus neoformans Am Rev Respir Dis* 132:189–191, 1985.

183 Perfect JR, Durack DT, Gallis HA: Cryptococcemia *Medicine (Baltimore)* 62:98–109, 1983

184. Kovacs JA, Kovacs AA, Polis M, et al Cryptococcosis in the acquired immunodeficiency syndrome *Ann Intern Med* 103:533–538, 1985

185. Zuger A, Louie E, Holzman RS, et al. Cryptococcal disease in patients with the acquired immunodeficiency syndrome; diagnostic features and outcome of treatment. *Ann Intern Med* 104:234–240, 1986

186 Drutz DJ, Huppert M: Coccidioidomycosis Factors affecting the host–parasite interaction. *J Infect Dis* 147:372–390, 1983

187. Deresinski SC, Stevens DA: Coccidioidomycosis in compromised hosts *Medicine (Baltimore)* 54:377–395, 1975

188 Craven PC, Graybill JR, Jorgensen JH, et al High-dose ketoconazole for treatment of fungal infections of the central nervous system *Ann Intern Med* 98:160–167, 1983

189 Howard PF, Smith JW: Diagnosis of disseminated coccidioidomycosis, by liver biopsy *Arch Intern Med* 143:1335–1338, 1983

190. Drutz DJ: Amphotericin B in the treatment of coccidioidomycosis, *Drugs* 26:337–346, 1983

191. Sarosi GA: Management of fungal diseases. *Am Rev Respir Dis* 127:250–253, 1983.

192. Catanzaro A, Einstein H, Levine B, et al: Ketoconazole for treatment of disseminated coccidioidomycosis. *Ann Intern Med* 96:436–440, 1982.

193. Galgiani JM: Ketoconazole in the treatment of coccidioidomycosis. *Drugs* 26:355–363, 1983

194. Wheat LJ, Slama TG, Zecfel ML: Histoplasmosis in the acquired immunodeficiency syndrome *Am J Med* 78:203–210, 1985.

195 Wheat LJ, Slama TG, Norton JA, et al Risk factors for disseminated or fatal histoplasmosis. *Ann Intern Med* 96:159–163, 1982.

196. Kaufman CA, Israel KS, Smith JW, et al: Histoplasmosis in immunosuppressed patients *Am J Med* 64:923–932, 1978.

197 Lehmann PF, Gibbons J, Senitzer D, et al T-lymphocyte abnormalities in disseminated histoplasmosis. *Am J Med* 75:790–794, 1983

198 Murray JJ, Heim GR: Hypercalcemia in disseminated histoplasmosis *Am J Med* 78:881–884, 1985

199. Schwarz J, Salfelder K Blastomycosis. A review of 152 cases, *Curr Top Pathol* 65:165–200, 1977

200 Bennett JE: Sporothrix schenckii In Mandell GC, Douglas GR, Bennett JE (eds): *Principles and Practice of Infectious Diseases* Wiley, New York, 1985, pp 1456–1458

201. Bennett JE Miscellaneous fungi In Mandell GC, Douglas GR, Bennett JE (eds) *Principles and Practice of Infectious Diseases.* Wiley, New York, 1985, pp 1502–1504

202. Yoo D, Lee HS, Kwong-Chung KJ: Brain abscesses due to *Pseudoallescheria boydii* associated with primary non-Hodgkin's lymphoma of the central nervous system: A case report and literature review. *Rev Infect Dis* 7:272–277, 1985.

203 Lutwick LI, Galgiani JN, Johnson RH, et al Visceral fungal infections due to *K. petriellidium boydii. Am J Med* 61:632–640, 1976.

204 Enggrano IL, Hughes WT, Kalwinsky DK, et al. Pseudoallescheria boydii in a patient with acute lymphoblastic leukemia *Arch Pathol Lab Med* 108:619–622, 1984

205 Shih L, Lee H: Disseminated petriellidiosis (allescheriasis) in a patient with refractory acute lymphoblastic leukemia. *J Clin Pathol* 37:78–82, 1984.

206. Blazar BR, Hurd DD, Snover DC, Alexander JW, McGlave PB. Invasive *Fusarium* infections in bone marrow transplant recipients. *Am J Med* 77:645–651, 1984.

207. Wheeler MS, McGinnis MR, Schell WA, et al. *Fusarium* infections in burned patients. *Am J Clin Pathol* 75:304–311, 1975

208. Young HA, Kwong-Chung KJ, Kubota TT, et al: Disseminated infection by fusarium moniliforme during treatment for malignant lymphoma *J Clin Microbiol* 77:589–594, 1978.

209. Schimpff SC, Young V Epidemiology and prevention of infection in the compromised host In Rubin RH, Young L (eds) *Clinical Approaches to Infection in the Compromised Host.* Plenum, New York, 1981, pp. 5–33.

210 Pizzo PA Empiric therapy and prevention of infection in the immunocompromised host. In Mandell GC, Douglas GR, Bennett JE (eds): *Principles and Practice of Infectious Diseases.* Wiley, New York, 1985, pp 1468–1477.

211 Shaikh B, Appelbaum P, Jones J, et al: Colonization of nasal ulcers as a source of *Candida parapsilosis* fungemia. *Arch Otolaryngol* 106:434–436, 1980

212. Schimpff S. Infection prevention during granulocytopenia. In Remington JS, Swartz M (eds). *Current Clinical Topics in Infectious Diseases.* McGraw-Hill, New York, 1980, pp. 85–106

213. Meunier-Carpentier F Chemoprophylaxis of fungal infections. *Am J Med* 76:652–666, 1984

214 DeGregorio M, Lee W, Ries C: Candida infections in patients with acute leukemia Ineffectiveness of nystatin prophylaxis and relationship between oropharyngeal and systemic candidiasis. *Cancer* 50:2780–2784, 1982.

215. Jones W, Kauffman C, McAuliffe L, et al. Efficacy of ketoconazole versus nystatin in prevention of fungal infection in neutropenic patients *Arch Intern Med* 144:549–551, 1984

216 Dekker A, Rozenberg-Arska M, Sixma J, et al. Prevention of infection by trimethoprim-sulfamethoxazole plus amphotericin B in patients with acute non-lymphocytic leukemia. *Ann Intern Med* 95:555–559, 1981.

217 Bodey G, Rosenbaum B. Effect of prophylactic measures on the microbial flora of patients in protected environment units, *Medicine (Baltimore)* 53:209–228, 1974

218. Schimpff S, Greene W, Young V, et al: Infection prevention

in non-lymphocytic leukemia *Ann Intern Med* **82**:351–368, 1975.

219. Schimpff S, Young V, Greene W, et al. Origin of infection in acute non-lymphocytic leukemia. Significance of hospital acquisition of potential pathogens. *Ann Intern Med* **77**:707–714, 1972.

220. Bodey G: The effect of amphotericin B on the fungal flora in feces. *Clin Pharmacol Ther* **10**:675–680, 1969

221. Ezdinli E, O'Sullivan D, Wasser L, et al. Oral amphotericin for candidiasis in patients with haematologic neoplasms. An autopsy study *JAMA* **424**:258–260, 1979

222. Bodey G, Rosenbaum B, Valdivieso M, et al: Effect of systemic antimicrobial prophylaxis on microbial flora. *Antimicrob Agents Chemother* **21**:367–372, 1982

223. Meunier-Carpentier F, Cruciani M, Klastersky J. Oral prophylaxis with miconazole or ketoconazole of invasive fungal disease in neutropenic cancer patients. *Eur J Cancer Clin Oncol* **19**:43–48, 1983

224. Kaufman C, Jones P, Bergman A, et al: Effect of prophylactic ketoconazole and nystatin on fungal flora. *Mykosen* **27**:165–172, 1983.

225. Estey E, Maksymiuk A, Smith T, et al: Infection prophylaxis in acute leukemia. *Arch Intern Med* **144**:1562–1568, 1984

226. Hann I, Prentice H, Corringham R, et al. Ketoconazole versus nystatin plus amphotericin B for fungal prophylaxis in severely immunocompromised patients *Lancet* **1**:826–829, 1982.

227. Acuna G, Winston D, Young L: Ketoconazole prophylaxis of fungal infections in the granulocytopenic patient *ICAAC* Abst no. 852, 1981.

228. DeJongh C, Finley R, Joshi J, et al. A comparison of ketoconazole to nystatin: Prophylaxis of fungal infection in neutropenic patients. *ICAAC* Abst. no. 497, 1982.

229. Shepp D, Klosterman A, Seigel M, et al: Comparison of patients treated in protective environment. *ICAAC* Abst no 1101, 1983.

230. Young L: The outlook for antifungal prophylaxis in the compromised host *J Antimicrob Chemother* **9**:338–340, 1982

231 Owens M, Nighingale C, Schweizer R, et al: Prophylaxis of oral candidiasis with clotrimazole troches *Arch Intern Med* **144**:290–293, 1984.

232. Meunier-Carpentier F: Prevention of fungal pneumonia in the immunocompromised host In Lode H, Kemmrich B, Klastersky J (eds). *Current Aspects of Bacterial and Non-Bacterial Pneumonias.* Thieme, Stuttgart, 1984, pp 176–183.

233. Wade J, Schimpff S, Hargadon M, et al: A comparison of trimethaprim-sulfamethoxazole plus nystatin with gentamicin plus nystatin in the prevention of infections in acute leukemia. *N Engl J Med* **304**:1057–1062, 1981

234. Meunier-Carpentier F, Snoeck R, Gerain J, et al Amphotericin B nasal spray as prophylaxis against aspergillosis in patients with neutropenia *N Engl J Med* **311**:1056, 1984.

235 Arnow PW, Andersen RL, Mainous D, et al: Pulmonary aspergillosis during hospital renovation. *Am Rev Respir Dis* **118**:49–53, 1978.

236. Poelvoorde J, Devroey C. Sources d'Aspergillus fumigatus en milieu hospitalier *Bull Soc Fr Mycol Med* **12**:85–88, 1983

237. Bodey GP, Johnston D. Microbiological evaluation of protected environment during patient occupancy. *Appl Microbiol* **22**:828–836, 1971.

238 Dreizen S: Oral candidiasis *Am J Med* **77**(4D):28–33, 1984

239 Ching M, Raymond K, Bury R, et al: Absorption of orally administered amphotericin B lozenges. *Br J Clin Pharm* **16**:106–108, 1983.

240 Kravetz H, Andriole V, Huber M, et al. Oral administration of solubilized amphotericin B. *N Engl J Med* **265**:183–184, 1961

241 Louria D Some aspects of the absorption, distribution and excretion of amphotericin B in man. *Antibiot Med Clin Ther* **5**:295–301, 1958.

242. Armstrong D, Gold J Treatment of opportunistic mycoses in the immunodepressed patient In Speller DCE (ed). *Antifungal Chemotherapy* Wiley, New York, 1980, pp 333–364

243. Medoff G, Kobayashi G Strategies in the treatment of systemic fungal infections *N Engl J Med* **302**:145–155, 1980

244. Meunier-Carpentier F. Combination of antifungal agents for systemic mycotic diseases In Klastersky J, Staquet M (eds)· *Combination Antibiotic Therapy in the Compromised Host* Raven, New York, 1982, pp 207–227

245 Drutz D: Newer antifungal agents and their use, including an update on amphotericin B and flucytosine. In Remington J, Swartz M (eds): *Current Clinical Topics in Infectious Diseases* Vol III. McGraw-Hill, New York, 1982, pp 97–135.

246. Burks L, Aisner J, Fortner C, et al. Meperidine for the treatment of shaking chills and fever. *Arch Intern Med* **140**:483–484, 1980.

247. Butler W, Bennett J, Hill G III, et al. Electrocardiographic and electrolyte abnormalities caused by amphotericin B in dog and man *Proc Soc Exp Biol Med* **116**:857–863, 1964

248. Utz J: Amphotericin B toxicity. Combined clinical staff conference at the NIH. General side effects *Ann Intern Med* **61**:334–340, 1964.

249 Craven PC, Gremillion DH Risk factors of ventricular fibrillation during rapid amphotericin B infusion *Antimicrob Agents Chemother* **27**:868–871, 1985.

250 Wright D, Robichaud K, Pizzo P, et al: Lethal pulmonary reactions associated with the combined use of amphotericin B and leukocyte transfusions *N Engl J Med* **304**:1185–1189, 1981

251. Bow E, Schroeder M, Louie T. Pulmonary complications in patients receiving granulocyte transfusions and amphotericin B *Can Med Assoc J* **130**:593–597, 1984

252 Dana B, Durie B, White R, et al Concomitant administration of granulocyte transfusions and amphotericin B in neutropenic patients. Absence of significant pulmonary toxicity *Blood* **57**:90–94, 1981

253. Ismail MA, Lerner SA Disseminated blastomycosis in a pregnant woman. *Am Rev Respir Dis* **126**:350–353, 1982

254 Posner J. Reservoirs for intraventricular chemotherapy *N Engl J Med* **288**:212–213, 1973

255 Bayer A, Edwards J, Guze E. Experimental intraabdominal candidiasis in rabbits Therapy with low total dose intravenous amphotericin B *Antimicrob Agents Chemother* **19**:179–184, 1982.

256 Wise G, Kozinn P, Goldberg P. Amphotericin B as a urologic irrigant in the management of noninvasive candiduria *J Urol* **124**:70–72, 1982

257 Rahko P, Davey P, Wheat J, et al: Treatment of Torulopsis glabrata peritonitis with intraperitoneal amphotericin B *JAMA* **249**:1187–1188, 1983.

258. Bayer A, Blumenkrantz M, Montgomerie J, et al. Candida peritonitis. Report of 22 cases and review of the English literature. *Am J Med* **61**:832–840, 1976

259 Bennett J. Flucytosine. *Ann Intern Med* **86**:319–322, 1977

260 White C, Traube J. Ulcerating enteritis associated with flucytosine therapy *Gastroenterology* **83**:1127–1129, 1982.

261. Wise G, Kozinn P, Goldberg P· Flucytosine in the management of genitourinary candidiasis· Five years of experience *J Urol* **124**:70–72, 1980

262 Wise G, Weinstein S, Goldberg P, et al. Flucytosine in urinary Candida infections *Urology* **3**:708–711, 1974

263. Diasio R, Lakings D, Bennett J Evidence for conversion of 5-FC to 5-FU in humans *Antimicrob Agents Chemother* **14**:903–908, 1978.

264 Kauffman C, Frame P. Bone marrow toxicity associated with 5-FC therapy *Antimicrob Agents Chemother* **11**:244–247, 1977

265 Fainstein V, Bodey G. Cardiorespiratory toxicity due to miconazole. *Ann Intern Med* **93**:432–433, 1980.

266 Deresinski S, Lilly R, Levine H, et al Treatment of fungal meningitis with miconazole *Arch Intern Med* **137**:1180–1185, 1977

267 Sung J, Grendahl J, Levine M. Intravenous and intrathecal miconazole therapy for systemic mycosis *West J Med* **126**:5–13, 1977

268 Lutwick LI, Rytel MW, Yanez JP, et al. Deep infections from *Petriellidium boydii* treated with miconazole *JAMA* **241**:272–273, 1979

269 Duarte P, Chow C, Simmons F, et al Fatal hepatitis associated with ketoconazole therapy *Arch Intern Med* **144**:1069–1070, 1984

270 Heiberg J, Svejgaard E. Toxic hepatitis during ketoconazole treatment *Br Med J* **283**:825–826, 1981

271 Horsburgh C, Kirkpatrick C, Teusch C Ketoconazole and the liver *Lancet* **1**:860, 1982

272 Lewis J, Zimmerman J, Benson G, et al Hepatic injury associated with ketoconazole therapy *Gastroenterology* **86**:503–513, 1984

273 Svejgaard E, Ramek L Hepatic dysfunction and ketoconazole therapy *Ann Intern Med* **96**:788–789, 1982.

274 Defelice R, Johnson D, Galgiani J Gynecomastia with ketoconazole *Antimicrob Agents Chemother* **19**:1073–1074, 1981

275 Grosso D, Boyden T, Parmentier R, et al. Ketoconazole inhibition of testicular secretion of testosterone and displacement of steroid hormones from serum transport proteins *Antimicrob Agents Chemother* **23**:207–212, 1983

276. Pont A, Williams P, Azhar S, et al. Ketoconazole blocks testosterone synthesis *Arch Intern Med* **142**:2137–2140, 1982

277. Schurmeyer T, Nieschlag E. Effect of ketoconazole and other imidazole fungicides on testosterone biosynthesis *Acta Endocrinol (Copenh)* **105**:275–280, 1984

278 Pont A, William P, Coose D, et al: Ketoconazole blocks adrenal steroid synthesis *Ann Intern Med* **97**:370–372, 1982.

279 Tucker WS, Snell BB, Island DP, et al. Reversible adrenal insufficiency induced by ketoconazole *JAMA* **253**:2413–24 4, 1985

279a. Meunier F: Serum fungistatic and fungicidal activity in volunteers receiving antifungal agents, *Eur J Clin Microb* **5**:103–109, 1986.

280 Engelhard D, Stutman HR, Marks MI. Interaction of ketoconazole with rifampin and isoniazid *N Engl J Med* **311**:1682–1683, 1984

281 Daneshemend T Ketoconazole–cyclosporin interaction, *Lancet* **2**:1342–1343, 1982

282 Ferguson R, Sutherland D, Simmons R, et al. Ketoconazole, cyclosporin metabolism and renal transplantation *Lancet* **2**:882–883, 1982

283 Morgenstern G, Powles R, Robinson B, et al Cyclosporin interaction with ketoconazole and melphalan *Lancet* **2**:1342, 1982

284 Brown MW, Maldonado AL, Meredith CG, et al. Effect of ketoconazole on hepatic oxidative drug metabolism *Clin Pharmacol Ther* **37**:290–297, 1985

285 Horsburgh C, Kirkpatrick C: Long-term therapy of chronic mucocutaneous candidosis with ketoconazole. Experience with twenty-one patients *Am J Med* **74**:23–29, 1983

286 Bennett JE: Antifungal agents In Mandell GC, Douglas GR, Bennett JE (eds) *Principles and Practices of Infectious Diseases* Wiley, New York, 1985, pp 263–270

286a. Meunier F: Prevention of mycoses in immunocompromised patients, *Rev Infect Dis* **9**: 408–416, 1987

287. Stein R, Kayser J, Klenher J. Clinical value of empirical amphotericin B in patients with acute myelogenous leukemia. *Cancer* **50**:2247–2251, 1982.

287a. Christiansens K, Bernard E, Gold J, et al Distribution and activity of amphotericin B in humans. *J Infect Dis* **152**:1037–1043, 1985.

288. Smego RA, Perfect JR, Durack DT Combined therapy with amphotericin B and 5-fluorocytosine for candida meningitis *Rev Infect Dis* **6**:791–801, 1984

288a. Horn R, Wong B, Kiehn T, et al. Fungemia in a cancer hospital. changing frequency, earlier onset and results of therapy, *Rev Infect Dis* **7**:646–656, 1985

289 Schaffner A, Frick PG. The effect of ketoconazole on amphotericin B in a model of disseminated aspergillosis *J Infect Dis* **151**:902–910, 1985

290 Merz W. Candida lusitaniae Frequency of recovery, colonization, infection and amphotericin B resistance *J Clin Microbiol* **20**:1194–1195, 1984

291 Merz W, Sandford G. Isolation and characterization of a polyene resistant variant of *C tropicalis* *J Clin Microbiol* **9**:677–680, 1979

292. Pappagianis D, Collins M, Hector R, et al: Development of resistance to amphotericin B in *Candida lusitaniae* infecting a human. *Antimicrob Agents Chemother* **16:**123–126, 1979.

293. Dick J, Merz W, Saral R: Incidence of polyene-resistant yeasts recovered from clinical specimens. *Antimicrob Agents Chemother* **18:**158–163, 1980.

294. Guinet R, Chanas J, Goullier A, et al: Fatal septicemia due to amphotericin B-resistant *C. lusitaniae, J Clin Microbiol* **18:**433–444, 1983.

295. Stiller R, Bennett J, Scholer H, et al: Susceptibility to 5-FC and prevalence of serotype in 402 *C. albicans* isolates in the US, *Antimicrob Agents Chemother* **22:**482–487, 1982

296. Stiller R, Bennett J, Scholer H, et al: Correlation of in vitro susceptibility test results with in vivo response. Flucytosine therapy in a systemic candidiasis model, *J Infect Dis* **147:**1070–1077, 1983.

297. Ruthe R, Andersen B, Epstein R: Efficacy of granulocyte transfusions in the control of systemic candidiasis in the leukopenic host, *Blood* **53:**493–498, 1978.

298. Swerdlow B, Deresinski S: Development of *Aspergillus* sinusitis in a patient receiving Amphotericin B treatment with granulocyte transfusions, *Am J Med* **76:**162–166, 1984.

299. Meunier-Carpentier F, Taterman J, Brassinne C, et al: In-vitro activity of amphotericin B encapsulated into liposomes. *ICAAC* Abst. no. 1020, 1984.

300. Meunier-Carpentier F, Coune A, Sculier JP, et al. Serum levels of amphotericin B, serum fungistatic and fungicidal activity in cancer patients receiving Fungizone[R] or amphotericin B encapsulated into liposomes. *ICACC* Abst. no. 1056, 1985.

300a. Sculier JP, Coune A, Meunier F, et al: Pilot study of amphotericin B entrapped into sonicated liposomes in cancer patients with mycotic complications, *ASCO Annual Meeting,* Abst. no. 964, 1986

301. Lopez-Bernstein G, Fainstein V, Hopfer R, et al: Liposomal amphotericin B for the treatment of systemic fungal infections in patients with cancer: A preliminary study *J Infect Dis* **151:**704–710, 1985.

302. Espinel-Ingroff A, Shadomy S, Gebhart RJ: In vitro studies with R–51,211 (Itraconazole). *Antimicrob Agents Chemother* **26:**5–9, 1984.

303. Van Cutsem J, Van Gerven F, Van de Ven MA, et al: Itraconazole, a new triazole that is orally active in aspergillosis. *Antimicrob Agents Chemother* **26:**527–534, 1984.

304. Humphrey M, Jevons S, Tarbit M. Pharmacokinetic evaluation of UK–49,858, a metabolically stable triazole antifungal drug, in animals and humans, *Antimicrob Agents Chemother* **28:**648–653, 1985.

305 Troke P, Andrews R, Brammer K, et al: Efficacy of UK–49,858 (Fluconazole) against Candida albicans experimental infections in mice, *Antimicrob Agents Chemother* **28:**815—818, 1985

9

Mycobacterial and Nocardial Infections in the Compromised Host

HARVEY B. SIMON

1. Introduction

Among the broad range of pathogenic and opportunistic microorganisms that can affect the immunologically impaired host are members of various mycobacterial and nocardial species. These organisms are often grouped together because of a common tinctorial property: both *Mycobacteria* and *Nocardia* spp. generally appear acid fast when stained with the traditional Ziehl-Neelson procedure or with modified acid-fast staining techniques. Despite this similarity, these organisms behave quite differently in biologic, clinical, and therapeutic terms, and as a result they require separate discussion here.

2. Mycobacteria

2.1. Classification and Microbiology

Tuberculosis is an ancient disease; unmistakable skeletal stigmata of tuberculosis have been identified in Egyptian mummies, and clinical descriptions date back to the writings of Aristotle and Hippocrates. With the isolation and identification of *M. tuberculosis* by Koch in 1882, the etiology of tuberculosis became clear. In the succeeding years numerous other mycobacterial species were identified from cultures of soil and water as well as from animal and human sources. Although *M. bovis* was quickly recognized as an important human pathogen, the potential pathogenicity of the other nontuberculous, or atypical, mycobacteria was not recognized until 1951. Since the introduction of Runyon's classification system in 1959, our understanding of the nontuberculous mycobacteria has progressed greatly. Although the prevalence of tuberculosis in the United States has declined greatly since the turn of the century, *M. tuberculosis* remains by far the most important mycobacterial pathogen both for normal and for immunosuppressed hosts. However, the nontuberculous mycobacteria are assuming increased importance in the compromised host; some of these organisms are pathogens that can produce clinical illness in normal or impaired hosts, whereas others are true opportunists that affect only the immunocompromised. In addition, it is becoming increasingly clear that various mycobacteria can produce nosocomial infections that may pose special hazards to the impaired host.

All mycobacteria share certain common properties: they are obligate aerobic bacilli that are nonmotile and nonsporulating. A distinctive feature of the mycobacteria is their high cell wall lipid content, which approaches 50% of the cell wall by weight. As a result of this high lipid content, mycobacteria are impermeable to conventional bacteriologic stains but are resistant to decolorization with acid alcohol after staining with carbol fuscin. Because of their lipid-rich cell walls, mycobacteria are hydrophobic, tend to clump together, and are difficult to work with in

HARVEY B. SIMON • Infectious Disease Unit, Massachusetts General Hospital; and Department of Medicine, Harvard Medical School, Boston, Massachusetts 02114 the laboratory. However, mycobacteria are very resistant to physical stress and can be subjected to digestion and concentration procedures that would kill ordinary bacteria. Although this can be an advantage in the diagnostic laboratory, mycobacteria can also survive many commonly employed hospital disinfectants, thereby posing the risk of nosocomial infection. Another feature common to most mycobacteria is their requirement for special enriched media to grow in the laboratory; the rapid growers of Runyon's group IV are an exception in that they can grow on some ordinary laboratory media such as MacConkey agar. These group IV organisms are also exceptions to the final important property of the mycobacteria: their slow rate of growth. For example, the generation time of M. tuberculosis is 12–18 hr in contrast to the 20-min division time for many ordinary bacteria. This slow rate of growth has two major consequences: in the laboratory, it takes 3–8 weeks to isolate most mycobacterial species, and in clinical terms, most mycobacterial infections progress at a subacute to chronic pace.

The mycobacteria can be subdivided into common or medically more important species and into the atypical mycobacteria. *Mycobacterium tuberculosis* is recognized in the laboratory on the basis of its slow rate of growth (15–40 days), by its heaped-up, nonpigmented or buff-colored, colonial morphology, and on the basis of the niacin test. *Mycobacterium tuberculosis* is unique among the mycobacteria in that it produces niacin, and a simple colorimetric test for niacin thus permits rapid laboratory identification of *M. tuberculosis*.

Mycobacterium bovis closely resembles *M. tuberculosis* in the laboratory but is niacin negative. Like *M. tuberculosis,* most strains of *M. bovis* are sensitive to INH and other antituberculous drugs. *Mycobacterium bovis* was once an important human pathogen causing pulmonary infection, lymphadenitis, osteomyelitis, enteritis, and other infections clinically identical to tuberculosis. With the slaughter of tuberculin-positive cattle and with the pasteurization of milk, *M. bovis* has become a clinical rarity in the United States. For example, between 1954 and 1968, the Mayo Clinic treated 2080 patients with infection caused by *M. tuberculosis* but only six with disease caused by *M. bovis*.[1]

Bacillus Calmette-Guérin (BCG) is a live attenuated strain of *M. bovis* that was selected by serial passage in the laboratory to serve as a vaccine against tuberculosis. Since its introduction in 1921, BCG has remained controversial; initially considered to be 80% effective in preventing tuberculosis,[2] more recent trials have failed to demonstrate efficacy.[3] BCG has little virulence for normal vaccines; it has been administered to an estimated 500 million people with fewer than 20 reported fatalities from disseminated BCG infection. However, BCG is now being administered in large doses to cancer patients as an immunologic adjuvant, and BCG infection in the compromised host is of growing concern.

Mycobacterium leprae is an uncommon pathogen in the United States, but leprosy remains an important problem in many parts of the world. *Mycobacterium leprae* has not been cultured in vitro, and relatively little is known about the organism. The most severe form of leprosy, lepromatous leprosy, results from a failure of cell-mediated immunity. Lepromatous leprosy has been reported in a renal transplant recipient.[4] However, leprosy is not a problem in the impaired host in the United States and is not considered further here.

The atypical mycobacteria, which are all niacin negative, were classified by Runyon into four groups based on their pigment production and rate of growth.[5]

Group I organisms produce pigmented colonies only when grown in the light and are hence called photochromogens. The most important member of group I is *M. kansasii,* which grows in 7–21 days, producing a yellow pigment in the light. *Mycobacterium kansasii* is an important cause of pulmonary disease, especially in urban areas of the midwest, and can disseminate in compromised hosts. Whereas most atypical mycobacteria are highly drug resistant, group I organisms are sensitive to most antituberculous drugs.

Group II organisms produce pigmented colonies whether grown in light or dark and are therefore called scotochromogens. These organisms also grow in 7–21 days and typically produce a yellow-orange pigment. The most important species is *M. scrofulaceum,* which causes cervical lymphadenitis in children.

Group III organisms are called nonchromogens because their colonies are nonpigmented. A member of this group, *M. avium-intracellulare* (formerly *M. battey*), is the most important of all the nontuberculous mycobacteria. *Mycobacterium avium-intracellulare* is most prevalent in rural areas of the southeast United States but is found in all regions of the country. *Mycobacterium avium-intracellulare* also grows in 7–21 days and is drug resistant. Pulmonary disease is the most common clinical manifestation of *M. avium-intracellulare* infection, but dissemination can occur occasionally both in normal and in impaired hosts. *M. avium-intracellulare* has been a particularly severe problem in patients with the acquired immunodeficiency disease (AIDS).

Group IV organisms are classified together as rapid growers because their colonies can be recognized in only 3–7 days. *Mycobacterium fortuitum* is the most important of the rapid growers, which are generally drug resistant. *Mycobacterium fortuitum* typically causes localized soft tissue abscesses but can disseminate in impaired hosts. Group IV organisms have been increasingly recognized as nosocomial pathogens.

2.2. Host Defenses

In order to understand which immunosuppressed patients are at greatest risk of mycobacterial infection, it is important to understand normal host-defense mechanisms against these organisms.[6] According to current immunologic dogma, the first step in immunity to tuberculosis involves the interaction of mycobacterial antigens with T lymphocytes. When exposed to tuberculoproteins, committed lymphocytes that recognize the antigen undergo blastogenesis, resulting in the establishment of a population of T lymphocytes sensitized to mycobacterial antigens. T lymphocytes are motile cells, and when further exposure to bacilli occurs, sensitized T cells will accumulate at the site of inflammation. The antigenetically stimulated lymphocyte in turn activates the host's macrophages,[7] probably by secreting soluable mediators (lymphokines) including chemotactic factor, migration inhibitory factor (MIF), macrophage activation factor (MAF), and others. The nodular accumulation of inflammatory cells that results is histologically recognizable as a granuloma. More importantly, the activated macrophages present in regions of granulomatous inflammation possess enhanced metabolic, phagocytic, and bactericidal potential. Tubercle bacilli are engulfed by

macrophages, and most of the bacteria are killed. However, a small number of bacilli are able to survive in a dormant state within host macrophages, and if immunity breaks down, clinical reactivation tuberculosis can result.

The implications for the immunosuppressed patient are clear: any process that interferes with the integrity of cell-mediated immunity increases the risk of dissemination of primary infection and of reactivation of latent mycobacterial infection. In clinical terms, the greatest potential risk is from human immunodeficiency virus (HIV) infection (as in AIDS) or prolonged corticosteroid therapy. Other settings in which cellular immunity may be impaired include Hodgkin disease and other neoplasia, debility and cachexia, old age, and treatment with antilymphocyte globulin, corticosteroids, and possibly with cytotoxic agents. By contrast, immunoglobulin deficiencies and granulocytopenia do not present a special risk for tuberculosis.

2.3. Skin Testing

Cell-mediated immunity to mycobacteria can be demonstrated clinically be means of delayed hypersensitivity skin testing. The tuberculin skin test is far more sensitive than the chest radiograph in detecting latent infection with *M. tuberculosis*. The Mantoux test using the intradermal injection of polysorbate 80-stabilized purified protein derivitive (PPD) is more reliable than multiple puncture tests such as the Tine test. Three strengths of PPD are available, the first strength containing 1 tuberculin unit (TU), the intermediate-strength 5 units, and the second strength 250 units. Intermediate-strength PPD is the standard test material. The tuberculin skin test should be interpreted at 48–72 hr after injection, and the diameter of induration rather than erythema determines the interpretation: 0–4 mm is a negative reaction; 5–9 mm is doubtful; and 10 mm or more is positive. First-strength PPD should be reserved for patients in whom a very strong reaction is anticipated; second-strength PPD should be reserved for individuals with negative reactions to a lower strength.

Skin testing can also be used to identify patients infected with nontuberculous mycobacteria. Whereas patients infected with *M. bovis* or BCG can be expected to react to intermediate PPD, patients infected with atypical mycobacteria typically have negative or very weak reactions. However, antigens can be prepared from each group of atypical mycobacteria (group I: PPD-Y; group II: PPD-G: group III: PPD-B; group IV: PPD-F), and patients infected with organisms from each group can be expected to have positive skin tests with the group-specific antigen. Unfortunately, the atypical mycobacterial antigens are not currently available for clinical use. However, a positive second-strength (250 TU) PPD test in the face of a negative or doubtful intermediate-strength (5 TU) test is suggestive of infection with atypical mycobacteria and resultant cross sensitization to PPD.

Obviously, whereas a positive skin test demonstrates previous mycobacterial infection, it does not by itself prove active disease. Conversely, negative reactions have been demonstrated in up to 70% of patients with active tuberculosis. There are three potential explanations for negative skin tests. The first is technical failure of the skin test itself because of inactive antigens, improper injection, or faulty interpretation. Technical failures have become much less prevalent since the introduction of bioassayed, polysorbate 80-stabilized PPD products. The second reason for negatie skin tests in patients with proven infection is the presence of an underlying disease or treatment that impaires cellular immunity. Except for viral infections (which produce only transient anergy) and sarcoidosis (which is only rarely complicated by infection), the problems responsible for anergy are precisely those encountered in the immunosuppressed host: AIDS, steroid therapy, Hodgkin disease and other neoplasia, cachexia, and treatment with antilymophocyte globulin and possibly certain cytotoxic agents. Finally, a third group of patients with active tuberculosis will have negative skin tests without underlying immunosuppressive conditions precisely because of the overwhelming nature of the mycobacterial infection itself. Miliary tuberculosis is the best example of this phenomenon. These patients generally recover tuberculin reactivity during the course of antituberculous therapy.

If intermediate and second-strength tuberculin skin tests are negative in the immunosuppressed patient with suspect mycobacterial infection, it is important to test for anergy with streptokinase-streptodornase, Candida, or mumps antigens. Although some workers have suggested that in vitro lymphocyte transformation in response to PPD may be pre-served in patients with negative skin tests,[8] other groups have found that the in vitro tests correlate well with cutaneous reactivity, so they are not diagnostically helpful.[9] The mechanism of anergy in tuberculosis was not well understood until the studies of Ellner demonstrated the presence of suppressor cell activity in the peripheral blood mononuclear cells of patients with pulmonary tuberculosis and negative PPD skin tests.[10]

2.4. Pathogenesis

With the elimination of bovine tuberculosis in the United States, virtually all cases of tuberculosis are acquired through person-to-person transmission via the aerosol route. Patients with active pulmonary infection shed infected droplets into the air; because most infectious patients discharge relatively few organisms, there is a low risk of infection in casual contacts, and most secondary cases occur in household members, schoolmates, or other close contacts of the index case. Infectivity is greatest in patients with cavitary disease, with tuberculosis of the larynx, and with thin, watery sputum; shedding is further enhanced by coughing. Once airborne, infected particles can remain aloft for many hours; thus, adequate ventilation is of prime importance for control of tuberculosis, particularly in the hospital setting. After the droplets have settled onto environmental surfaces, however, they are essentially noninfectious, although they may still contain viable bacilli.

Although a single tubercle bacillus is theoretically capable of causing infection, it must first bypass the upper airway defense mechanisms and lodge in the pulmonary alveoli; airborne particles 5–10 μm in diameter are thus most likely to transmit infection. Initial infection usually occurs in the lower lung fields because of both gravity and the greater ventilation of the lung bases. Once in the alveoli, tubercle bacilli multiply slowly, and because these organisms do not secrete any enzymes or toxins, they initially provoke little inflammatory reaction in the nonimmune host. By about 3 weeks, however, a single organism can potentially have given rise to over a million progeny, and these bacilli will have invaded lymphatics and spread to the draining regional nodes. With further multiplication, bacilli invade the bloodstream and can spread hematogenously to any organ. Even at this stage, the great majority of patients are completely asymptomatic, so that this truly is a silent bacillemia.[11] Although any tissue can be hematogenously seeded, organs with high blood flow tend to receive the most bacilli, and tissues with the highest Po_2 provide the most favorable environment for their multiplication; hence, the lung apices themselves are by far the most common repositories of organisms. Other frequently infected areas include the renal cortex, the vertebral column, and the metaphyseal ends of long bones.

By the time 6–8 weeks have passed, cell-mediated immunity is well established; the tuberculin skin test becomes positive at this time, but more importantly, granulomatous inflammation develops and contains the tubercle bacilli both in the lung and in regions of metastatic spread. As a result, most patients go on to healing of these initial tuberculous lesions, but if immunity is incomplete, progressive primary tuberculosis or even disseminated disease may develop. In patients who heal their primary lesions, the chest radiograph may be entirely normal or may show focal calcifications. The primary lower lobe lesion and its draining node may be recognized radiologically as the Ghon complex, whereas apical calcifications are termed Simon foci. It is essential to note, however, that healed or inactive granulomatous lesions contain small numbers of dormant but viable tubercle bacilli; inactive lesions can break down and result in reactivation infection.[12]

Reactivation of old tuberculous lesions occurs in no more than 3–5% of all infected individuals, with the remainder having positive skin tests but no clinical illness. At present, only 10% of all new tuberculosis diagnosed in this country result from primary infection, the great majority representing reactivation of latent endogenous infection. As many as one-fifth of patients with reactivation tuberculosis have histories of inadequately treated clinical tuberculosis. Reactivation is most likely to occur within the first few years after the initial infection or at times of lowered host resistance, such as in adolescence or during the postpartum period. However, reactivation can occur many decades after initial infection and, in fact, is now most common in the elderly. Not surprisingly, patients with tuberculosis tend to cluster in certain population groups, being more common in males, in the economically disadvantaged, in inner-city residents, and in members of certain minority groups. The majority of patients with active disease are above 50 years of age, and the proportion of

elderly patients appears to be increasing. Other population groups with a disproportionally high incidence of tuberculosis include immigrants, alcoholics, and patients with gastrectomies, neoplasia, and other debilitating diseases.

The atypical mycobacteria differ from *M. tuberculosis* in several important respects. First, whereas *M. tuberculosis* is highly adapted to humans and is spread by person-to-person transmission, the atypical mycobacteria live free in nature and spread from the environment to man. Person-to-person transmission of atypical mycobacteria does not occur; instead infection is acquired by inhalation of organisms from soil, by ingestion of organisms in milk or water, or by direct inoculation of organisms into the skin. Second, the atypical mycobacteria are much less virulent for man than is *M. tuberculosis*. Skin test surveys suggest that up to 40 million Americans have been infected with atypical mycobacteria, but only about one-third as many people have been infected with *M. tuberculosis*. However, because of the much greater virulence of *M. tuberculosis* and its greater potential for late reactivation, clinically active tuberculosis is much more common than atypical mycobacteriosis. About 25,000 new cases of mycobacterial infection are reported in the United States each year, but the atypical mycobacteria account for no more than 5% of this number.

Another clinically important difference between tuberculosis and the atypicals lies in the significance of a positive culture. Except for the occasional patient with very few organisms identified as a result of contaminated cultures,[13] the isolation of *M. tuberculosis* from a clinical specimen is sufficient to establish the diagnosis of active infection. Diagnosis of atypical mycobacterial infection is much more complex because these organisms can be present as saprophytes or even as laboratory contaminants. When dealing with immunosuppressed patients, the physician must maintain a particularly high index of suspicion about the significance of atypical mycobacteria. Clinical disease caused by an atypical *mycobacterium* should be suspected when the same species is repeatedly isolated from clinical specimens, when other potential pathogens are absent, and when the clinical, radiologic, and pathologic features are suggestive of atypical infection. Differential skin testing may be diagnostically helpful, but unfortunately many immunosuppressed patients are anergic. In all cases, the species of mycobacteria

TABLE 1. Relative Virulence of Certain Mycobacteria Encountered in Clinical Situations

Virulence	Organism (Runyon group)
Pathogens	*M. tuberculosis*
	M. bovis
	M. leprae
	M ulcerans (I)
Usually pathogenic	*M. marinum* (balnei) (I)
	M. kansasii (I)
	M. avium-intracellulare (battey) (III)
Sometimes pathogenic	*M. scrofulaceum* (III)
	M. fortuitum (IV)
	M. chelonei (IV)
Usually nonpathogenic	Bacillus Calmette–Guérin
	M gordonae (II)
Nonpathogenic or opportunistic	*M. gastri* (II)
	M. xenopi (III)
	M. terrae (III)
	M. smegmatis (IV)

isolated may provide important help since some species are much more likely to cause infection than are other low-virulence organisms. Table 1 classifies selected mycobacteria according to relative pathogenic potential. It must be remembered, however, that the compromised host is potentially vulnerable to organisms that are harmless for normal persons. Although diagnosis may be very difficult in these circumstances, it assumes great importance because of the final broad difference between tuberculosis and the atypicals: whereas most strains of *M. tuberculosis* are sensitive to many excellent chemotherapeutic agents, the atypical mycobacteria (except for group I) are generally drug resistant.

2.5. Epidemiology

These pathogenetic considerations are of particular importance in the case of the immunosuppressed host. In most cases, mycobacterial infection in the impaired host results from reactivation of latent endogenous infection. Although ordinary bacterial infections in these patients often originate from endogenous flora, mycobacterial infection differs in several respects. Vulnerability to reactivation can be predicted on the basis of a positive skin test (unless the patient is anergic), a history of previous tuberculosis, or radiographic evidence of old mycobac-

terial infection (Ghon complex, Simon focus). The potential for reactivation is life-long but is increased by factors that depress cellular immunity, such as corticosteroid therapy or cachexia. Thus, in addition to a careful history, physical examination, and chest radiograph, skin testing should be performed in all potentially immunosuppressed patients using PPD to determine tuberculin reactivity and one or more antigens to which most normal patients will react (streptokinase-streptodornase, *Candida*, or mumps) to test for anergy. This is particularly important because of the availability of chemoprophylaxis with isoniazid to prevent reactivation. The pros and cons of chemoprophylaxis are discussed in Section 2.7.

Although reactivation tuberculosis is the greatest risk in the immunocompromised patient, another epidemiologic factor has received insufficient attention: nosocomial infection. Many cases of tuberculosis are not recognized until late in the patient's hospitalization or even at postmortem; this is particularly true in the compromised host.[14] If patients with active pulmonary infection are not isolated appropriately, they may transmit disease to the hospitalized immunoimpaired patient. Finally, mycobacterial infection may even be iatrogenic—the problems of BCG infection and atypical mycobacterioses following surgery or dialysis will be discussed shortly.

Although these immunologic and pathophysiologic considerations provide many reasons why the immunosuppressed host should be more vulnerable to mycobacterial infection, the magnitude of this risk is far from clear. Indeed, with a few notable exceptions,[15] most major overviews of infection in the compromised host devote little attention to the mycobacteria.

Numerous case reports document the occurrance of significant mycobacterial infection in patients with neoplastic disease, but only a few large studies have examined this problem in detail. The association of pulmonary tuberculosis with carcinoma of the lung has long been known.[16] This relationship does not appear to be related to immunosuppression per se, since most of these lung cancer patients develop tuberculosis prior to antineoplastic therapy. In some persons, cachexia may impair host defenses. However, nonimmunologic factors such as smoking, alcohol intake, the occurrence of scar carcinomas in old inflammatory foci, and increased detection as a result of repeated chest radiographs probably account for this association. In fact, although miliary dissemination has occurred in lung cancer patients,[17] pulmonary infection is the rule. Moreover, infection in these individuals tends to behave in routine fashion, unlike the more serious processes encountered in compromised hosts. Pulmonary tuberculosis has also been reported in patients with mesotheliomas.[18]

In a study of cancer patients treated at Memorial Hospital in New York between 1950 and 1971, Kaplan et al.[19] detected 201 cases of active tuberculosis. Patients with lung cancer and lymphoproliferative disorders had the highest incidence of infection. An intermediate incidence was noted in patients with acute leukemias, head and neck malignancies, and stomach cancer. Patients with cancer of the breast, colon, and genitourinary tract had a significantly lower incidence of tuberculosis, but even in these cases, the incidence probably exceeded the risk of active tuberculosis in patients without tumors. In most cases, tuberculosis appeared to result from reactivation of old infection. Patients treated with corticosteroids, radiation, or chemotherapy had more severe forms of tuberculosis. As a group, these patients fared poorly with an overall mortality by tuberculosis of 17%. The prognosis was particularly poor in patients with lymphomas, who had a 48% mortality.

In a study of mycobacterial infections in cancer patients from the M. D. Anderson Hospital in Texas, 59 infections were discovered over a 5-year period.[20] Interestingly, 51% of these infections were caused by nontuberculosis mycobacteria, with *M. kansasii* and *M. fortuitum* being the most important. The geographic distribution of patients may account for the high incidence of atypical mycobacterial infections. The overall incidence of mycobacterial infections was about three times greater than the incidence in the general population of Texas. The median age of these 59 patients was 60 years; even when age adjustments were taken into account, the cancer patients had an incidence of mycobacterial infection about 50% higher than the general population. The most common malignancies in these patients were carcinomas of the head and neck and of the lung. Lymphoma and leukemia were also frequent. Neutropenia did not appear to be a significant factor in these infections, whereas chemotherapy did seem to predispose to infection, especially in the patients

with atypical mycobacterioses. In 80% of these cases, infection was confined to the lungs. Only three patients had miliary infection, and in all, the responsible organism was *M. tuberculosis*. Thirty-one of these 59 patients died, but most did not have autopsies, and it is unclear whether mortality was attributable to mycobacterial infection, the malignancy itself, or other processes. The authors of this study felt that infection was controlled in most patients who were diagnosed early enough to receive adequate antituberculous chemotherapy.

Although these studies of mycobacterial infection and malignancy derive from cancer hospitals, similar findings have been reported in a general hospital population.[21] The prevalence of mycobacterial infection was six times greater in patients with cancer than in the general hospital population. Lung cancer was the most common neoplasm in patients with mycobacterial infection, with hematologic malignancies ranking second. Many patients were receiving chemotherapy when the infection was diagnosed. Only 37% of patients with tuberculosis and cancer had positive tuberculin tests, whereas 70% of the infected patients without tumors were reactors. Nontuberculous mycobacteria were responsible for 27% of the infections, with *M. avium-intracellulare* and *M. kansasii* of equal importance.

Despite these studies, the precise incidence of tuberculosis in cancer patients is unknown. For example, a group of experienced investigators at the National Institutes of Health have not experienced an increased frequency of tuberculosis in patients with leukemia and lymphoma, although they do recognize the problem of disseminated infection in conjunction with chemotherapy.[22] By contrast, studies by the Atomic Bomb Casualty Commission in Hiroshima found an increased incidence of active tuberculosis in patients with chronic myelogenous leukemia and myelofibrosis but not in cases of acute leukemia or lymphoma.[23] The problem of disseminated mycobacterial infection in patients with aplastic anemia and leukemia has received a great deal of attention because of the controversies regarding the causal relationship between the infection and the hematologic abnormalities. This issue is discussed in Section 2.6.

These studies emphasize the importance of a high index of suspicion of tuberculosis in patients with malignant disease. In addition, it is important to remember that tuberculosis itself can present with clinical features which mimic cancer in patients without malignancies.[24] Most often, a tuberculous pulmonary lesion may be radiologically misinterpreted as lung cancer; similarly, tubercular lymphadinitis may be clinically misdiagnosed as lymphoma. Biopsy and culture should establish the correct diagnosis in these cases. Although corticosteroids are frequently cited as the factor most likely to be responsible for the reactivation of tuberculosis in immunosuppressed patients, the actual risk of tuberculosis in steroid-treated patients is unknown. In pharmacologic doses, corticosteroids, suppress inflammation and cause lymphocytopenia and monocytopenia. The direct effects of steroids on lymphocyte function are unclear, but adverse effects on monocyte–macrophage function have been recognized.[25] One result of the daily administration of prednisone is suppression of the delayed hypersensitivity skin test; about 2 weeks of steroid therapy will produce anergy in most patients.[26] By contrast, alternate-day prednisone therapy does not suppress delayed hypersensitivity.[27]

Because steroids suppress cell-mediated immunity, it is logical to expect that they should predispose to the reaction of tuberculosis in previously infected patients. Indeed, the American Thoracic Society recommends the administration of INH to tuberculin-positive patients who require steroid therapy.[28] By contrast, Schatz et al.[29] do not recommend INH prophylaxis because of their failure to detect active tuberculosis in 132 steroid-treated asthmatic patients. However, only 28% of their patients had positive 5-TU tuberculin skin tests, 59% were on alternate-day steroid schedules, and the mean prednisone dose in the patients receiving daily therapy was only 16 mg. Thus, it is far from clear that these patients were truly immunosuppressed, and the conclusions of this study are not necessarily applicable to patients receiving daily prednisone for the treatment of malignancies, transplantation, or inflammatory disease. The same qualifications apply to two large British studies of long-term corticosteroid therapy.[30,31] Although only one case of tuberculosis developed in a total of 786 steroid-treated patients, the great majority of these patients were on low-dose (≤10 mg prednisolone/day) or intermittent therapy, and the tuberculin status of the study population was not defined.

Although the incidence of tuberculosis in steroid-treated patients is unknown, the occurrence of this problem is well documented. Sohn and Lakshminaryan have reported 14 episodes of reactivation tuberculosis associated with corticosteroid therapy.[32] Most of these patients had underlying diseases with immunosuppressive effects, and four were receiving cytotoxic agents as well. Fever was absent in ten cases, suggesting that steroids can mask the symptoms of tuberculosis, making diagnosis difficult. Five patients had disseminated infection, but the response to chemotherapy was good. Because the population at risk was undefined, this study cannot estimate the incidence of tuberculosis in steroid-treated patients, and the authors quite properly refrain from firm recommendations as to the value of INH prophylaxis in steroid-treated patients.

Unfortunately, the incidence of tuberculosis in transplant recipients has not been fully defined. A number of case reports document pulmonary infection,[33,34] extrapulmonary infection,[35,36] and disseminated disease[35,37] caused by *M. tuberculosis*[37,38] and nontuberculous mycobacteria[39–42] in these patients. However, mycobacterial infections are uncommon in transplant recipients. For example, only three of 400 transplant recipients in Denver developed tuberculosis over a 10-year period,[37] and in Minneapolis there were only three cases in 845 recipients over a period of 12 years.[35]

Whereas the risk of tuberculosis in transplant recipients cannot be fully defined, Lichtenstein and MacGregor[43] estimated that it is at least 480 cases per 100,000 as compared with a tuberculosis rate of 131 per 100,000 in the general population. This study includes a number of interesting observations. Of the 47 renal transplant recipients with mycobacterial infection reported from various centers, 20 (43%) had disseminated disease and 16 (38%) had atypical mycobacteria. In two cases, tuberculin-negative recipients developed tuberculosis after receiving kidneys from tuberculin-positive donors, suggesting that infection may arise from reactivation of tubercle bacilli in the transplanted kidney.

Tuberculosis has also been reported in dialysis patients. Five cases of active tuberculosis were noted in one study of 136 dialysis patients;[44] none of the infected patients was receiving immunosuppressive therapy, and only one was a diabetic. The diagnosis of tuberculosis in these patients was difficult because of atypical features and concomitant uremic symptoms. The incidence of tuberculosis in this small group of patients is at least 15 times greater than in the general population and should raise the question of person-to-person transmission within the dialysis unit itself. The possibility of nosocomial infection was considered unlikely by Pradhan et al.,[44] but detailed epidemiologic data are not presented. Other dialysis centers have not reported a high incidence of tuberculosis, and the relevance of this single outbreak to other dialysis and transplant patients is unclear. However, nosocomial outbreaks of *M. chelonei* have been reported at several dialysis centers.[45,46] Clinical vigilance is mandatory, and the possibility of mycobacterial infection must be considered in transplant or dialysis patients with undiagnosed infections. In addition, routine PPD skin testing has been recommended for transplant recipients.[43,47,48] The administration of prophylactic INH to tuberculin-positive patients[43,48,49] has also been suggested but is controversial (see Section 2.7).

2.6. Clinical Features

Even in normal hosts, mycobacterial infections can produce an extremely diverse spectrum of clinical presentations, ranging from subtle disorders to overwhelming disease. In the immunocompromised host, this clinical spectrum is further expanded because, on the one hand, steroids and other medications may suppress fever and other symptoms, whereas, on the other hand, the immunosuppressed state may predispose to unusually fulminant infections. In addition, symptoms of the patient's underlying disorder may confuse the clinical presentation. Finally, the nontuberculous mycobacteria are more often pathogens in these patients, and in some cases patients may be simultaneously infected with mycobacteria and other organisms.

Because of this wide range of clinical presentations, it seems prudent first to review the usual features of tuberculosis and then to examine the unusual problems unique to impaired hosts, concentrating especially on disseminated infection and marrow involvement and on BCG and atypical mycobacteria.

2.6.1. Pulmonary Tuberculosis

2.6.1a. Primary Infection. More than 90% of patients are entirely asymptomatic at the time of pri-

mary infection and can be identified only through conversion of the tuberculin skin test from negative to positive. Most of these patients have normal chest radiographs, but fibrocalcific stigmata of old primary infection are radiographically demonstrable in others. In the past, primary infection occurred almost entirely in childhood, but as the incidence of tuberculosis has declined, primary tuberculosis is also seen in adults. Among symptomatic patients, four broad syndromes can be identified.[50] Most common is a picture not unlike atypical pneumonia with fever and nonproductive cough. Chest radiographs may show unilateral lower lobe patchy parenchymal infiltrates and/or paratracheal or hilar adenopathy. Although such patients should receive full antituberculous chemotherapy when diagnosed, most will go on to resolution of disease even without treatment.

The same is true for patients presenting with the second syndrome, tuberculous pleurisy with effusion. These individuals often have high fever, cough, and pleuritic chest pain and may be dyspneic. Chest radiographs reveal unilateral pleural effusions often without identifiable parenchymal lesions. The diagnosis should be suspected if there is a recent history of exposure to tuberculosis. Except in anergic patients, the tuberculin skin test is almost always strongly positive. Because cultures of sputum and/or gastric washings are positive in only about 30% of these patients, diagnosis depends on examination of the pleural fluid or on percutaneous needle biopsy of the pleura. Although primary tuberculous pleuritis will resolve spontaneously in most cases, up to 60% of these patients develop reactivation tuberculosis, so combined chemotherapy is indicated in all patients. Surgery is almost never needed, and complications are rare.

The third major syndrome of primary tuberculosis is direct progression to upper lobe disease. Finally, patients may develop extrapulmonary tuberculosis as a progression of primary infection. This was previously seen most commonly in young children who presented with cervical adenitis, miliary tuberculosis, or tuberculous meningitis but is now quite rare. Immunosuppressed patients may be at increased risk of miliary dissemination. In addition to these major manifestations, patients with primary tuberculosis may develop a variety of syndromes including erythema nodosum and other hypersensitivity reactions.

2.6.1b. Reactivation (Postprimary) Tuberculosis. This is the most common clinical form of tuberculosis and is seen most often in the elderly or debilitated patient. Symptoms usually begin insidiously and progress over a period of many weeks or months prior to diagnosis. Constitutional symptoms are often prominent including anorexia, weight loss, and night sweats. Most patients have low-grade fevers, but higher temperatures and even chills may be seen occasionally when the disease progresses more rapidly. Immunosuppressed patients are at greater risk of rapidly progressive pulmonary involvement. For example, nine of the 201 cancer patients with tuberculosis reported by Kaplan et al.[19] developed tuberculous pneumonia, which was uniformly fatal. One of these patients progressed from an inactive Ghon complex to fulminant tuberculous pneumonia, respiratory failure, and death in 6 days. Even in normal hosts, miliary tuberculosis can on rare occasion present with rapidly progressive diffuse interstitial infiltrates causing adult respiratory distress syndrome (ARDS).[51] Hence, although a subacute to chronic presentation is much more common, tuberculosis must also be considered in the differential diagnosis of rapidly progressive alveolar or interstitial infiltrates in the immunocompromised patient.

Most patients with postprimary tuberculosis present with pulmonary symptoms including cough and sputum production. Dyspnea is relatively uncommon in the absence of underlying chronic lung disease. A frequent complaint is hemoptysis, often in the form of bright red streaks of blood caused by bronchial irritation. Although physical examination is usually nondiagnostic, chest radiographs are highly suggestive of the diagnosis. Typical features include infiltration in the posterior–apical pulmonary segments, which may be unilateral or bilateral, progressing to frank cavitation. Apical lordotic views, chest tomography, and CT scans may be helpful in documenting cavitary disease. In occasional patients, the lower lung fields may be involved with postprimary tuberculosis, and in rare instances the chest radiograph may appear normal.[52,53]

The tuberculin skin test is positive in about 80% of patients with reactivation tuberculosis; patients with advanced disease are often malnourished and anergic. The diagnosis of pulmonary tuberculosis can be confirmed in most individuals by examination of the sputum. If patients are not able to produce sputum spontaneously, attempts should be made to induce sputum with the aid of pulmonary physiotherapy, IPPB, and mucolytic agents. Bronchoscopy may be necessary to obtain appropriate specimens. Although cultures are necessary for a positive diagnosis and are more sensitive than smears, sputum specimens should be examined microscopically either by the traditional Ziehl-Neelson acid-fast stain or by the newer Truant fluorescent stain. Sputum or bronchoscopic washings should be examined both directly and after concentration by centrifugation and digestion. Carefully collected individual specimens are preferred to a 24-hr pool of sputum and saliva. Cultures of first morning fasting gastric aspirates are also helpful. Because gastric acid is toxic to mycobacteria, the collection bottles should contain a buffer such as sodium bicarbonate. Smears of gastric juice are misleading because of the potential presence of saprophytic mycobacteria and should not be performed.

With combined chemotherapy, the prognosis of pulmonary tuberculosis is excellent. Without therapy, devastating complications may occur. Massive hemoptysis is one such complication. The vessels in the walls of tuberculous cavities are usually thrombosed and do not bleed, but if a pulmonary artery branch is patent, erosion into the vessel can produce a Rasmussen aneurysm and massive hemoptysis. Another complication is bronchogenic spread of infection to other pulmonary segments. In extreme cases, this can result in massive tuberculous pneumonia with hypoxia and an acute lethal course despite chemotherapy. Other complications of pulmonary tuberculosis include direct spread of infection to the pleural space, resulting in a bronchopleural fistula or tuberculous empyema, or to the upper airway, resulting in tuberculous laryngitis. Swallowed organisms can produce tuberculous enteritis. Tuberculous pericarditis may result from direct extension of an adjacent pulmonary focus. In other patients, late fibrosis may produce bronchial obstruction and/or mediastinal fibrosis. Bronchial obstruction may also be caused by extrinsic compression because of tuberculous lymphadenitis; such patients may develop secondary bacterial pneumonias. Still another complication of pulmonary tuberculosis is hematogenous dissemination with simultaneous extrapulmonary disease. Finally, the syndrome of inappropriate ADH is a not infrequent metabolic complication of pulmonary tuberculosis. Anemia is common in patients with advanced or longstanding disease. Diffuse hyperglobulinemia and elevated erythrocyte sedimentation rates are also common but nonspecific. Secondary amyloidosis is rare.

Illustrative Case 1: Pulmonary Tuberculosis

This 21-year-old woman was hospitalized in 1979 for neurologic reevaluation. She had been well until 1974 when she noted stumbling and right leg weakness. Over the next year she developed slurred speech, nystagmus, an obvious right-sided hemiparesis. She was hospitalized for study. Skull radiographs, a brain scan, and an EEG were unremarkable, but a pneumoencephalogram disclosed a mass lesion in the floor of the fourth ventricle with compression of the prepontine space The CSF was normal. Her chest radiograph, hemogram, and liver-function tests were normal A tuberculin skin test was not performed. She was considered to have a malignant brain stem tumor and was treated with 6000 rad and started on dexamethasone.

Over the ensuing 4 years, she remained on monthly CCNU injections. Several months prior to admission, she noted increased right leg weakness, and corticosteroid therapy was reinstituted. On presentation she was a frail, wasted dysarthic young woman with a right hemiparesis. She did not have a cushingoid habitus. She was afebrile and had no respiratory or constitutional symptoms. There was no history of exposure to tuberculosis.

The neurologic workup revealed a cystic brain stem lesion that subsequently proved to be a benign cyst. However, a routine admission chest radiograph revealed a cavitating lesion in the superior segment of the right lower lobe (Fig. 1). No sputum was available for examination. Her laboratory studies revealed a mild anemia with a normal white count and differential, a slightly elevated alkaline phosphatase and 5'-nucleotidase, and mild hyperglobulinemia. Intermediate strength (5 TU) PPD and SK–SD skin tests were negative.

Because of the peripheral location of the lesion, she underwent a percutaneous lung biopsy rather than a bronchoscopy Cytological examination revealed only inflammatory cells, and smears for acid-fast bacilli, bacteria, and fungi were negative Following the biopsy, she developed a 20% right pneumothorax that failed to resolve. Corticosteroids were discontinued. She became febrile to 103°F (39.4°C) and developed a mild nonproductive cough. After 6 weeks of incubation, her lung biopsy cultures became positive for *M tuberculosis* Therapy with INH, etham-

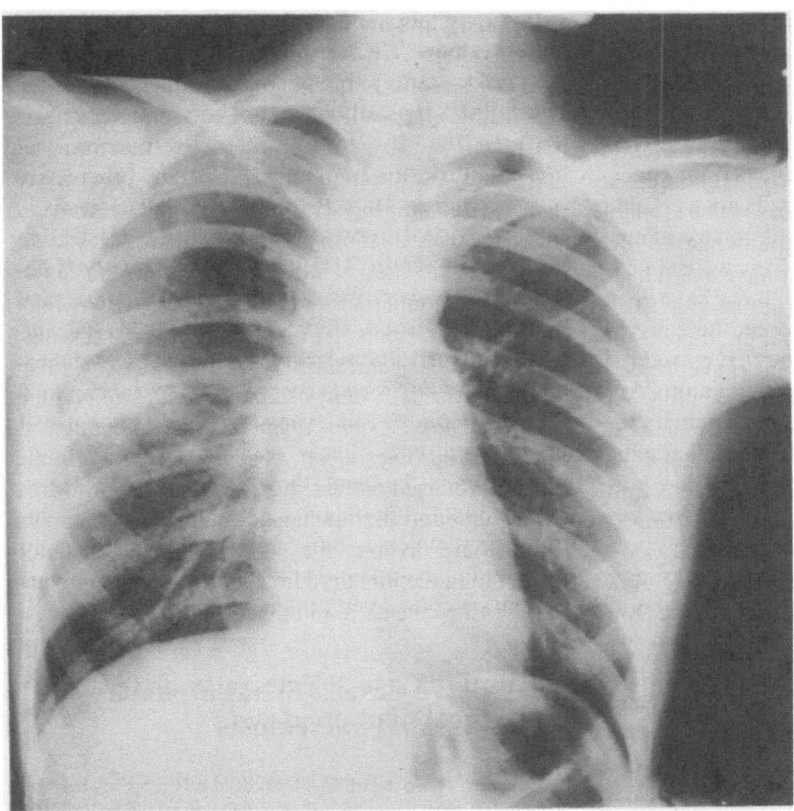

FIGURE 1. Chest radiograph from Illustrative Case 1 demonstrating a cavity lesion in the superior segment of the right lower lobe

butol, and streptomycin was instituted. Within 5 days she became afebrile, and her cough had ceased After 3 weeks of therapy, the pneumothorax resolved, and the infiltrate was appreciably smaller. After 6 weeks, streptomycin was discontinued, and she has continued to do well on INH and ethambutol.

Comment. Unfortunately, this young woman had received radiotherapy, chemotherapy, and corticosteroids for what eventually proved to be nonmalignant disease. Cutaneous anergy reflected the immunocompromised state that resulted from drug therapy and cachexia. Of interest was the fact that she was entirely free of both pulmonary symptoms and fever despite a large cavitary lesion, corticosteroids have been reported to mask the symptoms of tuberculosis in some patients, and this patient became febrile only when steroids were discontinued. This case demonstrates several points about the diagnosis of pulmonary tuberculosis when no sputum is available: invasive procedures such as lung biopsy or bronchoscopy may be necessary; cultures may be positive even when smears are negative, and persistent pneumothorax can complicate percutaneous lung biopsy in tuberculosis. Although many compromised hosts with tuberculosis fare poorly, this patient did very well, in part because it was possible to discontinue immunosuppressive therapy.

2.6.2. Extrapulmonary Tuberculosis

Approximately 10% of all newly recognized cases of tuberculosis in the United States are extrapulmonary; although the frequency of pulmonary tuberculosis is declining, the incidence of extrapulmonary disease is remaining relatively constant.[54] Although the clinical features of extrapulmonary tuberculosis vary widely, certain generalizations may be useful. Past history is not a reliable guide to the diagnosis of extrapulmonary tuberculosis; only about 25% of patients have a past history of tuberculosis, but virtually all of these have been inadequately treated. Except in children, there is typically a long latent period between the first episode of infection and the extrapulmonary presentation. Approximately 50% of patients with extrapulmonary tuberculosis have entirely normal chest radiographs; most of the others have stigmata of old inactive pulmonary disease, and a minority have coexisting active pulmonary infection. Although all organ systems can be involved with extrapulmonary disease, either singly or in various combinations, the most commonly involved areas are the genitourinary tract, the musculoskeletal system, and the lymph nodes.

Although generalizations are subject to many exceptions, I think it is clinically useful to divide extrapulmonary tuberculosis into three large categories. The first is subacute, progressive, life-threatening disease. These patients are generally febrile and

have prominent constitutional symptoms suggestive of infection. The tuberculin skin test may be negative in up to 20% because of the severity of the illness itself. Without therapy, they experience a progressive, downhill course with an extremely high mortality rate, often in a matter of weeks. Important examples of this fulminating type of extrapulmonary tuberculosis are miliary tuberculosis,[55,56] tuberculous meningitis,[57–59] and tuberculosis of the pericardium[60,61] and great vessels. Disseminated mycobacterial infection is a particular problem in immunosuppressed patients and is discussed separately (see Section 2.6.3).

The second category of extrapulmonary tuberculosis may be thought of as tuberculosis of the large serosal surfaces. These patients too have prominent constitutional symptoms including fever in almost all cases. As a rule, however, the tuberculin skin test is positive, the clinical course is longer, and the prognosis with or without therapy is better. Examples in this category include tuberculous pleuritis[62] and peritonitis.[63]

The third and most common type of extrapulmonary tuberculosis is infection of individual organ systems. These patients are most often afebrile and can be entirely free of constitutional complaints. Their illness typically pursues a very indolent course characterized by local organ dysfunction and eventually destruction rather than by progressive general decline. In fact, the differential diagnosis in these individuals more often suggests neoplastic disease then infection. Unless cellular immunity is depressed, the tuberculin skin test is positive in almost all of these patients. Clinical syndromes in this category include genitourinary tuberculosis,[64] tuberculous arthritis,[65] and osteomyelitis,[66] tuberculous lymphadenitis,[67] and many others. Although all these syndromes can occur in the immunocompromised patient, they are uncommon. Moreover, although the diagnostic features of these syndromes are diverse, they are not characteristically different in the impaired host; hence, these problems will not be considered in detail here.

Illustrative Case 2: Extrapulmonary (Meningeal) Tuberculosis

This 9-year-old girl was hospitalized because of fever and lethargy. Eighteen months earlier she was found to have Hodgkin disease, nodular sclerosing stage IIIB A complete remission had been induced and maintained with chlorambucil, vincristine, procarbazine, and prednisone. Twelve days prior to admission, she developed fevers to 102°F (38 9°C) and generalized headache. Seven days before admission she developed vomiting. Over the ensuing week, she remained febrile and became progressively lethargic. There was no history of exposure to tuberculosis

At the time of admission, she was drowsy but arousable and oriented. Aside from mild nuchal rigidity and a temperature of 103.2°F, her physical examination was normal. Laboratory studies included a Hct of 34% and a WBC count of 2700/mm^3 with 64% polys, 16% lymphocytes, and 20% monocytes. The platelets appeared normal on smear. The chest radiograph was normal, as was the urinalysis. Blood chemistries including liver function tests were normal. Blood and urine cultures were negative. Intermediate-strength PPD and *Candida* skin tests were negative

On the day of admission, a lumbar puncture revealed clear CSF under a pressure of 240 cm H_2O. The CSF contained six RBCs and 336 WBCs/mm^3, of which 97% were lymphocytes. The CSF protein was 116 mg/dl, and the sugar was 24 mg/dl with a simultaneous blood sugar of 96 mg/dl. Gram stain, AFB stain, and India ink preparations of the CSF were negative, as were cytologic examinations and a latex agglutination test for cryptococcal polysaccharide. No therapy was instituted. However, 48 hr later, the patient was more lethargic and was found to have bilateral sixth nerve palsies. Cultures of CSF for bacteria were negative. Therapy with INH, rifampin, and ethambutol was instituted. By the fifth day of treatment, she became afebrile, and her headache, stiff neck, and sixth nerve palsies resolved over the next 8–10 days. Cerebrospinal fluid cultures grew *M. tuberculosis*. The patient was maintained on all three drugs for 3 months and on INH and ethambutol for an additional 2 years. She remained free of tuberculosis, but her Hodgkin disease has relapsed.

Comment This child was clearly immunosuppressed as a result of Hodgkin disease and its chemotherapy. Like so many patients with extrapulmonary tuberculosis, she had neither a history of exposure to tuberculosis nor an abnormal chest radiograph. Her case illustrates the typical clinical features of tuberculous meningitis. This is the most rapidly progressive form of tuberculosis, and the history of fever, headache, and irritability progressing to lethargy and cranial nerve palsies over a period of about 3 weeks is highly characteristic. The CSF findings of a moderate lymphocytic pleiocytosis, low sugar, and elevated protein are also typical. This case also demonstrates that CSF cultures are more sensitive than acid-fast stains in the diagnosis of meningeal tuberculosis. Finally, her physicians proceeded appropriately in rapidly excluding bacterial, fungal, and neoplastic meningitis and in instituting antituberculous chemotherapy long before cultures became positive. Isoniazid, ethambutol, and rifampin all penetrate the CSF, and this girl's response to triple therapy was excellent

2.6.3. Disseminated Mycobacterial Infection and Hematologic Abnormalities

The problem of disseminated mycobacterial infection in patients with hematologic abnormalities is of particular interest. The Atomic Bomb Casualty Commission found an increased incidence of tuberculosis in patients with chronic myelogenous leukemia and myelofibrosis but not in patients with acute leukemia or lymphoma.[23] A more recent clinical series[68] found a 4.6% incidence of tuberculosis among 130 patients with hematologic diseases but only a 0.2% incidence among 13,930 patients without marrow disorders admitted to the same hospital during the same 18-month period. However, in a much larger autopsy series surveying 27,104 cases postmortem between 1925 and 1952, Lowther[69] found no evidence of an increased incidence of tuberculosis in leukemics.

If the risk of tuberculosis in patients with leukemia is unsettled, there is even more controversy about the significance of hematologic abnormalities in patients with tuberculosis. Most patients with miliary tuberculosis have some abnormality of the hemogram, which often includes anemia and which may include leukopenia, leukocytosis, and monocytosis.[70] In occasional patients, a dramatic leukemoid reaction can accompany miliary tuberculosis. However, in all these situations, the hematologic findings revert to normal during the course of effective antituberculous therapy.

In addition to these patients, numerous case reports describe the occurrence of either a frankly leukemic blood picture or of severe pancytopenia resembling aplastic anemia in patients with disseminated mycobacterial disease. On the basis of these reports, tuberculosis has sometimes been considered a "treatable" cause of leukemia or aplastic anemia. The careful study conducted by Glasser et al.[70] casts serious doubt on this proposition. From among 3507 tuberculosis patients, they studied 40 with miliary disease. Thirty-five had hematologic abnormalities, including anemia in 63% and leukopenia in 32%. Only three patients had a bacteriologic cure without full return to normal of the hematologic abnormalities, and of these patients with persistent abnormalities, one had clear-cut chronic lymphocytic leukemia, and two had only mild anemia. However, none of these patients had blood pictures resembling myeloproliferative disorders or aplastic anemia. In sharp contrast, this same study also identified 24 patients with leukemia, lymphoma, myeloma, or aplastic anemia and tuberculosis. None of these patients demonstrated hematologic recovery as a result of antituberculous therapy.

In reviewing the reported cases of leukemia or pancytopenia in patients with tuberculosis. Glasser et al.[70] point out that the vast majority of these cases have been fatal and that none of these patients has had documented marrow recovery as a result of antimicrobial therapy alone. They conclude that tuberculosis does not cause these severe marrow abnormalities but that patients with primary hematologic abnormalities may be unusually susceptible to disseminated and rapidly fatal mycobacterial infection because of their immunologic impairments. More recently, a patient with severe pancytopenia who survived miliary tuberculosis was reported.[71] However, although the patient was said to be "perfectly well" following therapy, no post-treatment hematologic data are presented. An additional patient with disseminated *M. kansasii* infection and pancytopenia recovered clinically and had recovery of normal marrow function after therapy.[72] Even granting marrow recovery in these patients, tuberculosis must be exceedingly rare as a bona fide cause of pancytopenia or of a truly leukemic blood picture.

Patients with leukemia or pancytopenia in whom mycobacterial infections develop may manifest either of two unique features of their infection. First is the occurrence of disseminated infection with atypical mycobacteria. Of 59 cancer patients with mycobacterial infection at M. D. Anderson, 51% were infected with nontuberculous mycobacteria.[20] Although none of these patients had disseminated disease, numerous case reports document the occurrence of disseminated atypical mycobacterial infection in patients with leukemia[73-80] or pancytopenia.[81-84] In many of these patients, *M. kansasii*, *M. avium-intracellulare*, or *M. chelonei* was the causative organism. Not surprisingly, these cases have almost all been fatal.

The second striking feature of tuberculous infection in patients with leukemia is the severity of the infection. In a postmortem series, Oswald[85] found that although tuberculosis was not more common in patients dying of leukemia than in those dying of other causes, there was a clear propensity for miliary dissemination in the leukemic patients. Among 262 patients dying with leukemia, 16 had inactive pulmonary tuberculosis, only three had active pulmonary infection, but 10 had miliary disease. Moreover, these infections were clinically fulminant, and many cases had a destructive pathologic picture of nonreactive tuberculosis. In nonreactive tuberculosis, lesions are more common in nodes and visceral organs and less common in the lungs and meninges than in ordinary miliary tuberculosis. The lesions themselves consist of areas of tissue necrosis teeming with acid-fast bacilli; there is little evidence of granuloma formation, although a polymorphonuclear exudate may be seen.[85,86] It seems clear that the immunologic deficiency of these patients impairs granuloma formation, thus allowing unchecked multiplication of bacilli and overwhelming infection in a situation analogous to lepromatous leprosy. Although nonreactive tuberculosis is rare, the diagnosis must be considered in leukemic or other immunosuppressed patients with overwhelming infection. In practical terms, it must be remembered that the absence of miliary lung lesions does not rule out disseminated mycobacterial infection and that even if biopsy specimens show only necrosis and acute inflammation without granulomas, acid-fast stains and mycobacterial cultures can still provide vital diagnostic information.

Illustrative Case 3: Occult Miliary Tuberculosis

This 65-year-old Polish-born gentleman was hospitalized in July 1969 because of recurrent fever There was no history of exposure to tuberculosis at any time. He had been entirely well except for head trauma sustained in an auto accident 3 years earlier. His only medications were phenytion (Dilantin) and phenobarbital. Three weeks before admission, he first experienced fevers to 104°F that recurred nightly. He admitted to rigors, drenching sweats, anorexia, and a 14-lb (6.4 kg) weight loss, but he denied other symptoms.

At the time of hospitalization he was an elderly, wasted, chronically ill man with a temperature of 104 6°F. His fundi were normal, and his neck was supple. His lungs were clear A soft systolic ejection murmur was audible at the cardiac apex. There was no hepatosplenomegaly or lymphadenopathy His admission laboratory studies included a Hct of 24%, a white WBC count of 1900/mm³ with 65% polys, 1% bands, 27% lymphocytes, 2% monocytes, and 5% eosinophils, and a platelet count of 69,000/mm³. The ESR was 69 mm/hr The urine was normal, as were the blood chemistries apart from an alkaline phosphatase of 8.7 BU (normal <4.5), an SGOT of 52 units (normal <40). Multiple cultures of blood and urine were negative The chest radiograph was normal.

In the hospital he had daily fevers, reaching 107°F on one occasion He grew progressively weaker. An IVP, a barium enema, and a UGI series were normal. Tuberculin skin tests with both 5 and 250 TU were negative, as were SK–SD and mumps skin tests. On the sixth hospital day, a bone marrow biopsy was performed, revealing reticulum cell sarcoma but no granulomas Before therapy could be instituted, he was found dead in bed on the ninth hospital day At autopsy, the patient was found to have reticulum cell sarcoma of the marrow, spleen, and paraaortic nodes In addition, there were multiple noncaseating granulomas in the liver (Fig. 2) and caseating granulomas in the marrow, spleen, and mediastinal lymph nodes but not in the lung. Acid-fast smears were negative, but cultures grew *M. tuberculosis.*

Comment. This case is unusual in that the patient was found to have a lymphoproliferative disease and miliary tuberculosis simultaneously. His fever, chills, weight loss, and pancytopenia could have been caused by the tumor, the tuberculosis, or both. He demonstrated cutaneous anergy, and his immunosuppressed state was probably caused by widespread lymphoma and cachexia.

This case demonstrates a number of features of miliary tuberculosis in the immunosuppressed patient. This diagnosis was not considered because of the normal chest radiograph, yet up to 10% of patients with miliary tuberculosis have normal chest radiographs Moreover, the involvement of liver, spleen, and nodes without pulmonary lesions appears to be more common in the immunosuppressed patient. This man had well-formed gran-

ulomas rather than the necrosis with acute inflammation sometimes seen in immunosuppressed hosts with fulminating nonreactive tuberculosis. This case also demonstrates that granulomas can be missed on marrow biopsy because of sampling error and that hepatic granulomas in tuberculosis are frequently noncaseating Finally, he illustrates the difficulty of determining whether pancytomenia is related to tuberculosis, tumor, or both The cause of this man's death was not determined, but even if chemotherapy had been instituted, the prognosis would have been very poor

Illustrative Case 4: Disseminated Nontuberculous Mycobacteriosis

This 48-year-old man was hospitalized in 1977 because of spiking fevers Two years earlier, a splenectomy and bone marrow biopsy were performed because of profound fatigue and severe

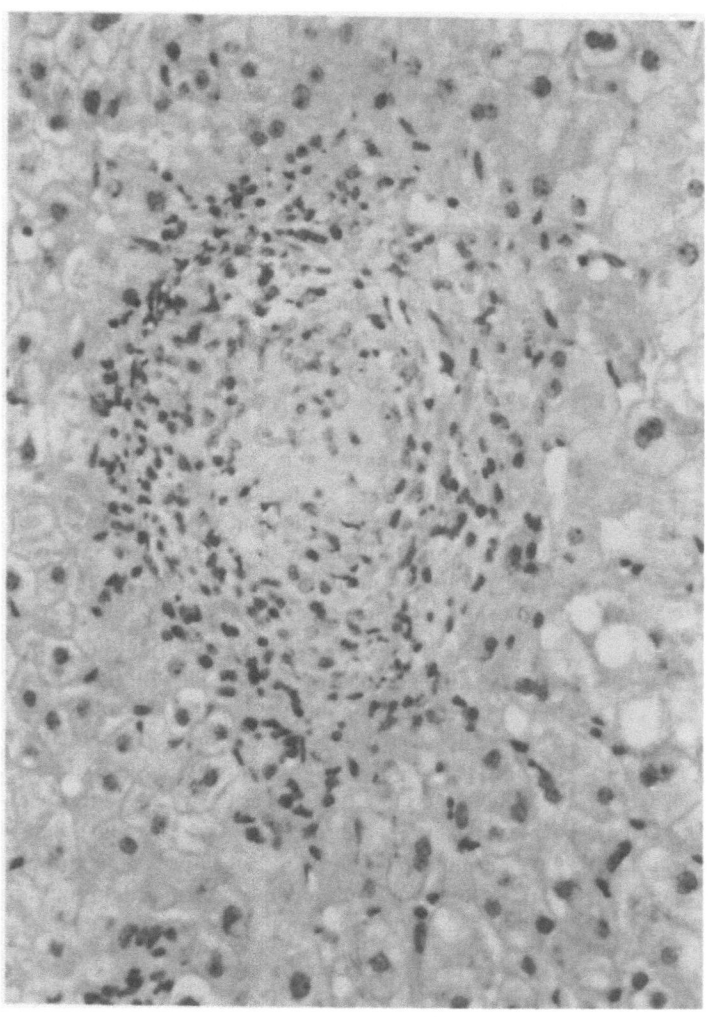

FIGURE 2. Liver biopsy from Illustrative Case 3 demonstrating granulomatous inflammation without caseation

pancytopenia He was found to have a malignant lymphoma of the poorly differentiated lymphocytic type He responded symptomatically to transfusions, prednisone, and cyclophosphamide Although there was no history of exposure to tuberculosis, his chest roentgenogram showed a calcified granuloma in the apical posterior segment of the left upper lobe An intermediate-strength PPD administered prior to therapy was positive Isoniazid was not prescribed.

Four months prior to admission, pancytopenia recurred His peripheral blood contained more than 50% mononuclear cells, many of which had hairy cytoplasmic borders Cyclophosphamide and prednisone were reinstituted He improved symptomatically, but 3 months later a temperature of 104 8°F as well as rigors and sweats developed He was hospitalized elsewhere. His physical examination was normal apart from fever. His chest radiograph showed hilar adenopathy Multiple blood and urine cultures were negative. Therapy with oxacillin, gentamicin, INH, ethambutol, prednisone, and indomethacin failed to control the fever, and he was transferred to the Massachusetts General Hospital

On admission, he was febrile to 103.4°F (39 7°C) He appeared acutely and chronically ill, and examination disclosed a cushingoid habitus, pallor, hepatomegaly, and mild confusion The Hct was 35%, the platelets 137,000/mm^3, and the WBC count 1700/mm^3 with 30% polys, 19% bands, 6% eosinophils, and 2% metamyelocytes. The urinalysis was normal, and the chest radiograph was unchanged. Blood chemistries included an SGOT that was elevated to 86 units and an alkaline phosphatase that was elevated to 17.7 Bodansky units Cultures of blood and urine remained sterile An attempted bone marrow aspiration yielded only a few mononuclear cells However, a liver biopsy revealed multiple noncaseating granulomas Acid-fast stains were negative, but culture grew *M avium-intracellulare* resistant to all antituberculous agents. The patient was treated with numerous medications including, at various times, INH, ethambutol, rifampin, streptomycin, pyrazinamide, and cycloserine. Nevertheless, his condition deteriorated with ongoing fevers, wasting, progressive hepatic dysfunction, and finally diffuse pulmonary infiltrates He died 4 months later Permission for an autopsy was denied

Comment. This patient demonstrates many of the features of disseminated mycobacterial infection that were evident in the preceding case The major difference is that this patient was infected with a group III atypical mycobacteria that were highly resistant to chemotherapeutic agents Disseminated infection with such organisms is rare in immunologically intact hosts but carries a grave prognosis in the impaired host. Although the diagnosis was made promptly in this case, therapy was ineffective, and the patient died of overwhelming *M avium-intracellulare* infection.

2.6.4. Bacillus Calmette-Guérin Vaccine in Immunocompromised Patients

Bacillus Calmette-Guérin (BCG) is a live attenuated strain of *M. bovis* that was introduced into clinical use in 1921. BCG remains controversial with estimates of its efficacy in providing protection against tuberculosis ranging from zero to 80%.[2,3,87]

Because of the low incidence of new tuberculous infection in the United States, BCG is not currently recommended for routine use.

Hundreds of millions of doses of BCG have been administered around the world. BCG is extremely safe when given intradermally to normal patients in doses recommended for the prevention of tuberculosis. Local reactions such as ulceration at the vaccination site and lymphadenitis are uncommon and are generally self-limited; BCG osteomyelitis is rare, and disseminated BCG infection is very rare.[2,87] Because most of these serious reactions have occurred in immunosuppressed patients, BCG should not be administered for the prevention of tuberculosis to patients with lymphoma, leukemia, or widespread cancer or to those receiving immunosuppressive drugs or radiotherapy.[2]

Over the past few years, however, BCG has been studied extensively as an immunotherapeutic agent in patients with melanoma, leukemia, lymphoma, and other malignancies.[88] The administration of BCG to cancer patients differs from the use of BCG as a vaccine against tuberculosis in several important respects.[89] Cancer patients are often given repeated doses of BCG, sometimes at intervals as short as 5 days. Extremely large doses may be given; in some protocols, organisms are injected directly into vascular tumor masses rather than into normal skin. Finally, the patients themselves are often immunosuppressed because of advanced malignancy, chemotherapy, or both.

Not surprisingly, cancer patients receiving BCG immunotherapy have experienced a variety of adverse reactions to the injection of viable mycobacteria. These complications can be divided into two broad categories. In immunocompetent patients, repeated injections can lead to hypersensitivity reactions, including local erythema and induration, regional lymphadenopathy, and constitutional reactions, including fever and even anaphylaxis and fatal shock with disseminated intravascular coagulation (DIC).[88] By contrast, in immunosuppressed patients, complications can be related to the unchecked spread of mycobacteria. These complications have been most pronounced following intratumor injection of BCG. Symptoms may include fever, chills, and an influenzalike syndrome in as many as 64% of patients receiving intralesional BCG.[90,91] Abnormal liver function tests are common in this setting, and hepatic dysfunction can be severe and persistent. Disseminated BCG infection can be documented by finding granulomas in the liver and bone marrow. BCG is sensitive to INH and to most other antituberculous agents. However, although some groups have found chemotherapy efficacious in the control of disseminated BCGosis in immunosuppressed patients,[90,91] others have been disappointed by the results of INH therapy.[91]

Another reported complication of BCG immunotherapy is the occurrence of radiographically evident pulmonary granulomas that mimic recurrent metastatic cancer.[90,105] These have occurred even after intradermal administration of BCG by the multiple-puncture technique. Although these patients are as a rule asymptomatic, the lesions can be clinically important if they are radiographically mistaken for malignancies.

In summary, BCG should not be given to immunosuppressed patients for the prevention of tuberculosis. When BCG is administered for the experimental immunotherapy of malignancies, both local and systemic reactions can occur. In immunocompetent patients, hypersensitivity reactions can range from local inflammation to life-threatening anaphylaxis. In immunosuppressed patients, disseminated BCGosis may occur with fever and hepatic dysfunction reflecting granulomatous lesions in liver, bone marrow, and lung. Pulmonary granulomas may be mistaken for tumor. Systemic BCG infections are generally seen in patients receiving intralesional injections. Although most patients recover spontaneously, morbidity can be prolonged. Antituberculous chemotherapy is indicated, but results have been variable.

2.6.5. Mycobacterial Infections in AIDS

Mycobacteria are among the many infectious agents that can cause serious disease in patients with AIDS (see Chapter 15). Both pathogenic (*M. tuberculosis*) and opportunistic (*M. avium-intracellulare* and other atypical forms) mycobacterial species can cause disease in these patients. Dissemination is the rule and the response to chemotherapy is generally poor; other infections are present simultaneously in most cases.

Tuberculosis was diagnosed in 27 of 45 Haitians with AIDS in Florida (92). In 22 (81%) of these patients, tuberculosis was discovered 1–17 months before the diagnosis of AIDS was established. Nineteen (70%) of these patients had extrapulmonary tuberculosis. Only one of these Haitians with AIDS had disseminated *M. avium-intracellulare* infection. Unfortunately, follow-up date were available in only a few of these patients, but all 10 patients with pulmonary tuberculosis who could be evaluated responded favorably to antituberculous chemotherapy, which included INH and rifampin in all cases.

In non-Haitians with AIDS, infection with *M. avium-intracellulare* appears to be more common than infection with *M. tuberculosis,* and the response to chemotherapy is much less favorable.[93–97] Disseminated infection is common, with organisms frequently present in the lungs, liver, spleen, and lymph nodes. Despite the presence of many mycobacteria in macrophages, well-formed granulomas are typically absent; this lepromatous histology reflects the profound impairment of cell-mediated immunity in these patients and explains their inability to contain the infection. Patients with AIDS may also exhibit an impaired humoral (antibody) response to *M. avium-intracellulare.*[98] When the newer blood culture techniques are utilized (65b), a high-grade *M. avium-intracellulare* bacillium can be demonstrated in many patients with AIDS.[99,100] Intestinal infection can often be documented by stool or colonic biopsy cultures.[101] *M. avium-intracellulare* may contribute to diarrhea in these patients. It is not known whether the GI tract is the portal of infection in these patients or whether the intestinal infection is a manifestation of dissemined infection from a pulmonary source.

Although multiple antituberculous drugs are used in these patients, the response to therapy is usually poor: cultures typically remain positive and clinical and radiographic evidence of atypical mycobacterial infection progresses. Because neoplasia and multiple viral, parasitic, bacterial, and fungal infections often coexist with mycobacterial infection in patients with AIDS, it is often difficult to determine how much the mycobacteria per se contributes to any patient's demise.

M. xenopi was isolated from the lung and liver of a patient with AIDS; cultures became negative on INH, rifampin, and pyrazinamide.[102]

Illustrative Case 5: Disseminated *M. Avium-intracellulare* in AIDS

This 38-year-old homosexual man developed cervical lymphadenopathy in December 1982. In February 1983, he noted weight loss, generalized lymphadenopathy, and oral candidiasis. Two months later, he was hospitalized with *Pneumocystis* pneumonia; a rash developed during therapy with trimethoprim–sulfamethoxazole, but the patient responded to pentamidine. Cutaneous Kaposi sarcoma developed in May 1983. Esophageal herpes simplex infection was documented by biopsy that same month, and ocular changes consistent with CMV infection developed shortly thereafter.

In July 1983, pancytopenia developed. A bone marrow biopsy revealed numerous acid-fast bacilli but no granulomas. Sputum smears revealed acid-fast bacilli, but the chest radiograph was clear. Sputum, blood, bone marrow, and stool cultures grew *M. avium-intracellulare*. The patient was treated with ansamycin, clofazamine, cycloserine, and isoniazid, which was discontinued after sensitivity testing revealed that the organisms were INH resistant.

Despite continued antituberculous therapy, blood, sputum, and stool cultures remained positive for *M. avium-intracellulare*. Diarrhea, profound weight loss, progressive lymphodenopathy, and hepatosplenomegaly were noted. Cutaneous lesions of Kaposi sarcoma progressed and nodular pulmonary lesions developed. By January 1984 the patient weighed only 66 lb (30 kg). A rapidly progressive encephalopathy developed, and the patient died.

Autopsy findings included Kaposi sarcoma of skin and lung, disseminated CMV, and diffuse encephalitis without organisms. The spleen and many lymph nodes were massively infiltrated with foamy macrophages laden with acid-fast bacilli. Similar macrophages were present in periportal areas of the liver, in the small bowel lamina propria, and in the subcutaneous fat. The bone marrow and lungs contained acid-fast bacilli. No granulomas were identified in any organ. Postmortem cultures were positive for *M. avium-intracellulare*.

Comment. In only 13 months, this young man lost 100 lb (45 kg). *Pneumocystis* pneumonia, oral candidiasis, esophageal herpes infection, and disseminated CMV were all important problems, but the dominant infection was disseminated *M. avium-intracellulare*. Despite ansamysin, clofazimine, and cycloserine, the infection progressed relentlessly. Kaposi sarcoma and AIDS encephalopathy combined with *M. avium-intracellulare* to cause death. Autopsy confirmed an enormous mycobacterial burden with a total absence of an appropriate granulomatous response, a situation reminiscent of lepromatous leprosy. When disseminated *M. avium-intracellulare* first becaue evident, the patient had a normal chest radiograph despite positive sputum smears and cultures. In 12% of patients with AIDS, chest radiographs are normal despite positive sputum cultures. The most common radiographic abnormality in this setting is hilar or mediastinal adenopathy (59%), localized infiltrates in the lower lung fields occur in 29%, but upper lobe infiltrates occur in only 18% [103]

2.7. Management of Mycobacterial Infections

The chemotherapy of tuberculosis in both normal and immunocompromised hosts involve two very different issues: isoniazid prophylaxis of patients who have been exposed to tuberculosis but are free of active disease, and combined chemotherapy of patients with active infection. Paradoxically, although there are many more patients who may be considered for chemoprophylaxis than there are patients with active tuberculosis, the guidelines for INH prophylaxis are more controversial than are the recommendations for chemotherapy. This is particularly true in the immunosuppressed host.

2.7.1. Chemoprophylaxis

The question of chemoprophylaxis is raised most commonly in patients with positive tuberculin skin tests. Except in patients who have received chemotherapy, a positive skin test implies the presence of a few dormant but viable tubercle bacilli that have the potential for reactivation. The overall risk of reactivation in patients with positive skin tests has been estimated at 3–5%. Although the risk of reactivation is always present, it is greatest within the first few years of initial infection, in childhood, in adolescence, and in patients who have had previous clinical tuberculosis but who have been inadequately treated by present standards.

In a sense, then, patients with positive tuberculin skin tests serve as their own reservoir for future clinical disease. It has been demonstrated that the administration of isoniazid (INH) daily for 1 year reduces the risk of subsequent tuberculosis by up to 80%.

A recent European study of 28,000 tuberculin-positive adults with fibrotic pulmonary lesions demonstrated that 52 weeks of INH chemoprophylaxis reduces the incidence of tuberculosis by 75%; a 24-week regimen produced a 65% reduction. The rate of hepatitis was only 0.5% among INH recipients as compared with 0.1% in placebo recipients. [104]

However, INH has its own potential toxicities and should therefore be used selectively. The major concern in the use of INH is its hepatotoxicity. This is quite rare below age 20 and occurs in no more than 0.3% between the ages of 20 and 34. On the other hand, among patients older than 50, up to 2.3% may develop INH hepatotoxicity. Based on the risk of reactivation and the risks of INH toxicity, risk–benefit ratios can be calculated to help select patients for INH chemoprophylaxis. Those who have converted a tuberculin skin test from negative to positive within 2 years should be considered for chemoprophylaxis. In addition, close contacts of patients with active pulmonary tuberculosis should be considered for INH therapy on epidemiologic grounds, particularly if they are children or adolescents. Older patients who have recovered from clinical tuberculosis but who have never received chemotherapy should be worked up to exclude active disease; if none is demonstrated, these persons too may benefit from INH. Finally, it can be argued that all persons below age 35 should be skin tested at the time of routine medical evaluations and that INH should be administered to positive reactors. The prevalence rate of positive reactions among 6-year-olds is now about 0.2% and among adolescents about 0.7%. Thus, a positive reaction in a young patient may indicate recent exposure. Additional arguments for the use of INH in young patients include the fact that the drug is well tolerated in this age group and that without chemoprophylaxis the risk of reactivation would persist for the life span of the individual.[106]

The question of chemoprophylaxis in the immunosuppressed patient is considerably more complex because of the lack of data in many critical areas. On the simplest level, the tuberculin skin test may be negative because of anergy in these patients. If possible, tuberculin skin testing should be performed prior to the institution of immunosuppressive therapy. When this is not possible, control skin tests should be applied at the same time as PPD is injected. If anergy is present, the immunosuppressed patient must still be considered at risk for reactivation tuberculosis if there is a history of previous PPD positivity, of close exposure to tuberculosis, or of previous clinical tuberculosis. Even if these are absent, the chest radiograph should be carefully reviewed for abnormalities compatible with previous tuberculous infection such as a Gohn complex, pleural abnormalities, or apical calcifications. Patients with these radiologic findings must also be considered at risk.

It is important to screen all immunosuppressed patients for previous tuberculosis exposure with skin tests, a detailed history, and chest radiographs. Patients with positive findings should be followed closely, and tuberculosis should be accorded a prominent position in the differential diagnosis of infectious processes in those patients, even if the features are atypical.

But apart from maintaining a high index of suspicion, can the clinician offer more to the immunosuppressed patient with previous tuberculosis exposure? Unfortunately, the data required to answer this question are incomplete. Although the immunosuppressed state is classically considered a predisposing factor to tuberculosis, the magnitude of the risk is unknown (see Section 2.5), and estimates run the gamut from a slight risk[28] to a major risk.[107] Moreover, the efficacy of INH in reducing this risk has not been studied comprehensively. On theoretical grounds, immunosuppression per se should not interfere with the action of INH, but tuberculosis has been reported in immunosuppressed patients receiving prophylactic INH.[32] In addition, if INH is to be administered, it is unknown whether 1 year of therapy is sufficient or if the drug should be given throughout the period of immunosuppression. Finally, concern has been voiced that INH may have a greater toxic potential in immunosuppressed patients. Although this point has not been demonstrated, it is clear that the interpretation of abnormal liver function tests in immunosuppressed patients is much more difficult because they are often receiving other potentially hepatotoxic drugs and because transfusions, dialysis, and organ transplantation increase the risk of viral hepatitis and CMV infection.[108–110]

Recommendations on the use of INH prophylaxis in the immunocompromised patient vary widely, with some groups advocating daily therapy as long as the immunologically impaired state exists,[107] others suggesting a year of therapy,[106,108] and still others advocating close clinical observation without therapy.[29] In view of the many unknowns, individualized decisions would seem preferable to blanket recommendations.

Factors favoring the use of INH in immunosuppressed patients would include recent tuberculin conversion, young age, previously active tuberculosis that had not been treated with appropriate drugs, normal liver function tests, and the absence of concurrent hepatotoxins, including both drugs and alcohol. Reliable patients who will cooperate with close follow-up and who can recognize symptoms of INH hepatitis are also better candidates for INH prophylaxis, as are patients who are clearly immunosupprssed but who are expected to survive their underlying disease for prolonged periods. The duration of therapy should also be individualized: 12 months of continuous daily INH should be the goal, but in the absence of toxicity, it is reasonable to continue treatment for longer periods if the patient remains immunosuppressed.

If INH chemoprophylaxis is recommended, the potential risks and benefits of INH should be explained. Patients who accept chemoprophylaxis should be instructed to discontinue the medication and report to the physician if adverse effects are noted, including skin rash, fever, symptoms of peripheral neuritis, or symptoms of hepatitis including fatigue, anorexia, abdominal distress, or jaundice.

The American Thoracic Society[106] does not recommend routine SGOT determinations in patients who are reliable and who are able to comply with these directions. However, immunosuppressed patients are much more complex and generally require close medical surveillance on other grounds, so periodic SGOT determinations would seem reasonable. The problem with SGOT determinations is that 10–20% of patients receiving INH can be expected to develop mild transient elevations in SGOT that will return to normal even during continued therapy and are of no clinical significance. Although precise data are lacking, a reasonable approach is to routinely determine the SGOT at monthly intervals for at least the first 3 months of therapy. In symptomatic patients with elevated SGOTs, the drug should be discontinued and LFTs monitored. In asymptomatic patients with mild elevations of SGOT (perhaps up to three times normal), the drug can be continued, but the patient should be monitored weekly. If the SGOT fails to return to normal in 3–4 weeks, it seems prudent to discontinue INH. On the other hand, even if a patient is asymptomatic, a single more substantial elevation of SGOT, perhaps above 200 units, may be grounds to discontinue the agent. Again, it must be emphasized that these are "rules of thumb" rather than precise guidelines.

2.7.2. Chemotherapy

The chemotherapy of active tuberculosis[111,112] is different from other antimicrobial programs and should proceed according to five basic principles. The first is the use of multiple drugs to prevent the emergence of drug-resistant organisms. A second principle of chemotherapy is that in treatment

failures, drugs should be changed in combination rather than singly; in such cases, drug sensitivity testing is mandatory. A third principle is that single daily dosages of drugs are preferred. The fourth principle is that prolonged chemotherapy is necessary. Standard regimens have employed multiple drugs for periods of 18–24 months. With combinations of newer agents, shorter regimens of 6–9 months have been found equally effective in normal hosts. No matter what regimen is chosen, it is important to follow patients closely to ensure compliance and to monitor drug efficacy and toxicity. For normal hosts, the currently recommended antituberculous regimens are so effective that following the conclusion of treatment, relapse is unlikely, and it is unnecessary to keep patients under prolonged surveillance. By contrast, immunosuppressed patients should be followed after therapy.

Finally, most patients with tuberculosis should be hospitalized for the initial phases of therapy. As little as 2 weeks of combined therapy will greatly decrease the infectiousness of patients with pulmonary tuberculosis, although a few mycobacteria may still be present on sputum smears or cultures. Hence, short-term admission to general hospitals is preferred, with early home care in patients who are reliable and clinically stable. Patients with extrapulmonary tuberculosis are much less infectious and can sometimes be managed entirely as outpatients if their clinical status permits. Immunocompromised patients may be sicker and may respond less rapidly to therapy, necessitating more prolonged hospitalization.

2.7.3. First-Line Antituberculous Agents

2.7.3a. Isoniazid. Introduced into clinical use during the early 1950s, Isoniazid remains the single most important antituberculous drug. INH is bactericidal against *M. tuberculosis*. Of importance also is the excellent tissue penetration of this small water-soluble molecule; the distribution of INH includes the CNS, tuberculous abscesses, and intracellular sites. The major metabolism of INH is by hepatic acetylation, with metabolites then excreted by the kidneys. Although metabolites are excreted by the kidney, it is not necessary to modify INH doses except in advanced renal failure. Isoniazid is available both orally and parenterally. The usual dose is 5 mg/kg body weight, which averages 300 mg/day for the adult. For initial therapy of life-threatening disease, doses of 10–15 mg/kg per day may be used. The major toxicities of INH include the following:

1. Neurologic toxicity ranging from peripheral neuropathy (prevented by administration of pyridoxine, 50 mg/day) to much less common manifestations including encephalopathies, seizures, optic neuritis, and personality changes.
2. Hypersensitivity reactions including fever, rash, and rheumatic syndromes with or without positive antinuclear antibodies (ANA) and lupus erythematosus preps.
3. Hepatitis including serious clinical hepatitis in less than 2%, but a transient clinically insignificant rise in SGOT in 10–20%.

Isoniazid is an inexpensive drug. We recommend the administration of pyridoxine in a daily dose of 50 mg to patients receiving INH.

2.7.3b. Rifampin. Rifampin is the newest of the major antituberculous agents; it rivals INH in efficacy. Rifampin is bactericidal against *M. tuberculosis*. Rifampin is a large fat-soluble molecule that achieves excellent tissue penetration, including the CNS. The drug is excreted by the liver; modification of dosage is not required in renal failure but may be necessary in patients with hepatic insufficiency. Although rifampin is available parenterally in Europe, only an oral preparation has been approved in the United States. Unlike INH and ethambutol, rifampin is actually a broad-spectrum antimicrobial agent, acting against some atypical mycobacteria, *M. leprae,* many bacteria (including staphylococci, meningococci, and various gram-negative bacilli), trachoma agents, and some viruses. The average dose in adults is 600 mg/day administered in a single dose. Patients should be cautioned to expect orange discoloration of urine, sweat, tears, and saliva, which is of no clinical significance. Toxicities include hypersensitivity reactions such as fever, rash, or eosinophilia, hematologic toxicities such as thrombocytopenia, leukopenia, and hemolytic anemia, and hepatitis, including elevated SGOTs in up to 10%. Drug interactions occur, so that rifampin antagonizes the effect of warfarin, oral contraceptives, and methadone. High-dose rifampin should never be used in intermittent therapy because toxic reactions, including hemolytic anemia, thrombocytopenia, and renal failure, occur frequently. Rifampin is an expensive drug.

2.7.4. Second-Line Antituberculous Agents

2.7.4a. Ethambutol. Ethambutol was introduced clinically in the United States in 1967 and represented a major advance in antituberculous chemotherapy. Ethambutol penetrates tissues well, including the CNS when the meninges are inflamed. A disadvantage of ethambutol is that it is only bacteriostatic against *M. tuberculosis*. The drug is excreted by the kidneys. Although a modification of drug dosage is required in patients with renal failure, a nomogram to calculate dosage is not available; serum ethambutol levels (available through the manufacturer) should be monitored in patients with renal failure who require the drug. Ethambutol is available only in an oral preparation. Many authorities recommend initial therapy with 25 mg/kg body weight per day for the first 6–8 weeks of therapy and then reduced doses of 15 mg/kg body weight per day for the remainder of the course. Good results have also been obtained with use of the lower dose throughout therapy. The major toxicities of ethambutol include hypersensitivity reactions, such as fever and rash and optic neuritis, which is dose related and is usually manifested first by a loss of color vision. Less common side effects include neuritis, GI intolerance, headache, and hyperuricemia. The cost of ethambutol is moderate.

2.7.4b. Streptomycin. Streptomycin was the first effective antituberculous agent and remains a useful member of the therapeutic arsenal. Like other aminoglycosides, streptomycin has only a fair tissue distribution, being inactive at an acid pH or in an anaerobic milieu and penetrating the CSF very poorly. The excretion of streptomycin is via the kidneys, and dosage should be reduced in patients with renal failure. Streptomycin must be given parenterally. The average adult dose is 1 g/day for the first 2–8 weeks of therapy followed by 1 g twice a week. Major toxicities include hypersensitivity reactions and eighth nerve toxicity, especially to the vestibular division, resulting in vertigo. The cost of streptomycin is moderate, averaging about $1.00 per day.

Streptomycin is active against a variety of organisms in addition to *M. tuberculosis,* although many gram-negative bacilli have now become resistant because of the widespread use of this drug over many years.

Pyrazinamide. One of the older antituberculous agents, pyrazinamide is receiving renewed attention because of its bactericidal action against dormant intracellular *M. tuberculosis* organisms. Pyrazinamide is well absorbed from the GI tract and achieves therapeutic serum levels and good tissue penetration. Metabolism and excretion are by both hepatic and renal routes. The average dosage of pyrazinamide is 20–35 mg/kg per day (3-g maximum) divided into three doses. Side effects include hyperuricemia and hypersensitivity reactions; hepatic toxicity may occur in 3–15%, which may cause confusion in patients who are also taking other drugs with hepatotoxic potential, including INH and rifampin.

2.7.5. Third-Line Antituberculous Agents

In addition to the five major drugs, five other agents are available in the United States for the treatment of tuberculosis. Three of these are administered orally including *p*-aminosalicylic acid (PAS), ethionamide, and cycloserine. For many years, PAS was considered a first-line drug, but its relatively weak tuberculostatic action and the very high incidence of GI intolerance have now relegated this drug to alternate status. Two other drugs are available parenterally including kanamycin, and capreomycin, both of which are pharmacologically similar to streptomycin. The third-line drugs tend to be both less effective and more toxic than the standard agents but occasionally are of critical importance in treating patients with drug-resistant tuberculosis or atypical mycobacterial infection or in patients who cannot tolerate the standard drugs.

2.7.6. Antituberculous Regimens

Many combinations of antituberculous agents are effective in the treatment of tuberculosis, and many different regimens have been advocated. For the chemoprophylaxis of tuberculin convertors or selected tuberculin reactors, isoniazid is the only drug that can be recommended. For patients with active tuberculosis ranging from minimal infection to moderately advanced pulmonary or extrapulmonary disease, two-drug therapy is efficacious.

Most authorities now recommend the use of INH and rifampin in these circumstances. Ethambutol may be substituted for rifampin if hepatotoxicity is a concern and if the patient does not have advanced tuberculosis; in immunologically impaired hosts, however, the concomitant use of INH and rifampin would seem preferable, and a third drug may even be advisable. In patients with advanced pulmonary tuberculosis, tuberculous meningitis, mililary tuberculosis, or tuberculous pericarditis, triple therapy with INH, rifampin, and ethambutol is advisable; ethambutol can be discontinued after 2–3 months if clinical improvement has occurred. Streptomycin or pyrazinamide may be substituted for one or more of these drugs in patients who are intolerant to the first-line drugs. The treatment of resistant organisms may requite other drug combinations.

Standard chemotherapy of tuberculosis requires daily administration of drugs for 18–24 months. In addition to these standard regimens, new approaches to the treatment of tuberculosis include short course[113,114] and intermittent[115] drug regimens. Although these programs can be very useful for normal hosts, they cannot be recommended for the immunocompromised patient with tuberculosis.

2.7.7. Ancillary Therapeutic Modalities

The availability of excellent chemotherapeutic agents has greatly reduced the role of surgery in the treatment of tuberculosis. In general, drugs are now used to erradicate infection per se, whereas surgery may be helpful occasionally to treat complications or to repair or remove damaged tissues. Corticosteroids are useful only in selected situations such as patients with tuberculous meningitis complicated by hydrocephalus or CSF block and possibly patients with tuberculous pericarditis. Elaborate programs of rest and diet have no place in the treatment of tuberculosis.

2.7.8. Atypical Mycobacteria

The treatment of atypical mycobacterial infections is often extremely difficult.[5] Whereas *M. kansasii* and *M. marinum* are sensitive to the usual antituberculous drugs, most other nontuberculous mycobacteria are highly drug resistant. Sensitivity testing is mandatory, and complex multidrug regimens are often needed. However, even these programs often fail, and surgical extirpation of localized disease may be necessary. The prognosis of disseminated atypical mycobacterial infection in the immunosuppressed host is extremely poor. Ansamycin, a compound related to rifampin, has shown promise in the treatment of *M. avium-intracellulare,* and is available on a compassionate investigational new drug basis from the Centers for Disease Control (404/329-3670). Clofazimine, an antileprosy drug, is also being studied in *M. avium-intracellulare* infections. Rapidly growing mycobacteria (Runyon group IV) may be susceptible to various antibiotics; amikacin, doxycycline, and sulfonamides have been used for *M. fortuitum,* and amikacin and cefoxitin have been used for *M. chelonei.*

3. *Nocardia*

Like many other opportunistic infections, nocardiosis has increased in prominence over the years from a medical curiosity to an important illness. Between the description of the causitive organism in 1888 and a review of nocardiosis in 1960,[116] only 174 cases were reported in the world's literature. By contrast, it has recently been estimated that as many as 500–1000 cases of nocardiosis occur in the United States annually.[118] It is not clear whether this apparent increase reflects more accurate recognition and reporting of this hard-to-diagnose infection or if the expanded population of immunosuppressed patients has contributed to a true increase in the incidence of nocardiosis. It is clear that an aggressive approach to the diagnosis of nocardiosis is vitally important, because the results of chemotherapy have been very encouraging even in the compromised host.

3.1. Classification and Microbiology

Nocardia species are often misclassified as fungi because of their branched, filamentous, hyphaelike morphology or as mycobacteria because of their acid fastness. In fact, the nocardias are true bacteria; unlike the fungi, they are prokaryotic (i.e.,

have no nuclear membrane), they lack cytoplasmic organelles, they are small (usually <1 μm in diameter), their cell walls contain muramic acid peptides characteristic of bacteria, and their cell membranes lack the sterols characteristic of fungi.

Three species of nocardia are clinically important. Of these, *N. asteroides* is by far the most important, accounting for at least 85% of the cases of pulmonary and disseminated nocardiosis[117] and for the great majority of nocardial infections in immunocompromised hosts. Although *N. caviae* and *N. brasiliensis* can cause identical clinical illnesses, the latter is most commonly encountered as the cause of chronic subcutaneous suppuration in tropical and semitropical regions. *N. brasiliensis* can cause pulmonary and disseminated disease in immunocompromised patients in the United States.[118] These three species of *Nocardia* are morphologically identical, and speciation can be difficult.

Nocardia appear as slender, filamentous, branching organisms that may fragment into coccobacillary forms. They stain gram positive, often in an irregular or beaded fashion. *Nocardia* are acid fast but are less resistant to decolorization than are the mycobacteria. Hence, they are best visualized with a modification of the Ziehl–Neelsen method, in which 1% sulfuric acid is substituted for acid alcohol as the decolorizing agent.[119] *Nocardia* may also be visualized in tissue with methenamine–silver stain, but they are not visible with hematoxylin and eosin or with periodic acid-Schiff (PAS) stains.

Nocardia can be grown in the laboratory on a variety of media, including the blood agar and thioglycollate broth generally used for bacteria, the Sabouraud agar generally used for fungi, and the Lowenstein–Jensen medium generally used for mycobacteria. These organisms grow aerobically, but their growth is slow: 3–5 days are often required to identify colonies, and final identification of *Nocardia* species can take 3 weeks or longer. Because of this, it is most important for the clinician to alert the laboratory when *Nocardia* is suspected, so that cultures will be held longer and scrutinized with particular care. Nocardial colonies may be orange pigmented or chalky white and have a characteristic wrinkled texture.

The nocardias are morphologically similar to the actinomyces, to which they are closely related. Actinomyces tend to be less acid fast and to form sulfur granules in tissues.[119] Actinomyces are unlike *Nocardia* in that they are commonly present as part of the normal human flora, they cause infections primarily in the normal host, and they are sensitive to penicillin. Laboratory differentiation is easy because the actinomyces are anaerobes, whereas the nocardias grow aerobically.

3.2. Epidemiology and Pathogenesis

Nocardiosis is a worldwide infection. Although the pulmonary and disseminated forms of the infection do not demonstrate any geographic concentration, the third type of nocardiosis is much more common in Central and South America. This process is a chronic granulomatous infection of the skin and of the subcutaneous tissue of the feet, called maduromycosis or mycetoma. Sinus tracts are commonly present, and this is the only form of nocardiosis in which sulfur granules (generally characteristic of actinomycosis) may be present in the purulent drainage. In some cases, bone may be involved. Maduromycosis is caused by direct inoculation of *N. brasiliensis* into the skin. Because this process is not characteristic of immunosuppressed patients, it is omitted from further consideration here.

The epidemiology of pulmonary and disseminated nocardiosis is not well understood. Nocardial species can be cultured from soil and decaying vegetable matter. It is presumed that they enter the body by inhalation of aerosolized organisms, but most patients do not have a history of soil or dust exposure. Person-to-person transmission is unknown. Cases may cluster together in hospitalized patients, and *N. asteroides* has been isolated from the air and dust in a renal transplant unit in which four cases of nocardiosis occurred,[120] but nosocomial infection has not been documented.

Males outnumber females with nocardiosis at a rate of about 2 : 1.[121] Patients of all ages have been infected. Serious underlying diseases are present in 50%[121] to 85%[117] of patients with nocardiosis. The most important predisposing conditions are those producing systemic immunosuppression, including leukemia, lymphoma, organ transplantation, and corticosteroid therapy. Nocardiosis can occur in patients with AIDS.[122] In the Stanford experience, heart transplant recipients were at unusually high

risk, a nocardiosis developed in 21 of 160 patients.[123] In other patients, nocardiosis is superimposed on underlying pulmonary diseases, including COLD, tuberculosis, and pulmonary alveolar proteinosis. Diabetes has also been cited as a predisposing factor. In occasional patients, trauma or chronic inflammatory diseases have been incriminated, but in up to 50% of patients with nocardiosis, no primary disorder can be identified.

The host response to *Nocardia* has not been well defined. Pathologically, an acute inflammatory response is present, often with areas of necrosis or even abscess formation. Although this picture is reminiscent of a pyogenic process, it has been suggested that cell-mediated immunity is important in host defense against nocardias.[124] Further studies will be required to clarify this issue.

3.3. Clinical Features and Diagnosis

The clinical picture of nocardiosis is extremely variable, ranging from inapparent infection to fulminating pulmonary and systemic disease. With the exception of primary cutaneous infection,[125] the lung is the portal of entry in most cases. *Nocardia* is not part of the normal human flora, and these organisms are uncommon as laboratory contaminants.[126] Because of this, the finding of a positive sputum culture is generally considered highly suggestive of active pulmonary infection. However, in Mayo Clinic experience with 25 cases of nocardiosis, nine had positive sputum cultures with negative chest radiographs; although these patients did not receive antimicrobial therapy, they remained free of clinical infection.[127] Hence, simple colonization or subclinical infection clearly represents one pole of the clinical spectrum of pulmonary nocardiosis. Moreover, in a review of nocardiosis in 22 patients, Young et al.[128] reported nine cases in which fever and respiratory symptoms were present but chest radiographs were negative. Despite multiple positive cultures for *Nocardia,* therapy was withheld. All nine patients recovered, suggesting that *Nocardia* can produce self-limited infection of the respiratory tract. *Nocardia* is also a rare cause of upper respiratory tract infection, including one interesting case of chronic sinusitis presenting as fever of unknown origin.[129]

Despite these milder presentations, most patients with nocardiosis present with symptomatic pulmonary and/or systemic disease. Here, too, the clinical and radiologic features are extremely variable.[130] Nocardiosis can produce solitary lung nodules, localized pneumonitis, or lung abscesses that may be single or multiple. A micronodular or miliary pattern is less common. Direct extension to the pleura or, rarely, the pericardium,[131] may occur. Although in many patients these infections are insidious in onset and indolent in progression, in some cases nocardiosis can produce an acute necrotizing pneumonia.[132] Not surprisingly, clinical findings vary widely from low-grade fever and cough to spiking fevers and chills, copious production of purulent or even bloody sputum, chest discomfort, and respiratory embarrassment. Malaise and weakness are often present, and weight loss can be prominent in chronic nocardiosis.

Hematogenous spread of infection is common in nocardiosis. The lungs are the initial site of infection in almost all patients, but in about 25%, the pulmonary focus is subclinical or has healed, so that it cannot be detected at the time of clinical presentation. The most frequent site of metastatic infection is the CNS. About 25% of all patients with nocardiosis develop CNS infection; brain abscess is the most common manifestation of metastatic nocardiosis.[121] The second most common type of extrapulmonary nocardiosis is infection of skin and subcutaneous tissues. On rare occasions, these soft tissue lesions can cause extensive local damage. But even in milder cases, subcutaneous abscesses can be very important clues to the diagnosis of nocardiosis because of their accessibility for biopsy and culture.[123] Virtually any other organ can be hematogenously seeded in the course of nocardiosis, including the eyes, the liver, spleen, lymph nodes, kidneys, bones, and joints.

The diverse clinical features of nocardiosis often make diagnosis difficult. This is particularly true in the immunosuppressed host, both because of the expanded differential diagnosis in these patients and because nocardiosis can develop simultaneously or in sequence with other pulmonary and systemic infections. An aggressive approach to the diagnosis of nocardiosis is mandatory because the prognosis without treatment is dismal, whereas with antimicrobial agents, the outlook is favorable.

Despite the prominence of pulmonary lesions, sputum smears and cultures will yield the diagnosis of nocardiosis in fewer than 30% of cases.[121] As a result, invasive studies are necessary in most cases, including procedures such as transtracheal aspiration, bronchoscopy with biopsy, bronchial brushings, and percutaneous or surgical lung biopsies. The choice of procedure depends on the type and location of the lesions, on the patient's ability to tolerate the studies, and on the expertise available at each institution. Interestingly, paratracheal abscesses have complicated transtracheal aspiration procedures in some patients with nocardiosis.[127] In the case of nocardial brain abscesses, scans and angiograms disclose nonspecific mass lesions. The CSF in such cases may be normal or may show a modest elevation of pressure and protein with a normal sugar and a mild lymphocytic pleiocytosis. Unless pulmonary lesions are present, cranitomy is generally required for diagnosis. If subcutaneous lesions are present, they provide excellent material for diagnostic studies. On rare occasions, positive blood cultures can lead to the diagnosis of nocardiosis.[133–135] In all cases, specimens should be examined by both Gram and modified acid-fast stains, and cultures should be examined closely for at least 5–7 days because of the slow rate of growth of this organism. Unfortunately, serologic and skin tests are not reliable for diagnosis.

Illustrative Case 6: Pulmonary Nocardiosis

This 41-year-old woman was hospitalized in 1978 because of cough and chest pain. Six months earlier, she had received a cadaver renal allograft, and she had been maintained on azathropine and prednisone. Five days before admission, a nonproductive cough and right-sided pleuritic chest pain had developed. She denied fever, chills, dyspnea, and hemoptysis

On examination, she was a cushingoid woman in moderate distress. She was afebrile, and her lungs were normal to examination. She had no lymphadenopathy, and there were no lesions of the skin or subcutaneous tissues. She was neurologically intact. Laboratory studies included a Hct of 26% and a WBC count of 11,400/mm³ with 77% polys, 11% bands, 5% lymphocytes, 2% myelocytes, and 5% metamyelocytes. The BUN was 26 mg/dl, the creatinine 1 8 mg/dl, and the blood sugar 83 mg/dl The results of liver function tests and arterial blood gas determinations were normal The chest radiograph demonstrated a 4-cm rounded density in the periphery of the right middle lobe Tomograms did not disclose either cavitation or calcification

A needle aspiration biopsy of the pulmonary lesion was performed; the material obtained contained many polys, but no organisms were visualized on Gram stain, fungal wet mounts, and acid-fast stain. After 5 days of incubation, aerobic and anaerobic cultures were negative, and an open lung biopsy was performed A

3-cm area of bronchopneumonia was found, with sheets of polys and areas of necrosis with abscess formation. Gram stain revealed slender, filamentous, branching gram-positive organisms (Fig. 3) that were acid fast when stained with the modified Ziehl–Neelson method. Culture grew *N asteroides*. The patient was treated with high-dose sulfisoxazole for 6 months and did well.

Comment. This case illustrates the need for an aggressive approach to the diagnosis of pulmonary infection in the immunosuppressed host. In this case, nocardiosis presented as pleuritic pain and a solitary lung nodule. In other patients, fever and productive cough dominate clinically, and rapid deterioration may occur. Radiographic findings are variable, including multiple nodules, necrotizing lesions, or both. Probably because of early diagnosis and vigorous therapy, there were no signs of hematogenous dissemination, and she responded well to treatment.

Illustrative Case 7: Nocardial Brain Abscess

This 79-year-old woman was hospitalized because of weakness and ataxia. Six years earlier, generalized lymphadenopathy had developed and she was found to have chronic lymphocytic leukemia. She was treated with prednisone and, in addition, received several courses of chlorambucil. She remained well until 2 days before admission when she developed weakness and loss of balance. She denied headache and fever.

On examination, she was afebrile and nontoxic. She was found to have cushiongoid facies, mild lymphodenopathy, and hepatosplenomegaly. The neurologic examination revealed proximal muscle weakness, a broad-based waddling gait, and absent

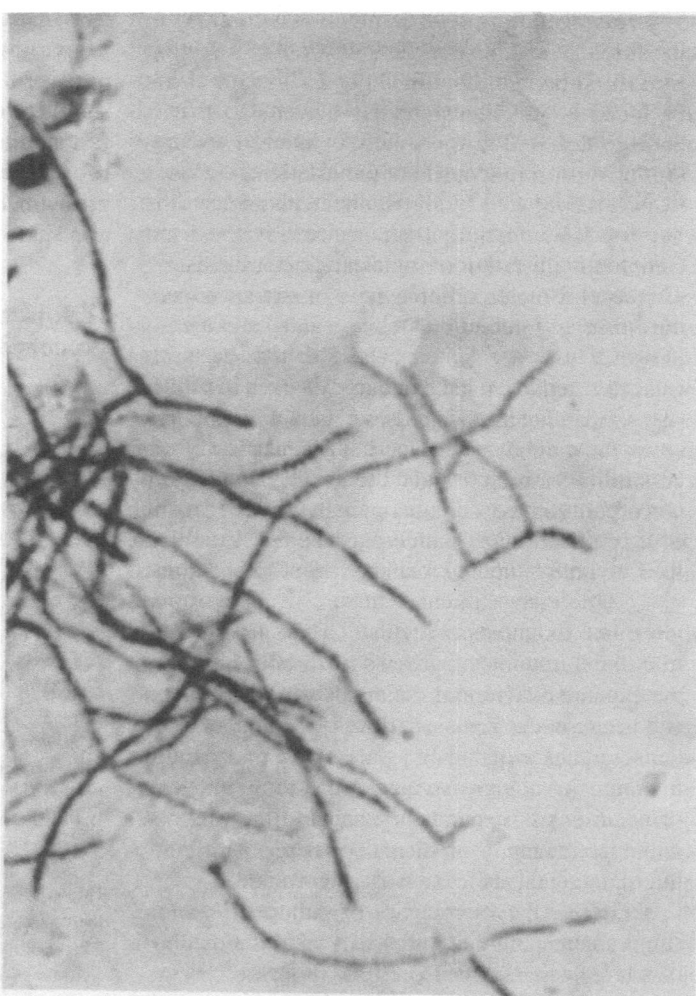

FIGURE 3. Gram stain of lung biopsy specimen from Illustrative Case 6 demonstrating the presence of slender, filamentous, branching gram-positive organisms.

ankle jerks bilaterally. Laboratory studies included a Hct of 30% and a WBC count of 19,000/mm^3 with 9% polys, 88% lymphocytes, 2% atypical lymphocytes, and 1% moncytes. Blood chemistries, including liver function tests, were normal. The chest radiograph revealed a patchy right lower lobe infiltrate, which had resolved when another film was obtained 4 days later.

Over the next 4 days, her gait deteriorated, and she developed incoordination of the arms and legs, an intention tremor, and mild dysmetria. Computed tomographic (CT) scan of the skull performed with contrast material disclosed a mass with surrounding edema and contrst enhancement. At craniotomy, a thick-walled abscess was found and excised. Histologically, acute inflammation was present. Gram stain revealed only rare short gram-positive bacillary forms that appeared weakly acid fast when stained with the modified Ziehl–Neelson technique. She was treated with high-dose steroids and intravenous sulfisoxazole and penicillin. Penicillin was omitted on the third postoperative day when cultures revealed organisms subsequently identified as *N asteroides* The patient was slowly improving neurologically, when she sustained a myocardial infarction and died on the sixth postoperative day.

Comment. This elderly woman was immunosuppressed by virtue of chronic lymphocytic leukemia and prolonged prednisone therapy. She presented with a progressive neurologic illness and was found to have a nocardial brain abscess The correct diagnosis was suspected on Gram stain even though only fragmented coccobacillary forms were seen. Her disease undoubtedly originated with hematogenous spread of infection from the lung to the brain. She had no pulmonary symptoms, but in retrospect, a transient pulmonary infiltrate had been present. The CNS is the most common site of extrapulmonary nocardiosis In patients who do not have concurrent pulmonary nocardiosis, cranitomy is required for diagnosis This patient was treated appropriately with surgical excision of the lesion and intravenously administered sulfasoxizole, but she died of unrelated causes

3.4. Therapy

Without therapy, nocardiosis is almost invariably fatal in the immunocompromised host. The overall survival rate at present is 58%[121] but, since these statistics include patients diagnosed late in their illness or even at autopsy, the results of early diagnosis and vigorous therapy should be more favorable. Adverse prognostic features include immunosuppression, acute onset of symptoms, dissemination of infection, and CNS involvement.

Sulfonamides have been the traditional treatment of choice for nocardiosis. High doses are required. Sulfisoxazole may be administered in a total daily dose of 6–10 g given in divided doses every 6 hr. In very sick patients, the drug should be administered intravenously, but as improvement occurs, the oral route may be used instead. Serum sulfonamide levels should be measured, and the drug dosage should be adjusted to achieve peak serum levels of 12–15 mg/dl. Other sulfonamides such as sulfadiazine or triple sulfonamides are also acceptable, but serum sulfa assays must be performed for the specific agent chosen.

The optimal duration of therapy for nocardiosis has not been established. However, relapses following cessation of treatment have been observed frequently, indicating the need for prolonged therapy. Antimicrobial agents should be administered for at least 6–8 weeks following clinical recovery, and many authorities suggest continuing treatment for 6–12 months.

A number of alternate antimicrobial regimens are now under study as a result of improved techniques for in vitro drug susceptibility testing.[136,137] Trimethoprim–sulfamethoxazole combinations are very active in some assays[136,137] but are less active in other test systems.[136,138] Only small numbers of patients have been treated with this combination,[139–141] but the results have been favorable; there have been no direct trials comparing trimethaprim–sulfamethoxazole with sulfonamides alone. Minocycline is active against the great majority of nocardial strains, and favorable results have been achieved with minocycline, 600 mg/day.[142,143] Combination therapy with ampicillin and erythromycin[142] was effective in a transplant patient who could not tolerate sulfonamides. Other antibiotics including amikacin are active against *Nocardia* in vitro,[135,136] but clinical experience with these drugs is scant.[144]

Although nocardial lung abscesses will generally resolve with antimicrobial therapy alone, brain abscesses require surgical excision as well. Similarly, other focal purulent infections may require surgical drainage in addition to medical therapy.

3.5. Infection Caused by Related Organisms

Immunocompromised hosts have repeatedly demonstrated their ability to contract infections with opportunistic organisms even before the microbiology of these organisms is well defined. The rhodocrous taxon is an incompletely defined genus of organisms that lies intermediate between group IV mycobacteria (rapid growers) and *Nocardia* species. Aerobic partially acid-fast members of the rhodochrous taxon are rare causes of pulmonary and disseminated infection in impaired hosts.[145] Optimal therapy of these infections has not been defined.

References

1 Karlson AG, Carr DT. Tuberculosis caused by *Mycobacterium bovis* Report of six cases 1954–1968 *Ann Intern Med* **73**:979, 1970.
2. BCG Vaccines. *MMWR* **28(21)**:241, 1979
3. BCG: Bad news from India (Editorial.) *Lancet* **1**:73, 1980.
4. Adu D, Evans DB, Millard PR, et al. Renal transplantation in leprosy. *Br Med J* **2**:280, 1973
5. Wolinsky E. Nontuberculous mycobacteria and associated diseases. *Am Rev Respir Dis* **119**:107, 1979.
6. Mackaness GB: Resistance to intracellular infection *J Infect Dis* **123**:439, 1971
7. Simon HB, Sheagren JN: Cellular immunity in vitro. Immunologically mediated enhancement of macrophage bactericidal capacity. *J Exp Med* **133**:1377, 1971.
8. Smith JA, Reichman LB: Lymphocyte transformation: An aid in the diagnosis of tuberculosis in patients with nonreactive skin tests. *Am Rev Respir Dis* **106**:194, 1972
9. Zeitz SJ, Ostrow JH, VanArsdel PP Jr: Humoral and cellular immunity in the anergic tuberculosis patient. *J Allergy Clin Immunol* **51**:20, 1974.
10. Ellner JJ: Suppressor adherent cells in human tuberculosis *J Immunol* **121**:2573, 1978
11. Stead WW, Bates JH: Evidence of a "silent" bacillemia in primary tuberculosis. *Ann Intern Med* **74**:559, 1971
12. Stead WW: Pathogenesis of the sporadic case of tuberculosis. *N Engl J Med* **277**:1008, 1967.
13. MacGregor RR, Clark LW, Bass F: The significance of isolating low numbers of mycobacterium tuberculosis in culture of sputum specimens. *Chest* **68**:518, 1975.
14. Rosenthal T, Pitlik S, Mitchaeli D: Fatal undiagnosed tuberculosis in hospitalized patients. *J Infect Dis* **131**:S51, 1975
15. Williams DM, Krick JA, Remington JS: Pulmonary infection in the compromised host Part II *Am Rev Respir Dis*, **114**:593, 1976.
16. Gopalakrishnan P, Miller JE, McLaughlin JS Pulmonary tuberculosis and coexisting carcinoma. A 10-year experience and review of the literature *Am Surg* **41**:405, 1975.
17. Neff TA, Ashbaugh DG, Petty TL. Miliary tuberculosis and carcinoma of the lung: Successful treatment with chemotherapy and resection. *Am Rev Respir Dis* **105**:111, 1972.
18. Roviaro GC, Sartori F, Calabro F, et al. The association of pleural mesothelioma and tuberculosis. *Am Rev Respir Dis* **126**:569, 1982.
19. Kaplan MH, Armstrong D, Rosen P. Tuberculosis complicating neoplastic disease. A review of 201 cases. *Cancer* **33**:850, 1974.
20. Feld R, Bodey GP, Groschel D: Mycobacteriosis in patients with malignant disease *Arch Intern Med* **136**:67, 1976
21. Ortbals DW, Marr JJ: A comparative study of tuberculous and other mycobacterial infections and their associations with malignancy *Am Rev Respir Dis* **117**:39, 1978.
22. Levine AS, Graw RG, Young RC: Management of infec-

tions in patients with leukemia and lymphoma. Current concepts and experimental approaches. *Semin Hematol* **9**:141, 1972
23. Morrow LB, Anderson RE Active tuberculosis in leukemia. *Arch Pathol Lab Med* **79**:484, 1965.
24. Pitlik SD, Fainstein V, Bodey GP Tuberculosis mimicking cancer—A reminder *Am J Med* **76**:822, 1984
25. Fauci AS, Dale DC, Balow JE· Glucocorticosteroid therapy. Mechanisms of action and clinical considerations. *Ann Intern Med* **84**:304, 1976.
26. Bovornkitti S, Kangsadal P, Sathirapat P, et al. Reversion and reconversion rate of tuberculin skin reactions in correlation with the use of prednisone. *Chest* **38**:51, 1960
27. MacGregor RR, Sheagren JN, Lipsett MB, et al· Alternate-day prednisone therapy *N Engl J Med* **280**:1427, 1969.
28. Busey JF, Fenger EPK, Hepper NG, et al: Adrenal corticosteroids and tuberculosis *Am Rev Respir Dis* **97**:484, 1968.
29. Schatz M, Patterson R, Kloner R, et al The prevalence of tuberculosis and positive tuberculin skin tests in a steroid-treated asthmatic population. *Ann Inter Med* **84**:261, 1976
30. Walsh SD, Grant WB. Corticosteroids in treatment of chronic asthma. *Br Med J* **2**:796, 1966.
31. Smyllie HC, Connolly CK. Incidence of serious complications of corticosteroid therapy in respiratory disease. *Thorax* **23**:571, 1968
32. Sahn, SA, Lakshminarayan S Tuberculosis after corticosteroid therapy. *Br J Dis Chest* **70**:195, 1976
33. Batata MA Pulmonary tuberculosis in a renal transplant recipient *JAMA* **237**:1465, 1977.
34. Kurzrock R, Zander A, Vellekoop L, et al: Mycobacterial pulmonary infections after allogenic bone marrow transplantation *Am J Med* **77**:35, 1984
35. Ascher NL, Simmons RL, Marker S, et al. Tuberculous joint disease in transplant patients. *Am J Surg* **135**:853, 1978.
36. Ortuno J, Teruel JL, Marcen R, et al: Primary intestinal tuberculosis following renal transplantation. *Nephron* **31**:59, 1982.
37. Neff TA, Hudgel DW. Miliary tuberculosis in a renal transplant recipient. *Am Rev Respir Dis* **108**:677, 1973
38. Rattazzi LC, Simmons RL, Spanos PK, et al. Successful management of miliary tuberculosis after renal transplantation *Am J Surg* **130**:359, 1975
39. Graybill JR, Silva J Jr, Fraser DW, et al. Disseminated mycobacteriosis due to *Mycobacterium abscessus* in two recipients of renal homografts *Am Rev Respir Dis* **109**:4, 1974
40. Fraser DW, Buxton AE, Naji A, et al: Disseminated *Mycobacterium kansasii* infection presenting as cellulitis in a recipient of a renal homograft, *Am Rev Respir Dis* **112**:125, 1975
41. Gombert ME, Goldstein EJ, Corrado ML, et al Disseminated *Mycobacterium marinum* infection after renal transplantation. *Ann Intern Med* **94**:486, 1981
42. Davis BR, Brumbach J, Sanders WJ, et al Skin lesions caused by *Mycobacterium haemophilum* *Ann Intern Med* **97**: 723, 1982
43. Lichtenstein IH, MacGregor RR. Mycobacterial infections in renal transplant recipients: Report of five cases and review of the literature *Rev Infect Dis* **5**:216, 1983

44 Pradhan RP, Katz LA, Nidus BD, et al· Tuberculosis in dialyzed patients JAMA 229:798, 1974

45 Band JD, Ward JI, Fraser DW, et al Peritonitis due to a Mycobacterium chelonei-like organism associated with intermittent chronic peritoneal dialysis J Infect Dis 145:9, 1982.

46 Nontuberculous mycobacterial infections in hemodialysis patients—Louisiana, 1982 MMWR 32(18):245, 1983

47 Raff, MJ, Waterman NG, Barnwell PA, et al. Infectious Diseases complicating renal transplantation. A survey and recommendations for prevention, recognition, and management South Med J 69:1603, 1976.

48 Duma RJ, Eickhoff TC, Remington JS, et al Panel discussion on infections in transplant patients Transplant Proc 4:717, 1972

49 Thomas PA Jr, Manko MA· Chemoprophylaxis for the prevention of tuberculosis in the immunosuppressed renal allograft recipient Transplantation 20:76, 1975.

50 Stead WW, Kerby GR, Schlueter DP, et al: The clinical spectrum of primary tuberculosis in adults. Ann Intern Med 68:731, 1968.

51 Huseby JS, Hudson LD: Miliary tuberculosis and adult respiratory distress syndrome Ann Intern Med 85:609, 1976

52 Miller WT, MacGregor RR. Tuberculosis: Frequency of unusual radiographic findings AJR 130:867, 1978.

53 Husen L, Fulkerson LL, DelVecchio E, et al: Pulmonary tuberculosis with negative findings on chest X-ray films. A study of 40 cases Chest 60:540, 1971.

54 Alvarez S, McCabe WR: Extrapulmonary tuberculosis revisited: A review of experience at Boston City and other hospitals. Medicine (Baltimore) 63:25, 1984

55 Sahn SA, Neff TA. Miliary tuberculosis. Am J Med 56:495, 1974

56 Munt PW. Miliary tuberculosis in the chemotherapy era with a clinical review in 69 American adults. Medicine (Baltimore) S1:139, 1972

57. Hinman AR. Tuberculous meningitis at Cleveland Metropolitan General Hospital 1959 to 1963 Am Rev Respir Dis 85:670, 1967

58 O'Toole RD, Thornton GF, Mukherjee DPH, et al: Dexamethasone in tuberculous meningitis Ann Intern Med 70:39, 1969.

59. Weiss W, Flippin HF· The prognosis of tuberculous meningitis in the isoniazid era Am J Med Sci 242:423, 1961

60 Rooney JJ, Crocco JA, Lyons HA Tuberculous pericarditis. Ann Intern Med 72:73, 1970.

61 Hageman JH, D'Esopo ND, Glenn WWL Tuberculosis of the pericardium N Engl J Med 270:327, 1964.

62 Berger HW, Mejia E: Tuberculous pleurisy Chest 63:88, 1973

63 Borhanmanesh F, Hekmat K, Vaezzadeh K, et al Tuberculous peritonitis Prospective study of 32 cases in Iran. Ann Intern Med 76:567, 1972.

64 Simon HB, Weinstein AJ, Pasternack MS, et al. Genitourinary tuberculosis Clinical features in a general hospital population Am J Med 63:410, 1977

65 Wallace R, Cohen AS Tuberculous arthritis A report of two cases with review of biopsy and synovial fluid findings Am J Med 61:277, 1976

66. Davidson PT, Horowitz I. Skeletal tuberculosis. A review with patient presentations and discussion. Am J Med 48:77, 1970

67 Iles PB, Emerson PA. Tuberculous lymphadenitis Br Med J 1:143, 1974.

68. Coburn RJ, England M, Samson DM, et al: Tuberculosis and blood disorders. Br J Haematol 25:793, 1973.

69. Lowther CP· Leukemia and tuberculosis Ann Intern Med 51:52, 1959.

70. Glasser RM, Walker RI, Herion JC: The significance of hematologic abnormalities in patients with tuberculosis Arch Intern Med 125:691, 1970

71 Jung A, Graziano M, Waldvogel F, et al: Unusual presentation of tuberculosis Br Med J 2:97, 1974.

72 Engstrom PF, Dewey GC, Barrett O. Disseminated Mycobacterium kansasii infection. Am J Med 52:533, 1972

73. Gruhl VR, Reese MH. Disseminated atypical mycobacterial disease presenting as "leukemia." J Clin Pathol 55:206, 1971

74 Manes JL, Blair OM: Disseminated Mycobacterium kansasii infection complicating hairy cell leukemia JAMA 236:1878, 1976

75. Grillo-Lopez AJ, Rivera E, Castillo-Staab M, et al: Disseminated M. kansasii infection in a patient with chronic granulocytic leukemia. Cancer 28:476, 1971.

76. McNutt DR, Fudenberg HH: Disseminated scotochromogen infection and unusual myeloproliferative disorder. Ann Intern Med 75:737, 1971.

77. Pottage JC Jr, Harris AA, Trenholme GM, et al. Disseminated Mycobacterium chelonei infection: A report of two cases Am Rev Respir Dis 126:720, 1982.

78. Pierce PF, DeYoung DR, Roberts GD: Mycobacteremia and the new blood culture systems Ann Intern Med 99:786, 1983

79. Wallace RJ Jr, Swenson JM, Silcox VA, et al: Spectrum of disease due to rapidly growing mycobacteria Rev Infect Dis 5:657, 1983.

80. Horsburgh CR Jr, Mason UG III, Farhi DC, et al. Disseminated infection with Mycobacterium avium-intracellulare A report of 13 cases and a review of the literature Medicine (Baltimore) 64:36, 1985.

81 Zamorano J, Tompsett R: Disseminated atypical mycobacterial infection and pancytopenia. Arch Intern Med 121:424, 1968.

82. Kilbridge TM, Gonnella JS, Bolan JT· Pancytopenia and death: Disseminated anonymous mycobacterial infection. Arch Intern Med 120:38, 1967.

83. Hagmar B, Kutti J, Lundin P, et al Disseminated infection caused by Mycobacterium kansasii Acta Med Scand 186:93, 1969.

84. Listwan WJ, Roth DA, Tsung SH, et al· Disseminated Mycobacterium kansasii infection with pancytopenia and interstitial nephritis Ann Intern Med 83:70, 1975

85 Oswald NC. Acute tuberculosis and granulocytic disorders. Br Med J 1:1489, 1963

86 Medd WE, Hayhoe FGJ: Tuberculosis miliary necrosis with pancytopenia. Q J Med 24:351, 1955

87. Eickhoff TC: The current status of BCG immunization against tuberculosis Annu Rev Med 28:411, 1977.

88. Bast RC, Zbar B, Borsos T, et al BCG and cancer. *N Engl J Med* **290:**1413, 1974

89 Aungst CW, Sokal JE, Jager BV Complications of BCG vaccination in neoplastic disease *Ann Intern Med* **82:**666, 1975

90 Sparks FC, Silverstein MJ, Hunt JS, et al. Complications of BCG immunotherapy in patients with cancer *N Engl J Med* **289:**827, 1973.

91. Rosenberg SA, Seipp C, Sears HF: Clinical and immunologic studies of disseminated BCG infection. *Cancer* **41:**1771, 1978

92. Pitchenik AE, Cole C, Russell BW, et al: Tuberculosis, atypical mycobacteriosis, and the acquired immunodeficiency syndrome among Haitian and non-Haitian patients in South Florida. *Ann Intern Med* **101:**641, 1984.

93. Greene JB, Sidhu GS, Lewin S, et al: *Mycobacterium avium-intracellulare:* A cause of disseminated life-threatening infection in homosexuals and drug abusers. *Ann Intern Med* **97:**539, 1982.

94. Poon M-C, Landay A, Prasthofer EF, et al. Acquired immunodeficiency syndrome with *Pneumocystis carinii* pneumonia and *Mycobacterium avium-intracellulare* infection in a previously healthy patient with classic hemophilia *Ann Intern Med* **98:**287, 1983.

95. Elliott JL, Hoppes WL, Platt MS, et al. The acquired immunodeficiency syndrome and *Mycobacterium avium-intracellulare* bacteremia in a patient with hemophilia. *Ann Intern Med* **98:**290, 1983

96. Fainstein V, Bolivar R, Mavligit G. Disseminated infection due to *Mycobacterium avium-intracellulare* in a homosexual man with Kaposi's sarcoma. *J Infect Dis* **145:**586, 1982

97. Zakowski P, Fligiel S, Berlin GW, et al. Disseminated *Mycobacterium avium-intracellulare* infection in homosexual men dying of acquired immunodeficiency *JAMA* **248:**2980, 1982.

98. Winter SM, Bernard EM, Gold JWM, et al Humoral response to disseminated infection by *Mycobacterium avium-intracellulare* in acquired immunodeficiency syndrome and hairy cell leukemia. *J Infect Dis* **151:**523, 1985.

99. Macher AM, Kovacs JA, Gill V, et al· Bacteremia due to *Mycobacterium avium-intracellulare* in the acquired immunodeficiency syndrome *Ann Intern Med* **99:**782, 1983

100. Wong B, Edwards FF, Kiehn TE, et al: Continuous high-grade *Mycobacterium avium-intracellulare* bacteremia in patients with acquired immune deficiency syndrome *Am J Med* **78:**35, 1985.

101. Damsker B, Bottone EJ. *Mycobacterium avium-intracellulare* from the intestinal tracts of patients with the acquired immunodeficiency syndrome: Concepts regarding acquisition and pathogenesis *J Infect Dis* **151:**179, 1985.

102. Eng RHK, Forrester C, Smith SM, et al: *Mycobacterium xenopi* infection in a patient with acquired immunodeficiency syndrome. *Chest* **86:**145, 1984

103. Pitchenik AE, Rubinson HA: The radiographic appearance of tuberculosis in patients with the acquired immuno deficiency syndrome (AIDS) and pre-AIDS. *Am Rev Respir Dis* **131:**393, 1985

104. International Union against Tuberculosis Committee on Prophylaxis: Efficacy of various durations of isoniazid preventive therapy for tuberculosis: Five years of follow-up in the IUAT trial *Bull WHO* **60:**555, 1982

105 Au FC, Webber B, Rosenberg SA Pulmonary granulomas induced by BCG. *Cancer* **41:**2209, 1978

106. Barlow PB, Black M, Brummer DL, et al: Preventative therapy of tuberculous infection *Am Rev Respr Dis* **110:**371, 1974

107. Millar JW, Horne NW. Tuberculosis in immunosuppressed patients. *Lancet* **1:**1176, 1979.

108. Thomas PA, Mozes MF, Jonasson O. Hepatic dysfunction during isoniazid chemoprophylaxis in renal allograft recipients *Arch Surg* **114:**597, 1979

109. Berne TV, Chatterjee SN, Craig JR, et al. Hepatic dysfunction in recipients of renal allografts *Surg Gynecol Obstet* **141:**171, 1975

110. Ware AJ, Luby JP, Eigenbrodt EH, et al: Spectrum of liver disease in renal transplant recipients *Gastroenterology* **68:**755, 1975.

111. Johnston RF, Wildrick KH. "State of the art" review. The impact of chemotherapy on the care of patients with tuberculosis. *Am Rev Respir Dis* **109:**636, 1974.

112. Bailey WC, Raleigh JW, Turner JAP: American Thoracic Society. Treatment of mycobacterial disease *Am Rev Respir Dis* **115:**185, 1977

113. Angel JH: Short-course chemotherapy in pulmonary tuberculosis. A controlled trial by the British Thoracic and Tuberculosis Association *Lancet* **2:**1102, 1976

114 Dutt AK, Moers D, Stead WW: Short-course chemotherapy for tuberculosis with mainly twice-weekly isoniazid and rifampin. *Am J Med* **77:**233, 1984.

115. Hudson LD, Sbarbaro JA. Twice weekly tuberculosis chemotherapy *JAMA* **223:**139, 1973

116. Murray JP, Finegold SM, Froman S, et al. The changing spectrum of nocardiosis. *Am Rev Respir Dis* **83:**315, 1961

117. Beaman BL, burnside J, Edwards B, et al Nocardial infections in the United States, 1972–1974 *J Infect Dis* **134:**286, 1976.

118 Smego RA Jr, Gallis HA. The clinical spectrum of *Nocardia brasiliensis* infection in the United States *Rev Infect Dis* **6(2):**164, 1984

119. Robboy SJ, Vickery AL Jr . Tinctorial and morphologic properties distinguishing actinomycosis and nocardiosis *N Engl J Med* **282:**593, 1970.

120. Stevens DA, Pier AC, Beaman BL, et al Laboratory evaluation of an outbreak of nocardiosis in immunocompromised hosts *Am J Med* **71:**926, 1981

121. Palmer DL, Harvey, RL, Wheeler JK Diagnostic and therapeutic considerations in nocardia asteroides infection, *Medicine (Baltimore)* **53:**391, 1974

122. Holtz HA, Lavery DP, Kapila R. Actinomycetales infection in the acquired immunodeficiency syndrome *Ann Intern Med* **102(2):**2–3, 1985

123 Simpson GL, Stinson EB, Egger MJ, et al. Nocardial infections in the immunocompromised host a detailed study in a defined population *Rev Infect Dis* **3:**492, 1981

124 Filice GA, Beaman BL, Remington JS Effects of activated macrophages on *Nocardia asteroides*. *Infect Immun* **27:**643, 1980.

125 Kahn FW, Gornick CC, Tofte RW Primary cutaneous

Nocardia asteroides infection with dissemination. *Am J Med* **70:**859, 1981.

126. Raich RA, Casey F, Hall WH: Pulmonary and cutaneous nocardiosis. *Am Rev Respir Dis* **83:**505, 1961.

127. Frazier AR, Rosenow EC, Roberts GD: Nocardiosis: A review of 25 cases occurring during 24 months. *Mayo Clin Proc* **50:**657, 1975.

128. Young LS, Armstrong D, Blevins A, et al: *Nocardia asteroides* infection complicating neoplastic disease. *Am J Med* **50:**356, 1971.

129. Katz P, Fauci AS: *Nocardia asteroides sinusitis*. Presentation as a trimethoprim-sulfamethoxazole responsive fever of unknown origin. *JAMA* **238:**2397, 1977

130. Balikian JP, Herman PG, Kopit S: Pulmonary nocardiosis. *Radiology* **126:**569, 1978.

131. Chavez CM, Causey WA, Conn JH: Constrictive pericarditis due to infection with *Nocardia asteroides Chest* **61:**79, 1972

132. Neu HC, Silva M, Hazen E, et al: Necrotizing nocardial pneumonitis. *Ann Intern Med* **66:**274, 1967

133. Roberts GD, Brewer NS, Hermans PE: Diagnosis of nocardiosis by blood culture. *Mayo Clin Proc* **49:**293, 1974

134. Avram MM, Nair SR, Lipner HI, et al: Persistent nocardemia following renal transplantation, *JAMA* **239:**2779, 1978.

135. Petersen DL, Hudson LD, Sullivan K: Disseminated *Nocardia caviae* with positive blood cultures. *Arch Intern Med* **138:**1164, 1978.

136. Bach MC, Sabath LD, Finland M: Susceptibility of *Nocardia asteroides* to 45 antimicrobial agents in vitro *Antimicrob Agents Chemother* **3:**1, 1973.

137. Wallace RJ JR., Septimus EJ, Musher DM, et al: Disk diffusion susceptibility testing of *Nocardia* species. *J Infect Dis* **135:**568, 1977.

138. Bennett JE, Jennings AE: Factors influencing susceptibility of *Nocardia* species to trimethoprim–sulfamethoxazole. *Antimicrob Agents Chemother* **13:**624, 1978

139. Maderazo EG, Quintilliani R: Treatment of nocardial infection with trimethoprim and sulfamethoxazole *Am J Med* **57:**671, 1974

140. Cook FV, Farrar WE Jr: Treatment of *Nocardia asteroides* infection with trimethoprim-sulfamethoxazole. *South Med J* **71:**512, 1978.

141. Wallace RJ Jr, Septimus EJ, Williams TW Jr, et al. Use of trimethoprim-sulfamethoxazole for treatment of infections due to *Nocardia*. *Rev Infect Dis* **4:**315, 1982.

142. Bach MC, Monaco AP, Finland M: Pulmonary nocardiosis: Therapy with minocycline and with erythromycin plus ampicillin. *JAMA* **224:**1378, 1973.

143. Petersen EA, Nash ML, Mammana RB, et al: Minocycline treatment of pulmonary nocardiosis. *JAMA* **250:**930, 1983

144. Yogev R, Greenslade T, Firlit CF, et al: Successful treatment of *Nocardia asteroides* infection with amikacin. *J. Pediatr* **96:**771, 1980.

145. Haburchak DR, Jeffery B, Higbee JW, et al. Infections caused by rhodochrous. *Am J Med* **65:**298, 1978.

10

Parasitic Diseases in the Compromised Host

JOEL RUSKIN

1. Introduction

In the United States, Western Europe, and the mature health care delivery systems of Asia and Africa, two parasitic diseases should be carefully considered in the evaluation of fever and possible infection in the immunocompromised host: toxoplasmosis and pneumocystosis. In addition, three other diseases—strongyloidiasis, giardiasis, and babesiosis—occasionally occur in patients who are immunosuppressed or splenectomized. The ongoing epidemic of acquired immunodeficiency syndrome (AIDS) has called our attention to two coccidial protozoa—*Cryptosporidium* and *Isospora belli*—as causes of diarrhea. These entities should be suspected in any patient with compromised cell-mediated immunity and symptoms of gastroenteritis. It should, however, be acknowledged that in many of the developing countries of the world a number of other common parasitic entities can be expected to afflict both immunosuppressed and normal hosts. Thus, malaria and Chagas disease are occasional causes of transfusion-associated infection, and the risk of hematogenous trypanosomiasis is sufficiently great that in Brazil serologic screening for evidence of infection is analogous to the mandatory requirements for hepatitis serological testing in the United States.[1]

JOEL RUSKIN • Department of Medicine, Infectious Diseases Service, Kaiser Permanente Medical Center, Los Angeles, California 90027; and University of California–Los Angeles School of Medicine, Los Angeles, California 90024.

Malaria has occasionally been reported in immunosuppressed patients in the United States who are presumably infected by the transfusion route[2]; fatal leishmaniasis (kala-azar) was observed in a renal transplant recipient who probably had reactivation of latent infection.[3] Clearly, a carefully taken history of travel or transfusion of blood products will be extremely important in ruling out unusual parasitic disorders. Not to be overlooked is the possibility of reactivation of disease initially acquired during travel to an endemic area but that remains quiescent for many years until host defenses are impaired.

2. *Pneumocystis carinii* Pneumonia

Few diseases of the immunocompromised host have proved as fascinating to the infectious disease clinician during the last decade than that associated with the presumed protozoan parasite, *Pneumocystis carinii*. During the more than 75 years that have elapsed since the description of the organism, numerous investigators have attempted in vitro cultivation of this pathogen. Successful cultivation in vitro has probably been achieved.[4] Nevertheless, the methods for propagation are quite complex and growth in vitro is not of the magnitude commonly obtained for commensal bacteria. Although Koch's postulates have not been fulfilled, and the disease remains a nosologic problem, effective chemotherapy and prophylaxis are now available. Reviews of recent developments in the biology and treatment of *Pneumocystis* infection have been published.[5,5a]

2.1. Historic Perspective

The first description of pneumocystosis in animals and humans should properly be attributed to Chagas, who observed cyst forms in the lungs of guinea pigs that were also infected with *Trypanosoma cruzi*.[6] Chagas interpreted these forms as the sexual stage or the sporogonia of the trypanosome. The following year, Carini, also working in Brazil, observed similar cysts in lungs of rats experimentally infected with another trypanosome, *T. lewisi*. Carini's observation became known to the husband-and-wife team, the Delanoes, who saw similar cysts in the lungs of Parisian sewer rats and gave these cysts the name *Pneumocystis carinii*. In 1913, Chagas also described in an autopsy of an adult the first probable case of pneumocystosis in man. Some 30 years subsequently elapsed before the description of additional human cases of pneumonic disease associated with the presence of these cysts in lung tissue. During World War II, Vandermeer and Brug observed such cases of pneumonitis in malnourished orphans.[7] During the two decades following the end of World War II, outbreaks of pneumocystosis in premature infants and institutionalized orphans in Europe and the Middle East were described. These illnesses were associated with prematurity and malnutrition. In a study of autopsied infants that was published in 1952, Vanek and Jirovec provided the strongest histopathologic evidence for the etiologic relationship between *Pneumocystis* organisms and interstitial plasma cell pneumonia.[8] For this reason, Frenkel has argued that the human parasite should be called *Pneumocystis jirovecii* in honor of Dr. Otto Jirovec rather than *Pneumocystis carinii*.[9] The latter is responsible for pneumonia in animals, and proof that the organisms causing disease in humans and animals are identical is lacking.

In 1958, Ivady and Paldy, working in Hungary, reported the first successful use of pentamidine in the treatment of pneumocystosis.[10] This agent was previously used successfully in the treatment of African sleeping sickness. Following this successful therapeutic approach and the recognition of cases in immunodeficient children in the United States,[11] the National Centers for Disease Control assumed responsibility for distribution of pentamidine in the United States.

During the mid-1960s, it was recognized that a combination of pyrimethamine and sulfadiazine was also effective in the treatment of human pneumocystosis. Whether or not this combination yields treatment results equivalent to or perhaps better than pentamidine has never been resolved. Recent therapeutic advances have been based on carefully designed studies of experimental corticosteroid-induced infections in rats.[12] Using this model, Hughes and collaborators reported in 1974 the effectiveness of trimethoprim–sulfamethoxazole (another antifolate–sulfonamide combination) in therapy and prophylaxis of rat pneumocystosis.[13] Thereafter, the safety and therapeutic effectiveness of trimethoprim–sulfamethoxazole was demonstrated in *Pneumocystis*-infected children[14] and adults.[15] More recently, trimethoprim–sulfamethoxazole was successfully employed in the prophylaxis of *Pneumocystis carinii* infection in leukemic children[16] and in bone marrow transplant recipients.[17]

There is increasing recognition that any patient who is immunosuppressed and has dyspnea or lung infiltrates should be considered a possible case of pneumocystosis. As a result of the AIDS epidemic we have come to appreciate that *P. carinii* is the most common cause of life-threatening opportunistic infection and is usually the presenting infection that establishes the diagnosis of AIDS.[18,19] Any patient with pneumonia who does not belong to one of the high-risk groups predisposed to AIDS should still be considered for the diagnosis if he or she has received a blood transfusion since 1980. The prognosis with treatment of the first episode is still fairly good but recrudescent disease is common. Therapeutic failures, toxicity, or hypersensitivity to available medications has spurred the search for alternative agents for treatment.[20] At the same time the AIDS epidemic has triggered research into the basic biology of the disease, improved methods for diagnosis, and renewed investigation of prophylactic approaches.[20a]

2.2. The Organism

There have been several reports of limited (short-term) passage of *Pneumocystis* organisms in tissue culture from lungs of animals or humans with pneumonitis.[4] The belief that the forms identified as *Pneumocystis* are viable and pathogenic is based on their presence and uniform morphology in the pulmonary alveolar spaces of patients and animals with pneumonitis, followed by their disappearance after treatment with folate antagonists—sulfonamides or pentamidine. Descriptions of the morphology of this microbe have been based on light and electron microscopy of pathologic material and study of organisms passed in tissue cultures. The organism appears to be a unicellular microbe with both cyst and trophozoite stages. The cystic unit contains up to eight oval bodies most often termed sporozoites. The cysts are best seen in silver-stained smears of infected fresh lung, whereas the sporozoites are better defined by Giemsa-stained imprint smears. Each sporozoite (or intracystic body) measures about 1–2 μm and has a deeply staining eccentric nucleus and a pale blue staining halo that is thought to be cytoplasm. However, the Giemsa stain is probably not the best technique for rapid recognition of pneumocysts, because it also stains background alveolar material and cell fragments rather than the characteristic cyst wall of the organism. Alternative methods for detecting *Pneumocystis* forms include the Gram–Weigert stain, which stains both cyst and sporozoite, and the toluidine blue stain, which delineates the cyst form but not the intracellular morphology.

The Gomori methenamine silver nitrate stain is, in our experience, the most reliable (but most time-consuming) procedure for identification of cyst forms in lung tissue. Pneumocysts identified by this silver stain have a thin, sometimes irregular gray/brown/black capsule and may appear almost round, disc-shaped, or crescentic in form (Fig. 1). These cysts are 4–6 μm in diameter and are almost as large as a red blood cell (RBC), often being mistaken for red cells if the silver stain is incorrectly carried out. Cysts often occur in clusters within the alveolar space. The internal structure of the cyst is variable. In lighter-stained round cysts, a pair of structures about 1 μm in length resembling opposed ''commas'' or parentheses is often seen, and these components are occasionally connected end to end by thin, delicate, strandlike structures. Other cysts contain only a marginal nodule. Some authorities suggest that the intracystic bodies may be thickened portions of the cyst wall.

In an urgent clinical situation such as following tracheal aspiration or lung biopsy, the Gram–Weigert, Giemsa, or toluidine blue stains may be used for rapid diagnosis.[21] Nonetheless, the silver

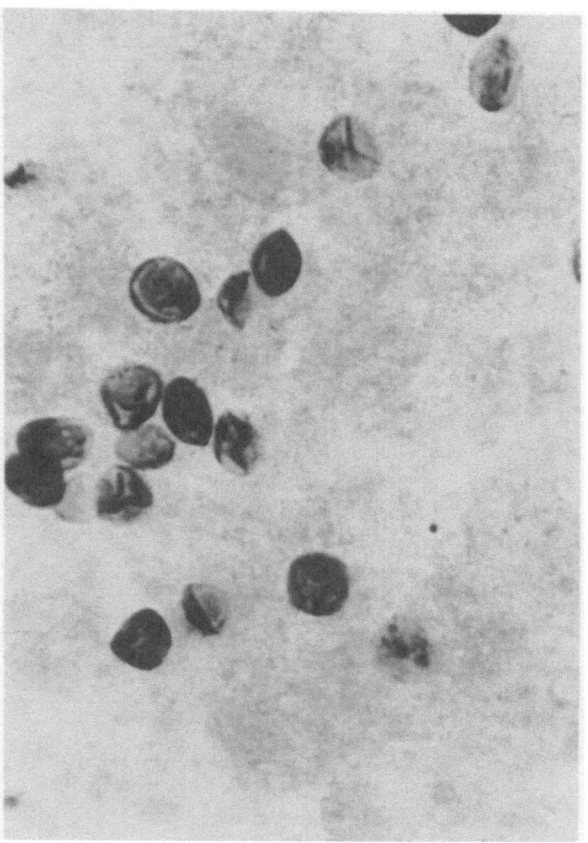

FIGURE 1. Gomori silver methenamine nitrate stain of impression smears of lung containing cysts of *Pneumocystis carinii.*

stain should always be carried out for confirmation, preferably with a positive and negative control (such as a slide with yeast forms and/or erythrocytes). Staining procedures vary, but a modification that produces a ''rapid silver stain'' (reliable results in a total of 2 hr) is used routinely in many laboratories and detailed in Table 1.

Electron microscopic evaluation reveals that the trophozoite is thin walled and has numerous evaginations of pseudopodlike projections called filopodia. These filopodia appear to anchor the organism to the alveolar septal wall and could explain the usual absence of pneumocysts in expectorated secretions. Although the smallest trophozoite form measures 1.5–2.0 μm in diameter, the cyst structure appears to be 3–5 μm in diameter. The mature cyst does not have filopodia but contains intracystic bodies measuring

TABLE 1. Rapid Methenamine Silver Stain

Solutions
  5% Chromic acid
    Chromic acid (CrO$_3$), 5 g
    Distilled water, 100 ml
  3% Methenamine
    Hexamethylenetetramine, USP [(CH$_2$)$_6$N$_4$], 3 g
    Distilled water, 100 ml
  Stock methenamine–silver nitrate
    Silver nitrate, 5% solution, 5 ml
    Methenamine, 3% solution, 1 dl
    A white precipitate forms but immediately dissolves on
      shaking. Clear solutions remain usable for months at
      refrigerator temperature.
  1% Sodium bisulfite
    Sodium bisulfite (NaHSO$_3$), 1 g
    Distilled water, 1 dl
  2% Sodium thiosulfate (hypo)
    Sodium thiosulfate (NaS$_2$O$_3$·5H$_2$O), 2 g
    Distilled water, 1 dl
  Working light green
    Light green, stock solution, 10 ml
    Distilled water, 40 ml
    This solution is stable for 1 month.
  5% Silver nitrate
    Silver nitrate (AgNO$_3$), 5 g
    Distilled water, 1 dl
  5% Borax
    Borax (photographic or USP, Na$_2$B$_4$O$_7$·10H$_2$O), 5 g
    Distilled water, 1 dl
  Working methenamine–silver nitrate
    Borax, 5% solution, 2 ml
    Distilled water, 25 ml
    Mix, and add Methenamine–silver nitrate, stock solution,
      25 ml
    Caution: This preparation (working methenamine–silver
      nitrate solution) must be prepared fresh each time the
      stain is run. Do not try to reuse even for a stain run
      immediately following.
  0 2% Gold chloride
    Gold chloride, 1% solution (AuCl$_3$·HCl·3H$_2$O), 10 ml
    Distilled water, 40 ml
    This solution may be used repeatedly. However, when
      toning begins to fail and the organisms come out too
      black, it should be changed.
    Note: 1% gold chloride solution is made from ampules
      and is diluted according to the directions accompanying
      it.
  Stock light green
    Light green, S.F. (yellow), 0.2 g

Distilled water, 1 dl
Glacial acetic acid (CH$_3$COOH), 0 2 ml
Preparation of smear for methenamine–silver stain
  Material to be stained is smeared on a slide and allowed to
    air dry. Tissue may be ground and then smeared on a
    slide. Impression smears from cut tissue may be prepared.
Fixation
  The air-dried smears are placed in absolute methyl alcohol
    for 5 min Fix a control smear (fungus or *Pneumocystis*)
    at the same time.
Staining procedure
  While slides are fixing, fill one Coplin jar (with a lid) with
    5% chromic acid In a screw-capped Coplin jar, prepare
    the working methenamine silver.
  Place fixed slides into chromic acid, and put both Coplin
    jars into a 48°C water bath. After 2 min, transfer the jar
    of chromic acid to a 56°C water bath for 10 min
  Wash the slides briefly in running tap water.
  Place the slides into 1% sodium bisulfite for 30 sec.
  Wash in running tap water for 15 sec
  Rinse slides in four changes of distilled water.
  Place the slides into the jar of working methenamine silver
    in the 48°C water bath for 2 min
  Transfer the jar to the 56° water bath for 25 min or less.
  Check control slide at 20 min to see if organisms have
    stained. To check control slide, remove control and
    patients slides to a water-filled Coplin jar. Leave the
    Coplin jar with the silver solution in the 56°C water bath.
    Coverslip control slide and quickly look for proper
    staining of the organisms: cytoplasms should be light
    brown with dark brown parentheses in the center. If so,
    proceed. If not, return the slides to the silver until they
    are stained.
  Rinse slides with four changes of distilled water
  Tone in 0.2% gold chloride for 1 min
  Rinse in 2 changes of distilled water
  Place slides into 2% sodium thiosulfate for 1 min.
  Wash slides in running tap water for 15 sec.
  Counter stain in working light green for 30 sec.
  Rinse in one change of distilled water.
  Dehydrate and clear for 1-min intervals in two changes each
    of 95% ethanol, 100% ethanol, and xylene
  Mount slides in Permount.
Interpretation
  Cyst walls are delicately stained brown or gray. Intracystic
    structures resembling "commas" or parentheses are often
    present and stain black. The cytoplasm is usually clear.
    Fungal structures, in contrast, are sharply delineated in
    black.

1–1.7 μm across and is enclosed by a double membrane that is partly connected to the inner layer of the cyst wall. Collapsed cysts are crescent shaped and are presumably the same forms seen by light microscopy of silver stain specimens.

From electron microscopic observations, a life cycle for *Pneumocystis carinii* has been postulated by Campbell[22]: the mature round cyst undergoes dissolution or "cracking" that permits escape of intracystic bodies. At that point, the intracystic bodies resemble a small trophozoite form. It appears that small trophozoites evolve to larger forms, their walls thicken, and a precyst develops which is devoid of intracystic bodies. The cycle is completed with the arrival of the mature cyst stage containing a quota of approximately eight daughter cysts. An alternative developmental cycle proposes that daughter cells form as well within thin-walled pneumocysts (i.e., trophozoites).[23]

2.3. Histopathology

Although the pathology of *Pneumocystis* pneumonia has been well studied, there still appears to be considerable confusion regarding the typical histologic pattern. The original descriptive term for pneumocystosis, interstitial plasma cell pneumonia, dates back to the pronounced plasma cell infiltration of the interalveolar septa documented almost exclusively in the newborns studied in nursery outbreaks occurring in Europe.[6] The alveolar walls are distended many times their normal thickness with resultant compression of alveolar spaces. In immunocompromised patients, thickened alveolar septa and cellular infiltration are less marked than in the plasma cell pneumonia of European description. Although some degree of interstitial mononuclear (lymphocyte or macrophage) infiltration has been observed, hyperplasia of alveolar lining cells appears most responsible for septal thickening. (Septal cell hyperplasia is a nonspecific reaction to infections of various etiologies, and it is quite common among immunosuppressed patients who have no evidence of *Pneumocystis* infection per se.) The predominant finding on hematoxylin and eosin staining is an intense eosinophilic foamy or honeycombed material rather than a plasma cell infiltrate that fills the alveolar spaces. This intraalveolar material is composed largely of inflammatory cells and degenerating bodies of pneumocysts, the latter staining bright red with the periodic acid–Schiff (PAS) stain because of their high carbohydrate content. Typical cysts or trophozoite forms of the parasite are seen only after application of a silver or Giemsa stain, respectively.

In a study of patients primarily with acute childhood lymphoblastic leukemia, three sequential stages of pneumocystosis were categorized by Hughes et al.[24] Stage 1 consists of isolated cysts in the alveolar septal wall with few cysts in the alveoli and little or no inflammation. Stage 2 is characterized

by the presence of cystic organisms within macrophages fixed to the alveolar wall and desquamation of these alveolar cells; trophozoite forms are found associated with cysts and also lying free in the alveolar space. There is only minimal septal inflammation at this time. The third and final stage is characterized by a reactive desquamative alveolitis with cysts appearing in alveolar macrophages in various states of degeneration. This so-called foamy exudate of pneumocystosis is neither edema fluid nor exudative inflammation but largely a coalescence of inflammatory cells (mainly macrophages) and organisms. It has been conjectured that spread of pneumocysts through pulmonary tissue does not occur by direct invasion through the interstitium or through vascular spaces. Rather, coughing may expectorate cysts from alveoli into larger airways, and organisms are then swept back into previously uninvolved alveolar areas. This hypothesis of intraairway transfer is supported by the usual finding of heaviest parasitic concentration in dependent portions of the lung.

Whether or not *Pneumocystis* infection can spread beyond the lung is a matter of controversy. Several cases of so-called generalized pneumocystosis in infants have been reported in which parasitemia and organ dissemination were demonstrable.[6] Although in some outbreaks, particles consistent with the sporozoite form have been seen in blood smears, the accuracy of these observations has been challenged. However, there have been a few well-documented cases of disseminated disease.[25–25b] Silver stain-positive cysts have been found to invade the bone marrow, splenic capsule, colon, liver, pancreas, retroperitoneal tissue, skin, and retina. Nonetheless, such cases appear to be exceedingly rare, and one series of some 200 patients had no instance of generalized infection.[26] In another study, using immunofluorescent techniques, no fragments or antigenic material derived from the cysts appeared in various sections of lymph nodes, liver, spleen, and kidney.[27]

2.4. Conditions Associated with Pneumocystosis in Humans and Animals

Table 2 summarizes the conditions associated with this disease in man and animals. Some of the earliest outbreaks of infantile disease in humans were associated with malnutrition and crowding. It is remarkable that even in the 1970s malnourished infants

TABLE 2. Pneumocystosis in Humans and Animals

Pneumocystosis in humans
  Malnutrition (epidemics)
  Crowding (epidemics)
  Immunodeficiency
    Primary
    Neoplasia plus therapy
    Transplantation-associated
    Acquired, secondary to retrovirus infection
    Drug related (cortisone, cyclosporine, antithymocyte
      globulin)
Pneumocystosis in Animals
  Natural
    Rats, mice, guinea pigs, rabbits, dogs, monkey, sheep,
      goats, horses
  Altered state
    Cortisone treatment
    Athymic (nude) mice

brought to the United States were found to have sporadic cases of *Pneumocystis* infection.[28] However,
the major association is clearly with compromised
host defenses of either a primary or acquired nature:
congenital immunodeficiency, neoplasia, cancer
chemotherapy, immunosuppression for collagen vascular disease, and corticosteroids or antithymocyte
globulin given to prevent graft rejection. The nature
of immunosuppressive therapy can be quite variable,
but corticosteroids are the most consistent component of drug regimens associated with this infection.
For instance, we have seen pneumocystosis complicating steroid treatment given for cutaneous inflammatory disorders such as pemphigus vulgaris or
secondary to attempted reduction of brain edema
with dexamethasone. On the other hand, patients
with severe asthmatic disorders rarely develop this
complication in spite of the tendency to use increasingly larger doses of cortisone to treat status
asthmaticus. Perhaps the otherwise intact nature of
host defenses in asthmatic states, the tendency to give
alternate-day therapy in asthma, or the fact that relatively low doses of cortisone or its congeners are used
may explain the lack of an association.

2.5. Predisposing Factors and Host-Defense Mechanisms

A precise appraisal of the relative importance of
the roles of specific components of host defenses

active against *Pneumocystis* infection cannot yet be
made. Although the disease has been reported rarely
in normal persons,[29] pneumocystosis usually
emerges in settings of both impaired lymphocyte and
humoral antibody function. That susceptibility to *P.
carinii* is related to a disorder of T-lymphocyte-mediated immune mechanisms is supported by the findings that overt disease is inducible in previously normal rabbits or rodents after conditioning with
corticosteroids or protein-calorie deprivation[12,13,30]
and that infection is transmissible from both experimentally infected rats and human lung material to
nude or athymic mice without corticosteroid conditioning.[31] The pattern of clinical disease in man suggests a T-lymphocyte abnormality inasmuch as the
three major disorders associated with pneumocystosis are Hodgkin disease, lymphatic leukemia, and AIDS. Hodgkin disease is the lymphoma
most often associated with pneumocystosis,[32] although it should be recognized that this association is
well documented only in the modern chemotherapeutic era when corticosteroids are important components of chemotherapy for this underlying disease.
Of the leukemias, pneumocystosis is most common
in lymphatic neoplasms, particularly the acute childhood type (for which steroids are now invariably employed), but it is uncommon in myelogenous leukemia unless corticosteroids are used. Recently, the use
of cyclosporine has been associated with increased
risk of clinically significant *Pneumocystis* infection.

There is, however, some evidence that *P. carinii* infection is secondary to a humoral immune disorder as well as a cellular abnormality. From in vitro
studies of pneumocyst–phagocytic cell interactions,[33] immune serum has been shown to enhance
the interiorization of cyst forms by alveolar macrophages. Among the earliest reported cases of
human disease are examples of patients with hypogammaglobulinemia or agammaglobulinemia. A review by the group at the Centers for Disease Control
(CDC) of the association between pneumocystosis
and primary immunodeficiency syndromes showed
that infected patients had decreased serum immunoglobulins, impaired antibody synthesis, or both.[34]

2.6. Epidemiology and Transmission

Knowledge of the epidemiology and transmission of *Pneumocystis* infection is based on careful

studies of experimentally infected animals and limited clinical and serologic investigations in humans. Naturally occurring epizootics of *Pneumocystis* infection have been documented in a colony of nude mice,[35] a finding again emphasizing the importance of T-lymphocyte-mediated immunity. Other studies demonstrate transmission of disease in experimental animals previously treated with cortisone. Hendley and Weller employed a model using steroid-treated rats obtained by cesarean section that were originally barrier sustained.[36] When exposed to an air supply from standard infected rats where the disease was engendered by cortisone treatment, evidence for airborne transmission was obtained. Airborne spread to non-steroid-treated nude mice was documented by Walzer and colleagues.[31] The evidence in humans in favor of a contagious process derives from the initial observations of epidemic disease that occurred in nurseries and foundling homes in central Europe and Iran.[6] In addition, there have been scattered reports of *Pneumocystis* infection occurring in roommates[37] and in family members.[38] In the United States, there have been three well-studied episodes of institutional outbreaks that occurred in cancer treatment centers. The largest of these studies, carried out at St. Jude Children's Cancer Research Hospital by Perera et al.[39] failed to confirm patient-to-patient spread. It was the conclusion of these investigators that the disease in most cases arose independently from reactivation of latent infection triggered by intensive antineoplastic drug protocols. By contrast, however, Singer et al. reported, in 1975, a small cluster of 11 cases that occurred over a 3-month interval at Memorial Sloan-Kettering Cancer Center.[40] The epidemiologic investigation, which included serologic studies of patients and hospital personnel, suggested interpersonal spread at the institution. A third outbreak occurring among childhood leukemia patients treated at the Riley Hospital in Indianapolis, Indiana involved 11 cases over 10-month period.[41] Here too, serological studies suggested involvement of nursing and medical personnel either as cases of inapparent infection or as actual carriers of disease.

Our concept of the epidemiology of *Pneumocystis* infection therefore encompasses the original postulates of Meuwissen et al.[42] and Hughes [43] that the infection is a common occurrence among young children. If individuals later become intensely immunosuppressed, the infection may become reactivated. Some normal adults may not have had childhood infection, experience mild or inapparent infections when exposed, and "contain" the process because of intact host defenses. These individuals, however, might be healthy nursing or medical personnel who demonstrate evidence of asymptomatic seroconversion. Still, they could transmit the disease to high-risk patients within the hospital environment. On the other hand, such instances are probably much less common than reactivation of latent infection, i.e., person-to-person spread is usually unlikely.

2.7. Clinical Features (Non-AIDS Related)

Clinical and epidemiologic information concerning *Pneumocystis carinii* infection has been derived from two excellent sources in the United States: (1) analyses of cases whose treatment was evaluated by the CDC[32,44] and (2) comprehensive longitudinal studies of children with neoplasms treated at the St. Jude Children's Cancer Research Hospital in Memphis, Tennessee.[5,45] The information is largely complementary, but the findings of these two groups must be evaluated in the context of the sources of the data. With the CDC assessments, the data base consists of report forms returned to the Parasitic Diseases Drug Service during the period when pentamidine, solely distributed by CDC, was the principal mode of treatment. The epidemiologic data from the CDC are valuable in discerning major trends. By drawing on a large sample of cases, the pitfalls of relying on information from a few major institutions are avoided. However, in such a series there could have been a systematic bias toward inclusion of patients in whom appropriate diagnostic procedures were attempted, such as those treated in large university-type referral centers. The St. Jude's experience benefits from having a well-defined population of children with malignancy that has been observed by excellent clinicians over a long period of time. Such a study proves highly reliable information on specific risk factors for pneumocystosis.

From the CDC data, the following observations may be made. The attack rate of pneumocystosis is highest in the age group less than 1 year (almost all affected patients in this group have a primary immunodeficiency) and progressively declines with advancing age.[46] Viewed in terms of numbers of patients, of some 194 patients with histologically confirmed *Pneumocystis* pneumonia, leukemia was the most common underlying disease and was present in 91 of the 194 cases. Of these, approximately two-thirds or 58 out of 91 were of the acute lymphatic type, and 18 of the 91 were of the chronic lymphatic type. Hodgkin disease and other lymphomas were the second largest group of underlying disease, followed by primary immunologic deficiency diseases. Recipients of organ transplants were the fourth largest group of patients. It was possible to calculate the attack rate of pneumocystosis for the different leukemias: 1.1% per year for acute lymphatic disease, 0.05% per year for chronic lymphatic disease, and 0.2% per year for acute myelocytic disease.[46] However, if these rates are expressed in terms of a lifetime risk, it is likely that patients with lymphatic leukemia, who now have a considerably longer survival than those with myelocytic leukemia, are at even greater risk of contracting pneumocystosis. Indeed, it is rare in our experience to encounter a case of pneumocystosis complicating myelocytic leukemia unless the patient has been given corticosteroid therapy. Since corticosteroids are not routinely employed in many of the common chemotherapeutic induction regimens for acute myelocytic leukemia, those relatively few cases of pneumocystosis in the latter group of patients may be more related to steroid therapy rather than to the leukemia per se.

In the CDC analysis, the most common symptom of *Pneumocystis* pneumonia was dyspnea, which was observed in 91% of patients (Table 3). Fever was present in two-thirds of patients, and cough was present in one-half. It is important to recognize that only 7% of patients had productive cough, and only two patients had hemoptysis. In the great majority of children, tachypnea with respiratory rate exceeding 40 per minute was present as well as a weak dry cough. Furthermore, an absence of characteristic rales has been occasionally noted even when severe pneumonitis is present radiographically. One of the more remarkable observations in the St. Jude's pediatric population was the finding that 21% of documented *Pneumocystis*-infected patients had mild to moderate diarrhea at the onset or during the course of pneumonitis.[45] Whether this finding might have resulted from antimicrobial therapy is not known.

The duration of symptoms in 153 patients with confirmed pneumocystosis in the CDC analysis ranged from less than 7 to greater than 90 days, with a

TABLE 3. Clinical Features of 168 Patients with Histologically Confirmed *Pneumocystis* Pneumonia[a]

Clinical features	Number of patients	Percent
Symptoms		
Dyspnea	152	91
Fever	110	66
Cough	79	47
Productive cough	12	7
Hemoptysis	3	2
Chest pain	11	7
Night sweats	1	1
Signs (respiratory)		
Cyanosis	66	39
Rales	56	33
Breath sounds		
Decreased	22	13
Bronchial/tubular	14	8
Dullness	9	5
Rhonchi	7	4
Wheezing	2	1
Signs (other)		
Hepatomegaly	59	35
Splenomegaly	32	19
Radiographic findings		
Infiltrate		
Diffuse and bilateral	164	98
Unilateral	4	2
Effusion	8	5
Adventitious air[b]	6	4

[a]From Walzer et al [32]
[b]Pneumothorax, pneumomediastinum, etc

median of approximately 12 days. The widespread belief that pneumocystosis is an acute fulminant pneumonitis may be, in part, a reflection of delayed diagnosis or at least dilatory management until the patient has deteriorated to the point where diagnostic measures became a medical emergency.

Illustrative Case 1

The patient was an 8-year-old white girl with a 1½-year history of acute lymphatic leukemia. After induction of remission with vincristine and prednisone, she relapsed and was successfully reinduced with vincristine, L-asparginase, prednisone, systemic methotrexate, and intrathecal methotrexate. She also received craniospinal radiation and 6-mercaptopurine. A month prior to this admission, she was admitted to the pediatric service of the hospital and given ampicillin 100 mg/kg IV q4h because of the 3-day history of cough, fever, and vomiting. A chest radiograph showed a right middle lobe infiltrate Sputum grew *Streptococcus viridans, Neisseria* species, *Staphylococcus edpidermidis,* a few yeastlike organisms, and a few *Hemophilus* species. However, the nature of the respiratory pathogen was not identified, and after 4 days in the hospital the patient was sent home on a gram of ampicillin a day. For the 2 weeks prior to admission, she had a productive cough, a rapid respiratory rate, decreased appetite, lethargy, fever to 101°F (38.3°C), but no cyanosis or dyspnea. Her prednisone dose (40 mg/day) was tapered, but admission was prompted by a progressive right middle lobe and newly documented left lower lobe infiltrate (Fig. 2A). Physical examination revealed a tachypneic, irritable young white girl with a blood pressure of 120/50 mm Hg, respiratory rate 40, pulse 140, temperature 100.4°F (38°C). Physical examination of the lungs revealed diffuse inspiratory wheezes and rales greater on the left than on the right and greater at the bases than the apices. Complete blood count (CBC) revealed a hemoglobin (Hb) of 12.2 mg/dl hematocrit (Hct) 35%, white blood cell (WBC) 1600 with 68% segmented forms, 4% band forms, 18% lymphocytes, 10% mononuclear cells, and 140,000 platelets. A cold agglutinin titer was negative and a venous blood gas showed a pH 7.45 P_{CO_2} 40 mm Hg, P_{O_2} 33 mm Hg, with 66% saturation.

The patient was started on carbenicillin, gentamicin, oxacillin, trimethoprim–sulfamethoxazole, and erythromycin. The trimethoprim–sulfamethoxazole was initially given orally. Her respiratory status continued to deteriorate over the next several days, and she was given 35% O_2 by mask. She also developed a vesicular rash in the distribution of T 7–8 dermatone consistent with herpes zoster, and adenine arabinoside was started. At this point, she was taken to the operating room where under general anesthesia an open-wedge biopsy of the left lower lobe was performed. *Pneumocystis carinii* was detected in the lung biopsy, and the patient was started on intravenous trimethoprim–sulfamethoxazole. Blood levels of trimethoprim exceeded 5 μg/ml, 1 hr postinfusion. Varicella pneumonia was not excluded at the time, but subsequently cultures of lung tissue were negative for varicella. Thereafter, the patient showed gradual clinical improvement, although she demonstrated evidence of the inappropriate ADH syndrome. Her arterial blood P_{O_2} gradually rose from 55 mm Hg to 90 mm Hg on room air. A total of 14 days of intravenous trimethoprim–sulfamethoxazole was given, and the chest radiograph returned to normal over the next 4 weeks (Fig. 2B).

Comment. This case illustrates many of the typical findings of *Pneumocystis* infection complicating childhood leukemia: (1) the disease occurs during bone marrow remission, often when steroids are being tapered; (2) the duration of respiratory symptoms (particularly tachypnea) can be weeks, (3) there can be concurrent infections (in lung and other sites) like herpes zoster, (4) but appropriate therapy will result in complete radiologic resolution Furthermore, this case illustrates the problems with orally administered, empirical trimethoprim–sulfamethoxazole. Absorption may be incomplete, and the question of drug failure versus inadequate dosage remains. An aggressive diagnostic approach led to identification of the pulmonary pathogen (it was not varicella) and a more reliable therapeutic approach; intravenous trimethoprim–sulfamethoxazole was then used. Clearly, we do not condone the delay in undertaking a diagnostic procedure as occurred in this case (see Section 2 9), nor do we advocate empirical therapy in patients

able to undergo a biopsy procedure. It is fortunate that residual evidence of *Pneumocystis* infection was present in the biopsy specimen.

Relevant to our case is that one-fourth of the CDC-analyzed patients with confirmed pneumocystosis had another documented infection.[46] The simultaneous occurrence of cytomegalovirus infection with *Pneumocystis* pneumonia has been particularly common in recipients of organ transplants.[47]

An interesting comparison and contrast between the incidence of varicella–zoster and *Pneumocystis carinii* pneumonia in leukemic children has also been reported.[48] Whereas one-quarter of patients given the most intense chemotherapy regimen developed pneumocystosis, there was really no increased risk of varicella–zoster virus (VZV) infection. Twenty percent of patients who failed to achieve remission had VZV infections, and 30% in this category also developed pneumocystosis.

In related studies, Hughes and collaborators documented the risk of *Pneumocystis* pneumonia in relation to the phase and type of antileukemic therapy.[48] During a phase when treatment consisted of prednisone, vincristine, and L-asparginase over a 4-week cycle, no patient out of a total of 149 developed pneumocystosis During a succeeding phase that included intrathecal methotrexate and central nervous system (CNS) irradiation, this same group of 149 patients experienced a 4% incidence of pneumocystosis. Subsequent attempts at consolidation of remission over a 2–3-year period involved randomization into four treatment groups. Those patients maintained on methotrexate or methotrexate plus 6-mercaptopurine and cyclophosphamide experienced about a 5% incidence of pneumocystosis. By contrast, when cytosine arabinoside was added to methotrexate, 6-mercaptopurine, and cyclophosphamide, 10 of 41 children, or 22.4%, developed *Pneumocystis carinii* pneumonia The incidence of *Pneumocystis* in acute lymphocytic leukemia thus appeared to be a reflection of the intensity of chemotherapy. Extent of the neoplastic disease and mediastinal irradiation could have been additive factors.

2.8. Radiologic Findings

The typical radiologic pattern in biopsy-proven pneumocystosis, observed in almost 100% of the CDC-reported cases, is a diffuse bilateral alveolar infiltrate.[32] Only 5% of patients in the CDC series were found to have a pleural effusion. Consistent with this experience, 78 out of the 80 patients studied at St. Jude had diffuse alveolar disease, and the two patients who had normal chest radiographs died within 48 hr, at which time pneumocysts were found in the lung at autopsy.[45] Several interesting reports suggest that the appearance of pulmonary infiltrates may be delayed and lag behind the abrupt onset of dyspnea.[49,50] Thus, dyspnea alone could be an important clinical clue in patients at high risk of developing pneumocystosis. Persons who suddenly experience tachypnea and are found to be hypoxic even in the absence of pulmonary infiltrates should be carefully

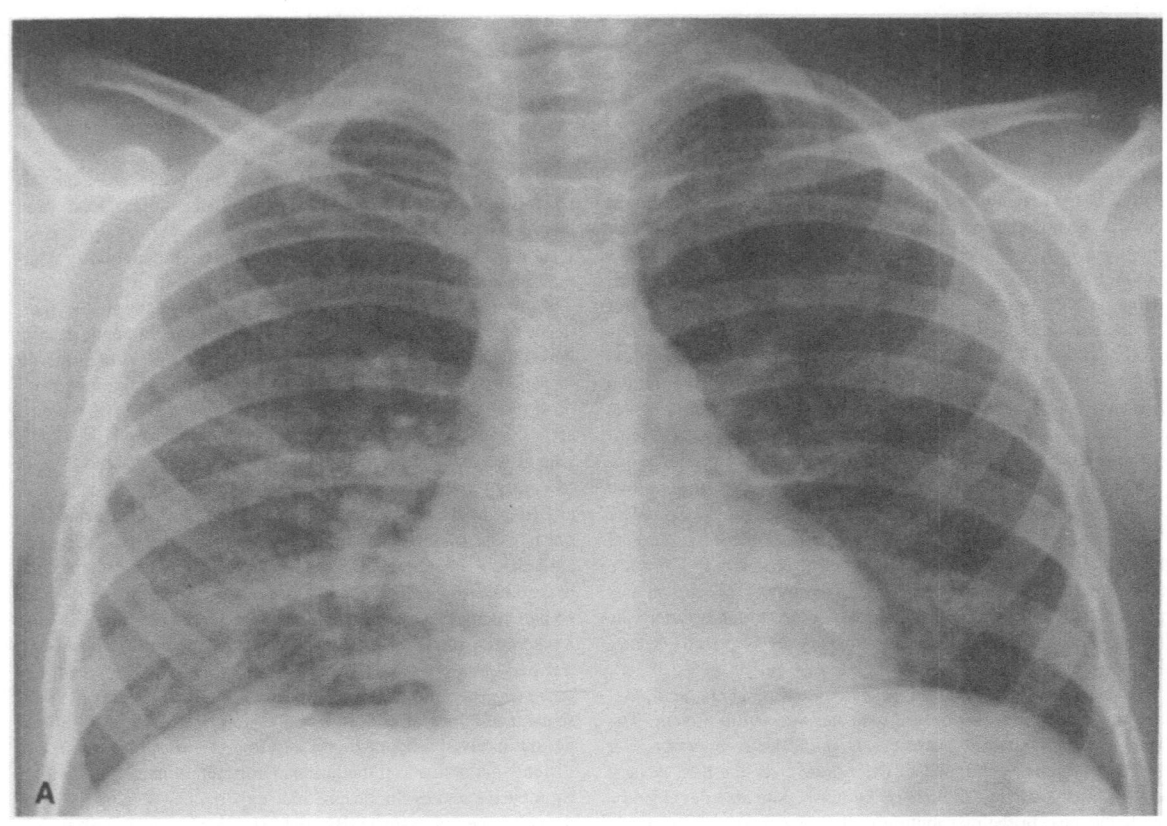

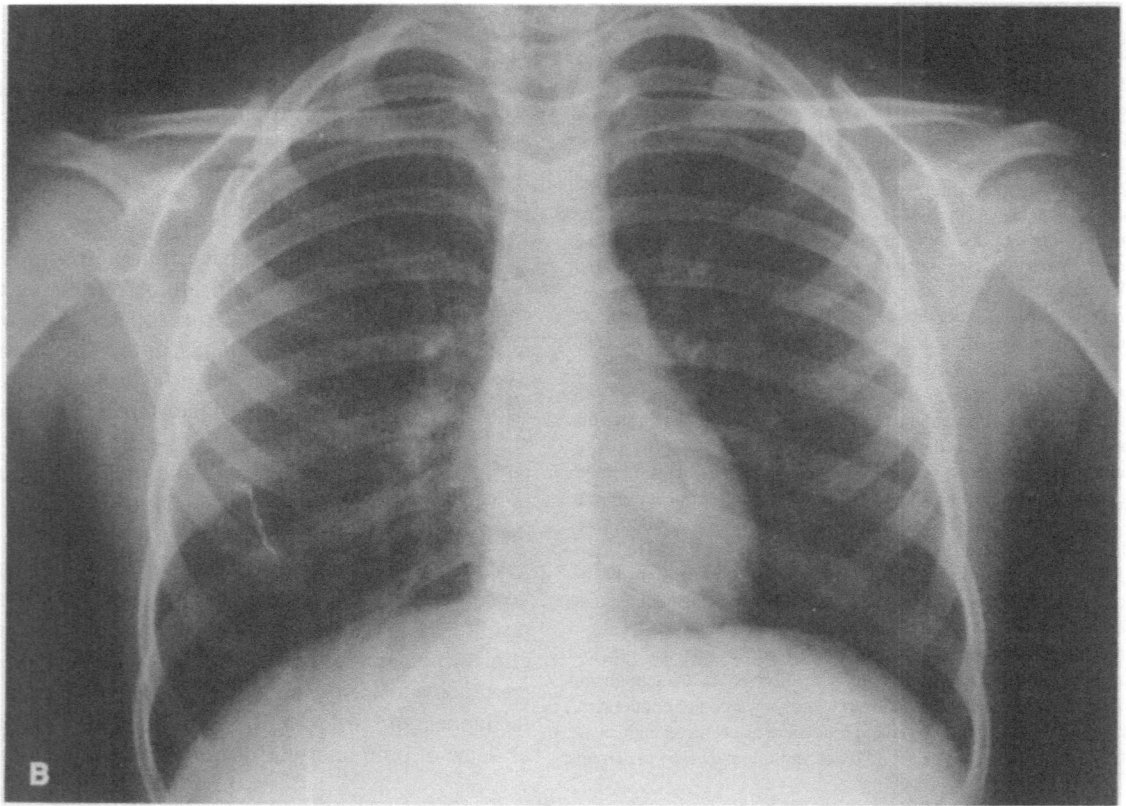

evaluated and have daily chest radiographs, because the infiltrates may appear later. Furthermore, there are several reports that a lung scan, particularly with gallium,[50,51] may identify lung involvement prior to the radiograph (but is not specific for pneumocystosis). In several reported cases, the chest radiograph has remained normal despite severe dyspnea and hypoxemia.[52]

Another study of the radiologic features of *Pneumocystis carinii* pneumonia involved 30 patients with confirmed disease.[53] It was emphasized that the typical radiographic picture is an acute perihilar and basilar infiltrate progressing to diffuse alveolar consolidation within 3–5 days, usually unassociated with hilar adenopathy or pleural changes. However, in this study the incidence of atypical radiographic findings was appreciable, with 17 of 30 patients showing at least one atypical finding. Such findings included sparing of the apices of the lung, unilateral appearance of the infiltrate, lobar or segmental consolidation (in addition to diffuse involvement), and a pseudonodular pattern that could be confused with metastatic processes. Additional reports document that pneumocystosis may even cause "coin" lesions[54] or pneumatoceles.[55] Although pleural effusion is exceedingly unusual in pneumocystosis, this observation must be tempered by the recognition that pleural effusions can be a part of an underlying disease such as neoplasm or collagen vascular disorder that predisposes to *Pneumocystis* infection. Similarly, a finding of a mediastinal mass does not militate against the diagnosis of *Pneumocystis* infection of the lung. Although it is common to attribute a mediastinal mass to progression of underlying disease (lymphoma or leukemia), 43% of patients with mediastinal masses in the St. Jude Hospital series had *Pneumocystis* infection.[48] In summary, therefore, no radiologic finding per se completely excludes the diagnosis of *Pneumocystis*.

2.9. Diagnostic Approaches to Suspected *Pneumocystis carinii* Infection

The diagnosis of pneumocystosis still involves controversial issues: (1) What are the indications and value of attempting an invasive procedure to diagnose *Pneumocystis* infection? (2) Should patients with suspected infection initially receive an empirical trial of antimicrobial therapy that will "cover" this organism (as in the case illustrated)? (3) What diagnostic procedure is best or most expedient in different hosts? Much time is spent at the bedside or on ward rounds in debating these issues. Our working principles are that every reasonable attempt should be made to establish a specific diagnosis and that empirical therapy should be avoided if possible. Furthermore, we believe that open lung biopsy still represents the most reliable means of confirming diagnosis but is unquestionably the most invasive procedure. Patients with *Pneumocystis* infection are often critically ill and, in addition to being tachypneic and hypoxic, often are receiving antiinflammatory agents that impair wound healing. Some may have a marked bleeding diathesis. Obviously diagnostic procedures such as thoractomy or transbronchial biopsy may aggravate hypoxia and add to the risk of hemorrhage. Whether there can be compromises in the diagnostic approaches, i.e., less invasive procedures of equal sensitivity and specificity, is an issue that still remains unresolved.

The major argument in the past in favor of making a specific diagnosis was based on the observation that almost 50% of patients treated with pentamidine experienced a significant untoward reaction.[32] Thus, a proven diagnosis made pentamidine treatment a justifiable hazard, whereas a negative biopsy avoided toxic empirical therapy. With the availability of trimethoprim–sulfamethoxazole, an alternative argument has been raised: namely, that therapy is relatively nontoxic (at least in non-AIDS patients) and all clinically suspected cases should be given a therapeutic trial. If the patient improves, a possibly dangerous diagnostic procedure is averted. Walzer et al.[32] have no quarrel with this argument, nor do they object to the empirical use of trimethoprim–sulfamethoxazole in the patient in whom it is not possible, for good reasons, to attempt an invasive diagnostic procedure. On the other hand, trimethoprim-sulfamethoxazole is not specific for *Pneumocystis carinii*, and clinical improvement cannot be ascribed to the specific therapy directed against this protozoan parasite. That would be of little practical concern to

FIGURE 2. (A) Chest radiograph taken immediately prior to lung biopsy of Illustrative Case 1, subsequently proven to have pneumocystosis (B) Chest radiograph following successful completion of course of intravenous trimethoprim–sulfamethoxazole.

the improving patient, but the dilemma begins if the patient does not improve.

It has been amply demonstrated in a number of series, perhaps the best of which is from the National Cancer Institute, that *Pneumocystis* accounts for probably no more than one-third of the etiologies of diffuse pulmonary infiltrates.[56] To treat empirically with trimethoprim–sulfamethoxazole alone would delay the chance of identifying other treatable diseases (tuberculosis, aspergillosis, cryptococcosis, or interstitial pneumonitis secondary to anticancer drugs) where different therapy would obviously be indicated. The recent recognition of new, potentially treatable pulmonary infections is an important reminder of the value of making a specific diagnosis. Moreover, if a diagnostic procedure is carried out after a course of empirical therapy has been initiated, it may not be possible to identify the original provocative agent. The clinician is then left to deliberate if the initial therapy were correct, whether the patient might harbor a strain morphologically altered by therapy but resistant to the drugs given, or whether cysts were missed simply because of sampling error. Thus, early empirical therapy with trimethoprim–sulfamethoxazole may obfuscate the nature of underlying infection (whether caused by *Pneumocystis* or by other microbes); if a biopsy is obtained at a later point, the quality of the information derived is likely to be less reliable.

Perhaps a more trenchant question is whether benefit always accrues to the patient in whom a specific diagnosis of infection is made by lung biopsy. From an intellectual and protocol-oriented view, there is no argument about the desirability of determining the etiology of a patient's pulmonary infection. Unfortunately, some of the better retrospective studies of open lung biopsy have failed to discern a difference in mortality between patients who had a specific diagnosis made and those who did not or between those whose treatment was altered because of diagnosis and those in whom the results of biopsy did not affect treatment.[57] Yet, it is not possible to conclude from such a study that open lung biopsy is completely without value, since patients with specific diagnoses may constitute a higher risk group whose mortality rate might even be higher if they were undiagnosed or inappropriately treated. In fact, other studies[58,59] have reported lower mortality rates for patients who had a specific diagnosis established

than for those who did not. Thus, a definite conclusion about the value of establishing a diagnosis can be made only in patients with a specific diagnosis prospectively randomized into treatment and nontreatment groups, and it is doubtful that such a study will ever be carried out.

Since survival statistics for immunosuppressed patients who develop pulmonary infiltrates are depressingly poor and mortality rates of many of the underlying diseases are also substantial, it is only reasonable to adopt an approach to the diagnosis of pulmonary pathology that is tempered by clinical circumstances. In patients who have failed to respond to conventional therapy and in whom the chances of experimental therapy working are bleak (refractory neoplasm), empirical anti-*Pneumocystis* therapy may be justified. We also favor empirical therapy if the patient has an uncorrectable bleeding diathesis that precludes invasive diagnostic measures. By contrast, aggressive diagnostic approaches are clearly indicated in dealing with new pulmonary infiltrates in young patients whose leukemias or lymphomas may be in remission.

An important question is whether nonspecific polypharmacy might lead to better patient survival and cost effectiveness than diagnostic open biopsy. It can be argued that by empirical use of a number of antimicrobial agents, most of the infectious problems found in immunosuppressed patients could be treated. The reservations about this approach include the following: (1) patients with undiagnosed neoplastic or drug-induced pulmonary infiltrates would not be correctly treated; (2) multiple drugs may interact in ways to potentiate organ toxicity (e.g., nephrotoxicity) or in ways we cannot anticipate; (3) dosage of empirical therapy may not be adequate or "pushed" with the confidence that exists when a diagnosis is established. In one study, two-thirds of patients having an underlying malignancy were found to have the same neoplastic process responsible for pulmonary infiltrates. Hospital mortality rate was only 8%,[60] emphasizing the importance of directed radiation/chemotherapy in these patients. Thus, a specific diagnosis is highly desirable whenever there is a strong suspicion of disseminated malignancy.

Fully 40% of the patients in Hughes's trial of trimethoprim–sulfamethoxazole versus pentamidine did not initially respond to the agent of first choice, and the total of 80% beneficial responses included approximately 20% of the patients who were crossed over to the alternative regimen.[49] Whether these patients would have improved if they had been maintained on the initial agent selected is open to question. We have certainly seen patients who did not respond to pentamidine for up to 8 days when pentamidine was the only parenteral agent that could be used for treatment of *Pneumocystis* infection (see Section 2.10). An even more important question, however, is whether or not there may be differing susceptibility of *Pneumocystis* strains for the different antimicrobial agents that are available at this time. Without establishing a specific diagnosis, particularly of *Pneumocystis*, empirical therapy may thus miss those patients who could be failing on one regimen and could potentially benefit by a switch to the other or in whom the dose of one of the agents could be increased.

Two studies carried out in oncology centers[61,62] document the superiority of open lung biopsy over less invasive diagnostic procedures: simultaneous sampling was performed in each of these studies and, not surprisingly, the yield of specific diagnoses was greatest with open lung biopsy. Unfortunately, nonspecific or idiopathic pneumonitis was found in a disturbingly large proportion of cases in both series. In the final analysis, local experience and expertise should be the basis for selection of a diagnostic procedure. The yield from examination of expectorated sputum is low except in patients with AIDS, in whom the number of cyst forms appears to be high.[63]

Transtracheal aspiration in certain selected cases has readily yielded the diagnosis and is an approach that we would favor providing the patient's platelet count were in excess of 40,000 mm³.[64] We do not advocate transtracheal aspiration solely as a means for making a diagnosis of pneumocystosis. It is recommended as a valuable means of diagnosing infectious pulmonary disease and has been particularly helpful in documenting nosocomial gram-negative bacillary and anaerobic lung infection.[65] In fact, in our hands, the successful identification of *Pneumocystis* by transtracheal aspiration has been a dividend of attempts to diagnose tuberculosis or other bacterial infection in the lung. Transtracheal aspiration may also be attempted as a prelude to fiberoptic bronchoscopy. Transbronchial biopsy or fiberoptic bronchoscopy with brushing are now readily available in a number of centers, but a major problem with

endoscopic techniques is that material insufficient for all of the desired microbiologic as well as histopathologic studies is often obtained.

In some centers, particularly those oriented to pediatrics, percutaneous thoracic closed needle aspiration under fluoroscopic guidance has been carried out, usually without complication.[66] Perhaps in young children the lung seems to "seal" better after puncture, but our experience with needle aspiration or biopsy in the adult has not been so salutary. Indeed, puncture of the lung in an adult with a bleeding diathesis or thrombocytopenia may lead to both pneumothorax and uncontrolled bleeding.

Our recommendation is that transtracheal aspiration and either fiberoptic bronchoscopy with brushing or transbronchial biopsy be performed initially, but neither of the latter two techniques reliably diagnoses aerobic and anaerobic bacterial infection, hence the added value of transtracheal aspiration (TTA).

A variation of the bronchoscopic procedure is bronchoalveolar lavage, where the catheter is wedged into a bronchus and a fairly large amount of saline (200 ml) rapidly introduced and reaspirated.[67] The recovered fluid is concentrated for culture and examination, using such tools as monoclonal antibody staining for herpes viruses. While these procedures are being planned and executed, we see no harm in giving an IV dose of furosemide (100 mg) to those patients in whom congestive heart failure has not been excluded with a Swan Ganz type of pulmonary outflow catheter. This can lead to dramatic relief of dyspnea within hours and, coupled with radiologic improvement, might lead to postponement of more invasive procedures. If TTA and bronchoscopic procedures do not yield a diagnosis, we would unhesitatingly proceed to open lung biopsy. Thus, the basic approach must be a commitment to an escalating tempo of diagnostic evaluation. If one procedure fails to lead to a specific diagnosis, the next step should be undertaken immediately without delay.

The diagnostic evaluation does not end with the surgical procedure. It does no good to carry out an open lung biopsy on an emergency basis if the proper services within the hospital are not mobilized to process such specimens rapidly. Bacteriologic, mycologic, and acid-fast studies are mandatory, but culture of the specimen for anaerobes and viruses is also clearly indicated. We believe that rapid methods for staining cysts or trophozoites—Giemsa, toluidine blue, and Gram–Weigert stains—are valuable methods for making the diagnosis, but a definitive diagnosis rests on the identification of material by silver stain. Permanently fixed tissue sections take longer to process than impression smears of biopsy specimens, but silver stains of both materials should be performed using procedures such as those outlined in Table 1.

Some success has been reported in skilled and experienced hands by using an immunofluorescent technique for the detection of *Pneumocystis* in sputum or tracheal aspirates.[68] Monoclonal antibodies specific for *Pneumocystis* have been developed and these may be of diagnostic value.[69]

Serologic tests have been evaluated for more than a decade both in Europe and in the United States.[42,70] The value of a complement fixation test reported by some European workers has not been borne out when subject to critical scrutiny. An indirect immunofluorescence test for detecting circulating antibody using cysts prepared from either human lung or from animals has been reported to be positive in perhaps one-third of cases.[71] We believe, in fact, that the sensitivity and specificity of the test can be increased, but in our hands no more than two-thirds of patients are positive at time of presentation. If serologic tests are positive, they are suggestive of *Pneumocystis* infection. This may be an interesting way to recoup the diagnosis in patients who were treated empirically and whose serial antibody titers might be followed along the course of recovery.

Preliminary efforts at cultivating the parasite have been reported by several groups, but these techniques cannot be applied for diagnostic purposes.[4] In one report, cyst antigen harvested from in vitro passage has been used to produce antiserum which has been used in countercurrent immunoelectrophoretic tests to detect circulating *Pneumocystis* antigen. However, a positive test result seems more suggestive of pneumonitis rather than *Pneumocystis* infection.[72] Considerable debate has arisen regarding such antibody tests[73,74] and at present they cannot be considered of any diagnostic value.

2.10. Treatment

There are three regimens that have proven effective for therapy of *Pneumocystis* infection: pentami-

dine isethionate, the fixed combination of trimethoprim–sulfamethoxazole, and the combination of pyrimethamine and a sulfonamide. A variation of the latter two regimens is to substitute the sulfonamide with a sulfone such as diaminodiphenyl sulfone (Dapsone). Clinical experience has been greatest with pentamidine and trimethoprim–sulfamethoxazole. The numbers of cases treated with pyrimethamine and sulfadiazine is small, and no studies have been carried out to compare the latter regimen with trimethoprim–sulfamethoxazole. Pentamidine and trimethoprim–sulfamethoxazole have been evaluated in a comparative manner in at least one study in leukemics and found to be equivalent.[49] Pentamidine has been compared with pyrimethamine-sulfadiazine in a very small series where the preliminary results were similar. However, pyrimethamine–sulfadiazine was difficult to administer in severely ill patients.[76] No information is available on the relative effectiveness of the individual components of the two-drug combinations, that is, whether trimethoprim or pyrimethamine alone might be effective in the treatment of pneumocystosis. The latter question could be clinically important in the patient who has well-documented sulfonamide allergy. Many other agents have been tried over the years, including *p*-aminosalicylic acid, isoniazid, and amphtericin B, but no convincing evidence for their effectiveness has been presented. Another folate sulfonamide combination, pyrimethamine–sulfadoxine (Fansidar), is a long-acting combination that was effective prophylactically in studies carried out in Iran.[77]

Despite the availability of clinically effective agents, important questions still remain about the use of any of the three acceptable therapeutic approaches. One issue is that of pharmacokinetics and of the adequacy of some of the presently recommended dosage regimens. The second consists of potential cumulative toxicity when agents such as pentamidine are used with other nephrotoxic compounds such as aminoglycosides and amphotericin. Because of inability to achieve long-term cultivation of the causative agent, questions about drug resistance remain as yet unanswered. Since the folate antagonists bind dihydrofolate reductase, the site of action for some anticancer drugs such as methotrexate, treatment or prophylaxis with folate antagonists could potentiate chemotherapy aimed at an underlying neoplasm. An unanswered issue in man is whether or not two or more of the effective regimens, e.g., pentamidine and trimethoprim–sulfamethoxazole, might be better than one alone. (There is no support for this in experimental animal studies.[78]) Finally, important bedside questions are duration of therapy and the clinical guidelines for adhering to one form of treatment before switching to alternative treatment.

2.10.1. Pentamidine

Pentamidine isethionate (Lomidine), 4-4′-diamidinodiphenoxypentane di-β-hydroxyethanesulfonate, is a diamidine compound with antiprotozoal and antifungal activity. Originally, this agent was synthesized as a hypoglycemic agent, and the problem of hypoglycemia persists as a potential complication of pentamidine therapy. Prior to the availability of pentamidine, the mortality from *Pneumocystis* pneumonitis was approximately 50% in the pediatric cases observed during European epidemics and close to 100% in immunodeficient children and adults.[76,77] In 1958, Ivady and Paldy first reported that pentamidine therapy of infantile *Pneumocystis* infection lowered mortality from 50% to 3%.[10] Several hundred cases of the epidemic disease in nurseries in Hungary were treated successfully with dose of 4 mg/day of pentamidine IM for 12–14 days. Clinical responses were usually apparent 4–6 days after the initiation of treatment, but radiographic improvement was often delayed for several weeks. Other investigators in Europe have reported comparable results in smaller series of children.

Pharmacologic effects of pentamidine vary depending on the route of administration.[75] In animals, a precipitous transitory fall in blood pressure has been noted immediately after injection, and renal toxicity has followed repeated administration. To avoid immediate toxic reactions associated with intravenous administration, IM injection is preferred, but in markedly thrombocytopenic patients, consideration must still be given to the intravenous route. Some evidence exists that pentamidine inhibits dihydrofolate reductase in tissues. In addition, pentamidine interacts and forms water-insoluble products with specific nucleotides and nucleic acids. Alternatively, it has been proposed that pentamidine acts through interference with aerobic glycolysis. There is no question that megaloblastosis of the bone

marrow has been reported in patients treated with pentamidine, and this is paralleled by lower serum folate levels. Nonetheless, it has not been shown that pretreatment with folinic acid influences the therapeutic efficacy of pentamidine in rats infected with *Pneumocystis*.

Administration and Dosage. Each suspension of pentamidine isethionate must be freshly prepared with sterile distilled water. Under no circumstances should normal saline be used as a diluent because of the insolubility of the drug in such material. Pentamidine must be given parenterally because it is poorly absorbed via the oral route.

The dose for *Pneumocystis carinii* peneumonia is 4 mg/kg given IM once a day for 12–14 days, but in some circumstances (patients with AIDS) therapy may have to be continued for more than 2 weeks. For large adults (>80 kg), doses in excess of 200 mg may be considered.

The calculated daily dose should be dissolved in no more than 3 ml sterile distilled water in order to reduce the volume of injection. Solutions showing turbidity or slight crystalline remnants are still suitable for intramuscular but not intravenous injections. Such solutions seem to possess no more toxicity or loss of activity. However, it should be borne in mind that sterile abscesses can result from too large a volume of injection and from irritation from the drug itself. In situations in which IM injections are considered hazardous, administration via the intravenous route can be attempted providing that the patient is under constant observation, preferably in an intensive care setting. The total dose to be administered is dissolved in 25–50 ml of sterile distilled water and infused by drip infusion over a 30–60 mm period. A V- or Y-type intravenous line is employed with intravenous glucose solution running and the pentamidine dripped into the IV line. Blood pressure determinations should be taken at 10-min intervals during the administration of the drug. If a significant fall in blood pressure is observed, the infusion should be terminated and the blood pressure allowed to return to pretreatment levels. An attempt at reinfusion at one-half the prior rate may be undertaken if circumstances permit, i.e., the patient is stable enough and will also remain under constant observation.

A variety of side effects has been reported following intravenous administration of pentamidine.

These include hypotension, rapid pulse, flushing, dizziness, salivation, sweating, headache, nausea, vomiting, dyspnea, syncope, incontinence, epileptiform activity, and facial edema. Even following intramuscular injection, hypotension, tachycardia, nausea, and vomiting are commonly encountered.

In the experience accumulated by the CDC, 42% of all patients treated with pentamidine and 63% of those treated for 9 or more days recovered.[32] Adverse reactions were noted in 189 (47%) of 404 patients who received the drug for either confirmed or suspected infection. Fully 24% of patients developed impaired renal function; liver dysfunction was observed in 10%, hypoglycemia in 6%, hematologic disturbances in 4%, injection-site reactions (usually sterile abscesses) in 18%, hypotension in 2%, skin rashes in 2%, and hypocalcemia in 1%.

In other centers where there has not been a large preponderance of older and more debilitated patients, i.e., pediatric leukemia therapy centers, the therapeutic recovery rates have approached 80%, but the adverse effects have been similar to those reported by the CDC.[49]

2.10.2. Pyrimethamine and a Sulfonamide

For almost two decades, evidence has existed that the combination of pyrimethamine and a sulfonamide is effective in the treatment of *Pneumocystis* pneumonia. The first evidence came from animal studies of cortisone-treated rats carried out by Frenkel and colleagues.[9] Scattered case reports attest to the efficacy of this approach, but as noted previously, limited comparisons have been made to other forms of therapy such as pentamidine or trimethoprim–sulfamethoxazole.[76,77,79] In addition, Post and colleagues reported effective prophylaxis of the epidemic infantile infections with sulfadoxine plus pyrimethamine.[80] The adult dose of pyrimethamine and sulfadiazine, the latter being available in the United States, is 25–50mg/day pyrimethamine with 4 g/day sulfadiazine.

2.10.3. Trimethoprim–Sulfamethoxazole

Because of the success in experimental therapy obtained with pyrimethamine and a sulfonamide, it was only logical that somewhat similar drugs such as trimethoprim and sulfamethoxazole would be se-

lected for study. Using the cortisone-induced rat model of pneumocystosis, Hughes and collaborators demonstrated that this fixed combination was as effective as pentamidine in the treatment of *Pneumocystis* pneumonitis.[13] In addition, when administered prophylactically, the combination successfully prevented the infection. Following the initial studies in animals, many trials have been reported, including pediatric[14,49] and adult patients.[15,81,82]

Some comments about the dosage of trimethoprim–sulfamethoxazole used in the human clinical studies of pneumocystosis are warranted. Pediatric trials carried out by Hughes used two doses, a low-dosage form (10 mg trimethoprim and 50 mg sulfamethoxazole/kg) and a higher-dosage form (20 mg trimethoprim and 100 mg sulfamethoxazole/kg) administered daily. The latter was found to be more effective. It is important to recognize that this dosage is three times that recommended for the treatment of bacterial infections in adults. Hughes and colleagues definitively compared trimethoprim–sulfamethoxazole and pentamidine in a randomized controlled study of 37 children with *Pneumocystis carinii* infections.[49] The basic study design involved a crossover from the initial drug regimen to the alternative regimen if patients failed to improve. Of 18 patients treated with pentamidine, 11 recovered, one died after receiving the drug alone, and six others required crossover to trimethoprim–sulfamethoxazole; three of these recovered. Of 19 patients treated with trimethoprim–sulfamethoxazole, 13 recovered after initial therapy, whereas six required crossover, of whom two recovered. The overall recovery rates (assuming that the initial agent was most effective and expressed in terms of the initial agent) were 78% with pentamidine and 79% with the combination of trimethoprim and sulfamethoxazole. This conclusion indicates that pentamidine and trimethoprim–sulfamethoxazole are equivalent in effect when used in appropriate dosage. On the other hand, our preference is for trimethoprim and sulfamethoxazole because of the lower incidence of serious side effects. No significant side effects were encountered in either the adult or pediatric studies that would have led to alteration of drug therapy or to termination of treatment.

Several issues of major importance are still unresolved. Can we be sure, for instance, that a failure to respond within 3 days represents a clinical failure and is an indication for crossover? The first case illustrated in this review did not show clinical improvement until after the seventh day of treatment. We have observed that clinical improvement on either pentamidine or trimethoprim–sulfamethoxazole may be slow and take up to 5–11 days. If there are concurrent pathogens such as the mixture of CMV with a *Pneumocystis* infection, following radiologic changes per se might be a misleading way to evaluate treatment of pneumocystosis. Our present policy is to recommend that patients be given at least 72–96 hr of therapy with trimethoprim–sulfamethoxazole. If blood gases, respiratory rate, and chest radiography remain stable, we would still maintain them on this therapy for an additional 3 days. If, during this initial 72–96-hr period of observation, the patient has worsened in terms of blood gases and chest radiography, we would cross over to pentamidine. The most important clinical principle at this juncture is to consider other possible (simultaneous) infectious processes.

Considerations of dosage are one of the unresolved issues in trimethoprim–sulfamethoxazole treatment.[82] Some preliminary results of early passage of putative cysts in tissue culture have suggested that a concentration of trimethoprim of 5 μg/ml is necessary to inhibit the parasite. Indeed, the preliminary goal of our clinical studies has been to exceed this blood level at least in the postinfusion or posttreatment dose, i.e., 2 hr after ingestion of oral medication or $\frac{1}{2}$ hr to 45 min after the completion of an infusion given over 1 hr. A more serious clinical problem is the question of adequacy of absorption of orally administered drug in critically ill patients. Patients who are intubated, tracheostomized, or in a state of altered consciousness may not be able to take either the tablet or liquid form of trimethoprim–sulfamethoxazole. Those who have undergone open lung biopsy may develop a postsurgical ileus in which the absorption of either component of the fixed combination will be variable.

For these reasons, we recommend the parenteral form of trimethoprim–sulfamethoxazole, for any patient in whom there is a question about the adequacy of absorption of the drug from the gastrointestinal (GI) tract. One problem with this preparation is the relatively large volume of diluent recommended for the infusion of each ampule of trimethoprim–sulfamethoxazole. Originally, the manufacturer recommended that for each infusion some 200 ml of 5% dextrose in water (D_5W) also given, but it has now been shown that the total volume required for the infusion can be as little as 70 ml. The recommended oral dose for an adult is 20 mg/kg, in 3 divided dosages; the daily IV dose may be lower (12–15 mg/kg).

A valid question is whether physicians should really be concerned about a maximum dosage of the parenteral form of trimethoprim–sulfamethoxazole, since the primary aim of therapy in the initial stages of the disease is arrest of the growth of the parasite in the lung. We have obtained blood levels of trimethoprim as high as 15 μg/ml, three times the target goal, with no evidence of toxicity. It would seem prudent, therefore, that in the early stages of the disease, blood levels could be monitored to ensure adequacy of therapy but that there appears little danger of an initial therapeutic overshoot. After 7–10 days of trimethoprim–sulfamethoxazole therapy, the question of antagonism of folate synthesis becomes important but manageable. In *Toxoplasma gondii*, folate antagonists such as pyrimethamine fail to antagonize the mammalian dihydrofolate acid reductase. This is probably the case with *Pneumocystis*. Replacement therapy with folinic acid would be beneficial to mammalian cells but should not promote the growth of the parasite.

We feel that general reluctance to use large doses of trimethoprim–sulfamethoxazole in the early stages of the disease is actually a moot point. The effect of folate antagonism will not manifest itself for perhaps a week during which time the infection should come under control. At that point, there would apparently be little risk of giving the patient folinic acid to obviate an adverse effect on hematopoietic stem cells.

With regard to the issue of safety, trimethoprim–sulfamethoxazole has been associated with hypersensitivity reactions but rarely organ toxicity such as damage to liver or kidneys. Most (but perhaps not all) reported reactions appear linked to the sulfonamide: fever, diffuse erythematous or maculopopular rash, and rarely a picture of vasculitis or Stevens–Johnson syndrome (erythema multiforme). Such reactions have occurred in patients with hematologic malignancies (generally fewer than 10% of treated patients) but appear to be much more common in AIDS patients (up to 80% in patients with *Pneumocystis*). Most reactions can be managed by discontinuation of drug. Mild reactions may require no treatment at all, allowing the patient to complete a course of therapy. However, a severe reaction may require corticosteroid therapy for a few days.

2.10.4. *Pneumocystis* in AIDS

While the clinical features, radiologic manifestations, and laboratory findings are similar in patients with or without AIDS in whom *P. carinii* infection develops, some important differences have been noted in some reviews,[83,84] as summarized in Table 4. The principal observations are that (1) the disease appears associated with a much heavier burden of organisms, (2) it can be more insidious in onset but more slow to respond, (3) clinical response may not correlate with eradication of organisms (as determined by repeat bronchoscopy), (4) clinical infection is associated with a high rate of recurrence, and (5) there is a high incidence of side effects to treatment, particularly with a sulfonamide.[85] Despite the high rate of reactions to trimethoprim–sulfamethoxazole the response rates are not significantly different from that obtained with pentamidine, and we still would recommend that an AIDS patient be started on trimethoprim–sulfamethoxazole unless a reaction to the latter compound has occurred previously. In those patients with a history of a sul-

---

TABLE 4. Some Differences between *Pneumocystis* Infection in AIDS Patients versus Those without AIDS

1. AIDS patients have longer clinical prodromes
2. Recovery of pneumcysts from sputum is easier, more invasive studies show a heavier cyst burden, and cysts often persist in lung secretions after treatment in AIDS patients
3. AIDS patients may take 5–11 days to respond to trimethoprim–sulfamethoxazole and require therapy longer than 14 days.
4. Incidence of hypersensitivity reactions to trimethoprim–sulfamethoxazole (e.g., maculopapular rashes) is much higher in AIDS patients—up to 80% in some series—and these characteristically occur after 7–10 days of treatment
5. Pentamidime appears to have less renal and hepatic toxicity in AIDS patients but is associated with occasional precipitous neutropenia and hypoglycemia.
6. Rate of recrudescence is high—in carefully followed AIDS patients not receiving prophylaxis. This rate exceeds 50%, as compared with much lower recurrence rates in leukemic patients.

---

fonamide reaction, initial therapy should consist of pentamidine.

Patients with AIDS being treated for an initial episode of pneumocystosis should be given a course of trimethoprim–sulfamethoxazole for 4–6 days. If they are not deteriorating the trimethoprim–sulfamethoxazole could be continued for up to a total of 9 days before crossover to pentamidine—but the crossover could be on day 4 if the patient's condition is deteriorating (rapid fall in oxygenation requiring intubation). Generally speaking, the mortality in patients who are crossed over[18] approaches 90% and may exceed this figure in those who are intubated. A first episode of *P. carinii* pneumonia has a good prognosis, with more than 75% of patients responding clinically. The response to successive episodes of the same infection is generally poorer, possibly because of other concomitant infections that cause fever and add to the picture of clinical deterioration. Alternative infectious etiologies should obviously be sought in the febrile deteriorating patient with persistent lung infiltrates, but whether the other possible co-pathogens, e.g., mycobacteria and cytomegalovirus (CMV) can really be effectively treated has not been established.

Pentamidine is not innocuous in AIDS patients. Newer insights into its pharmacology show it can persist and accumulate in the body[86] thus triggering the toxic reactions of neutropenia and hypoglycemia (and occasionally azotemia and liver function abnormalities). After the fourth day of treatment, clinicians should be alert to this agent's complications: alternate-day measurements of WBC, blood sugar, and creatinine are strongly recommended. Large amounts of intravenous glucose can reverse the hypoglycemia, but such infusions may have to be maintained for a few days. The neutropenia can be quite severe and may predispose the AIDS patient to acute bacterial septicemia such as caused by *Pseudomonas aeruginosa*. These toxic reactions are almost always reversible if the patient receives vigorous supportive care.

2.10.5. New Therapy for *Pneumocystis* Infections

The AIDS epidemic, in which *Pneumocystis* infection has figured prominently as the most important opportunistic infection, has triggered a search for more effective, less toxic treatment. Some approaches include Dapsone plus trimethoprim[87] or the folate antagonist trimetrexate with leucovorin rescue.[88] Clinical results appear satisfactory with the former, but clear-cut superiority or reduction in side effects compared with trimethoprim–sulfamethoxazole is not striking. The ornithine decarboxylase inhibitor, α-difluoromethylornithine (DFMO), has been used on a compassionate clearance basis in the United States.[89] Evaluation of results with DFMO following pentamidine failure is difficult to interpret because of the long half-life of the latter. Results of therapy with DFMO are now being assessed in pilot studies. Used in large doses, DFMO can cause precipitous thrombocytopenia. Other experimental agents continue to be assessed in animal models of pneumocystosis and one class of compounds, sulfonylurea drugs, appears promising.[90]

2.10.6. Other Supportive Measures in Caring for the Patient during Active *Pneumocystis* Infection

Although we have detailed the pharmacologic therapy of pneumocystosis, the nature and quality of ancillary supportive measures in determining recovery cannot be overemphasized. Intubation and, if necessary, a tracheostomy may be required for adequate ventilation. Frequent monitoring of blood gases and adjustment of positive end-expiratory pressure (PEEP) mandates that these patients be managed in either centers for therapy of respiratory failure or intensive care units. Clinicians must be alert to bacterial superinfection and the dangers of oxygen toxicity.

One of the many unresolved issues about the management of *Pneumocystis* infection is whether high–dose corticosteroid therapy or therapeutic lung lavage has any role in the management of the refractory disease. From histopathologic sections of diseased lung, there is no question that the threat to the survival of the patient comes from the hypoxia secondary to the dense intraalveolar exudate. Anecdotal reports of the benefits of steroids or lung lavage in a manner analogous to the management of pulmonary alveolar proteinosis have been made available to the author, but these approaches need formal study. They might be considered in the desperately ill patient who is not improving in the face of apparently optimal pharmacologic therapy.

Another crucial factor affecting survival relates to the nature of the underlying disease. As has been repeatedly observed with the neoplastic disorders, recovery from infection is ultimately related to the ability to achieve a hematologic remission or some improvement in the status of the disease that initially predisposed to infection.

One situation where a major therapeutic decision must often be made occurs with proven *Pneumocystis* infection in the renal transplant recipient. There is no problem in supporting a patient who has received a renal homograft because of the ability to dialyze such a patient and maintain him in an acceptable state of renal function. The clinician therefore has the alternative of allowing the patient to reject his graft, which immediately results in a diminution if not a total withdrawal of immunosuppression, and thereby enhances the ability of the patient's own host defenses to combat this infection. This would appear to be an advisable approach if the renal transplant patient is not responding to an initial 3–5 days of therapy. In other transplant states such as cardiac or bone marrow transplantation, that "luxury" of allowing rejection to occur is not available.

2.11. Patient Isolation and Prophylaxis of *Pneumocystis* Infection

In general, we recommend that patients with pneumocystosis be placed in single-room isolation for the initial 3 days of therapy. Prudent measures such as handwashing before and after patient contact should obviously be employed, but mask and gown precautions seem unnecessary. Prophylaxis of medical personnel and contacts is not indicated, and prophylaxis of other patients in the hospital will depend on the clinical and epidemiologic circumstances.

Several combinations of folate antagonists with sulfonamides may serve as effective prophylactic agents, but the only medication studied extensively in the United States is trimethoprim–sulfamethoxazole. Widespread prophylactic use of this agent might well favor the emergence of resistant strains, something that, at this point, we would be unable to detect and could only suspect after clinical failures had occurred. On the other hand, in certain defined populations of leukemic children or organ transplant recipients, in whom a high incidence of pneumocystosis has been observed, carefully administered prophylaxis appears justified. The threshold for instituting prophylaxis seems to be an annual incidence of 5% of cases of underlying disease per year. The evidence for the efficacy of prophylaxis comes from the peerless studies of Hughes and collaborators who, for 2 years, followed a group of 80 leukemic children, half of whom received placebo and half of whom received up to two tablets of trimethoprim–sulfamethoxazole (160 mg trimethoprim) on a twice-daily basis.[16] No *Pneumocystis* infections were documented in the prophylaxis group, and a significantly larger number were found in those individuals who were given placebo. After the code was broken in this double-blind study, all patients at that institution were maintained on trimethoprim–sulfamethoxazole, and a negligible incidence of *Pneumocystis* infection has been encountered.

Similarly, the risk of pneumocystosis in marrow transplant recipients has also been reduced to very low levels with prophylactic trimethoprim–sulfamethoxazole (see Chapter 20). Our preference as outlined in a study by Winston et al. of marrow transplant patients is to give intermittent prophylaxis.[17] The specific regimen calls for an administration to adults of three tablets of trimethoprim–sulfamethoxazole (240 mg trimethoprim) twice a day on 2 consecutive days of the week, scheduled in such a way as not to interfere with methotrexate administration. Methotrexate is usually given in marrow transplant recipients to prevent graft-versus-host disease, and the cumulative effect of trimethoprim–sulfamethoxazole and methotrexate may be a sudden precipitous fall in white count. Intermittent prophylaxis has also been recently proven efficacious in children with acute lymphatic leukemia.[90a]

Because of all the other confounding variables, the lowest amount of drug that will produce a prophylactic effect, as appears to have occurred in our bone marrow transplant series, would appear to be the most advisable regimen at this time. As marrow transplant patients recover from their immune deficiency, the risk of *Pneumocystis* appears to decrease, and prophylaxis may not be indicated after half a year post-transplant. In leukemic children, duration of prophylaxis may well be related to the duration that maintenance therapy is given in remission. Evidence now points to the need for a minimum of 5 months of prophylaxis, particularly during the phase of consolidating chemotherapy and the tapering of steroid dose.[41,91]

Second attacks of histologically proven *Pneumocystis* infection have been well documented.[92] We believe it prudent to give continuous prophylaxis to leukemic patients undergoing chemotherapy who have a history of proven pneumocystosis. Indications for prophylaxis of the renal transplant recipient are summarized in Chapter 21. Those with urinary tract infection will probably be treated for that condition with trimethoprim–sulfamethoxazole for 4 months irrespective of risk of pneumocystosis. It also seems prudent to give prophylaxis to those patients with active CMV infection in view of the association of that opportunistic infection with pneumocystosis.

Recommendations for patients with AIDS and an initial episode of pneumocystosis are summarized in Section 2.13.

We have no hesitation about using pentamidine in a patient who develops a histologically proven *Pneumocystis* infection after trimethoprim–sulfamethoxazole prophylaxis. On the other hand, a really careful history is important, since patients may not take their medication, and, indeed, it would be crucial to verify the history before designating such an example as a failure of prophylaxis.

2.12. Postinfection Fibrosis

With increasing numbers of patients surviving documented pneumonitis, the question has been raised as to whether some patients may develop pulmonary fibrosis as a result of this infection. Since repair of lung tissue is mediated by type II pneumocytes, the proliferative and repair response of this cell might actually cause lung damage. The following case history suggests that some patients may develop this postinfection fibrosis. Pulmonary infiltrates may take many weeks to resolve. An increasing number of patients in our experience have some residual changes as seen radiographically. If they eventually come to autopsy, pulmonary fibrosis may be observed. In our experience, this is more likely if the patient is an adult, has received either radiation to the lung or other agents known to injure the lung such as alkylating agents or bleomycin, and if the patient has an underlying disease that can lead to pulmonary fibrosis per se, e.g., a collagen vascular disease. There is no established method for averting these long-term sequelae.

Illustrative Case 2

This patient was a 44-year-old white man with a long-standing history of ankylosing spondylitis, status postfusion of the spine, who had been receiving long-term corticosteroid therapy because of his rheumatologic disorder He had many manifestations of advanced disease including bilateral ulnar deviation, "swan neck" deformity of the fingers, and flexion contractures of his knees and toes. Outpatient therapy consisted of prednisone, 75 mg alternating with 120 mg every day. In addition, he had been treated with cyclophosphamide, 150 mg/day, PO, until 2 weeks prior to admission. During the addition of cyclophosphamide to his treatment, his prednisone dosage was gradually tapered to a level of 40 mg/day. Beginning 6 weeks prior to admission, the patient complained of symptoms of a mild cold accompanied by shortness of breath and low-grade fever. One month prior to admission he was seen in the emergency room and was treated with oral ampicillin for upper respiratory infection. A week later, however, he had more pronounced shortness of breath but was found to have a normal chest radiograph. Arterial blood gases (ABGs) at that time revealed a pH of 7.48, $Paco_2$ 31 mm Hg, Pao_2 65 mm Hg (3 weeks prior to admission) He was treated with intermittent positive-pressure respiration and bronchodilators and was discharged because the chest radiograph was within normal limits. However, in the ensuing 2 weeks, he had progressive shortness of breath and fever which intensified in the week prior to admission. He was admitted to the hospital with severe shortness of breath.

On admission, ABGs revealed pH 7.48, Pao_2 on room air of 30 mm Hg, $Paco_2$ 30 mm Hg, and a bicarbonate of 21 mg/dl. Chest examination revealed diffuse inspiratory rales, bronchial breath sounds, and tubular breath sounds. Chest radiography indicated bilateral interstitial and alveolar infiltrates (Fig. 3). The patient was subsequently intubated and eventually required tracheostomy Fiberoptic bronchoscopy performed through the tracheostomy tube yielded bronchial brushings that were diagnostic for *Pneumocystis carinii* on silver stain Intravenous trimethoprim–sulfamethoxazole was immediately begun at an initial dose of 14 mg trimethoprim/kg per day IV. The dose was divided into four doses given q6h intravenously. Initial peak trimethoprim levels were 4.8 μg/ml with a valley of 3.4 μg/ml. A week after therapy was initiated, peak trimethoprim levels stabilized in the range of 9 7–10.4 μg/ml, and valley levels were found to be in the range of 7 5–9.1 μg/ml

A host of medical complications were encountered during management in the respiratory intensive care unit (ICU) The patient became intermittently hypotensive, had persistent intermittent fevers, developed an upper GI hemorrhage, and experienced a cardiac arrest. Other medications such as aminoglycosides and cephalosporins were given for the possibility of a bacterial component to his pulmonary disease. His ABGs improved after treatment with a decrease in FIo_2 from 100% to 30% to maintain adequate

oxygenation. One seizure was observed on the 14th day of trimethoprim–sulfamethoxazole therapy The patient became afebrile with a gradual improvement in blood gases, Pao_2 rising from 30 mm Hg on room air to 90 mm Hg on a 40% FIo_2. Repeat suctioning of tracheobronchial secretions from the tracheostomy tube failed to reveal forms consistent with *P. carinii*. Despite defervescence and increase in Pao_2, the patient's chest radiograph did not clear, and he required intensive care for a subsequent 3 months. His overall condition gradually deteriorated, he became hypoxic once again and he expired with recurrent fevers possibly caused by bacterial infections (although the etiology was never documented). His chest radiograph continued to show diffuse, persistent pulmonary infiltrates. A postmortem examination revealed findings consistent with 26 years of ankylosing spondylitis involving the entire spine. He was found to have diffuse amyloidosis, and the sections of lung revealed consolidation and extensive fibrosis but no *Pneumocystis carinii*

Comment. This case demonstrates many points. Although the patient did not have a neoplasm, he was treated with high doses of corticosteroids for a rheumatologic disorder, and cyclophosphamide had been recently discontinued before the intense flare of his symptoms. In addition, there was significant reduction of corticosteroid dosage prior to the exacerbation of his respiratory symptoms. Of considerable interest was the observation that the patient had approximately 6 weeks of symptoms with normal chest radiographs prior to the development of fulminant pneumonitis. The effect of corticosteroids in suppressing the inflammatory response coupled with exacerbation of disease when the dosage was tapered were considered important features of Case 2. This patient improved clinically, as has been our experience with the great majority of patients treated with intravenous trimethoprim–sulfamethoxazole, but pulmonary infiltrates failed to clear. An adequate dosage of trimethoprim–sulfamethoxazole was given, and the patient gradually became afebrile with increasing Po_2; therefore, no consideration was given to changing treatment to pentamidine.

From a diagnostic point of view, material adequate for establishing the diagnosis was obtained from fiberoptic bronchoscopy and brushing once an endotracheal tube had been inserted. This approach may be valuable in patients with marked hypoxia and demonstrates the ability to establish a diagnosis even if the patient requires intubation. On the other hand, the disturbing finding was that this patient gradually manifested a downhill course, dying in respiratory failure after approximately 3 months in the hospital. At autopsy, a diffuse fibrotic process but not *Pneumocystis carinii* was found in the lung. Many investigators believe that infection with *Pneumocystis* may cause extensive alveolar damage and pulmonary fibrosis. This case may be such an example. On the other hand, this patient had received cyclophosphamide and had amyloidosis secondary to this rheumatic disorder Oxygen toxicity may have contributed to postinfectious fibrosis. Death in this case cannot be attributed to pneumocystosis but perhaps to postinflammatory fibrosis that was an inexorable sequel to the infection. Postinfectious fibrosis has been rarely seen in children but may be more common in the adult form of the disease.

Clinically, patients have persistent pulmonary infiltrates, remain hypoxic, and may be suspected of having drug-resistant pneumocystosis. Our policy has been to maintain the initially se-

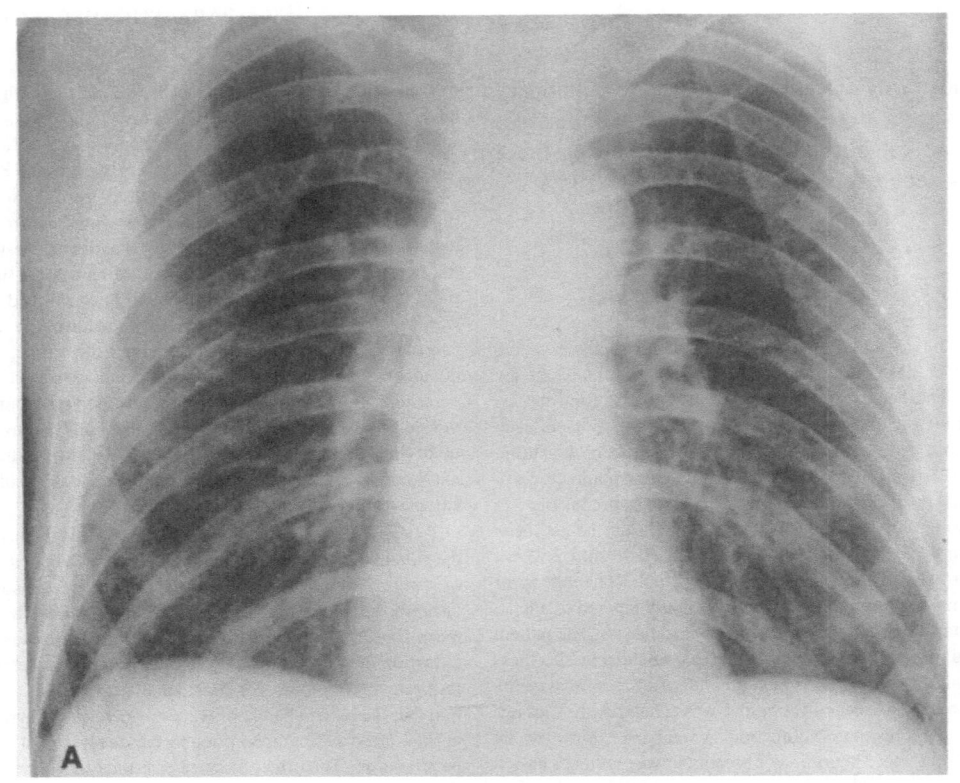

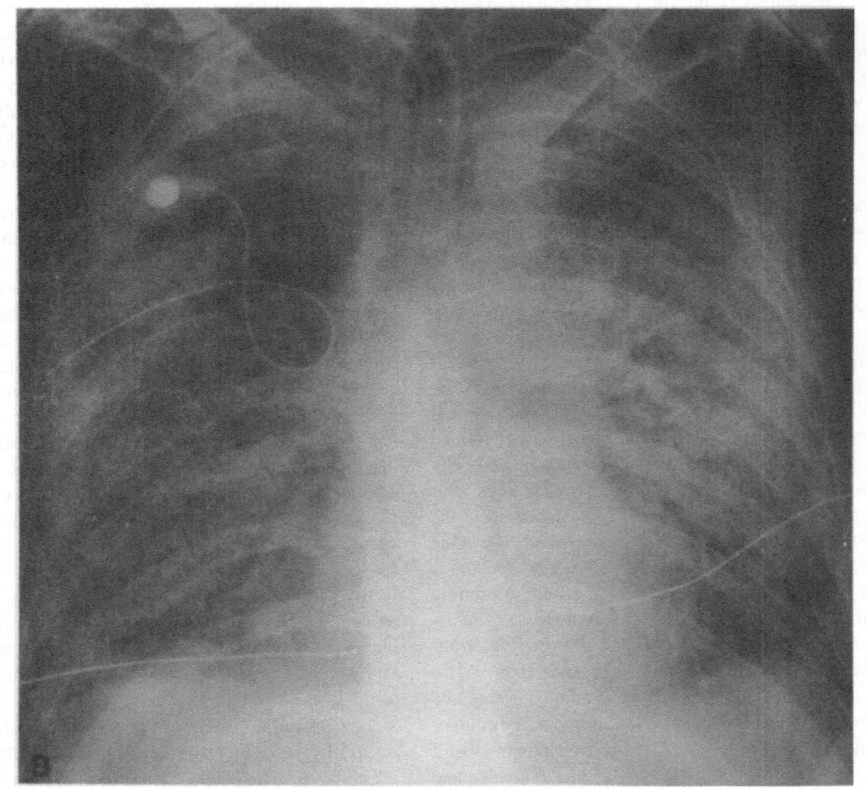

lected medication if the patient is stable and experiences some defervescence.

2.13. Overview of Therapeutic and Prophylactic Approaches

Considerable progress in the management of *Pneumocystis* infection has been made during the past decade, but the experience during the current epidemic of AIDS indicates that newer, safer forms of therapy and prophylaxis are badly needed. The advent of trimethoprim–sulfamethoxazole has led to an oral and parenteral form of therapy which, although not convincingly superior to pentamidine, appears to be easier to give and is associated with fewer side effects except in AIDS patients. On the other hand, the seeds of a real clinical problem may be seen by the ready availability of an oral preparation, since we will not know if resistance develops unless we are confronted by a convincing set of clinical failures. Whereas trimethoprim–sulfamethoxazole is an excellent antibacterial agent for many gram-negative rods and most gram-positive cocci (with the exception of *Enterococcus* and *Pseudomonas*), its prophylactic use in the immunocompromised patient population should probably be restricted to patients treated in a program experiencing a high incidence of *Pneumocystis* infection.

What criteria should be applied in making the decision to institute routine prophylaxis? At the present time, prophylaxis would seem to be indicated in recipients of organ transplants and in leukemic children if their calculated annual incidence of pneumocystosis exceeds 5%. This recommendation is based on a review of the available literature and is not meant to be dogma: clearly, individual circumstances, magnitude of problem, ease of diagnosis of infection, and clinical success rate after the documentation of proven infection are all factors to be considered before prophylaxis is given.

In leukemic patients, prophylaxis can probably be stopped several months after the cessation of all chemotherapy (including corticosteroids) and the achievement of a solid remission.

For patients with AIDS, controlled data on prophylactic use have been difficult to marshall. The high documented recurrence rate mandates that some prophylactic measure be given, but perhaps most AIDS patients have had a hypersensitivity reaction to trimethoprim–sulfamethoxazole. Those who can tolerate this medication should continue to receive 160 mg trimethoprim (with a corresponding amount of sulfamethoxazole) twice a day, though less frequent dosing may suffice. One group has found that most patients reacting to trimethoprim–sulfamethoxazole can tolerate pyrimethamine–sulfadoxine (Fansidar), 25 mg : 500 mg, in a dose of one tablet of the fixed combination per week orally.[93] The reason that this preparation is generally well tolerated is unknown but might be related to the lower dose of the long-acting sulfonomide. Occasional severe reactions, not unlike Stevens–Johnson syndrome have been observed. Thus, this form of prophylaxis must be initiated with care: we advise it be started after all evidence of a previous drug reaction has subsided—either 2 weeks after trimethoprim–sulfamethoxazole or 4 weeks after pentamidime. The risk of a reaction must be judged against the risk of recurrent pneumocystosis and a severe reaction should be treated with a short course of corticosteroids.

For the AIDS patients who cannot tolerate a sulfonomide containing preparation, a single intramuscular dose of pentamidime can be given every 2–4 weeks on an outpatient basis. This appears to be effective; studies are now under way to evaluate aerosal administration of pentamidime as a way of avoiding the systemic toxicity of that agent.

3. Babesiosis

More than 70 species of protozoan parasites belonging to the genus *Babesia* have been isolated and identified throughout the world. Only within the last two decades has it become apparent that these species are pathogenic for man, and, remarkably, three of the first four human cases reported in the literature died

---

FIGURE 3. (A) Chest radiograph of Illustrative Case 2 for symptoms of cough and dyspnea several weeks before documentation of *Pneumocystis* infection. (B) Despite defervescence and clinical improvement, bilateral diffuse pulmonary infiltrates persist in Case 2 during trimethoprim–sulfamethoxazole treatment.

of acute disease.[94] All these first four patients had been splenectomized, a procedure that presumably rendered them susceptible to this infection. Although cases of human babesiosis are apparently uncommon, the worldwide distribution of these protozoan parasites and the results of epidemiologic studies indicating that mild and subclinical infections occur form a sufficient basis to recommend that disease caused by *Babesia* species should be considered among the diagnostic possibilities in immunocompromised febrile patients.

It is likely that epidemics of babesiosis date back to biblical times, when devastating epizootics occurred among cattle and domestic animals. The protozoan parasite was first described by Babes in 1888 who identified an intraerythrocytic agent which he mistakenly took for a bacterium.[94] Five years later, however, Theobald Smith and F. L. Kilborne investigated an epidemic of fever in cattle and established that the pathogen was both protozoan and transmitted by a blood-sucking tick.[95] *Babesia* species subsequently have been isolated from sheep, goats, horses, swine, dogs, cats, rodents, and many other warm-blooded animals. A number of species of ticks have been shown to transmit babesiosis including the common *Ixodes* and *Dermacentor* ticks. Thus, a history of tick bite can be a particularly important clue in establishing the diagnosis of babesiosis. Clearly, however, a tick bite may be an easily overlooked part of the history and an experience that the patient may readily forget or even be unaware of, so the apparent absence of tick contact does not exclude the diagnosis.

The occurrence of babesiosis in animals is worldwide, and thus, the potential for human disease must be viewed in this light. The first case was described in the Balkans, the second in California, and the third case in Ireland. Seroepidemiologic studies suggest that the disease occurs in Europe and Central and South America. More recently, a series of interesting reports of human disease has emanated from the Martha's Vineyard, Nantucket, and the eastern Long Island portions of the United States.[96-98] Careful epidemiologic studies have suggested that this infection is more common than the scattered appearance of cases with clinical disease. Furthermore, although many of these cases have been associated with bovine ticks, epidemiologic studies have failed to implicate tick contact in some patients. Noteworthy about the outbreaks in the Massachusetts area has been that the majority of cases have been in patients with intact spleens. It now appears that although splenectomy increases susceptibility to babesiosis, it is not the only factor predisposing to clinical disease.

3.1. Clinical Features

Although babesiosis is recognized as having a broad spectrum of manifestations from inapparent infection to a fulminating illness, perhaps the most important factor to remember is that it can present as a malarialike illness. Indeed, an examination of blood smears can result in the identification of morphologic forms that may be easy to confuse with *Plasmodium* species.

The severe clinical forms of babesiosis have a predilection for individuals without spleens, and four such cases have proven to be fatal with a clinical course terminating in about a week. One recent case report describes a patient splenectomized for Hodgkin disease who developed fatal infection caused by *B. divergens*.[99] High fever, chills, anemia, jaundice, hemoglobinemia, hemoglobinuria, hypotension, anuria, and coma have been serial clinical manifestations. The anemia clearly appears to be of a hemolytic type comparable to that observed with malaria. Serious illnesses have lasted about 1 month in those persons who have recovered, and even following recovery, patients have required prolonged convalescence because of postinfection asthenia.

It appears from careful documentation of the history of tick feeding that the incubation period ranges from 7 to 21 days, with a median of approximately 2 weeks.

Those individuals with moderate to severe illness usually have had intact spleens and have tended to be older than 40 years of age. There is some indication that although exposure may be the same for persons of all ages, clinical disease has a predilection for the elderly. The best-studied cases of this form of babesiosis have been summarized in the report of the Nantucket cases by Ruebush et al.[97] In decreasing order of frequency, symptoms have included fever, fatigue, myalgia, arthralgia, mental depression, drenching sweats, shaking chills, nausea and vomiting, hyperaesthesia, and splenomegaly. Lymph node enlargement, rash, and abnormal neurologic signs were absent. Temperature elevations were as high as 106°F. Following clinical infection, some of these patients have experienced long periods of low-grade fever and lassitude with symptoms lasting for up to 2 years.

Subclinical and mild infection have been documented by retrospective serologic studies and/or microscopic examinations of blood films. An epidemiologic survey carried out by Ruebush and colleagues included the study of a total of 964 specimens, 577 from Nantucket, 154 from Martha's Vineyard, and 100 from Cape Cod.[97] Twenty-one specimens were considered positive with a titer by indirect immunofluorescence of 1:64 or greater. Eleven of the 577 samples were collected from patients at the Nantucket Hospital for routine diagnostic tests, and ten of 133 specimens were obtained from Nantucket residents and visitors who had a history of tick bite or fever. Of the 19 seropositive patients who could be contacted, six had a febrile illness in the previous 6 months and had been hospitalized, but all were well at the time of blood specimen collection, and none had a history of malaria. Of the hospitalized patients, one had had a short febrile illness with recovery followed by relapse. Of the three hospitalized patients, one was found to have a blood smear showing *Babesia,* whereas blood from the other two was inoculated in hamsters. *Babesia microti,* the most common species found in the Eastern United States, was isolated in both instances. Similar documentation of mild or innapparent infections have occurred in low gulf coast areas of Mexico, Nigeria, and Georgia.

The potential for transmission of babesiosis has been raised during the evaluation of putative cases of transfusion-associated malaria. Healy and colleagues identified a case of probable babesiosis while attempting to trace the source of a case that was diagnosed as *P. vivax* infection.[100] One of five blood donors had light parasitemia; the clinical disease in both the donor and the recipient of the transfusion could either have been malaria or babesiosis. The serologic evidence favored babesiosis. Thus, the potential for human infection caused by transmission of blood from donor to immunocompromised host remains as much a possibility with this organism as it does with malaria. Moreover, in the United States,

the reservoir for *Babesia* infection would appear to be far larger than that for malaria.

3.2. Laboratory Diagnosis

Human infection has been documented with three relatively small *Babesia* species, *bovis, divergens,* and *microti.* A presumptive diagnosis of babesiosis can be made by identification of the parasite in host erythrocytes. Thin blood films are stained by the Giemsa technique as for the identification of malarial parasites (Fig. 4). In severe infections, up to 50% of patients' erythrocytes may be parasitized. The merozoites appear to be pear-shaped, round, or oval, varying in size from 1 to 5 μm in length. All species of *Babesia* invade and propagate in erythrocytes only. They are easily mistaken for *Plasmodium* species, either *falciparum* or *vivax.* However, unlike *falciparum* parasites, *Babesia* species do not leave residual hemozoin pigment after they ingest vacuole-stored hemoglobin. Therefore, the absence of pigment in the parasitized blood cell is a hallmark of babesial infection. *Babesia* multiply by forming two or four or more merozoites, and in heavy infections, these forms may be seen outside of the erythrocytes. Tetrad forms ("Maltese crosses") may be produced by budding. The presence of these tetrad forms will reliably distinguish *Babesia microti* from the *Plasmodium* species.

Next to direct visualization of *Babesia* in blood smears, serologic techniques are the most important means for diagnosis and are crucial for epidemiologic studies. Serodiagnosis is the only practical means for identifying subclinical infection, since positive blood smears are usually obtained only from patients with clinical disease. An indirect immunofluorescent antibody test has been developed and evaluated by Chisholm and co-workers at the CDC.[101] The antigen is a strain of *Babesia microti* harvested from hamsters. After an initial incubation of this antigen with human serum, antihuman immunoglobulin labeled with fluorescein is added. A diagnostic titer is considered to be 1:64 or greater. It is not unusual for acute-phase specimens to have titers equal to or greater than 1:1024. Seropositive samples may cross-react with a number of species of *Babesia* and three species of *Plasmodium* including *vivax, falciparum,* and *brasilianum.* However, titers

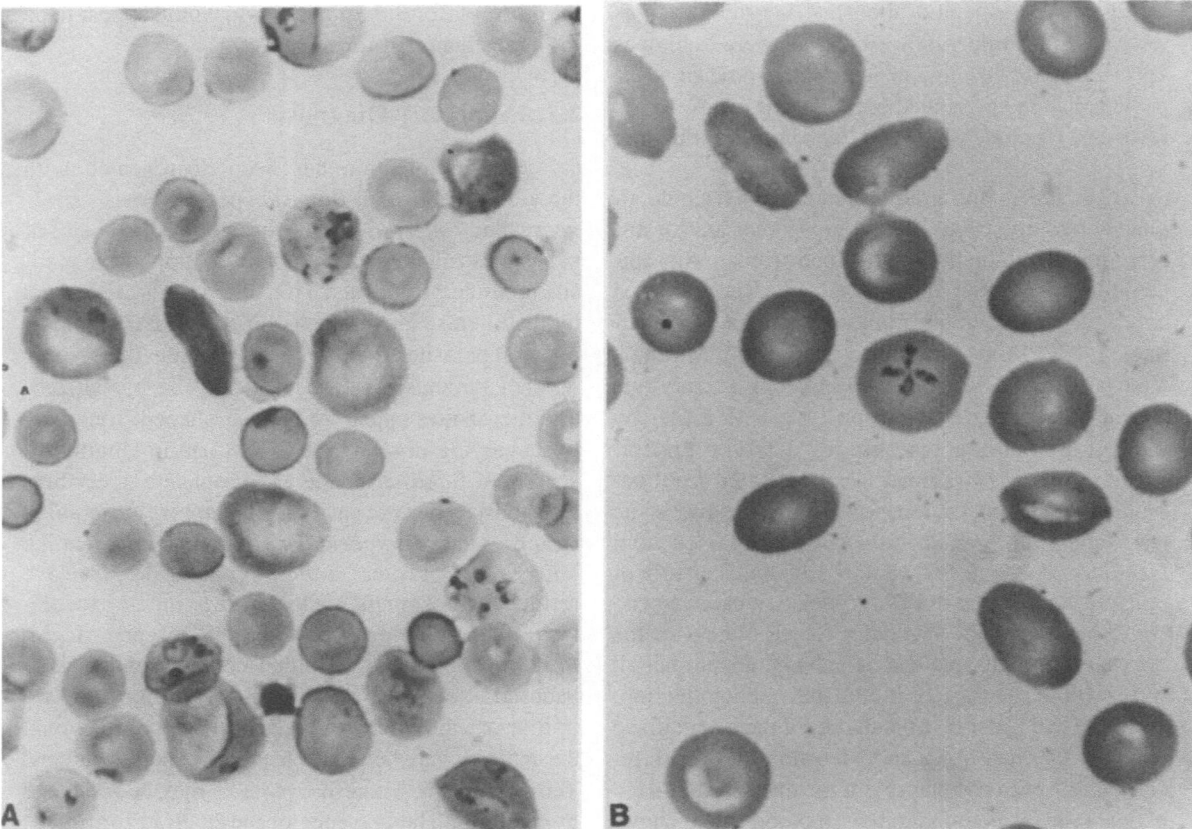

FIGURE 4. (A) Wright-stained smears of peripheral blood demonstrating numerous ring forms from case of human babesiosis. These forms are easily confused with *Plasmodium* species (B) Classic tetrad form ("Maltese cross") that distinguishes *Babesia* infection from malaria.

against the infecting *Babesia* species are higher than to the other *Babesia* and plasmodial antigens tested.

Physicians should be aware of the identity between the ticks that are the carriers of Rocky Mountain spotted fever and *Babesia* species. Clinically, other diseases that must be considered in differential diagnosis are Weil disease, leptospirosis, and brucellosis. Dammin reviewed the histopathologic laboratory findings in the mild and severe cases.[94] Cases of fatal disease have been deeply jaundiced and showed marked congestion of abdominal viscera, lungs, and brain. This is the result of plugging of capillaries by parasitized erythrocytes in a manner that resembles malarial infections.

3.3. Treatment

It is logical that chloroquine would be one of the first agents to be used for the treatment of babesiosis because of the initial confusion of this entity with malaria. Studies reported by Ruebush and Spielman demonstrate that chloroquine phosphate, 1.5 g initially and 0.5 g/day for 2–12 weeks, results in symptomatic improvement and abatement of fever within 3–7 days.[96] However, parasitemia persisted for more than a month in three patients, and convalescence was prolonged. Indeed, there is no definite relationship between chloroquine therapy and reduction of parasitemia in humans and animals.[102] The blood of patients receiving chloroquine will still infect experimental animals, and the major effect of this agent may be to suppress inflammation. Conversely, symptomatic improvement in the absence of chloroquine has occurred. It appears that most persons infected with *Babesia microti* can clear the infection without specific antiparasitic therapy if they have intact host-defense mechanisms.

Several alternatives to chloroquine treatment are available. A number of tetracyclines reduce parasitemia. Pentamidine and diminazene (as Berenil available from the Parasitic Diseases Drug Service of the CDC) reduce and suppress parasitemia, but parasitemia recurs after discontinuation of these drugs. Diminazene is effective therapy in animals, but its use in one case of human infection was associated with Guillain–Barré syndrome.[96] Diminazene or pentamidine should be considered only if heavy parasitemia is documented. Some authorities suggest the use of trimethoprim–sulfamethoxazole to treat active infection,[94] but the clinical experience is limited.

The most promising therapeutic approach now appears to be the combination of clindamycin, 600 mg qid, and quinine, 650 mg tid.[103] Treatment should be considered with this regimen if parasitemia is documented in immunocompromised hosts.

In summary, it appears that babesiosis has had a minor effect on public health of the world's population despite the fact that there are few places in the world that are free of *Babesia*. Patients with impaired host defenses, such as following splenectomy, or recipients of blood transfusions should be evaluated for the possibility of this infection if they develop fever, chills, hemolysis, and jaundice.

4. Giardiasis

Giardia lamblia has received increased attention as an important cause of diarrhea and malabsorption in both the normal host and patients with immunodeficiency. Like many other modern opportunistic pathogens, it was often regarded as a nonpathogenic commensal organism until the past decade.[104] However, several recent lines of evidence have now established *G. lamblia* as an important cause of GI disease.

1. Although there is a high rate of inapparent infection, *G. lamblia* has been shown to be a major etiologic agent of diarrhea in individuals returning from the Soviet Union, Southeast Asia, and other geographic areas of high endemicity.[104–106]
2. Numerous well-studied epidemics of waterborne diarrheal disease in the United States have been linked to this organism. Indeed, *G. lamblia* is the most frequently documented cause of water-borne epidemic diarrheal disease in the United States.[104,107–109]
3. *G. lamblia* has been convincingly associated with diarrhea and malabsorption in patients with a variety of types of hypogammaglobulinemia.[104,110,111]

4.1. The Organism

Approximately 50 species of *Giardia* have been isolated from primates, other mammals, and even amphibians. In the past, it was assumed that each host species harbored its own *Giardia* species, and hence, each was given its own name and species designation. However, recent studies demonstrating cross-infectivity between human *Giardia* strains in the beaver, the dog, and other nonhuman hosts have led to serious doubts about species specificity.[104,109]

The human strain, *G. lamblia*, may take one of two forms. The motile form, or trophozoite, is responsible for the disease manifestations in the upper small intestine. Cysts, the more hardy infective form, develop as organisms, traverse the bowel, and are subjected to increasing degrees of dehydration. The trophozoite is a $13-19 \times 8-11$ μm piriform-shaped structure whose most important anatomic feature is a large, bilobed concave sucking disc by which the organism becomes attached to the upper small intestinal epithelium. The cyst forms are thick-walled, oval structures measuring $8-12 \times 7-10$ μm. Trophozoites may occasionally be found in the stool of patients with a very watery diarrhea and, presumably, a very rapid intestinal transit time. Otherwise, only cysts will be observed in the stool, and duodenal intubation is necessary to demonstrate the trophozoites.[104]

4.2. Epidemiology

The most important means of transmission of *G. lamblia* is by ingestion of contaminated drinking water. Municipal water supplies, rural streams, and individual wells have been implicated as sources of infection. Cysts may remain viable in fresh water for months and are not destroyed by usual chlorination procedures. It has previously been assumed that the source of water contamination was infected human feces. However, increasing evidence suggests that contamination with animal excreta may play a role in the transmission of infection to humans. Only beavers have been definitely implicated as playing such a role. In addition, direct person-to-person transmission may occur via the fecal–oral route and is particularly important among young children, institutionalized subjects, and male homosexuals.[104,108,109,112–114]

The inapparent infection rate appears quite high. Children will manifest symptoms more frequently than will adults with a similar parasite load. Previous exposure may enhance protection against reinfection in immunologically intact individuals.[104,115,116]

4.3. Pathogenesis

Data from both experimental *Giardia* infection and from investigation of water-borne epidemics in which small numbers of *Giardia* cysts were found in quantitative stool studies suggest that the ingestion of as few as 100 cysts will reliably establish infection.[117] After ingestion, excystation takes place in the upper GI tract, yielding the disease-causing trophozoites. An unexplained paradox is that although a low pH appears to be necessary for excystation to occur in vitro, individuals with achlorhydria appear to be at increased risk of symptomatic infection. Once excystation occurs, the motile flagellated trophozoites replicate, move along the surface of the small bowel, and attach themselves directly to the mucosa via their bilobed sucking discs. These events result in shortening and flattening of the villi, elongation of crypts, and increased mitotic activity of the epithelial cells. Electron microscopic studies reveal thinning of the surface coat of the brush border and a variety of changes in the microvilli. The structural abnormalities observed in the microvilli are reflected in the functional defects that are observed in symptomatic individuals: disaccharidase deficiency (the clinically most important being an acquired lactase deficiency) and evidence of protein, fat, and vitamin malabsorption. Only in the minority of the most heavily infected persons do trophozoites actually penetrate the bowel wall. Even without such penetration, however, an inflammatory response may be observed in the underlying submucosa, consisting of variable numbers of polymorphonuclear leukocytes, plasma cells, and lymphocytes.[104,118–122]

Susceptibility to infestation with *Giardia* appears to be increased not only in patients with achlorhydria, but also in those with pancreatic dysfunction[123] and protein-calorie malnutrition.[104] This last may be secondary to immune deficits created by the malnourished state. Overgrowth of the small bowel with colonic flora may occur in giardiasis, and it has been hypothesized that this may play a role in the pathogenesis of the diarrhea, the bacteria causing bile salt deconjugation or, perhaps, direct injury to the small bowel mucosa.[124]

Why some individuals with giardial infestation develop symptomatic disease and others do not is poorly understood. Three observations point toward immunologic factors:

1. Epidemiologic studies indicate that attack rates are higher in children than in adults and in newcomers rather than long-term residents of endemic areas.[104,115]
2. Studies in human subjects suggest an increased incidence and severity of giardiasis in patients with nodular lymphoid hyperplasia of the small bowel, a variety of dysgammaglobulinemias, and hypogammaglobulinemic sprue.[104,110,111,121] This appears to underscore the importance of antibody production in the protection against giardial infection, particularly local secretory antibody in the intestine itself.
3. Studies in the mouse model of giardiasis have demonstrated that resistance to reinfection follows an initial infection that clears. By contrast, athymic mice neither clear their initial infection nor acquire resistance. Resistant mice can transfer resistance to their progeny through breast milk in which anti-

trophozoite antibodies of the IgA and IgG class can be demonstrated.[104,116,125–127]

Thus, although the precise mechanisms of resistance to giardial infection are incompletely understood, there is already ample evidence that specific local and systemic humoral immune mechanisms are involved.

4.4. Clinical Manifestations

An estimated 20–50% of infected individuals develop clinical symptoms 1–3 weeks after initial infection. Characteristically, there is an abrupt onset of midabdominal cramps, watery, foul-smelling diarrhea, abdominal distention, nausea, and flatulence. Chills and/or low-grade fevers may occur at the beginning of the illness but should not persist for longer than a few days. Vomiting, headache, belching, and a generalized malaise are not uncommon. After the first 3–4 days, a variety of patterns of illness may be observed in the untreated patient: in the majority of individuals either persistent or recurring symptoms of moderate severity will occur, with brief episodes of foul-smelling diarrhea, abdominal distention, flatulence, belching, and substernal discomfort being noted. Some patients experience symptoms over weeks to months and have as the major manifestations malabsorption, weight loss, and a general failure to thrive. The last is the major pattern of disease seen in the immunocompromised patient. It is important to emphasize that, particularly in ethnic groups with a predisposition to lactase deficiency, chronic symptoms of diarrhea, flatulence, abdominal distention, and malabsorption may persist for months even after effective therapy has been administered. A lactose-free diet will correct these abnormalities.[104]

4.5. Giardiasis in the Compromised Host

The most firmly established relationship of giardiasis to a host defense defect is that with dysgammaglobulinemias such as occur with the variable immunodeficiency syndrome.[110,111,121] In the best study of this relationship, Ament et al.[111] carefully studied clinical symptoms, multiple small intestinal biopsies, stool samples, and a variety of GI function assays in a group of 39 patients with primary immunodeficiency syndromes with altered γ-globulin pro-

duction. Their findings are as follows: *Giardia lamblia* was found in eight of nine patients with symptoms of diarrhea, weight loss, vomiting, and anorexia, but in only three of 30 patients who were free of gastrointestinal complaints. Pathologic and functional abnormalities included mild to severe villus abnormalities, malabsorption (often severe) of folic acid and vitamin B_{12}, steatorrhea, lactose intolerance, generalized disaccharidase deficiency, and protein-losing enteropathy. Virtually all these abnormalities were reversed following treatment with metronidazole and eradication of the parasite. Of these eight patients, one had infantile X-linked agammaglobulinemia, and seven were classified as having the variable immunodeficiency syndrome. An extremely important observation was the difficulty encountered in establishing the diagnosis of giardiasis. Stool examination yielded the diagnosis in only 30% of cases; multiple intestinal biopsies revealed the patchy nature of the involvement. Examination of such biopsies and/or Giemsa-stained smears of mucus adhering to the biopsies was required to make the diagnosis in most instances.

Whether other immunocompromised patients have an increased incidence and/or severity of giardiasis remains unclear. Clearly, any diarrheal syndrome in patients with known dysgammaglobulinemias, particularly of the variable type, should lead the clinician to suspect giardial infection. Although it has been suggested that apparently normal individuals with giardiasis have a deficiency in intestinal production of IgA,[128] current evidence is against this hypothesis.[129] Therefore, in an apparently normal adult, the diagnosis of giardial infection by itself should not lead to an elaborate evaluation for immunodeficiency. We have observed several cases of symptomatic giardiasis in renal transplant patients, but these instances could have been chance events rather than reflecting increased susceptibility to this infection.

4.6. Diagnosis

The diagnosis of giardiasis can usually be made rather easily by examination of several stool specimens in patients with acute disease. Using direct smear and formol–ether concentration techniques on stool specimens from patients with giardiasis, the diagnosis can be made on 76% of patients after one stool examination, 90% after two, and 97.6% after three.[104] With more chronic disease, diagnosis by stool examination may be more difficult, particularly since cyst excretion may be episodic. Purging does not appear to increase diagnostic yield. In such instances, particularly in patients with dysgammaglobulinemias in whom stool examinations notoriously give low yields,[111] examination of small bowel contents for trophozoites should be carried out.

The combination of small bowel biopsy and duodenal intubation are the definitive techniques for diagnosing giardial infection. An alternative method is the use of the Entero-test. With this technique, a fasting patient swallows a capsule containing one end of a long string, the other end of which is taped to the patient's face. Over the course of 4 hr, the capsule dissolves, and the string reaches the duodenal–jejunal junction. The string is then withdrawn, and the distal 20–30 cm which is coated with a bile-stained mucus is then examined microscopically for the presence of trophozoites.[130]

In some patients with highly compatible histories, appropriate epidemiologic exposure, and/or an underlying dysgammaglobulinemia, a therapeutic trial of antigiardial therapy is indicated.

4.7. Treatment

Any patient harboring G. lamblia with or without symptoms should be treated for the disease. The treatment regimen of choice is quinacrine hydrochloride (Atabrine) at a dose of 100 mg three times a day for 7 days. Possible adverse effects of this regimen include skin rash, GI disturbances, fever, and psychosis. On the whole, however, this regimen is quite well tolerated and is effective in at least 95% of persons. An alternative drug, particularly useful in children because it is available as an oral suspension, is furazolidone, although experience with this agent is much less.[104]

A more controversial form of effective therapy involves use of metronidazole (Flagyl). Metronidazole at a dosage of 750 mg three times a day for 10 days is probably as effective as quinacrine.[131] A simpler regimen consisting of a single dose of 2 g/day for 3 days as a single daily dose appears to be almost as effective.[132] Of concern, however, are reports that metronidazole may be carcinogenic in mice[133] and mutagenic in bacteria.[134] One long-term follow-up study in women who had received this drug for treatment of Trichomonas vaginalis infection failed to reveal any excess incidence of tumors.[135] The issue must be regarded as unsettled at the present time.

Whatever regimen is used, the clinician must be aware that relapse rates of 5–20% have been noted. Hence, close clinical follow-up and reexamination of stool and/or small bowel contents may be necessary in patients with only partial or temporary responses to therapy.[104]

5. Toxoplasmosis

Clinical and epidemiologic interest in toxoplasmosis as a disease of the immunocompromised host has paralleled interest focused on Pneumocystis carinii pneumonia. Fewer cases of toxoplasmosis relative to pneumocystosis have been reported in the recent literature, but the possibility of toxoplasmosis is often raised in the very same patients suspected of having pneumocystosis. However, P. carinii infection is almost always confined to the lung, whereas the causative agent of toxoplasmosis, Toxoplasma gondii, infrequently causes pneumonitis alone. More commonly, T. gondii affects multiple organ systems and has a special predilection for the central nervous system (CNS) in the immunologically impaired host. The special predilection of clinical toxoplasmosis for the CNS has been borne out by the current AIDS epidemic.[136,137]

Impressive progress in recent years has been made in understanding the epidemiology of toxoplasmosis.[138] Unlike P. carinii, which cannot be cultivated in vitro, abundant taxonomic and microbiologic information is available on this common protozoan parasite.

Toxoplasma gondii has been implicated in several clinical problems that are not covered extensively in this chapter: (1) as an infectious agent that can trigger recurrent abortions in humans (a role that is debated); (2) as the cause of a congenital infectious syndrome characterized by encephalitis, mental retardation, and microcephaly; and (3) as an ocular infection, usually retinochoroiditis. In the area of diagnosis, there are still major problems in interpreting serologic test results. The problems with diagnosis are most important in the immunocompromised host where, like pneumocystosis, *Toxoplasma* infections can be life-threatening medical complications. Many cases of toxoplasmosis in immunosuppressed patients have been diagnosed only at necropsy. This is unfortunate inasmuch as effective therapy for the infection has been available for 30 years and consists of the use of one folate antagonist, pyrimethamine, combined with a sulfonamide such as sulfadiazine.

5.1. History

It is likely that the first description of toxoplasmosis in man dates back to the work of Samuel Darling, a pathologist and parasitologist in Panama who described a case of a young male with an acute illness characterized by fever, headache, and joint stiffness, who had encysted organisms in a muscle biopsy suspected of containing *Trichinella* or *Sarcosporidia*.[139] This report of probable toxoplasmosis published in 1908 took place in the same year that Nicolle and Manceaux identified *Toxoplasma* in a North African rodent, the gondii, and Splendore made the same observations in rabbits in Brazil.[140] Some 15 years later, Janku described retinal parasites in sections taken from a baby who apparently had expired of congenital toxoplasmosis.[141] This was the first suggestion of a relationship between a human illness and the parasitic forms identified in various mammalian and avian species in different continents. It has subsequently become apparent that strains of toxoplasmosis obtained from human and animal sources differ from country to country. In 1939, Wolf and colleagues demonstrated *Toxoplasma* by inoculation into animals of tissues taken from a baby with neonatal encephalitis.[142] Sabin subsequently showed that antibodies to *Toxoplasma* could be demonstrated by mixing organisms with the sera of patients and injecting the mixture into the skin of the rabbit.[143] This was a complex and cumbersome technique for measuring antibodies to *Toxoplasma*. In 1948, Sabin and Feldman described what has become the reference serologic test for detection of antibodies against *Toxoplasma*.[144] The basis for the test is the observation that *Toxoplasma* trophozoites do not stain with methylene blue dye in the presence of specific anti-body. Subsequently, complement fixation, indirect hemagglutination, immunofluorescence, and an enzyme-linked immunoabsorbent assay (ELISA) of antibodies have been described.

The identification of *Toxoplasma* as an important etiologic agent of uveitis was initially documented in histopathologic studies. The lymphadenopathic form of toxoplasmosis was described during the early 1950s by Siim[145] and by Gard and Magnusson,[146] and there has been widespread recognition that this is the most common clinical manifestation of toxoplasmosis in man. It has been concluded that approximately 15% of otherwise unexplained lymphadenopathy is caused by toxoplasmosis.[147] Confusion of this finding with lymphoma has been well described, as have cases of coexistent toxoplasmosis and lymphoma.

5.2. The Organism

Toxoplasma gondii are obligate intracellular protozoan parasites. They are considered to be coccidian because of an enteroepithelial cycle and are presently classified among the sporozoa in the suborder *Eimerina*. Three forms exist in nature: trophozoites, tissue cysts, and oocysts. The trophozoites are crescent to oval in shape and are on the order of 3–7 μm in size. They are well stained by readily available Wright or Giemsa stains. This form is present in the acute stage of infection, having the capability of penetrating all mammalian cells except nonnucleated RBCs. Division continues until the host cell lyses or a tissue cyst forms. These trophozoites can be propagated intraperitoneally in a variety of warm-blooded animals, in tissue cultures, or in embryonated eggs (Fig. 5). Tissue cysts vary in size from 10 to 100 μm and may contain thousands of organisms. Tissue cysts are present in the chronic or latent phase of *Toxoplasma* infection and can be identified by PAS stain. These cysts are infective after oral ingestion because disruption of their walls by gastric juice and digestive enzymes frees viable trophozoites that survive long enough to penetrate GI mucosa. Freeze-thawing, heating in excess of 60°C, or desiccation will destroy tissue cysts.

Oocysts are oval structures 10–12 μm in diameter found only in feline hosts. Following ingestion of either tissue cysts or oocysts, protozoan forms of *T.*

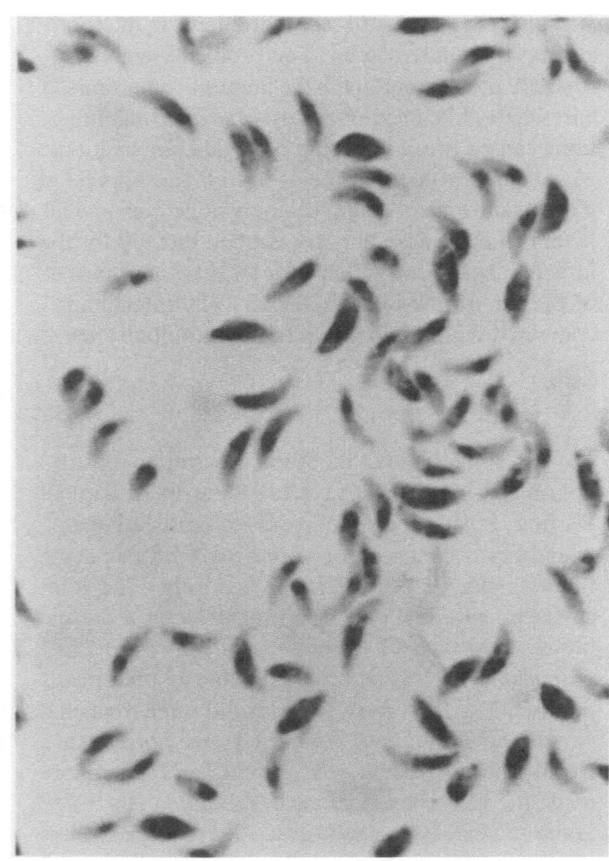

FIGURE 5. Trophozoites of *Toxoplasma gondii* as readily stained by either the Wright or Giemsa technique.

gondii invade the GI tract of the cat, and an asexual cycle (schizogony) is followed by a sexual cycle (gametogony) that results in the development of a noninfectious, nonsporulated oocyst. Cats excrete vast numbers, in excess of millions, of oocysts for approximately 2 weeks. Sporogony occurs outside of the feline host over a period of approximately 5 days and results in an infectious oocyst. These oocysts are highly resistant to physical destruction and remain infectious for more than a year. Ingestion of oocysts has been shown to transmit toxoplasmosis, and oocysts probably play an important role in orally acquired infection. Feline animals, including both domestic and feral cats, appear to be the definitive hosts in the life cycle of the *Toxoplasma* organism, and no other animal has been found to shed oocysts. Transmission between cats and a wide variety of omnivorous, herbivorous, and carnivorous animals occurs via the ingestion of oocysts or ingestion of cysts

present in meat. Animals such as cattle, pigs, and birds (including poultry) thus are intermediate hosts that are infected either by congenital transmission, ingestion of oocysts, or through the ingestion of other animals whose flesh contain cysts. Humans acquire the infection primarily by eating the flesh of animals that contain cysts or ingestion of cat excreta contaminated with oocysts.

Surveys of meat available in butcher shops have demonstrated that as many as 10% of mutton, 25% of pork, and less than 1% of beef samples contain tissue cysts that can serve as source of infection if consumed raw or poorly cooked. It is possible that man becomes infected by oocysts through the contamination of human food by coprophagous insects such as cockroaches and flies. The congenital form of disease results when women acquire the acute infection during pregnancy, with the fetus acquiring infection pari passu by the transplacental route. It does not appear that toxoplasmosis acquired prior to pregnancy can lead to congenitally infected offspring. A small number of infections have been definitely traced to laboratory accidents or by transfusion of whole blood or WBCs. By a variety of serologic techniques, it has been demonstrated that the acquisition of antibodies by humans increase with age, and by midlife an average 50% and as many as 93% of patients surveyed in certain geographic areas have evidence of infection.[140]

Following the usual acquisition of infection by the oral route, *T. gondii* spreads hematogenously to all major organs and tissues. In normals, the generation of host immune response coincides with the disappearance of trophozoites from tissue, and the tissue cyst forms of *T. gondii* take place, i.e., encystation occurs. These cysts contain organisms that are viable for the remainder of the life of the host. Preferred sites of encystment include skeletal and cardiac muscles as well as brain, but tissue cysts may be found in just about every organ. Some investigators believe that monocytes or macrophages can act as a sanctuary for viable trophozoites.

5.3. Pathogenesis

The basic mechanisms underlying host susceptibility to toxoplasmosis have become more clearly defined as a result of both experimental and in vitro studies.[148,149] Evidence for the importance of T-cell-mediated delayed hxpersensitivity immune mechanisms has been presented by Frenkel who demonstrated the ease of infecting nude or congenitally athymic mice with *Toxoplasma*.[150] Unquestionably, therapy with agents that impair T-cell function such as glucocorticoids can reactivate latent *Toxoplasma* infection. Three decades ago Frenkel demonstrated that corticosteroids and irradiation exacerbate *Toxoplasma* infection in hamsters.[151] Such animals develop multifocal central nervous system lesions similar to that observed in immunocompromised humans. Subsequent studies by Strannegard and Lycke have shown that antilymphocyte serum prolongs parasitemia in mice and decreases survival time of infected animals.[152]

These experiments parallel what is observed in man: the tendency for toxoplasmosis to reactivate in patients with Hodgkin disease or AIDS whose T-cell function is especially impaired. More than one-third of patients summarized in Table 5 had Hodgkin disease. Moreover, disseminated disease caused by *T. gondii* appears to occur almost exclusively in patients with underlying hematologic malignancy, recipients of immunosuppressive therapy, or patients with AIDS. Tumors infiltrating tissues that contain cysts seem to have little risk of reactivating infection. Interestingly, some antineoplastic/immunosuppressive agents such as the corticosteroids and cyclophosphamide seem more able to cause recrudescence of latent *Toxoplasma* infection than others, such as vinblastine or bleomycin.

The state of knowledge about specific components of host defense mechanisms against *Toxoplasma* has been enhanced by recent in vitro studies of monocyte–macrophage T-cell interactions. Both experimental mice and humans infected with *Toxoplasma* have stimulated ("activated") macrophages that inhibit or kill *Toxoplasma* in vitro.[153–155] Human monocytes and monocyte-derived macrophages from normal (unsensitized, nonactivated) or chronically infected patients are unable to kill *Toxoplasma* in vitro. The mechanism by which these macrophages become microbicidal is now being defined. A variety of lymphokines or cytokines, such as γ-interferon (IF_γ) and interleukin-2 (IL-2) are potent activators of mononuclear phagocytes to kill *Toxoplasma*.[156,157] The actual microbicidal mechanisms can be oxygen dependent or independent, depending on specific cell type.[158] The intrinsic susceptibility of the nude mouse to toxoplasmosis gives credence to the primary role of the lymphocyte in the immune process.[150]

It is not known whether the armed or activated macrophage is solely responsible for the efferent limb of the immune process. Stimulated mouse macrophages kill different organisms (other than *Toxoplasma*) equally well, so there is evidence that the efferent process is non-organism-specific. The presence of *Toxoplasma* organisms intracellularly prevents fusion of the phagolysosome in both normal and stimulated macrophages; therefore, such fusion does not account for inhibition or killing of *Toxoplasma* organisms. Furthermore, macrophage stimulation does not always correlate in time with protection of the host.[159] Attempts to enhance cell-mediated immune function by bacille Calmette-Guérin (BCG) immunization or transfer factor are of undetermined validity in prophylaxis or treatment of toxoplasmosis, and other approaches toward immu-

TABLE 5. Cases of Toxoplasmosis in the Compromised Host—Excluding AIDS[a]

Underlying condition	Cases	Major neurologic presentation or pathology	Treated	Improved
Hodgkin disease	38	25	12	10
Non-Hodgkin lymphoma	10	6[b]	1	0
Leukemia	15			
Acute lymphocytic leukemia	4	1	3	2
Chronic lymphocytic leukemia	4	2	1	1
Acute myelogenous leukemia	2	1	1	1
Chronic myelogenous leukemia	5	1	2	2
Myeloid metaplasia	1	0		
Multiple myeloma	2	2		
Carcinoma				
Breast	3	2	1	1
Ovary	1	0		
Lung	1	1		
Seminoma	1[c]	1[c]		
Melanoma	1	1		
Chromophobe adenoma	1	1		
Neuroblastoma	1	0		
Thymoma	1	1		
Collagen–vascular				
Systemic lupus erythematosus	3	3		
Scleroderma	2	2	2	2
Autoimmune hemolytic anemia	1	0		
Organ transplant				
Bone marrow	9	8	2	1
Kidney	8	6		1
Liver	1	0		
Heart	5	1	3	1[d]
Total	120	65	28	22

[a]Updated from Ruskin and Remington 162
[b]Includes one case with uveitis
[c]This patient also had chronic lymphocytic leukemia
[d]This patient improved secondary to withdrawal of immunosuppression

nologic stimulation or reconstitution have not been investigated.

Toxoplasma infection does not seem to be as common in congenital immunodeficiency syndromes as *Pneumocystis carinii,* and it is not as common in multiple myeloma as in Hodgkin disease despite the tendency to use corticosteroids so commonly in myeloma. This underscores the apparent importance of cell-mediated immune function in defense against this intracellular parasite. The proclivity for *Toxoplasma* to infect the central nervous system in immunocompromised patients suggests that host factors active against *Toxoplasma* are poorly operative in the CNS.

5.4. Signs and Symptoms of Toxoplasmosis in Immunologically Intact Patients

There are three well-recognized forms of toxoplasmosis in the normal host: lymphadenitis, uveitis, and congenital infection. Without doubt, the great majority of congenital and acquired infections in patients without immunodeficiency is inapparent. Clinical disease results from either newly acquired infection or from reactivation of latent infection, since organisms remain viable for the life of the host. The latter mechanism appears to be quite common in the uveitis syndrome. Uveitis in the immunologically intact adult is almost always the result of reactivation of congenital infection rather than of acquisition of a new infection.

In congenital toxoplasmosis, the maternal infection is usually inapparent. Furthermore, not all mothers who acquire toxoplasmosis during pregnancy produce infected offspring; recently published studies suggest that no more than one-third of maternal infections result in congenital infection. There is good evidence that transplacental passage increases with gestational age, but the incidence of clinical disease appears to decrease. Infants with congenital toxoplasmosis may overcome their infection without sequelae, but others may develop chorioretinitis, ocular muscle problems, epilepsy, blindness, psychomotor seizures, and mental retardation. Clinical manifestations of neonatal infection include chorioretinitis, hydrocephalus, microcephaly, cerebritis with sequelae of complications and convulsions, lymphadenopathy, fever, hepatosplenomegaly, jaundice, rash, cerebrospinal fluid (CSF) pleocytosis, and elevated protein.

Asymptomatic lymphadenitis is the most common clinical manifestation of acquired toxoplasmosis. Nontender, discrete lymph nodes are most often enlarged in the cervical areas, but generalized enlargement may be present. Symptoms such as fever, sore throat, myalgias, and malaise may lead to confusion with infectious mononucleosis. A maculopapular rash and hepatosplenomegaly may mimic cytomegalovirus (CMV) infection. Much less common involvement includes pneumonitis, encephalitis, hepatitis, and polymyositis. Pericarditis is possibly more common than myocarditis, and the latter is actually quite rare.[160]

The lymphadenopathic form of toxoplasmosis, when accompanied by systemic symptoms of fever, malaise, and the findings of hepatosplenomegaly, is often suggestive of a lymphoma. There are many anecdotal accounts of patients referred to major cancer treatment centers for therapy of lymphoma or actually started on antineoplastic chemotherapy who were subsequently found to have only toxoplasmosis. Enlarged lymph nodes should be biopsied unless there is an obvious contraindication. Dorfman and Remington believe that lymph nodes, when infected with *Toxoplasma*, exhibit virtually pathognomonic architectural changes.[161] These changes include (1) reactive hyperplasia associated with irregular clusters of epithelioid histocytes in cortical and paracortical zones, and (2) focal distention of subcapsular and trabecular sinuses by monocytoid cells. In a series of cases studied by these investigators, every patient who had *Toxoplasma* lymphadenitis by histologic criteria also had serologic findings (including Sabin–Feldman dye tests, IgM immunofluorescent antibodies, or both) that corroborated the histopathologic diagnosis.[161]

5.5. Toxoplasmosis in the Compromised Host

Infection in the immunocompromised host can clearly result from reactivation of latent infection, but exogenous or neoacquisition of the organism can produce an equally devastating illness. In a previous review, some 81 published and unpublished cases of toxoplasmosis occurring up to 1975 in patients with neoplasia, collagen vascular disease, and recipients of organ transplants were summarized.[162] Table 5 is an attempt to update that summary with additional cases reported during the ensuing 9 years.[163–175] In both the original analysis and in this updated table, it is apparent that neurological manifestations predominate in more than half the patients.

In patients with AIDS, the major clinical findings are almost exclusively limited to the CNS.[136,137] Lymphadenopathy as part of AIDS itself or the clinical prodrome known as AIDS-related complex (ARC) is rarely caused by toxoplasmosis. Toxoplasmosis has been increasingly recognized in recipients of bone marrow transplants[176–178] and in these intensely immunosuppressed patients parasitemia has been documented.[176] In the compromised host, clinical manifestations include diffuse encephalopathy, meningoencephalitis, enlarging central mass lesions, or a combination thereof. Focal signs, seizures, motor impairment, and impaired consciousness are common clinical findings. Examination of the spinal fluid has shown mild reactive pleocytosis with a predominance of mononuclear forms and only a modest elevation in protein. Many patients have had concurrent infections with DNA viruses, and such individuals have usually been more severely ill. Toxoplasmosis may coexist with a neoplastic disorder (particularly lymphoma) and may be confused with a metastatic process in the liver, spleen, lungs, or CNS.[173,174] Noninvasive techniques such as radionuclide scanning,[175] computed tomography (CT), or magnetic resonance imaging (MRI) are expeditiously required to establish the possibility of infection mimicking tumor. Rarely, now, is arteriography required to distinguish between a vascular mass such as a tumor, and a toxoplasmic abscess. In our experience, mediastinal lymphadenopathy and eosinophilia are not useful in distinguishing lymphoma (e.g., Hodgkin disease) from toxoplasmosis.

Besides newly acquired (per oral) infection or reactivation of dormant infection, toxoplasmosis can be acquired by transfusion of blood products. Siegel and associates described four patients with acute leukemia who developed acute toxoplamosis after receipt of leukocytes from donors with chronic myelogenous leukemia.[179] On the basis of retrospective serologic studies, evidence was obtained implicating donor leukocytes as the source of the parasite. In vitro studies indicate that T. gondii remains viable in banked blood for up to 50 days at refrigerated temperatures and that the parasite can be isolated from the buffy coat of totally asymptomatic individuals. Other than the experience of Siegel and colleagues,[179] there are no other well-documented examples of hematogenous or transfusion-associated toxoplasmosis. On the other hand, Raisanen and colleagues have described an experimental model wherein whole human blood inoculated with Toxoplasma and stored up to 28 days caused lethal infections in rabbits after transfusion.[180] Thus, transfusion-associated toxoplasmosis appears to be real, but the risk of disease seems very small. It seems impractical at this time to recommend screening of blood products for evidence of prior or recent Toxoplasma infection. Correspondingly, some authors have suggested that only Toxoplasma-antibody-negative subjects serve as donors of organ allografts to antibody-negative recipients but that such a policy would not appear to be judicious if the recipient had evidence of prior infection (i.e., seropositivity). Toxoplasmosis involving both donor and recipient hearts has been reported after heterotopic cardiac transplantation.[181]

There is little specific information on the incidence of uveitis in the immunocompromised host, and no solid data on the proportion of cases caused by Toxoplasma. The differential diagnosis of uveitis in the immunocompromised patient really does not differ from that in the patient with intact host defenses.

Thus, in patients with appropriate geographic background, histoplasmosis must be considered high on the list of infectious etiologies causing similar fundoscopic and clinical findings. It can be stated with certainty that uveitis appears to be relatively less common than intracerebral involvement in the cases reviewed in Table 5.

5.6. Toxoplasmosis in AIDS Patients

It is well established that patients with AIDS have a predilection for the development of toxoplasmic encephalitis.[136,137] The risk of CNS disease in patients with positive toxoplasma serology may be as high as 12%.[137] In a study of AIDS patients by Snider and colleagues, T. gondii accounted for 38% of known CNS infections and 36% of focal intracerebral lesions.[182] In another hospital study, toxoplasmic encephalitis was the leading cause of death among Haitian patients who were autopsied.[183] In Haitian patients, concomitant infection due to M. tuberculosis is common, as are a host of other infectious problems. Other conditions that may be confused with T. gondii involving the central nervous system are infections due to Candida, Aspergillus, Cryptococcus neoformans, Mycobacteria, progressive multifocal leukoencephalopathy, intracerebral lymphoma, or Kaposi sarcoma. Focal abnormalities are present in most patients and seizures either of a generalized or focal nature may be a presenting finding. Most patients with AIDS have infection localized to the brain, but disseminated disease has also been reported. The presence of intracerebral mass lesions, particularly in the basal ganglia region are quite suggestive of the diagnosis. Since there may be a number of absolute or relative contraindications to brain biopsy, many authorities recommend empiric treatment for toxoplasmosis of CNS mass lesions, even if the diagnosis of Toxoplasma infection is not firmly established. The rationale for this recommendation is that the other entities likely to cause a mass lesion(s) are probably not as readily treated and will not respond quickly to therapy. Once successful treatment of the acute episode occurs (and the response may occur within days, particularly when accompanied by a short course of corticosteroids to decrease cerebral edema), it would seem prudent to place the patient on chronic suppressive therapy with pyrimethamine (25 mg/day) and probably a sulfonamide preparation (2–4 g/day) if the patient can tolerate one of the latter group of agents.

Serodiagnosis of *Toxoplasma* encephalitis in AIDS patients presents a major challenge. Most patients with proven disease do not have elevated *Toxoplasma* titers and seroconversion is infrequent, in marked contrast to the situation in nonimmunosuppressed patients. Parasitemia has been documented in AIDS patients.[184] Some have reported that the *Toxoplasma* agglutination test is a more sensitive indicator of acute infection, particularly in patients with low dye test titers. Remington and colleagues recommend that sera from patients in high-risk groups for AIDS be stored to facilitate specific diagnosis if CNS disease develops later. At that point, changes in titers can be sought.[185] When used in conjunction with the dye test, titers obtained by the agglutination test seem to be the most useful noninvasive indicator of toxoplasmic encephalitis.[186]

5.7. Diagnosis

There are several pitfalls in the accurate diagnosis of clinically significant toxoplasmosis in both the immunocompromised and normal host. Stringent, unequivocal criteria on which to base such a diagnosis include (1) demonstration of trophozoite forms in body fluids or tissues and/or (2) the finding of *Toxoplasma* antibodies of specific type and titer in serums (and/or body fluid).

Tissue culture isolation techniques have been used to document parasitemia in patients with toxoplasmosis complicating marrow transplantation[176] and AIDS,[184] and this would provide strong evidence of disseminated disease. However, isolation per se of the parasite following inoculation of human tissue into a susceptible laboratory animal or tissue culture does not provide definitive proof of acute infection because cysts remain viable in such tissues as lymph node, muscle, heart, and brain for life. However, in view of the rarity of cyst forms in enlarged lymph nodes, the isolation of viable *Toxoplasma* from such nodes might be meaningful when combined with the data from serologic studies. Organisms may even be recoverable from blood of asymptomatic patients more than 1 year after initial infection. By the same token, histologic demonstration of the cyst form of the parasite in tissue does not altogether eliminate the possibility that infection is still acute. During the course of active disease, there may be coexistence of cyst forms with trophozoites in the same organs.

There is a growing literature on the serodiagnostic approaches to *Toxoplasma* infection, but no consensus about the most reliable test. Table 6 sum-

TABLE 6. Serodiagnostic Tests for Toxoplasmosis

Test	Acute	Chronic/latent	Comment	Reference
Agglutination	≥1 : 100	1 : 16–1 : 256	For IgG antibodies	186
Complement fixation	≥1 : 32	neg—1 : 8		187
Enzyme-linked immunosorbent-assay (ELISA)	≥1 : 512	≤1 : 256		188
IgM capture	>1 : 256	neg—1 . 64	Lower titers in infants	189
IgM immunoabsorbent				190
Fluorometric immunoassay	>100 signal units			191
Hemagglutination, indirect	≥1 : 100	1 : 16–1 : 256		192
Immunofluorescence				
Antiglobulin second antibody	≥1 : 1000	1 : 8–1 : 1000		193
Anti-IgM second antibody	≥1 : 80[a]	neg after 4 months	Earliest positive, correlates best with acute infection	194
Sabin–Feldman dye uptake	≥1 : 1000[b]	1 : 4–1 : 1000	Requires viable organisms	144

[a]IgM titers ≥1 80 highly suggestive of acute infection
[b]IgG titers 1 16,000 suggestive of acute infection

marizes the commonly used serologic tests for toxoplasmosis with a summary of the ranges of titers in acute disease and the titer ranges seen in chronic or latent infection.[185-194] As with all serologic tests, the most important principle is that the diagnosis of acute toxoplasmosis is established by a rising titer in serial specimens: either from negative to positive or at least a fourfold rise in titer. One of the major problems with the commonly available serodiagnostic methods (Sabin–Feldman dye test, indirect immunofluorescence, indirect hemagglutination, and ELISA), is that titers may remain elevated years after acute infection. Although some advocates of the complement-fixation test claim that titers of 1:16 or greater reflect acute disease, we believe that elevated titers in this range may also persist for years.

Often a patient may be tested for evidence of toxoplasmosis after the peak of symptoms. It may be of value to perform several serodiagnostic tests simultaneously. The earliest test to become positive is one that detects IgM-specific anti-*Toxoplasma* antibodies, followed by the Sabin–Feldman dye test, the indirect hemagglutination test, and the complement fixation test. The IgM–IFA test has been proposed as the most accurate test of acute infection,[193] but problems with this assay have been encountered by several other laboratories. These interlaboratory variations could be because of differences in the fluoroscein-labeled anti-IgM antiserum.

IgM detecting methodologies have also been proposed as the most reliable means for distinguishing acute from chronic infection,[189,190,194] but there are notable exceptions to this premise.[185] Patients with AIDS or a disseminated neoplasm may not mount a humoral antibody response.[195] The converse of this conclusion is that some compromised hosts (e.g., heart transplant recipients) may demonstrate significant rises in IgM antibody titers without clinical evidence of active infection.[185] The best working principle is that a detectable immune response, particularly a change in antibody concentrations, is one piece of evidence in establishing a diagnosis, but the absence of change in antibody levels does not exclude the diagnosis of toxoplasmosis.

Several experimental tests have been described that report the detection of free *Toxoplasma* antigens in serum[196,197] or body fluids.[198] Such approaches could be immensely helpful in clarifying confusing clinical and laboratory findings.

Studies for mononuclear–lymphocyte reactivity as well as tests of delayed hypersensitivity have no value in the diagnosis of acute infection in the immunocompromised host. Although lymphocyte transformation occurs in congenitally infected infants,[199] skin tests become positive months after infection and therefore cannot diagnose newly acquired acute infection. Furthermore, such tests are not helpful in evaluating reactivated disease and could well become negative secondary to the effects of immunosuppressive treatment.

5.8. Summary of Diagnostic Approach to Possible CNS Toxoplasmosis

Since CNS involvement is a life-threatening complication, the following steps are reasonable diagnostic measures to be undertaken with celerity.

1. Lumbar puncture should be taken for (a) routine studies (the cell count should be primarily mononuclear, the protein may be modestly elevated, but the glucose may be normal); (b) cytology (the CSF sediment or better yet a cytocentrifuge preparation should be stained with Giemsa and examined by immunofluorescence using *Toxoplasma*-specific antibodies; (c) CSF inoculation into mice (fresh or refrigerated samples should be inoculated into mice intraperitoneally; freezing of the sample will kill trophozoites and should be avoided); and (d) serology (which should be performed and compared to serum titer).
2. Serum serology should be compared with CSF titer. Desmonts[200] proposed a method for assessing antibody activity in the aqueous humor of the eye (for diagnosing ocular toxoplasmosis) by factoring for IgG concentration. The following equation was used.

$$C = \frac{\text{aqueous humor titer}}{\text{serum titer}} \times \text{globulin concentration} \left(\frac{\text{serum}}{\text{aqueous humor}} \right)$$

If $C \geq 8$, antibody production is local. Applied to CSF (in place of aqueous humor), the diagnosis of toxoplasmosis in the CSF should be considered if the titer/IgG is greater in CSF than in serum.

3. CT scan of brain and/or brain scan should be performed.

Definitive diagnosis would be established by brain biopsy if the patient has a mass lesion in an accessible area and there are no contraindictions to surgery. Examination of the specimens by both light and electron microscopy and by immunoperoxidase staining is desirable. However, we would be inclined to initiate empiric therapy (see Section 5.9), depending on the clinical situation (essentially, how unstable the patient's overall condition is) and on the basis of positive serology.

5.9. Therapy

The decision to treat must obviously be based on the constellation of clinical findings, the underlying severity of the patient's illness and a careful weighing of the benefits of drug therapy in view of the limitations and toxic effects of the agents that can be used. There is little question, however, that few clinicians should hold back in therapy if the patient demonstrates CNS involvement, pericarditis, hepatosplenomegaly, or pneumonitis in the presence of elevations in any of the antibody titers listed on Table 6. A more important issue, however, is whether empirical anti-*Toxoplasma* therapy should be started in patients who are awaiting confirmation of the diagnosis by serology, since such specimens are often referred to specialized laboratories, and delay in obtaining results may be experienced. Our policy has been to start empiric therapy in the patient with underlying lymphoma, in recipients of high-dose corticosteroid therapy, and in the individual with AIDS who has evidence of a CNS mass lesion that does not appear to be a tumor by noninvasive studies. There would appear to be little risk associated with pyrimethamine and sulfadiazine in this situation (which would also "cover" infections such as *Nocardia*), and if the patient were to have a brain abscess, the cure would likely require surgical extirpation.

No antimicrobial agent is effective against a tissue cyst form of *T. gondii*. Pyrimethamine, a di-aminopyrimidine, and sulfonamide are both active against the trophozoite form and interact synergistically when used in combination. These agents are antagonists of dihydrofolic acid reductase and *p*-aminobenzoic acid, respectively. Both agents are readily absorbed from the GI tract and penetrate lipids and lipid cells in the central nervous system. There is conflicting information about the efficacy of trimethoprim plus sulfamethoxazole as an anti-*Toxoplasma* agent, but recent studies in animals and in tissue culture suggest that it is effective.[201] Unfortunately, human clinical data are lacking, and at this point we do not advise that this agent be used for confirmed *Toxoplasma* infection. The author has seen *Toxoplasma* encephalitis develop in AIDS patients who had recently been given trimethoprim-sulfamethoxazole for pneumocystosis.

For seriously ill patients, a loading dose of 100–200 mg pyrimethamine is recommended during the initial day of treatment in adults followed by a maintenance daily dosage of 1 mg/kg per day. For children, 2 mg/kg should be given as a loading dose for the first 3 days of treatment. There is no problem with the administration of folinic acid (calcium leukovorin) orally or intramuscularly in doses of 2–10 mg/day in conjunction with pyrimethamine to obviate the effect of pyrimethamine on bone marrow DNA synthesis. Fortunately, neither folinic acid nor Baker's yeast (unlike folic acid) inhibits the action of pyrimethamine on *T. gondii*, making this an ideal form of chemotherapy. Reservations about giving folinic acid stem from the concern that in some hematologic malignancies (e.g., leukemia) it might cause proliferation of neoplastic cells. Sulfadiazine or a triple sulfa mixture are the most active sulfonamides against *T. gondii*, whereas other sulfonamides such as sulfisoxazole are less active, and their use should be avoided. Dosage of sulfadiazine in adults is 100 mg/kg per day divided into four hourly doses after a loading dose of 50 mg/kg. For infants, the dosage is 100–140 mg/kg per day PO in four equal portions after a loading dose of 100 mg/kg.

There is little information on optimal duration of pyrimethamine–sulfa therapy, but a month may be adequate. Patients with chronically impaired host defenses, such as AIDS, may require life-long suppressive therapy.

A number of other antimicrobial agents have been investigated for anti-*Toxoplasma* activity, and two, clindamycin and spiramycin, have been found active.[185] There are now several reports of successful use of the combination of clindamycin in very high dose (e.g., 1200 mg 3–4 times per day) plus pyrimethamine in the usual dose to treat patients with AIDS.[185] This approach remains experimental and should only be attempted as a last resort in patients with severe hypersensitivity to sulfonamides.

For the patient with uveitis, the additional benefit of corticosteroids given either topically or systematically has been debated, with proponents advocating their use for the antiinflammatory effects and detractors arguing that their use further aggravates host immune defects. Certainly, it is folly to use steroids alone in the treatment of uveitis,[202] and if steroids are employed, they should be given as an adjunct to appropriate anti-*Toxoplasma* treatment.

5.10. Prevention

For seronegative patients perhaps the most appropriate measure is adequate cooking of meat to temperatures in excess of 60°C. Avoidance of cats or areas contaminated with cat feces is probably commendable but of dubious practicality. Also, the determination of the antibody seropositivity of a pet cat is valueless in excluding a potential hazard. Theoretically, avoidance of donors of blood products who are seropositive may be desirable, but is not likely to be feasible; this also applies to selection of donors of organ transplants. Long-term antimicrobial prophylaxis of toxoplasmosis has not been studied in the immunocompromised host, and, indeed, there are appropriate concerns about the effects of such agents on the bone marrow in certain underlying diseases. Prophylaxis might be considered in a clinical situation characterized by high risk of active infection as has been defined for pneumocystosis, but such a situation has not presented itself for study to date.

An unanswered but important question is whether or not all patients with lymphoma or leukemia or prospective organ transplant recipients should be screened for anti-*Toxoplasma* antibodies and possibly given "preventive therapy" if seropositive. Such serologic screening should be part of a routine initial procedure prior to therapy or transplantation (if only to establish a baseline for future comparison). If a patient has elevated or equivocally elevated titers, preventative therapy will probably be of little risk but

remains of unproven efficacy. Many patients with neoplastic diseases, recipients of organ transplants, and patients with AIDS receive prophylaxis with trimethoprim–sulfamethoxazole against *P. carinii* infection, and it will be interesting to see whether this has any impact on the incidence of toxoplasmosis.

6. Coccidial Infections

Two agents belonging to the subclass Coccidia within the class of sporozoal parasites have become prominent since 1980 as infectious complications occurring in immunocompromised hosts. These agents are *Cryptosporidia* and *Isospora belli*. Technically, these intracellular parasites are related to the *Toxoplasma* group—tissue cyst-forming coccidial organisms that belong to the suborder *Eimeria*. Both agents can now be readily identified by modified acid-fast staining of fecal specimens (such as the Kinyoun stain), but other more elaborate identification techniques are available.[203] In fact, together they constitute the only acid-fast staining parasites of any clinical significance. The two species can be readily distinguished. Features for *I. belli* include its large size (15 × 25 μm), which characteristically contain two sporoblasts (Fig. 6). In contrast, *Cryptosporidia* oocysts are much smaller (average 5 μm in diameter) and they contain four sporozoites (Fig. 7). However, the small size of *Cryptosporidia* is one reason that they may escape detection unless a special effort is made at diagnosis.

Most clinical attention has been focused on *Cryptosporidia,* a protozoan parasite that completes its life cycle closely adherent to the intestinal surface epithelium of mammals, birds, and reptiles. Cryptosporidiosis was first noted as a human infection following symptoms of overwhelming watery diarrhea in an immunosuppressed host.[204] The clinical prominence of this organism, as well as that of *I. belli,* has been mainly due to the role both have played as causes of severe diarrhea in patients with AIDS. Typically, the diarrhea is watery, profuse, associated with cramps and bloating, and results in severe malabsorption. Perhaps the first report of cryptosporidial disease in an AIDS patient was published in 1981.[205] It concerned a 48-year-old homosexual man treated in December 1979. This patient may well have been one of the earliest cases of AIDS, and the relationship

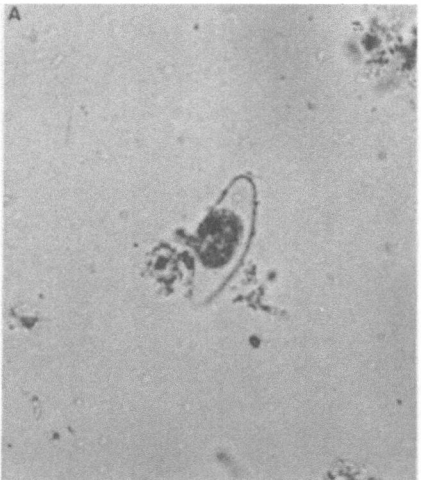
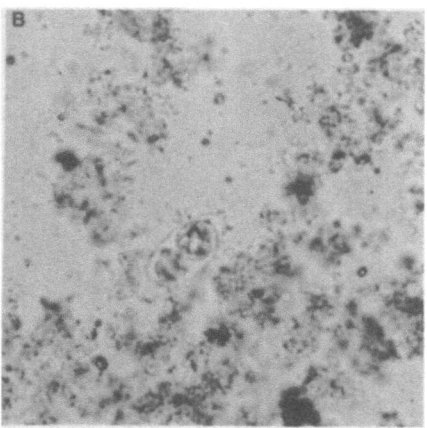

FIGURE 6. The oocysts of *Isospora bella* have a large, distinctive oval shape (25 × 15 μm) containing two intracellular sporoblasts. (A) The latter structures overlap. (B) The latter structures are distinct. (Photos courtesy of Lynne Garcia, UCLA Clinical Microbiology Laboratory.)

of the pathogen to the underlying immunopathologic disorder was not appreciated at the time. As with many subsequent cases, that patient's illness could not be controlled with a variety of antibacterial, antimalarial, and other antiprotozoal medications. Terminally, the patient developed a disseminated CMV infection and died.

Subsequent to the description of cryptosporidiosis in AIDS patients, worldwide attention has focused upon the disease as it occurs in animals.[206] By far and away, this seems to be its greatest importance, particularly in terms of economic ramifications. Besides patients with AIDS, individuals with other types of therapeutic immunosuppression or underlying disorders characterized by defects in cell-mediated immunity are now being described as having cryptosporidiosis: transplant recipients, patients receiving corticosteroids, and patients with IgA nephropathy.[207] With increasing interest focused on this pathogen, more extensive studies of diarrheal illnesses have been carried out with a specific interest in this pathogen. Not surprisingly, this organism has been increasingly detected in stool specimens of normal healthy patients.[208,209] Cryptosporidial disease now appears to be a common cause of diarrhea in developing countries,[210,211] but the reason it has not been more prominent in the clinical literature now seems clear.

First, the normal host is able to overcome or control the infection and the illness is short and self-limited. Recurrent disease has actually been documented in veterinarians,[212] and the evidence for a lasting immunity to this infection has not been established. Secondly, the diagnosis has not been frequently made before the current epidemic of AIDS because the organism is rather small and has not been readily detected by many of the procedures previously used to screen stool specimens. However, when appropriate techniques are used, the organism is identified without difficulty. Extraintestinal cryptosporidiosis has been reported. Ma and colleagues[213] reported three cases of interstitial pneumonia with this pathogen, but such occurrences are uncommon.

Illustrative Case 3

The patient was a 42-year-old homosexual man who had been in generally good health all his life, except for several episodes of gonorrhea and one episode of hepatitis B. Following a slow convalescence from hepatitis B, the patient then began to notice an onset of increasing watery diarrhea, weight loss, and low-grade fever. Over a period of 6 weeks he became severely anorectic with bloating, diffuse abdominal cramps, and severe anorexia. Except for clear liquids and gelatinlike foods, he was unable to eat. After approximately 3 months of watery diarrhea and a 30-lb weight loss, he sought medical attention. Several examinations of the stool revealed the acid-fast oocyst of *Cryptosporidia* species. The

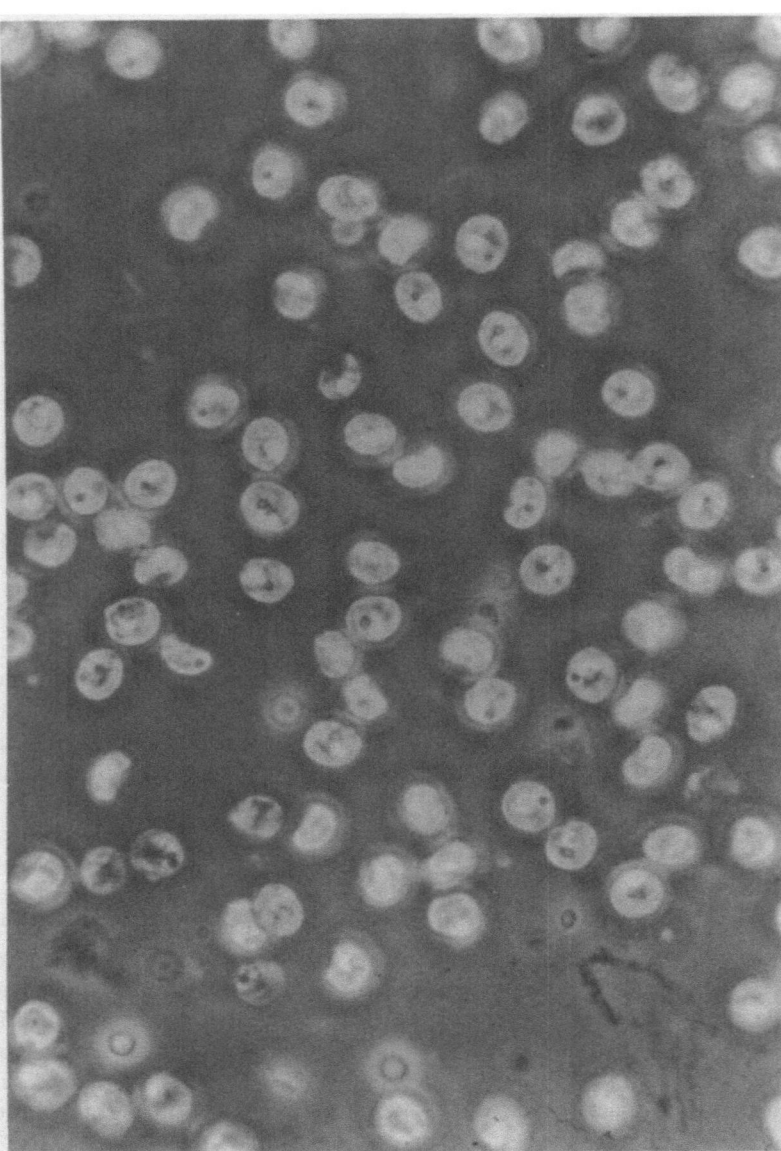

FIGURE 7. Like *Isospora, Cryptosporidia* are acid-fast but much smaller (4–6 μm in diameter) and roundly shaped. They may be tightly adherent to intestinal epithelial surfaces. (Photo courtesy of Lynne Garcia, UCLA Clinical Microbiology Laboratory.)

patient was treated with a variety of antidiarrheal agents, including bismuth-containing compounds, and opiate-containing medications without success. A program of systemic hyperalimentation through a Hickman catheter was initiated. This had no effect on the diarrhea (characterized by production of up to 20 thin, watery, explosive, diarrheal stools per day) but did result in some modest gain in weight. Serum albumin gradually rose and liver function tests, improved slightly. In an attempt to control the diarrhea, a variety of medications were used. This included chloroquine and clindamycin plus quinine. There was modest response to the latter combination but the latter two agents were extremely unpalatable. The dose of quinine and clindamycin was varied somewhat, but the

patient was unable to take his medications consistently. Finally, naproxen was given in a dosage of 200 mg four times per day. Within about 24 hr there was a dramatic reduction in stool output. The patient was able to gain considerable symptomatic relief with naproxen and subsequent stool examination using a modified acid-fast stain identified no cryptosporidial organisms. Some half-dozen follow-up stool examinations were carried out. When naproxen was discontinued, however, there was a return of watery diarrhea, cramping and bloating. Despite some stabilization on naproxen and hyperalimentation, the patient continued to lose weight and then developed low-grade fevers and lung infiltrates. The infiltrates were consistent with *Pneumocystis carinii* pneumonitis, and the patient was treated empirically with tri-methoprim–sulfamethoxazole. Lung infiltrates responded to this empiric therapy. Subsequently, however, he developed disseminated infection due to *Cryptococcus neoformans* with meningitis and positive blood cultures. The patient subsequently expired while being treated with amphotericin B, and no autopsy was obtained.

Comment. This patient presents with a fairly typical clinical progression of infections as seen in AIDS patients. Other patients with cryptosporidial or *I. belli* infection that we have encountered since the beginning of the outbreak have had marked weight loss, fluid and electrolyte loss, and severe inanition. The organism was missed on initial stool examinations but was subsequently identified with an acid-fast stain. The case report demonstrates that the major clinical management problem is fluid and electrolyte loss and it may become necessary to begin hyperalimentation simply in order to keep that patient alive

With regard to therapy, a variety of symptomatic and perhaps more specific antiparasitic medications were used in this unfortunate patient. Clindamycin plus quinine was tried because of its reported success in other protozoan infections.[103] Interestingly, *Cryptosporidia* were not seen in stool after the clindamycin plus quinine therapy, but a small bowel biopsy and autopsy examination were not performed in order to validate clinical efficacy Unfortunately, this is a major problem of evaluating response to therapy in patients with AIDS or similar immunologic disorders. What did give the patient symptomatic relief was a prostaglandin inhibitor, naproxen. Other medications such as indomethacin had been used with similar success. As has occurred in so many AIDS patients, one serious life-threatening infection such as cryptosporidiosis was supplanted by several other processes and the actual cause of death could not be precisely determined.

With regard to therapy of cryptosporidiosis, there has been some reported success with an experimental macrolide, spiramycin, in terminating the cryptosporidial diarrhea of AIDS patients.[214] However, the overall prognosis is extremely poor Therapeutic responses are somewhat better in patients with *I belli* infection Trimethoprim–sulfamethoxazole therapy is usually rapidly effective with termination of diarrhea in 48 hr,[215] and treatment should be continued for 2–4 weeks Nonetheless, there is a high rate of recurrence, and while long-term suppressive therapy has been advocated for AIDS patients, this may not be feasible because of drug intolerance. Alternative medications include metronidazole and pyrimethamine–sulfadiazine

7. Strongyloidiasis

In healthy subjects, infection caused by the intestinal threadworm *Strongyloides stercoralis* is usually clinically inapparent or manifested by mild GI symptoms of epigastric pain and diarrhea. As with toxoplasmosis, infection can rapidly progress to a fatal outcome in immunocompromised hosts. The causative organism is fairly common throughout the world, and the diagnosis should be suspected in pa-tients with diffuse pneumonitis, eosinophilia, and GI symptoms. Some of the most severe systemic infections caused by this parasite are also associated with sustained or unexplained bacteremia caused by *Enterobacteriaceae* or *P. aeruginosa*. However, the parasitic organism may not be found in routine stool examinations, and infected patients may not have eosinophilia.

7.1. The Organism

Strongyloides stercoralis is an intestinal nematode with a complex life cycle. Three different life cycles may occur at various times. The parasitic female lives in the intestine in a parthenogenic state. Eggs are released and hatched in the mucosa, and rhabdoid larvae are passed in the feces. Similar to what occurs in hookworm, rhabdoid larvae develop in the soil into filariform larvae that can penetrate human skin on contact, migrate through the bloodstream, and pass into the lungs. In the lungs, the larvae break out of the capillaries into the alveoli, migrate up the tracheobronchial tree to the pharynx, and are swallowed, whereby they again colonize the GI tract. A second life cycle involves the transformation of rhabdoid larvae in the soil into free living male and female adults which mate; these eggs hatch into larvae which may become infective for man. The third or so-called autoinfection cycle can take place entirely within the gastrointestinal tract of the host. Rhabdoid larvae molt and change into filariform larvae which are invasive. These filariform larvae can penetrate the intestinal mucosa or the skin of the perianal areas as they are passed in the stool. By this mechanism, clinical systemic infection can occur many decades after a patient leaves an endemic area.

7.2. Clinical Manifestations

Disseminated, occasionally fatal strongyloidiasis may occur in subjects whose immune mechanisms are presumably intact. But the most common setting for systemic infection is one of immunodeficiency resulting from either an underlying neoplastic disease or from immunosuppressive treatment. In those infections initiated by penetration of the skin by filariform larvae, the presence of a rash characterized by erythematous, maculopapular, or serpiginous lesions associated with pruritis is an early manifestation of infection. Urticaria may also be present. This pruritic reaction occurs directly at the site of larval skin penetration and usually appears within 24 hr. In those patients with autoinfection secondary to GI carriage, such lesions may be seen in the area of the lower abdomen, buttocks, perineum, or upper thighs. These lesions contain filariform larvae. During the early stage of active infection, blood eosinophilia is a common but not necessarily consistent finding. With persistence of the infection, eosinophilia may disappear, but in chronic strongyloidiasis associated with eosinopenia, the prognosis has been poor. Granulomatous reactions of pseudotumors around degenerating larvae or adult worms have been described in the intestine of animals and humans.

In the intestinal phase of strongyloidiasis, the major clinical manifestations are burning or colicky abdominal pain associated with diarrhea. The stool may be watery and contain mucus or blood. In severe infections, a malabsorption syndrome may develop as the patient loses large amounts of fat and protein in the feces. Bowel lesions resembling ulcerative colitis may develop and lead to systemic manifestations including systemic toxicity and fever. Severe malabsorption, dehydration, electrolyte imbalance, and paralytic ileus may ensue. Immunosuppressive therapy and corticosteroids in particular may inhibit cell-mediated immune mechanisms against invading larvae or suppress the humoral antibody response to these antigens. The mechanical effect of a paralytic ileus resulting from other therapy or from an obstructing tumor may alter the host–parasite relationship in favor of the parasite. Massive intestinal infection with *Strongyloides* may itself cause paralytic ileus. Decreased intestinal motility from any cause may result in the 24–48-hr time interval required for the transformation of rhabditiform to invasive filariform larvae which then migrate out of the gut into the bloodstream.

Overwhelming infection by *Strongyloides* has received relatively little attention in the current literature on opportunistic infection. Scowden et al. have reviewed this subject comprehensively and pointed out more than 20 conditions associated with systemic strongyloidiasis, including Hodgkin disease, acute and chronic leukemias, leprosy, nephrotic syndrome, renal transplants, lupus erythematosus, protein-calorie malnutrition, and chronic renal fail-

ure.[216] Scowden et al. use the term hyperinfection syndrome to designate massive invasion of the gastrointestinal tract and lungs, whereas disseminated strongyloidiasis is used to refer to extensive parasitic invasion of other tissues. Hyperinfection is an exaggeration of the normal life cycle of the parasite, and patients present with a combination of respiratory and gastrointestinal symptoms. Disseminated strongyloidiasis implies involvement of organs not part of the ordinary life cycle of the parasite. In such an extension of disease, involvement by large filariform larvae can cause direct injury to heart, liver, skeletal muscle, adrenals, pancreas, kidney, and CNS. Because of the ready availability of chest radiography, perhaps the most commonly recognized site of involvement in both the hyperinfection syndrome and disseminated disease is the lung. Hemorrhagic pulmonary infiltrates or diffuse bilateral alveolar infiltrates with or without GI complaints have been reported.[217] Strongyloidiasis has also been associated with the onset of the adult respiratory distress syndrome (ARDS).[218]

In the gastrointestinal tract, severe ulcerating hemorrhagic enterocolitis may serve as a port of entry for bacterial and fungal superinfection. Both the hyperinfection syndrome and disseminated disease may be associated with sustained gram-negative bacteremia, and bacteremic pneumonia may be confused with parasitic infection in the lungs. This pattern of sustained bacteremia should be a clue to consider the diagnostic possibility of strongyloidiasis, particularly in the patient with eosinophilia or abdominal symptoms. Similarly, gram-negative bacillary meningitis can be an important concomitant process. It is not certain, however, that the parasitic infection always directly involves the brain. Meningitis probably results from bacteremia, but several authors have speculated that bacteria are (1) transported through the circulation and the brain in a piggyback fashion, i.e., adherent to the worm itself, and (2) excreted by migrating larvae. The manifestations of CNS disease can range from abnormalities in mental status to stupor and deep coma.

Illustrative Case 4

A 57-year-old Puerto Rican man was diagnosed as having polyarteritis nodosa in 1971. He was maintained on an average daily dose of 60 mg prednisone for the next 7 years He then developed diarrhea and both a *Salmonella* species, group E, was isolated from stool, and larvae of *Strongyloides stercoralis* was detected in the same specimen. The *Salmonella* was untreated and the *Strongyloides* treated with 1.5 g thiabendazole bid for 2 days. Five months later, he experienced return of fevers and polyarthralgias, and his stool was again positive for *Strongyloides*. A lumbar puncture was performed after mild headache developed and the CSF found to contain 4030 WBC/mm^3 of which half were neutrophils. The protein content of this sample was 180 mg/dl, and the glucose 77 mg/dl. All cultures and serologic tests on the CSF were negative. The patient was treated with 18 million units of penicillin, and his condition gradually improved. On two subsequent occasions, the patient was found to have larvae of *Strongyloides* swarming in his stools. With the second of these episodes, blood cultures were positive for *Escherichia coli* and *Pseudomonas aeruginosa* and the latter was isolated from CSF, which showed an elevated protein and WBC count. The patient responded to intravenous gentamicin and carbenicillin. Before therapy was completed, the patient developed progressive back pain and was found to have compression fractures of the L4 and L5 vertebrae. Tomograms revealed erosive lesions of both vertebral bodies, and bone scan showed increased radionuclide uptake. The diagnosis of vertebral osteomyelitis was confirmed by an open biopsy and recovery of a *P. aeruginosa* with the same antibiogram as the blood isolate.

Comment. Although there is no proof of systemic invasion by the round worm, this case represents a probable example of disseminated infection caused by *Strongyloides stercoralis*. In retrospect, the first episode of bacteriologically sterile meningitis may have represented invasion of the meninges by *Strongyloides*. Polymicrobial gram-negative bacillemia and metastatic bone infection are commonly associated with disseminated *Strongyloides* infection in immunosuppressed hosts.[216] In patients with repeatedly positive stool examinations containing *Strongyloides* and systemic bacterial infections, long-term intermittent suppressive therapy is recommended (Section 7.4)

7.3. Diagnosis

The unambiguous diagnosis of *Strongyloides* involves detection of rhabdoid larvae in feces, secretions (e.g., sputum), or tissue. Freshly passed feces may contain active rhabdoid larvae, but stool may be negative in more than 70% of cases despite careful examination.[217] Refrigeration of stool causes rapid disappearance of larvae. Ova can rarely be detected in stools, and multiple repeat stool examinations may be necessary, since larvae may only appear several weeks after institution of immunosuppressive therapy.[218] Caution must be urged in the examination of older clinical specimens because any hookworm eggs present in the feces for any length of time could hatch and yield rhabdoid larvae that are morphologically similar. If stools are negative, but a strong clinical

suspicion remains, aspirated duodenal contents should be examined for the presence of larvae. Recently, greatly improved detection has been observed using the Entero-test method for sampling of duodenal contents (this procedure is described in Section 4.6).

Larvae have also been reported present in sputum, peritoneal fluid, and urine. Tracheal or transtracheal aspiration may be necessary for detection in respiratory secretions, and sputum specimens should preferably be concentrated. Filariform larvae may be present in biopsies of skin lesions. Larvae have also been identified in pleural fluid, peritoneal fluid, lymph nodes, and urine and are best identified by a wet-mount examination and/or Giemsa stain. Eosinophilia exceeding 30% is common in infection with *Strongyloides* in intact hosts and has been present in perhaps half of immunosuppressed patients.[216] Patients with disseminated disease receiving corticosteroids, however, may not have this valuable laboratory clue. Other aspects of laboratory diagnosis, including skin testing and serologic methods, have not been helpful, particularly in immunocompromised hosts.

Radiologic studies of the small intestine may suggest the diagnosis.[219,220] Findings consistent with the diagnosis of Strongyloidiasis include dilated loops of bowel with thickened mucosal folds. These findings reflect worm penetration of the intestinal mucosa, lymphatic obstruction, and allergic edema of bowel wall.

7.4. Treatment

Patients with intact host defenses still have the potential for accelerated autoinfection, and it has been recommended that every patient with *Strongyloides* infestation be treated. This is no less urgent than in the patient with altered host defenses. Because the results of treatment of disseminated strongyloidiasis in the compromised host have varied from fair to poor, every effort to make the diagnosis in patients who have appropriate geographic histories prior to the start of immunosuppressive therapy is indicated. Although definitive proof is lacking, early and appropriate treatment in these hosts may avert a potentially catastrophic bacterial or fungal superinfection.

The agent of choice for *Strongyloides* is thiabendazole in doses of 25 mg/kg twice daily for 2–3 days in normal hosts. An alternative agent may be mebendazole, given in doses of 100 mg bid for 3 days. These agents are quite effective in normal hosts with only minimal adverse reactions consisting of nausea and GI upset. In the treatment of the immunosuppressed host, a significantly longer course of therapy seems necessary, and the agent has been given as long as 15 days with a mean of about 7 days. There is little danger of drug toxicity. More often, shorter but multiple courses of therapy are given. For those patients with repetitive episodes of sepsis–meningitis, it may be best to give thiabendazole 25 mg/kg 2–3 days every month.[216] Another method of suppression is to give a 5-day course of thiabendazole followed by a 3-day course of mebendazole. This appears to interrupt the cycle of recurrent systemic larval infection. The best guide to adequacy of treatment is the careful serial monitoring of feces or duodenal aspirates as well as following the course of extraintestinal manifestations (e.g., the chest radiograph). Persistent or recurrent disease has been associated with anatomic bowel abnormalities such as blind loops or diverticula and may require longer therapy or direct instillation of drug. Eosinophilia may take a longer period of time to resolve, perhaps as long as 2 months. Corticosteroids should be avoided, even in the face of high blood eosinophil counts. When polymicrobial infection is present, such as characterized by recurrent or breakthrough bacteremia, the bacteremia may cease only after effective antiparasitic treatment is given.

References

1. Weinstein RA, Young LS: Other procedure-related infections. In Bennett JV, Brachman PS (eds) *Hospital Infections.* Little, Brown, Boston, 1979, pp 489–505

2. Tapper ML, Armstrong D: Malaria complicating neoplastic disease. *Arch Intern Med* **136**:807–810, 1976

3. Ma DDF, Concannon AJ, Hayes J. Fatal leishmaniasis in renal-transplant patients. *Lancet* **2**:311–312, 1979

4. Smith JW, Bartlett MS. In Vitro cultivation of Pneumocystis In LS Young (ed): *Pneumocystis carinii Pneumonia.* Dekker, New York, 1984, pp. 107–138

5. Young LS (ed): *Pneumocystis carinii Pneumonia* Dekker, New York, 1984.

5a. Ruskin J, Spotkov J: Pneumocystis infection. In Spittell JA, Jr (ed): *Clinical Medicine*, Vol. 3 Harper and Row, New York, 1986, pp. 1–18

6. Dutz W. *Pneumocystis carinii* pneumonia *Pathol Annu* **5**:309–341, 1970.

7. Van der Meer G, Brug SL· Infection par pneumocystis chez l'homme et chez les animaux. *Ann Soc Belg Med Trop* **22**:301–307, 1942

8. Vanek J, Jirovec O. Parasitare penumonie. "Interstitielle" plasmazell pneumonie der frugeburten verursach durch *Pneumocystis carinii.* *Zentralbl Bakteriol* **158**:120–127, 1952.

9. Frenkel JK *Pneumocystis jiroveci* n. sp. In Robbins JB, Devita VT Jr, Dutz W (eds). *Symposium on Pneumocystis carinii Infection*, NCI Monograph #43. National Cancer Institute, Washington, D.C., 1976, pp. 13–30

10. Ivady G, Paldy L. Ein neues Behandlung sverfarhren der interstitiellen plasmazelligen Pneumonie fruhgeborener mit funtwertigen Stibium und aromatischen Diamidinen. *Monatsschr Kinderheilkd* **106**:10–14, 1958

11. Gajdusek DC. *Pneumocystis carinii*—etiologic agent of interstitial plasma cell pneumonia of young and premature infants. *Pediatrics* **19**:543–545, 1957

12. Frenkel JK, Good JT, Shultz JA: Latent pneumocystic infection of rats, relapse, and chemotherapy *Lab Invest* **15**:1559–1577, 1966

13. Hughes WT, McNabb PC, Makres, TD, et al: Efficacy of trimethoprim and sulfamethoxazole in the prevention and treatment of *Pneumocystis carinii* pneumonitis *Antimicrob Agents Chemother* **5**:289–293, 1974.

14. Hughes WT, Feldman S, Sanyal SK. Treatment of *Pneumocystis carinii* pneumonitis with trimethoprim/sulfamethoxazole. *Can Med Assoc J* **112**:47S–50S, 1975

15. Lau WK, Young LS: Trimethoprim–sulfamethoxazole treatment of *Pneumocystis carinii* pneumonia in adults. *N Engl J Med* **295**:716–718, 1976.

16. Hughes WT, Kuhn S, Chaudhary S, et al. Successful chemoprophylaxis of *Pneumocystis carinii* pneumonitis *N Engl J Med* **297**:1419–1426, 1977

17. Winston DJ, Gale RP, Meyer DV, et al: Infectious complications of human bone marrow transplantation. *Medicine (Baltimore)* **58**:1–31, 1979

18. Murray JF, Felton CP, Garay SM, et al. Pulmonary complications of the acquired immunodeficiency syndrome: Report of a National Heart, Lung and Blood Institute workshop. *N Engl J Med* **310**:1682–1688, 1984

19. Zakowski PC, Gottlieb MS, Groopman J: Acquired immunodeficiency syndrome (AIDS), Kaposi's sarcoma, and *Pneumocystis carinii* pneumonia. In LS Young (ed): *Pneumocystis carinii pneumonia* Dekker, New York, 1984, pp 195–226.

20 Hughes WT, Smith BL. Efficacy of diaminodiphenyl sulfone and other drugs in murine *Pneumocystis carinii* pneumonitis. *Antimicrob Agents Chemother* **26**:436–440, 1984.

20a Ruskin J: Newer developments in diagnosis and treatment of pneumocystis infections. In Remington JS, And Swartz MN (eds): *Current Clinical Topics in Infectious Diseases*, Vol. 7 McGraw-Hill, New York, 1986, pp. 194–215.

21 Smith JW, Bartlett MS Diagnosis of pneumocystis pneumonia *Lab Med* **10**:430–435, 1979.

22. Campbell WG. Ultrastructure of pneumocystis in human lung. *Arch Pathol Lab Med* **93**:312–324, 1972

23. Vossen MEMH, Beckers PJA, Meuwissen JHETL, et al: Developmental biology of *Pneumocystis carinii*, an alternative view on the life cycle of the parasite. *Z Parasitenkd* **55**:101–118, 1978.

24. Hughes WT, Price RA, Kim HK, et al: *Pneumocystis carinii* pneumonitis in children with malignancies. *J Pediatr* **82**:404–415, 1973.

25. Awen C, Baltzan M: Systemic dissemination of *Pneumocystis carinii* pneumonia. *Can Med Assoc J* **104**:809–812, 1971.

25a. Coulman CU, Greene I, Archibald RWR: Cutaneous pneumocystis. *Ann Intern Med* **106**: 396–398, 1987.

25b. Kwok S, O'Donnell JJ, Wood IS: Retinal cotton-wool spots in a patient with *Pneumocystis carinii* infection. *N Engl J Med* **307**: 184–185, 1982.

26. Barnett RW, Hull JG, Vortel V, et al: *Pneumocystis carinii* in lymph nodes and spleen. *Arch Pathol Lab Med* **88**:175–181, 1969.

27. Brzosko WJ, Nowoslawski A: Identification of *Pneumocystis carinii* antigens in tissues. *Bull Acad Pol Sci* **13**:49–54, 1965.

28. Redman JC: *Pneumocystis carinii* pneumonia in an adopted Vietnamese infant. *JAMA* **230**:1561–1563, 1973.

29. Lyons, HA, Vinijchaikul K, Hennigar GR: *Pneumocystis carinii* pneumonia unassociated with other disease. *Arch Intern Med* **108**:173–180, 1961.

30. Hughes WT, Price RA, Sisko F, et al: Protein calorie malnutrition. A host determinant for *Pneumocystis carinii* infection. *Am J Dis Child* **128**:44–50, 1974.

31 Walzer PD, Schnelle V, Armstrong D, et al: Nude mouse: A new experimental mode for *Pneumocystis carinii* infection *Science* **197**:177–179, 1977.

32. Walzer PD, Perl DP, Krogstad DJ, et al. *Pneumocystis carinii* pneumonia in the United States: Epidemiologic, diagnostic, and clinical features. *Ann Intern Med* **80**:83–93, 1974

33. Masur H, Jones TC: The interaction in vitro of *Pneumocystis carinii* with macrophages and L-cells *J Exp Med* **147**:157–170, 1978

34. Walzer PD, Schultz MG, Western KA: *Pneumocystis carinii* pneumonia and primary immune deficiency disease of infancy and childhood. *J Pediatr* **82**:416–422, 1973.

35. Veda K, Goto Y, Yamazaki S, et al. Chronic fatal pneumocystosis in nude mice *Jpn J Exp Med* **47**:475–482, 1977

36 Hendley JO, Weller TH. Activation and transmission in rats of infection with pneumocystis *Proc Soc Exp Biol Med* **137**:1401–1404, 1971

37. Brazinsky JH, Phillips JE. Pneumocystis pneumonia transmission between patients with lymphoma *JAMA* **209**:1527, 1969

38. Watanabe JM, Chinchinian H, Weitz C, et al: *Pneumocystis carinii* pneumonia in a family. *JAMA* **193**:119–120, 1965.

39. Perera DR, Western KA, Johnson HD, et al: *Pneumocystis carinii* pneumonia in a hospital for children *JAMA* **214**:1074–1078, 1970.

40. Singer C, Armstrong D, Rosen PP, et al. *Pneumocystis carinii* pneumonia A cluster of eleven cases *Ann Intern Med* **82**:772–777, 1975

41 Ruebush TK II, Weinstein RA, Baehner RL, et al: An outbreak of pneumocystis pneumonia in children with acute lymphocytic leukemia *Am J Dis Child* **132**:143–148, 1978

42. Meuwissen JHET, Tauber I, Leeuwenberg ADEM, et al: Parasitologic and serologic observations of infection with pneumocystis in humans *J Infect Dis* **136**:43–49, 1977

43 Stagno S, Pifer LL, Hughes WT, et al: *Pneumocystis carinii* pneumonitis in young, immunocopetent infants. *Pediatrics* **66**:56–62, 1980.

44. Western KA, Perera DR, Schultz MG: Pentamidine isethionate in the treatment of *Pneumocystis carinii* pneumonia. *Ann Intern Med* **73**:695–702, 1970.

45. Hughes WT, Sanyal SK, Price RA: Signs, symptoms and pathophysiology of *Pneumocystis carinii* pneumonitis. In Robbins JB, De Vita VT Jr, Dutz W (eds). *Symposium on Pneumocystis carinii Infection*. NCI Monograph #43 National Cancer Institute, Washington, DC, 1976, pp 77–88.

46. Walzer PD, Perl DP, Krogstad DJ, et al: *Pneumocystis carinii* pneumonia in the United States. Epidemiologic, diagnostic and clinical features In Robbins JB, DeVita VT Jr, Dutz W (eds): *Symposium on Pneumocystis Carinii Infection*. NCI Monograph #43. National Cancer Institute, Washington, DC, 1976, pp 55–63.

47 Wang NS, Huang SN, Thurlbeck WM: Combined *Pneumocystis carinii* and cytomegalovirus infection. *Arch Pathol Lab Med* **90**:529–535, 1970.

48. Hughes WT, Feldman S, Aur RJA, et al: Intensity of immunosuppressive therapy and the incidence of *Pneumocystis carinii* pneumonitis. *Cancer* **36**:2004–2009, 1975.

49. Hughes WT, Feldman S, Chaudhary SC, et al: Comparison of pentamidine isethionate and trimethoprim–sulfamethoxazole in the treatment of *Pneumocystis carinii* pneumonia. *J Pediatr* **92**:285–291, 1978.

50. Turbiner EH, Yeh SDJ, Rosen PP, et al: Abnormal gallium scintigraphy in *Pneumocystis carinii* pneumonia with a normal chest radiography. *Radiology* **127**:437–438, 1978

51. Levenson SM, Warren RD, Richman SD, et al. Abnormal pulmonary gallium accumulation in *P. carinii* pneumonia *Radiology* **119**:395–398, 1976.

52 Sirotzky L, Memoli V, Roberts JL, et al: Recurrent pneumocystis pneumonia with normal chest roentgenograms. *JAMA* **240**:1513–1515, 1978

53. Doppman JL, Geelhoed GW. Atypical radiographic features in *Pneumocystis carinii* pneumonia. In Robbins JB, DeVita VT Jr, Dutz W (eds): *Symposium on Pneumocystis carinii Infection*. NCI Monograph #43. National Cancer Institute, Washington, DC, 1976, pp 89–97.

54. Cross AS, Steigbigel RT: *Pneumocystis carinii* pneumonia presenting as localized nodular densities. *N Engl J Med* **291**:831–832, 1974.

55. Luddy RE, Champion LAA, Schwartz AD: *Pneumocystis carinii* pneumonia with pneumatocoele formation. *Am J Dis Child* **131**:470–471, 1977.

56 Goodell B, Jacobs JB, Powell RD, et al: *Pneumocystis carinii* The spectrum of diffuse interstitial pneumonia in pa-

tients with neoplastic disease. *Ann Intern Med* 72:337–340, 1970.

57. Rossiter SJ, Miller DC, Churg AM, et al: Open lung biopsy in the immunosuppressed patient. *J Thorac Cardiovasc Surg* 77:338–345, 1979.

58. Greenman RL, Goodall PT, King D: Lung biopsy in immunocompromised hosts. *Am J Med* 59:488–496, 1975

59. Pennington JE, Feldman NT: Pulmonary infiltrates and fever in patients with hematologic malignancy: Assessment of transbronchial biopsy. *Am J Med* 62:581–587, 1977

60. Fishman NH: Discussion. *J Thorac Cardiovasc Surg* 77:344, 1979.

61. Springmeyer SC, Silvestri RC, Sale GE, et al: Role of transbronchial biopsy for the diagnosis of diffuse pneumonia in immunocompromised marrow transplant recipients. *Am Rev Respir Dis* 126:763–765, 1982.

62. Burt ME, Flye WW, Webber BL, Wesley RA: Prospective evaluation of aspiration needle, cutting needle, transbronchial, and open lung biopsy in patients with pulmonary infiltrates. *Ann Thorac Surg* 32:146–153, 1981.

63. Bigby PD, Margolskee D, Curtis J, et al: Usefulness of induced sputum in diagnosis of pneumonia in patients with Acquired Immunodeficiency Syndrome. *Am Rev Respir Dis* 133:515–518, 1986.

64. Lau WK, Young LS, Remington JS: *Pneumocystis carinii* pneumonia. Diagnosis by examination of pulmonary secretions. *JAMA* 236:2399–2402, 1976.

65. Lorber B, Swenson RM: Bacteriology of aspiration pneumonia: A prospective study of community and hospital acquired cases. *Ann Intern Med* 81:329–331, 1974.

66. Chaudhary S, Hughes WT, Feldman S, et al: Percutaneous transthoracic needle aspiration of the lung. *Am J Dis Child* 131:902–907, 1977.

67. Stover DE, Zaman ME, Hadju SI, Lange M, et al: Bronchoalveolar lavage in the diagnosis of diffuse pulmonary infiltrates in the immunocompromised host. *Ann Intern Med* 101:1–6, 1984.

68. Lim SK, Eveland WC, Porter RJ: Direct fluorescent-antibody method for the diagnosis of *Pneumocystis carinii* pneumonitis from sputa or tracheal aspirates from humans. *Appl Microbiol* 27:144–149, 1974.

69. Kovacs JA, Gill V, Swan JC, et al: Prospective evaluations of a monoclonal antibody in diagnosis of *Pneumocystis carinii* pneumonia. *Lancet* 2:1–3, 1986.

70. Meuwissen JHET, Leeuwenberg ADEM: A microcomplement fixation test applied to infection with *Pneumocystis carinii*. *Trop Georgr Med* 24:282–291, 1972

71. Norman L, Kagan IG: Some observations on the serology of *Pneumocystis carinii* infections in the United States *Infect Immunol* 8:317–321, 1973.

72. Meyer JD, Pifer LL, Sale GE, et al: The value of *Pneumocystis carinii* antibody and antigen detection for diagnosis of *Pneumocystis carinii* pneumonia after marrow transplantation. *Am Rev Respir Dis* 120:181–182, 1979.

73. Pifer LL: Serodiagnosis of *Pneumocystis carinii*. *Chest* 87:698–700, 1985.

74. Hughes WT: Recent advances in serodiagnosis of *Pneumocystis carinii*. *Chest* 89:764–765, 1986.

75. Waalkes TP, Makulu DR: Pharmacologic aspects of pentamidine. In Robbins JB, DeVita VT Jr, Dutz W (eds). *Symposium on Pneumocystis carinii Infection*. NCI Monograph #43. National Cancer Institute, Washington, DC, 1976, pp 171–177.

76. Young RC, DeVita VT Jr: Treatment of *Pneumocystis carinii* pneumonia. In Robbins JB, DeVita VT Jr, Dutz W (Eds): *Symposium on Pneumocystis carinii Infection*. NCI Monograph #43. National Cancer Institute, Washington, DC, 1976, pp. 193–198.

77. Dutz W, Post C, Jennings-Khodadad E, et al. Therapy and prophylaxis of *Pneumocystis carinii*. In Robbins JB, Devita VT Jr, Dutz W (eds): *Symposium on Pneumocystis carinii Infection*. NCI Monograph # 43 National Cancer Institute, Washington, DC, 1976, pp. 179–185.

78. Kluge RM, Spaulding DM, Spain JA: Combination of pentamidine and trimethoprim–sulfamethoxazole in the therapy of *Pneumocystis carinii* pneumonia in rats. *Antimicrob Agents Chemother* 13:975–978, 1978.

79. Whisnant JK, Buckley RH. Successful pyrimethamine–sulfadiazine therapy of pneumocystis pneumonia in infants with X-linked immunodeficiency with hyper IgM. In Robbins JB, DeVita VT Jr, Dutz W (eds): *Symposium on Pneumocystis carinii Infection*. NCI Monograph #43. National Cancer Institute, Washington, DC, 1976, pp. 211–216.

80. Post C, Fakoughi T, Dutz W, et al: Prophylaxis of epidemic infantile pneumocystosis with a 20 : 1 sulfadoxine and pyrimethamine combination. *Curr Ther Res* 13:273–279, 1971.

81 Winston DJ, Lau WK, Gale RP, et al: Trimethoprim–sulfamethoxazole for the treatment of *Pneumocystis carinii* pneumonia *Ann Intern Med* 92:762–769, 1980

82 Young LS: Treatment of *Pneumocystis carinii* pneumonia in adults with trimethoprim/sulfamethoxazole. *Rev Infect Dis* 4:608–613, 1982.

83. Haverkos HW: PCP Therapy Project Group Assessment of therapy for *Pneumocystis carinii* pneumonia. *Am J Med* 76:501–508, 1984.

84. Kovacs JA, Hiemenz JM, Macher AM, et al: *Pneumocystis carinii* pneumonia: A comparison between patients with the acquired immunodeficiency syndrome and patients with other immunodeficiencies. *Ann Intern Med* 100:495–499, 1984.

85. Wharton JM, Coleman DL, Wofsy CB, et al: Trimethoprim–sulfamethoxazole or pentamidine for *Pneumocystis carinii* pneumonia in the acquired immunodeficiency syndrome. *Ann Intern Med* 105:37–44, 1986.

86. Bernard EM, Donnelly JH, Maher MP, et al: Use of a new bioassay to study pentamidine pharmacokinetics. *J Infect Dis* 152:750–754, 1985.

87. Leoung GS, Mills J, Hopewell PC, et al: Dapsone–Trimethoprim for *Pneumocystis carinii* in the acquired immunodeficiency syndrome. *Ann Intern Med* 105:45–48, 1986.

88. Allegra CJ, Kovacs JA, Chabner BA, et al: Potent in vivo and in vitro activity of a lipid soluble antifolate, trimetrexate against *Pneumocystis carinii* *Clin Res* 34:674A, 1986.

89 Golden JA, Sjoerdsma A, Santi DV. *Pneumocystis carinii* pneumonia treated with alpha-difluoromethylornithine. *West J Med* 141:613–623, 1984.

90. Hughes WT, Smith-McCain BL: Effects of sulfonyl urea

compounds on Pneumocystis carinii. *J Infect Dis* **153**:944–947, 1986

90a. Hughes WT, Rivera GK, Schell MJ, et al: Successful intermittent chemoprophylaxis for *Pneumocystis carinii* pneumonitis. *N Engl J Med* **316**:1627–1632, 1987.

91. Hughes WT: Limited effect of trimethoprim sulfamethoxazole prophylaxis on *Pneumocystis carinii*. *Antimicrob Agents Chemother* **16**:333–335, 1979.

92. Hughes WT, Johnson WW: Recurrent *Pneumocystis carinii* pneumonia following apparent recovery. *J Pediatr* **79**:755–759, 1971.

93. Gottlieb M, Knight S, Mitsuyasu R, et al: Prophylaxis of *Pneumocystis carinii* infection in acquired immunodeficiency syndrome (AIDS) with pyrimethamine/sulfadoxine (Fansidar). *Lancet* **2**:398–399, 1984.

94. Dammin GJ: Babesiosis. In Weinstein L, Fields BN (eds): *Seminars in Infectious Diseases.* Vol 1. Stratton International, New York, 1978, pp 169–199.

95. Healy GR: Babesia infections in man. *Hosp Prac* **13**:107–116, 1979.

96. Ruebush TK II, Spielman A: Human babesiosis in the United States. *Ann Intern Med* **88**:263, 1978.

97. Ruebush TK II, Cassaday PB, March HJ, et al: Human babesiosis on Nantucket Island: Clinical features. *Ann Intern Med* **86**:6–9, 1977

98. Ruebush TK II, Juranek DD, Chisholm ES, et al: Human babesiosis on Nantucket Island: Evidence for self-limited and subclinical infections. *N Engl J Med* **297**:825–827, 1977.

99. Entrican JH, Williams H, Cook IA, et al: Babesiosis in man: A case from Scotland. *Br Med J* **2**:474, 1979.

100. Healy GR, Walzer PD, Sulzer AJ: A case of asymptomatic babesiosis in Georgia. *Am J Trop Med Hyg* **25**:376–378, 1976.

101. Chisholm ES, Ruebush TK II, Sulzer AJ, et al. *Babesia microti* infection in man: Evaluation of an indirect immunofluorescent antibody test. *Am J Trop Med Hyg* **7**:14–19, 1978.

102. Miller LH, Neva FH, Gill F: Failure of chloroquine in human babesiosis (*Babesia microti*). *Ann Intern Med* **88**:200–202, 1978.

103. Rowin KS, Tanowitz HB, Wittner M: Therapy of experimental babesiosis. *Ann Intern Med* **97**:556–558, 1982.

104. Stevens, DP, Mahmoud AAF: Giardiasis: The rediscovery of an ancient pathogen. In Remington JS, Swartz MN (eds): *Current Clinical Topics in Infectious Disease,* McGraw-Hill, New York, 1980, pp. 195–207.

105. Brodsky RE, Spencer HC, Schultz MG: Giardiasis in American travelers in the Soviet Union. *J Infect Dis* **130**:319–323, 1974.

106. Butler T, Middleton FG, Earnest DL, et al: Chronic and recurrent diarrhea in American servicemen in Vietnam *Arch Intern Med* **132**:373–377, 1973

107. Shaw PK, Brodsky RE, Lyman DO, et al: A community-wide outbreak of giardiasis with documented transmission by municipal water. *Ann Intern Med* **87**:426–432, 1977

108. Horwitz MA, Hughes JM, Craun GF: Outbreaks of waterborne disease in the United States, 1974. *J Infect Dis* **133**:588–593, 1976.

109 Dykes AC, Juranek DD, Lorenz RA: Municipal water-borne giardiasis: An epidemiologic investigation: Beavers implied as a possible reservoir. *Ann Intern Med* **92**(part I):165–170, 1980.

110. Hermans PE, Huizenga KA, Hoffman HN, et al: Dysgammaglobulinemia associated with nodular lymphoid hyperplasia of the small intestine *Am J Med* **40**:78–89, 1966.

111. Ament ME, Ochs HD, Davis SD: Structure and function of the gastrointestinal tract in primary immunodeficiency syndrome: A study of 39 patients. *Medicine (Baltimore)* **52**:227–248, 1973.

112. Barbour AG, Nichols CR, Fukushima T: An outbreak of giardiasis in a group of campers. *Am J Trop Med* **25**:384–389, 1976.

113. Black RE, Dykes AC, Sinclair SP, et al: Giardiasis in day-care centers: Evidence of person-to-person transmission *Pediatrics* **60**:486–491, 1977.

114. Schmerin MJ, Jones TC, Klein H, et al: Giardiasis: Association with homosexuality. *Ann Intern Med* **88**:801–803, 1978.

115. Keysteon JS, Krajden S, Warren MR. Person-to-person transmission of *Giardia lamblia* in day care nurseries. *Can Med Assoc J* **119**:241–248, 1978.

116. Roberts-Thomson IC, Stevens DP, et al: Acquired resistance to infection in an animal model of giardiasis. *J Immunol* **117**:2036–2037, 1976.

117. Rendtorff RC: The experimental transmission of human intestinal protozoan parasites: *Giardia lamblia* cysts given in capsules. *Am J Hyg* **59**:209–220, 1954.

118. Saha TK, Ghosh TK: Invasion of small intestinal mucosa by *Giardia lamblia* in man. *Gastroenterology* **72**:402–405, 1977.

119. Hoskins LC, Winawer SJ, Broitman SA, et al: Clinical giardiasis and intestinal malabsorption. *Gastroenterology* **53**:265–279, 1967.

120. Morecki R, Parker JG: Ultrastructural studies of the human *Giardia lamblia* and subjacent jejunal mucosa in a subject with steatorrhea. *Gastroenterology* **52**:51–164, 1967.

121. Ament ME, Rubin CE: Relation of giardiasis to abnormal intestinal structure and function in gastrointestinal immunodeficiency syndromes. *Gastroenterology* **62**:216–226, 1972.

122. Erlandsen SL, Chase DG: Morphological alterations in the microvillous border of villous epithelial cells produced by intestinal microorganisms. *Am J Clin Nutr* **27**:1277–1286, 1974.

123. Sheehy TW, Holley HP Jr: *Giardia*-induced malabsorption in pancreatitis. *JAMA* **233**:1373–1375, 1975.

124. Tandon BN, Tandon RK, Satpathy BK, et al: Mechanism of malabsorption in giardiasis: A study of bacterial flora and bile salt deconjugation in upper jejunum. *Gut* **18**:176–181, 1977

125. Stevens DP, Frank DM, Mahmoud AAF: Thymus dependency of host resistance to *Giardia muris* infection: Studies in nude mice. *J Immunol* **120**:680–682, 1978

126. Roberts-Thomson IC, Mitchell GF: Giardiasis in mice. I. Prolonged infections in certain mouse strains and hypothymic (nude mice). *Gastroenterology* **75**:42–50, 1978

127. Stevens DP, Frank DM: Local immunity in murine giardiasis. Is milk protective at the expense of material gut? *Trans Assoc Am Physicians* **91**:268–272, 1978.

128. Zinneman HH, Kaplan AP: The association of giardiasis with reduced intestinal secretory immunoglobulin A *Am J Dig Dis* **17**:793–797, 1972.

129. Jones EG, Brown WR: Serum and intestinal fluid immunoglobulin in patients with giardiasis, *Am J Dig Dis* **19**:791–796, 1974.

130. Bezjak B: Evaluation of a new technique for sampling duodenal contents in parasitologic diagnosis. *Am J Dig Dis* **17**:848–850, 1972.

131 Roe FJ: Metronidazole: Review of uses and toxicity *J Antimicrob Chemother* **3**:205–212, 1977

132. Knight R, Wright SG: Progress report. Intestinal protozoa *Gut* **19**:940, 1978

133. Rustia M, Shubik P. Induction of lung tumors and malignant lymphomas in mice by metronidazole, *J Natl Cancer Inst* **48**:721–726, 1972.

134 Voogd CE, Van der Steel JJ, Jacobs JA: The mutagenic action of nitroimidazoles: I. Metronidazole, dimetridazole and ronidazole. *Mutation Res* **26**:483–490, 1974.

135. Beard CM, Noller KL, O'Fallon WM, et al. Lack of evidence for cancer due to use of metronidazole. *N Engl J Med* **301**:519, 1979.

136. Luft BJ, Brooks RG, Conley FK, et al: Toxoplasmic encephalitis in patients with acquired immune deficiency syndrome. *JAMA* **252**:913–917, 1984

137. Wong B, Gold JWM. Brown AE, et al: Central-nervous-system toxoplasmosis in homosexual men and parenteral drug abusers. *Ann Intern Med* **100**:36–42, 1984

138. Feldman HA. Toxoplasmosis. *N Engl J Med* **279**:1370–1375, 1431–1437, 1968

139 Remington JS: Toxoplasmosis in the adult. *Bull NY Acad Med* **50**:211–227, 1974

140. Feldman HA; Toxoplasmosis: An overview *Bull NY Acad Med* **50**:110–127, 1974.

141 Janku J: Pathogenesis and pathologic anatomy of coloboma of macula lutea in eye of normal dimensions, and in microophthalmic eye with parasites in return. *Cas Lek Clsk* **62**:1021–1027, 1923.

142 Wolf A, Cowen D, Paige B. Human toxoplasmosis. Occurrence in infants as an encephalomyelitis. Verification by transmission to animals. *Science* **89**:226–227, 1939.

143. Sabin AV, Ruchman I: Characteristics of toxoplasma neutralizing antibody. *Proc Soc Exp Biol Med* **51**:1–6, 1942.

144. Sabin A, Feldman HA: Dyes as microchemical indicators of a new immunity phenomenon affecting a protozoan parasite (Toxoplasma). *Science* **108**:660–663, 1978

145. Siim JC. Acquired toxoplasmosis. Report of seven cases with strongly positive serologic reactions. *JAMA* **147**:1651–1645, 1951

146. Gard S, Magnusson JH: Glandular form of toxoplasmosis in connection with pregnancy *Acta Med Scand* **141**:59–64, 1951

147. World Health Organization: *Toxoplasmosis*. Technical Report Series 431. The World Health Organization, Geneva, 1969.

148. Anderson SE Jr, Remington JS: Toxoplasmosis. In Hoeprich

PD (ed): *Infectious Diseases*. Harper & Row, Hagerstown, Maryland, 1977, pp. 967–976.

149 McLeod R, Remington JS. Influence of infection with toxoplasma on macrophage function, and role of macrophages in resistance to toxoplasma *Am J Trop Med Hyg* **26**:170–186, 1977.

150. Lindberg RE, Frenkel JK: Toxoplasmosis in nude mice. *J Parasitol* **63**:210–221, 1977.

151. Frenkel JK. Effects of cortisone, total body radiation and nitrogen mustard on chronic latent toxoplasmosis *Am J Pathol* **33**:618–619, 1957.

152. Strannegard O, Lycke E. Effect of antithymocyte serum on experimental toxoplasmosis in mice. *Infect Immun* **5**:769–774, 1972.

153. Remington JS, Krahenbuhl JL, Mendenhall JW: A role for activated macrophages in resistance to infection with toxoplasma. *Infect Immun* **6**:829–834, 1972.

154. Jones TC, Len L, Hirsch J: Assessment in vitro of immunity against toxoplasma gondii. *J Exp Med* **171**:466–482, 1975.

155. Anderson SE Jr, Remington JS: Effect of normal and activated human macrophages on *Toxoplasma gondii*. *J Exp Med* **139**:1154–1174, 1974.

156. Murray HW, Gellene RA, Libby DM Activation of tissue macrophages from AIDS patients: In vitro response of AIDS alveolar macrophages to lymphokines and interferon-gamma. *J Immunol* **135**:2374–2377, 1985

157. Nathan CF, Pendergast, Weiber ME, et al: Activation of human macrophages Comparison of other cytokines with gamma interferon macrophages. *J Exp Med* **160**:600–609, 1984

158 Catteral JR, Sharma SD, Remington JS. Oxygen independent killing by alveolar macrophages. *J Exp Med* **163**:1113–1120, 1986.

159 Swartzberg JE, Krahenbuhl, JL, Remington JS: Dichotomy between macrophage activation and degree of protection against *Listeria monocytogenes* and *Toxoplasma gondii* in mice stimulated with *Corynebacterium parvum*. *Infect Immun* **12**:1037–1043, 1975.

160 Leak D, Meghji M. Toxoplasmic infection in cardiac disease *Am J Cardiol* **43**:841–849, 1979

161 Dorfman R, Remington J: Value of lymph-node biopsy in the diagnosis of acute acquired toxoplasmosis *N Engl J Med* **289**:878–881, 1973.

162 Ruskin J, Remington JS: Toxoplasmosis in the compromised host. *Ann Intern Med* **84**:193–199, 1976

163 Ryning FW, McLeod R, Maddox JC, et al. Probable transmission of *Toxoplasma gondii* by organ transplantation *Ann Intern Med* **90**:47–49, 1979

164 Ghatak NR, Sawyer DR A morphologic study of opportunistic cerebral toxoplasmosis *Acta Neuropathol* **42**:217–221, 1978

165 Powell HC, Gibbs CJ Jr, Lorenzo AM, et al. Toxoplasmosis of the central nervous system in the adult. Electron microscopic observations *Acta Neuropathol* **41**:211–216, 1978

166 McLeod R, Berry PF, Marshall WH, et al: Toxoplasmosis presenting as brain abscess *Am J Med* **67**:711–714, 1979.

167. Frenkel JK, Amare M, Larsen W. Immune competence in a patient with Hodgkin's disease and relapsing toxoplasmosis *Infection* **6**:84–91, 1978

168 Slavick HE, Lipman IJ: Brain stem toxoplasmosis complicating Hodgkin's diesease. *Arch Neurol* **34:**636–637, 1977.

169 Whiteside JD, Begent RHJ: Toxoplasma encephalitis complicating Hodgkin's disease. *J Clin Pathol* **28:**443–445, 1975.

170. Nicholdon DH, Wolchok EB. Ocular toxoplasmosis in an adult receiving long-term corticosteroid therapy. *Arch Ophthalmol* **94:**248–257, 1976.

171. Kersting F, Newmann J: "Malignant Lymphoma" of the brain following renal transplantation. *Acta Neuropathol* **6**(suppl VI)**:**131–133, 1975.

172. Herb HM, Jontofsoh R, Loffler HD, et al: Toxoplasmosis after renal transplantation *Clin Nephrol* **8:**529–532, 1978

173. Schulkof LA, Russell JR: Intracerebral toxoplasmosis presenting as a mass lesion *Surg Neurol* **4:**9–11, 1975.

174. Barlotta FM, Odhoa M Jr, Neu HC, et al: Toxoplasmosis, lymphoma or both? *Ann Intern Med* **70:**517–528, 1979

175. Menges HW, Fischer E, Valavanis A, et al: Cerebral toxoplasmosis in the adult. *J Comput Assist Tomogr* **3:**413–416, 1979.

176. Shepp DH, Hackman RC, Conley FK, et al: *Toxoplasma gondii* reactivation identified by detection of parasitemia in tissue culture. *Ann Intern Med* **103:**218–221, 1985.

177. Jehn V, Fink M, Gundlach P: Lethal cardiac and cerebral toxoplasmosis in a patient with acute myeloid leukemia after successful allogenic bone marrow transplantation. *Transplantation* **38:**430–433, 1984.

178 Hirsch R, Burke BA, Kersey JH: Toxoplasmosis in bone marrow transplant recipients. *J Pediatr* **105:**426–428, 1984

179. Siegel S, Lunde M, Gelderman A, et al: Transmission of toxoplasmosis by leukocyte transfusion *Blood* **37:**388–394, 1971.

180 Raisanen S: Toxoplasmosis transmitted by blood transfusions. *Transfusion* **18:**329–332, 1978.

181 Rose AG, Uys CJ, Novitsky D, et al: Toxoplasmosis of donor and recipient hearts after heterotopic cardiac transplantations. *Arch Pathol Lab Med* **107:**368–373, 1983

182 Snider WD, Simpson DM, Nielsen S, et al. Neurological complications of acquired immunodeficiency syndrome. Analysis of 50 patients. *Ann Neurol* **14:**403–418, 1983.

183 Moskowitz LB, Kory P, Chan JC. et al: Unusual causes of death in Haitians residing in Miami High prevalence of opportunistic infections *JAMA* **250:**1187–1191, 1983.

184 Hofflin JM, Remington JS. Tissue culture isolation of toxoplasma from blood of a patient with AIDS. *Arch Intern Med* **145:**925–926, 1985.

185. Luft BJ, Remington JS. Toxoplasmosis of the central nervous system. In Remington JS, Swartz M (eds). *Current Clinical Topics in Infectious Disease.* Vol 5 McGraw-Hill, New York, 1985, pp. 315–358

186. McCabe RE, Gibbons D, Brooks RG, et al: Agglutination test for diagnosis of toxoplasmosis in AIDS *Lancet* **2:**680, 1983

187 Cooney MK, Kimball AC, Bauer H Studies on toxoplasmosis I. Complement fixation tests with peritoneal exudate antigen. *J Immunol* **81:**177–186, 1958

188. Walls KW, Bullock SL, English DK: Use of the enzyme-linked immunosorbent assay (ELISA) and its microadapta-

tion for the serodiagnosis of toxoplasmosis, *J Clin Microbiol* **5:**273–277, 1977.

189. Siegel JP, Remington JS: Comparison of methods for quantitating antigen specific immunoglobulin M antibody with a reverse enzyme linked immunoabsorbent assay. *J Clin Microbiol* **18:**63–70, 1983

190. Wielaard F, van Gruighuigsen H, Duermeyer W, et al: Diagnosis of acute toxoplasmosis by an enzyme immunoassay for specific immunoglobulin M antibodies *J Clin Microbiol* **17:**981–987, 1983.

191. Gordon MA, Duncan RA, Kingsley LC. Automated immunofluorescence test for toxoplasmosis *J Clin Microb* **13:**283–285, 1981.

192. Jacobs L, Lunde MN: A hemagglutination test for toxoplasmosis. *J Parasitol* **43:**308–314, 1957

193. Remington JS, Miller MJ, Brownlee I: IgM antibodies in acute toxoplasmosis. II. Prevalence and significance in acquired cases. *J Lab Clin Med* **71:**855–866, 1968.

194. Welch PC, Masur H, Jones TC, et al: Serologic diagnosis of acute lymphadenopathic toxoplasmosis. *J Infect Dis* **142:**256–264, 1980.

195. Hakes TB, Armstrong D: Toxoplasmosis. Problems in diagnosis and treatment. *Cancer* **52:**1535–1540, 1983.

196. Araujo FG, Remington JS: Antigenemia in recently acquired acute toxoplasmosis. *J Infect Dis* **141:**144–150, 1980.

197. Brooks RG, Sharma SD, Remington JS: Detection of *Toxoplasma gondii* antigens by a dot-immunobinding technique. *J Clin Microbiol* **21:**113–116, 1985

198. Rollins DF, Tabbara KF, O'Conner GR, et al. Detection of toxoplasma antigen and antibody in ocular fluids in experimental ocular toxoplasmosis *Arch Ophthalmol* **101:**455–457, 1983.

199. Wilson CB, Desmonts G, Couvreur J, et al Lymphocyte transformation in the diagnosis of congenital toxoplasma infection. *N Engl J Med* **302:**785–788, 1980.

200. Desmonts G. Definitive serologic diagnosis of ocular toxoplasmosis *Arch Ophthalmol* **76:**839–851, 1966

201. Grossman P, Remington J: The effect of trimethoprim and sulfamethoxazole on toxoplasma gondii in vitro and in vivo *Am J Trop Med Hyg* **28:**445–455, 1979.

202. O'Connor GR, Frenkel JK. Dangers of steroid treatment in toxoplasmosis. *Arch Ophthalmol* **94:**213, 1976

203. Ma P, Soave R: Three-step stool examination for cryptosporidiosis in 10 homosexual men and protracted watery diarrhea. *J Infect Dis* **147:**824–828, 1983.

204. Meisel JL, Perera DR, MeLigro C, et al. Overwhelming watery diarrhea associated with a cryptosporidium in an immunosuppressed patient *Gastroenterology* **70:**1156–1160, 1976

205. Weinstein L, Edelstein SM, Madara J, et al. Intestinal cryptosporidiosis complicated by disseminated cytomegalovirus infection. *J Am Gastroenterol Assoc* **81:**584–591, 1981

206 Tzipori S: Cryptosporidiosis in animals and humans. *Microbiol Rev* **47:**84–96, 1983.

207. Weisburger WR, Hutcheon DF, Yardley JH, et al: Cryptosporidiosis in an immunosuppressed renal-transplant recipient with IgA deficiency *Am J Clin Pathol* **72:**473–478, 1979.

208. Wolfsor JS, Richter JM, Waldron MA, et al. Cryp-

tosporidiosis in immunocompetent patients. *N Engl J Med* **213**:1278–1282, 1985

209. DuPont HL: Cryptosporidiosis and the healthy host. *N Engl J Med* **312**:1319–1320, 1985.

210. Bogaerts J, Lepage P, Rouvroy D, et al: Cryptosporisium spp., a frequent cause of diarrhea in central Africa. *J Clin Microb* **20**:874–876, 1984.

211. Soave R, Ma P: Cryptosporidiosis—Traveler's diarrhea in two families. *Arch Intern Med* **145**:70–72, 1985.

212. Current WL, Reese NC. Ernst JV, et al: Human cryptosporidiosis in immunocompetent and immunodeficient persons: Studies of an outbreak and experimental transmission. *N Engl J Med* **308**:1252–1257, 1983.

213. Ma P, Villanueva TG, Kaufman D, et al: Respiratory cryptosporidiosis in the acquired immune deficiency syndrome: Use of modified cold Kinyoun and Hemacolor stains for rapid diagnoses. *JAMA* **252**:1298–1301, 1984.

214. Portnoy D, Whiteside ME, Buckely III E, et al: Treatment of intestinal cryptosporidiosis with spiramycin *Ann Intern Med* **101**:202–204, 1984.

215. DeHovitz JA, Pape, JW, Boncy M, et al. Clinical manifestations and therapy of *Isospora belli* infection in patients with the acquired immunodeficiency syndrome. *N Engl J Med* **315**:87–90, 1986

216. Scowden EB, Schaffner W, Stone WJ: Overwhelming strongyloidiasis: An unappreciated opportunistic infection. *Medicine (Baltimore)* **57**:527–544, 1978.

217. Rassiga AL, Lawry JL, Forman WB: Diffuse pulmonary infection due to strongyloides stercoalis. *JAMA* **230**:426–430, 1974.

218. Scoggin CH, Call NB: Acute respiratory failure due to disseminated strongyloidiasis in a renal transplant recipient. *Ann Intern Med* **87**:456–458, 1977.

219. Kuberski TT, Gabor EP, Boudreaux D: Disseminated strongyloidiasis—A complication of the immunosuppressed host. *West J Med* **122**:504–508, 1975.

220. Rivera E, Maldonado N, Velez-Garcia E, et al: Hyperinfection with strongyloides stercoralis. *Ann Intern Med* **72**:199–204, 1970.

11

Legionellosis in the Compromised Host

NEIL M. AMPEL and EDWARD J. WING

1. Introduction

Legionella pneumophila was first described in early 1977 by McDade et al.[1] They recognized that this organism was the causative agent for the outbreak of acute pneumonia that occurred during the state American Legion convention in Philadelphia that previous summer. Further epidemiologic investigation led to the discovery that these organisms were also responsible for earlier outbreaks of acute disease for which no cause could be found.[2,3] Since these initial studies, much has been learned about *Legionellae* and the diseases caused by them, but our knowledge remains incomplete. Currently, at least seven species are definitely associated with human illness (Table 1),[1,4-9] but the number of recognized species is continuing to expand.[10]

As our knowledge has increased, it has become clear that compromised hosts, especially patients on cytotoxic drugs and corticosteroids, are at increased risk for acquiring *Legionella* pneumonia.[11-14] Indeed, the overwhelming majority of all cases of infection due to *L. micdadei* occur in hospitalized patients receiving immunosuppressive therapy.[15-18] In addition, *Legionella* species may be responsible for a significant proportion of nosocomial-acquired pneumonia.[19-22]

NEIL M. AMPEL • Department of Medicine, Section of Infectious Diseases, Veterans Administration Medical Center, Arizona Health Sciences Center, Tuscon, Arizona 85724. EDWARD J. WING • Department of Medicine, Division of Infectious Diseases, Montefiore Hospital, University of Pittsburgh School of Medicine, Pittsburgh, Pennsylvania 15213.

Despite the recognition of newer species, *L. pneumophila* still accounts for more then 80% of all infections[23] (Table 1) and remains the most thoroughly studied organism. *L. micdadei* is responsible for about 6% of all cases[23] but has a special predilection for the compromised host. Although much less is known about the other species, in general they cause disease similar to that due to *L. pneumophila*.[5-8,24] This discussion is therefore limited for the most part to *L. pneumophila* and *L. micdadei*.

Epidemiologic studies have indicated that infection due to *Legionellae* occurs in two distinct patterns. The first is an acute pneumonia that affects a small percentage of those exposed, has an incubation period of 2-10 days, and has a case-fatality rate of 20%. The second pattern, called Pontiac fever, is a benign, self-limited flulike illness with an incubation period of 1-2 days and affects up to 95% of those exposed.[25] For reasons that remain unclear, both patterns can be produced by the same organism.[26] To date, Pontiac fever has not been a major cause of illness among compromised patients and is not discussed further in this chapter. In the following sections, the term legionellosis refers generally to any infection caused by *Legionella* species and, in particular, to the acute pneumonia caused by these organisms.

2. Microbiology

2.1. Classification

The *Legionellae* are formally classified according to the Centers for Disease Control (CDC) as be-

TABLE 1. Recognized species of *Legionella*[a,b]

Species and serogroup	Percent of total causing clinical illness
L. pneumophila, serogroups 1–9[c]	85
L. micdadei[c]	6
L. bozemanii, serogroups 1–2[c]	3
L. dumoffii[c]	1
L. longbeachae, serogroups 1–2[c]	<1
L. wadsworthii[c]	<1
L. feeleii[d]	<1
L. jordanis[e]	—
L. gormanii	—
L. oakridgensis	—
L. sainthelensis	—

[a]Data from refs 1, 4, 5–9, 23
[b]As of January of 1985
[c]Associated with clinical pneumonia
[d]Associated with Pontiac fever only
[e]Serologically associated with human disease

longing to the family Legionellaceae and to the single genus *Legionella*. As of January 1985, there were 11 recognized species (Table 1), but work in progress indicates the existence of at least 10 more.[10,27]

At the genus level, *Legionellae* are gram-negative aerobic bacilli distinguished by their ability to grow on buffered charcoal–yeast extract agar containing iron and cysteine but not on media deficient in these substances. Identification can be confirmed by finding a high percentage of cellular branched-chain fatty acids using gas–liquid chromatography (GLC).[27–29]

Although new *Legionella* species may be tentatively identified by their phenotypic and biochemical characteristics and by their inability to react with currently available antisera, definitive speciation depends on DNA homology studies. In general, the DNA relatedness between strains within the same species is 70% or more.[27,30] Strains closely related by DNA hybridization to a previously recognized species but that fail to react to antisera against that species are considered new serogroups. Currently, there are at least nine recognized serogroups of *L. pneumophila*[31] and two serogroups each for *L. bozemanii*[32] and *L. longbeachae*.[33] Other species have only one recognized serogroup. New strains not closely related to previously known species by DNA hybridization and not reactive to antisera represent new species.[27]

2.2. Morphology

L. pneumophila is a rod about 2.0 μm in length with tapering ends and the ultrastructural characteristics of a gram-negative bacillus, including triple-layered inner and outer membranes and a dense polysaccharide capsule.[34,35] Other species have a similar morphologic appearance, although *L. micdadei* differs by having an additional layer of material adjacent to the outer membrane.[35,36] A single polar flagellum has been identified on all species except *L. oakridgensis*.[9,37,38]

Legionellae eluded initial identification because of their inability to stain by common methods. They are not distinguishable after staining by the Giemsa, acid-fast, and hemotoxylin–eosin methods.[39] Despite their ultrastructural resemblance to gram-negative rods, *Legionellae* in clinical specimens have only rarely been distinguishable after Gram staining,[39–41] although they will stain when grown on artificial media. *L. micdadei* is unique among the *Legionellae* in that it is weakly acid fast and can be readily seen in clinical specimens by using a modified acid-fast stain.[15,16] This property is lost after culture on artificial media.[42] *Legionellae* can be seen in formalin-fixed paraffinized tissue using Dieterle silver-impregnation stain. For samples not embedded in paraffin, the Gimenez stain is useful.[39] As fully discussed in Section 6.3, organisms may be easily identified in clinical specimens using direct fluorescent-antibody staining techniques.

2.3. Cultural and Biochemical Characteristics

Early attempts at in vitro cultivation of *Legionellae* led to the discovery of important cultural characteristics. *Legionellae* were found to be obligate aerobes that demonstrated enhanced growth in an atmosphere containing 5% CO_2. Optimal growth occurred when a source of amino acids, iron, and L-cysteine was present at a pH level of 6.9–7.0 and a temperature of 37°C.[40] Growth could be enhanced if the medium contained charcoal, possibly because charcoal absorbs toxic oxygen products produced by the yeast extract.[43] Currently, the most widely used culture medium is a buffered charcoal–yeast extract agar supplemented with α-ketoglutarate.[44,45]

Growth of *Legionella* species on artificial media is slow, usually requiring at least 3 days of incubation before colonies are visible. Colonies are small, gray, and glistening. When observed under a microscope, they have a characteristic ground-glass appearance.[40] Most species of *Legionella*, when cultured on media containing L-tyrosine or L-phenylalanine, produce a soluble brown pigment[7,38,46-48] due to the conversion of these substances to melanin. Under long-wave ultraviolet (UV) light, most species also manifest a dull yellow fluorescence,[8,9,49,50] but certain species are able to fluoresce a blue-white color.[49]

Legionellae are unable to reduce nitrates, to split urea, or to ferment carbohydrates.[40] However, all 11 species produce catalase,[9,35,42,47] and all but *L. feeleii* produce gelatinase.[9,35] *L. pneumophila, L. jordanis, L. longbeachae,* and *L. micdadei* are oxidase positive,[7,9,35,42,47] while all species except *L. micdadei*[42,47] and *L. feeleii*[9] produce β-lactamase. A potentially useful test that differentiates *L. pneumophila* from other species is its ability to hydrolyze hippurate.[51] However, *L. feeleii* also has a weak activity in this regard.[9] A unique property of *Legionellae* is that 80% or more of their cellular fatty acids are branched-chain moieties containing 14–17 carbon atoms (C_{14}–C_{17}).[28] Among species, differences exist in the composition of these fatty acids. In addition, *Legionella* species contain unusual ubiquinones, which also vary according to species.[52] In the future, the combination of cellular fatty acid analysis and tests for ubiquinones may allow for rapid chemical differentiation of *Legionella* species in the clinical laboratory.[52]

3. Pathology, Pathogenesis, and Immunology

3.1. Pathology and Pathogenesis

Pathologically, *L. pneumophila* pneumonia is most commonly a bronchopneumonia. Less frequently, a lobar pattern with red and gray hepatization suggestive of pneumococcal pneumonia is demonstrated. Occasionally, a distinctly nodular, well-demarcated peripheral lesion is found; rarely, frank abscesses are seen. There is no apparent predilection for any particular lobe or segment and bilateral disease is frequent. In most autopsy cases, a small pleural effusion is present.[24,53]

Microscopically, there is an intraalveolar inflammatory exudate containing a mixture of polymorphonuclear leukocytes, macrophages, red blood cells (RBCs), fibrin, and proteinaceous material.[24,53] A particular finding of *Legionella* pneumonia is the presence of degenerating inflammatory cells within the exudate, called leukocytoclasis by Winn and Myerowitz.[24] Organisms appear to abound within the exudate both extracellularly and within phagocytic cells but are especially evident within alveolar macrophages.[53-55]

Pneumonia due to other *Legionella* species is similar to that of *L. pneumophila,* although nodular lesions and small abscesses are more commonly observed with *L. micdadei* infection.[24] Pathologic manifestations of *Legionella* pneumonia do not appear to differ between normal and immunocompromised hosts.[53]

Once *Legionellae* gain access to the respiratory tract, their primary site of infection appears to be the terminal alveolus. From there, secondary spread to the larger airways and to the interstitium and lymphatics occurs.[56] Organisms have been found to spread to hilar and mediastinal lymph nodes as well as to the liver, spleen, and kidneys.[57-59] Bacteremia has been documented on several occasions,[60-62] and extrapulmonary infection, although rare, is becoming increasingly recognized[63-69] (see Section 5.5). In most cases, extrapulmonary legionellosis appears to be a consequence of bacteremic spread from a primary pulmonary nidus.

Despite the frequency of nonpulmonary symptoms during *Legionella* pneumonia, pathologic findings outside the lungs are few. For example, although symptoms of central nervous system (CNS) dysfunction occur commonly in patients with *L. pneumophila* pneumonia, specific pathologic abnormalities have not been found.[70,71] Similarly, a variety of hematologic,[72-75] renal,[76-78] and musculoskeletal[78,79] abnormalities have been reported without any evidence of direct bacterial invasion of the involved organs. This has led to the conclusion that toxins may play an important role in the pathogenesis of legionellosis. *L. pneumophila* has been found to produce an endotoxinlike substance[80,81] as well as a variety of extracellular products,[82-84] some of which appear to inhibit the function of phagocytic cells.[85,86]

Animal studies have increased our understanding of the pathogenesis of acute *Legionella* pneumonia. Guinea pigs exposed to aerosols of *L. pneumophila* develop pneumonia that pathologically resembles the human disease.[87] Using this model, Davis et al.[88] were able to follow the intrapulmonary inflammatory events of *Legionella* pneumonia over time. Bacteria grew exponentially in the lung during the first 24 hr, during which time viable bacteria were found in close association with resident alveolar macrophages. Subsequently, the number of organisms reached a plateau and, in animals that survived, began to decrease 6 days after aerosol exposure. The plateau and decrease in the number of intrapulmonary bacteria occurred in parallel with an influx of polymorphonuclear leukocytes and macrophages and with the development of specific antibody. These investigators believed that initial exponential growth of *L. pneumophila* occurred within the resident alveolar macrophage, a notion supported by other observers.[89]

3.2. Immunology

Clinical studies indicate that immunocompromised patients, particularly those with defects in cellular immunity, appear to be at increased risk for legionellosis. Renal transplant recipients[4,12] and patients receiving corticosteroids[11,14,90–92] are especially susceptible. In our experience during an outbreak of nosocomial pneumonia due to *L. micdadei,* 88% of the those involved were receiving corticosteroids and 65% were receiving both corticosteroids and cytotoxic drugs.[18] Animal studies have supported this impression. Widen et al.[93] showed that the lethal infectious dose of *L. pneumophila* given to mice, animals usually highly resistant to infection by this organism, is reduced by 2 log after treatment with cyclophosphamide.[93] Myerowitz et al.[94] were able to protect nonimmune guinea pigs from *L. micdadei* pneumonia by adoptively transferring spleen cells from immune animals. These observations suggest that cell-mediated immunity is important in the defense against *Legionellae.*

In vitro studies by Horwitz and Silverstein and their co-workers have demonstrated that *L. pneumophila* is a facultative intracellular parasite with the ability to replicate exponentially within human monocytes[95] and human alveolar macrophages.[96] The organism is resistant to the bactericidal effects of serum containing high titers of specific antibody,[97] and antibody in the presence of complement increases the uptake of the organism by monocytes without inhibiting their intracellular multiplication.[98] Polymorphonuclear leukocytes ingest *L. pneumophila* only in the presence of both antibody and complement but kill very few bacteria.[97] Horwitz and Silverstein have presented in vitro evidence that cell-mediated immunity may be active in the defense against *L. pneumophila* infection. Human monocytes, exposed to supernatants either from mitogen-stimulated lymphocytes[99] or from antigen-stimulated lymphocytes obtained from immune patients,[100] were able to inhibit the intracellular growth of the organism markedly. *L. micdadei* also grows exponentially in monocytes[101] and alveolar macrophages.[102] Polymorphonuclear leukocytes will ingest *L. micdadei* in the presence of complement alone, but no intracellular killing occurs.[103]

The mechanism by which *Legionellae* are able to evade intracellular killing by phagocytic cells is unknown. Horowitz[104] showed that live *L. pneumophila* appears to inhibit phagosome–lysosome fusion; in this way, it may avoid the toxic intracellular milieu caused by the release of lysosomal enzymes. Although *L. pneumophila* is sensitive to the oxygen-dependent microbicidal substances generated after phagocytosis, including hydrogen peroxide and the products of myeloperoxidase,[105,106] it appears to release a low-molecular-weight peptide toxin capable of blocking the generation of these toxic oxygen metabolites[85] by selectively inhibiting the phagocyte superoxide-generating complex.[107]

The role of humoral immunity in the protection against legionellosis is unclear. Freidman et al.[108] demonstrated that the in vitro lymphocyte blastogenic response to *L. pneumophila* antigen is caused predominantly by B cells; Rolstad and Berdal[109] were able to protect rats from infection by administering syngeneic immune serum. On the other hand, a killed vaccine did not protect guinea pigs from aerosolized *L. pneumophila* infection despite the development of high titers of specific serum antibody,[110] and passive transfer of antisera from immune guinea pigs failed to protect nonimmune animals from challenge with *L. micdadei.*[94]

4. Epidemiology

4.1. General Considerations

Infection due to *Legionella* species has been reported from most areas of the continental United States and has worldwide distribution. Sporadic illness tends to be more common during the summer months.[13] Overall, *L. pneumophila* accounts for 80–85% of all *Legionella* infections; another 6% are due to *L. micdadei,* and the remainder are caused by other species.[23] The precise incidence of disease is unknown, but several studies have suggested that the incidence of community-acquired *Legionella* pneumonia requiring hospitalization is 6–15%.[21,111,112] Outbreaks of nosocomial infection due to *L. pneumophila* have occurred in numerous hospitals throughout the United States,[19,20,113,114] and most cases of pneumonia due to *L. micdadei* have occurred in hospitalized patients.[15–18]

Legionellosis is an illness with a predilection for the compromised host. England et al.[13] reviewed the first 1005 cases of sporadic legionellosis reported to the CDC and found that a variety of underlying diseases, including renal dialysis or transplantation, chronic lung disease, diabetes mellitus, cancer, immunosuppressive therapy, and smoking, appeared to increase the risk of acquiring the disease. In the outbreak at the Wadsworth Veterans Administration Medical Center, 20 of the first 49 cases were in patients with underlying diseases and 18 were receiving either corticosteroids or cytotoxic drugs.[12] In our experience, during an outbreak of nosocomial pneumonia due to *L. micdadei,* 26 of 27 patients had an underlying disease, including chronic renal failure, collagen vascular disease, carcinoma, and hematologic malignancy.[18] Renal transplant recipients appear to be at particular risk for legionellosis,[1,13,14,115,116] but patients undergoing bone marrow transplantation[117] and cardiac transplantation[118] have also been reported. Although children generally have a low incidence of symptomatic pneumonia due to *Legionellae,*[13,119] infection has occurred in those with cancer undergoing chemotherapy.[120,121] Treatment with corticosteroids is a particular risk factor for the nosocomial acquisition of infection with either *L. pneumophila*[11,14,91,92] or *L. micdadei.*[15–18] Currently, only a small number of

AIDS patients with infection due to *Legionellae* have been reported.[68,122]

4.2. Ecology

Legionella species are widely distributed within environmental waters. Fliermans et al.[123] sampled the water from 67 lakes and rivers in the Southern and Eastern United States and found *Legionellae* in virtually all samples. The densities were low, representing fewer than 1% of the total bacterial population. Organisms were isolated from aquatic habitats with a wide range of physiochemical parameters, including temperatures of 5.7°–63°C. However, there was seasonal variation, with more organisms being isolated during the summer months, when water temperatures were warmer. Environmental sampling during an outbreak of legionellosis at the Memorial Union at Indiana University disclosed the presence of *Legionellae* in the Union cooling tower water, as well as from the waters and banks of a nearby river.[124] The ubiquity of these fastidious organisms within environmental waters has been speculated to be due to their ability to proliferate in and around free-living aquatic organisms. Blue-green algae are able to provide extracellular factors that promote the growth of *L. pneumophila,*[125] and *Legionellae* have been shown to grow within a variety of protozoans, including *Naegleria,*[126] *Acanthamoeba,*[126,127] and *Tetrahymena.*[128]

4.3. Nosocomial Legionellosis

Nosocomial outbreaks of legionellosis have been linked to two sites of environmental contamination. Most cases have been associated with contamination of the potable water supply of the hospital, but at least one outbreak has been related to the growth of *Legionellae* within cooling tower water.

Nosocomial disease associated with contaminated potable water was first identified by Tobin et al.[115] in 1980, when they isolated similar strains of *L. pneumophila* from two renal transplant recipients with pneumonia and from the shower water from the postoperative cubicle that housed both patients. The following year, Cordes et al.[116] identified *L. pneumophila* in shower water specimens from three hospitals with outbreaks of nosocomial infection. Yu et al.[111] found *L. pneumophila* to be ubiquitous within their water system just prior to a major outbreak of nosocomial disease. When these workers eradicated the organism from the water supply, the number of nosocomial cases dropped.[129] Other nosocomial outbreaks due to *L. pneumophila* have also appeared to end after eradication of the organism from the potable water supply.[114,130,131]

It is likely that *L. pneumophila*, present in low numbers in the main water supply, proliferates within the sediment at the bottom of large hot-water tanks, where the temperature is often cool enough to allow for growth of the organism.[132] From there, it is dispersed throughout the water system, secondarily contaminating plumbing fixtures and pipes.[111,132] There is also evidence that *L. pneumophila* is able to grow on certain types of water fittings, leading to secondary proliferation after leaving the hot-water tank.[133] The mere presence of organisms within the potable water supply of a hospital does not mean that there are necessarily nosocomial cases of legionellosis. *Legionellae* have been isolated from the water system of a number of hotels and hospitals in which there was no known association with disease.[134,135]

The association of potable water and nosocomial infection due to *L. micdadei* is less clear. Although *L. micdadei* can be isolated from the same sites within the water system as *L. pneumophila*, it is found in much lower numbers.[136] *L. micdadei* has been isolated from the couplant water of an ultrasonic nebulizer, but no cases of pneumonia were associated with the use of this device.[137] During the evaluation of the first 26 cases of nosocomial pneumonia due to *L. micdadei* in our hospital, environmental sampling of the potable water supply initially demonstrated large numbers of *L. pneumophila* but only rare *L. micdadei*. Furthermore, when organisms were markedly reduced in the plumbing system through heating and flushing, complete eradication of cases did not occur.[138]

A second mechanism associated with nosocomial outbreaks of legionellosis is airborne spread of organisms from contaminated cooling towers. Dondera et al.[113] described an outbreak within and around a Memphis hospital of 44 cases of pneumonia due to *L. pneumophila* associated with the use of an auxiliary cooling tower subsequently found to be colonized by *L. pneumophila*. Those at highest risk for acquiring the illness were in rooms in which ven-

tilation intake was in the direct path of the drift from the tower.

5. Clinical Manifestations

5.1. Symptoms

Although the symptoms seen in patients with pneumonia due to *L. pneumophila* vary widely, several features occur in most patients that may suggest the diagnosis (Table 2).[19,139–142] The onset of illness is often influenzalike, with malaise, myalgias, and a general toxic state. Virtually all patients present with fever, which increases with time and is associated with recurrent chills and even frank rigors. A dry cough occurs early in most patients and subsequently becomes productive of nonpurulent or minimally purulent sputum in more than one-half of cases. The same number will develop pleuritic chest pain during the course of their illness. Almost one-half of these patients have diarrhea, which is characteristically watery and not associated with abdominal pain. Headache is an early feature of illness and may be severe. Studies that have compared the symptoms of patients with confirmed *L. pneumophila* pneumonia

TABLE 2. Common Symptoms and Signs of Pneumonia Due to *L. pneumophila* and *L. micdadei*[a]

	Percentage of total	
	L. pneumophila	*L. micdadei*
Symptoms		
Fever	99	100
Cough	89	78
Chills	78	—
Headache	50	—
Dyspnea	48	74
Diarrhea	45	—
Chest pain	45	56
Signs		
Temperature		
>39.4°C	79 (65)	50 (27)
>38.2°C	71	—
Neurologic abnormalities	37	67 (27)
Rales	80 (123)	89 (27)

[a]Based on 231 patients[19,139,140,142] for *L. pneumophila* and on 44 patients[17,18] for *L. micdadei* (except where indicated by numbers in parentheses)

with those with pneumonia due to other causes have found that patients with legionellosis present significantly more often with headache and diarrhea and usually lack a preceding history of an upper respiratory tract infection.[140,141]

5.2. Signs

Upon examination (Table 2), the patient with *L. pneumophila* pneumonia appears acutely ill and toxic, with fever, tachypnea, and diaphoresis. The fevers are high, almost always > 38.9°C, and nonremitting. Relative bradycardia, with a heart rate below 100 beats/min in the face of a temperature of > 39.4°C, has been considered a suggestive sign of *L. pneumophila* infection.[19] A variety of neurologic abnormalities have been described, but changes in mental status, including confusion, disorientation, and lethargy, are the most frequent and have been reported to occur in more than one-third of patients (see Section 5.51).[70,71,139,143] Localized moist rales are the most common pulmonary finding followed by signs of consolidation and, less commonly, by a pleural friction rub or by signs of a plueral effusion.[139,143] Occasionally, diffuse abdominal tenderness is elicited, but specific findings, particularly enlargement or tenderness of the liver or spleen, are distinctly uncommon.[139] The rest of the physical examination is usually within normal limits.

In our experience with 27 patients, 26 of whom were immunocompromised, with nosocomial acquired pneumonia due to *L. micdadei*, there was a characteristic presentation (Table 2).[18] Patients developed an abrupt fever, a dry cough, and dyspnea without any prodrome. More than 50% complained of pleuritic chest pain. On physical examination, high-spiking temperatures were common and one-half of the patients had temperature elevations of > 39.4°C. In addition, more than 60% exhibited changes in mental status, including lethargy, confusion, agitation, and stupor. Tachycardia was common and appropriate to the elevation in temperature. Otherwise, findings were limited to the chest and included localized rales and, later in the course, signs of consolidation. As compared with patients with nosocomial pneumonia due to other causes, patients with *L. micdadei* pneumonia more commonly had a productive cough, dyspnea, and pleuritic chest pain; they also more often displayed changes in mental

status and had significantly higher temperatures. Similar findings were noted in another outbreak of nosocomial *L. micdadei* pneumonia.[17]

5.3. Laboratory Findings

Multiple abnormalities of routine laboratory tests have been reported in patients with infection due to *L. pneumophila,* suggesting multisystem involvement. A leukocyte count of > 10,000/mm³ has been seen in most cases, and a shift to the left is common.[19,139,143] Hyponatremia (serum sodium < 130 mEq/ml) is present in 30–67% of patients.[17,20,139,143] Renal abnormalities including elevated BUN and creatinine, proteinuria, pyuria, and hematuria have been reported by some authorities[139,143] but not by others.[20] Hypophosphatemia and liver function abnormalities have also been noted occasionally.[19,143] We found no specific laboratory abnormalities associated with *L. micdadei* pneumonia. In particular, abnormalities in liver function, electrolytes, serum phosphate, and urinary sediment reflected the patients' underlying diseases and were no more common than in patients with pneumonia due to other causes.[18]

5.4. Radiographic Findings

The most common chest radiographic abnormality in patients with legionella pneumonia is a unilobar patchy alveolar infiltrate, usually present at the initial radiographic evaluation.[144–146] As the disease progresses, the infiltrate tends to enlarge and consolidate. Less commonly, noncontiguous areas in the same or opposite lung become involved.[144] Multilobe pulmonary involvement was seen in 85% of 26 immunocompromised patients with *L. micdadei* infection.[18] Abscess formation and cavitation are uncommon but not rare complications of both *L. pneumophila*[147] and *L. micdadei*[18] pneumonia and occur in both normal[145,148,149] and immunocompromised patients (Fig. 1).[11,18,150] About one-third of all patients will develop small pleural effusions, but these are not a prominent part of the radiologic picture.[144,145,151] Rapidly expanding peripheral nodules have been reported as the radiographic presentation for some cases of *L. micdadei*[16,152] and *L. pneumophila*.[151] These lesions may suggest the diagnosis of septic pulmonary embolism. Overall, there

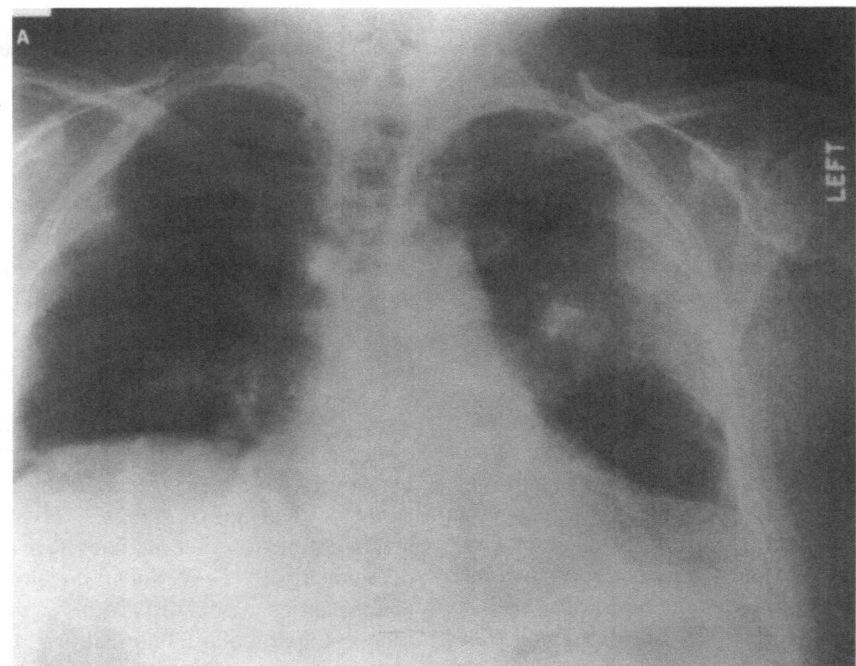

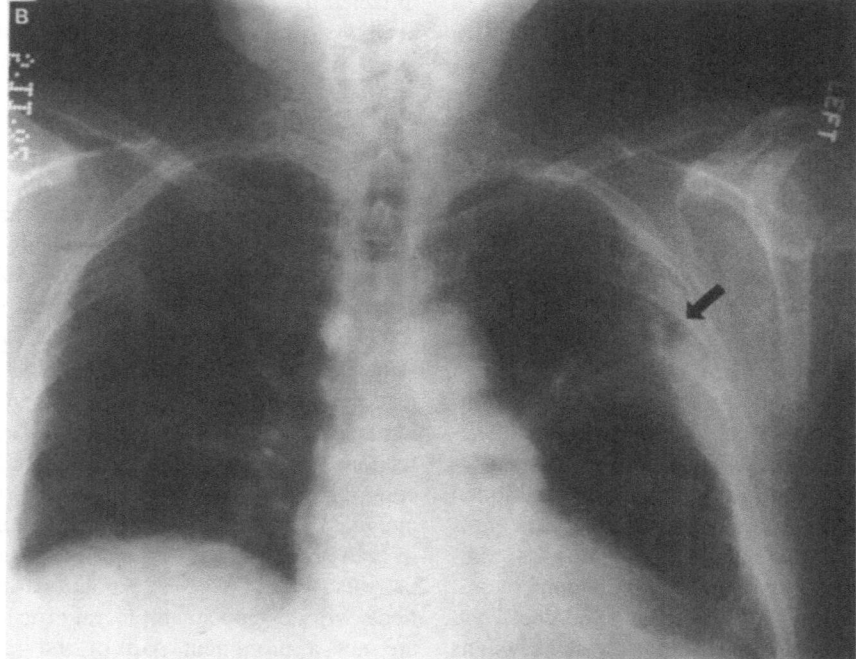

FIGURE 1. (A) Chest radiograph of a patient at the time of presentation with *Legionella* pneumonia Note the pleural based right upper and left upper lobe infiltrates. (B) After 1 week of therapy, the radiographic picture has evolved. Despite clinical improvement, a definite cavity (arrow) is present in the left upper lobe consolidation. (C) After 1 month of therapy, the chest radiograph has improved, but pleural thickening and parenchymal scarring remain

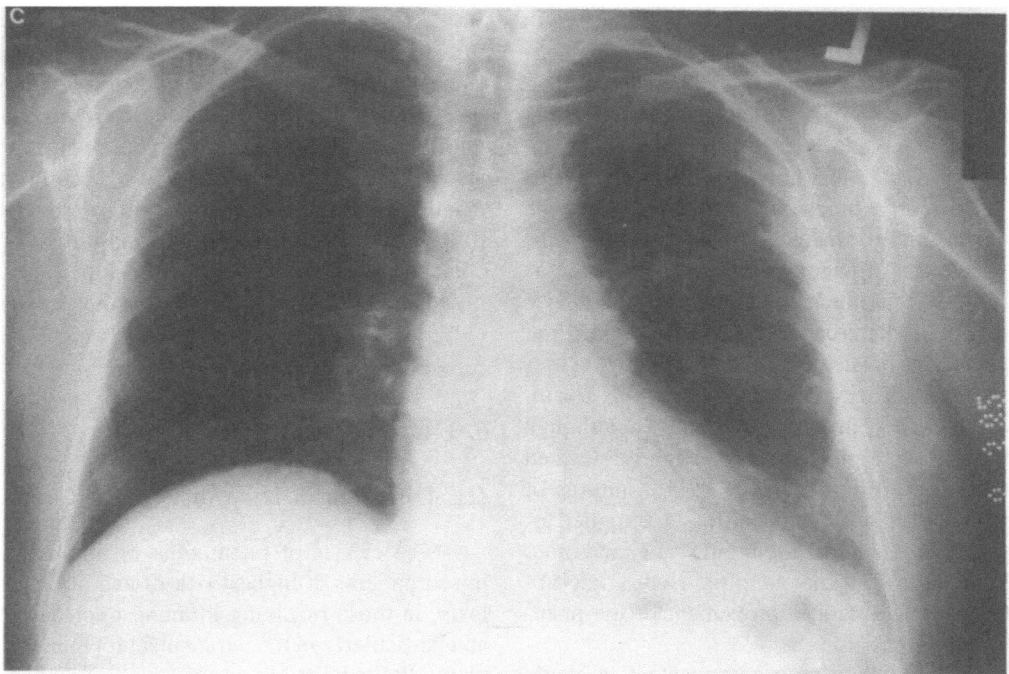

FIGURE 1. (*Continued*)

appear to be no major radiologic differences between *Legionella* pneumonia in the compromised and normal host.[146,153]

Illustrative Case 1

A 61-year-old woman was admitted to the hospital for evaluation of chronic active hepatitis. Her medications included predisone, 15 mg/day, and chlorambucil, 4 mg/day. On the twelfth hospital day, she became abruptly lethargic and developed a temperature of 40°C. There was no cough, chest pain, or dyspnea, but a chest radiograph demonstrated a new right basilar infiltrate. Because the patient could not produce sputum, a transtracheal aspirate was performed. The aspirate contained faintly staining gram-negative rods that were acid fast, using a modified Kinyoun stain. Direct fluorescent antibody (DFA) stain of this material was positive for *L. micdadei*, this same organism was isolated on buffered charcoal–yeast extract (BCYE) agar several days later She was treated with erythromycin, 2 g/day orally, and over the next week her mental status improved, her fever subsided and there was resolution of her pulmonary infiltrate

Comment This case demonstrates several important clinical points. The patient, with her underlying illness and immunosuppressive drug therapy, was clearly a highly compromised host The time course indicates that she acquired her pneumonia nosoco-

mially. Her presentation, with mental status changes and high fever, was nonspecific but suggestive of legionellosis. Because clinical suspicion was high, respiratory secretions were sampled promptly by a route that bypassed the oropharynx. The finding of acid-fast bacteria on a modified acid-fast stain was a definite clue of infection with *L. micdadei;* this was confirmed by the positive DFA stain and culture for this organism. With appropriate therapy, the patient improved.

5.5. Extrapulmonary Complications

It has become increasingly recognized that pneumonia due to *Legionellae* is often accompanied by nonpulmonary complicatons. These complications are of two types: those not directly due to infection of the involved area and those associated with actual bacterial invasion.

5.5.1. Noninfectious Extrapulmonary Complications

Abnormalities of CNS function are the most common nonpulmonary complications of *Legionella* pneumonia and are seen in at least one-third of patients.[18,70,71] Changes in mental status are most prominent and include lethargy with decreased alertness, confusion, disorientation, and behavioral or personality alterations.[18,71] Such changes are greater than can be accounted for by concurrent hypoxemia, azotemia, or metabolic abnormalities. Decreased mental status can progress to obtundation and even coma. Occasionally, changes in mental function may precede the onset of pneumonia.[71] Other neurologic abnormalities occur much less frequently and include ataxia and gait disturbances, seizures, dysarthria, and cranial nerve palsies.[70,71] Diagnostic procedures have for the most part yielded normal results. Examination of the CSF is usually unremarkable, although a modest leukocyte pleocytosis or slightly elevated protein has been observed.[70,71,139,143] Cultures of cerebrospinal fluid (CSF) are sterile.[71] Computed tomography (CT), radionuclide brain scans, and other specialized studies are not helpful. Neurologic abnormalities resolve with improvement of the pneumonia.[71,139]

Renal dysfunction may complicate *Legionella* pneumonia. Of 123 patients from the original outbreak of Legionnnaires' disease in Philadelphia, 14 developed oliguric renal failure. Six of these occurred in the absence of shock.[139] Three cases of renal failure due to acute tubular necrosis in association with elevated serum creatine phosphokinase (CPK) values have been reported.[76,78,79] In one of these, myoglobinuria with rhabdomyolysis of skeletal muscle was documented at autopsy.[79] Several hematologic complications of legionellosis have been noted. These include thrombotic thrombocytopenic purpura,[72] disseminated intravascular coagulation (DIC),[73] and autoimmune hemolytic anemia.[74] In general, these conditions improve with successful treatment of the pneumonia.

5.5.2. Infectious Extrapulmonary Complications

Direct invasion of nonpulmonary tissue is an increasingly recognized complication of legionella pneumonia. Instances of purulent pericarditis,[66] pyelonephritis,[63] hemodialysis fistulae infection,[64] sinusitis,[68] and rectal abscess[65] have been reported in patients with *L. pneumophila* pneumonia. There have been two instances of nonpulmonary infection due to *L. pneumophila* in the absence of pneumonia.

In the first, a case of prosthetic valve endocarditis, the source of the bacterium was not determined.[67] The second instance was an infection of a prosthetic hip wound acquired directly from contaminated whirlpool water.[154] Extrapulmonary infection can also be caused by *L. micdadei*. We recently cared for a patient receiving high-dose corticosteroids for necrotizing vasculitis, in whom a cellulitis and frank cutaneous abscess of the leg developed due to this organism. The source of the infection was presumably the lung.[69]

6. Diagnosis

6.1. Differential Diagnosis

The causes of pneumonia in immunocompromised patients at highest risk of acquiring legionellosis, in those receiving immunosuppressive drugs, and particularly in renal transplant recipients[11,13] are many. Potential etiologic agents include cytomegalovirus (CMV), a variety of bacteria including *Enterobacteriaceae, Staphylococcus aureus, Pseudomonas aeruginosa,* and *Nocardia asteroides,* fungi such as *Aspergillus* spp. and *Cryptococcus neoformans,* and the protozoan *Pneumocystis carinii.* Noninfectious etiologies, such as pulmonary emboli and pulmonary edema, must also be considered.[155]

Certain clinical and laboratory findings may point toward the diagnosis of legionellosis. A Gram stain of respiratory secretions showing only inflammatory cells without organisms is suggestive, although on rare occasions *Legionellae* have been seen in clinical specimens as gram-negative rods.[11,41] For *L. micdadei,* the finding of acid fast organisms on a modified acid-fast stain of respiratory secretions is a definite clue.[15,16] The failure of penicillins, cephalosporins, or aminoglycosides as treatment for a pneumonia due to unknown causes also suggests the diagnosis of legionellosis.[141,156] However, pneumonia due to a variety of other pathogens also will fail to respond to these drugs. Several studies have found that the association of headache, encephalopathy and diarrhea in a patient with pneumonia is suggestive of *L. pneumophila* infection.[140–142] In our experience, the abrupt onset of fever, pleuritic chest pain, and decreased mental status in a hospitalized immunocompromised patient with multiple pulmonary infiltrates was typical of *L. micdadei* pneumonia.[18] However, many patients with *Legionella* infections do not have distinguishing clinical and laboratory characteristics.[11,17,20,90]

6.2. Dual Infection

Simultaneous pulmonary infection with *Legionella* species and other pathogens is not rare.[11,18,90,143,157,158] Compromised hosts, particularly those receiving corticosteroids, are particularly represented in these cases. *Klebsiella pneumoniae* and other gram-negative bacilli, *Streptococcus pneumoniae,* and *Hemophilus influenzae* are among organisms that have been isolated from normally sterile pulmonary secretions in patients with well-documented legionellosis. Failure to recognize dual infection may lead to a delay in the use of appropriate therapy and increased risk for the patient. Although not as serious a treatment problem, simultaneous infection with *L. pneumophila* and *L. micdadei* has also been reported.[73,159]

6.3. Specific Diagnosis

Because of these problems, infection due to *Legionellae* may not be correctly identified using clinical findings and general laboratory testing alone. Specialized methods are necessary in order to establish a specific diagnosis.

The diagnosis of *Legionella* pneumonia can be directly made through the examination and culture of respiratory secretions. The most rapid method, the DFA technique, involves the staining of clinical material with fluorescein-labeled antibody directed against various *Legionella* strains. Stained smears are read under a fluorescent microscope and scored; a finding of five or more forms structurally typical of *Legionellae* is considered positive.[160] A positive DFA can supply an immediate diagnosis of infection due to *Legionellae* and can remain positive for up to 3 days after specific treatment is instituted.[157] However, there are several caveats in its use. First, it is a subjective test, and experienced laboratory personnel are required for interpretation of the smears. Second, although rare, false-positive tests may occur.[161] Finally, the sensitivity of the DFA in detecting documented *Legionella* infection is no more than 50%.[157,162,163] Thus, a negative DFA in no way precludes the diagnosis of legionellosis.

With the development of media that support the growth of *Legionellae,* it is now possible for the microbiology laboratory to isolate and identify these organisms from clinical specimens. Currently, the standard medium consists of buffered charcoal yeast–extract agar containing supplemental α-ketoglutarate (BCYE).[44,45] Culture of respiratory specimens using this medium appears to be significantly more sensitive than the DFA in the diagnosis of legionellosis,[157,162,163] and the specificity is virtually 100%. The addition of inhibitory antibiotics to media has allowed for the isolation of *Legionellae* from contaminated sites. One such medium, containing polymyxin B, anisomycin, and vancomycin, has been shown to improve the isolation of *Legionellae* from sputum, although it does not appear to aid the isolation of the organism from specimens obtained from normally sterile areas, such as from a transtracheal aspirate.[162,163] In some cases, dyes have been added to media to permit more rapid identification of these organisms and even differentiation from one another.[164] There are drawbacks in the use of culture as a diagnostic tool. The first is time. Visible growth of the organism from clinical samples requires an average of 3–5 days of incubation.[157] As well, even with the use of media containing inhibitory antibiotics, overgrowth by less fastidious organisms may mask the growth of *Legionellae* when samples are obtained from or through areas that are not normally sterile.

Respiratory secretions obtained by a variety of means may be used in the diagnosis of legionella pneumonia. With the use of culture media containing inhibitory antibiotics and special procedures such as acid treatment of the specimen,[162] the use of sputum for identifying *Legionellae* has greatly improved. However, techniques that bypass the oropharynx appear to be optimal. In a prospective pneumonia study, material obtained by transtracheal aspirate (TTA) was the most useful for early diagnosis with a culture sensitivity of 83%.[163] We have found that both TTA and percutaneous pulmonary aspiration are useful techniques in diagnosing pneumonia due to *L. micdadei* in the compromised host.[165] These methods offer the additional advantage of correctly identifying dual infection, due to either *Legionellae* and other organisms[157,158] or to *L. pneumophila* and *L.*

micdadei.[73] The role of specimens obtained by bronchoscopy is less clear because of the inherent risk of oropharyngeal contamination. However, Kohorst et al.[166] were able to identify nine cases of *Legionella* pneumonia in compromised patients through the use of bronchoalveolar lavage. This technique may be the one of choice in patients not able to undergo invasive procedures because of thrombocytopenia or coagulopathy. Open-lung biopsy has been shown to be a successful technique for identifying *Legionella* pneumonia in immunocompromised patients[90] and is recommended if other methods fail. Occasionally, these organisms have been identified in pleural fluid[18] and, when appropriate media is used, they have been cultured from blood.[60]

In the past there has been a heavy reliance on the use of serology, specifically the indirect fluorescent-antibody (IFA) test, for establishing the diagnosis of legionellosis. In this test, antigen prepared from killed bacteria is exposed to various dilutions of the serum to be tested. Antibodies in the serum that remain bound to antigen after washing are stained with fluorescein-labeled anti-human immunoglobulin and can be seen using a fluorescent microscope. The titer is the reciprocal of the highest serum dilution that demonstrates fluorescence. A fourfold rise to ≥ 128 in a convalescent serum sample is consistent with recent infection, while a single titer of ≥ 256 suggests infection at an undetermined time.[167]

As a diagnostic tool, the IFA test has several pitfalls. First, because of the delay from initial clinical presentation to development of significant antibody titers, the test is generally retrospective. Zuravleff et al.[163] found that only 27% of patients with documented *L. pneumophila* pneumonia had an elevated serologic titer during the first week of illness. Second, while the IFA test has been reported to be positive in 75–91% of documented infections,[157,168] new strains of pathogenic legionellae not antigenically cross-reactive with currently recognized strains are being increasingly recognized. Such antigenic complexity may seriously reduce the sensitivity of the test. In one study using 29 separate *Legionella* antigens to perform the IFA, Wilkinson et al.[169] found that no single antigen detected even one-half of the total number of positive sera. Third, although the specificity of serologic testing for *Legionellae* has been reported as greater than 95%,[168,169] cross-reactions to a variety of gram-negative organisms, including *Bacteroides fragilis*[161] and, in patients with cystic fibrosis, *Pseudomonas aeruginosa*,[170] have been reported. Finally, because serodiagnosis depends on the immunocompetence of the host, the sensitivity of this test may be lower than anticipated when used in the compromised patient. For all these reasons, serologic testing in the compromised host should be used only in conjunction with other techniques.

One test that may find increased use in the future is the detection of *Legionella* antigen in the urine. This test is rapid and noninvasive and in clinical evaluation was found to have a sensitivity of $> 80\%$ with rare false-positive results in the diagnosis of infection due to *L. pneumophila* serogroup 1.[171–173] However, further confirmation with other *Legionella* strains is needed before this test can be used clinically.

6.4. Diagnostic Approach

We suggest the following approach for the diagnosis of *Legionella* pneumonia in the compromised patient. Every effort should be made to obtain adequate respiratory secretions for examination by DFA staining and culture. Initial attempts to identify the organism can be made using sputum. If this appears inadequate, however, more invasive techniques should be tried. For maximum yield, the DFA and culture should be performed using specimens obtained by techniques that bypass the oropharynx. In particular, the TTA appears to be the method of choice. Open lung biopsy should be considered if other techniques fail to provide a diagnosis. All three methods—culture, DFA staining, and serum IFA—should be used in order to optimize the yield. The IFA should be obtained initially and every 2 weeks thereafter. A fourfold rise to ≥ 128 in the appropriate clinical setting is diagnostic. A single titer of ≥ 256 is only suggestive of *Legionella* infection. Reagents used in the DFA and IFA tests for *L. pneumophila* serogroups 1 and 6 and for *L. micdadei* are available from the CDC. BCYE agar and reagents for other *Legionella* species and serogroups are available commercially. Finally, if any clinical suspicion for legionellosis exists in a patient, specific therapy should be started without waiting for test results.

Illustrative Case 2

An 82-year-old man with pancytopenia due to aplastic anemia was transferred from another hospital on antibiotic therapy for presumed *Pseudomonas* pneumonia. On admission, he was afebrile, alert, and in no distress. A chest radiograph revealed consolidative infiltrates in the right upper and right lower lobes. The patient had < 1000 circulating granulocytes/mm³, and the platelet count was 27,000/mm³. Antibiotics were continued and high-dose corticosteroids administered. On the eleventh hospital day, he developed a temperature of 39.7°C. New right, middle, and left lower lobe infiltrates were seen on the chest radiograph. The patient could not bring up sputum and, on the next day, a bronchoscopy was performed. Gram stain of the fluid obtained revealed no inflammatory cells and a few gram-negative bacilli and gram-positive cocci. DFA stain for *Legionellae* was negative. The following day, the fluid was reported to be growing *Klebsiella pneumoniae, Pseudomonas aeruginosa,* and *Staphylococcus aureus.* Appropriate antibiotics were given, but the patient failed to improve. Four days after bronchoscopy, the culture of the lavage fluid was positive for *L. pneumophila,* serogroup 5 Erythromycin therapy was started. However, the patient remained febrile, developed increasing hypoxia, and died 5 days later. Autopsy revealed a bilateral bronchopneumonia that was positive by DFA stain and culture for *L. pneumophila,* serogroup 5.

Comment. This highly immunocompromised patient acquired a nosocomial *Legionella* infection during the course of pseudomonas pneumonia. Invasive biopsy techniques were contraindicated because of thrombocytopenia,[50] respiratory secretions were obtained by bronchoscopy. Although it is possible that results from this procedure represent oropharyngeal contamination, it is more likely that the patient had simultaneous infection with *Legionellae* and the other organisms isolated from the lavage fluid. This case illustrates the fact that a negative DFA stain does not preclude legionellosis. Diagnosis was delayed until the culture became positive. Subsequent therapy with erythromycin failed to eliminate the organism from the lung.

7. Treatment

7.1. Retrospective Studies

Because there are no prospective clinical studies on the effectiveness of antimicrobial therapy of legionellosis, information must be obtained retrospectively. In the 1976 Philadelphia outbreak, case fatalities were lowest in those patients who received either erythromycin or tetracycline. The highest mortality was seen in those treated with cephalosporins and was intermediate in those receiving penicillins, aminoglycosides, and chloramphenicol. However, these differences were not statistically significant.[139] In cases evaluated during the outbreak at the Wadsworth VA Medical Center, erythromycin was clearly the most effective agent. This was especially true for immunocompromised patients, in whom the case–fatality rate of those treated with erythromycin was 24%, compared with 80% for those receiving other regimens.[19] Erythromycin also appears to be effective for the treatment of *L. micdadei* infection.[18,174] There is scant clinical information on the effectiveness of other agents. The combination of erythromycin and rifampin has been used successfully in compromised patients who failed therapy with erythromycin alone.[11,90] Kirby et al. noted a clinical response to therapy with trimethaprim–sulfamethoxazole in a renal transplant recipient,[19] and we have treated two patients with *L. micdadei* pneumonia who failed to improve with erythromycin therapy but responded to trimethaprim–sulfamethoxazole.[18,175] The data on tetracylines are unclear. Although they have been effective in occasional cases,[158] several treatment failures have been reported and patients have acquired legionellosis while on these agents.[19]

7.2. Animal Studies

Animal models have provided the only means of prospectively studying the antimicrobial treatment of legionellosis. Because of its susceptibility, the guinea pig has been used almost exclusively as the study animal. In one model, using intraperitoneal inoculation of *L. pneumophila* at a lethal dose, Fraser et al.[176] found both erythromycin and rifampin highly effective in preventing mortality, while penicillin, gentamicin, tetracycline, and chloramphenicol were not. Using a similar model, Plouffe et al.[177] showed that trimethaprim–sulfamethoxazole is also effective.

Intratracheal inoculation of *L. pneumophila* reliably produces a pneumonia in guinea pigs that closely resembles the disease in humans.[178] Edelstein et al.[179] used this model to study a variety of antimicrobial agents. No effect on mortality, histologic changes, or bacterial clearance was seen in animals treated with either gentamicin or cefoxitin as compared with untreated controls. Erythromycin, rifampin, doxycycline, and trimethaprim–sulfamethoxazole were all highly effective in preventing mortality, but rifampin acted far more quickly than other agents in reducing bacterial counts within the lungs. Treatments combining rifampin with other antimicrobials were no more effective than treatments using single agents. Similar results have been noted using the guinea pig model for experimental pulmonary infection due to *L. micdadei*.[180]

7.3. Factors Determining Antimicrobial Efficacy

The results of in vitro testing of antimicrobials against *Legionellae* have correlated only partially with clinical results and animal testing. Using the agar-dilution technique, *L. pneumophila* appears to be most sensitive to rifampin but is also inhibited by erythromycin, aminoglycosides, chloramphenicol, and trimethaprim–sulfamethoxazole.[181] It is generally resistant to all β-lactam antibiotics with the exception of cefoxitin[181,182] and is highly resistant to vancomycin[181,183] and clindamycin.[183] Tetracyclines have shown only moderate activity against these organisms[181,182] but may be inactivated by the charcoal yeast extract agar.[182] The in vitro susceptibility of *L. micdadei* to antimicrobial agents appears to be similar to that of *L. pneumophila*, with the exception of an increased sensitivity to β-lactams due to its lack of a β-lactamase.[183,184]

There are at least two reasons for the discrepancy between the in vitro activity and the in vivo efficacy of various antimicrobials against *Legionellae*. *Legionellae* are facultative intracellular parasites with the ability to replicate within phagocytic cells.[45] Hence, for an antibiotic to be active, it must penetrate intracellularly. Johnson *et al.*[185] showed that while penicillins and cephalosporins enter cells very poorly, both rifampin and erythromycin achieve intracellular concentrations far in excess of their extracellular levels. Gentamicin and tetracycline enter in levels equivalent to their extracellular concentrations. The intracellular growth of *L. pneumophila* in cell culture has been shown to be markedly inhibited by the addition of erythromycin or rifampin to the cell culture media,[186,187] but the bacteria will continue to grow in the presence of penicillins and cephalosporins and are only slightly inhibited by chloramphenicol, tetracycline, and gentamicin.[187] The second, probably less important, factor affecting antimicrobial efficacy in legionellosis is the penetration of the agent into the lung tissue. Both erythromycin and rifampin appear to maintain prolonged intra-

pulmonary concentrations at therapeutic levels, while other agents, such as gentamicin, do not.[188]

7.4. Recommendations

On the basis of these data, erythromycin and rifampin are the most active agents for the treatment of legionellosis. Trimethaprim–sulfamethoxazole and the tetracyclines are potentially useful agents, but experience with them remains too limited to advocate their general use. Penicillins, cephalosporins (including cefoxitin and other newer agents), aminoglycosides, chloramphenicol, vancomycin, and clindamycin are ineffective against legionellosis.

For initial therapy, we recommend erythromycin, 2–4 g/day. Oral therapy with erythromycin has been associated with failures in immunocompromised patients,[90] and intravenous therapy should be used if the patient is severely ill. If there is evidence of treatment failure, consideration should be given to adding rifampin, 1200 mg/day, to the regimen. Because of the theoretical possibility of emergence of resistance, rifampin should not be given alone.[189] Alternatively, trimethaprim–sulfamethoxazole may be given at a dosage of 80 mg trimethaprim with 400 mg sulfamethoxazole[175] to 400 mg trimethaprim with 2000 mg sulfamethoxazole[19] every 8 hr. The length of antimicrobial therapy has not been established. There has been at least one relapse in a renal transplant recipient who received a 3-week course of erythromycin.[190] We therefore suggest therapy for the compromised patient be given for at least this long. If possible, immunosuppressive therapy should be reduced.

7.5. Course

In general, patients respond promptly to treatment with erythromycin. In the Wadsworth experience with *L. pneumophila* pneumonia, subjective improvement occurred within 2 days after therapy was started, and temperature returned to normal after about 4 days.[19] In our experience with immunocompromised patients and *L. micdadei* pneumonia, about one-third of patients displayed clinical improvement within 2 or 3 days after erythromycin therapy. However, another one-third required up to 2 weeks to respond, and six of 25 patients died despite the prompt use of erythromycin.[18] In patients who die, progressive respiratory insufficiency and hypotension usually occur.

Radiologic resolution may lag well behind clinical improvement. Radiographic progression may even occur during the first few days of therapy despite clinical improvement (Fig. 1).[144] Cavitary pneumonia, especially in immunocompromised patients, may respond very slowly and may require 4 or more weeks of therapy.[150] One patient with cavitary legionellosis had evidence of *Legionella* in respiratory secretions 18 days after initiation of erythromycin.[147]

8. Prevention and Control

Both animal[191] and clinical[192] studies have indicated that person-to-person transmission of legionellosis does not occur, nor is there evidence of oropharyngeal carriage.[193] Consequently, patients with *Legionella* pneumonia need not be placed in respiratory isolation. In addition, there is no evidence that prophylactic use of antimicrobial agents will prevent disease.

Because nosocomial outbreaks of legionellosis have often been associated with contaminated potable water,[111,114,130,131] it is reasonable to culture the hot-water tanks and other sites in the event of hospital-acquired cases of legionellosis. If *Legionellae* are found within the potable water in association with clinical cases, they should be eliminated. Two methods of sterilization appear to be efficacious. These are hyperchlorination[131] and heating and flushing the potable water supply intermittently.[129] In some instances, it may be necessary to replace the plumbing fixtures.[133] A more complete discussion of these issues may be found elsewhere.[189,194]

References

1 McDade JE, Shepard CC, Fraser DW, et al. Legionnaires' disease Isolation of a bacterium and demonstration of its role in other respiratory disease. *N Engl J Med* 297:1197–1203, 1977.

2 Thacker SB, Bennett JV, Tsai TF, et al: An outbreak in 1965 of severe respiratory illness caused by the Legionnaires' disease bacterium. *J Infect Dis* 138:512–519, 1978.

3 Terranova W, Cohen ML, Fraser DW. 1974 Outbreak of Legionnaires' disease diagnosed in 1977 *Lancet* 2:122–124, 1978

4 Pasculle AW, Myerowitz RL, Dowling JN New bacterial agent of pneumonia isolated from renal-transplant recipients. *Lancet* 2:58–61, 1979.

5. Thomason BM, Harris PP, Hicklin MD, et al: A *Legionella*-like bacterium related to WIGA in a fatal case of pneumonia. *Ann Intern Med* 91:673–676, 1979.

6. Lewallen KR, McKinney RM, Brenner DJ, et al: A newly identified bacterium phenotypically resembling, but genetically distinct from, *Legionella pneumophila* An isolate in a case of pneumonia. *Ann Intern Med* 91:831–834, 1979

7 McKinney RM, Porschen RK, Edelstein PH, et al *Legionella longbeachae* species nova, another etiologic agent of human pneumonia *Ann Intern Med* 94:739–743, 1981.

8 Edelstein PH, Brenner DJ, Moss CW, et al: *Legionella wadsworthii* species nova. A cause of human pneumonia. *Ann Intern Med* 97:809–813, 1982

9. Herwaldt LA, Gorman GW, McGrath T, et al. A new *Legionella* species, *Legionella feeleii* species nova, causes Pontiac fever in an automobile plant. *Ann Intern Med* 100:333–338, 1984

10. Brenner DJ, Steigerwalt AG, Gorman GW, et al. Ten new *Legionella* species. In *Twenty-fourth Interscience Conference on Antimicrobial Agents and Chemotherapy, Washington, DC, October 8–10, 1984.* (abst. 160)

11. Gump DW, Frank RO, Winn WC Jr, et al: Legionnaires' disease in patients with associated serious disease *Ann Intern Med* 90:538–542, 1979.

12. Haley CE, Cohen ML, Halter J, et al. Nosocomial Legionnaires' disease: A continuing common-source epidemic at Wadsworth Medical Center *Ann Intern Med* 90:583–586, 1979.

13 England AC III, Fraser DW, Plikaytis BD, et al: Sporadic legionellosis in the United States: The first thousand cases. *Ann Intern Med* 94:164–170, 1981

14. Arnow PM, Chou T, Weil D, et al: Nosocomial Legionnaires' disease caused by aerosolized tap water from respiratory devices. *J Infect Dis* 146:460–467, 1982

15. Myerowitz RL, Pasculle AW, Dowling JN, et al: Opportunistic lung infection due to "Pittsburgh Pneumonia Agent." *N Engl J Med* 301:953–958, 1979.

16. Rogers BH, Donowitz GR, Walker GK, et al: Opportunistic pneumonia. A clinicopathological study of five cases caused by an unidentified acid-fast bacterium. *N Engl J Med* 301:959–961, 1979

17 Muder RR, Yu VL, Zuravleff JJ: Pneumonia due to the Pittsburgh Pneumonia Agent: New clinical perspective with a review of the literature. *Medicine (Baltimore)* 62:120–128, 1983

18. Rudin JE, Wing EJ: A comparative study of *Legionella micdadei* and other nosocomial acquired pneumonia *Chest* 86:675–680, 1984.

19. Kirby BD, Snyder KM, Meyer RD, et al: Legionnaires' disease· Report of sixty-five nosocomially acquired cases and review of the literature *Medicine (Baltimore)* 59:188–205, 1980

20. Yu VL, Kroboth FJ, Shonnard J, et al: Legionnaires' disease: New clinical perspective from a prospective pneumonia study *Am J Med* 73:357–361, 1982

21. Muder RR, Yu VL, McClure JK, et al: Nosocomial Legion-

naires' disease uncovered in a prospective pneumonia study. *JAMA* **249:**3184–3188, 1983.

22. Meyer RD: Legionnaires' disease. Aspects of nosocomial infection. *Am J Med* **76:**657–663, 1984.

23. Reingold AL, Thomason BM, Brake BJ, et al: Legionella pneumonia in the United States: The distribution of serogroups and species causing human illness. *J Infect Dis* **149:**819, 1984.

24. Winn WC Jr, Myerowitz RL: The pathology of the legionella pneumonias. *Human Pathol* **12:**401–422, 1981

25. Fraser DW: Legionnaires' disease: Four summers' harvest. *Am J Med* **68:**1–2, 1980.

26. Girod JC, Reichman RC, Winn WC Jr, et al: Pneumonic and nonpneumonic forms of legionellosis. *Arch Intern Med* **142:**545–547, 1982.

27. Brenner DJ: Classification of legionellae. In Thornsberry C, Balows A, Feeley JC, Jakubowsky W (eds): *Legionella. Proceedings of the Second International Symposium.* American Society for Microbiology, Washington, DC, 1984, pp. 55–60.

28. Moss CW, Weaver RE, Dees SB, et al. Cellular fatty acid composition of isolates from Legionniares disease. *J Clin Microbiol* **6:**140–143, 1977

29. Moss CW, Dees SB: Further studies of the cellular fatty acid composition of Legionnaires disease bacteria. *J Clin Microbiol* **9:**648–649, 1979.

30. Brenner DJ, Steigerwalt AG, McDade JE: Classification of the Legionnaires' disease bacterium: *Legionella pneumophila,* genus novum, species nova, of the Family *Legionellaceae. Ann Intern Med* **90:**656–658, 1979.

31. Edelstein PH, Bibb WF, Gorman GW, et al: *Legionella pneumophila* serogroup 9: A cause of human pneumonia *Ann Intern Med* **101:**196–198, 1984

32. Tang PW, Toma S, Moss CW, et al: *Legionella bozemanii* serogroup 2: A new etiological agent. *J Clin Microbiol* **19:**30–33, 1984.

33 Bibb WF, Sorg RJ, Thomason BM, et al: Recognition of a second serogroup of *Legionella longbeachae. J Clin Microbiol* **14:**674–677, 1981.

34. Chandler FW, Cole RM, Hicklin MD, et al: Ultrastructure of the Legionnaires' disease bacterium. *Ann Intern Med* **90:**642–647, 1979.

35. Hebert GA, Callaway CS, Ewing EP: Comparison of *Legionella pneumophila, L. micdadei, L. bozemanii,* and *L dumoffii* by transmission electron microscopy *J Clin Microbiol* **19:**116–121, 1984.

36. Gress FM, Myerowitz FL, Pasculle AW, et al: The ultrastructural morphologic features of Pittsburgh Pneumonia Agent. *Am J Pathol* **101:**63–78, 1980.

37. Chandler FW, Roth IL, Callaway CS, et al. Flagella on Legionnaires' disease bacteria. *Ann Intern Med* **93:**711–714, 1980.

38. Orrison LG, Cherry WB, Tyndall RL, et al: *Legionella oakridgensis.* Unusual new species isolated from cooling tower water. *Appl Environ Microbiol* **45:**536–545, 1983.

39. Chandler FW, Hicklin MD, Blackmon JA: Demonstration of the agent of Legionnaires' disease in tissue. *N Engl J Med* **297:**1218–1220, 1977

40. Isenberg HD: Microbiology of Legionnaires' disease bacterium *Ann Intern Med* **90:**502–505, 1979.

41. Liu F, Wright DN. Gram stain in Legionnaires' disease *Am J Med* **77:**549–550, 1984.

42. Hebert GA, Thomason BM, Harris PP, et al. ''Pittsburgh Pneumonia Agent''. A bacterium phenotypically similar to *Legionella pneumophila* and identical to the TATLOCK bacterium. *Ann Intern Med* **92:**53–54, 1980.

43. Hoffman PS, Pine L, Bell S: Production of superoxide and hxdrogen peroxide in medium used to culture *Legionella pneumophila.* Catalytic decomposition by charcoal *Appl Environ Microbiol* **45:**784–791, 1983.

44. Pasculle AW, Feeley JC, Gibson RJ, et al. Pittsburgh Pneumonia Agent. Direct isolation from human lung tissue. *J Infect Dis* **141:**727–732, 1980.

45. Edelstein PH. Improved semiselective medium for isolation of *Legionella pneumophila* from contaminated clinical and environmental specimens. *J Clin Microbiol* **14:**298–303, 1981

46. Baine WB, Rasheed JK: Aromatic substrate specificity of browning by cultures of the Legionnaires' disease bacterium. *Ann Intern Med* **90:**619–620, 1979.

47. Orrison LH, Cherry WB, Fliermans CB, et al: Characteristics of environmental isolates of *Legionella pneumophila. Appl Environ Microbiol* **42:**109–115, 1981.

48. Cherry WB, Gorman GW, Orrison LH, et al: *Legionella jordanis:* A new species of *Legionella* isolated from water and sewage. *J Clin Microbiol* **15:**290–297, 1982.

49. Morris GK, Steigerwalt AG, Feeley JC, et al: *Legionella gormanii* sp. nova. *J Clin Microbiol* **12:**718–721, 1980.

50. Campbell J, Bibb WF, Lambert MA, et al: *Legionella sainthelensi.* A new species of *Legionella* isolated from water near Mt St. Helens. *Appl Environ Microbiol* **47:**369–373, 1984.

51. Hebert GA: Hippurate hydrolysis by *Legionella pneumophila. J Clin Microbiol* **13:**240–242, 1981.

52. Karr DE, Bibb WF, Moss CW: Isoprenoid quinones of the genus *Legionella. J Clin Microbiol* **15:**1044–1048, 1982.

53. Hernandez FJ, Kirby BD, Stanley TM, et al· Legionnaires' disease. Postmortem pathologic findings of 20 cases. *Am J Clin Pathol* **73:**488–495, 1980.

54. Chandler FW, Blackmon JA, Hicklin MD, et al. Ultrastructure of the agent of Legionnaires' disease in the human lung. *Am J Clin Pathol* **71:**43–50, 1979.

55 Glavin FL, Winn WC Jr, Craighead JE: Ultrastructure of lung in Legionnaires' disease. *Ann Intern Med* **90:**555–559, 1979.

56. Hicklin MD, Thomason BM, Chandler FW, et al: Pathogenesis of acute Legionnaires' disease pneumonia. *Am J Clin Pathol* **73:**480–487, 1980.

57 Watts JC, Hicklin MD, Thomason BM, et al. Fatal pneumonia caused by *Legionella pneumophila,* serogroup 3: Demonstration of the bacilli in extrathoracic organs. *Ann Intern Med* **92:**186–188, 1980

58. Weisenburger DD, Helms DM, Renner ED. Sporadic Legionnaires' disease. A pathologic study of 23 fatal cases *Arch Pathol Lab Med* **105:**130–137, 1981.

59 Evans CP, Winn WC Jr: Extrathoracic localization of

Legionella pneumophila in Legionnaires' pneumonia. *Am J Clin Pathol* **76**:813–815, 1981.

60. Edelstein PH, Meyer RD, Finegold SM: Isolation of *Legionella pneumophila* from blood. *Lancet* **1**:750–751, 1979.

61. Rodgers FG: Isolation of *Legionella pneumophila* from blood. *Lancet* **1**:925, 1979

62 MacRae AD, Greaves PW, Platts P: Isolation of *Legionella pneumophila* from blood culture. *Br Med J* **2**:1189–1190, 1979

63. Dorman SA, Hardin NJ, Winn WC Jr: Pyelonephritis associated with *Legionella pneumophila*, serogroup 4. *Ann Intern Med* **93**:835–837, 1980.

64. Kalweit WH, Winn WC Jr, Rocco TA, et al: Hemodialysis fistula infections caused by *Legionella pneumophila*. *Ann Intern Med* **96**:173–175, 1982.

65. Arnow PM, Boyko EJ, Friedman EL: Perirectal abscess caused by *Legionella pneumophila* and mixed anaerobic bacteria. *Ann Intern Med* **98**:184–185, 1983.

66. Mayock R, Skale B, Kohler RB: *Legionella pneumophila* pericarditis proved by culture of pericardial fluid. *Am J Med* **75**:534–536, 1983.

67. McCabe RE, Baldwin JC, McGregor CA, et al: Prosthetic valve endocarditis caused by *Legionella pneumophila*. *Ann Intern Med* **100**:525–527, 1984.

68. Schlanger G, Lutwick LI, Kurzman M, et al: Sinusitis caused by *Legionella pneumophila* in a patient with the acquired immune deficiency syndrome. *Am J Med* **77**:957–959, 1984.

69. Ampel NM, Ruben FL, Norden CW: Cutaneous abscess caused by *Legionella micdadei*. *Ann Intern Med* **102**:630–631, 1985.

70. Pendlebury WW, Perl DP, Winn WC Jr, et al: Neuropathic evaluation of 40 confirmed cases of *Legionella* pneumonia. *Neurology (NY)* **33**:1340–1344, 1983.

71 Johnson JD, Raff MJ, Van Arsdall JA: Neurologic manifestations of Legionnaires' disease. *Medicine (Baltimore)* **63**:303–309, 1984.

72. Riggs SA, Wray NP, Waddell CC, et al: Thrombotic thrombocytopenic purpura complicating Legionnaires' disease. *Arch Intern Med* **142**:2275–2280, 1982.

73. Dowling JN, Kroboth FJ, Karpf M, et al: Pneumonia and multiple lung abscesses caused by dual infection with *Legionella micdadei* and *Legionella pneumophila* *Am Rev Respir Dis* **127**:121–125, 1983.

74. Strikas R, Seifert MR, Lentino JR: Autoimmune hemolytic anemia and *Legionella pneumophila* pneumonia. *Ann Intern Med* **99**:345, 1983.

75. Knudsen F, Nielsen AH, Hansen KB, et al: *Legionella micdadei* (Pittsburgh Pneumonia Agent) may cause non-pneumonic legionellosis. *Lancet* **1**:708, 1983.

76 Williams ME, Watanakunakorn C, Baird IM, et al: Legionnaires' disease with acute renal failure *Am J Med Sci* **279**:177–183, 1980.

77. Saleh F, Rodichok LD, Satya-Murti S, et al: Legionnaires' disease. Report of a case with unusual manifestations. *Arch Intern Med* **140**:1514–1516, 1980.

78. Hall SL, Wasserman M, Dall L, et al: Acute renal failure secondary to myoglobinuria associated with Legionnaires' disease. *Chest* **84**:633–635, 1983.

79. Posner MR, Caudill MA, Brass R, et al: Legionnaires' disease associated with rhabdomyolysis and myoglobinuria. *Arch Intern Med* **140**:848–850, 1980.

80. Wong KH, Moss CW, Hochstein DH, et al: "Endotoxicity" of the Legionnaires' disease bacterium. *Ann Intern Med* **90**:624–627, 1979.

81 Johnson W, Elliott JA, Helms CM, et al: A high molecular weight antigen in Legionnaires' disease bacterium. Isolation and partial characterization. *Ann Intern Med* **90**:638–641, 1979.

82. Thorpe TC, Miller RD: Extracellular enzymes of *Legionella pneumophila*. *Infect Immun* **33**:632–635, 1981.

83 Thompson MR, Miller RD, Iglewski BH: In vitro production of an extracellular protease by *Legionella pneumophila* *Infect Immun* **34**:299–302, 1981.

84. Winn WC Jr, Chandler FW: Role of virulence factors in *Legionella* infections. *Arch Pathol Lab Med* **106**:105–107, 1982.

85. Friedman RL, Lochner JE, Bigley RH, et al: The effects of *Legionella pneumophila* toxin on oxidative processes and bacterial killing of human polymorphonuclear leukocytes. *J Infect Dis* **146**:328–334, 1982.

86. Friedman M, Klein TW, Friedman H. *Legionella pneumophila*-induced suppression of macrophage spreading in vitro. *Infect Immun* **42**:421–423, 1983.

87. Davis GS, Winn WC Jr, Gump DW, et al: Legionnaires' pneumonia after aerosol exposure in guinea pigs and rats. *Am Rev Respir Dis* **126**:1050–1057, 1982.

88 Davis GS, Winn WC Jr, Gump DW, et al: The kinetics of early inflammatory events during experimental pneumonia due to *Legionella pneumophila* in guinea pigs. *J Infect Dis* **148**:823–835, 1983.

89. Katz SM, Hashemi S: Electron microscopic examination of the inflammatory response to *Legionella pneumophila* in guinea pigs. *Lab Invest* **46**:24–32, 1982.

90. Saravolatz LD, Burch KH, Fisher E, et al: The compromised host and Legionnaires' disease. *Ann Intern Med* **90**:533–537, 1979.

91. Glazier MC, Kohler RB, Campbell RL: Legionnaire's disease in postoperative neurosurgical patients *J Neurosurg* **59**:596–600, 1983.

92. Lin RY, DeCotis A, Krey PR. Legionnaires' disease complicating steroid therapy in systemic lupus erythematosus. *J Rheumatol* **11**:375–376, 1984.

93. Widen R, Klein T, Friedman H: Enhanced susceptibility of cyclophosphamide-treated mice to infection with *Legionella pneumophila*. *J Infect Dis* **149**:1023–1024, 1984.

94. Myerowitz RL, Dowling JN, Pasculle AW. Immunity to Pittsburgh Pneumonia Agent in guinea pigs. In *Twentieth Interscience Conference on Antimicrobial Agents and Chemotherapy, New Orleans, Louisiana, 1980*. (abst 497.)

95. Horwitz MA, Silverstein SC. Legionnaires' disease bacterium (*Legionella pneumophila*) multiples intracellulary in human monocytes. *J Clin Invest* **66**:441–450, 1980.

96. Nash TW, Libby DM, Horwitz MA: Interaction between the Legionnaires' disease bacterium (*Legionella pneumophila*)

and human alveolar macrophages. Influence of antibody, lymphokines, and hydrocortisone. *J Clin Invest* **74**:771–782, 1984.

97. Horwitz MA, Silverstein SC: Interaction of the Legionnaires' disease bacterium *(Legionella pneumophila)* with human phagocytes I *L. pneumophila* resists killing by polymorphonuclear leukocytes, antibody, and complement. *J Exp Med* **153**:386–397, 1981.

98. Horwitz MA, Silverstein SC: Interaction of the Legionnaires' disease bacterium *(Legionella pneumophila)* with human phagocytes. II. Antibody promotes binding of *L pneumophila* to monocytes but does not inhibit intracellular multiplication. *J Exp Med* **153**:398–406, 1981.

99. Horwitz MA, Silverstein SC: Activated human monocytes inhibit the intracellular multiplication of Legionnaires' disease bacteria. *J Exp Med* **154**:1618–1635, 1981

100. Horwitz MA: Cell mediated immunity in Legionnaires' disease. *J Clin Invest* **71**:1686–1697, 1983.

101. Weinbaum DL, Benner RR, Dowling JN, et al: Interaction of *Legionella micdadei* with human monocytes. *Infect Immun* **46**:68–73, 1984.

102. Levi M, Pasculle AW, Dowling JN, et al: Multiplication of *Legionella micdadei* and *Legionella pneumophila* in cultured alveolar macrophages from susceptible and immune guinea pigs. In Thornsberry C, Balows A, Feeley JC, Jakubowski W (eds). *Legionella. Proceedings of the Second International Symposium.* American Society for Microbiology, Washington, DC, 1984, pp. 171–173.

103. Weinbaum DL, Bailey J, Benner RR, et al: The contribution of human neutrophils and serum to host defense against *Legionella micdadei J Infect Dis* **148**:510–517, 1983.

104. Horwitz MA: The Legionnaires' disease bacterium *(Legionella pneumophila)* inhibits phagosome-lysosome fusion in human monocytes. *J Exp Med* **158**:2108–2126, 1983

105. Locksley RM, Jacobs RF, Wilson CB, et al. Susceptibility of *Legionella pneumophila* to oxygen-dependent microbicidal systems *J Immunol* **129**:2192–2197, 1982.

106. Lochner JE, Friedman RL, Bigley RH, et al: Effect of oxygen-dependent antimicrobial systems on *Legionella pneumophila. Infect Immun* **39**:487–489, 1983.

107. Lochner JE, Bigley RH, Iglewski BH· Defective triggering of polymorphonuclear leukocyte oxidative metabolism by *Legionella pneumophila* toxin. *J Infect Dis* **151**:42–46, 1985.

108. Friedman H, Widen R, Klein T, et al: *Legionella pneumophila*-induced blastogenesis of murine lymphoid cells in vitro. *Infect Immun* **43**:314–319, 1984

109. Rolstad B, Berdal BP: Immune defenses against *Legionella pneumophila* in rats. *Infect Immun* **32**:805–812, 1981.

110. Eisenstein TK, Tamada R, Meissler J, et al: Vaccination against *Legionella pneumophila:* Serum antibody correlates with protection induced by heat-killed or acetone-killed cells against intraperitoneal but not aerosol infection in guinea pigs. *Infect Immun* **45**:685–691, 1984.

111. Stout J, Yu VL, Vickers RM, et al: Ubiquitousness of *Legionella pneumophila* in the water supply of a hospital with endemic Legionnaires' disease. *N Engl J Med* **306**:466–468, 1982.

112. MacFarlane JT, Finch RG, Ward MJ, et al: Hospital study of adult community-acquired pneumonia. *Lancet* **2**:255–258, 1982.

113. Dondero TJ, Rendtorff RC, Mallison GF, et al: An outbreak of Legionnaires' disease associated with a contaminated air-conditioning cooling tower. *N Engl J Med* **302**:365–370, 1980.

114. Helms CM, Massanari RM, Zeitler R, et al: Legionnaires' disease associated with a hospital water system: A cluster of 24 nosocomial cases. *Ann Intern Med* **99**:172–178, 1983.

115. Tobin JO, Beare J, Dunnill MS, et al: Legionnaires' disease in a transplant unit: Isolation of the causative agent from shower baths. *Lancet* **2**:118–121, 1980

116. Cordes LG, Wiesenthal AM, Gorman GW, et al Isolation of *Legionella pneumophila* from hospital shower heads *Ann Intern Med* **94**:195–197, 1981

117. Kugler JW, Armitage JO, Helms CM, et al: Nosocomial Legionnaires' disease. Occurrence in recipients of bone marrow transplants. *Am J Med* **74**:281–288, 1983

118. Copeland J, Wieden M, Feinberg W, et al: Legionnaires' disease following cardiac transplantation *Chest* **79**:669–671, 1981

119. Andersen RD, Lauer BA, Fraser DW, et al. Infections with *Legionella penumophila* in children. *J Infect Dis* **143**:386–390, 1981.

120. Ryan ME, Feldman S, Priutt B, et al: Legionnaires' disease in a child with cancer *Pediatrics* **64**:951–953, 1979

121. Kovatch AL, Jardine DS, Dowling JN, et al: Legionellosis in children with leukemia in relapse *Pediatrics* **73**:811–815, 1984

122. Murray JF, Felton CP, Garay SM, et al· Pulmonary complications of the acquired immunodeficiency syndrome *N Engl J Med* **310**:1682–1688, 1984

123. Fliermans CB, Cherry WB, Orrison LH, et al: Ecological distribution of *Legionella pneumophila Appl Environ Microbiol* **41**:9–16, 1981

124. Politi BD, Fraser DW, Mallison GF, et al A major focus of Legionnaires' disease in Bloomington, Indiana. *Ann Intern Med* **90**:587–591, 1979.

125. Tison DL, Pope DH, Cherry WB, et al: Growth of *Legionella pneumophila* in association with blue-green algae (cyanobacteria) *Appl Environ Microbiol* **39**:456–459, 1980

126. Tyndall RL, Domingue EL: Cocultivation of *Legionella pneumophila* and free-living amoebae *Appl Environ Microbiol* **44**:954–959, 1982.

127. Holden EP, Winkler HH, Wood DO, et al Intracellular growth of *Legionella pneumophila* within *Acanthamoeba castellanii* Neff *Infect Immun* **45**:18–24, 1984

128. Fields BS, Shotts EB, Feeley JC, et al. Proliferation of *Legionella pneumophila* as an intracellular parasite of the diliated protozoan *Tetrahymena pyriformis Appl Environ Microbiol* **47**:467–471, 1984

129. Best M, Yu VL, Stout J, et al. *Legionellaceae* in the hospital water-supply. *Lancet* **2**:307–310, 1983

130. Fisher-Hoch SP, Bartlett CLR, Tobin JO, et al. Investigation and control of an outbreak of Legionnaires' disease in a district general hospital *Lancet* **1**:932–936, 1981

131. Shands KN, Ho JL, Meyer RD, et al: Potable water as a source of Legionnaires' disease. *JAMA* **253**:1412–1416, 1985.

132. Wadowsky RM, Yee RB, Mezmar L, et al: Hot water systems as sources of *Legionella pneumophila* in hospital and nonhospital plumbing fixtures. *Appl Environ Microbiol* **43**:1104–1110, 1982.

133. Colbourne JS, Pratt DJ: Water fittings as sources of *Legionella pneumophila* in a hospital plumbing system. *Lancet* **1**:210–213, 1984.

134. Tobin JO, Swann RA, Bartlett CLR: Isolation of *Legionella pneumophila* from water systems: Methods and preliminary studies. *Br Med J* **282**:515–517, 1981.

135. Dennis PJ, Taylor JA, Ritzgeorge RB, et al: *Legionella pneumophila* in water plumbing systems. *Lancet* **1**:949–951, 1982.

136. Stout J, Yu VL, Vickers RM, et al: Potable water supply as the hospital reservoir for Pittsburgh Pneumonia Agent. *Lancet* **1**:471–472, 1982.

137. Gorman GW, Yu VL, Brown A, et al: Isolation of Pittsburgh Pneumonia Agent from nebulizers used in respiratory therapy. *Ann Intern Med* **93**:572–573, 1980.

138. Rudin JE, Wing EJ: An ongoing outbreak of *Legionella micdadei*. In Thornsberry C, Balows A, Feeley WC, Jakubowski W (eds): *Legionella. Proceedings of the Second Symposium.* American Society for Microbiology, Washington, DC, 1984, pp. 227–229.

139. Tsai TF, Finn DR, Plikaytis BD, et al: Legionnaires' disease: Clinical features of the epidemic in Philadelphia. *Ann Intern Med* **90**:509–517, 1979.

140. Helms CM, Viner JP, Sturm RH, et al: Comparative features of pneumococcal, mycoplasmal, and Legionnaires' disease pneumonias. *Ann Intern Med* **90**:543–547, 1979

141. Broome CV, Goings SAJ, Thacker SB, et al: The Vermont epidemic of Legionnaires' disease. *Ann Intern Med* **90**:573–577, 1979.

142. Sharrar RG, Friedman HM, Miller WT, et al: Summertime pneumonias in Philadelphia. An epidemiologic study. *Ann Intern Med* **90**:577–580, 1979.

143. Kirby BD, Snyder KM, Meyer RD, et al: Legionnaires' disease: Clinical features of 24 cases. *Ann Intern Med* **89**:297–309, 1978.

144. Kirby BD, Peck H, Meyer RD: Radiographic features of Legionnaires' disease. *Chest* **76**:562–565, 1979.

145. Fairbank JT, Mamourian AC, Dietrich PA, et al: The chest radiograph in Legionnaires' disease. *Radiology* **147**:33–34, 1983.

146. Kroboth FJ, Yu VL, Reddy SC, et al. Clinicoradiographic correlation with the extent of Legionnaire disease *AJR* **141**:263–268, 1983.

147. Edelstein PH, Meyer RD, Finegold SM. Long-term followup of two patients with pulmonary cavitation caused by *L. pneumophila*. *Am Rev Respir Dis* **124**:90–93, 1981.

148. Lake KB, Van Dyke JJ, Gerberg E, et al. Legionnaires' disease and pulmonary cavitation. *Arch Intern Med* **139**:485–486, 1979.

149. Lewin S, Brettman LR. Goldstein EJC, et al: Legionnaires' disease. A cause of severe abscess-forming pneumonia *Am J Med* **67**:339–342, 1979.

150. Gombert ME, Josephson A, Goldstein EJC, et al: Cavitary Legionnaires' pneumonia: Nosocomial infection in renal transplant recipients. *Am J Surg* **147**:402–405, 1984.

151. Dietrich PA, Johnson RD, Fairbank JT, et al: The chest radiograph in Legionnaires' disease. *Radiology* **127**:577–582, 1978.

152. Pope TL Jr, Armstrong P, Thompson R, et al: Pittsburgh Pneumonia Agent: Chest film manifestations. *AJR* **138**:237–241, 1982.

153. Muder RR, Reddy SC, Yu VL, et al. Pneumonia caused by Pittsburgh Pneumonia Agent. Radiographic manifestations. *Radiology* **150**:633–637, 1984.

154. Brabender W, Hinthorn DR, Asher M, et al: *L. pneumophila* wound infection. *JAMA* **250**:3091–3092, 1983.

155. Ramsey PG, Rubin RH, Tolkoff-Rubin NE, et al: The renal transplant patient with fever and pulmonary infiltrates: Etiology, clinical manifestations, and management. *Medicine (Baltimore)* **59**:206–222, 1980.

156. Fraser DW, Tsai TR, Orenstein W, et al. Legionnaires' disease. Description of an epidemic of pneumonia *N Engl J Med* **297**:1189–1197, 1977.

157. Edelstein PH, Meyer RD, Finegold SM. Laboratory diagnosis of Legionnaires' disease. *Am Rev Respir Dis* **121**:317–327, 1980.

158. Meyer RD, Edelstein PH, Kirby BD, et al· Legionnaires' disease: Unusual clinical and laboratory features *Ann Intern Med* **93**:240–243, 1980

159. Muder RR, Yu VL, Vickers RM, et al. Simultaneous infection with *Legionella pneumophila* and Pittsburgh Pneumonia Agent. Clinical features and epidemiologic implications. *Am J Med* **74**:609–614, 1983.

160. Broome CV, Cherry WB, Winn WC Jr, et al: Rapid diagnosis of Legionnaires' disease by direct immunofluorescent staining. *Ann Intern Med* **90**:1–4, 1979

161. Edelstein PH, McKinney RM, Meyer RD, et al Immunologic diagnosis of Legionnaires' disease: Cross-reactions with anaerobic and microaerophilic organisms and infections caused by them. *J Infect Dis* **141**:652–655, 1980.

162. Buesching WJ, Brust RA, Ayers LW. Enhanced primary isolation of *Legionella pneumophila* from clinical specimens by low-pH treatment. *J Clin Microbiol* **17**:1153–1155, 1983.

163. Zuravleff JJ, Yu VL, Shonnard JW, et al: Diagnosis of Legionnaires' disease. An update of laboratory methods with new emphasis on isolation by culture. *JAMA* **250**:1981–1985, 1983.

164. Vickers RM, Brown A, Garrity GM: Dye-containing buffered charcoal-yeast extract medium for differentiation of members of the family *Legionellaceae J Clin Microbiol* **13**:380–382, 1981.

165. Wing EJ, Schafer FJ, Pascule AW: The use of tracheal and pulmonary aspiration to diagnose *Legionella micdadei* pneumonia. *Chest* **82**:705–707, 1982

166. Kohorst WR, Schonfeld SA, Macklin JE, et al. Rapid diagnosis of Legionnaires' disease by bronchoalveolar lavage. *Chest* **84**:186–190, 1983.

167. Wilkinson HW· Serodiagnosis of legionellosis. *Legionella pneumophila, L. bozemanii, L micdadei,* and *L gormanii* as indirect immunofluorescence antigens In Schlessinger D

(ed): *Microbiology 1981*. American Society for Microbiology, Washington, DC, 1981, pp 165–168.

168. Wilkinson HW, Crude DD, Broome CV: Validation of *Legionella pneumophila* indirect immunofluorescence assay with epidemic sera. *J Clin Microbiol* **13**:139–146, 1981.

169. Wilkinson HW, Reingold WL, Brake BJ, et al. Reactivity of serum from patients with suspected legionellosis against 29 antigens of legionellaceae and *Legionella*-like organisms by indirect immunofluorescence assay *J Infect Dis* **147**:23–31, 1983.

170. Collins MT, McDonald J, Hoiby N, et al: Agglutinating antibody titers to members of the family *Legionellaceae* in cystic fibrosis patients as a result of cross-reacting antibodies to *Pseudomonas aeruginosa. J Clin Microbiol* **19**:757–762, 1984.

171. Kohler RB, Zimmerman SE, Wilson E, et al. Rapid radioimmunoassay diagnosis of Legionnaires' disease *Ann Intern Med* **94**:601–605, 1981.

172. Sathapatayavongs B, Kohler RB, Wheat LJ, et al: Rapid diagnosis of Legionnaires' disease by urinary antigen detection. Comparison of ELISA and radioimmunoassay *Am J Med* **72**:576–582, 1982.

173. Kohler RB, Winn WC Jr. Wheat LJ: Onset and duration of urinary antigen excretion in Legionnaires' disease. *J Clin Microbiol* **20**:605–607, 1984

174. Wing EJ, Schafer FJ, Pasculle AW: Successful treatment of *Legionella micdadei* (Pittsburgh Pneumonia Agent) pneumonia with erythromycin. *Am J Med* **71**:836–840, 1981

175. Rudin JE, Evans TL, Wing EJ. Failure of erythromycin in treatment of *Legionella micdadei* pneumonia. *Am J Med* **76**:318–320, 1984

176. Fraser DW, Wachsmuth IK, Bopp C, et al Antibiotic treatment of guinea pigs infected with agent of Legionnaires' disease. *Lancet* **1**:175–177, 1978.

177. Plouffe JF, Para MF, Bollin GE: Sulfamethoxazole–trimethaprim treatment of guinea pigs infected with *Legionella pneumophila. J Infect Dis* **150**:780–782, 1984.

178. Winn WC Jr, Davis GS, Gump DW, et al. Legionnaires' pneumonia after intratracheal inoculation of guinea pigs and rats. *Lab Invest* **47**:568–578, 1982

179. Edelstein PH, Calarco K, Yasui VK: Antimicrobial therapy of experimentally induced Legionnaires' disease in guinea pigs. *Am Rev Respir Dis* **130**:849–856, 1984.

180. Pasculle AW, Dowling JN. Antimicrobial therapy of experimental *Legionella micdadei* pneumonia in guinea pigs *Interscience Conference on Antimicrobial Agents and Chemotherapy, Miami Beach, Florida, 1982.* (abst. 95)

181. Thornsberry C, Baker CN, Kirven LA. In vitro activity of antimicrobial agents on Legionnaires' disease bacterium *Antimicrob Agents Chemother* **13**:78–80, 1978

182. Edelstein PH, Meyer RD. Susceptibility of *Legionella pneumophila* to twenty antimicrobial agents *Antimicrob Agents Chemother* **18**:403–408, 1980

183. Pasculle AW, Dowling JN, Weyant RS, et al Susceptibility of Pittsburgh Pneumonia Agent *(Legionella micdadei)* and other newly recognized members of the genus *Legionella* to nineteen antimicrobial agents *Antimicrob Agents Chemother* **20**:793–799, 1981

184. Dowling JN, Weyant RS, Pasculle AW. Bactericidal activity of antibiotics against *Legionella micdadei* (Pittsburgh Pneumonia Agent). *Antimicrob Agents Chemother* **22**:272–276, 1982.

185. Johnson JD, Hand WL, Francis JB, et al· Antibiotic uptake by alveolar macrophages *J Lab Clin Med* **95**:429–439, 1980.

186. Horwitz MA, Silverstein SC. Intracellular multiplication of Legionnaires' disease bacteria *(Legionella pneumophila)* in human monocytes is reversibly inhibited by erythromycin and rifampin *J Clin Invest* **71**:15–26, 1983

187. Yoshida S-I, Mizuguchi Y: Antibiotic susceptibility of *Legionella pneumophila* Philadelphia-1 in cultured guinea-pig peritoneal macrophages *J Gen Microbiol* **130**:901–906, 1984

188. Gibson DH, Fitzgeorge RB· Persistence in serum and lungs of guinea pigs of erythromycin, gentamicin, chloramphenicol and rifampicin and their in-vitro activities against *Legionella pneumophila. J Antimicrobial Chemother* **12**:235–244, 1983.

189. Meyer RD. Legionella infections: A review of five years of research. *Rev Infect Dis* **5**:258–278, 1983.

190. Sanders KL, Walker DH, Lee TJ Relapse of Legionnaires' disease in a renal transplant recipient. *Arch Intern Med* **140**:833–834, 1980

191. Katz SM, Habib WA, Hammel JM, et al. Lack of airborne spread of infection by *Legionella pneumophila* among guinea pigs *Infect Immun* **38**:620–622, 1982.

192. Yu VL, Zuravleff JJ, Gavlik L, et al. Lack of evidence for person-to-person transmission of Legionnaires' disease. *J Infect Dis* **147**:362, 1983

193. Bridge JA, Edelstein PH: Oropharyngeal colonization with *Legionella pneumophila J Clin Microbiol* **18**:1108–1112, 1983.

194. Bartlett CLR: Potable water as reservoir and means of transmission In Thornsberry C, Balows A, Feeley WC, Jakubowski W (eds): *Legionella Proceedings of the Second Symposium.* American Society for Microbiology, Washington, DC, 1984, pp. 210–215

12

Viral Hepatitis in the Compromised Host

JULES L. DIENSTAG

1. Introduction

Four categories of viral hepatitis have been recognized: hepatitis A, hepatitis B, non-A, non-B hepatitis, and hepatitis B-associated delta hepatitis. Although all four have the potential to produce similar illnesses, clinical severity and outcome as well as the contribution of immunologic mechanisms to the clinical expression of infection and illness appear to differ among the various types. Observations of viral hepatitis in immunosuppressed persons have taught us important lessons about the biology of these viral agents, on the one hand, and about the approach to immunologically compromised patients with hepatitis, on the other. Unlike susceptibility of immunosuppressed persons to opportunistic infections, susceptibility to viral hepatitis per se is not increased in the immunosuppressed; however, because patients with immunologic derangements are very likely to require transfusions of blood products, the frequency of viral hepatitis in this group of patients is increased. In addition, severity of acute illness, likelihood of chronic infection, infectivity, and the early and late consequences of chronic infection differ distinctly between immunocompetent and immunosuppressed hosts.

Among the four categories of viral hepatitis, only hepatitis B and non-A, non-B hepatitis agents appear to be more frequent and to alter clinical expression in immunocompromised persons. Hepatitis A is primarily an enterically spread virus, unassociated with appreciable viremia, chronic infection, or chronic hepatitis. Although the frequency of infection with hepatitis A virus (HAV) is high in persons with Down syndrome in whom immunologic deficiencies have been documented, the frequency of serologic markers of HAV infection is just as high in institutionalized persons with other forms of mental retardation, unassociated with compromised immune function.[1] Moreover, the clinical features and benign outcome of acute HAV infection in institutionalized mentally retarded persons are indistinguishable from those of comparably-aged normal, immunocompetent persons. In other categories of immunocompromised persons, such as those requiring chronic hemodialysis, neither the prevalence nor the incidence of HAV infection is higher than those found in immunocompetent persons.[2] As far as the recently described hepatitis B-associated delta hepatitis agent,[3] observations in immunosuppressed persons have yet to be described. Moreover, clinical and histologic observations exist which suggest that both HAV and the delta agent are directly toxic to hepatocytes and, unlike hepatitis B and non-A, non-B hepatitis agents, do not require participation by the host–immune system for cytopathology.[4,5] In considering viral hepatitis in the immunocompromised host, attention should therefore be drawn to hepatitis B and non-A, non-B hepatitis.

JULES L. DIENSTAG • Gastrointestinal Unit, Medical Services, Massachusetts General Hospital, and Department of Medicine, Harvard Medical School, Boston, Massachusetts 02114

2. Role of Immunologic Mechanisms in the Pathogenesis of Viral Hepatitis

2.1. Hepatitis B

Hepatitis B virus (HBV) is a DNA virus that belongs to the hepadnavirus group, characterized by three morphologic forms: a 42-nm genome-containing virion and 22-nm spherical and tubular forms composed of the virion surface protein, hepatitis B surface antigen (HBsAg); an association with acute and chronic liver disease; and a DNA genome with a single-stranded region. Within the virion is the nucleocapsid, on the surface of which is expressed hepatitis B core antigen (HBcAg) and on the inside of which is the DNA, DNA polymerase, and hepatitis B e antigen (HBeAg), a nonparticulate, internal nucleocapsid protein. In persons infected with HBV, serologic markers detectable routinely include HBsAg, HBeAg, their respective antibodies, anti-HBs and anti-HBe, and antibody to HBcAg (anti-HBc). In general, those with current HBV infection have circulating HBsAg and anti-HBc, whereas those who have recovered have circulating anti-HBc and anti-HBs. When current infection is accompanied by circulating HBeAg, the levels of replication and infectivity are high; in those with HBsAg in serum who are anti-HBe positive, virus replication and infectivity are quite limited. Among the several HBV antibodies, anti-HBs is considered the protective antibody; the goal of immunoprophylaxis is to provide the susceptible host with circulating anti-HBs. The three primary modes of hepatitis B transmission are via percutaneous–transmucosal inoculation, intimate contact, and perinatal exposure.

In immunocompetent persons infected with HBV, clinical expression of infection is quite variable. In most cases, infection is accompanied by liver cell necrosis and followed by virus elimination and recovery. In rare instances, most or all hepatocytes are destroyed, leading to fulminant hepatitis, with a mortality rate of approximately 80%. In about 10% of those with clinically apparent acute hepatitis B, infection remains chronic. Some in this category remain free of liver morphologic abnormalities and are classified as chronic carriers, while others continue to have liver cell necrosis and inflammation; those with chronic inflammatory activity may have mild to severe chronic hepatitis. In addition, both the level of viral replication and the rate of progression may vary considerably among persons with chronic hepatitis B. Because asymptomatic chronic hepatitis B carriers have normal liver morphology despite ongoing virus replication in liver cells, liver cell necrosis in hepatitis B appears not to be the result of a direct cytopathic injury by HBV. The differences in expression and outcome of HBV infection have therefore been attributed to variability in host-immune responsiveness.[6,7]

Observations that support the contribution of immunologic mechanisms include the following:

1. Chronic hepatitis B carriage is more likely to follow acute HBV infection in those with immunologic immaturity (e.g., neonates) or with immunologic deficiencies (e.g., persons with Down syndrome, lepromatous leprosy, chronic renal failure, and those receiving cytotoxic or immunosuppressive chemotherapy).[8-11]
2. Chimpanzees treated with cyclophosphamide during acute experimental infection with HBV remain chronically infected with the virus.[12]
3. A close spatial relationship exists between necrotic hepatocytes and mononuclear inflammatory cells, presumed to be the immunologic effectors of hepatocytolysis.
4. When cytotoxic chemotherapy is withdrawn in immunosuppressed persons with circulating HBsAg, massive hepatocellular necrosis and severe hepatitis may occur,[13] presumably as a result of the restoration of immune competence.
5. Similarly, in patients with chronic hepatitis B, immunosuppressive therapy allows an increase in the level of HBV replication, and a transient elevation in serum aminotransferase levels may follow withdrawal of immunosuppressive therapy.[14-16]

Cellular, rather than humoral, immune responsiveness has been postulated to be the major contributor to the immunopathogenesis of viral hepatitis. In chronically hemodialyzed patients and in those with lepromatous leprosy and Down syndrome, cellular immune defects are thought to be paramount. In addition, in patients with chronic hepatitis B, manipulation of humoral immunity by infusion of large doses of anti-HBs does not lead to hepatocellular necrosis,[17,18] while cellular immune stimulation or reconstitution is followed by elevation of aminotransferase levels, a reflection of liver cell injury.[18-20] Also cited to acquit humoral immune responses in the pathogenesis of liver injury in viral hepatitis is the observation that both acute and chronic hepatitis, often quite severe, can occur in the absence of intact humoral immune responsiveness, e.g., in patients with agammaglobulinemia.[21]

Current understanding of the immunopathogenesis of liver injury in hepatitis B is incomplete. Recent evidence has accumulated that suggests that cytolytic T cells directed at HBcAg expressed at the liver cell surface play a central role and that competition between these cytolytic T cells and circulating anti-HBc for HBcAg on the liver-cell membrane can modulate the cytolytic attack.[22,23] The data to support this hypothesis are inconclusive, and other mechanisms, perhaps at the immunoregulatory level, must be involved as well. What is more, a case of typical acute viral hepatitis B with complete recovery was recently documented in a patient with an underlying lifelong T-cell defect.[24] The occurrence of hepatocytolysis and the resolution of infection in the absence of T cell integrity weigh against the importance of cellular immune mechanisms in hepatitis B, and new evidence appears to support the role of nonimmunologic factors.[6] Adding even more to the complexity of the issue is the detection of HBV DNA and HBsAg in bone marrow cells and peripheral blood lymphocytes from patients with hepatitis B,[25] suggesting that HBV may have a direct effect on immunologic competence, mediated by infection of immunocytes. Still, despite uncertainties about how crucial immunologic factors are, clinical experience has taught us that immunologically impaired hosts respond differently than immunocompetent hosts do when infected with hepatitis B. Similarly, there is a predictable increase in the level of HBV replication in immunocompetent persons treated with immunosuppressive drugs.[14,15] In managing immunologically compromised patients, therefore, we have to remain cognizant of the relationship between immunologic integrity and response to hepatitis B.

2.2. Non-A, Non-B Hepatitis

Non-A, non-B hepatitis is the designation used to classify cases of viral hepatitis in which HAV and HBV, as well as other identifiable viruses, can be excluded serologically. Despite many reports to the contrary, no virus-specific agent or serologic marker has been identified. Cross-challenge studies in chimpanzees and studies of physicochemical properties, however, suggest that there are at least two blood-borne non-A, non-B agents. Although epidemiologic studies are limited by the absence of serologic markers, observations generated over the last decade suggest that HBV and non-A, non-B hepatitis are transmitted by similar routes of infection.[26,27]

Because of the many clinical and epidemiologic similarities between HBV and non-A, non-B hepatitis, these two types of viral hepatitis have been postulated to share similar pathophysiologic mechanisms. Although a limited number of immunologic observations have been described in patients with non-A, non-B hepatitis, this area of investigation has been handicapped by the absence of identifiable viral antigens. Thus, although laboratory evidence for a role of immunologic mechanisms is wanting, the occurrence of asymptomatic carriers with normal liver histology suggests that the virus agent(s) are not directly cytopathic to hepatocytes. As is the case for hepatitis B, immunologic properties of the host probably affect the clinical expression and outcome of non-A, non-B hepatitis infection, on the one hand, and, on the other, infection with non-A, non-B hepatitis appears to impair the host's immunologic competence.

3. Viral Hepatitis in the Immunocompromised Host

Following the identification of HBsAg, then known as Australia antigen, by Blumberg and associates,[28] the first patients found to have a high frequency (11%) of antigenemia were leukemics, and for a brief time, the antigen was even thought to be a leukemia antigen. When the frequency of chronic HB$_s$ antigenemia in other patient groups was tested, Blumberg and colleagues found that not only leukemics, but also institutionalized persons with Down syndrome (30%), patients with Hodgkin's disease

(8%), patients with lepromatous leprosy (20%), and chronically hemodialyzed patients with chronic renal failure (10%) had high HBsAg prevalences.[8-10] In each of these patient groups, cellular immune defects have been postulated or documented.[28,29]

In addition to the categories just listed of immunocompromised patients whose response to viral hepatitis differs from the norm are neonates. Immunologic immaturity is postulated to account for the unique clinical expression of HBV infection in the newborn and infants. Whereas acute infection in neonates tends to be asymptomatic, such infection early in life also tends to remain chronic, a feature of HBV infection in other immunocompromised patients. Even more reminiscent of the response to HBV infection in the immunosuppressed is that seen in persons with Down syndrome. In this population, defects in cellular immune function have been invoked to explain their high frequency of infections in general and of chronic infection after acute hepatitis B in particular.[30] As in neonates and other immunosuppressed persons, in those with Down syndrome, acute HBV infection is almost invariably subclinical. Chronicity has followed acute infection in 20–38% of persons with Down syndrome.[31-36] Although persons with this chromosomal aberration are not sufficiently immunocompromised to merit consideration as immunosuppressed patients for clinical purposes, their responses to HBV infection illustrate a pattern expressed in other immunosuppressed groups. Not only are they more likely to be exposed because of circumstances of their care (institutionalization at an early age), to have subclinical acute HBV infections, and to harbor infection chronically, but they are also more likely to support higher levels of virus replication and, therefore, to be more infectious for others. In a comparison by Szmuness et al.,[37] persons with Down syndrome and chronic HBV infection were found to have a higher prevalence of HBeAg than that of HBsAg-positive blood donors or HBsAg-positive persons with non-Down types of mental retardation (Table 1). The frequency of HBeAg in Down syndrome was even higher, 61%, in a study from Australia,[32] figures comparable to the HBeAg prevalence found by Szmuness et al.[37] in hemodialysis patients (Table 1). The important point is that those with Down syndrome not only experience a high risk of HBV infection themselves but also serve as a reservoir for dissemination of infection to others institu-

TABLE 1. Frequency of Replicative Hepatitis B Virus Infection in HBsAg Carrier Populations, as Reflected by HBeAg Status[a]

Carrier population	Percent with HBeAg
Volunteer blood donors	9
Mentally retarded persons	
Down syndrome	39
Other mentally retarded	10
Hemodialysis patients	71

[a]Adapted from Szmuness et al [37]

tionalized with them and to those who care for them; they become a focus for the amplification of HBV infection.

Most reports on viral hepatitis in immunocompromised persons represent observations about hepatitis B, but the importance of non-A, non-B hepitatis is also being recognized. Generalizations such as those reviewed for persons with Down syndrome appear to apply also to other groups with naturally acquired or immunosuppressive therapy-induced immunodeficiencies. They are more likely to require blood products and to be exposed to the blood-borne hepatitis viruses, HBV and non-A, non-B hepatitis. Once infected, immunocompromised persons are less likely to have clinically recognizable or severe acute illnesses but are more likely to remain chronically infected than they are to clear their infections. Moreover, they have a higher likelihood of supporting high levels of virus replication and of being infectious for their contacts. Thus, immunosuppressed persons with viral hepatitis, because of blunted clinical expression on the one hand but increased virus replication on the other, are more likely to pose a risk of infection to their health providers and to serve as foci for perpetuation of infection among others hospitalized with them. Infection with these hepatitis agents, in turn, appears to lead to more profound immunosuppression in these already immunocompromised hosts, an effect with the potential for beneficial as well as detrimental consequences.

From a practical perspective, clinically significant immunosuppression and hepatitis are likely to overlap and to be encountered primarily in three categories of patients, hemodialyzed patients with chronic renal failure, recipients of organ transplants, and patients with lymphoproliferative and myeloproliferative malignancies.

3.1. Hemodialyzed Patients with Chronic Renal Failure

3.1.1. Hepatitis B in Hemodialysis Units

During the late 1960s and early 1970s, hepatitis B was recognized as a major hazard for patients and staff of hemodialysis units.[38,39] A substantial body of literature documented the high risk observed during that period, the tendency for HBsAg to be of subtype *ay* rather than the more prevalent *ad,* and the mechanisms of transmission in such units. In a study by Szmuness et al.,[40] the point prevalence of current or past HBV infection was 50% in patients and 34% in staff. During the first year in hemodialysis units, the incidence of new infections ranged between 40 and 47% in patients and staff. Recognition soon emerged of the relationship between duration of treatment and intensity of blood exposure in dialysis units and hepatitis B. In these units, extracorporeal blood is present almost continuously, and little imagination is required to comprehend that HBV can be transmitted via blood leaks in dialysis machines as well as via contamination by blood of gloves, clamps, other instruments, dialysis machine surfaces and control knobs, and other environmental surfaces.[41] These observations do not distinguish those in dialysis units from immunologically competent persons. Indeed, although the modes of inoculation differed, the risks to patients (exposed via blood transfusion and contaminated instruments and surfaces) and staff (exposed primarily via needlesticks and other percutaneous–transmucosal penetrations) were quite comparable. Here the similarities ended, however.

On the one hand, hemodialysis patients were much more likely than hemodialysis staff to have an asymptomatic, anicteric acute illness associated with HBV infection, while, on the other hand, hemodialysis patients were substantially more susceptible to chronic infection (Table 2).[38,42–46] Once chronically infected, hemodialysis patients were also more likely to remain HBeAg-positive, i.e., to have high levels of ongoing viral replication and to be infectious (Table 2).[37,47,48] Thus, although specific im-

TABLE 2. Hepatitis B Virus Infection in Hemodialysis Units: Comparison between Patients and Staff

	Patients (%)	Staff (%)
Prevalence of current or past infection[2,40,42]	50–67	34
Incidence of new infections during first year[2,40]	40	47
Clinically apparent acute illness[38]	32	85
Remain chronically infected[43–46]	60–90	10
HBeAg-positive chronic infection[37,47,48]	53–61	10

munologic defects have not been demonstrated consistently in hemodialysis patients with chronic HBV infection,[43,44] hemodialysis patients do have evidence of depressed cellular immune function[29] and do respond to HBV infection as immunosuppressed hosts do—with failure to destroy virus-infected hepatocytes and, therefore, with a paucity of hepatitis symptoms; with failure to clear infection; and with failure to contain virus replication and infectivity. Therefore, once HBV infection is introduced into a dialysis unit, unless steps are taken to control or eliminate it (see Section 4), dialysis patients who are infected tend to be very infectious and to propagate the cycle of infection within the hemodialysis unit to other patients and staff and to amplify the spread of infection outside the unit to family and other household contacts.[40,49,50]

Limited information is available about the long-term consequences of chronic HBV infection in hemodialysis patients. Many come eventually to renal transplantation, which may have a dramatic impact on their clinical courses (see Section 3.2), and few studies have been done to assess hepatic morphology and the course of liver disease in hemodialysis patients who do not receive renal homografts. What data exist indicate that histologic progression is quite variable in this group of HBsAg-positive patients.[51,52] Clinical expression of HBV infection, however, remains silent. In one study for example,[52] liver histology ranged from normal to chronic persistent hepatitis to chronic lobular hepatitis to chronic active hepatitis. Follow-up biopsies done in a limited number of these patients showed progression from the milder forms of chronic hepatitis (chronic persistent and chronic lobular hepatitis) to chronic active hepatitis with fibrosis, despite the absence of necrosis and inflammation. Despite such progression, symptoms were minimal or absent, and aminotransferase levels were no higher than 1.5–3 times the upper limits of normal. Thus, as observed in other immunosuppressed patients (see Section 3.2), histologic liver lesions that are nonprogressive in immunocompetent hosts may deteriorate silently to more severe lesions in hemodialysis patients with chronic HBV infection.[53]

3.1.2. Non-A, Non-B Hepatitis in Hemodialysis Units

Control measures have reduced substantially the risk of HBV infection in hemodialysis units (see Section 4). As the risk of hepatitis B has declined, however, the occurrence of non-A, non-B hepatitis in patients and staff of dialysis units has been recognized with increasing frequency. Attention to hemodialysis-associated non-A, non-B hepatitis was generated initially by Galbraith et al.,[54] who described two outbreaks in a London hospital of HBsAg-negative hepatitis in 1966–1967 and 1968–1970 involving 29 hemodialysis patients. Originally labeled incorrectly as cases of hepatitis A,[55] these illnesses were shown by retrospective serologic analysis to be classified as cases of non-A, non-B hepatitis. Seven patients had two discrete episodes of non-A, non-B hepatitis, and in eight, chronic liver disease developed. Another dramatic outbreak of hemodialysis-associated hepatitis occurred in Edinburgh in 1969–1978.[56] Lasting 14 months, this outbreak involved 29 cases of clinical hepatitis, five asymptomatic HBV infections, and 13 clinical cases in staff. The high frequency of cases, the exceptionally high mortality of 24% in patients and 31% in staff, and the high frequency of hepatic failure (coagulopathy or encephalopathy) even in survivors led to a year-long closing down of the dialysis program to new patients. Many of the cases were HBsAg-positive, but non-A, non-B hepatitis appears to have been involved as well. Although the reason for the very high mortality could not be established with certainty, a clue emerged from a study in an experimental animal. Serum from one of the HBsAg-positive patients who was implicated in transmitting hepatitis to six staff members, including three who succumbed, was inoc-

ulated in a chimpanzee. The hepatitis B that developed was very mild, but there was a prolonged period of liver biochemical abnormalities in the animal in the absence of HBV antigens in liver tissue. This analysis suggested that dual infection with HBV and a non-A, non-B hepatitis agent was responsible for the alarming severity observed. Other outbreaks and sporadic cases of non-A, non-B hepatitis have been reported from other hemodialysis units.[57,58]

Studies have been undertaken as well to assess the prevalence and incidence of non-A, non-B hepatitis in dialysis units. Koretz et al.[59] found elevated aminotransferase levels in 16% of patients in a hemodialysis unit in Los Angeles, a substantial proportion of which cases could not be attributed serologically to current HBV infection. Similarly, in an HBV-free hemodialysis unit in a teaching hospital in Boston, 15% of patients were found to have elevated aminotransferase activities in the absence of serologic evidence for current infection with hepatitis A or B or cytomegalovirus (CMV).[60] Studies of the incidence of new non-A, non-B hepatitis cases in hemodialysis units have shown an annual attack rate of approximately 5% for patients and approximately 1% for staff.[61,62] In one study, the risk of non-A, non-B hepatitis for patients was associated significantly with recent transfusion, while, for staff, the most important risk factor was recent needlestick.[60] The importance of these modes of transmission and the absence of secondary cases among family members of affected patients and staff (in contrast to hemodialysis-associated hepatitis B) provide compelling evidence for predominantly percutaneous transmission of non-A, non-B hepatitis in dialysis units and the requirement of direct percutaneous exposure for efficient transmission of non-A, non-B hepatitis (in contrast to hepatitis B, which may rely in addition on nonpercutaneous routes for its spread). An important observation is that, as is true for hepatitis B in hemodialysis units, severity of dialysis-associated non-A, non-B hepatitis was found to be less pronounced and jaundice less frequent but the likelihood of chronicity higher in patients than in staff.[60]

3.2. Hepatitis in Recipients of Organ Transplants

Hepatitis occurs in recipients of transplanted kidneys, livers, hearts, and bone marrow, but adequate study has been undertaken and reported only in recipients of renal transplants. In liver transplant recipients, other factors, such as graft rejection, are a cause for abnormal biochemical tests and for histologic changes that obscure the presence of suspected transplantation-associated viral hepatitis. Therapy with immunosuppressive drugs such as azathioprine and cyclosporin A, not to mention other potentially hepatotoxic drugs, may also contribute to impaired liver function in transplant recipients. On the other hand, evidence points to a role for viral hepatitis agents in a substantial proportion of the hepatic dysfunction seen in transplanted patients. Data generated in the study of renal transplant patients should be applicable to recipients of other organ transplants as well.

3.2.1. Hepatitis B in Renal Transplant Recipients

Exposure to hepatitis B is common among renal transplant recipients. Hemodialysis preceding transplantation, intentional pretransplantation blood transfusions, and additional exposure in the peritransplant period contribute to the potential for HBV infection. Rarely, the transplanted organ may derive from an HBsAg-positive donor.[63,64] Among these risk factors, pretransplantation hemodialysis is considered the largest contributor by some investigators,[65] but others find that the frequencies of pretransplantation and post-transplantation HBV infection are similar.[66] In 1974, Luby et al.[67] followed 45 consecutive renal transplant recipients prospectively and identified nine cases (20%) of hepatitis B. In addition to the natural immunosuppression of the chronic renal failure and hemodialysis that antedate transplantation, transplant recipients are subjected to pharmacologic immunosuppression with high-dose corticosteroids and azathioprine or cyclosporin A, not to mention occasional requirements for other forms of immunosuppressive therapy, all designed to abrogate cellular immune function sufficiently to prevent allograft rejection. As expected, like other immunosuppressed patients, once infected with HBV, they are less likely to experience a recognizable acute icteric illness, but they are more likely to remain chronically infected, to retain high levels of virus replication, and to be very infectious for their contacts.[51] The presence of HBsAg in their urine is

quite common[68] and has also been linked circumstantially to HBV exposure in their family contacts.[69] There are even reports of *reactivation* of hepatitis B after renal transplantation in a number of patients who became HBsAg positive after transplantation but who had anti-HBc in an earlier serum sample[16,70,71] or reactivation of viral replication in those with nonreplicative HBV infection at the time of transplantation.[71] These patterns have been observed more commonly in oncology patients receiving cytotoxic chemotherapy (see Section 3.3). Although their frequency in transplant recipients is unknown, their occurrence raises the possibility that some apparent de novo cases of hepatitis B after transplantation may actually represent reactivation.

In addition, several investigators have found differences in graft and patient survival that are influenced by the recipient's response to HBV. London et al.[72,73] found that patients with chronic HBV infection (HBsAg positivity) prior to transplantation appear to have a higher rate of allograft survival, while transplant patients, primarily females, with pretransplantation anti-HBs and who receive male donor kidneys have an increased rate of allograft rejection, independent of donor–recipient HLA status or of the status of the donor (cadaver vs. living–related) (Fig. 1).[72] To explain these differences, London and colleagues proposed the hypothesis that an antigenic determinant on certain strains of HBV cross-reacts with an antigen on the tissues of some males. No cross-reactivity could be found with the male Y antigen, however, and although London's group made the same observation in a second cohort of transplant recipients, other investigators have not been able to confirm the original observation. Although slight decreases in graft survival among anti-HBs-positive renal transplant recipients have been observed by others,[74] the differences have not always been significant, and others detect no difference[42] in or even an increase in graft survival among anti-HBs-positive patients; most investigators have not been able to detect any difference in graft survival (i.e., no increase in graft tolerance) in HBsAg-positive recipients,[73] except, perhaps, among those who acquire their HBV infections after transplantation.[75]

The other controversy in the literature relates to the effect of HBV infection on patient survival after renal transplantation. Pirson et al.[76] reported that, whether HBsAg was present at the time of transplan-

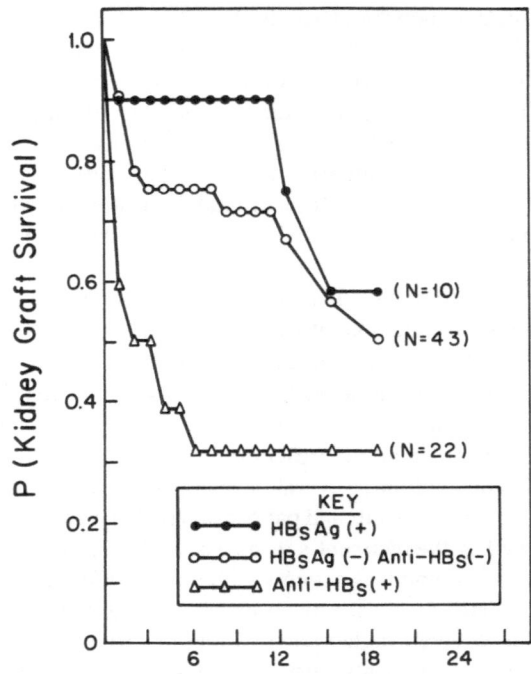

FIGURE 1. Renal-allograft survival curves for patients who were known HBsAg carriers, who had no hepatitis B markers, or who had anti-HBs prior to transplantation. The numbers in parentheses represent the numbers of patients in each category. (From London et al.[72], with permission.)

tation or acquired thereafter, mortality, resulting from progressive liver disease, was fivefold higher between 6 months and 4 years after transplantation in HBsAg-positive renal allograft recipients. Similarly, Hillis et al.[77] found that renal transplant recipients who were HBsAg positive at the time of transplantation had a dramatically reduced survival; those who acquired the infection after transplantation also had a higher mortality rate. In this series, however, most deaths were not related to liver disease but to other factors, primarily other infections and cerebrovascular accidents. Many other investigators, however, have been unable to detect any increase in patient mortality, whether from hepatic or nonhepatic causes, in HBsAg-positive renal transplant recipients.[75,78-82] Some have attempted to attribute the differences between the two conflicting experiences to the confounding effect of differences in immunosuppressive protocols, in superimposed non-A,

non-B hepatitis and/or CMV infection, or in the background frequency of HBV infection in the transplanted populations; however, differences in these variables fail to explain the conflicting observations. Potentially, HLA differences between HBsAg-positive and HBsAg-negative patients could affect the outcome of transplantation, and Hillis et al.[83] found an increased freqency of HLA Bw15, Bw17, and Bw35 in HBsAg-positive patients with end-stage renal failure. These observations have not been confirmed, however.[84]

The data generating the most concern were reported recently by Parfrey et al.[85] In a prospective study of 22 immunosuppressed renal transplant recipients with HBsAg in serum, approximately two-thirds of whom were documented to have acquired their HBV infections within the first 6 months after transplantation, these investigators found, as expected, that none lost their circulating HBsAg during a 1–8-year follow-up. Despite relatively benign histologic diagnoses on initial biopsy (normal histology or chronic persistent hepatitis), progression was quite common. Ultimately, by the end of the observation period, seven (32%) had cirrhosis and six (27%) had chronic active hepatitis. Eight of the 13 with chronic active hepatitis or cirrhosis had clinical evidence of jaundice, portal hypertension, and/or liver failure; three died of liver failure, and two died of hepatocellular carcinoma. Most of the deaths resulted from liver disease, and the rate of liver-related deaths in the HBsAg-positive renal transplant group was 5% per patient-year. By contrast, a cohort of 10 HBsAg-positive patients with chronic renal failure followed in the same way but, managed with maintenance hemodialysis instead of transplantation, experienced no liver-related deaths, and four ultimately lost their HBsAg. Another case of hepatocellular carcinoma 10 years after renal transplantation was reported in a woman who became HBsAg-positive four months after transplantation and remained persistently infected with HBV.[86] These ominous findings led Parfrey et al.[85] to suggest that transplantation of HBsAg-positive patients with end-stage chronic renal failure may be inadvisable. Because of the contradictory observations in the literature, however, current data are insufficient to support such a policy.

As noted above for hemodialysis patients, and as emphasized by the findings of Parfrey et al.,[85] transplant recipients with chronic hepatitis B may have insidiously progressive chronic active hepatitis and cirrhosis in the absence of symptoms.[51,87] Degos et al.[65] found that in 25% of patients with chronic persistent hepatitis at the time of transplantation, their histologic lesions evolved to the more severe and progressive chronic active hepatitis; Parfrey et al.[85] found that 42% of patients with normal liver histology or chronic persistent hepatitis on initial biopsy progressed to chronic active hepatitis or cirrhosis.

Other factors besides HBV may contribute to hepatic dysfunction in renal transplant patients and should be included in differential diagnostic considerations. Azathioprine may be hepatotoxic[88,89]; other hepatotropic (non-A, non-B hepatitis agents) and systemic virus infections, especially herpes simplex and zoster and CMV[90] may cause liver dysfunction; sepsis, too, can result in secondary hepatocellular dysfunction. As hepatitis B has been reduced in hemodialysis populations by control measures, so too has the role of HBV in posttransplant hepatic disease declined. Current data suggest that non-A, non-B hepatitis agent(s) are the cause of most cases of transplantation-associated hepatitis.

3.2.2. Non-A, Non-B Hepatitis in Renal Transplant Recipients

Non-A, non-B hepatitis can cause appreciable morbidity and even mortality in renal transplant recipients. Ware et al.[91] described 72 episodes of acute hepatitis or elevations in serum aminotransferase activity in 62 (38%) of 162 renal transplant recipients. Although drug hepatotoxicity and infections with CMV, HBV, Epstein-Barr virus (EBV), or varicella zoster could be incriminated in as many as 74% of the 34 cases of acute hepatitis, drug hepatotoxicity or infection with these agents was not linked to the chronic liver disease encountered in this group of patients. Of the 38 cases of chronic liver disease, 27 (71%) were attributed by serologic exclusion to non-A, non-B hepatitis agent(s). Sixteen of the patients with chronic liver disease, most of whom had non-A, non-B hepatitis, had progressive deterioration; cirrhosis ultimately developed in 11, four experienced a transition from chronic persistent to chronic active hepatitis, and one died of liver failure 1 year after the onset of disease. At least 18% of cases of chronic liver disease in a renal transplant unit in Spain were

classified as non-A, non-B hepatitis, and the proportion would have been even higher if any of the cases had been included that were associated with antibodies to, but not necessarily caused by, cytomegalovirus or HBV.[92] In all likelihood, many of the other unexplained cases of liver disease described in renal transplant recipients[90,93] are also related to non-A, non-B hepatitis agent(s).

Degos et al.[65] found that most cases of liver disease in renal transplant recipients began prior to transplantation and were acquired during hemodialysis. By contrast, analyses by others have shown that most of the liver disease that occurs in renal transplant recipients occurs after transplantation. In a report by LaQuaglia et al.,[94] the 10-year experience of 405 consecutive renal transplant recipients at the Massachusetts General Hospital was reviewed. Despite reliance on frozen washed red blood cells (RBCs) as the exclusive source of transfused blood, biochemical or clinical evidence of acute hepatitis occurred after transplantation in 10.4%, 62% of whom (or 6.5% of the total) were categorized by serologic and clinical exclusion as having non-A, non-B hepatitis. Five cases were caused by HBV, but all five occurred during the first 3 years of the observation period, 1970–1973, a trend that has been recognized almost universally in American transplantation programs. Therefore, the relative population of non-A, non-B hepatitis cases during the last 7 years of observation was even higher. After acute infection, chronicity was very common; chronic hepatitis developed in 93% of those whose acute hepatitis occurred during the first year after transplantation and in 64% of those affected after the first year. Not only was chronicity likely, but morbidity and mortality were unexpectedly common. Those with hepatitis had a significantly higher mortality rate (45%) than patients without hepatitis (16%) (Fig. 2). The surprising finding about this high mortality was that death in approximately 80% of fatal cases was due not to liver disease (only one patient died of liver failure) but to extrahepatic sepsis. Similarly, even among survivors, life-threatening extrahepatic infections were significantly more common in patients with hepatitis (52%) than in patients without hepatitis (20%) and a substantial cause of morbidity (Table 3). In addition to the increased frequency of serious infections in the patients with hepatitis, there was a significantly increased 1-year allograft survival in the

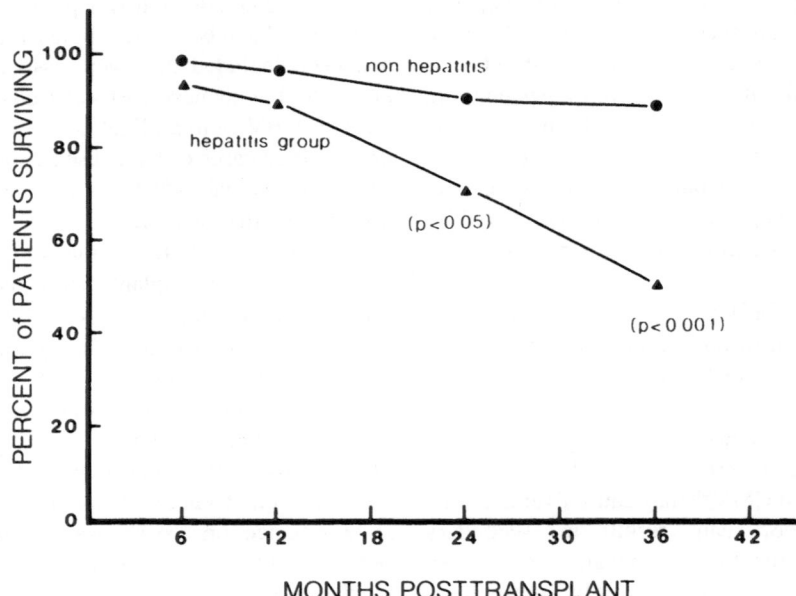

FIGURE 2. Survival of patients with and without hepatitis following renal transplantation. (From LaQuaglia et al.[94])

patients with hepatitis (73%) compared with that in patients without hepatitis (50%) (Table 3). These observations suggested that non-A, non-B hepatitis infection, like infection with CMV, had an immunosuppressive effect on transplant recipients.

On the basis of this observation and in an attempt to prevent this increase in life-threatening infections, this group has adopted a protocol of reducing the doses of immunosuppressive drugs in renal transplant patients with hepatitis and has not experienced an increase in organ rejection during such reductions.

TABLE 3. Impact of Non-A, Non-B Hepatitis on Renal Transplant Recipients[a]

Clinical feature	Hepatitis (%)	No hepatitis (%)
Graft survival	73	50
Mortality	45	16
Life-threatening infections among survivors	52	20

[a]From LaQuaglia et al [94]

Illustrative Case 1

A 62-year-old male executive presented for evaluation of gout; after administration of intravenous contrast material during a pyelogram, renal failure developed precipitously. Recovery was incomplete, and chronic renal failure followed, necessitating hemodialysis for more than 1 year before a cadaver kidney became available for transplantation in mid-1982. His immediate posttransplant course was uncomplicated, and maintenance immunosuppressive therapy consisted of standard doses of prednisone and azathioprine. His liver biochemical tests remained normal during hemodialysis but became abnormal within several months after transplantation; his aminotransferase levels ran in the mid-100 to mid-300 range. All serologic tests for hepatitis A and B viruses remained undetectable. Two years after transplantation, he noted swelling of his right elbow, and he was found to have staphylococcal olecranon bursitis. Antibiotic therapy with nafcillin was complicated by disseminated rash and an acute icteric hepatitislike exacerbation in his liver biochemical tests. Percutaneous liver biopsy during his hepatitislike episode revealed underlying cirrhosis and a histologic pattern, remarkable for polymorphonuclear and eosinophilic infiltration, consistent with a superimposed acute toxic hepatitis, i.e., presumably a drug reaction to nafcillin. The course was complicated also by bilateral pneumonitis, which resolved without definitive diagnosis. Recovery and convalescence were slow, but he returned home and did well except for an episode 3 months later of acute cholecystitis. Cholecystectomy was performed without incident. Three months later, however, he was admitted with arthritis of his left thumb and both ankles. A diagnosis of pseudogout was made when arthrocentesis yielded positively birefringent crystals. As he was being treated with a nonsteroidal antiinflammatory drug for his arthritis, necrotizing cutaneous lesions, fever, and renal deterioration developed. A skin biopsy was consistent with septic vasculitis, but neither broad-spectrum antibiotics nor corticosteroids arrested the process, and he succumbed. At postmortem examination, his lungs were studded with white nodules; both these and his cutaneous lesions, as well as his small bowel, were found to contain *Legionella*.

Comment. This patient's course provides an example of acute liver dysfunction presenting after transplantation and progressing within 2 years to postnecrotic cirrhosis. By serologic exclusion, he was believed to have non-A, non-B hepatitis. His clinical course beginning 2 years after transplantation, while on maintenance immunosuppressive therapy, was dominated by life-threatening infections, first *Staphylococcus* bursitis, then disseminated legionellosis, which was his cause of death. Although the organism found at autopsy was a surprise, the case is a good example of the type of extrahepatic life-threatening infections to which patients with non-A, non-B hepatitis after transplantation are at increased risk.

The report by LaQuaglia et al.[94] was based on a 10-year experience, but most of the morbidity and mortality (associated with extrahepatic sepsis) was observed during the first 3 years of follow-up in individual patients. Since the publication of this study, however, many of the patients with chronic non-A, non-B hepatitis have reached a follow-up interval of 5–10 years. Whereas the early morbidity and mortality were unrelated to hepatic decompensation, the late morbidity and mortality have shifted to hepatic deterioration. After 5–10 years of asymptomatic low-level elevations of aminotransferase activity, several of these patients have presented with new-onset ascites, hepatic encephalopathy, or bleeding from esophageal varices. In fact, the same slow, insidious, late deterioration has been observed 5–10 years after the onset of transfusion-associated non-A, non-B hepatitis in immunocompetent persons.[95] Whether the frequency of late hepatic deterioration differs between immunosuppressed and immunocompetent persons remains to be determined. The important point is that in immunosuppressed transplant recipients, subtle progression of chronic liver disease does occur, and the absence of symptoms or of clinical evidence of hepatic inflammation and necrosis belie the severity of the disease.

Illustrative Case 2

A 50-year-old woman underwent uneventful HLA-identical, living-related-donor renal transplantation in 1975 for chronic renal failure resulting from membranous glomerulonephritis. She had been hemodialyzed for 3 months prior to transplantation, but her liver tests were normal at the time of transplantation. She was maintained on a standard maintenance regimen of alternate-day prednisone and azathioprine. Eleven months after transplantation, she was noted to have minor elevations (1.5 × the upper limit of normal) in her serum aminotransferase level. Thereafter, her liver tests hovered in the normal to near-normal range, with aminotransferase levels ranging between normal and twice normal and bilirubin usually in the normal range, never exceeding 1.8 mg/dl, she had no symptoms of liver disease, and all serological tests for infection with hepatitis A and B viruses were negative. Ten years after transplantation, at the age of 60, she presented with upper gastrointestinal (GI) bleeding and was found to have esophageal varices. Her SGOT was normal, and her bilirubin was 1.3 mg/dl. She underwent sclerotherapy, which controlled her bleeding, but three months later she experienced massive variceal bleeding again and required emergency portasystemic shunt. At the time of surgery, she was found to have portal vein thrombosis, and she was anticoagulated. Shortly thereafter, she had another episode of upper GI bleeding. This was the result of a gastric ulcer, and endoscopic biopsy revealed plasmacytoma. She died 3 months after her shunt of complications of her malignancy and liver failure.

Comment. This is an example of slow, insidious, late progression of chronic non-A, non-B hepatitis to end-stage chronic liver disease and its complications. The important observation was the fact that the patient had no symptoms of liver disease and only subtle abnormalites in her liver biochemical tests. Similar cases have been observed in which the presenting manifestations of end-stage liver disease 5–10 years after transplantation were new-onset ascites or hepatic encephalopathy.

Non-A, non-B hepatitis, including fatal cases, is being recognized with increasing frequency at renal transplantation centers. Although generally obscured by other potential causes of liver dysfunction in liver transplant recipients, non-A, non-B hepatitis has been observed in this group of organ recipients as well. An example is a case described of severe acute non-A, non-B hepatitis progressing to cirrhosis and death in a liver transplant recipient.[96]

3.3. Hepatitis in Oncology Patients

3.3.1. Hepatitis B in Oncology Patients Receiving Chemotherapy

Hepatitis B has been shown to be a hazard for oncology patients who require immunosuppressive therapy.[9,10,13,97–106] Reports of the frequency of circulating HBsAg in oncology patients with leukemia and lymphoma ranged from a low of 1% to a high of 33%; the frequency of antibodies to HBV in these patients has been reported in the range of 19–55%.[9,10,99,100,107–110] Therefore, total current or past exposure to HBV has been observed in 29–69% of patients with myeloproliferative and lymphoproliferative malignancies. In patients with solid tumors, the frequencies are lower; HBsAg has been found in approximately 1% and HBV antibodies in an additional 1–16%.[100,110,111] These high frequencies of HBV infection result from the exposure of such patients to blood products—especially when bone marrow is replaced by malignant cells and during therapy-induced marrow aplasia—and high-risk hospital environments. Moreover, their immunosuppressed status subjects them to a high likelihood of remaining chronically infected with HBV.

During cytotoxic chemotherapy, immunosuppression allows an often dramatic increase in the level of circulating viremia, as reflected by substantial rises in the titer of HBsAg during therapy and return to pretreatment titers when the marrow is repopulated,[100] conversion from nonreplicative (HBeAg/DNA polymerase/HBV DNA negative) to replicative (HBeAg/polymerase/HBV DNA positive) HBV infection (Fig. 3),[104] and, even occasionally, reexpression of hepatitis B surface antigenemia in patients whose blood contained anti-HBs prior to chemotherapy,[100,101,107,112] i.e., a reactivation of HBV infection.[100,104,113] Because levels of viremia are high, and because most of the infections are subclinical, these patients provide a poorly appreciated reservoir of HBV infection and serve as a source of infection for the medical personnel who care for them as well as family members.[101,107,114] Falls in the

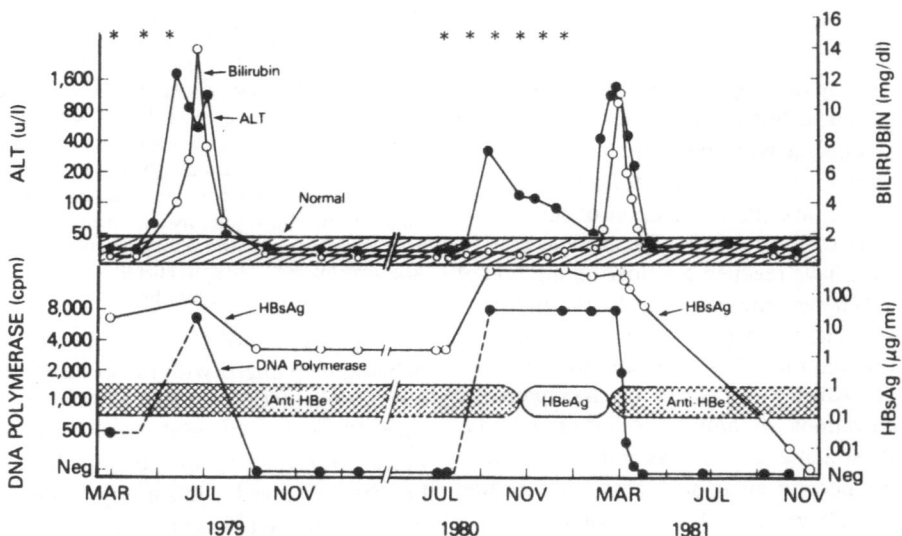

FIGURE 3. Clinical, biochemical, and serologic findings in a 35-year-old HBsAg-positive patient with lymphoma who underwent chemotherapy. Asterisks (∗) indicate courses of chemotherapy. Clinical and histologic evaluation prior to chemotherapy suggested that the patient was an asymptomatic HBsAg carrier. Prior to chemotherapy, she lacked serum HBV DNA and had circulating anti-HBe, but she had low-level DNA polymerase activity. During the third course of combination chemotherapy with cyclophosphamide, vincristine, prednisone, and procarbazine, she became icteric, and serum alanine aminotransferase (ALT) increased dramatically During her severe episode of acute hepatitis, her HBsAg titer and DNA polymerase level increased, HBV DNA became detectable in serum, and her prothrombin time increased to 4 sec above that of control With recovery from this severe episode of hepatitis, her ALT, bilirubin, and HBsAg titer fell to prechemotherapy levels, and both HBV DNA and DNA polymerase became undetectable Approximately 1 year later, when her lymphoma recurred and she was treated again with chemotherapy, she had an increase in expression of HBV replication, reflected by an asymptomatic increase in HBsAg titer, reappearance in serum of HBV DNA and DNA polymerase, and coversion from anti-HBe positive to HBeAg positive. Chemotherapy was discontinued after six cycles, and 3 months later, severe hepatitis recurred, with high ALT and bilirubin, coagulopathy (prothrombin time 12 sec above control), and encephalopathy At the same time, markers of high HBV replication disappeared Prednisone therapy was instituted, and the severe hepatitis resolved Nine months later, her HBsAg became undetectable. HBsAg, hepatitis B surface antigen, HBeAg, hepatitis B e antigen. (From Hoofnagel et al [104])

level of anti-HBs have also been observed during chemotherapy-induced marrow aplasia in these patients,[100] and many oncology patients who are immunosuppressed fail to mount any antibody response (anti-HBs or anti-HBc) to HBV.[107]

The interesting observation of high virus replication during cytotoxic chemotherapy and low or undetectable virus replication before and after chemotherapy, the pattern observed by most investigators, is difficult to reconcile with the conflicting and difficult-to-understand observation reported by Vergani et al.[105] These investigators could not detect HBV markers in serum in a small group of Italian children with acute leukemia in whom HBV antigens could be detected in hepatocytes. Moreover, the levels of HBsAg in these children increased (a reflection of increased virus replication) and became detectable after chemotherapy was completed. The discrepancy between this sole report on the one hand and all the other reports on the other has not been explained satisfactorily.

Concern for these patients has been raised by the observation that withdrawal of chemotherapy in asymptomatic HBsAg carrier oncology patients has been associated with acute hepatitislike exacerbations. Although in some patients, this may be followed by recovery and elimination of the virus,[104] in others, massive hepatic necrosis with fulminant, often fatal hepatitis, rarely chronic active hepatitis, follows within 1–6 weeks,[13,115,116] up to 3 months in one case.[104] These events have been interpreted as a reflection of the absence of a direct cytopathic effect of HBV during periods of intense virus replication in the permissive environment of chemotherapy but recurrence of presumably immunologically mediated lysis of an abundance of HBV-infected and virus-antigen-expressing hepatocytes once immune competence is restored by withdrawal of immunosuppressive therapy.

The response of HBsAg-positive oncology patients to chemotherapy is not uniform, however; the acute, severe hepatitis described in oncology patients receiving chemotherapy does not always occur as chemotherapy is being withdrawn. Included in reports of this observation are instances of acute severe hepatitis, acute hepatitislike events, and biochemical evidence of hepatocellular damage that begin *during* chemotherapy, at a time of active virus replication and peak immunosuppression.[100,102–105] Thus, two

points can be made. First, acute HBV infection is not always asymptomatic in immunosuppressed oncology patients. Second, acute hepatitis can occur either during chemotherapy or after its withdrawal. Because the course of events in HBsAg-positive oncology patients receiving chemotherapy is unpredictable, both administration and withdrawal of chemotherapy should be accompanied by careful monitoring of aminotransferase levels. Some have suggested that in these patients withdrawal of chemotherapy be done gradually rather than abruptly and that immunosuppressive chemotherapy be reinstituted at the first sign of acute hepatitis during withdrawal; it remains to be determined whether this strategy is effective.

Chronicity of hepatitis B after acute infection, the expected pattern,[117] is not invariable either. Of six children with acute leukemia in whom HBsAg became detectable, all six cleared their antigenemia,[107] and 86% of a group of oncology patients with acute hepatitis B following injections with an HBV-contaminated tumor vaccine recovered completely and cleared their HBsAg.[102]

In summary, then, the frequency of HBV infection in oncology patients is increased primarily as a result of exposure through transfused blood products. During chemotherapy, levels of HBV replication tend to increase, and withdrawal of chemotherapy may be associated with severe acute hepatitis as immunologic competence is restored and virus-expressing hepatocytes are destroyed. As a rule, acute HBV infection acquired during chemotherapy-induced or disease-induced immunosuppression tends to be mild and asymptomatic, and chronicity of HBV infection can be anticipated in such patients. Finally, exceptions to all these generalizations occur with some regularity.

3.3.2. Non-A, Non-B Hepatitis in Oncology Patients

Non-A, non-B hepatitis occurs in oncology patients, primarily as a result of exposure through transfusions[105,106,117–119] but is less well characterized in this group of patients than hepatitis B. An important but controversial observation has been made in these patients, however. The question of the effect of hepatitis on remission and survival was raised by Barton and Conrad.[119] These investigators reported that among 50 patients with acute myelogenous leukemia (AML) who survived 6 weeks, those with hepatitis, defined as aminotransferase levels >50 on at least two occasions, had a higher remission rate (21/23, 91%) and mean ±SD duration of survival (76 ± 11 weeks) than those in whom hepatitis did not develop (8 of 13, 62% remission rate and duration of survival of 39 ± 5 weeks). Foon et al.[120] made similar observations in 47 patients with AML, as have other investigators treating patients with AML[121,122] and other malignancies.[123,124] Although some of the hepatitis cases were caused by HBV, most were thought to be cases of transfusion-associated non-A, non-B hepatitis. These improvements in survival and remission have been postulated to represent either a direct beneficial effect of hepatitis virus infection on the malignancies (e.g., by destruction of leukemic stem cells), a reflection of greater immunologic competence in the hepatitis group (which permits virus-induced but immunologically mediated hepatocytolysis to be expressed and which is associated with an improved prognosis in leukemia), an increased sensitivity of hepatocytes and leukemic cells to the toxicity of chemotherapeutic agents (i.e., the patients may not have viral hepatitis at all), or a facilitation by hepatitis viruses of entry into leukemic cells (and hepatocytes) of antitumor drugs.[119,120,125]

Others have failed to confirm the apparent beneficial effect of viral hepatitis on leukemia. Wade et al.[106] found that mild hepatitis, predominantly type non-A, non-B, developed in 73% of 94 consecutive patients treated for nonlymphocytic leukemia. No consistent effect on remission or survival was observed in those with hepatitis, however. Similarly, no difference in response to therapy of leukemia between patients with and without hepatitis was observed by several other groups.[126,127]

Whether unidentified confounding factors account for the differences in observations, whether definitions of hepatitis are adequate or comparable in these studies, even the potential benefit of hepatitis on leukemia does not necessarily outweigh the potentially high likelihood of the chronic liver disease that may result. Malone and Novak[117] found that in more than one-half of a group of 31 children with acute leukemia and acute transfusion-associated hepatitis (18 type non-A, non-B, 13 type B) chronic hepatitis, primarily chronic active hepatitis, developed. Hepatitis is undesirable in these patients not only because

of the high frequency of chronic liver disease, but also because of the resulting limitation on the amount of additional chemotherapy that can be given.

Another point is worth considering in a discussion of non-A, non-B hepatitis among oncology patients receiving chemotherapy. Not every instance of apparent hepatitis in the absence of HBV serologic markers represents non-A, non-B hepatitis. Included in the differential diagnosis of jaundice and hepatocellular dysfunction during chemotherapy are hepatotoxicity of the chemotherapeutic agents (e.g., adriamycin), hepatitis resulting from infection with a nonhepatotropic virus,[128] as well as the hepatic manifestations of sepsis in the marrow-suppressed patient.[129]

4. Prevention

An increased exposure to blood-borne hepatitis viruses and a high likelihood of chronic infection and of high-replicative infection and infectivity are themes that have emerged often during the consideration of hepatitis in immunosuppressed persons. These observations translate into a high risk of infection among immunosuppressed patients and their contacts, primarily health workers and family members. A simple program of education, serologic surveillance, and common-sense precautionary measures can reduce markedly the frequency of new hepatitis virus infections in both staff and patients. For example, in hemodialysis units, recommended procedures include patient and staff education about the risks of hepatitis and its potential avenues of spread within high-risk units; periodic (every 1–3 months) screening of staff and patients for HBsAg and anti-HBs as well as for elevations of serum aminotransferase levels; segregation of HBsAg-positive from HBV-susceptible patients and designation of a separate dialysis machine, or even dialysis unit, for HBsAg-positive patients; assignment of anti-HBs-positive, i.e., immune personnel to care for HBsAg-positive patients; adherence to strict standards of personal and environmental hygiene; and chemical disinfection (with formalin, gluteraldehyde, hypochlorite, or iodophors) of surfaces contaminated by spilled blood or secretions. Although this approach cannot prevent all cases of non-A, non-B hepatitis, it has been credited with markedly reducing the frequency of hepatitis B as a hemodialysis-acquired infection.[41,130-132] Every attempt should be made to avoid sharing of secretions with or ungloved-hand exposure to blood and body fluids from patients with hepatitis. This admonition applies in the hospital and in the home of such patients. It goes without saying that organ donors should be screened for HBsAg and that organs from HBsAg-positive donors should not be transplanted except in very unusual circumstances (e.g., the recipient is already a HBsAg carrier).

Still, although precautions and physical barriers have made an important contribution to limiting the spread of HBV in high-risk areas (hemodialysis, transplantation, and oncology units), occasional cases of hepatitis B continue to surface. In addition to general hygienic measures, immunoprophylaxis of susceptible patients, staff, and family members to prevent hepatitis B infection is recommended. Hepatitis B vaccine, prepared from the plasma of HBsAg carriers, has been shown to be safe, immunogenic, and protective against HBV infection. Its use is recommended preexposure for patients and staff of hemodialysis, transplantation, and oncology units as well as for family members who share a household with a chronic HBsAg carrier. Three intramuscular (deltoid, not gluteal) injections of 1 ml, containing 20 μg of HBsAg, are administered at time 0, 1, and 6 months to immunocompetent adults; half-dose injections are recommended for infants and children under the age of 10. In immunosuppressed persons, a double-dose regimen, in which each injection consists of 40 μg of HBsAg (2 ml of vaccine), is recommended.[133]

Unfortunately, despite the higher vaccine dose, immunocompromised persons do not respond optimally to hepatitis B vaccine. Whereas 95–97% of immunocompetent children and adults acquire protective anti-HBs after vaccination with 20 μg of vaccine and are protected, the immunogenicity of the vaccine is substantially reduced in hemodialysis patients, approximately 60–80%, given double the dose.[134-137] Conflicting results have emerged from studies of the protective efficacy of hepatitis B vaccine in hemodialysis patients. The French (Pasteur)[138] and Dutch (Netherlands Red Cross)[139] vaccines were shown to be protective in controlled trials, while the vaccine prepared in the United States (Merck Sharp & Dohme) was not effective in this group of patients.[135] The discrepancy and failure to demonstrate

vaccine efficacy in the American study may have resulted in part from the much lower than anticipated hepatitis B attack rate among placebo recipients in the participating American hemodialysis units or, perhaps, from the increased immunogenicity of the European vaccines, which are not subjected to as many inactivation steps as the American vaccine.[140] An adequate explanation for the differences in outcomes of the two sets of studies, however, is not apparent. Certainly immunogenicity is lower in hemodialysis patients, and, therefore, protection of nonresponders to the vaccine would not be expected. In the same vein, the argument could be advanced that the European vaccines are slightly more immunogenic in hemodialysis patients and therefore more protective. In the United States study, however, hepatitis B surface antigenemia and even clinical hepatitis B occurred in vaccine responders with circulating anti-HBs documented prior to HBV infection.[135] In all likelihood, suboptimal immunogenicity and protective efficacy of currently available hepatitis B vaccines in hemodialysis patients should be anticipated. In these patients, even naturally acquired anti-HBs may not be protective.[56]

Similarly, in renal transplant recipients, only 18–32% have been shown to acquire anti-HBs after double-dose vaccination, and the levels of anti-HBs achieved are substantially lower than those in immunocompetent persons. Moreover, the appearance of anti-HBs is often delayed and of limited duration.[136,140] An important point emanating from studies of hepatitis B vaccine in renal transplant patients, however, is the safety of vaccination in this group. Data from some transplant centers have suggested that anti-HBs-positive hemodialysis patients had an increased rate of graft rejection. Studies of hepatitis B vaccine in renal transplant recipients, although limited to date, have shown no association between vaccine-induced anti-HBs and graft rejection.[141]

In oncology patients, immunosuppressed both by their underlying diseases and by immunosuppressive, cytotoxic chemotherapy, responsiveness to hepatitis B vaccine appears to be linked with survival. Among surviving adults with solid tumors, the anti-HBs response rates to three 40-μg doses of vaccine have been shown to approach 70%; however, responsiveness was negligible, 9%, among those who did not survive, and even among survivors, antibody levels tended to be low and poorly sustained.[111]

Similarly, only 25% of children with solid tumors have responded to three 40-μg doses of hepatitis B vaccine, four times the recommended dose in this age group.[142] Expected immunogenicity rates to hepatitis B vaccine in immunosuppressed groups compared to immunocompetent controls are shown in Fig. 4.[111,135,141,143] Whether vaccinated oncology patients in whom anti-HBs appears will be protected remains to be seen. Occasionally, even naturally acquired anti-HBs can become undetectable in oncology patients during cytotoxic chemotherapy.[100,107]

Despite these limitations, however, and because of the consequences of HBV infection in immunosuppressed persons and the absence of therapy once infection is established, most authorities recommend prophylactic administration of three 40-μg doses of hepatitis B vaccine in these patients. Adequate prevention of hepatitis B in immunosuppressed hemodialysis and renal transplant patients will probably require vaccination of patients with chronic renal failure prior to transplantation, preferably even before initiating hemodialysis, as renal failure evolves. In oncology patients, the earlier vaccine is administered the better; for those who are likely to acquire exposure to blood products during the course of their therapy, the first dose of vaccine should be given before chemotherapy is begun.

For unvaccinated health workers without natural immunity to HBV in dialysis, transplant, and oncology units who sustain a percutaneous or trans- mucosal exposure to HBsAg-positive material, a combination of passive and active immunization is recommended (postexposure prophylaxis). Passive immunization with high-anti-HBs-titer hepatitis B immune globulin (HBIG), 0.06 ml/kg IM, should be accomplished as soon after the accidental exposure as possible. This should be accompanied or followed shortly thereafter by initiation of a complete course of hepatitis B vaccine.[133,144] Similarly, when immunosuppressed patients suffer an accidental, identifiable percutaneous HBV exposure, HBIG should be administered.

5. Summary

Because they are exposed to blood products, immunosuppressed patients have an increased risk of infection with blood-borne hepatitis viruses, hepatitis B virus and non-A, non-B agents. Included in the category of immunocompromised patients most likely to be encountered by clinicians are chronically hemodialyzed persons with end-stage renal failure, organ transplant recipients, and oncology patients receiving cytotoxic chemotherapy. Although the precise pathogenesis of viral hepatitis has not been defined, most evidence points toward a central role for cytolysis of virus-infected hepatocytes by host cellular immune mechanisms. Deficient in cellular immune competence, these patients are more likely not only to be exposed and infected, but also to remain

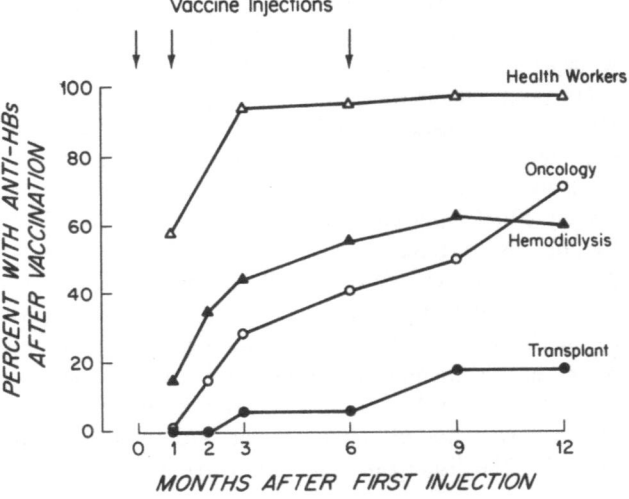

FIGURE 4. Relative immunogenicity of triply inactivated, plasma-derived hepatitis B vaccine (Heptavax-B, Merck Sharp & Dohme) in renal transplant recipients,[141] oncology patients receiving chemotherapy,[111] and hemodialysis patients[135] who received three 40-μg injections, compared with immunocompetent health workers[143] who received three 20-μg injections.

chronically infected after acute infection, to maintain high levels of virus replication, and to be highly infectious for their contacts. Despite the fact that acute infection may not be accompanied by severe illness, late life-threatening consequences of chronic hepatitis are observed in immunosuppressed patients. Even chronic persistent hepatitis, which is benign and nonprogressive in immunocompetent persons, can deteriorate to the more severe and progressive chronic active hepatitis in the immunosuppressed patient. Moreover, reactivation of hepatitis virus replication and clinical hepatitis can occur in immunocompromised persons. This can be especially severe during withdrawal of cytotoxic chemotherapy in oncology patients who are hepatitis B carriers, presumably as a result of sudden restoration of cellular immune cytotoxic potential. In renal transplant recipients, controversy exists over the impact of hepatitis B infection and immunity on graft and patient survival; however, chronic non-A, non-B hepatitis appears to have an immunosuppressive effect, reflected in higher rates of life-threatening extrahepatic infections and increased graft survival. Prevention of viral hepatitis in patients, their household contacts, and health workers is based on programs of mechanical intervention, education, surveillance, and other common-sense hygienic precautions. In addition, preexposure immunoprophylaxis with hepatitis B vaccine and postexposure immunoprophylaxis with a combination of hepatitis B immune globulin and vaccine for accidental inoculation are recommended.

References

1 Szmuness W, Purcell RH, Dienstag JL, et al. Antibody to hepatitis A antigen in institutionalized mentally retarded patients. *JAMA* **237:**1702–1705, 1977.

2. Szmuness W, Dienstag JL, Purcell RH, et al: Hepatitis type A and hemodialysis: A seroepidemiologic study in 15 U S. centers. *Ann Intern Med* **87:**8–12, 1977.

3. Rizzetto M: The delta agent. *Hepatology* **3:**729–737, 1983

4. Popper H, Thung SN, Gerber MA, et al: Histologic studies of severe delta agent infection in Venezuelan Indians. *Hepatology* **3:**906–912, 1983

5 Friedman LS, Dienstag JL: The disease and its pathogenesis. In Gerety RJ (ed): *Hepatitis A*, Academic, Orlando, Florida, 1984, pp. 55–79.

6 Dienstag JL, Bhan AK, Klingenstein RJ, et al: Immunopathogenesis of liver disease associated with hepatitis B In Szmuness W, Alter HJ, Maynard JE (eds): *Viral Hepatitis–1981 International Symposium*, Franklin Institute, Philadelphia, 1982, pp. 221–236.

7 Dienstag JL: Immunologic mechanisms in chronic viral hepatitis. In Vyas GN, Dienstag JL, Hoofnagle JH (eds): *Viral Hepatitis and Liver Disease*. Grune & Stratton, Orlando, Florida, 1984, pp. 135–166.

8. Blumberg BS, Sutnick AI, London WT: Australia antigen as a hepatitis virus: Variation in host response. *Am J Med* **48:**1–8, 1970.

9. Blumberg BS, Gerstley BJS, Hungerford DA, et al: A serum antigen (Australia antigen) in Down's syndrome, leukemia and hepatitis. *Ann Intern Med* **66:**924–931, 1967.

10. Blumberg BS, Sutnick AI, London WT: Hepatitis and leukemia: Their relation to Australia antigen. *Bull NY Acad Med* **44:**1566–1586, 1968.

11. Szmuness W, Harley EJ, Ikram H, et al: Sociodemographic aspects of the epidemiology of hepatitis B. In Vyas GN, Cohen SN, Schmid R (eds). *Viral Hepatitis*. Franklin Institute, Philadelphia, 1978, pp. 297–320.

12. Markenson JA, Gerety RJ, Hoofnagle JH, et al: Effects of cyclophosphamide on hepatitis B virus infection and challenge in chimpanzees. *J Infect Dis* **131:**79–87, 1975.

13. Galbraith RM, Eddleston ALWF, Williams R, et al: Fulminant hepatic failure in leukemia and choriocarcinoma related to withdrawal of cytotoxic drug therapy. *Lancet* **2:**528–530, 1975.

14. Sagnelli E, Manzillo G, Maio G, et al: Serum levels of hepatitis B surface and core antigens during immunosuppressive treatment of HBsAg-positive chronic active hepatitis. *Lancet* **2:**395–397, 1980

15. Scullard GH, Smith CI, Merigan TC, et al: Effects of immunosuppressive therapy on viral markers in chronic active hepatitis B. *Gastroenterology* **81:**987–991, 1981.

16. Villa E, Theodossi A, Portmann B, et al: Reactivation of hepatitis B virus infection in two patients: Immunofluorescence studies of liver tissue, *Gastroenterology* **80:**1048–1053, 1981.

17. Reed WD, Eddleston ALWF, Cullens H, et al: Infusion of hepatitis B antibody in antigen-positive active chronic hepatitis. *Lancet* **2:**1347–1451, 1975.

18. Kohler PF, Trembath J, Merrill DA, et al: Immunotherapy with antibody, lymphocytes and transfer factor in chronic hepatitis B. *Clin Immunol Immunopathol* **2:**465–471, 1974

19 Thomas HC, Chadwick RG, Jain S, et al: Levamisole therapy for HBs antigen positive chronic liver disease *Gastroenterology* **73:**A52, 1977 (abst.)

20. Jain, S, Thomas HC, Sherlock S: Transfer factor in the attempted treatment of patients with HBsAg-positive chronic liver disease. *Clin Exp Immunol* **30:**10–15, 1977.

21. Good RA, Page AR. Fatal complications of virus hepatitis in two patients with agammaglobulinemia. *Am J Med* **29:**804–810, 1960.

22. Mondelli M, Mieli Vergani G, Alberti A, et al: Specificity of T lymphocyte cytotoxicity to autologous hepatocytes in chronic hepatitis B virus infection: Evidence that T cells are directed against HBV core antigen expressed on hepatocytes. *J Immunol* **129:**2773–2778, 1982.

23. Naumov NV, Mondelli M, Alexander GJM, et al: Relationship between expression of hepatitis B virus antigens in

isolated hepatocytes and autologous lymphocyte cytotoxicity in patients with chronic hepatitis B virus infection. *Hepatology* 4:63–68, 1984.

24. Ceuppens JL, Stevens E, Fevery J, et al: Complete recovery from hepatitis B and associated hemolysis in a patient with underlying T-cell deficiency. *Gastroenterology* 86:937–940, 1984.

25. Romet-Lemonne JL, McLane MF, Elfassi E, et al: Hepatitis B virus infection in cultured human lymphoblastoid cells. *Science* 221:667–669, 1983.

26. Dienstag JL: Non-A, non-B hepatitis. I. Recognition, epidemiology, and clinical features. *Gastroenterology* 85:439–462, 1983.

27. Dienstag JL: Non-A, non-B hepatitis. II. Experimental transmission, putative virus agents and markers, and prevention. *Gastroenterology* 85:743–768, 1983.

28. Blumberg BS, Alter HJ, Visnich S: A "new" antigen in leukemia sera. *JAMA* 191:541–546, 1965.

29. Goldblum SE, Reed WP: Host defenses and immunologic alterations associated with chronic hemodialysis. *Ann Intern Med* 93:597–613, 1980.

30. Agarwal SS, Blumberg BS, Gerstley BS, et al: DNA polymerase activity as an index of lymphocyte stimulation: Studies in Down's syndrome. *J Clin Invest* 49:161–169, 1970.

31. Boughton CR, Hawkes RA, Schroeter DR, et al: The epidemiology of hepatitis B in a residential institution for the mentally retarded. *Aust NZ J Med* 6:521–529, 1976.

32. Hawkes RA, Boughton CR, Schroeter DR, et al: Hepatitis B infection in institutionalized Down's syndrome inmates. A longitudinal study with five hepatitis B virus markers. *Clin Exp Immunol* 40:478–486, 1980.

33. Madden DL, Dietzman DE, Matthew EB, et al: Epidemiology of hepatitis B virus in an institution for mentally retarded persons. *Am J Ment Defic* 80:369–375, 1976.

34. Chaudhary RK, Perry E, Cleary TE: Prevalence of hepatitis B infection among residents of an institution for the mentally retarded. *Am J Epidemiol* 105:123–126, 1977.

35. Szmuness W, Pick R, Prince AM: The serum hepatitis virus specific antigen (SH): A preliminary report of epidemiologic studies in an institution for the mentally retarded. *Am J Epidemiol* 92:51–61, 1970.

36. Hollingsworth DR, Hollingsworth JW, Roeckel I, et al: Immunologic reactions and Australia antigenemia in Down's syndrome. *J Chron Dis* 27:483–490, 1974.

37. Szmuness W, Neurath AR, Stevens CE, et al: Prevalence of hepatitis B "e" antigen and its antibody in various HBsAg carrier populations. *Am J Epidemiol* 113:113–121, 1981.

38. Garibaldi RA, Forrest JN, Bryan JA, et al: Hemodialysis-associated hepatitis. *JAMA* 225:384–389, 1973.

39. Snydman DR, Bryan JA, Hanson B: Hemodialysis-associated hepatitis in the United States—1972 *J Infect Dis* 132:109–113, 1975.

40. Szmuness W, Prince AM, Grady GF, et al: Hepatitis B infection: A point-prevalence study in 15 US hemodialysis centers. *JAMA* 227:901–906, 1974.

41. Centers for Disease Control: Hepatitis—Control measures for hepatitis B in dialysis centers. Viral hepatitis investigations and control series. U.S. Department of Health, Education and Welfare, Phoenix, November 1977, pp. 1–9

42. Szmuness W: Large-scale efficacy trials of hepatitis B vaccines in the USA: Baseline data and protocols. *J Med Virol* 4:327–340, 1979.

43. Sengar DPS, Rashid A, McLeish WA, et al: Hepatitis B surface antigen (HBsAg) infection in a hemodialysis unit. II. Factors affecting host immune response to HBsAg. *Can Med Assoc J* 113:945–948, 1975.

44. London WT, Drew JS, Lustbader ED, et al: Host responses to hepatitis B infection in patients in a chronic hemodialysis unit. *Kidney Int* 12:51–58, 1977.

45. Snydman DS, Bregman D, Bryan JA: Hemodialysis-associated hepatitis in the United States, 1974. *J Infect Dis* 135:687–691, 1977.

46. Ribot S, Rothstein M, Goldblat M, et al: Duration of hepatitis B surface antigenemia (HBsAg) in hemodialysis patients *Arch Intern Med* 139:178–180. 1979.

47. Gahl GM, Hess G, Arnold W, et al: Hepatitis B virus markers in 97 long-term hemodialysis patients. *Nephron* 24:58–63, 1979.

48. Beorchia S, Trepo C, Betuel H, et al: Interest of HBeAg in the study of immunogenetic factors influencing HBV infection in hemodialysed and kidney transplanted patients. In Touraine JL, Traeger J, Betuel H, et al (eds): *Transplantation and Clinical Immunology*. Vol 10. Excerpta Medica, Amsterdam, 1979, pp. 44–49.

49. Snydman DR, Bryan JA, Macon EJ, et al: Hemodialysis-associated hepatitis: Report of an epidemic with further evidence on mechanisms of transmission. *Am J Epidemiol* 104:563–570, 1976.

50. Garibaldi RA, Hatch FE, Bisno AL, et al. Nonparenteral serum hepatitis. Report of an outbreak *JAMA* 220:963–966, 1972.

51. Coughlin GP, Van Deth AG, Disney APS, et al: Liver disease and the e antigen in HBsAg carriers with chronic renal failure *Gut* 21:118–122, 1980.

52. Degott C, Degos F, Jungers P, et al: Relationship between liver histopathological changes and HBsAg in 111 patients treated by long-term hemodialysis. *Liver* 3:377–384, 1983.

53. Jungers P, Naret C, Degott C, et al: Histological and immunological survey of chronic active hepatitis in 650 hemodialyzed patients In Touraine JL, Traeger J, Betuel H, et al (eds). *Transplantation and Clinical Immunology*. Vol 10 Excerpta Medica, 1979, pp. 38–43.

54. Galbraith RM, Dienstag JL, Purcell RH, et al. Non-A non-B hepatitis associated with chronic liver disease in a hemodialysis unit. *Lancet* 1:951–953, 1979.

55. Galbraith RM, Portmann B, Eddleston ALWF, et al. Chronic liver disease developing after outbreak of HBsAg-negative hepatitis in haemodialysis unit. *Lancet* 2:886–890, 1975.

56. Marmion BP, Burrell CJ, Tonkin RW, et al. Dialysis-associated hepatitis in Edinburgh, 1969–1978. *Rev Infect Dis* 4:619–637, 1982.

57. Coursaget P, Maupas P, Dubois F, et al. Hepatites non-A, non-B chez six malades hemodialyses *Nouv Presse Med* 7:3515–3519, 1978.

58. Mery JP, Simon N, Courouce AM: Hepatite non-A, non-B chez les hemodialyses chroniques: 5 observations. *Nouv Presse Med* 8:3973, 1979.

59. Koretz RL, Stone O, Brezina M, et al: Chronic hepatitis in the dialysis unit: Etiologic considerations. *Gastroenterology* **78:**1198, 1980 (abst).

60. Dienstag JL, Stevens CE, Szmuness W: The epidemiology of non-A, non-B hepatitis: Emerging patterns. In Gerety JR (ed): *Non-A, non-B Hepatitis.* Academic, New York, 1981, pp. 119–137.

61. Simon N, Mery JP, Trepo C, et al: A non-A, non-B hepatitis epidemic in a HB antigen-free hemodialysis unit. Demonstration of serological markers of non-A, non-B virus, *Proc Eur Dial Transplant Assoc* **17:**173–178, 1980.

62. Avram MM, Feinfeld DA, Gan AC: Non-A, non-B hepatitis: A new syndrome in uraemic patients. *Proc Eur Dial Transplant Assoc* **16:**141–147, 1979.

63. Wolf JL, Perkins HA, Schreeder MT, et al: The transplanted kidney as a source of hepatitis B infection. *Ann Intern Med* **91:**412–413, 1979.

64. Lutwick LI, SyWassink JM, Corry RJ, et al: The renal transplant as a source of hepatitis B virus (HBV). *Clin Res* **29:**258A, 1981 (abst.).

65. Degos F, Degott C, Bedrossian J, et al: Is renal transplantation involved in post-transplantation liver disease? A prospective study. *Transplantation* **29:**100–102, 1980.

66. Toussaint C, Thiry L, Kinnaert P, et al: Prognostic significance of hepatitis B antigenemia in kidney transplantation. *Nephron* **17:**335–342, 1976.

67. Luby JP, Burnett W, Hull AR, et al: Relationship between cytomegalovirus and hepatic function abnormalities in the period after renal transplant. *J Infect Dis* **129:**511–518, 1974.

68. Kaiser L, Kelly TJ, Patterson MJ, et al: Hepatitis B surface antigen in urine of renal transplant recipients. *Ann Intern Med* **94:**783–784, 1981.

69. Mayor GH, Kelly TJ, Hourani MR, et al: Intermittent hepatitis B surface antigenuria in a renal transplant recipient. *Am J Med* **68:**305–307, 1980.

70. Nagington J, Cossart YE, Cohen BJ: Reactivation of hepatitis B after transplantation operations. *Lancet* **1:**558–560, 1977.

71. Dusheiko G, Song E, Bowyer S, et al: Natural history of hepatitis B virus infection in renal transplant recipients—A fifteen-year follow-up. *Hepatology* **3:**330–336, 1983.

72. London WT, Drew JS, Blumberg BS, et al: Association of graft survival with host response to hepatitis B infection in patients with kidney transplants. *N Engl J Med* **296:**241–244, 1977.

73. London WT, Jarvinen H, Jasko L, et al: Hepatitis B virus infection in kidney transplant recipients. In Bianchi L, Gerok W, Sickinger K, et al (eds): *Virus and the Liver.* MTP Press, Lancaster, 1980, pp. 267–276.

74. Jarvinen H, Shofer FS, Burke JF, et al: Antibody to hepatitis B surface antigen and kidney graft survival. *Transplant Proc* **15:**1094–1098, 1983.

75. Toussaint C, Cappel R, Vereerstraeten P, et al: Graft survival and response to hepatitis-B virus in kidney recipients. *Transplant Proc* **11:**89–92, 1979.

76. Pirson Y, Alexandre GPJ, van Ypersele de Strihou C: Long-term effect of HBs antigenemia on patient survival after renal transplantation. *N Engl J Med* **296:**194–196, 1977.

77. Hillis WD, Hillis A, Walker WG: Hepatitis B surface antigenemia in renal transplant recipients: Increased mortality risk. *JAMA* **242:**329–332, 1979.

78. Chatterjee SN, Payne JE, Bischell MD, et al: Successful renal transplantation in patients positive for hepatitis B antigen. *N Engl J Med* **291:**62–65, 1974.

79. Berne TV, Fitzgibbons TJ, Silberman H: The effect of hepatitis B antigenemia on long-term success and hepatic disease in renal transplantation. *Transplantation* **24:**412–415, 1977.

80. Fine RN, Malekzadeh MH, Pennisi AJ, et al: HBs antigenemia in renal allograft recipients. *Ann Surg* **185:**411–416, 1977.

81. Ponticelli C, De Vecchi A, Cantaluppi A, et al: Hepatitis and renal transplants. (Letter.) *N Engl J Med* **296:**1170, 1977.

82. Rashid A, Sengar D, Couture R, et al: Hepatitis and renal transplants. (Letter.) *N Engl J Med* **296:**1170–1171, 1977.

83. Hillis WD, Hillis A, Bias WB. et al: Association of hepatitis B surface antigenemia with HLA locus B specificities. *N Engl J Med* **296:**1310–1314, 1977.

84. Opelz G. Terasaki PI: Graft survival rates and HLA antigen frequencies in renal cadaver transplant recipients with hepatitis B antigenemia. *Transplantation* **25:**159–161, 1978.

85. Parfrey PS, Forbes RDC, Hutchinson TA, et al: The clinical and pathological course of hepatitis B liver disease in renal transplant recipients. *Transplantation* **37:**461–466, 1984.

86. Schroter GPJ, Weill R III, Penn I, et al: Hepatocellular carcinoma associated with chronic hepatitis B virus infection after kidney transplantation. (Letter.) *Lancet* **2:**381–382, 1982.

87. Anuras S, Piros J, Bonney WW, et al: Liver disease in renal transplant recipients. *Arch Intern Med* **137:**42–48, 1977.

88. Strom TB: Hepatitis B, transfusions, and renal transplantation—five years later. (Editorial.) *N Engl J Med* **307:**1141–1142, 1982.

89. Berne TV, Chatterjee SN, Craig JR, et al: Hepatic dysfunction in recipients of renal allografts. *Surg Gynecol Obstet* **141:**171–175, 1975.

90. Mozes MF, Ascher NL, Balfour HHJ, et al: Jaundice after renal allotransplantation. *Ann Surg* **188:**783–790, 1978.

91. Ware AJ, Luby JP, Hollinger B, et al: Etiology of liver disease in renal-transplant patients. *Ann Intern Med* **91:**364–371, 1979.

92. Alvarez V, Plaza JJ, Carreno V, et al: Viral infections and liver damage in renal transplant patients. *Gastroenterology* **79:**1001, 1980 (abst.).

93. Fennell RS III, Andres JM, Pfaff WW, et al: Liver dysfunction in children and adolescents during hemodialysis and after renal transplantation. *Pediatrics* **67:**855–861, 1981.

94. LaQuaglia MP, Tolkoff-Rubin NE, Dienstag JL, et al: Impact of hepatitis on renal transplantation *Transplantation* **32:**504–507, 1981.

95. Alter HJ, Hoofnagle JH: Non-A, non-B: Observations on the first decade. In Vyas GN, Dienstag JL, Hoofnagle JH (eds): *Viral Hepatitis and Liver Disease.* Grune & Stratton, Orlando, 1984, pp. 345–354.

96. Wyke RJ, Williams R: Clinical aspects of non-A, non-B hepatitis infection. *J Virol Methods* **2:**17–29, 1980.

97. Sutnick AI, London WT, Blumberg BS, et al: Australia

antigen (a hepatitis associated antigen) in leukemia. *J Natl Cancer Inst* **44:**1241–1249, 1970.

98. Sutnick AI, Levine PH, London WT, et al: Frequency of Australia antigen in patients with leukemia in different countries. *Lancet* **1:**1200–1202, 1971.

99. Grange MJ, Erlinger S, Teilletd F, et al: A possible relationship to treatment between hepatitis-associated antigen and chronic persistent hepatitis in Hodgkin's disease. *Gut* **14:**433–437, 1973.

100. Wands JR, Chura CM, Roll FJ, et al: Serial studies of hepatitis-associated antigen and antibody in patients receiving antitumor chemotherapy for myeloproliferative and lymphoproliferative disorders. *Gastroenterology* **68:**105–112, 1975.

101. Wands JR, Walker JA, Davis TT, et al: Hepatitis B in an oncology unit. *N Engl J Med* **291:**1371–1375, 1974.

102. Schulman AN, Fagen ND, Brezina M, et al: HBe-antigen in the course and prognosis of hepatitis B infection: A prospective study. *Gastroenterology* **78:**253–258, 1980.

103. Trinchet JC, Beaugrand M, Hecht Y, et al: Hépatite fulminante à virus B survenue au cours d'un traitement immunodepresseur. *Gastroenterol Clin Biol* **4:**59–62, 1980.

104. Hoofnagle JH, Dusheiko GM, Schafer DF, et al: Reactivation of chronic hepatitis B virus infection by cancer chemotherapy. *Ann Intern Med* **96:**447–449, 1982.

105. Vergani D, Locasciulli A, Masera G, et al: Histological evidence of hepatitis-B-virus infection with negative serology in children with acute leukemia who develop chronic liver disease. *Lancet* **1:**361–364, 1982.

106. Wade JC, Gaffey M, Wiernik PH, et al: Hepatitis in patients with acute nonlymphocytic leukemia, *Am J Med* **75:**413–422, 1983.

107. Locasciulli A, Santamaria M, Masera G, et al: Hepatitis B virus markers in children with acute leukemia: The effect of chemotherapy. *J Med Virol* **15:**29–33, 1985.

108. Cowan DH, Kouroupis GM, Leers W-D: Occurrence of hepatitis and hepatitis B surface antigen in adult patients with acute leukemia. *Can Med Assoc J* **112:**693–697, 1975.

109. Sauerbruch T, Frosner G, Theml H, et al: Hepatitis B-virusmarker und rotelnantikorper bei patienten mit hodgkin-, non-hodgkin-lymphomen und allgemein internistischen erkrankungen. *Blut* **40:**259–266, 1980.

110. Tabor E, Gerety RJ, Mott M, et al: Prevalence of hepatitis B in a high risk setting: A serlogic study of patients and staff in a pediatric oncology unit. *Pediatrics* **61:**711–715, 1978

111. Weitberg AB, Weitzman SA, Watkins E, et al: Immunogenicity of hepatitis B vaccine in oncology patients receiving chemotherapy. *J Clin Oncol* **3:**718–722, 1985.

112. Schulman AN, Fagen ND, Ling CM, et al: Repeated type B hepatitis infections: Ten case studied prospectively. *Gastroenterology* **72:**1182, 1977 (abst).

113. Lightdale CJ, Ikram H, Pinsky C: Primary hepatocellular carcinoma with hepatitis B antigenemia: Effects of chemotherapy. *Cancer* **46:**1117–1122, 1980.

114. Steinberg SC, Alter HJ, Leventhal BG: The risk of hepatitis transmission to family contacts of leukemia patients. *J Pediatr* **87:**753–757, 1975.

115. Wands JR: Subacute and chronic active hepatitis after withdrawal of chemotherapy. (Letter.) *Lancet* **2:**979, 1975.

116. Thung SN, Gerber MA, Klion F, et al: Massive hepatic necrosis after chemotherapy withdrawal in a hepatitis B virus carrier. *Arch Intern Med* **145:**1313–1314, 1985

117. Malone W, Novak R: Outcome of hepatitis in children with acute leukemia. *Am J Dis Child* **134:**584–587, 1980.

118. Locasciulli A, Alberti A, Barbieri R, et al: Evidence of non-A, non-B hepatitis in children with acute leukemia and chronic liver disease. *Am J Dis Child* **173:**354–356, 1983.

119. Barton JB, Conrad ME: Beneficial effects of hepatitis in patients with acute myelogenous leukemia. *Ann Intern Med* **90:**188–190, 1979

120. Foon KA, Yale C, Clodfelter K, et al. Posttransfusion hepatitis in acute myelogenous leukemia. Effect on leukemia *JAMA* **244:**1806–1807, 1980.

121. Rotoli B, Formisano S, Martinelli V: Long-term survival in acute myelogenous leukemia complicated by chronic active hepatitis. (Letter.) *N Engl J Med* **307:**1712–1713, 1982

122. Cacciola E, Giustolisi R. Acute myelogenous leukemia and hepatitis. (Letter.) *Ann Intern Med* **92:**127–128, 1980.

123. Brody SA, Russell WG, Krantz SB, et al: Beneficial effect of hepatitis in leukemic reticuloendotheliosis. *Arch Intern Med* **141:**1080–1081, 1981.

124. Shepard KV, Levin B, Faintuch J, et al: Hepatitis as a beneficial prognostic factor in patients receiving intra-arterial chemotherapy for metastatic colorectal carcinoma. *Clin Res* **31:**779A, 1983 (abst.).

125. Rosner F: Hepatitis and leukemia. (Letter.) *Ann Intern Med* **90:**853, 1979.

126. van den Ouweland FA, Holdrinet RSG, de Pauw BE, et al: Transaminase, hepatitis B, and prognosis in acute nonlymphoblastic leukemia. (Letter.) *N Engl J Med* **309:**990, 1983.

127. Julia A, Font L: Hepatitis and leukemia. (Letter) *Ann Intern Med* **93:**780, 1980.

128. Carmichael GP, Zahradnik JM, Moyer GH, et al. Adenovirus hepatitis in an immunosuppressed adult patient. *Am J Clin Pathol* **71:**352–355, 1979.

129. Katz ME, Cassileth PA: Hyperbilirubinemia during induction therapy of acute granulocytic leukemia. *Cancer* **40:**1390–1392, 1977.

130. Public Health Laboratory Service Survey: Hepatitis B in retreat from dialysis units in United Kingdom in 1973. *Br Med J* **1:**1579–1581, 1976.

131. Postic B, Schreiner DP, Hanchett JE, et al: Containment of hepatitis B virus infection in a hemodialysis unit. *J Infect Dis* **138:**884–889, 1978.

132. Najem GR, Louria DB, Thind IS, et al: Control of hepatitis B infection: The role of surveillance and an isolation hemodialysis center. *JAMA* **245:**153–157, 1981.

133. Immunization Practices Advisory Committee: Recommendations for protection against viral hepatitis. *MMWR* **34:**313–324, 329–335, 1985.

134. Stevens CE, Szmuness W, Goodman AI, et al: Hepatitis B vaccine: Immune response in hemodialysis patients. *Lancet* **2:**1211–1213, 1980.

135. Stevens CE, Alter HJ, Taylor PE, et al: Hepatitis B vaccine in patients receiving hemodialysis: Immunogenicity and efficacy. *N Engl J Med* **311:**496–501, 1984.

136. Grob PJ, Binswanger U, Zaruba K, et al: Immunogenicity of

a hepatitis B subunit vaccine in hemodialysis and in renal transplant recipients *Antiviral Res* **3**:43–52, 1983.

137. Bergamini F, Zanetti AR, Ferroni P, et al: Immune response to hepatitis B vaccine in staff and patients in renal dialysis units. *J Infect* **7** (Suppl. 1):35–40, 1983.

138. Crosnier J, Jungers P, Courouce A-M, et al: Randomized placebo-controlled trial of hepatitis B surface antigen vaccine in French haemodialysis units. II. Haemodialysis patients. *Lancet* **2**:797–800, 1981.

139. Desmyter J, Colaert J, De Groot G, et al: Efficacy of heat-inactivated hepatitis B vaccine in hemodialysis patients and staff: Double-blind placebo-controlled trial. *Lancet* **2**:1323–1327, 1983.

140. Desmyter J, Colaert J: Comparative immunogenicity of MSD, Pasteur and CLB hepatitis B vaccines in 245 hemodialysis patients (abst). In Vyas GN, Dienstag JL, Hoofnagle JH (eds): *Viral Hepatitis and Liver Disease*. Grune & Stratton, Orlando, 1984, pp. 709–710.

141. Jacobson IM, Jaffers G, Dienstag JL, et al: Immunogenicity of hepatitis B vaccine in renal transplant recipients. *Transplantation* **39**:393–395, 1985.

142. Arnold W, Baumann W: Vaccination of children with malignant diseases with alum-adsorbed hepatitis B vaccine—Immunogenicity studies. *Scand J Infect Dis* **38**(Suppl):33–36, 1983.

143. Dienstag JL, Werner BF, Polk BF, et al: Hepatitis B vaccine in health care personnel: Safety, immunogenicity, and indicators of efficacy. *Ann Intern Med* **101**:34–40, 1984.

144. Centers for Disease Control: Postexposure prophylaxis of hepatitis B: Recommendations of the Immunization Practices Advisory Committee. *Ann Intern Med* **101**:351–354, 1984.

13

Herpes Group Virus Infections in the Compromised Host

MARTIN S. HIRSCH

1. Introduction

Disorders of cell-mediated immunity are frequently associated with herpesvirus infections that are occasionally severe and prolonged. Such infections can be primary, as when the renal transplant recipient who is seronegative for cytomegalovirus (CMV) is grafted with a kidney from a seropositive donor. More often, they result from reactivation of latent virus, as when the patient with Hodgkin disease develops zoster following irradiation and chemotherapy.

　　All members of the human herpes virus group— herpes simplex virus (HSV), cytomegalovirus (CMV), Epstein–Barr virus (EBV), and varicella-zoster virus (VZV)—are detected more frequently in immunocompromised hosts than in immunologically intact individuals. They can cause a spectrum of syndromes ranging from subclinical or trivial infection to fulminating lethal disease. This chapter will attempt to summarize current concepts regarding epidemiology, pathogenesis, diagnosis, and therapy of herpes virus infections in immunocompromised patients.

2. Herpes Simplex Virus

Illustrative Case 1

　　A 24-year-old man was admitted to the Massachusetts General Hospital because of respiratory distress 6 months after transplan-

MARTIN S. HIRSCH • Infectious Disease Unit, Massachusetts General Hospital, and Department of Medicine, Harvard Medical School, Boston, Massachusetts 02114.

tation of a cadaveric kidney. He had been maintained on prednisone and azathioprine in high doses for persistent evidence of active rejection. Impetigenous and ulcerative lesions developed on his upper lip 2 months before admission. A biopsy of an ulcer disclosed changes consistent with herpes simplex infection, and cultures were positive for HSV-1. Several weeks before admission, a low-grade fever developed with progressive cough, dyspnea, anorexia, and weight loss.

　　On admission, the temperature was 100.6°F (38.1°C), the pulse 140, and the respiration rate 30. The patient was dyspneic on minimal exertion, with a frequent, nonproductive cough. Clusters of ulcerative lesions were present about the nose and upper lip (Fig. 1). Shallow ulcerations were also observed in the pharynx. Crackling inspiratory rales were heard at both lung bases. The hematocrit (Hct) was 35, the white blood cell (WBC) count 4300 with 55% neutrophils, 6% band forms, 28% lymphocytes, 2% monocytes, 7% eosinophils, and 2% basophils. The BUN was 80 mg/dl, and creatinine 3.6 mg/dl. Gram stains of tracheal secretions were unimpressive, but cytologic examination disclosed multinucleated cells with intranuclear inclusions (Fig. 2). Chest radiographs revealed diffuse haziness in both lung fields. A specimen of arterial blood drawn with the patient breathing room air had a Pao_2 of 87 mm Hg, $Paco_2$ of 32 mm Hg, and pH 7.47. Over the next week, progressive respiratory failure developed with superimposed gram-negative bacteremia, and the patient died.

　　At autopsy, the lungs were 2.5 times normal weight. Microscopic examination showed multiple foci of a necrotizing bronchopneumonia with multinucleated giant cells and eosinophilic intranuclear inclusion bodies characteristic of herpetic infection. Herpetic infection was also found throughout the tracheobronchial tree and larynx, where it produced diffuse necrosis and ulceration of mucosa. Diffuse intraalveolar *Pneumocystis carinii* pulmonary infection was also observed. Bacterial cultures were negative, but viral cultures of lung tissue grew HSV-1. Numerous herpetic ulcers of the esophagus were also found, but herpes infection was not observed elsewhere. The fatal progression in this patient was clearly related to progressive herpetic bronchopneumonia complicated by *Pneumocystis carinii* alveolar involvement.

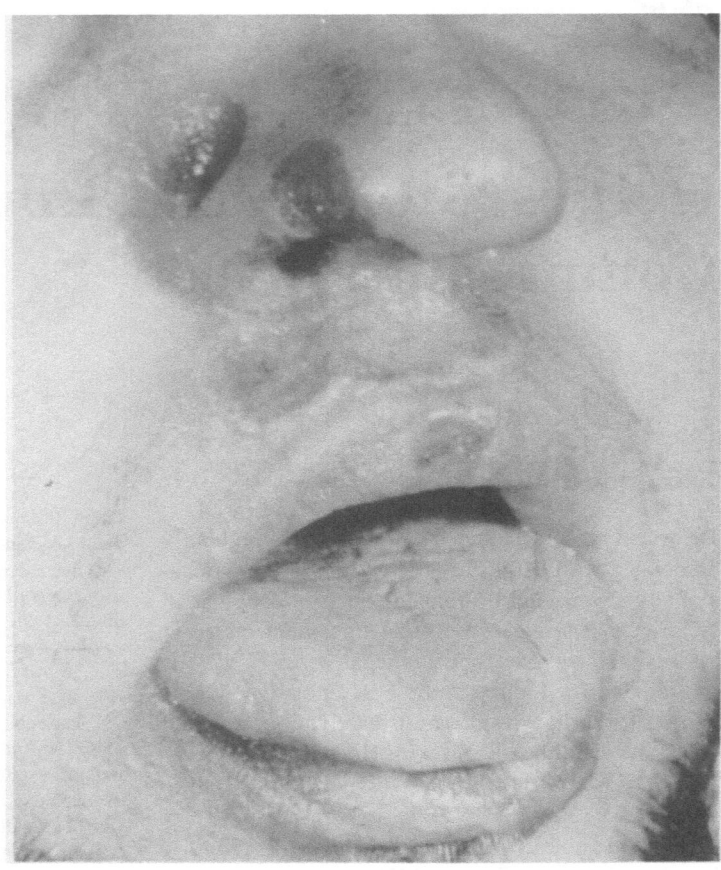

FIGURE 1. Severe herpetic ulcerations on lips and nose of renal transplant recipient. This HSV-1 infection ultimately resulted in fatal pneumonitis.

2.1. Clinical Epidemiology and Patterns of Infection

Fortunately, the progressive respiratory failure described in Illustrative Case 1 is a rare event, occurring only in severely compromised patients. Even in moderately suppressed individuals, HSV infection, though often severe, is usually self-limited.

Herpes simplex infections are worldwide in distribution. HSV-1 frequently infects children between the ages of 2 and 10; occasionally, primary infection is delayed to adolescence or young adulthood. It is transmitted primarily by contact with oral secretions and is chiefly responsible for perioral, ocular, and encephalitic infections in adults. HSV-2 is spread by genital contact; thus, major periods of infection follow puberty. It is a major cause of penile vesicular lesions, cervicovaginitis, and proctitis, as well as neonatal disseminated disease.

Recurrent infection occurs frequently with both HSV-1 and HSV-2. The majority of recurrences are secondary to endogenous reactivation of virus, although exogenous reinfection can occur. Recurrences tend to be milder than the primary infection.

Individuals with defects in cell-mediated immunity or breaks in the natural mucocutaneous barrier are susceptible to more serious or unusual forms of HSV infection. This population at risk includes organ transplant recipients,[1-5] recipients of cytotoxic agents for malignancy,[6,7] the severely malnourished,[8] patients with certain skin disorders,[9] burn patients,[10] and those with congenital or acquired cellular immune defects.[9,11,12]

Most immunosuppressed patients have localized and self-limited herpes simplex infections that differ little from infections in intact hosts. It is unclear whether the frequency of symptomatic infections or asymptomatic excretion is increased in im-

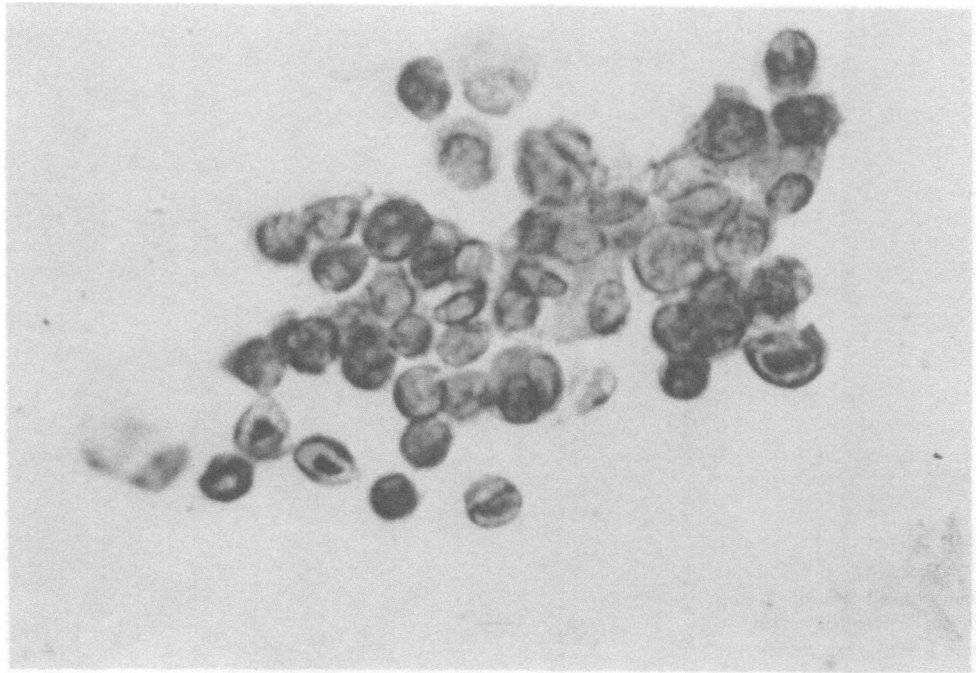

FIGURE 2. Sputum cytology from patient with HSV-1 pneumonia. Multinucleated giant cells and intranuclear inclusions are seen

munodeficient hosts. Our own studies in renal transplant recipients indicate that shortly following grafting, approximately 80% of seropositive recipients begin to excrete HSV in throat washings[5] Two-thirds of the excretors will develop lesions shortly after excretion is detected.

Lesions in immunosuppressed patients may be more severe and protracted than in normal individuals. Chronic, large ulcerated lesions (herpes phagenda) may persist for weeks to years (Fig. 3) and have been most commonly described in patients with acquired immunodeficiency syndrome (AIDS),[12] hematologic malignancies[6] and after transplantation.[1] Such lesions may affect both nasolabial and anogenital sites.

Eczema herpeticum (Kaposi varicelliform eruption) is a widely distributed cutaneous dissemination of HSV usually developing in sites of preexistent skin disease. It is classically associated with atopic eczema but is also seen with Darier disease, certain forms of pemphigus, and the Wiskott–Aldrich syndrome.[9] Eczema herpeticum has also been described in patients with lymphoreticular malignancies in-

volving the skin.[6] Visceral dissemination may occur, and mortality varies from 10 to 50%. This complication in burn patients is difficult to appreciate clinically, as the lesions may be atypical and appear in areas of partial healing.

Involvement of the tracheobronchial tree may occur as part of local or disseminated disease. Focal pneumonias appear to result from contiguous spread of virus, often secondary to local trauma induced by endotracheal intubation.[13] Diffuse interstitial pneumonitis may be a manifestation of hematogenous dissemination. A high prevalence of HSV antibodies in sera prior to pneumonia and identical restriction endonuclease patterns between mucosal and lung isolates suggest that most cases of HSV pneumonia result from endogenous reactivation.[14]

Esophagitis is another condition that is more common than clinically appreciated in the compromised host. In one autopsy review, 25% of cases of esophagitis were attributable to HSV.[15] Superficial, punched-out lesions are seen in the upper two-thirds of the esophagus with confluence in the lower one-third. *Candida* esophagitis is frequently coexistent.

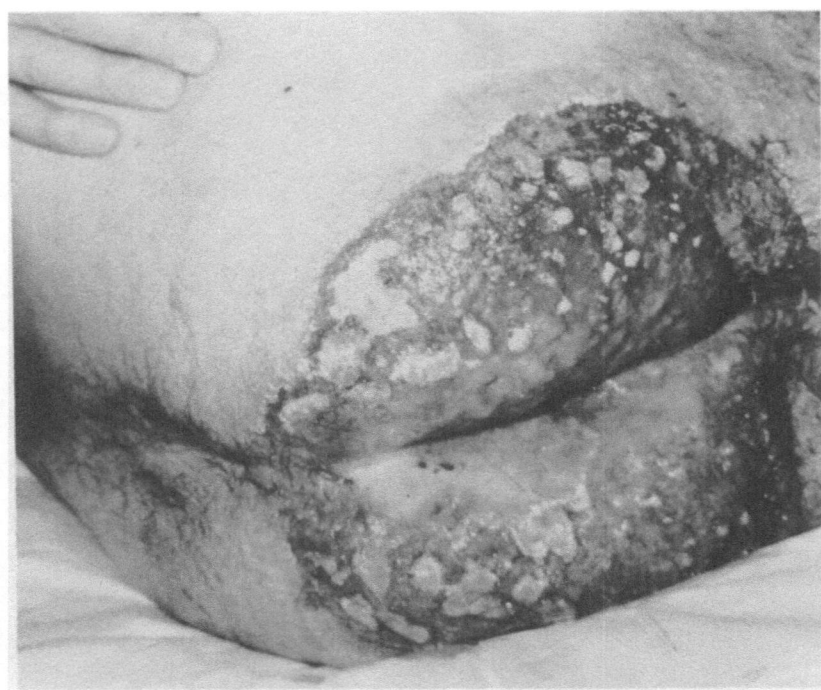

FIGURE 3. Ulcerative HSV-2 infection of buttocks and perineum in a patient with chronic lymphocytic leukemia. These lesions were partially responsive to both adenine arabinoside and human leukocyte interferon.

Predisposing factors include immunosuppressive therapy and the presence of a nasogastric tube. Although the pathogenesis of this condition has been thought to represent tracking of virus from oral sites, the isolation of HSV from the vagus ganglia of humans[16] suggests that this may represent a site directly affected by reactivation of latent virus. Esophagitis may be seen in association with herpetic pneumonia or hepatitis and may well serve as a site for visceral dissemination.

Widespread visceral involvement of liver, lungs, adrenals, gastrointestinal (GI) tract, central nervous system (CNS), and skin can occur in the immunocompromised host. The factors that determine whether severe localized disease, cutaneous dissemination, or visceral dissemination will occur in a given individual are as yet not well defined. Disseminated intravascular coagulation may accompany visceral spread, and when this occurs, mortality approaches 100%.

2.2. Pathogenesis

Primary infections of skin and mucous membranes are produced by viral invasion of epithelial cells. With viral replication, cell death, and concomitant inflammatory responses, the characteristic vesicle on an erythematous base is produced. Further virus replication may result in viremia and visceral dissemination if host responsiveness is compromised.

Several host responses are involved in limitation of virus replication. In both murine and human models, monocyte/macrophage maturity and interferon production may help determine whether virus remains localized or disseminates.[17,18] Subsequently, other defense mechanisms, e.g., the production of antibodies, natural killer (NK) cells, and sensitized T lymphocytes, are elicited to help prevent spread of infection.

Humoral antibody alone is not a major mediator of resistance, as recurrent and even fatal disease can occur in the presence of high titers of neutralizing antibodies. Although these antibodies do not protect against recurrent disease, they may be important in modulating its severity, particularly as a cofactor in antibody-dependent cell-mediated cytotoxicity (ADCC).[19] Local humoral factors, e.g., secretory IgA neutralizing antibody and interferon, may be of importance in containing infection. Although neutralizing IgA antibodies have not been demonstrated in secretions of individuals with herpes labialis, intravesicular interferon production appears to correlate with crusting and healing.[20] In addition, exogenous interferon in high-risk patients may reduce the incidence of HSV excretion and lesion development.[21]

Compelling evidence for the importance of T-cell-mediated immunity in the control of HSV infections comes from clinical observations and animal studies. Disorders of T-cell function are those most frequently complicated by HSV infections.[1-7,9,11] Potent suppressors of cell-mediated immunity (CMI) in animals, e.g., antithymocyte globulin (ATG), are also potent enhancers of HSV-associated morbidity and mortality.[22] In vitro studies of CMI in humans have not given consistent results, although there is some suggestion that specific T-lymphocyte proliferative and cytotoxic responses may be diminished between attacks in individuals subject to frequent recurrences.[23,24] Similarly, lymphocyte production of interferon may be reduced in patients with recurrent infections.[25] Both diminished lymphocyte transformation and interferon production in response to HSV antigens have been demonstrated during the early post-transplant period.[3,4] These deficiencies correlate well with the peak incidence of clinical and asymptomatic HSV infections among such patients.

2.3. Diagnosis and Therapy

Significant mucocutaneous HSV infections are not generally difficult to diagnose. Visceral involvement, e.g., pneumonitis, hepatitis, and encephalitis, may present diagnostic problems. Appropriate specimens should be examined for characteristic multinucleated giant cells by cytologic or histologic techniques using a variety of stains (e.g., Giemsa, hematoxylin–eosin, Wright, Papanicalaou). Immunofluorescence for demonstration of herpes antigens may be a useful adjunctive assay. The virus grows readily on a variety of cell cultures, and diagnosis by characteristic cytopathic changes can frequently be made within 24–48 hr. Specimens should be collected early after onset of lesions and promptly inoculated into tissue cultures. If delay is unavoidable, specimens can be stored in appropriate carrying media at 4–9°C. for a few hours, but for longer periods they should be stored below −70°C. Serologic techniques are rarely of value in the diagnosis of HSV infections.

Acyclovir is the drug of choice for both prophylaxis and therapy of HSV infections in high-risk immunocompromised patients. Both intravenous and oral acyclovir are useful in prophylaxis in a variety of settings, including bone marrow transplant recipients and patients with leukemia undergoing intensive chemotherapy[26-29]. Oral doses of 1–2 g/day appear adequate for prophylaxis in HSV-seropositive individuals susceptible to frequent reactivation. Not all seropositive, immunocompromised patients require prolonged prophylaxis; it should be reserved for those with severe compromise who are subject to repeated clinical recurrences.

Acyclovir is also effective therapy against mucocutaneous HSV infections in the immunosuppressed host. Intravenous regimens (750 mg/m^2 per day) have been used successfully to treat infections in bone marrow and cardiac transplant recipients in controlled trials.[30,31] Oral acyclovir has also been effective in the control of mucocutaneous infections among other immunocompromised patients,[32] although controlled trials are lacking. Topical 5% acyclovir ointment applied six times daily to mucocutaneous lesions has also demonstrated efficacy in double-blind placebo-controlled studies[33]; lesion healing, pain resolution, and virus clearance were all accelerated. Thus, the choice of which acyclovir preparation to employ will depend largely on such factors as the likelihood of organ involvement, cost, and toxicity. Localized mucocutaneous HSV infections can often be successfully managed with topical acyclovir, whereas disseminated infection requires circulating drug levels achievable by the intravenous or oral routes.

3. Varicella-Zoster Virus

Illustrative Case 2

A 55-year-old man with Hodgkin disease was admitted to the Massachusetts General Hospital because of right-sided facial pain of 2 days' duration and vesicular eruption of 6-hr duration. His Hodgkin disease had been classified stage IIIA 4 years previously, and he had received extensive radiation and chemotherapy. For 5 months prior to admission, the patient had been receiving vinblastine, procarbazine, CCNU, and prednisone intermittently.

On admission, the patient was afebrile but in considerable pain. Zosteriform eruptions involving all three divisions of the right trigeminal nerve were observed, with concentration of vesicular, erythematous lesions greatest over areas supplied by the ophthalmic and maxillary divisions (Fig 4). No dissemination outside this dermatome was observed. Laboratory studies were within normal limits. A Tzanck preparation of vesicular scrapings was positive for multinucleated giant cells (Fig. 5). He was enrolled into a placebo-controlled study of adenine arabinoside for zoster. Over the next few days, fever developed, and some increase in local spread of lesions was observed VZV virus was isolated from a vesicle aspirate. On day 5 following admission, dissemination of vesicles was noted on the trunk and extremities, and the temperature rose to 102°F. After discussion with the study coordinators, the randomized code was broken, and it was determined that the patient had received placebo. Adenine arabinoside 10 mg/kg per day, was instituted. On day 7, he was observed to be less responsive and more confused. On neurologic examination, incomplete right eye abduction and adduction were noted, as were myoclonic movements of fingers and toes Delirium and hallucinations developed. Lumbar puncture was performed, cerebrospinal fluid (CSF) contained 88 red blood cells (RBCs) and 109 white blood cells/mm³. Cerebrospinal fluid protein was 122 mg/dl, glucose 55 mg/dl (with simultaneous serum glucose of 66 mg/dl) Gram, Ziehl–Nielsson, and fungal smears were negative, as was a test for cryptococcal antigen. Cerebrospinal fluid cultures for bacteria, fungi, and viruses were negative Electroencephalogram (EEG) showed generalized delta slowing. Over the next 2 weeks, the patient's obtundation increased, and fever persisted. Repeat lumbar puncture showed decreased protein (100 mg/dl) and WBCs (10/mm³) Electroencephalogram demonstrated progressive slowing. By the 25th hospital day, the patient was comatose and hypo-

tensive. Cardiac arrhythmias appeared on this day, and the patient expired. No autopsy was performed.

3.1. Clinical Epidemiology and Patterns of Infection

The immunocompromised host can develop a variety of syndromes related to VZV infection. Primary varicella with visceral dissemination and death is not uncommon in children with cancer who are on chemotherapy.[34,35] Estimates are that 20–35% of varicella in such children will be associated with visceral dissemination and a mortality rate of 7–30%. Dissemination appears to be related to low peripheral blood lymphocyte counts (<500/mm³) early in the course of infection. Primary varicella may also be particularly severe in transplant recipients, particularly children who have received bone marrow grafts.[36] Certain cell-mediated immunodeficiency disorders of childhood have been associated with visceral, sometimes fatal attacks of varicella; these include cartilage–hair hypoplasia and Nezeloff syndrome.[37]

When visceral involvement occurs during primary varicella, the lung is the major target organ,

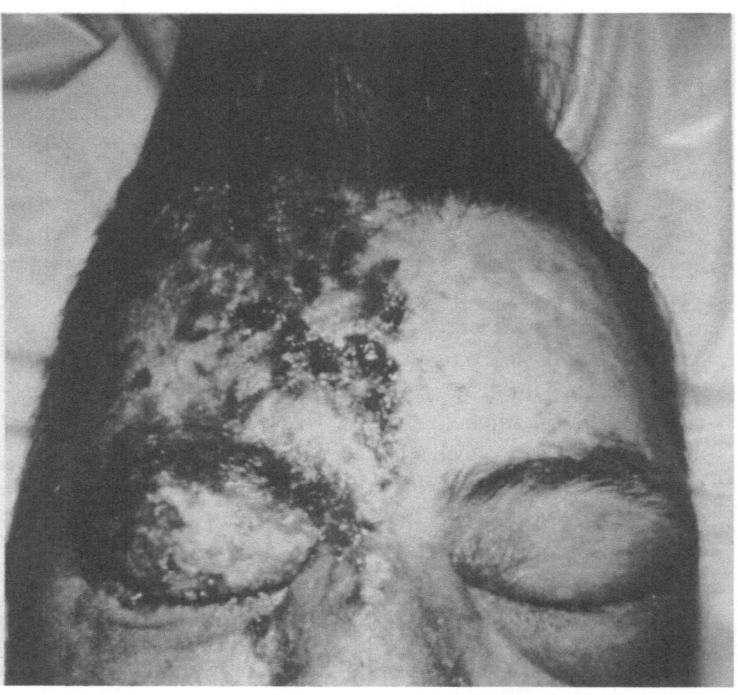

FIGURE 4. Ophthalmic zoster in a patient with Hodgkin disease. This infection ultimately resulted in fatal encephalitis

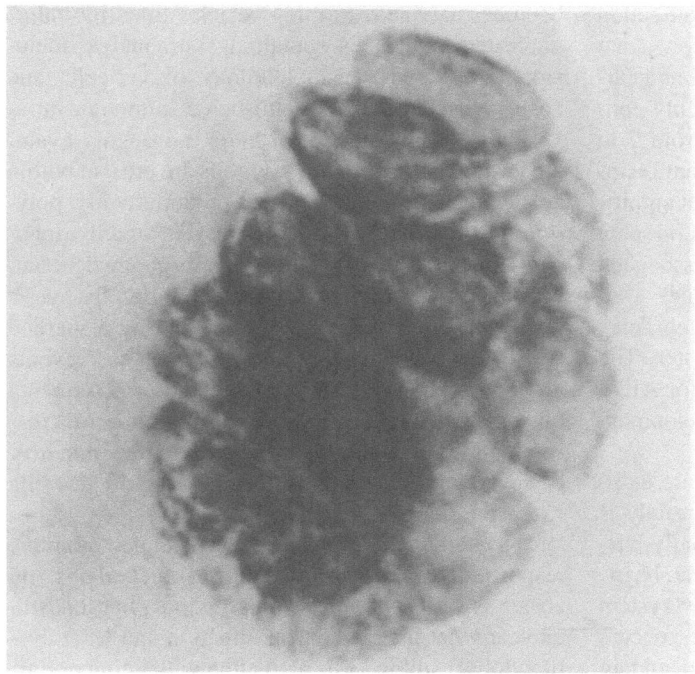

FIGURE 5. Tzanck preparation of vesicular lesion positive for multinucleate giant cells and compatible with VZV or HSV infection

with liver and brain involved less commonly. Varicella pneumonia usually occurs 3–7 days after onset of skin lesions. Pneumonitis can be rapidly progressive over a few days or may linger with gradual improvement over 2–4 weeks. Secondary bacterial infection, either cutaneous or bacteremic, may occur. Neurologic complications occur most frequently 4–8 days after onset of rash and often indicate a poor prognosis.

Among immunodeficient adults, herpes zoster is a more common complication than primary varicella. Hodgkin disease patients appear particularly susceptible to both localized and disseminated zoster. Review of several large series encompassing more than 1600 Hodgkin disease patients indicates that the risk of developing zoster is 13–15%, compared with 7–9% for non-Hodgkin lymphoma patients, and 1–3% for patients with solid tumors.[38–44] Approximately 15–30% of Hodgkin disease patients with zoster will demonstrate significant dissemination. However, mortality rates in adults with malignancy and localized or disseminated zoster are much lower than in children with malignancy and varicella. Several conclusions based on clinical studies of zoster in malignancy are possible.

1. Localized zoster is more common during advanced stages (III–IV) of disease than in less advanced disease or during remission. Dissemination is also more likely in advanced disease.
2. Because of the widespread use of more intensive therapy, the frequency of zoster as a complication of malignancy has been increasing over the past several years.
3. Zoster develops more frequently at areas of regionalized tumor and/or localized radiation therapy.
4. Patients receiving combination chemotherapy or radiation plus chemotherapy have a higher incidence of zoster than those receiving radiation alone or no therapy.
5. Most zoster infections occur within the first 12 months after onset of radiation therapy.
6. Visceral dissemination is associated with decreased survival.

Several points regarding zoster in malignancy are unclear or controversial: these include the risk factor of splenectomy, the prognostic implications of zoster, and the immunologic abnormalities underlying susceptibility. The latter is discussed in Section 3.2.

The risk of clinical zoster among renal and cardiac transplant recipients has been remarkably constant in several series[3,45–47] and ranges from 7 to 9%. The course of infection among transplant recipients is generally uncomplicated and without significant dissemination. Syndromes of unilateral pain without a skin eruption have also been associated with rises in antibody to VZV in this group.[48]

Patients with AIDS or AIDS-related complex (ARC) also appear at increased risk for zoster. The appearance of zoster in individuals at risk for AIDS appears to be a bad prognostic sign for development of AIDS.[48a,b]

Dissemination of zoster generally occurs 6–10 days after onset of localized lesions and usually is limited to cutaneous involvement. Occasionally, visceral dissemination develops, with CNS, lung, heart, and GI tract involvement. Central nervous system involvement, as described in our patient, occurs more commonly in the immunosuppressed and in those with ophthalmic zoster and is often associated with cutaneous dissemination.[49]

Second cases of chickenpox among immunologically intact hosts are exceedingly rare. However, among the immunosuppressed, they are not uncommon and are often referred to as atypical disseminated zoster or varicelliform zoster.[38,42,44,50] These eruptions occur in individuals with a previous history of chickenpox and do not have a dermatomal distribution. Rarely, second attacks of chickenpox have been associated with pneumonitis,[34] but more often they are mild and self-limited.

3.2. Pathogenesis

Early events in VZV pathogenesis are obscure. The initial site of virus entry and replication is unknown, although the respiratory tract, skin, or conjunctiva are likely possibilities. Following local replication, virus is carried via the bloodstream to focal cutaneous and visceral sites. Viremia appears to be intermittent and associated with leukocyte carriage of virus.[51] Subsequent localization of virus in the stratum germinativum and the stratum spinosum is followed by virus replication, vacuole formation, ballooning degeneration of epithelial cells, and accumulation of edema fluid. The stratum corneum becomes elevated, forming vesicles lined by multinucleated giant cells containing intranuclear inclusion bodies. The histopathology of varicella and zoster vesicles is indistinguishable, although intravesicular events have been more thoroughly evaluated in zoster.[52] Initially, few cells are present within zoster vesicles, and they are predominantly polymorphonuclear (PMNL); monocytes and lymphocytes are sparse at all stages. Polymorphonuclear leukocyte counts subsequently increase abruptly over a 1–2-day period and are accompanied by a marked rise in intravesicular interferon titers. These events are temporally correlated with clouding and crusting of vesicles and, in zoster, with termination of dissemination. Surrounding inflammatory reaction may be severe in zoster and result in scarring; in varicella extensive scarring is unusual.

Systemic humoral and cell-mediated immune responses have been studied during chicken pox and zoster as well as in intervening periods, but it is still unclear what factors control infection and what dysfunctions result in virus activation with aging or during periods of immunosuppression. VZV antibodies appear more rapidly and reach higher titers during episodes of zoster than during chickenpox,[53] suggesting anamnestic response following reactivation or reexposure. In a group of renal transplant recipients followed sequentially over several years, complement-fixing (CF) antibody titer fluctuations were observed in asymptomatic individuals, suggesting that subclinical virus release and antigenic stimulation may be involved in maintaining prolonged immunity.[48]

By contrast, subclinical primary infections appear rare to nonexistent if sensitive serologic assays are employed.[54] Antibody may have a protective role in prophylaxis of high-risk groups against varicella, e.g., children with leukemia, lymphoma, and immunodeficiency syndromes, as demonstrated by several studies of exogenously administered zoster immune globulin (ZIG) or plasma (ZIP).[55–59] Antibody administered late in incubation or during clinical infection has not been found to be helpful. Similarly, the presence of circulating antibody does not appear to protect against the activation or dissemination of endogenous VZV.[53,60] Once the virus is within susceptible target cells in skin or ganglia, it would not be expected that this strongly cell-bound virus would be significantly altered by circulating antibodies unless

ADCC mechanisms were important in such protective host responses.

Within recent years, several groups have studied the role of cell-mediated immune responses in VZV infections. The impetus for these studies is the increased morbidity associated with disorders of cell-mediated immunity such as Hodgkin disease and congenital T-cell disorders. Various assays of both afferent and efferent limbs of the cell-mediated immune response have been studied, including lymphocyte transformation to VZV antigens,[41,61,62] production of lymphokines such as interferon,[61,63] in vitro inactivation of VZV,[64] and skin-test reactivity to VZV antigens.[65]

Although assay conditions have varied among investigators, lymphocyte transformation to viral antigens appears to be a reliable indicator of past exposure to VZV,[63] as does skin test reactivity to inactivated VZV.[65] The time course of reactivity following primary infection has not been well established, but skin-test conversion in susceptible individuals occurs 5–7 days after administration of live varicella virus vaccine.[60] During zoster, VZV-specific lymphocyte proliferative responses are diminished early after onset of disease in contrast to nonspecific lymphocyte responses which may be normal.[62–64] Such specific hyporesponsiveness may, in fact, contribute to VZV activation. Subsequent limitation of infection is correlated with increased cell-mediated responsiveness as manifest by lymphocyte transformation, interferon production, and inhibition of in vitro virus replication. A variety of cell types appears to be involved in these responses. T lymphocytes are necessary for proliferative responses, whereas non-T lymphocytes appear more important for interferon production.[63,66] Both lymphocytes and monocytes are necessary for virus inhibition in vitro.[64] Patients with increased susceptibility to clinical zoster secondary to lymphoma or renal transplantation may have diminished cellular responses to VZV while demonstrating normal humoral responsiveness.[3,64] In addition, delayed local interferon production is related to dissemination of VZV in immunosuppressed patients.[52]

3.3. Diagnosis and Therapy

The diagnosis of uncomplicated chickenpox or herpes zoster can usually be made with confidence on clinical grounds alone. Rarely, HSV infection in the immunosuppressed patient can produce varicelliform or zosteriform eruptions distinguishable only by culture of fresh vesicles. VZV in culture has a much narrower host cell range, is more labile, and grows more slowly than HSV. It usually is lost upon freezing and must be cultured fresh, preferably on human fibroblast monolayers. Distinctive cytopathic effects usually appear in 3–10 days. VZV infections can be distinguished from other causes of vesicular lesions, e.g., vaccinia, variola, rickettsialpox, and enterovirus infections, by distribution of lesions, associated clinical findings, or Tzanck smear of scrapings taken from the base of a newly formed vesicle. Confirmatory serologic studies should be performed on acute and convalescent sera.

During VZV pneumonia, virus can also be cultured from sputum, and sputum cytologic examination may show multinucleated giant cells with intranuclear inclusions. It should be remembered that other opportunistic infections such as *Pneumocystis carinii* may coexist with VZV and that not all pneumonias with evident varicella or zoster are caused by VZV. Thus, lung biopsy or bronchial brushing may be necessary in selected patients for accurate diagnosis.

Similarly, encephalitis occurring in this setting may be difficult to diagnose. In zoster encephalitis, as demonstrated by our patient, VZV is not ordinarily isolated from CSF.[49,67] The diagnostic utility of brain biopsy in this situation has not been established, but levels of VZV membrane antibody (FAMA) in CSF may be useful.[49,68]

Immunosuppressed children without a history of varicella should receive varicella–zoster immune globulin (VZIG) if heavily exposed to either chickenpox or zoster.[55–59] To be maximally effective, VZIG must be administered soon after exposure. Current dose regimens are 1.25 ml/10 kg up to a maximum of 6.25 ml; this single dose is protective for approximately 4 weeks. Commercial immune serum globulin (ISG) is ineffective prophylaxis. Accepted criteria for release of VZIG are shown in Table 1.

A live attenuated VZV vaccine has been produced and is widely used in immunosuppressed and normal children in Japan.[69] Neutralizing, complement-fixing, and fluorescent antibodies to membrane antigens were induced by vaccination. The vaccine

TABLE 1. Criteria for Varicella–Zoster Immune Globulin Prophylaxis of Varicella as Suggested by the Centers for Disease Control

1 One of the following underlying illnesses or conditions.
   Leukemia or lymphoma
   Congenital or acquired immunodeficiency
   Under immunosuppressive medication
   Newly born of mother with varicella
   Premature infants (>28 weeks) whose mother lacks a
     history of chickenpox.
   Premature infant (<28 weeks or <1000 g) regardless of
     maternal history
2. One of the following types of exposure to varicella or
   zoster patient:
   Household contact
   Playmate contact (>1 hr play indoors)
   Hospital contact (in same two–four-bed bedroom or
     adjacent beds in a large ward)
   Newborn contact (newborn whose mother contracted
     varicella 5 days or less before delivery or within 48 hr
     after delivery)
3 Susceptible to VZV infection[a]
4. The request for treatment must be initiated within 96 hr of
   exposure

[a]By history if under age 15, if over age 15, it is advisable to check VZV
serologic status

has had extensive clinical trials in children with malignancy. If chemotherapy was suspended in these patients, there was minimal immediate risk associated with vaccination, and protection against subsequent exposure was demonstrated. Preliminary trials of VZV vaccine in the United States have also been very promising.[69–71] It appears likely that this vaccine will be a valuable addition to the armamentarium against varicella in the immunosuppressed child.

Important strides have also been made in the chemotherapy of VZV infections in immunosuppressed hosts. Vidarabine (adenine arabinoside, ara-A) and acyclovir both have demonstrated efficacy against varicella in immunocompromised hosts.[72,73] Vidarabine (10 mg/kg per day) reduces time of new lesion formation, fever, and visceral complications. Although acyclovir has not been as well evaluated in chickenpox, a small study demonstrated a reduction in pneumonitis (15 mg/kg per day).

Two well-controlled studies comparing vidarabine with placebo have been conducted in immunocompromised patients with acute herpes

zoster.[74,75] If begun within the first 72 hr of lesion formation, healing time was shortened and both cutaneous and visceral dissemination were reduced by vidarabine. Resolution of postherpetic neuralgia was also accelerated.

Intravenous acyclovir also retards the spread of cutaneous zoster in immunosuppressed patients, and reduces the likelihood of visceral zoster.[76] In a randomized comparison of intravenous acyclovir and vidarabine, acyclovir recipients had diminished dissemination and shortened healing time.[76a] Thus, intravenous acyclovir is now the treatment of choice for herpes zoster in this setting.

Intramuscular α-interferon (IF_α) has demonstrated benefit in both varicella and zoster as well, but is not currently licensed for these indications.[77,78]

4. Cytomegalovirus

Illustrative Case 3

A 15-year-old boy was admitted to the Massachusetts General Hospital for increasing renal failure and suspected rejection 5 weeks following the transplantation of a three-antigen-match kidney from a living related donor. He had been receiving 50 mg prednisone and 25 mg azathioprine daily On admission, he was afebrile but was noted to have mild pharyngeal injection and a slightly enlarged spleen. Following two 1-g bolus doses of methyl prednisolone sodium succinate, his renal function improved. Shortly thereafter, he developed leukopenia (WBC 1400/mm³), atypical lymphocytosis (6%), thrombocytopenia (36,000/mm³), and fever (104°F, or 40°C). Pharyngitis increased and was accompanied by nonproductive cough, headache, and malaise. Chest radiography demonstrated diffuse interstitial reticulonodular pulmonary infiltrates (Fig. 6) despite minimal clinical signs of respiratory embarassment. Physical examination was unchanged, and a specimen of arterial blood, drawn with the patient breathing room air, demonstrated a Pao_2 value of 88 mm Hg, a $Paco_2$ value of 37 mm Hg, and pH 7 40. Bronchial brushings were negative for bacteria, fungi, or *Pneumocystis carinii*. However, both bronchial and urine cultures were positive for CMV. Over the ensuing 3 weeks, pulmonary infiltrates, fever, thrombocytopenia, and leukopenia gradually resolved. Complement-fixation antibody to CMV rose during this period from <8 to 32

4.1. Clinical Epidemiology and Patterns of Infection

The ubiquity of CMV infections has become apparent within recent years, and the role of CMV as a major cause of congenital malformations[79,80] and heterophil-negative mononucleosis is well established. In patients with disordered cell-mediated im-

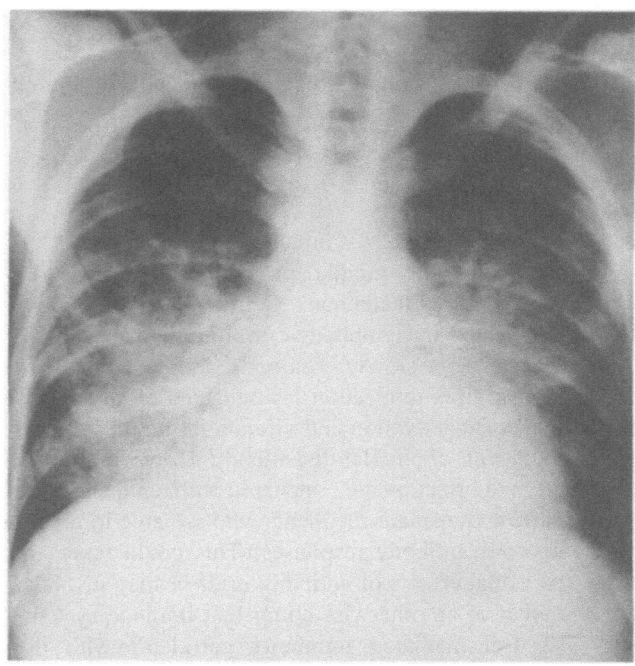

FIGURE 6. Chest radiograph of renal transplant recipient with CMV pneumonia. Bilateral interstitial infiltrates are seen.

munity, CMV is frequently isolated and can cause a variety of clinical syndromes, including pneumonitis, colitis, hepatitis, mononucleosis, retinitis, and possibly encephalitis.[4,5,47,81—96]

Among renal, hepatic, and cardiac transplant recipients, CMV is the most common opportunistic pathogen detected and is an important cause of morbidity and mortality. It can cause a variety of syndromes by itself (see Illustrative Case 3), can predispose to severe fungal and bacterial superinfection, and may be related to enhanced graft dysfunction. The occurrence of such complications corresponds in time with CMV viremia, excretion, and seroconversion, usually 1–4 months following transplantation. The relative risk appears to be greater in primary CMV infections, i.e., when seronegative recipients receive grafts from seropositive donors.[81,88,89] However, since this population is a minority of all patients transplanted, the overall morbidity from reactivation infection in seropositive recipients may be equally high. Patients receiving certain immunosuppressive agents, e.g., antithymcyte globulin may be more likely to have severe infections than those receiving other agents, e.g., cyclosporin.

Prolonged fever associated with malaise, anorexia, fatigue, night sweats, myalgias, and arthralgias is frequently found in CMV-infected transplant recipients. Transient abnormalities in liver function tests, depression in WBC and/or platelet counts, and atypical lymphocytosis may be seen during these febrile episodes. Occasionally, a dry hacking cough and tachypnea become superimposed on this syndrome, suggesting respiratory involvement. Radiologic examination may demonstrate a symmetric bilateral interstitial pneumonitis, as seen in the illustrative case, usually beginning in the periphery of the lower lobes and spreading centrally and superiorly; less commonly, unilateral lobar consolidation is demonstrated.[83]

If CMV-associated illnesses are prolonged and associated with leukopenia ($<1500/mm^3$) and viremia, superinfection with fungal, protozoan, and bacterial pathogens may occur. These infections take on the characteristics of the superinfecting organism and are frequently severe.

Clinical CMV infections in the transplant patient may be recurrent[97] or progressive.[98] Progressive CMV infection is characterized by prostration, orthostatic hypotension, and mild hypoxemia, progressing to severe pulmonary and hepatic dysfunction, muscle wasting, CNS depression, and death. In this rare complication, CMV CF antibody responses are minimal.[89]

Asymptomatic CMV excretion in the transplant recipient is common and is sometimes prolonged for months or years. Viremia may also be prolonged and asymptomatic.[99] However, it has become clear that viremic individuals are more likely to develop renal dysfunction and superinfection.[93,100] The renal dysfunction associated with viremia may result from a CMV-induced glomerulopathy.[93,100] Thus, what has been described as CMV-enhanced rejection is often actually renal dysfunction induced by a nonrejection mechanism.

The bone marrow transplant recipient is at particular risk for developing severe CMV pneumonitis.[90] Approximately one-half of marrow graft recipients develop interstitial pneumonia, usually after successful engraftment; nearly one-half of these cases are associated with CMV infection. The attack rate is higher for those with underlying malignancy than for those with aplastic anemia, and the mortality rate approaches 90%. The occurrence of CMV interstitial pnemonia appears closely linked with the presence of graft-versus-host reactions (GVHR) and serological hyporesponsiveness to CMV antigens. In addition, recipients of marrow from CMV-seropositive donors appear more likely to develop CMV pneumonia than recipients of marrow from seronegative donors. The incidence of significant CMV infections may also be increased in recipients of granulocyte transfusions.[90]

The frequency and importance of CMV infections among patients with neoplasms are not well defined. Leukemia and lymphoma patients may excrete the virus asymptomatically or may have syndromes characterized by prolonged fever, mononucleosis, or interstitial pneumonia.

CMV is also an important pathogen in patients with AIDS.[94–96] Syndromes of fever, leukopenia, and pneumonitis are common. CMV retinitis often begins with small opaque white areas of granular necrosis that spread in a centrifugal manner, later accompanied by hemorrhages, vessel sheathing, and edema.[95,96] Gastrointestinal involvement may be localized or extensive. Ulcers of the esophagus, stomach, small intestine, or colon may result in bleeding or perforation. Chronic encephalitis or subacute encephalopathy in patients with AIDS has also been associated with CMV infection. Fatal infections are often characterized by persistent viremia and multiple organ system involvement, including adrenal necrosis.[101]

4.2. Pathogenesis

Following CMV infection in normal hosts, humoral antibodies rapidly appear and can be measured by a variety of techniques. Cell-mediated immunity, as detected by lymphocyte proliferative responses, appears more slowly. Antibody does not suffice to abolish virus replication, as indicated by the occurrence of reactivation and viremia in the presence of high levels of circulating antibody. However, modulation of infection does appear in both renal and bone marrow transplant recipients who are able to mount vigorous antibody responses. This could represent the actual effects of antibody itself or may just be a marker of an otherwise competent immune system.

Cell-mediated immunity correlates with the presence of circulating antibody in normal individuals who have recovered from primary CMV infection. However, cell-mediated immunity appears to be lost for several months following transplantation.[102] It is likely that loss of specific T-cell function or the diminished production of cell-associated mediators such as interferon is reflected in the increased morbidity of CMV infections during the early posttransplant period. Recovery of cell-mediated immune responses is associated with a decreased incidence of severe CMV infections.

In murine models of CMV infection, the use of T-cell-active immunosuppressive agents, e.g., antithymocyte globulin (ATG), is associated with activation of severe CMV infections. Murine CMV infection, in turn, can suppress the normal cell-mediated host response to other microbes and increase the severity of subsequent *Candida albicans* and *Pseudomonas aeruginosa* infections.[102a,b] As mentioned previously, human CMV infections in immunosuppressed hosts can also increase the severity of fungal and bacterial superinfections.[93] Human CMV infection suppresses lymphocyte reactivity to both mitogens and antigens but does not appear to interfere with function of polymorphonuclear leukocytes.[103] The combination of absolute leukopenia and T-cell dysfunction may account for the enhanced susceptibility to superinfection.

The sites of CMV latency in man are not certain but may well include peripheral blood leukocytes, kidney, salivary glands, and lung. The mechanisms by which latent CMV becomes activated following transplantation are also unclear but may represent a combination of both allogeneic activation and iatrogenic immunosuppression.

4.3. Diagnosis and Therapy

Virus excretion or viremia can be readily detected by culture of appropriate specimens on human fibroblast monolayers. A major problem, however, is the length of time required in culture before viral cytopathic effects appear, often extending beyond 2–3 weeks. An urgent need is the development of techniques for rapid diagnosis of CMV infections.

Recent advances in molecular biology have allowed DNA–DNA hybridization techniques to be used for rapid detection of CMV in urine and buffy coat specimens with a sensitivity and specificity of approximately 90%.[104,105] To date, these techniques are experimental and require the use of ^{32}P-labeled probes. It is hoped that the use of nonradioactive stable probes will permit this promising technique to become more generally available. Another rapid technique that will be increasingly employed is detection of CMV antigens in specimens by immunofluorescence or immunoperoxidation using monoclonal antibodies directed against CMV-specific antigens.[106]

A variety of serologic assays—complement fixation, immunofluorescence, indirect hemagglutination, and enzyme-linked immunosorbent assay (ELISA)—are available to detect antibody rises to CMV antigens. Antibody rises may not be detectable for up to 4 weeks after primary infection and titers often remain high for years after infection. Thus, single sample antibody determinations are not of value in assessing the acuteness of infection.

Several avenues of prophylaxis and therapy of CMV infections in high-risk groups are under investigation. Primary infections can be reduced by protective matching of donor or recipient pairs in transplant situations,[81,89] by using only blood products from seronegative donors, or by using only frozen-thawed and deglycerolized blood for transfusions. These, at best, are approaches with only limited value. Live attenuated CMV vaccines and CMV immune globulins may also be of value in seronegative organ transplant recipients.[107-109]

Prophylactic α-interferon (IF$_\alpha$) 3×10^6 units, three times per week for 6 weeks and then twice per week for 8 weeks, prevented reactivation of CMV syndromes and delayed CMV excretion in high-risk kidney transplant recipients, i.e., those receiving cadavar organs and antithymocyte globulin.[110] Interferons have not been successful in the therapy of ongoing CMV syndromes, however, either in transplant recipients or in patients with AIDS.[111]

Nucleoside derivatives, including vidarabine and acyclovir, have also been unsuccessful in the treatment of CMV infections. Newer compounds, particularly 9-1-(1,3-dihydroxy-2-propoxymethyl)guanine (DHPG), also known as ganciclovir, show considerable activity against CMV in vitro. Preliminary clinical trials demonstrate reversal of CMV retinitis and colitis by DHPG, although prolonged maintenance therapy is required in patients with AIDS.[112,113]

5. Epstein–Barr Virus

Illustrative Case 4

A 52-year-old homosexual man presented with a 3-month history of bilateral generalized lymphadenopathy, fever, weight loss, and diarrhea. HIV antibody was present, and the TH/TS ratio was 0.1. Two purple skin lesions were observed. Biopsies of a skin lesion and a cervical lymph node demonstrated Kaposi sarcoma. High-dose IF$_\alpha$ was instituted with resolution of skin lesions and adenopathy. However, skin lesions recurred once interferon was discontinued, and treatment with doxyrubicin, vinblastine, and bleomycin was begun. Cryptococcal meningitis developed 1 week later, requiring therapy with amphotericin B and 5-fluorocytosine.

Three weeks later, GI bleeding was noted, and gastroscopy demonstrated multiple 0.5–2.0-cm polypoid nodules of the stomach, assumed to be Kaposi sarcoma. Treatment with vincristine, bleomycin, and cis-platin was instituted, but *Klebsiella* bacteremia, hypotension, and renal failure ensued. He died 13 months after the initial diagnosis of AIDS.

At autopsy, tumor nodules were noted on the skin, stomach, small intestine, colon, mesentery, liver, and pleura. Microscopically, the nodules were composed primarily of sheets of immature lymphoid cells with interspersed histiocytes and were classified as undifferentiated lymphoma, non-Burkitt, or small noncleaved cell type. Foci of Kaposi sarcoma were also observed in the stomach, intestine, and skin.

DNA extracted from bowel, lymph node, and spleen was assayed for EBV DNA by nucleic acid hybridization, using Southern blot analysis. A radiolabeled probe was employed, containing the Bam H1K fragment of the EBV genome. Bowel tumor contained EBV genomic information, while normal spleen and lymph node did not. Premortem serum had demonstrated EBV antibodies (VCA IgG 1 : 1280, EBNA 1 : 5), compatible with prior EBV infection.

5.1. Clinical Epidemiology and Patterns of Infection

In the normal host, EBV is the principal cause of heterophile antibody-positive infectious mononucleosis and has been implicated in a variety of neurologic and neoplastic syndromes.[114-117] Among immunodeficient individuals, its importance as a pathogen is unclear.

As with other members of the herpes group, EBV excretion is increased among immunosuppressed populations such as renal transplant recipients and patients with lymphoproliferative diseases.[118-121] Primary EBV infection in transplant recipients may present as pneumonia resembling that caused by CMV or as heterophile-positive mononucleosis.[122] Reactivation EBV infection occurs commonly in transplant recipients.[118,119,121,123] Approximately 50–60% of renal transplant recipients will become EBV excreters. Most of these infections appear to be asymptomatic, are associated with virus excretion in throat washings, and may or may not be accompanied by concurrent antibody rises.

The incidence of EBV excretion in other disorders associated with immunosuppression is also higher than that seen in the general community. Excretion rates in patients with connective tissue diseases on immunosuppressive therapy were 47%; in patients with Hodgkin disease 16–23%; and in other lymphomas, leukemias, and cancers 25–58%.[118-120] These compare with rates of 75–90% in patients with infectious mononucleosis and 0–25% in healthy adults. No discrete clinical syndromes attributed to EBV have been demonstrated in these immunosuppressed patients.

Recent reports indicate that EBV may induce B-cell lymphoproliferative syndromes in a wide variety of immunocompromised hosts, including organ transplant recipients, patients with AIDS, and children with certain congenital immune deficiencies.[124-129] The incidence of lymphoproliferative syndromes or lymphomas in transplant recipients appears to vary with the nature of the allograft and the type or degree of immunosuppression, reaching a maximum of 13% in cardiac transplant recipients receiving high-dose cyclosporine.[124,125] Most of the lymphomas in these settings are multiclonal or oligoclonal B-cell neoplasms, and nearly all contain EBV genetic information. Sometimes, polyclonal B-cell proliferation may undergo transition to a monoclonal lymphoma.[125] B-cell lymphomas are also an increasingly frequent manifestation of AIDS[127,128] and, as demonstrated in our illustrative case, are often EBV genome positive.

One familial EBV-associated syndrome deserves particular comment. Several families with an apparent X-linked immunodeficiency syndrome have developed an EBV-linked B-lymphocyte proliferative disorder that can present either as a neoplasm (Burkitt lymphoma, immunoblastic sarcoma, plasmacytoma) or as an aproliferative syndrome (agammaglobulinemia, agranulocytosis, aplastic anemia).[129,130]

5.2. Pathogenesis

Initial EBV replication appears to take place in epithelial cells of the nasopharynx.[131] Thereafter, B lymphocytes become infected and transformed or immortalized. By contrast, T lymphocytes have not been found to have EBV receptors. Although different strains of EBV may induce transformed cells with different biologic and antigenic characteristics, infection of human umbilical cord lymphocytes generally results in stimulation of cellular DNA synthesis, development of EBV nuclear antigen (EBNA), and lymphoblastoid transformation, all within the first week of culture.[132] With longer time in culture, the number and percentage of cells positive for EBNA increase. The presence of EBNA, unlike the EBV-induced early antigen (EA) or VCA, is compatible with cell proliferation. By contrast, early antigen or VCA production signals entry into a productive lytic cycle and rarely occurs following exogenous EBV infection. The surface representation of nonviral antigens, e.g., histocompatibility (HLA) antigens, may also be altered by EBV infection and transformation.

The sequence of events that follows in vivo infection with EBV is less clear. The incubation period between exposure and clinical manifestations of infectious mononucleosis in normal hosts varies between 30 and 50 days. Among the abnormalities that may occur during the course of infectious mononucleosis are an atypical lymphocytosis in the peripheral blood, production of heterophile and autoantibodies, and a diminution in cell-mediated responsiveness to certain antigens despite an increase in spontaneous DNA synthesis among T-cell populations. Most of the atypical lymphocytes present in peripheral blood are T lymphocytes, although a small proportion of early atypical cells appear to be B lymphocytes.[133] During the acute phase of infectious mononucleosis, cells specifically cytotoxic for B-cell lines transformed by EBV can be found in peripheral blood. At this time, intense lymphoproliferative changes are also found in thymus-dependent paracortical zones of lymph nodes. The intense T-cell response against EBV-infected cells may result in a state of temporary anergy against other encountered antigens. It is possible that the syndrome of infectious mononucleosis may be the result of this vigorous T-lymphocyte-mediated rejection reaction against EBV-altered B lymphocytes. The EBV-infected B cells may, in turn, be responsible for the production of heterophile and autoantibodies characteristic of this syndrome.

Following recovery from mononucleosis, both EBNA-positive B lymphoblasts and T lymphoblasts cytotoxic for EBNA-positive cells disappear from peripheral blood. In seropositive normal persons, there may be intermittent asymptomatic oropharyngeal excretion of EBV. Neutralizing antibodies and antibodies against VCA and EBNA persist for prolonged periods together with minute numbers of latently infected cells in the peripheral blood.

Little is known concerning the sequence of events that is associated with EBV infection in the immunosuppressed host. However, it is likely that depression of T-lymphocyte-mediated responses allows expression of EBV from cells in the nasopharynx and possibly from B lymphoid cells in tissues and peripheral blood. Certain immunosuppressive agents, e.g., antithymocyte globulin, appear to be associated with an increased expression of EBV, as manifest by elevated VCA antibody titers and greater virus excretion.[116] Cyclosporin recipients appear to have a dose-dependent deficiency of cytotoxic T cells specific for EBV-infected B cells.[134] The high incidence of EBV-associated B-cell lymphoproliferative disorders in some renal transplant and AIDS patients suggests that this association should be further explored.

Certain patients appear to manifest a particularly severe genetically controlled lymphoproliferative syndrome related to progressive EBV infection.[129,130] Although specific immunologic defects are unclear, various immunoregulatory defects have been described.[135–137] If EBV replication is abortive but transformed B-cell proliferation is unchecked, a lymphoproliferative syndrome may ensue. Alternatively, if EBV replication is not controlled, production of infectious virus might result in widespread B-cell destruction and an agammaglobulinemic syndrome. In rare fatal cases of infectious mononucleosis, EBV antigens may be found in many organs.[138]

5.3. Diagnosis and Therapy

The overwhelming majority of immunosuppressed persons infected with EBV will not demonstrate the characteristic markers of infectious mononucleosis, i.e., heterophile antibodies and peripheral blood atypical lymphocytosis. EBV isolation from throat washings is a tedious and time-consuming process not currently performed by most virus diagnostic laboratories. The most useful diagnostic tests currently available are serologic assays for specific EBV antibodies.

A variety of EBV-associated antigens are expressed during infection or reactivation. The most sensitive marker of ongoing infection in renal transplant recipients appears to be change in the titer of antibodies to EBV viral capsid antigen (VCA) measured by immunofluorescence. Titer rises often occur to VCA in the absence of rises to other EBV antigens. Preliminary studies from our institution suggest that antibodies to other EBV antigens (EA-R or EBNA) may more accurately reflect severe EBV syndromes manifest by fever and leukopenia.[121] In pediatric patients with Hodgkin disease under therapy, titers to VCA were also increased, as were titers to the diffuse component of the early antigen (EA-D), whereas titers to nuclear antigen (EBNA) were depressed.[120]

Therapy of EBV infections in immunosuppressed patients does not appear necessary in most situations. Interferon, adenine arabinoside, acyclovir, and DHPG are inhibitory in vitro,[139–143] but no comparable studies have been done in human subjects. In our prophylactic study of human leukocyte interferon in renal transplant recipients, patients receiving interferon had fewer episodes of EBV infection, as manifest by virus excretion, than did placebo recipients.[116] Acyclovir has also demonstrated some activity against EBV infection in vivo, and DHPG may undergo clinical trials in the near future.

6. Other Human Herpesviruses

A new herpesvirus, called human B lymphotropic virus (HBLV) by one group, has been isolated from peripheral blood leukocytes of 6 persons with a variety of lymphoproliferative disorders.[144] Similar viruses have been isolated by others (C. Lopez, unpublished observations). These newly isolated viruses replicate preferentially in lymphocytes and do not cross-react with other human herpesviruses. Their association with disease is unclear.

References

1. Crosby DL, Jones JH, Sussman M: Herpetic naso-oral ulcers after renal transplantation. *Lancet* 2:1191, 1969.
2. Anuras S, Summers R: Fulminant herpes simplex hepatitis in an adult: Report of a case in a renal transplant recipient. *Gastroenterology* 70:425–428, 1976.
3. Rand KH, Rassmussen LE, Pollard RB, et al: Cellular immunity and herpesvirus infections in cardiac transplant patients. *N Engl J Med* 296:1372–1377, 1977.
4. Pass RF, Long WK, Whitley RJ, et al: Productive infection with cytomegalovirus and herpes simplex virus in renal transplant recipients. Role of source of kidney. *J Infect Dis* 137:556–563, 1978
5. Cheeseman SH, Rubin RH, Stewart JA, et al: Controlled clinical trial of prophylactic human leukocyte interferon in renal transplantation: Effects on cytomegalovirus and herpes simplex virus infections. *N Engl J Med* 300:1345–1349, 1979.
6. Muller SA, Herrman EC Jr, Winkelmann RK: Herpes simplex infections in hematologic malignancies. *Am J Med* 52:102–114, 1972.
7. Faden HS, Bybee BL, Overall JC Jr, et al: Disseminated herpes virus hominis infection in a child with acute leukemia. *J Pediatr* 90:951–953, 1977
8. Becker WB, Kipps A, McKenzie D. Disseminated herpes simplex virus infection—its pathogenesis based on virological and pathological studies in 33 cases. *Am J Dis Child* 115:1–8, 1968.
9. Wheeler CE Jr, Abele DC: Eczema herpeticum, primary and recurrent. *Arch Dermatol* 93:162–173, 1966.
10. Foley FD, Greenawald KA, Nash G, et al: Herpes virus infections in burned patients. *N Engl J Med* 282:652–656, 1970.
11 Sutton AL, Smithwick EM, Seligman SJ, et al: Fatal disseminated herpesvirus hominis type 2 infection in an adult with associated thymic dysplasia. *Am J Med* 56:545–553, 1974.
12. Siegal EP, Lopez C, Hammer GS, et al: Severe acquired immunodeficiency in male homosexuals, manifested by chronic perianal ulcerative herpes simplex lesions. *N Engl J Med* 305:1439–1444, 1981
13. Nash G: Necrotizing tracheobronchitis and bronchopneumonia consistent with herpetic infection. *Hum Pathol* 3:283–291, 1972.
14. Ramsey PG, Fife KH, Hackman RC, et al: Herpes simplex virus pneumonia—clinical, virologic, and pathologic features in 20 patients. *Ann Intern Med* 97:813–820, 1982.
15. Nash G, Ross JS: Herpetic esophagitis—a common cause of esophageal ulceration. *Hum Pathol* 5:339–345, 1974.
16. Warren KG, Brown SM, Wroblewska Z, et al: Isolation of latent herpes simplex virus from the superior cervical and vagus ganglions of human beings. *N Engl J Med* 298:1068–1070, 1978.
17. Hirsch MS, Zisman B, Allison AC: Macrophages and age-dependent resistance to herpes simplex virus in mice. *J Immunol* 104:1160–1165, 1970
18. Linnavuori K, Hovi T: Restricted replication of herpes simplex virus in human monocyte cultures: Role of interferon *Virology* 130:1–9, 1983.
19. Shore SL, Milgrom H, Wood PA, et al: Antibody-dependent cellular cytoxicity to target cells infected with herpes simplex viruses: Functional adequacy in the neonate *Pediatrics* 59:22–28, 1977.
20. Rasmussen LE, Jordan GW, Stevens DA, et al: Lymphocyte interferon production and transformation after herpes simplex infections in humans. *J Immunol* 112:728–736, 1974.
21. Pazin GJ, Lam MT, Armstrong JA, et al. Interferon prevention of HSV reactivation. *N Engl J Med* 301:225–230, 1979.
22. Zisman B, Hirsch MS, Allison AC: Effects of anti-lymphocyte serum, anti-macrophage serum and silica on herpes simplex virus infection of mice *J Immunol* 104:1155–1159, 1970.
23. Thong YH, Vincent MM, Hensen SA, et al: Depressed specific cell mediated immunity to herpes simplex virus type 1 in patients with recurrent herpes labialis *Infect Immunol* 12:76–80, 1975.
24. Kirchner H, Schwenteck M, Northoff H, et al: Defective in vitro lymphoproliferative responses to hepes simplex virus in patients with frequently recurring herpes infections during the disease-free interval. *Clin Immunol Immunopathol* 11:267–274, 1978.
25 Rasmussen LE, Jordan GW, Stevens DA: Lymphocyte interferon production and transformation after herpes simplex infections in humans *J Immunol* 112:728–736, 1974
26. Saral R, Burns WH, Laskin OL, et al: Acyclovir prophylaxis of herpes-simplex virus infections: A randomized, double-blind controlled trial in bone-marrow-transplant recipients. *N Engl J Med* 305:63–67, 1981
27 Saral R, Ambinder RF, Burns WH, et al: Acyclovir prophylaxis against herpes simplex virus infection in patients with leukemia—a randomized, double-blind, placebo-controlled study. *Ann Intern Med* 99:773–776, 1983.
28. Gluckman E, Lotsberg J, Devergie A, et al: Prophylaxis of

herpes infections after bone-marrow transplantation by oral acyclovir. *Lancet* **2**:706–708, 1983.

29. Wade JC, Newton B, Fluornoy N, et al: Oral acyclovir for prevention of herpes simplex virus reactivation after marrow transplantation. *Ann Intern Med* **100**:823–828, 1984.

30. Wade JC, Newton B, McLaren C, et al: Intravenous acyclovir to treat mucocutaneous herpes simplex virus infection after marrow transplantation. *Ann Intern Med* **96**:265–269, 1982.

31. Chou S, Gallagher JG, Merigan TC: Controlled clinical trial of intravenous acyclovir in heart-transplant patients with mucocutaneous herpes simplex infections. *Lancet* **1**:1392–1394, 1981.

32. Straus SE, Seidlin M, Takiff H, et al: Oral acyclovir to suppress recurring herpes simplex virus infections in immunodeficient patients. *Ann Intern Med* **100**:522–524, 1984

33. Whitley RJ, Levin M, Barton N, et al: Infections caused by herpes simplex virus in the immunocompromised host. Natural history and topical acyclovir therapy. *J Infect Dis* **150**:323–329, 1984.

34. Feldman S, Hughes WT, Daniel CB: Varicella in children with cancer: Seventy-seven cases. *Pediatrics* **56**:388–397, 1975.

35. Reboul F, Donaldson SS, Kaplan HS: Herpes zoster and varicella in children with Hodgkin's disease—an analysis of contributing factors. *Cancer* **41**:95–99, 1978.

36. Atkinson MK, Storb R, Prentice RL, et al: Analysis of late infections in eighty-nine long-term survivors of bone marrow transplantation. *Blood* **53**:720–731, 1979.

37. Lux SE, Johnston RB Jr, August CS, et al: Chronic neutropenia and abnormal cellular immunity in cartilage–hair hypoplasia. *N Engl J Med* **282**:231–236, 1970.

38. Sokal JE, Firat D: Varicella–zoster infection in Hodgkin's disease. *Am J Med* **39**:452–463, 1965.

39. Goffinett DR, Glatstein EJ, Merigan TC: Herpes zoster-varicella infections and lymphoma. *Ann Intern Med* **76**:235–240, 1972

40. Monfardini S, Bajetta E, Arnold CA, et al. Herpes zoster-varicella in malignant lymphomas. *Eur J Cancer* **11**:51–57, 1975.

41. Ruckdeschel JS, Schimpff SC, Smyth AC, et al: Herpes zoster and impaired cell-associated immunity to the varicella–zoster virus in patients with Hodgkin's disease. *Am J Med* **62**:77–85, 1977.

42. Schimpff S, Serpick A, Stoler B, et al: Varicella–zoster infection in patients with cancer *Ann Intern Med* **76**:241–254, 1972.

43. Wilson JF, Marsa GW, Johnson RE: Herpes zoster in Hodgkin's disease. *Cancer* **29**:461–465, 1972.

44. Mazur MH, Dolin R: Herpes zoster at the NIH: A 20 year experience *Am J Med* **65**:738–744, 1978.

45. Rifkind D: The activation of varicella–zoster virus infections by immunosuppressive therapy. *J Lab Clin Med* **68**:463–474, 1966.

46. Spencer ES, Anderson HK: Clinically evident, non-terminal infections with herpes viruses and the wart virus in immunosuppressed renal allograft recipients. *Br Med J* **3**:251–254, 1970.

47. Naraqi S, Jackson GG, Jonasson O, et al: Prospective study of prevalence, incidence, and source of herpesvirus infections in patients with renal allografts. *J Infect Dis* **136**:531–540, 1977.

48. Luby JP. Ramirez-Ronda C, Rinner S, et al. A longitudinal study of varicella–zoster virus infections in renal transplant recipients. *J Infect Dis* **135**:659–663, 1977.

48a. Friedman-Kien AE, Lafleur FL, Gendler E, et al: Herpes zoster: A possible early clinical sign for development of acquired immunodeficiency syndrome in high-risk individuals. *J Am Acad Dermatol* **14**:1023–1028, 1986

48b. Melbye M, Grossman RJ, Goedert JJ, et al. Risk of AIDS after herpes zoster. *Lancet* **i**:728–731, 1987.

49. Jemsek J, Greenberg SB, Taber L, et al. Herpes zoster associated encephalitis. Cliniopathologic report of 12 cases and review of the literature. *Medicine (Baltimore)* **62**:81–97, 1983.

50. Dolin R, Reichman RC, Mazur MH, et al: Herpes zoster-varicella infections in immunosuppressed patients. *Ann Intern Med* **89**:375–388, 1978.

51. Feldman S, Chaudary S, Ossi M, et al: A viremic phase for herpes zoster in children with cancer. *J Pediatr* **91**:597–600, 1977.

52. Stevens DA, Ferrington RA, Jordan GW, et al: Cellular events in zoster vesicles: Relation to clinical course and immune parameters. *J Infect Dis* **131**:509–515, 1975.

53. Miller LH, Brunell PA: Zoster, reinfection or activation of latent virus? *Am J Med* **49**:480–483, 1970.

54. Gershon AA, Krugman S: Seroepidemiologic survey of varicella: Value of specific fluorescent antibody test. *Pediatrics* **56**:1005–1008, 1975.

55. Brunell PA, Gershon AA, Hughes WT, et al: Prevention of varicella in high risk children: A collaborative study. *Pediatrics* **56**:718–722, 1972.

56. Meyers JD, Witte JJ: Zoster immune globulin in high-risk children. *J Infect Dis* **129**:616–618, 1974.

57. Wisnes R: Efficacy of zoster immunoglobulin in prophylaxis of varicella in high-risk patients. *Acta Paediatr Scand* **67**:77–82, 1978.

58. Orenstein WA, Heymann DL, Ellis RJ, et al: Prophylaxis of varicella in high-risk children. Dose–response effect of zoster immune globulin. *J Pediatr* **98**:368–373, 1981.

59. Varicella–zoster immune globulin for the prevention of chicken pox—recommendations of the immunization practices advisory committee (ACIP). *MMWR* **33**:84–100, 1984.

60. Uduman SA, Gershon AA, Brunell PA: Should patients with zoster receive zoster immune globulin? *JAMA* **234**:1049–1051, 1975.

61. Jordan GW, Merigan TC: Cell-mediated immunity to varicella-zoster virus: In vitro lymphocyte responses. *J Infect Dis* **130**:495–501, 1974

62. Russell AS, Maini RA, Bailey M, et al: Cell-mediated immunity to varicella–zoster antigen in acute herpes zoster (shingles). *Clin Exp Immunol* **14**:181–185, 1972.

63. Arvin AM, Pollard RB, Rasmussen LE, et al: Selective impairment of lymphocyte reactivity to varicella–zoster virus antigen among untreated patients with lymphoma. *J Infect Dis* **137**:531–539, 1978.

64. Gershon AA, Steinberg M, Smith M: Cell-mediated immu-

nity to varicella–zoster virus demonstrated by viral inactivation with human leukocytes. *Infect Immunol* **13**:1549–1553, 1976.

65. Kamiya H, Ihara T, Hattori A, et al: Diagnostic skin test reactions with varicella virus antigen and clinical application of the test *J Infect Dis* **136**:784–788, 1977.

66 Kirchner H: Herpes simplex virus and lymphocytes. In Proffitt M (ed)· *Virus–Lymphocyte Interactions. Implications for Disease.* Elsevier, New York, 1979, pp. 259–266.

67. Norris FH Jr, Leonards R, Calanchini PR, et al: Herpes-zoster meningoencephalitis. *J Infect Dis* **122**:335–338, 1970.

68. Gershon A, Steinberg S, Greenberg S, et al: Varicella-zoster-associated encephalitis: Detection of specific antibody in cerebrospinal fluid. *J Clin Microbiol* **12**:765–767, 1980.

69. Brunell P, Shehab Z, Geiser C, et al: Administration of live varicella vaccine to children with leukemia. *Lancet* **2**:1069–1072, 1982.

70. Gershon AA, Steinberg SP, Gelb L, et al: Live attenuated varicella vaccine: Efficacy for children with leukemia in remission. *JAMA* **255**:355–362, 1984.

71 Weibel RE, Neff BJ, Kuter BJK, et al: Live attenuated varicella virus vaccine-efficacy trial in healthy children. *N Engl J Med* **310**:1409–1415, 1984

72. Whitley R, Hilty M, Haynes R, et al: Vidarabine therapy of varicella in immunosuppressed patients. *J Pediatr* **101**:125–131, 1982.

73. Prober CG, Kirk LE, Keeney RE: Acyclovir therapy of chicken pox in immunosuppressed children—a collaborative study *J Pediatr* **101**:622–625, 1982.

74 Whitley RJ, Soong SJ, Dolin R, et al. Early vidarabine therapy to control the complications of herpes zoster in immunosuppressed patients. *N Engl J Med* **307**:971–975, 1982.

75. Whitley RJ, Chien LT, Dolin R, et al: Adenine arabinoside therapy of herpes zoster in the immunosuppressed. NIAID Collaborative Antiviral Study. *N Engl J Med* **294**:1193–1194, 1976.

76. Balfour HH Jr, Bean B, Laskin OL, et al: Acyclovir halts progression of herpes zoster in immunocompromised patients. *N Engl J Med* **308**:1448–1453, 1983.

76a. Shepp DH, Dandliker PS, Meyers JD: Treatment of varicella-zoster virus infection in severely immunocompromised patients. *N Engl J Med* **314**:208–212, 1986.

77. Merigan TC, Rand KH, Pollard RB, et al: Human leukocyte interferon for the treatment of herpes zoster in patients with cancer. *N Engl J Med* **298**:981–987, 1978.

78. Arvin AM, Kushner JH, Feldman S, et al: Human leukocyte interferon for the treatment of varicella in children with cancer. *N Engl J Med* **306**:761–765, 1982.

79 Ho M: *Cytomegalovirus—Biology and Infection.* Plenum, New York, 1982

80. Plotkin SA, Michelson S, Pagano JS, Rapp F (eds): *CMV: Pathogenesis and Prevention of Human Infection.* Liss, New York, 1984.

81. Betts RF, Freeman RB, Douglas RG Jr, et al: Clinical manifestations of renal allograft derived primary cytomegalovirus infection *Am J Dis Child* **131**:759–763, 1977

82. Luby JP, Burnett W, Hull AR, et al. Relationship between cytomegalovirus and hepatic function abnormalities in the period after renal transplantation *J Infect Dis* **129**:511–518, 1974.

83. Rubin RH, Cosimi AB, Tolkoff-Rubin NE, et al: Infectious disease syndromes attributable to cytomegalovirus and their significance among renal transplant recipients. *Transplantation* **24**:458–464, 1977

84 Broughton WL, Cupples HP, Parver LM. Bilateral retinal detachment following cytomegalovirus retinitis. *Arch Ophthalmol* **96**:618–619, 1978.

85. Murray HW, Know DL, Green WR, et al: Cytomegalovirus retinitis in adults. *Am J Med* **63**:574–584, 1977.

86. Dorfman LJ: Cytomegalovirus encephalitis in adults. *Neurology (NY)* **23**:136–144, 1973.

87. Simmons RL, Lopez C, Balfour H, et al. Cytomegalovirus: Clinical virological correlations in renal transplant recipients. *Ann Surg* **180**:623–632, 1974.

88 Suwansirikul S, Rao N, Dowling JN, et al: Primary and secondary cytomegalovirus infection. Clinical manifestations after renal transplantation *Arch Intern Med* **137**:1026–1029, 1977.

89. Rubin RH, Levin M, Cohen C, et al: Summary of workshop on cytomegalovirus infections during organ transplantation. *J Infect Dis* **139**:728–734, 1979

90. Meyers JD: Cytomegalovirus infection following marrow transplantation: Risk, treatment, and prevention. In Plotkin SA, Michelson S, Pagano JS, et al (eds): *CMV: Pathogenesis and Prevention of Human Infection.* Liss, New York, 1984, pp. 101–117.

91. Pollard RB, Egbert PR, Gallagher JG, et al: Cytomegalovirus retinitis in immunosuppressed hosts. I Natural history and effects of treatment with adenine arabinoside. *Ann Intern Med* **93**:655, 1980.

92. Glenn J: Cytomegalovirus infections following renal transplantation. *Rev Infect Dis* **3**:1151–1178, 1981

93 Schooley RT, Hirsch MS, Colvin RB, et al: Association of herpesgroup virus infections with T-lymphocyte subset alterations, glomerulopathy, and opportunistic infections following renal transplantation. *N Engl J Med* **308**:307–313, 1983.

94. Macher AM, Reichert CM, Straus SE, et al: Death in the AIDS patient: role of cytomegalovirus. *N Engl J Med* **309**:1454, 1983.

95. Friedman AH, Orellana J, Freeman WR, et al. Cytomegalovirus retinitis: A manifestation of the acquired immune deficiency syndrome (AIDS). *Br J Ophthalmol* **67**:372–380, 1983.

96. Holland GN, Pepose JS, Pettit TH, et al: Acquired immune deficiency syndrome—ocular manifestations. *Ophthalmology* **90**:859–873, 1983.

97 Friedman HM, Grossman RA, Plotkin SA, et al: Relapse of pneumonia caused by cytomegalovirus in two recipients of renal transplants *J Infect Dis* **139**:465–473, 1979.

98. Simmons RL, Matas AJ, Rattazzi LC, et al: Clinical characteristics of the lethal cytomegalovirus infection following renal transplantation. *Surgery* **82**:537–546, 1977.

99 Cheeseman SH, Stewart JA, Winkle S, et al:

Cytomegalovirus excretion two to fourteen years after renal transplantation. *Transplant Proc* **9**:71–74, 1979.

100. Richardson WP, Colvin RB, Cheeseman SH, et al. Glomerulopathy associated with cytomegalovirus viremia in renal allografts. *N Engl J Med* **305**:57–63, 1981.

101. Tapper ML, Rotterdam HZ, Lerner CW, et al: Adrenal necrosis in the acquired immunodeficiency syndrome. *Ann Intern Med* **100**:239–241, 1984.

102. Quinnan GV Jr, Rook AH: The importance of cytotoxic cellular immunity in the protection from cytomegalovirus infection. In Plotkin SA, Michelson S, Pagano JS, et al (eds): *CMV. Pathogenesis and Prevention of Human Infection.* Liss, New York, 1984, pp. 245–261.

102a. Hamilton JR, Overall JC Jr, Glasgow LA: Synergistic infection with murine cytomegalovirus and *Candida albicans* in mice. *J Infect Dis* **135**:918–924, 1977.

102b. Hamilton JR, Overall JC Jr.. Synergistic infection with murine cytomegalovirus and *Pseudomonas aeruginosa* in mice *J Infect Dis* **137**:775–782, 1978.

103. Hirsch MS: Cytomegalovirus–leukocyte interactions. In Plotkin SA, Michelson S, Pagano JS, et al (eds): *CMV: Pathogenesis and Prevention of Human Infection.* Liss, New York, 1984, pp. 161–173.

104. Chou S, Merigan TC: Rapid detection and quantitation of human cytomegalovirus in urine through DNA hybridization. *N Engl J Med* **308**:921–925, 1983.

105. Spector SA, Rua JA, Spector DH: Detection of human cytomegalovirus in clinical specimens by DNA–DNA hybridization. *J Infect Dis* **150**:121–126, 1984

106. Volpi A, Whitley RJ, Ceballos R: Rapid diagnosis of pneumonia due to cytomegalovirus with specific monoclonal antibodies. *J Infect Dis* **147**:1119–1120, 1983.

107. Winston DJ, Pollard RB, Ho WG, et al: Cytomegalovirus immune plasma in bone marrow transplant recipients. *Ann Intern Med* **97**:11–18, 1982.

108. Meyers JD, Leszczynski J, Zaia JA, et al. Prevention of cytomegalovirus infection by cytomegalovirus immune globulin after marrow transplantation. *Ann Intern Med* **98**:442–446, 1983.

109. Plotkin SA, Smiley ML, Friedman HM, et al: Towne-vaccine-induced prevention of cytomegalovirus disease after renal transplants. *Lancet* **1**:528–530, 1984.

110. Hirsch MS, Schooley RT, Cosimi AB, et al: Effects of interferon alpha on cytomegalovirus reactivation syndromes in renal transplant recipients—results of a placebo controlled trial. *N Engl J Med* **308**:1489–1493, 1983.

111. Meyers JD, McGuffin RW, Bryson YJ, et al: Treatment of cytomegalovirus pneumonia after marrow transplant with combined vidarabine and human leukocyte interferon. *J Infect Dis* **146**:80–84, 1982.

112. Felsenstein D, D'Amico D, Hirsch MS, et al: Treatment of cytomegalovirus retinitis with 9-[2-hydroxy-1-(hydroxymethyl)ethoxymethyl]guanine (BWB759U). **103**:377–80, 1985.

113. Collaborative DHPG Treatment Study Group: Treatment of serious cytomegalovirus infections with 9-(1,3 dihydroxy-2-propoxymethyl)guanine in patients with AIDS and other immunodeficiencies. *New Engl J Med* **314**:801–805, 1986.

114. Grose C, Henle W, Henle G, et al: Primary Epstein-Barr virus infections in acute neurologic diseases *N Engl J Med* **292**:392–395, 1975.

115. Klein G: The relationship of the virus to nasopharyngeal carcinoma. In Epstein MA, Achong BG (eds): *The Epstein-Barr Virus.* Springer-Verlag, Berlin, 1979, pp. 339–350.

116. Epstein MA, Achong BG: The relationship of the virus to Burkitt's lymphoma. In Epstein MA, Achong BG (eds): *The Epstein-Barr Virus.* Springer-Verlag, Berlin, 1979, pp. 321–37.

117. Hochberg FH, Miller G, Schooley RT, et al: Central nervous system lymphoma related to Epstein-Barr virus *N Engl J Med* **309**:745–748, 1983.

118. Strauch B, Siegel N, Andrews LL, et al: Oropharyngeal excretion of Epstein-Barr virus by renal transplant recipients and other patients treated with immunosuppressive drugs *Lancet* **1**:234–237, 1974.

119. Chang RS, Lewis JP, Reynolds RD, et al: Oropharyngeal excretion of Epstein-Barr virus by patients with lymphoproliferative disorders and by recipients of renal homografts. *Ann Intern Med* **88**:34–40, 1978.

120. Lange B, Arbeiter A, Hewetson J: Longitudinal study of Epstein-Barr virus antibody titers and excretion in pediatric patients with Hodgkin's disease. *Int J Cancer* **22**:521–527, 1978.

121. Cheeseman SH, Henle W, Rubin RH, et al. Epstein-Barr virus infection in renal transplant recipients. Effects of antithymocyte globulin and interferon. *Ann Intern Med* **193**:39–42, 1980.

122. Grose C, Henle W, Horwitz MS: Primary Epstein-Barr virus infection in a renal transplant recipient. *South Med J* **70**:1276–1278, 1977.

123. Marker SC, Ascher NL, Kalis JM, et al: Epstein-Barr virus antibody responses and clinical illness in renal transplant recipients. *Surgery* **85**:433–440, 1978.

124. Crawford DH, Thomas JA, Janossy G Epstein-Barr virus nuclear antigen-positive lymphoma after cyclosporin-A treatment in patients with renal allograft. *Lancet* **1**:1355–1356, 1980.

125. Cleary ML, Sklar J: Lymphoproliferative disorders in cardiac transplant recipients are multiclonal lymphomas. *Lancet* **2**:489–494, 1984.

126. Hanto DW, Frizzera G, Gajl Peczalska KJ, et al: Epstein-Barr virus induced B-cell lymphoma after renal transplantation. Acyclovir therapy and transition from polyclonal to monoclonal B-cell proliferation. *N Engl J Med* **306**:913–918, 1982.

127. Ziegler JL, Miner RC, Rosenbaum E, et al: Outbreak of Burkitt's-like lymphoma in homosexual men *Lancet* **1**:631–633, 1982.

128. Ziegler JL, Beckstead JA, Volberding PA, et al: Non-Hodgkin's lymphoma in 90 homosexual men: relationship to generalized lymphadenopathy and the acquired immunodeficiency syndrome *N Engl J Med* **311**:565–570, 1984.

129. Sullivan JL, Byron JS, Brewster FE, et al. X-linked lymphoproliferative syndrome: natural history of the immunodeficiency. *J Clin Invest* **71**:1765–1778, 1983.

130. Purtilo DT, Sakamoto KB, Barnabei V, et al: Epstein-Barr

virus-induced diseases in boys with the X-linked lympho-proliferative syndrome—update on studies of the registry. *Am J Med* **73**:49–56, 1982.

131. Sixbey JW, Nedrud JG, Raab-Traub N, et al: Epstein-Barr virus replication in oropharyngeal epithelial cells. *N Engl J Med* **310**:1225–1230, 1984.

132. Robinson J, Miller G: Assay for Epstein-Barr virus based on stimulation of DNA synthesis in mixed leukocytes from human umbilical cord blood. *J Virol* **15**:1065–1071, 1975.

133. Pattengale PK, Smith RW, Perlin E: Atypical lymphocytes in acute infectious mononucleosis. *N Engl J Med* **291**:1145–1148, 1974.

134. Crawford DH, Sweny P, Edwards JMB, et al: Long-term T-cell-mediated immunity to Epstein-Barr virus in renal allograft recipients receiving cyclosporin A. *Lancet* **1**:10–13, 1981.

135. Sullivan JL, Byron KS, Brewster FE, et al: Deficient natural killer cell activity in X-linked lymphoproliferative syndrome. *Science* **210**:543–545, 1980.

136. Lindsten T, Seeley JK, Ballow M, et al: Immune deficiency in the X-linked lymphoproliferative syndrome. II. Immunoregulatory T cell defects. *J Immunol* **129**:2536–2540, 1982.

137. Ochs HD, Sullivan JL, Wedgwood RJ, et al: X-linked lymphoproliferative syndrome: Abnormal antibody responses to bacteriophage. *Birth Defects* **19**:321–323, 1983.

138. Britton S, Andersson-Anvret M, Gergely P: Epstein-Barr virus immunity and tissue distribution in a fatal case of infectious mononucleosis. *N Engl J Med* **298**:89–92, 1978.

139. Adams A, Strander H, Cantell K. Sensitivity of the Epstein-Barr virus transformed human lymphoid cell lines to interferon. *J Gen Virol* **28**:207–217, 1975.

140. Coker-Vann M, Dolin R: Effect of adenine arabinoside on Epstein-Barr virus in vitro. *J Infect Dis* **135**:447–453, 1977.

141 Datta AK, Colby BM, Shaw JE, et al: Acyclovir inhibition of Epstein-Barr virus replication. *Proc Natl Acad Sci USA* **77**:5163–5166, 1980

142. Garner JG, Hirsch MS, Schooley RT: Prevention of Epstein-Barr virus-induced B-cell outgrowth by interferon alpha *Infect Immun* **43**:920–924, 1984.

143 Lin JC, Smith MC, Pagano JS: Prolonged inhibitory effect of 9-(1,3-dihydroxy-2-propoxy methyl)guanine against replication of Epstein-Barr virus *J Virol* **50**:50–55, 1984.

144. Salahuddin SZ, Ablashi Dv, Markham PD, et al. Isolation of a new virus, HBLV, in patients with lymphoproliferative disorders. *Science* **234**:596–601, 1986.

14

Morbidity in Compromised Patients Due to Viruses Other Than Herpes Group and Hepatitis Viruses

ROBERT T. SCHOOLEY

1. Introduction

The past decade has witnessed greatly increased awareness of the multiple roles played by viral agents in immunocompromised patients. This interest, which has been stimulated by the development of effective antiviral chemotherapy for herpes group viruses, in particular, has been greatly facilitated by the development of more direct approaches to diagnosis using molecular biologic and monoclonal antibody technology. Lessened reliance on standard serologic techniques for viral diagnosis has been especially useful in immunocompromised patients in whom humoral responses may be delayed or absent.

It has become increasingly apparent that viral agents may contribute to morbidity in immunocompromised patients by several mechanisms in addition to traditional cytopathology and end-organ damage. Immunomodulation, which has been extensively studied in the herpes group virus system, is a feature of other viral agents, such as measles and mumps. In addition, immunocompromised patients may prove to be the population in which the biologic relevance of our increasing understanding of the transforming properties of several viral agents, such as BK virus, adenoviruses, and papillomaviruses, is tested. This chapter attempts to outline the morbidity due to viruses other than herpes group and hepatitis viruses in immunocompromised patients. Although immunocompromised patients are susceptible to the same spectrum of infections that cause morbidity for the general populations, certain agents appear to be particularly devastating to immunocompromised individuals. Only agents for which increased morbidity and mortality in immunocompromised patients have been clearly demonstrated are discussed (Table 1).

2. DNA Viruses

2.1. Adenoviruses

Adenoviruses are a common cause of acute febrile illness in immunocompetent adults. In children, however, up to 10% of hospitalizable pneumonias may be due to adenovirus infection.[1] Over the past decade, it has become apparent that adenoviruses may cause major morbidity in immunocompromised patients.[2-5] Adenovirus-associated morbidity has been reported in patients with both cellular and humoral immune defects with predisposing conditions that have included severe combined immunodeficiency, malignancy, and solid organ or bone marrow allograft transplantation.

Illustrative Case 1

A 19-year-old man with renal failure due to focal sclerosing glomerulonephritis received a renal allograft from a cadaveric do-

ROBERT T. SCHOOLEY • Infectious Disease Unit Massachusetts General Hospital; and Harvard Medical School, Boston, Massachusetts 02114

TABLE 1. Organ System Involvement with Viruses Other Than Herpes Group and Hepatitis Viruses in Immunocompromised Patients

Virus	CNS	Pulmonary	Hepatic	GI	Renal	Musculoskeletal	Skin
Adenovirus	+	+ +	+ + +	+ +	+		
Papovaviruses							
JC	+						
BK					+		
Papillomaviruses							+ +
Vaccinia							+ + +
Polio	+ +						
Echo	+ +						+ +
Coxsackie	+			+			
Measles	+ +	+ +					+
RSV		?					
Rotavirus				+ +			

nor.[6] Eight weeks after transplantation, fever, leukopenia, and thrombocytopenia developed. Cytomegalovirus (CMV) was isolated from his saliva. An eightfold rise in complement-fixation antibody titers to CMV was documented. The syndrome resolved spontaneously over 2–3 weeks. Six months later, he returned to hemodialysis due to recurrent focal sclerosis.

One year after the initial transplantation procedure, a second allograft from a cadaveric donor was implanted. He received prednisone, azathioprine, and antithymocyte globulin but progressive azotemia, hypertension, and oliguria developed. Two weeks following transplantation, fever and dyspnea developed. Bilateral basilar rales were present. A chest radiograph revealed diffuse interstitial pulmonary infiltrates. Leukopenia with a relative lymphocytosis was noted. The immunosuppressive regimen was rapidly tapered. Hemodialysis was reinstituted 3 weeks following transplantation. With withdrawal of the immunosuppressive regimen, the fever and pulmonary interstitial infiltrates resolved over a 2-week period. Adenovirus type 34 and CMV were isolated from three urine specimens. Adenovirus antibodies measured by hemagglutinin inhibition rose from <8 to 32 in conjunction with the clinical syndrome. The CMV antibody titer did not rise.

This patient with a previous renal allograft procedure which had been complicated by CMV reactivation developed fever, leukopenia, and interstitial pneumonitis in conjunction with isolation of adenovirus type 34 and CMV from urine. The brisk humoral immune response to adenovirus type 34 coupled with the lack of an antibody titer rise to CMV suggests the febrile illness during the second post-transplant period was due to adenovirus rather than CMV. Management consisted of supportive care and of withdrawal of immunosuppressive therapy

Adenovirus hepatitis is the most frequently recognized clinical entity in this group of patients. Patients with adenovirus hepatitis present with fever, anorexia, nausea, and vomiting. The hepatitis may be fulminant with rapidly rising hepatocellular en-

zymes, and swiftly deteriorating hepatic synthetic function, but with very little cholestasis. Hepatic tissue obtained by biopsy or at autopsy generally reveals necrotic hepatocytes with amphophilic or basophilic nuclear inclusion bodies. Portal tracts and hepatic blood vessels are usually spared, as compared with the marked hepatocellular involvement. Electron microscopy of hepatic tissue reveals crystalline arrays of hexagonal adenovirus virions.[2–4] Although some patients with adenovirus-associated hepatitis recover, many succumb to hepatic or extrahepatic involvement with the virus.

Pneumonia is also frequently recognized as a manifestation of adenovirus infection in the immunocompromised host.[4–12] Although patients may present with isolated pneumonia, many patients have hepatic involvement as well. In most cases, the pneumonia is bilateral and interstitial, although cases of unilateral involvement have been reported.[2] Pleural effusions may appear in up to 20% of cases.[2,9] Lung biopsy reveals interstitial pneumonia with intranuclear inclusions. The course of adenovirus pneumonia is variable and may be dependent on the degree of immunosuppression of the host, the prior experience of the host with adenoviruses, and perhaps the serotype of the isolate. Patients have been reported with rapidly progressive pneumonia with hypoxemia and death; others have manifested a much more indolent course.[2,9]

A number of patients have been reported in whom the predominant clinical manifestation of adenovirus infection was gastroenteritis.[13] Adenovirus was isolated from the stools of 12 of 78 bone marrow allograft recipients participating in a prospective study of gastrointestinal (GI) pathogens during the early post-transplant period. In nine of these patients, adenovirus was the sole viral pathogen. These patients presented with vomiting (8 of 9), diarrhea (5 of 9), and abdominal cramps (4 of 9). Four also had respiratory symptoms. Among this group of patients there were four deaths. Most of the adenovirus isolates were recovered during a 3-month period, during which adenovirus was prevalent among the pediatric population of the hospital, suggesting that patients acquired the pathogen from hospital visitors and staff.

Isolation of adenovirus from the urine of a renal transplant recipient has been associated with hemorrhagic cystitis.[14] Renal parenchymal involvement by adenovirus has also been documented in one large carefully performed study of bone marrow allograft recipients.[12] In this study, comprising 1051 patients over a 5-year period, 6 adenoviruses were isolated from 51 patients. In all but 10 patients, either no clinical manifestations were apparent in conjunction with adenoviral isolation, or other clinical problems, including herpes group virus activity, precluded attribution of clinical findings to the isolated adenovirus. Adenoviruses were isolated from renal parenchyma of 5 of the 10 patients for whom organ damage in association with adenovirus infection could be documented. Four of the five patients developed renal impairment; three required dialysis. Although each of the five patients received potentially nephrotoxic drugs, the demonstration of adenovirus inclusions in association with tubular epithelial necrosis in two of the patients supports the hypothesis that the virus also contributed to renal functional impairment. In addition to hepatic, pulmonary, and GI involvement, adenovirus may occasionally involve the central nervous system (CNS) in immunocompromised patients.[15] This complication appears to be relatively infrequent even in patients with disseminated adenoviral infection.

Diagnosis is greatly facilitated by a familiarity with the clinical syndromes associated with adenovirus infection in the immunocompromised, and by attention to ongoing viral activity in the community. Definitive diagnosis rests with the demonstration of virus in an involved organ by viral isolation, by

electron microscopy, by demonstration of adenoviral antigens in infected cells or by the demonstration of a fourfold rise in adenovirus-specific antibodies during the clinical episode. No specific therapy is available for adenovirus infection. Although immunoglobulin (Ig) therapy has been advocated for patients with humoral immune deficiency,[10] there is no convincing evidence from controlled trials that this approach is beneficial. As in other situations in which the degree of immunosuppression can be manipulated, it would be prudent to decrease the exogenous immunosuppression to as great a degree as possible during acute infection. Because adenoviruses are relatively highly contagious and infection can have significant consequences for immunocompromised persons, respiratory and enteric isolation should be employed for patients with recognized adenoviral infection in units with immunosuppressed patients.

2.2. Papovaviruses

The relatively recently described human papovaviruses, BK and JC, have received increasing attention as pathogens in immunosuppressed patients. Serologic surveys have demonstrated that these agents are ubiquitous in the adult population, with up to 90% of adults having evidence of prior BK virus infection and 70% of adults having evidence of prior JC virus infection.[16–18] There have been reports of morbidity in association with these viruses in immunocompetent patients.

2.2.1. JC Virus

Illustrative Case 2

A 68-year-old man developed renal failure in December 1981 due to rapidly progressive glomerulonephritis despite a course of therapy with prednisone and cyclophosphamide. He received a cadaveric renal allograft in November 1982 following 6 months of hemodialysis. His early post-transplant course was characterized by repeated bouts of acute rejection, for which he received three courses of antithymocyte globulin in addition to azathioprine and prednisone.

Seven months after transplantation, his family noted the onset of forgetfulness and emotional lability. Progressive dementia was noted over the ensuing 6 weeks. He returned for evaluation following a grand mal seizure. On examination, he was an afebrile elderly man in no acute distress. His general physical examination was remarkable for a cushingoid habitus and a nontender renal allograft in the right iliac fossa. He had no focal neurologic findings. Short-term memory was markedly impaired. Long-term memory was moderately impaired. He could name the three most recent presidents but could not perform serial 7 subtractions

A computed tomographic (CT) study of the cranium revealed an area of decreased density with indistinct margins in the left frontal lobe. No mass effect was noted (Fig. 1). The initial radiographic interpretation was that the CT scan was most compatible with an infarct of several weeks duration, although a low-grade infiltrating tumor could not be ruled out. A lumbar puncture revealed a normal opening pressure Two lymphocytes were present. The glucose and protein were normal. An electroencephalogram (EEG) was diffusely abnormal, with slowing throughout both hemispheres

A biopsy of the left frontal lobe lesion revealed replacement of normal brain tissue with large, bizarre astrocytes surrounded by degenerating oligodendrocytes. Electron microscopy, which revealed papovavirus particles within nuclei of the degenerating oligodendrocytes, established the diagnosis of progressive multifocal leukoencephalopathy.

A second CT study revealed the development of additional areas of decreased attenuation within the white matter of the brain. Following the brain biopsy, the dementia progressed rapidly. No antiviral therapy was administered. Increasing seizure activity led to the development of aspiration pneumonia. The patient died 10 months following transplantation, after a 4-month course of progressive multifocal leukoencephalopathy.

JC virus, a member of the human polyomavirus group, is the etiologic agent for the vast majority of cases of progressive multifocal leukoencephalopathy (PML). This exceedingly rare clinical entity, initially described by Richardson and co-workers[19] in 1958 has, to date, been reported in fewer than 250 patients. Almost all patients have demonstrable immunologic defects, with cellular immune defects being much more common than defects in humoral immunity. The combination of the immunocompromised patient population in which the disease was initially recognized, and the morphology of involved oligodendrocytes led Richardson to suggest a viral etiology for this clinical entity.[19,20] Following a decade during which viral particles compatable with polyomavirus were demonstrated in oligodendrocytes by electron microscopy,[21] two groups reported the iso-

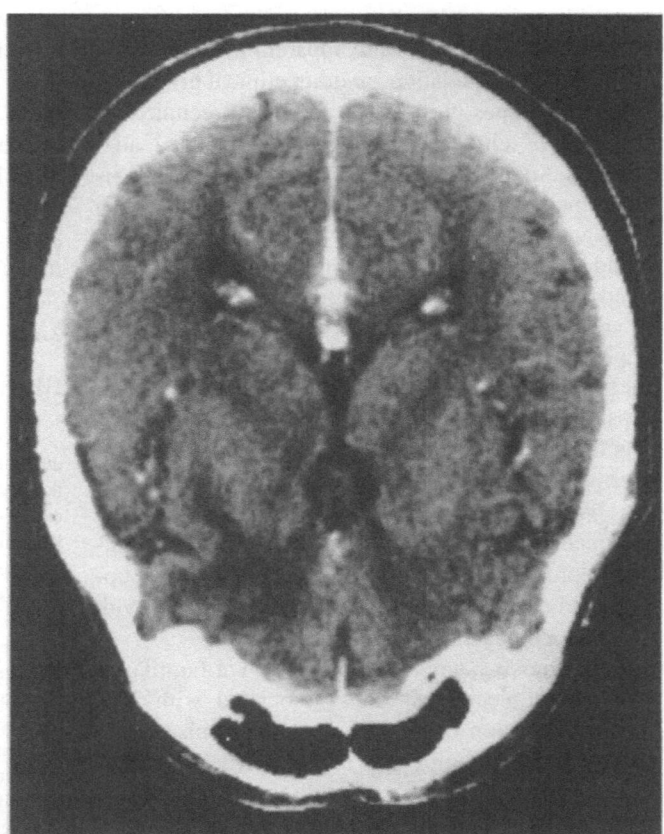

FIGURE 1. Computed tomographic (CT) study from patient 1 demonstrating areas of decreased attenuation, particularly involving the left frontal lobe.

lation of viral agents from PML brains in tissue culture.[22,23] One group isolated a polyomavirus, designated JC virus, from a PML brain, using primary human fetal glial cell cultures; a second group reported the isolation of a virus identical to, or very closely related to Simian virus 40 (SV40) using an independent technique. All subsequent isolates have been of the JC type.

Serologic studies have demonstrated that JC virus is a ubiquitous agent, Antibodies to JC virus can be demonstrated in sera from 70% of the adult population.[17] Primary infection occurs most frequently during the second decade of life and is generally subclinical. Following primary infection, the virus is thought to remain within the host in latent form. With immunosuppression such as that used in renal transplantation, or in pregnancy, reactivation of JC virus is evident in some persons by both serologic changes and by shedding of the virus in the urine.[24,25] In general, these bouts of reactivation are also clinically inapparent. For reasons that are unclear, JC virus invades the CNS of a very small minority of patients and results in PML.[26,27]

Patients with PML have generally experienced defects in cellular immunity for months to years prior to onset of neurologic symptoms. The chronicity of the cellular immune defect associated with human immunodeficiency virus (HIV) infection places patients with AIDS at particular risk for PML.[28-30] It was recently demonstrated that HIV is itself neurotropic.[31,32] A number of neurologic syndromes, including dementia, aseptic meningitis, peripheral neuropathy, and vacuolar myelopathy, have been reported in association with HIV infection.[31-33] Thus, not all neurologic syndromes in acquired immune-deficiency syndrome (AIDS) patients clinically compatible with PML are due to JC virus. Presentation is usually insidious, with neurologic signs reflecting the multifocal nature of the process.[20,26,27] In most patients, progression is relatively rapid with early deterioration in cognitive function, speech, and vision. Motor deficits, cortical blindness, and sensory abnormalities follow shortly thereafter. Patients rarely complain of headaches or exhibit fever or seizures. Occasional cases have been described in which involvement of the spinal cord has been clinically prominent, but these cases are very uncommon. Most patients succumb to the illness within 6 months of the onset of neurologic signs.

Definitive diagnosis requires brain biopsy. Nonetheless, in the appropriate setting. an extremely strong clinical diagnosis can be established without resorting to an invasive procedure. Lumbar puncture usually reveals a normal opening pressure with a normal glucose and protein level. A few lymphocytes may be present, but in general the hallmark of this illness in both the cerebrospinal fluid (CSF) and the brain is the lack of inflammatory reaction. EEGs are diffusely abnormal but nondiagnostic. The individual lesions are usually too small to be detectable by radionuclide scanning. Pneumoencephalography and cerebral angiography are usually normal. Computed tomography, however, is often capable of demonstrating multiple demyelinative lesions. The ubiquity of antibodies to JC virus in the adult population and the relative frequency of serologic evidence of JC virus activity in immunocompromised hosts in the absence of PML[34] make serologic diagnosis impossible.

In atypical cases, brain biopsy may be required to rule out other treatable entities. The central pathologic feature of PML is demyelination, which occurs as a result of lytic infection of oligodendrocytes by JC virus. In contrast to multiple sclerosis, very few inflammatory cells are demonstrable. With disease progression, confluent demyelination results in widely distributed plaques of increasing size. Electron microscopic evaluation of involved oligodendrocytes reveals crystalline arrays of papovavirus particles.[35] Viral antigens can also be demonstrated by other techniques, such as immunofluorescence or immunoperoxidase staining. Late in disease, as oligodendrocytes are progressively depleted, viral particles and antigen become more difficult to demonstrate. JC virus can be isolated in tissue culture, using primary human fetal glial cells. Typical cytopathic effects of loss of contact inhibition, destruction of spongioblasts, and the appearance of multinucleate astrocytes are usually apparent 10–12 days after initiation of the culture.

There is no effective treatment for PML. There have been a number of reports of therapy with nucleoside analogues, including IUDR, cytosine arabinoside, and adenine arabinoside.[36-48] Although occasional case reports have maintained that stabilization or improvement was coincident with the use of these agents, these observations are uncontrolled and anecdotal. One case has been reported with apparent spontaneous remission. Treatment is thus largely supportive.

2.2.2. BK Virus

BK virus was initially isolated from the urine of a renal allograft recipient with ureteral stenosis.[49] Subsequent case reports have also made note of the association between BK virus infection and ureteral stenosis.[50] One carefully performed pathologic study documented the presence of papovavirus inclusions in ureteral epithelial cells in an area of ureteral stenosis in two renal allograft recipients. BK virus excretion is much more frequently observed, however, than is ureteral stenosis.[51,52] As in the case of CMV, BK virus may be transmitted to BK-seronegative allograft recipients by kidneys from BK-seropositive donors.[52] An association between BK virus excretion and the development of pancreatitis postrenal transplantation has also been demonstrated.[53] Whether this association implies an etiologic relationship and whether it might be generalizable to other clinical settings is unclear. Outside the setting of renal transplantation, reports of BK virus-associated morbidity have been sparse. One 6-year-old boy was reported with tubulointerstitial nephritis associated with BK virus infection.[54] This child with congenital dysgammaglobulinemia developed renal failure and subsequently died after a series of infections including *Cryptococcus neoformans* and *Enterobacter cloacae sepsis*. At postmortem examination, renal glomeruli were relatively normal, but renal tubular cells were focally necrotic with large amounts of polyomavirus antigen in both tubular lining cells and cast material. DNA hybridization studies revealed a disseminated BK virus infection with BK sequences in kidney lymph nodes, spleen, and lungs. It is likely from the data generated since the initial description of BK virus 15 years ago that this agent will be increasingly implicated as a pathogen in immunocompromised persons in vitro. Neither seroconversion nor viral excretion was affected by prophylactic interferon-α (IF_α) therapy in a randomized study of renal allograft recipients.[53]

2.2.3. Papillomavirus

For several hundred years, warts have been postulated to be of an infectious etiology. Human inoculation experiments in the first decade of the twentieth century established the viral etiology of human warts, but further progress was greatly hampered by the lack of suitable tissue culture techniques for propagation of the etiologic agents. The recent application of molecular biologic techniques to the study of human warts has confirmed the viral etiology of these common skin tumors and has provided insight into the plurality of animal papillomaviruses. These agents have been shown to be small DNA viruses and are included in the same family (Papovaviridae) as polyomaviruses. These recent studies have also delineated the associations of specific strains of papillomavirus with specific clinical types of warts.[55] Twenty-five types of human papillomavirus have been delineated.

Clinicians have long been aware of the increased frequency and severity of warts in patients with immunodeficiency states.[56-59] This increased frequency has been noted in patients with a wide variety of primary and secondary immunodeficiency states but is most notable in patients with defects in cellular immunity. It has been the impression of many clinicians that warts are particularly likely to be induced by sun exposure. Scattered reports of possible degeneration of warts to squamous cell tumors have appeared.[60] Therapy is generally based on local destruction of the involved area by cryosurgery or electrodessication. These modes of therapy are much less likely to meet with success in immunocompromised persons than in immunologically normal hosts. Current clinical trials are under way in which the potential value of interferons is being addressed in the management of warts. If these studies suggest that interferons are useful in immunologically normal persons, extension of the studies to immunocompromised patients appears likely.

2.3. Vaccinia

Prior to the cessation of routine smallpox vaccination, vaccinia necrosum was a major cause of morbidity and mortality with immunocompromised vaccines.[61] This entity, also known as progressive vaccinia, occurred when patients with predominantly cellular immune defects were inadvertently vaccinated for smallpox with vaccinia virus.[61-64] The vaccination site initially appears normal but, rather than resolution, progressive destruction is observed at the site of vaccination. Eventually metastatic cutaneous lesions are evident. In general, very little lymphadenopathy or local reaction is noted in the absence of bacterial superinfection. Treatment has included vaccinia immune globulin and thiosemicarbazone.[65,66]

3. RNA Viruses

3.1. Picornaviruses

3.1.1. Poliomyelitis

Paralytic poliomyelitis has become an extremely rare disease in industrialized countries. In the United States, cases of paralytic poliomyelitis declined 20-fold with the introduction of the Salk vaccine in 1955, and an additional 100-fold with the widespread use of the live attenuated (Sabin) vaccine.[67] The gains in control of paralytic poliomyelitis for the general population with the Sabin vaccine have been complicated by the fact that the live attenuated strains capable of inducing lasting immunity in the immunocompetent host, can induce paralytic poliomyelitis in the immunocompromised host.[68,69] This is particularly true for the type 2 vaccine strain. Since 1969, 7% of cases of paralytic poliomyelitis in the United States were in immunocompromised persons in association with live attenuated vaccine strains.[68] The risk of paralytic poliomyelitis following administration of oral poliovaccine strain is increased approximately 10,000-fold in hypogammaglobulinemics.[69] By contrast, paralysis is seen in association with much more comparable proportions (about 2.5%) of immunocompetent and immunocompromised persons in association with infection with wild-type strains.

An analysis of cases of paralytic poliomyelitis in immunocompromised patients in association with live attenuated vaccine strains has revealed that patients with humoral, cellular defects, and combined effects are at increased risk from oral polio vaccine.[70–77] Nonetheless, not all immunodeficient patients without prior immunity who receive oral polio vaccine develop paralytic poliomyelitis; it has been estimated that the risk for hypogammaglobulinemics is that 1 in 40 will develop paralytic disease following exposure to the oral vaccine.[69] The incubation period between vaccination and onset of paralytic manifestations is typically prolonged in immunocompromised persons but ranged from 2 weeks to 7 months in one survey.[68] The disease in immunodeficient persons is frequently characterized by a stuttering prolonged onset of neurologic symptoms, which include both upper and lower motor neuron signs. Gastrointestinal shedding of virus frequently becomes chronic in immunodeficient persons.

Vaccination with live attenuated polio vaccine of patients with known or suspected immunodeficiency of any variety should be avoided. Vaccination of family members living with such persons with live attenuated vaccine should also be avoided given the demonstrable spread of vaccine strains among family members and contacts as the result of focal shedding of virus. Once neurologic manifestations have become apparent, no effective therapy is available. An excellent case can be made however, for long-term immunoglobulin therapy of hypogammaglobulinemic patients following inadvertent exposure to live attenuated vaccine if the exposure is recognized prior to the onset of neurologic manifestations. Because of the prolonged fecal shedding of virus by immunocompromised persons, care should be exercised to prevent nosocomial spread if such patients are hospitalized among other immunodeficient persons.

3.1.2. Coxsackie and Echo Viruses

In addition to being at increased risk for paralytic poliomyelitis in association with live attenuated polio vaccine, hypogammaglobulinemic patients are at increased risk for chronic meningoencephalitis from other enteroviruses.[78–85] Chronic meningoencephalitis is most frequently associated with echovirus infections (types 2, 3, 5, 9, 11, 19, 24, 25, 30, 33) but has occasionally been reported in association with Coxsackie B infection.[86] The onset may be relatively acute but is frequently insidious. Severity ranges from subclinical involvement, to more obvious neurologic findings including headaches, nuchal rigidity, cognitive dysfunction, lethargy, seizures, tremor, motor weakness, or ataxia. Many, but not all, patients also manifest a prominent dermatomyositis-like syndrome. The pathogenesis of the myositis is not certain, but isolation of virus from muscle of one of these cases suggests that direct muscle involvement by virus may contribute to this aspect of the illness in some patients.[84]

Cerebrospinal fluid usually includes a predominantly lymphocytic pleocytosis and a mildly elevated protein with a normal glucose. Virus can be isolated from CSF repeatedly or intermittently but is usually not isolatable from extraneural sites.

No specific antiviral therapy for echoviruses or Coxsackie viruses is currently available. Although most hypogammaglobulinemic patients with chronic meningoencephalitis due to enteroviruses are receiving supplemental immunoglobulin therapy at presentation, clinical improvement has been reported in several patients in association with therapy with immunoglobulin preparations with neutralizing activity to the specific implicated enterovirus.[80-84]

In addition to the occasional involvement of the CNS of hypogammaglobulinemic patients by Coxsackie virus, two recent reports have implicated Coxsackie viruses in the causation of acute gastroenteritis among hospitalized immunocompromised patients.[87,88] Both reports involved the same bone marrow transplant unit.

Illustrative Case 3

A 9-year-old boy with renal failure due to obstructive uropathy received four renal allografts between 1976 and 1979. The first three allografts were lost to rejection. He underwent splenectomy in January 1981 in preparation for a fourth allograft procedure. He received a cadaveric allograft in July 1982. Immunosuppression consisted of cyclophosphamide, prednisone, and total lymphoid irradiation. During the first 3 months following transplantation, he had several episodes of rejection that were managed with boluses of solumedrol. Antithymocyte globulin was added to the immunosuppressive regimen in the fourth postoperative month.

In November 1982, he awoke one morning with a headache, fever, and vomiting. He was initially managed with Tylenol. That evening, he awoke with a temperature of 103°F (39.4°C) and had a grand mal seizure similar to seizures he had experienced with bouts of fever in the past. In the emergency room, he was found to be febrile to 102.6°F (39.2°C) and to have a blood pressure of 200/100. The fundi were benign. The neck was supple. The abdomen was distended, with active bowel sounds. No localized tenderness or rebound was appreciated. Stool was guaiac negative. The neurologic examination was normal.

Laboratory studies included a serum sodium level of 138 mEq/liter, a potassium level of 4.8 mEq/liter, a chloride level of 111 mEq/liter, and a bicarbonate level of 21 mEq/liter. The BUN and creatinine were unchanged from the previous week at 30 and 1.3 mg/dl, respectively. The hematocrit was 24%, the white blood cell (WBC) count 4500/mm³ with 67% polymorphonuclear cells, 4 bands, 8 lymphocytes, 16 monocytes, and 5 basophils. A traumatic lumbar puncture revealed 8800 red blood cells (RBCs)/mm³, and 8 WBCs/mm³, of which 80% were lympho-

cytes and 20% were polymorphonuclear cells. The CSF glucose was 64 mg/dl; the protein was 79 mg/dl. CSF was sent for bacterial, fungal, and viral cultures and for cryptococcal antigen.

Over the next several days, his headache resolved, but he remained febrile to 101°–102°F. Vomiting ceased but he had several loose stools per day that were trace guaiac positive. A percutaneous renal biopsy revealed acute and chronic rejection. Allograft irradiation was added; the ATG was continued. A lumbar puncture performed 4 days after admission revealed a 10 RBCs/mm³, and 22 WBCs/mm³. Twenty percent of the WBCs were polymorphonuclear cells; the remainder were mononuclear cells. The CSF glucose was 55 mg/dl; the protein had fallen to 34 mg/dl.

By the tenth hospital day he was afebrile. His headaches, nausea, and diarrhea had resolved. Following discharge, cytopathic effect consistent with that induced by an enterovirus was identified in viral cultures of the initial CSF sample. During hospitalization, three other patients in the transplant unit experienced unexplained bouts of diarrhea.

In summary, this heavily immunosuppressed renal allograft recipient experienced a bout of fever, headaches, nausea, vomiting, and diarrhea at a time during which enterovirus was isolated from cerebrospinal fluid. The possibility of nosocomial spread was raised by the simultaneous occurance of unexplained diarrhea in three other concurrently hospitalized allograft recipients.

In one of the two reports, 7 of 14 patients transplanted during a 3-week period developed gastroenteritis due to Coxsackie virus, type A1.[87] Infected patients had significantly larger stool volumes than noninfected patients. Six of the seven infected patients died. At postmortem examination, pronounced GI lymphoid atrophy was evident. This was associated with overlying foamy vacuolated GI epithelium. The extremely high mortality rate led to closing of the bone marrow transplantation unit to new admissions and to the institution of enteric precautions for all patients. These maneuvers were associated with cessation of the outbreak.

3.2. Paramyxoviruses

3.2.1. Measles

Measles (rubeola) is generally a self-limited disease of childhood that has decreased in incidence by 95% since widespread vaccination began in 1961.[89] It is, however, not infrequently associated with major morbidity in immunocompromised hosts. In addition to the direct effects on the host, measles virus has the potential to induce more profound immunosuppression in a fashion analogous to that documented for the herpesviruses.[90-92]

The most frequently encountered forms of excess morbidity associated with measles infection in immunocompromised hosts are giant cell pneumonia[93,94] and encephalitis.[95,96] The association between measles virus and giant cell pneumonia in immunocompromised children was first proved by Enders and colleagues, who isolated the virus from the lungs of three immunocompromised children with fatal pneumonia. The pathologic hallmark of this illness is the multinucleated giant cells, which are widespread in lungs and other organs. It should be noted that these patients do not, in general, exhibit rash. Diagnosis is facilitated by the recognition of the clinical syndrome of fever and diffuse interstitial pneumonia in an immunocompromised person who has no history of measles vaccination, particularly if a history of exposure to measles is elicited.

Subclinical involvement of the CNS in up to 50% of immunocompetent patients with measles is suggested by the frequent observation of abnormal EEGs in acute measles.[97] The occasional isolation of measles virus from the brain of patients with fatal measles encephalitis and the demonstration of the association between measles and subacute sclerosing panencephalitis (SSPE)[98–101] further strengthens the evidence that the CNS may be targeted by measles virus in the normal host. Measles encephalitis in immunocompromised patients has been increasingly recognized over the past two decades.[95–96,100–104] Measles encephalitis in immunocompromised patients may initially present as a focal process with motor deficits or focal seizures, but progression over a relatively brief period of time is quite common. In contrast to patients with measles virus-associated giant cell pneumonia, immunocompromised patients with measles encephalitis usually manifest a viral exanthem that may precede the onset of neurologic findings by several days to up to 6 months. Initial CSF examination may reveal a normal glucose and protein level and few or no cells. Most patients succumb to this complication of measles virus infection. Although IF_α therapy was associated with a brief stabilization of one patient,[105] failure of IF_α therapy has also been reported.[106] No other specific antiviral has been shown to be effective for either the pneumonia or encephalitis associated with measles in immunocompromised individuals. The reports of convulsions and pneumonia in immunocompromised patients receiving the live attenuated measles vaccine underscores the rationale for avoiding this live vaccine in immunocompromised patients.[107]

3.2.2. Respiratory Syncytial Virus

Respiratory syncytial virus (RSV) is the most frequent cause of pneumonia, bronchiolitis, or tracheobronchitis among young children.[108] Among persons over the age of 3, RSV infection is usually manifest as only tracheobronchitis or, more commonly, as an upper respiratory illness.[109] RSV infection has been well recognized as a nosocomial pathogen[110–112] and has been demonstrated to be associated with significantly increased mortality in infants with congenital heart disease.[113] Although animal models have demonstrated prolonged RSV shedding in immunosuppressed animals,[114] only scattered reports of increased morbidity due to RSV among immunosuppressed children have appeared.[115,116] The extent of the increased morbidity due to RSV among immunosuppressed adults appears to be extremely limited, if such increased morbidity exists.

3.3. Rotaviruses

Rotaviruses are a major cause of infantile diarrhea of worldwide distribution. Clinical manifestations range from mild diarrhea to a severe dehydrating illness that may be fatal.[117,118] Although most cases of outbreaks of viral gastroenteritis among adults and school-age children appear to be due to Norwalk-like agents, experimental transmission of rotavirus to adults has been associated with diarrhea.[119] With the increasingly frequent application of the enzyme-linked immunosorbent assay (ELISA) for detection of rotavirus antigen in stool, the agent is becoming increasingly recognized as a pathogen for immunocompromised children and adults.

Rotavirus-associated diarrhea in immunocompromised patients may present as a relatively chronic process, or the onset may be more acute.[88,120,121] Rotavirus infection was documented in 9 of 78 hospitalized bone marrow allograft recipients.[88] In 8 of these patients, rotavirus was the only viral pathogen isolated in association with gastroenteritis. Although not as striking as with Coxsackie A1-associated gastroenteritis patients investigated in the same unit, rotavirus-infected patients exhibited increased mortality, as compared with patients who did not experience viral gastroenteritis.

Rotavirus does not grow efficiently using conventional tissue culture techniques. Although rotavirus can be demonstrated in stool by conventional or immune electron microscopy, the development of ELISA and radioimmunoassay (RIA) has greatly facilitated diagnosis of rotavirus gastroenteritis.[122-126] The value of serologic responses to rotaviruses has not yet been demonstrated in immunocompromised individuals.

Therapy is primarily supportive. In immunocompetent infants most of the severe morbidity is directly attributable to fluid and electrolyte imbalance.[118] The mechanism by which rotavirus infection appears to contribute to increased mortality in bone marrow allograft recipients is unclear. Although one could hypothesize that additional insults to the GI mucosa could potentiate the development of bacteremia, this was not documented in the bone marrow transplant prospective study.[88] In infants with severe combined immunodeficiency, oral therapy with human milk containing antibodies to rotavirus may be useful.[120] As in the situation with other outbreaks of nosocomial diarrhea, rotavirus-associated diarrhea should result in the institution of enteric precautions, particularly in settings in which other immunocompromised patients are present. Although most immunocompetent adults do not develop diarrhea in association with rotavirus exposure, serologic responses of adult contacts of children with rotavirus diarrhea, and the occasional outbreak of rotavirus diarrhea in settings such as nursing homes, suggest that hospital staff may facilitate nosocomial spread.[127-129]

3.4. Human T-Lymphotropic Viruses

At the time of this writing, more than 14,000 cases of AIDS have been reported in the United States.[130] It has been estimated that between 0.5 and 1 million persons are infected with the etiologic agent for AIDS, i.e., HIV.[130] The current case definition of AIDS excludes patients who have received immunosuppressive therapy or who are immunosuppressed by other known ongoing disorders (e.g., Hodgkin disease). Thus, by definition, organ allograft recipients cannot fulfill diagnostic criteria for AIDS no matter how severe the opportunistic infection and no matter how trivial the exogenous immunosuppressive therapy. Nonetheless, the demonstration of HIV in a wide variety of organs and fluids (blood, semen, urine, saliva, tears, breast milk, female genital secretions) coupled with the increasing prevalence of the agent in the US population suggests that this virus will soon be recognized as a major problem in organ transplantation. Current technology allows serologic identification of the vast majority of HIV infected persons. It is clear that organ procurement teams should follow the same procedure of deferring procurement of organs from high-risk donors and of serologic testing of donors prior to organ transplantation to recipients. We have recently observed the failure of one patient with primary HIV infection who was receiving cytotoxic therapy to manifest a detectable antibody response to HIV. Thus, serologic studies may prove inadequate in identifying HIV infection in immunocompromised persons. The role of HIV in organ allograft transplantation may not become clear for the next decade, but it is highly likely that, as increasing numbers of latently infected individuals donate and receive organs, HIV-associated morbidity will begin to be recognized in this patient population (see Chapter 21).

References

1 Chanock RM: Impact of adenovirus in human disease. *Prev Med* 3:466–472, 1974.

2. Zahradnik JM, Spencer MJ, Parker DD. Adenovirus infection in the immunocompromised patient. *Am J Med* 68:725–732, 1980.

3. Carmichael GP, Zahradnik JM, Moyer GM, et al: Adenovirus hepatitis in an immunosuppressed adult patient. *Am J Clin Pathol* 71:352–355, 1979.

4. Rodriguez FH, Liuzza GE, Gohd RH: Disseminated adenovirus serotype 31 infection in an immunocompromised host. *Am J Clin Pathol* 82:615–618, 1979.

5. Myerowitz RL, Stadler H, Oxman MN, et al: Fatal disseminated adenovirus infection in a renal transplant recipient *Am J Med* 59:591–598, 1975.

6. Keller EW, Rubin RH, Black PH, et al: Isolation of adenovirus type 34 from a renal transplant recipient with interstitial pneumonia. *Transplantation* 23:188–191, 1977.

7. Neiman PE, Reeves W, Ray G, et al: A prospective analysis of interstitial pneumonia and opportunistic viral infections among recipients of allogeneic bone marrow grafts. *J Infect Dis* 136:754–767, 1977.

8. Lecatsas G, Van Wyk JAC: DNA viruses in urine after renal transplantation. *S Afr Med J* 53:787–788, 1978.

9. Wigger HJ, Blanc WA: Fatal hepatic and bronchial necrosis in adenovirus infection with thymic alymphoplasia. *N Engl J Med* 275:870–874, 1968.

10. Dagan R, Schwartz RH, Insel RA, et al: Severe diffuse adenovirus 7a pneumonia in a child with combined immunodeficiency: Possible therapeutic effect of human serum immune globulin containing specific neutralizing antibody *Pediatr Infect Dis* 3:246–249, 1984.

11. Siegal FP, Dikman SH, Arayatu RB, et al: Fatal disseminated adenovirus pneumonia in an agammaglobulinemic patient. *Am J Med* 71:1062–1067, 1981.

12. Shields AF, Hackman RC, Fife HK,et al: Adenovirus infection in patients,undergoing bone marrow transplantation. *N Engl J Med* 312:529–533, 1985.

13. Yolken RH, Bishop CA, Townsend TR, et al: Infectious gastroenteritis in bone marrow transplant recipients. *N Engl J Med* 306:1009–1012, 1982.

14. Lecatsas G, Prozesky OW, Van Wyk J: Adenovirus type 11 associated with hemorrhagic cystitis after renal transplantation. *S Afr Med J* 48:1932–1935, 1974.

15. Chou SM, Roos R, Burrell R, et al: Subacute focal adenovirus encephalitis. *J Neuropathol Exp Neurol* 32:34–50, 1973.

16. Shah KV, Daniel RW, Warszawski RM: High prevalence of antibodies of BK virus, on SV 40 related papovavirus, in residents of Maryland. *J Infect Dis* 127:784–787, 1973.

17. Padgett B, Walker D: Natural history of human polyomavirus infections. In Stevens JG, Todaro GJ, Fox CF (eds): *Persistent Viruses*. Academic, New York, 1978, pp. 751–758.

18. Shah KV, Daniel RW, Zeigel KK, and Murphy GP. Search for BK and SV 40 virus reactivation in renal transplant recipients. *Transplantation* 17:131–134, 1974.

19. Astrom KE, Mancall EL, Richardson EP Jr: Progressive multifocal leukoencephalopathy: hitherto unrecognized complication of chronic lymphatic leukemia and Hodgkin's disease. *Brain* 81:93–111, 1958.

20. Richardson EP Jr: Progressive multifocal leukoencephalopathy. *N Engl J Med* 265:815–823, 1961.

21. ZuRhein GM, Chow SM: Particles resembling papovaviruses in human cerebral demyelinating disease. *Science* 148:1477–1479, 1965.

22. Padgett BL, Walker DL, ZuRhein GM, et al: Cultivation of papova-like virus from human brain with progressive multifocal leukoencephalopathy. *Lancet* 1:1257–1260, 1971.

23. Weiner LP, Herndon RM, Narayan O, et al: Isolation of virus related to SV40 from patients with progressive multifocal leukoencephalopathy. *N Engl J Med* 286:385–390, 1972.

24. Hogan T, Borden E, McBain J, et al: Human polyomavirus infections with JC virus and BK virus in renal transplant patients. *Ann Intern Med* 92:373–378, 1980.

25. Coleman D, Wolfendale M, Daniel R, et al: A prospective study of human polyomavirus infection in pregnancy. *J Infect Dis* 142:1–8, 1980.

26. Lyon LW, McCormick WF, Schochet SS Jr: Progressive multifocal leukoencephalopathy. *Neurology (NY)* 21:72–77, 1971.

27. Horte-Barbosa L, Hamilton R, Fucillo DA, et al: Progressive multifocal leukoencephalopathy. *N Engl J Med* 286:1060, 1972.

28. Miller JR, Barrett RE, Britton CB: Progressive multifocal leukoencephalopathy in a male homosexual with T-cell immune deficiency. *N Engl J Med* 307:1436–1438, 1982.

29. Snider WD, Simpson DM, Nielsen S, et al: Neurological complications of acquired immune deficiency syndrome: Analysis of 50 patients. *Ann Neurol* 14:403–417, 1983.

30. Levy RM, Bredesen ED, Rosenblum ML: Neurological manifestation of the acquired immune deficiency syndrome (AIDS): Experience at UCSF and the review of the literature. *J Neurosurg* 62:475–495, 1985.

31. Shaw GM, Harper ME, Hahn BH. et al: HTLV-III infection in brains of children and adults with AIDS Encephalopathy. *Science* 227:177–181, 1985.

32. Ho DD, Rota TR, Schooley RT, et al. Isolation of HTLV-III from CSF and neural tissues of patients with AIDS related neurological syndromes. *N Engl J Med* 313:1493–1497, 1985.

33. Petito CK, Navia BA, Cho E-S, et al: Vacuolar myelopathy pathologically resembling subacute combined degeneration in patients with the acquired immune deficiency syndrome. *N Engl J Med* 312:874–879, 1985.

34. Hogan TF, Borden EC, McBain JA, et al: Human polyomavirus infections with JC virus and BK virus in renal transplant patients. *Ann Intern Med* 92:373–378, 1980.

35. Woodhouse MA, Dayan AD, Burston J, et al: Progressive multifocal leukoencephalopathy: Electron microscope study of four cases. *Brain* 90:863–870, 1967.

36. ZuRhein GM, Varakis J: Progressive multifocal leukoencephalopathy in a renal allograft recipient. *N Engl J Med* 291:798, 1974.

37. Bauer WR, Turel AP, Johnson KP: Progressive multifocal leukoencephalopathy and cytarabine: Remission with treatment. *JAMA* 226:174–176, 1973.

38. Smith CR, Sima AAF, Salit IE, et al: Progressive multifocal leukoencephalopathy: Failure of cytarabine therapy. *Neurology (NY)* 32:200–203, 1982.

39. Conomy JP, Beard NS, Matsumoto H, et al: Cytarabine treatment of PML. *JAMA* 229:1313–1316, 1974.

40. VanHorn G, Bastian FO, Moate JL: Progressive multifocal leukoencephalopathy: Failure of response to transfer factor and cytarabine. *Neurology (NY)* 28:744–747, 1978.

41. Peters ACB, Vertsteeg J, Bots GTA, et al: Progressive multifocal leukoencephalopathy: Immunofluorescent demonstration of SV 40 antigen on CSF cells and response to cytarabine therapy. *Arch Neurol* 37:497–501, 1980.

42. Rand RH, Johnson KP, Rubenstein LJ, et al: Adenine arabinoside in the treatment of progressive multifocal leukoencephalopathy: Use of virus containing cells in the urine to assess response to therapy. *Ann Neurol* 1:458–462, 1977.

43. Rockwell D, Ruben FL, Windlestein A, et al. Absence of immune deficiency in a case of progressive multifocal leukoencephalopathy. *Am J Med* 61:433–436, 1976.

44. Marriott PS, O'Brien MD, MacKenzie IC, et al. Progressive multifocal leukoencephalopathy: Remission with cytarabine. *J Neurol Neurosurg Psychiatry* 38:205–209, 1975.

45. Castleman G, Scully RE, McNeeley BU: Clinicopathological conference. *N Engl J Med* **286**:1047–1054, 1972.

46. Tarsy D, Holden EM, Segarra JM, et al: 5-Iodo-2'-deoxyuridine given intraventricularly in the treatment of progressive multifocal leukoencephalopathy. *Cancer Chemother Rep* **57**:73–78, 1973.

47. Hedley Whyte ET, Smith BP, Tyler HR, et al. Multifocal leukoencephalopathy with remission and five year survival. *J Neuropathol Exp Neurol* **25**:107–116, 1966.

48. Holden EM, Tarsy D, Calabresi P, et al: Use of 5-iodo-2'-deoxyuridine in progressive multifocal leukoencephalopathy. *Neurology (NY)* **21**:448, 1971.

49. Gardner SD, Field AM, Coleman DV, et al: New human papovavirus (BK) isolated from urine after renal transplantation. *Lancet* **1**:1253–1257, 1971.

50. Coleman DV, MacKenzie EFD, Gardner SD, et al: Human polymavirus (BK) infection and ureteric stenosis in renal allograft recipients. *J Clin Pathol* **31**:338–347, 1978.

51. Lecatsas A, Prozesky OW, Van Wyk J, et al: Papovavirus in urine after renal transplantation. *Nature (Lond)* **241**:343–344, 1973.

52. Andrews C, Shah KV, Rubin RH, et al: BK papovavirus in renal transplant recipients: Contribution of donor kidneys. *J Infect Dis* **145**:276, 1982.

53. Cheeseman SH, Black PH, Rubin RH, et al: Interferon and BK papovavirus. Clinical and laboratory studies. *Infect Dis* **41**:157–161, 1980.

54. Rosen S, Harmon W, Krensky AM, et al: Tubulointerstitial nephritis associated with polyomavirus (BK type) infection. *N Engl J Med* **308**:1192–1196, 1983.

55. Gross G, Pfister H, Hagedorn M, et al. Correlation between human papillomavirus (HPV) type and histology of warts. *J Invest Dermatol* **78**:160–164, 1982.

56. Morrison WL: Viral warts, herpes simplex, and herpes zoster in patients with secondary immune deficiencies and neoplasms *Br J Dermtol* **92**:625–630, 1975

57. Barnett N, Mak H, Winkelstein J: Extensive verrucosis in primary immunodeficiency diseases. *Arch Dermatol* **119**:5–7, 1983.

58. Spencer ES, Anderson HK: Clinically evident, non-terminal infections with herpesviruses and the wart virus in immunosuppressed renal allograft recipients. *Br Med J* **3**:251–254, 1970.

59. Perry TL, Harman L Jr: Warts in diseases with immune defects. *Cutis* **13**:359–362, 1974.

60. Mullen DL, Silverberg SG, Penn I, et al: Squamous cell carcinoma of the skin and lip in renal homograft recipients. *Cancer* **37**:729–734, 1976.

61. Lane JM, Ruben FL, Abrutyn E, et al: Deaths attributable to smallpox vaccination 1959 to 1966, and 1968, *JAMA* **212**:441–444, 1970.

62. Lane JM, Ruben FL, Neff JM, et al: Complications of smallpox vaccination, 1968. II Results of the ten statewide surveys. *J Infect Dis* **122**:303–308, 1970.

63. Lane JM, Ruben RL, Neff JM, et al: Complications of smallpox vaccination, 1968: 1. National surveillance in the United States. *N Engl J Med* **281**:1201–1208, 1969.

64. Neff JM, Lane JM, Pert JH, et al: Complications of smallpox vaccination. I. National surveillance in the United States, 1963. *N Engl J Med* **276**:125–132, 1967.

65. Turner W, Bauer DJ, Nimmo-Smith RH: Eczema vaccinatum treated with N-methylisatin β-thiosemicarbazone. *Br Med J* **1**:1317–1319, 1962.

66. Brainerd HD, Hanna L, Jawetz E: Methisazone in progressive vaccinia. *N Engl J Med* **276**:620–622, 1967.

67. Centers for Disease Control. Poliomyelitis Surveillance Summary. 1980–1981. CDC, Atlanta, Georgia, 1982.

68. Moore M, Katona P, Kaplan JE, et al. Poliomyelitis in the United States, 1969–1981. *J Infect Dis* **146**:558–563, 1982

69. Wyatt HV: Poliomyelitis in hypogammaglobulinemics. *J Infect Dis* **128**:802–806, 1973

70. Chang TW, Weinstein L, MacMahon HE. Paralytic poliomyelitis in a child with hypogammaglobulinemia: Probable implications of type I vaccine strain. *Pediatrics* **37**:630–636, 1966.

71. Riker JB, Brandt CD, Chandra R, et al: Vaccine-associated poliomyelitis in a child with thymic abnormality. *Pediatrics* **48**:923–929, 1971.

72. Feigin RD, Guggenheim MA, Johnson SD: Vaccine related paralytic poliomyelitis in an immunodeficient child. *J Pediatr* **79**:642–647, 1971

73. Saulsbury FT, Winkelstein JA, Davis LE, et al: Combined immunodeficiency and vaccine related poliomyelitis in a child with cartilage hair hypoplasia. *J Pediatr* **86**:868–872, 1975.

74. Centers for Disease Control: Neurotropic Disease Surveillance. Annual Summary 1969. U S. Department of Health, Education and Welfare, Public Health Service, Washington, DC, 1969.

75 Lopez C, Biggar WD, Park BH, et al: Nonparalytic poliovirus infections in patients with severe combined immunodeficiency disease. *J Pediatr* **84**:447–502, 1974

76. Davis LE, Bodian D, Price D, et al: Chronic progressive poliomyelitis secondary to vaccination of an immunodeficient child. *N Engl J Med* **297**:241–245, 1977.

77 Wright PF, Hatch MH, Kasselberg AG, et al. Vaccine associated poliomyelitis in a child with sex linked agammaglobulinemia *J Pediatr* **91**:408–412, 1977.

78. Ziegler JB, Penny R: Fatal echo 30 virus infection and amyloidosis in X-linked hypogammaglobulinemia. *Clin Immunol Immunopathol* **3**:347–352, 1975.

79. Bardelas JA, Winkelstein JA, Seto DSY, et al: Fatal ECHO 24 infection in a patient with hypogammaglobulinemia: Relationship to dermatomyositis-like syndrome *J Pediatr* **90**:396–399, 1977.

80. Wilfert CM, Buckley RH, Mohanakumar T, et al: Persistent and fatal central nervous system echovirus infections in agammaglobulinemia. *N Engl J Med* **296**:1485–1489, 1977.

81. Webster ADB, Tripp JH, Hayward AR, et al: Echovirus encephalitis and myositis in primary immunoglobulin deficiency. *Arch Dis Child* **53**:33–37, 1978.

82. Bodensteiner JB, Morris HH, Howell JT, et al: Chronic echo type 5 virus meningoencephalitis in X-linked hypogammaglobulinemia. Treatment with immune plasma *Neurology (NY)* **29**:815–819, 1979

83 Weiner LS, Howell JT, Langford MP, et al: Effect of specif-

ic antibodies on chronic echovirus type 5 encephalitis in a patient with hypogammaglobulinemia. *J Infect Dis* **140:**858–863, 1979.

84. Mease PJ, Ochs HD, Wedgewood RJ: Successful treatment of echovirus meningoencephalitis and myositis-fascitis with intravenous immune globulin therapy in a patient with X-linked agammaglobulinemia. *N Engl J Med* **304:**1278–1281, 1981.

85. Hodes DS, Espinoza DV: Temperature sensitivity of isolate of echovirus type II causing chronic meningoencephalitis in an agammaglobulinemic patient. *J Infect Dis* **144:**377, 1981.

86. Cooper JB, Pralt WR, English BK, et al: Coxsackievirus B3 producing fatal meningoencephalitis in a patient with X-linked agammaglobulinemia. *Am J Dis Child* **137:**82–83, 1983.

87. Townsend TR, Yolken RH, Bishop CA, et al: Outbreak of coxsackie A1 gastroenteritis: A complication of bone marrow transplantation. *Lancet* **1:**820–823, 1982.

88. Yolken RH, Bishop CA, Townsend TA, et al: Infectious gastroenteritis in bone marrow transplant recipients. *N Engl J Med* **306:**1009–1012, 1982.

89. Krugman S. Present status of measles and rubella immunization in the United States: A medical progress report. *J Pediatr* **90:**1–12, 1977.

90. Smithwick EM, Berkovich S: *In vitro* suppression of lymphocyte response to tuberculosis by live measles virus. *Proc Soc Exp Biol Med* **123:**276–278, 1966.

91. Schooley RT, Hirsch MS, Colvin RB, et al: Association of herpesvirus infections with T-lymphocyte subset alterations glomerulopathy, and opportunistic infections after renal transplantation. *N Engl J Med* **308:**313–318, 1983.

92. Blumberg RS, Schooley RT· Lymphocyte markers and infectious diseases. *Semin Hematol* **22:**81–114, 1985

93. Enders JF, McCarthy K, Mitus A, et al: Isolation of measles virus at autopsy in cases of giant cell pneumonia without rash. *N Engl J Med* **261:**875–881, 1959.

94. Breitfeld V, Hashida Y, Sherman FE, et al: Fatal measles infection in children with leukemia. *Lab Invest* **29:**279–291, 1973.

95. Aicardi J, Goutieres F, Arseni-Nunes ML, et al: Acute measles encephalitis in children with immunosuppression. *Pediatrics* **59:**232–239, 1977.

96. Simpson R, Eden OB: Possible interferon response in a child with measles encephalitis during immunosuppression. *Scand J Infect Dis* **16:**315–319, 1984.

97. Gibbs FA, Gibbs EL, Carpenter PR, et al: Electrocephalographic changes in uncomplicated childhood diseases. *JAMA* **171:**1050–1059.

98. Meulen VT, Muller D, Kackell Y, et al: Isolation of infectious measles virus in measles encephalitis. *Lancet* **2:**1172–1175, 1972.

99 Shaffer MF, Rake G, Hodes HL: Isolation of virus from a patient with fatal encephalitis complicating measles. *Am J Dis Child* **64:**815, 1982.

100. Connolly JH, Allen IV, Hurwitz LJ, et al: Measles virus antibody and antigen in subacute sclerosing panencephalitis. *Lancet* **1:**542–544, 1967.

101. Barbosa LH, Fucciloo DA, Sever JL, et al. Subacute sclerosing panencephalitis: Isolation of measles virus from a brain biopsy. *Nature (Lond.)* **221:**974, 1969.

102. Editorial: Measles encephalitis during immunosuppressive treatment. *Br Med J* **1:**1552, 1976.

103. Murphy JV, Yunis EJ: Encephalopathy following measles infection in children with chronic illness. *J Pediatr* **88:**937–942, 1976.

104. Agamarolis DP, Tun JS, Parker DL: Immunosuppressive measles encephalitis in a patient with a renal transplant. *Arch Neurol* **36:**686–690, 1979.

105. Pullen CR, Noble TC, Scott DJ, et al: Atypical measles infections in leukaemic children on immunosuppressive treatment. *Br Med J* **1:**1562–1565, 1976

106. Olding-Stenkvist E, Forsgren M, Henley D, et al: Measles encephalopathy during immunosuppression: Failure of interferon treatment. *Scand J Infec Dis* **14:**1–4, 1982.

107. Mitus A, Holloway A, Evans AE, et al: Attenuated measles vaccine in children with leukemia. *Am J Dis Child* **103:**243–248, 1962.

108. Glezen WP, Denny FW: Epidemiology of acute lower respiratory disease in children. *N Engl J Med* **288:**498–505, 1973.

109. Hall CB, Geiman JM, Biggar R, et al: Respiratory syncytial virus infections within families. *N Engl J Med* **294:**414–419, 1976.

110. Hall GB, Douglas RG Jr: Modes of transmission of respiratory syncytial virus. *J Pediatr* **99:**100–103, 1981.

111. Hall CB: Nosocomial viral respiratory infections. Perennial weeds on pediatric wards. *Am J Med* **70:**670–767, 1981.

112. Sims DG, Downham MAPS, Webbs JKG, et al: Hospital cross-infection on children's wards with respiratory syncytial virus and the role of adult carriage. *Acta Paediatr Scand* **64:**541–545, 1975.

113. MacDonald NE, Hall CB, Suffin SC, et al: Respiratory syncytial viral infection in infants with congenital heart disease. *N Engl J Med* **307:**397–400, 1982.

114. Johnson RA, Prince GA, Suffin SC, et al: Respiratory syncytial virus infection in cyclophosphamide-treated cotton rats. *Infect Immun* **37:**369–373, 1982.

115. Milder JE, McDearmon SC, Walzer PD: Presumed respiratory syncytial virus pneumonia in an adolescent compromised host. *South Med J* **72:**1195–1198, 1979

116. Hall CB. MacDonald NE, Klemperer MR, et al: Respiratory syncytial virus in immunosuppressed children. *Pediatr Res* **15:**613, 1981.

117. Rodriguez WJ, Kim HW, Arrobio JO, et al: Clinical features of acute gastroenteritis associated with human reovirus like agent in infants and young children *J Pediatr* **91:**188–193, 1977.

118. Carlson JAK, Middleton PJ, Ssymanski MT, et al: Fatal rotavirus gastrointeristis. An analysis of 21 cases. *Am J Dis Child* **132:**477–479, 1978.

119. Kapikian AZ, Wyatt RG, Levin MM, et al. Oral administration of human rotavirus to volunteers: Induction of illness and correlates of resistance. *J Infect Dis* **147:**95–106, 1983.

120. Saulsbury FT, Winklestein JA, Yolken RH: Chronic ro-

tavirus infection in immunodeficiency. *J Pediatr* **97**:61–65, 1980.

121. Jarvis WR, Middleton PJ, Gilford EW: Significance of viral infections in severe combined immunodeficiency disease *Pediatr Infect Dis* **2**:187–192, 1983.

122. Flewett TH, Bryden AS, Davies H: Virus particles in gastroenteritis. *Lancet* **2**:1497, 1973.

123. Kapikian AZ, Kim HW, Wyatt RG, et al: Reovirus like agent in stools: association with infantile diarrhea and development of serologic tests. *Science* **185**:1049–1053, 1974.

124. Brendt CD, Kim HW, Rodriguez WJ, et al: Comparison of direct electron microscopy, immune electron microscopy, immune electron microscopy, and rotavirus enzyme linked immunosorbent assay for detection of gastroenteritis viruses in children. *J Clin Microbiol* **13**:976–988, 1981.

125. Middleton PJ, Holdaway MD, Petore M, et al: Solid phase radioimmunoassay for the detection of rotavirus. *Infect Immun* **16**:439–444, 1977.

126. Yolken RH, Kim HW, Clem T, et al: Enzyme linked immunosorbent assay (ELISA) for detection of human reovirus-like agent of infantile gastroenteritis. *Lancet* **2**:263–267, 1977.

127. Kim HW, Brandt CD, Kaoikain AZ, et al. Human reovirus like agent (HRLVA) infection Occurrence in adult contacts of pediatric patients with gastroenteritis. *JAMA* **238**:404–407, 1977

128. Halvrsrud J, Ostavik I: An epidemic of rotavirus associated gastroenteritis in a nursing home for the elderly. *Scand J Infect Dis* **12**:161–164, 1980.

129. Holzel H, Cubett DW, McSwiggan DA, et al: An outbreak of rotavirus infection among adults in a cardiology ward. *J Infect* **2**:33, 1980.

130. Curran JW, Morgan WM, Hardy AM, et al. The epidemiology of AIDS: Current status and future prospects. *Science* **229**:1352–1357, 1985.

15

Acquired Immunodeficiency Syndrome

MICHAEL S. GOTTLIEB

1. Introduction

Acquired immunodeficiency syndrome (AIDS) is a clearly characterized clinical syndrome secondary to impaired function of T lymphocytes that increases susceptibility to opportunistic infections.[1-6] Compelling evidence implicates recently described human T-lymphotropic retroviruses in the etiology and pathogenesis of AIDS.[7,8] Human T-lymphotropic virus strain III (HTLV-III) and lymphadenopathy-associated virus (LAV) have been involved in clinical circumstances ranging from an asymptomatic carrier state to fully developed AIDS. These viruses appear to be identical and have been renamed human immunodeficiency virus (HIV). The previously healthy status of most patients and the ever-increasing case for viral factors in pathogenesis clearly establish AIDS and related syndromes as acquired, i.e., secondary immune-deficiency states.

2. Epidemiology

2.1. Case Definition

Subsequent to the initial reports in June 1981 of Pneumocystis pneumonia and Kaposi sarcoma in previously healthy homosexual males, the Centers for Disease Control (CDC) established surveillance criteria for AIDS in the United States, defined in 1982 (Table 1).[9] Additional exclusion criteria (Table 2) are listed for children, in whom various congenital immune deficiencies and infections must be considered and ruled out.[9a] However, prior to June 1985, laboratory criteria were not incorporated into the AIDS case surveillance definition. Despite early recognition of a characteristic lymphopenia and deficiency of helper T cells, a clinical definition was deliberately employed to minimize bias in the surveillance reports. Since the publication of the case definition in 1982, a wider spectrum of illness associated with the AIDS epidemic has evolved.[10,11] A wide array of signs, symptoms, hematologic disorders, and less severe infections were observed, and linkage with HIV exposure was established. Persistent generalized lymphadenopathy, fevers, sweats, idiopathic thrombocytopenic purpura, oral candidiasis, and *Herpes zoster* are common features of these conditions. The general term AIDS-related complex (ARC) was historically applied to these illnesses, although a precise definition was neither successfully formulated nor generally accepted.[12] Serological testing for HIV is expected to improve clinical diagnosis of the AIDS-relatedness of illnesses not meeting the current surveillance definition (Table 3). As a component of the revised (June 1985) CDC case definition (Table 3), the detection of HIV antibody will add specificity and permit a diagnosis of AIDS in specific disease states, e.g., high-grade non-Hodgkin lymphoma.[13]

The advent of testing for serum antibodies to HIV is a step toward better understanding of the ex-

MICHAEL S. GOTTLIEB • Department of Medicine, University of California–Los Angeles, Los Angeles, California 90024

TABLE 1. Surveillance Definition of AIDS[a,b]

1. The presence of a reliably diagnosed disease at least moderately predictive of cellular immunodeficiency,
2. The absence of an underlying cause for the immunodeficiency or of any defined cause for reduced resistance to the disease. Diseases at least moderately predictive of cellular immunodeficiency:
   - A. Cancers
     1. Kaposi sarcoma
     2. Primary lymphoma of brain
   - B. Protozoal and helminthic infections
     1. Cryptosporidiosis, intestinal: causing diarrhea for more than 1 month
     2. *Pneumocystis carinii* pneumonia
     3. Strongyloidosis: pneumonia, CNS infection, or disseminated infection
     4. Toxoplasmosis: pneumonia or CNS infection
   - C. Fungal infection
     1. Aspergillosis: CNS or disseminated infection
     2. Candidiasis: esophagitis
     3. *Cryptococcus:* pulmonary, CNS, or disseminated infection
   - D. Bacterial infection
     1. Atypical mycobacteriosis (species other than *M tuberculosis* or *M. leprae*): disseminated infection
   - E. Viral infection
     1. Cytomegalovirus: pulmonary, gastrointestinal tract, or CNS infection
     2. Herpes simplex virus
        a. Chronic mucocutaneous ulcers persisting more than 1 month,
           or
        b. Pulmonary, gastrointestinal tract, or disseminated infection
     3. Progressive multifocal leukoencephalopathy (presumed papovavirus)

[a]From Centers for Disease Control (1982)[9]
[b]Within each category, the diseases are listed in alphabetical order Disseminated infection is involvement of lungs and multiple lymph nodes or other internal organs

tent of this epidemic. Although a seronegative HIV culture positive state has been described,[14] the percentage of such persons among those infected appears rare. The sensitivity of these tests in symptomatic members of AIDS risk groups ranges from 85% to 95% using enzyme-linked immunosorbent assays (ELISA) to whole disrupted HIV virus.[15] Current serologic tests are being improved, with a goal toward minimizing false-positive tests. Although ELISA specificity exceeds 90%, a confirmatory test is considered mandatory. This is usually accomplished by electrophoresis/transfer immunoblotting techniques (Western blot technique). Ongoing

seroepidemiologic surveys of the recognized risk groups, blood donors, and the general population are expected to provide an accurate approximation of the extent of exposure in countries where the application of this technology is economically feasible. Cultures of blood or body fluids have little role in routine evaluation of patients.

2.2. AIDS in the United States and Europe

Since the initial recognition of AIDS in the United States in 1981, the number of cases in the United States and Western Europe has surpassed 30,000, with the number of cases doubling every 12–18 months. The distribution by risk group in the United States is summarized in Table 4. The highest proportion have occurred among homosexual and bisexual men (73%), followed by intravenous drug users (17%). A history of intravenous drug use was also positive in approximately 15% of homosexual/bisexual men with AIDS. Among women, 54% of cases were associated with intravenous drugs, 14% with sexual contact with members of known risk groups, and 9% with blood transfusions. Of all cases, 6% were not associated with known risk factors; however, 22% of women had no known risk factor, in contrast to 5% of men. Among men, 79% had a

TABLE 2. Provisional Case Definition of AIDS in Children[a]

For the limited purposes of epidemiologic surveillance, the CDC defines a case of pediatric autoimmunodeficiency syndrome (AIDS) as a child who has had:
1. A reliably diagnosed disease at least moderately indicative of underlying cellular immunodeficiency
2. No known cause of underlying cellular immunodeficiency or any other reduced resistance reported to be associated with that disease

The diseases accepted are the same as for adults (Table 1) after the exclusion of congenital infections, e g., toxoplasmosis or herpes simplex virus infections in the first month after birth or cytomegalovirus infection in the first 6 months after birth. Specific conditions that must be excluded in a child include.
1. Primary immune deficiency diseases severe combined immunodeficiency, DiGeorge syndrome, Wiskott–Aldrich syndrome, ataxia–telangiectasia, graft-versus-host disease, neutropenia, neutrophil function abnormality, agammaglobulinemia, or hypogammaglobulinemia with raised IgM
2. Secondary immune deficiency associated with immunosuppressive therapy, lymphoreticular malignancy, or starvation

[a]See Ref 9a

**TABLE 3. Revisions on CDC Case Definition
of AIDS**[a]

1. That the case definition of AIDS used for national reporting
   continue to include only the more severe manifestations of
   HTLV-III/LAV infection
2. That CDC develop more inclusive definitions and classifica-
   tions of HTLV-III/LAV infection for diagnosis, treatment,
   and prevention, as well as for epidemiologic studies and
   special surveys
3. That the following refinements be adopted in the case definition of AIDS used for national reporting.
   a. In the absence of the opportunistic diseases required by
      the current case definition, any of the following diseases
      will be considered indicative of AIDS if the patient has
      a positive serologic or virologic test for HTLV-III/LAV
      i. Disseminated histoplasmosis (not confined to lungs
         or lymph nodes), diagnosed by culture, histology,
         or antigen detection
      ii. Isosporiasis, causing chronic diarrhea (over 1
          month), diagnosed by histology or stool microscopy
      iii. Bronchial or pulmonary candidiasis, diagnosed by
           microscopy or by presence of characteristic white
           plaques grossly on the bronchial mucosa (not be
           culture alone)
      iv. Non-Hodgkin lymphoma of high-grade pathologic
          type (diffuse, undifferentiated) and of B-cell or
          unknown immunologic phenotype, diagnosed by bi-
          opsy
      v. Histologically confirmed Kaposi sarcoma in patients
         who are 60 years old or older at diagnosis
   b. In the absence of the opportunistic diseases required by
      the current case definition, a histologically confirmed
      diagnosis of chronic lymphoid interstitial pneumonitis in
      a child (under 13 years of age) will be considered indi-
      cative of AIDS unless test(s) for HTLV-III/LAV are
      negative.
   c. Patients who have a lymphoreticular malignancy diag-
      nosed more than 3 months after the diagnosis of an
      opportunistic disease used as a marker for AIDS will no
      longer be excluded as AIDS cases
   d. To increase the specificity of the case definition, pa-
      tients will be excluded as AIDS cases if they have a
      negative result on testing for serum antibody to HTLV-
      III/LAV, have no other type of HTLV-III/LAV test
      with a positive result, and do not have a low number of
      T-helper lymphocytes or a low ratio of T-helper to T-
      suppressor lymphocytes In the absence of test results,
      patients satisfying all other criteria in the definition will
      continue to be included.

[a]Centers for Disease Control (1985) [13]

homosexual or bisexual risk factor. AIDS in children
occurred most commonly (75%) in families in which
a parent had AIDS or among population groups at
increased risk for AIDS, usually intravenous drug
users or bisexual males. Blood or clotting factor

transfusion was implicated in 14% of pediatric AIDS
cases. From the beginning of the epidemic, the epidemiologic pattern of AIDS was consistent with an
infectious agent transmitted chiefly through sexual
contact, shared needle use, and blood or blood product transfusions (40). Transmission to infants is likely to be intrauterine or during delivery. Evidence for
horizontal transmission is lacking.

Cases of AIDS have been reported from 18
countries in Europe.[16] The homosexual/bisexual risk
factor was implicated in 70%, and 12% of European
cases were of African origin.

2.3. AIDS in Africa and the Caribbean

In 1982 AIDS was recognized in Belgium and
France among patients of African origin primarily
presenting with opportunistic infections.[17,18] Retrospective analysis indicates sporadic cases dating
from 1976–1978. Epidemiologic studies from Zaire
and Ruwanda indicate a high incidence of the syndrome; however, case recognition has been complicated by their lack of diagnostic techniques compared
to the United States and Europe. Cryptococcal meningitis has been the most conspicuous opportunistic
infection in African cases; however, no centralized
case registry for AIDS in African countries has been
established.

In African nations, where AIDS appears to be
epidemic, a modified, more sensitive case definition
may be required to understand the extent of the problem. For example, bronchoalveolar lavage or laboratory support to document *Pneumocystis* as the cause
of pneumonias is not routinely available. Some epi-
demiologists studying AIDS epidemic areas of Africa have already modified the case definition to include cases with chronic diarrheal illness or weight
loss for which other causes could not be established.[17] Among Africans, the balance of AIDS
cases between the sexes is relatively even, and the
disease occurs among all socioeconomic classes.
Heterosexual promiscuity is the major conspicuous
risk factor identified thus far. A high prevalence of
antibody to HIV has been reported among female
prostitutes in Zaire and Ruwanda.[19]

AIDS is prevalent among Haitians residing both
in their country and in the United States.[20–22] Cases
have occurred predominantly in Florida and New
York owing to their large Haitian immigrant commu-
nities. Most cases have been in males aged 20–40.

TABLE 4. Acquired Immunodeficiency Syndrome: U.S. Report Cases
to CDC as of January 13, 1986, by Risk Groups

Group	Males N	Males Percent	Females N	Females Percent	Total cases N	Total cases Percent
Adult/adolescent						
Homosexual or bisexual	11,910	79	—	—	11,910	73
Intravenous (IV) drug user	2,195	14	571	54	2,766	17
Hemophilia/coagulation disorder	120	1	4	10	124	1
Heterosexual contact	28	0	154	14	182	1
Transfusion with blood/blood products	163	1	98	9	261	2
None of the above/other	745	5	239	22	984	6
Total	15,161	100	1,066	100	16,227	100
Pediatric						
Hemophilia/coagulation disorder	11	9	0	0	11	5
Parent with AIDS or at increased risk for AIDS	88	69	86	83	174	75
Transfusion with blood/blood product	22	17	11	11	33	14
None of the above/other	6	5	7	6	13	6
Total	127	100	104	100	231	100

The profile of opportunistic infections among Haitians often includes disseminated *Mycobacterium tuberculosis* and cerebral toxoplasmosis as well as *Pneumocystis* pneumonia and oral/esophageal candidiasis.[20,21] In Haiti, Pape et al.[20] studied 177 previously healthy Haitians who developed AIDS during the period between June 1979 and September 1984: 27 had Kaposi sarcoma, and 150 had opportunistic infections. Risk factors included bisexuality (32%), blood transfusions (14%), and heterosexual promiscuity among males and females. The factors accounting for this well-circumscribed focus in the Caribbean remain obscure.

3. Etiology and Pathogenesis

3.1. Human T-Lymphotropic Retroviruses

Although the AIDS syndrome was first delineated in 1981, specific etiologic factors were lacking. Rapid progress toward understanding the clinical, immunologic, and epidemiologic features of AIDS ensued when human retroviruses were isolated from lymphoid cells of these patients.[7,23] The characteristic depletion of T cells in AIDS, particularly the helper/inducer subset bearing the T4 surface antigen, was an early clue.[1,24] The two previously described human retroviruses were known to preferentially infect this cell type, engendering the hypothesis that a T-cell tropic retrovirus might be an etiologic factor in AIDS.[22]

A retrovirus encodes its genetic information as RNA, employing a unique viral enzyme (reverse transcriptase) to transcribe its RNA genome into DNA, which then integrates within the host cell genome in a form termed a provirus. The typical retrovirus contains three genes coded for the viral internal core proteins (*gag*), the polymerase or reverse transcriptase gene (*pol*), and the gene for the envelope glycoprotein (*env*). The transcription-initiation signals for a retrovirus lie within long terminal repeat nucleic acid sequences at the 3' and 5' ends of the genome. In some animal retroviruses, certain viral genes are replaced by a cell-drived sequence known as an *onc* gene, which allows these viruses to transform target cells acutely.

Animal retroviruses, such as feline leukemia

virus, had previously been linked unequivocally to cancers and immunodeficiency states. It was not until 1980 that the first retrovirus of humans, human T-cell leukemia/lymphoma virus strain I (HTLV-I), was isolated from occasional patients with T-cell lymphoma[22,25,26] and a distinct syndrome of adult T-cell leukemia.[26] HTLV-I is also endemic in certain regions of Africa and the Caribbean basin. A second T lymphotropic virus (HTLV-II) was isolated in 1982 from a patient with a T cell variant of hairy cell leukemia.[27] The remarkable ability to culture human retroviruses followed directly from the advances in cell culture, specifically the ability to maintain long-term growth of mature human T cells using T-cell growth factor, interleukin-2 (IL-2), first described in 1976.[23]

In the years prior to the association of human retroviruses with AIDS, characterization of the biologic agents involved progressed rapidly. The genes for HTLV-I and HTLV-II have been cloned and analyzed in detail; these studies have become the foundation for subsequent advances in the detection, isolation, and detailed characterization of HIV.

Cumulative evidence for HIV as etiologic in AIDS is persuasive. In early studies at the National Cancer Institute (NCI), more than 95 isolates of HIV from blood or lymph node cells were made. During that same period, no viral isolates were obtained from healthy heterosexual donors. Circulating antibodies to HIV are present in more than 90% of patients with AIDS or related syndromes using ELISA with whole disrupted virus.[15] Binding to specific viral proteins has been confirmed by Western blot electrophoresis. In extensive studies conducted during the process of licensing test reagents for blood screening, antibodies were detected in less than 0.1% of healthy blood donors. The major population groups in which AIDS occurs evidence a prevalence of antibody to HIV indicative of previous exposure, and in most cases, ongoing viral replication. Studies in selected cases of AIDS related to blood transfusion indicated at least one blood donor with antibody to HIV in every instance.[28] Nevertheless, Koch's postulates are not completely satisfied. HIV infection and seroconversion have been observed following experimental inoculation of primates, although the clinical AIDS syndrome has not been reproduced.

HIV is quite distinct genetically from HTLV-I and HTLV-II. In contrast to HTLV-I and HTLV-II, HIV is genetically polymorphic by restriction endonuclease analysis.[22,29] HIV major core and envelope proteins do not cross-react with those of HTLV-I and HTLV-II.[22] Nevertheless, these exogenous retroviruses have features in common, the most striking of which is a relative tropism for T4 antigen bearing lymphocytes (T tropic). Studies suggest that the T4 molecule on the surface of helper T cells may be the receptor for viral attachment.[30-32]

The T4 molecule also plays an important role in the formation of the characteristic multinucleated giant cells, which develop following the fusion of neighboring T4-positive cells, requiring the presence of the T4 molecule.[33] Once infection of the T4-positive cells occurs, cellular destruction may not occur. In vitro studies have shown that whereas unstimulated HIV-infected T4 cells may remain alive for prolonged periods, immunologic activation results in rapid cell depth. This observation may explain how repeated episodes of immune stimulation with other infectious agents or allogeneic blood or semen could modulate the clinical course of HIV infection.[34]

Besides lymphocytes, HIV infects mononuclear phagocytes.[35] The predominant cell types infected within the brain and lungs of patients with HIV infection are cells of the monocyte/macrophage series. These are almost assuredly the critical elements in the production of the devastating central nervous system (CNS) effects of HIV infection and the lymphocytic intestinal pneumonitis syndrome seen particularly in pediatric AIDS patients. It is also likely that other cells of monocyte/macrophage lineage at other sites are infected. These include the dendritic cells in lymph nodes and the Langerhans cells in the dermis of the skin. Infected macrophages produce larger quantities of virus for longer periods of time than do infected T cells and thus may serve as an important reservoir of virus for other cells and tissues in an infected person. HIV isolates from T cells appear to have a lesser ability to infect macrophages in vitro than T cells; conversely, macrophage isolates appear to be more adapted to these cells than T cells. Thus, the genomic variation of different HIV isolates may be correlated with a tropism of a particular isolate for particular cell types, and thus account for very different clinical effects.[36-40]

A model has been proposed in which virally encoded factors coincidentally interact with regulatory sequences of cellular genes leading to uncontrolled growth (leukemia or lymphoma) induced by HTLV-I and HTLV-II, and cytopathic effects (T-helper cytopenia) induced by HIV.[41–43] HIV replicates rapidly in vivo in contrast to HTLV-I and HTLV-II, which exist for prolonged periods in unexpressed proviral (DNA) form. This rapid replication may contribute to the observed cytopathic effects of HIV on T4-positive lymphocytes.

Environmental cofactors may contribute to the clinical outcome of HIV infection. While infection with this virus is considered necessary, infection alone may not be sufficient for the development of the AIDS syndrome. Specific manifestations of AIDS may be associated with specific cofactor, as in the case of Kaposi sarcoma, which is strongly associated with homosexuality.[8,44,45] Among homosexual or bisexual men with AIDS, 43% develop Kaposi sarcoma, compared with fewer than 11% of patients who have other risk factors. However, the cofactors accounting for the difference have not been identified.

3.2. Immunologic Features

3.2.1. AIDS with Opportunistic Infections and/or Kaposi Sarcoma

The nature of the opportunistic pathogens in AIDS (protozoan, viral, fungal, and mycobacterial) led to an early focus on defects in T-cell-mediated immunity. However, other components of the immune system (notably humoral immunity and natural killer cell function) are abnormal. The scope of the immune defects in AIDS have been grouped by Fauci[46] into three categories: (1) defects characteristic of the syndrome; (2) defects secondary to a primary lesion of helper/inducer cells; and (3) nonspecific defects that are probably epiphenomena.

The tropism of HIV has a central role in the pathogenesis of the syndrome. Most patients with CDC-defined AIDS have marked depletion of absolute numbers of circulating T cells with the OKT4/Leu 3 (T helper/inducer) phenotype. OKT8/Leu 2 (T suppressor/cytotoxic) cell numbers are usually normal or elevated, although possibly reduced in individuals with severe lymphopenia.[24] In AIDS, the remaining OKT4/Leu 3-positive cells are functionally abnormal.[47]

Lymphocytes from AIDS patients have im-paired specific cytotoxic and natural killer mechanisms for tumor targets as well as herpes virus-infected target cells.[4] Immaturity of the T-cell lineage or activation in AIDS is evidenced by increased numbers of circulating cells bearing surface markers for HLA-DR or OKT10.[48]

Abnormalities of humoral immunity are prominent in AIDS and in ARC.[47] Both adults and children typically have polyclonal hypergammaglobulinemia of the IgG and IgA classes. Functional studies have revealed a state of in vivo B-cell activation. Primary and secondary antibody responses may be impaired, a factor that probably contributes to the higher frequency of septicemias and localized bacterial infections in infants and children with AIDS. A correlate of these observations is that immunizations may be ineffective.

Leukopenia and neutropenia are common findings, particularly in patients with the febrile prodrome of AIDS or who present with opportunistic infection. Leukopenias are frequently exacerbated by trimethoprim–sulfamethoxazole or pentamidine therapy of *Pneumocystis carinii* pneumonia.[46] Moreover, defects in monocyte–macrophage function have been reported.[46,49]

In most patients with CDC-defined AIDS, serial studies of immune cell phenotype and function indicate persistent deficiency of helper T cells and a progressive general lymphopenia. In accordance with this observation, patients who survive a first opportunistic infection experience major morbidity due to a cascade of subsequent infections.

The presentation of AIDS with *Pneumocystis carinii* pneumonia tends to be followed by a several-months period of improvement marked by weight gain and increased sense of well-being. However, sustained clinical or immunologic improvement is rarely, if ever, observed; survival beyond 2 years is unusual. The prognosis for tumor response and survival is better for a subset of patients with Kaposi sarcoma, in whom immune function is relatively preserved at presentation.[50] Occasional patients with Kaposi sarcoma maintain normal absolute numbers of helper T lymphocytes; this finding has a favorable prognosis.

3.2.2. AIDS-Related Complex

The most common HIV-related syndrome not meeting the initial CDC definition of AIDS has been referred to as AIDS-related complex (ARC). This syndrome is also associated with prominent immunologic aberrations, but its definition is imprecise. Major symptoms include lymphadenopathy, fever, sweats, weight loss, and malaise.[51] The term persistent generalized lymphadenopathy (PGL) describes a subset of ARC.[52,53] In most cases, lymph node biopsies reveal intense follicular hyperplasia.[54] Occasionally, mycobacterial infection (usually *M. tuberculosis*) may be discovered in biopsies among population groups with a high tuberculosis exposure. Other biopsy findings have included visceral Kaposi sarcoma, lymphoma,[55] atypical mycobacteriosis, and histoplasmosis. Less severe infections associated with T-cell immunity are common in this patient group, including Herpes zoster[56–58] as well as chronic oral and cutaneous candidiasis.[51,52,59]

In patients with ARC there is considerable diversity of the T-cell phenotypic profile.[24,59–61] Helper T-cell numbers are often below the fifth percentile. HIV can be isolated from a large percentage of ARC or PGL cases, and the vast majority have serum antibody to the virus.[15,29,62] In several series of homosexual males with ARC, progression to AIDS has been observed at a rate of 25%/year.[12,52,63] Studies with ARC patients at UCLA have linked progression to AIDS with lower absolute helper T-cell numbers and lower helper/suppressor T-cell ratios.[12]

Illustrative Case 1

A 23-year-old white male homosexual presented with a 3-month history of fever, night sweats, and generalized adenopathy. His sexual practices included both insertive and receptive anal intercourse, fisting, and the use of such drugs as amyl nitrate, cocaine, and marijuana. Past medical history included treatment for gonorrhea on three occasions, syphilis, shigellosis, and hepatitis B. He had remained generally well until the past 3 months, during which time he began to note intermittent temperature elevations as high as 102°F (38.9°C), without rigors, as well as frequent night sweats, and a 20-lb (g-kg) weight loss. Over the past month, he had noted symmetric enlargement of cervical and axillary lymph nodes.

On physical examination, the patient was a thin, anxious white man with an oral temperature of 100.6°F (38.1°C). The general physical examination was remarkable for the presence of nontender, somewhat shotty 2 × 2 cm lymph nodes bilaterally in the anterior cervical, axillary, and inguinal regions.

Laboratory data included hematocrit (Hct) 38, white blood cell (WBC) count 3100/mm³ with 90% polys, 5% lymphs, 2% eosinophils, and 3% monocytes. The T4/T8 ratio was 0.3. Serum

heterophile and HBsAg studies were negative. Antibody tests to both hepatitis B and cytomegalovirus (CMV) were positive. Lymph node biopsy revealed nonspecific reactive hyperplasia. HIV antibody testing by ELISA and Western blot techniques was positive.

Comment. This is a very typical nonspecific prodrome of an individual with HIV infection. The epidemiologic history, including the previous infections and sexual practices, is very common for persons contracting HIV infection. It is now apparent from prospective studies in uninfected gay males that acute HIV infection results in a mononucleosis-like syndrome that may be self-limited. Alternatively, as in this patient, a more prolonged febrile illness, associated with generalized adenopathy may occur. Some 20–30% of such persons will develop full-blown AIDS over a 2–3-year period.

The immunologic findings in asymptomatic HIV-seropositive persons are varied, and in many the T-cell profile is entirely normal. In others, there is an increase in absolute number of OKT8/Leu 2 cells (T suppressor/cytotoxic), yet other patients have deficient OKT4/Leu 3 cells (T helper/inducer). Preliminary studies of the natural history of HIV infection indicate that increased T suppressor/cytotoxic cell numbers may represent the earliest change in T-cell phenotype following seroconversion.

The immune deficiency in AIDS and ARC is probably compounded by secondary opportunistic infections. Cytomegalovirus, other viruses, and disseminated mycobacterial infection are known to produce immunosuppression and may be cofactors with HIV for the full expression of the syndrome. Thus, treatment for these complicating infections may be required as components of multiagent antiviral and immunotherapy regimens.

4. Risk Groups for AIDS and HIV Infection

The highest incidence of AIDS has occurred in several well-defined population groups listed in Table 4, an epidemiologic pattern related to transmission of HIV by sexual contact, shared needle use, and receipt of blood or clotting factor products. Evidence also favors maternal–fetal transmission in utero or during the peripartum period, but there is no evidence for horizontal transmission in households. Although the virus has been cultured from some saliva and tear specimens, epidemiologically the disease does not suggest transmission of infection by aerosol. Experience to date with the hepatitis B vaccine, hepa-

TABLE 5. Infectious Disease Syndromes and Etiologic Agents in AIDS

Pulmonary disease

Bacteria
 Streptococcus pneumoniae
 Mycobacterium tuberculosis
 Mycobacterium avium complex
Protozoa
 Pneumocystis carinii
 Cryptosporidium

Fungi
 Cryptococcus neoformans
 Histoplasma capsulatum
 Coccidiodes immitis
Viruses
 Cytomegalovirus

Neurologic disease

Bacteria
 Listeria
 Mycobacterium tuberculosis
Protozoa
 Toxoplasmosis
Fungi
 Cryptococcal meningitis

Viruses
 Cytomegalovirus encephalitis
 HIV encephalitis
 Progressive multifocal leukoencephalopathy (J–C virus)
 Vasculitis presumed secondary to herpes
  zoster
 Cerebrovascular accident (CVA) or transient ischemic attack (TIA) attributed
  to nonbacterial thrombotic endocarditis
  (etiology unknown)

Gastrointestinal disease

Bacteria
 Salmonella enteritis
 Mycobacterium avium complex enteritis
Protozoa
 Cryptosporidium enteritis
 Isospora belli enteritis
 Entamoeba histolytica colitis

Fungi
 Candida esophagitis
Viruses
 Cytomegalovirus colitis
 Herpes simplex colitis

titis B immune globulin, and both intramuscular as well as intravenous preparations of immunoglobulin indicates that these materials do not cause HIV infection.

5. Clinical Features

5.1. General

The patient with AIDS or other HIV-related syndromes challenges the diagnostic acumen of both the generalist and specialist, inasmuch as multiple organ systems are potential targets for infectious, neoplastic, and autoimmune complications. During the 1980s, HIV infection and AIDS have replaced syphilis as a primer of medicine for house officers.[64] In the United States and Europe, most patients have presented in one of several ways:

Fever and weight loss followed by opportunistic infection (febrile prodrome): In approximately 73%

of the first 10,000 cases, AIDS was diagnosed by the presence of an opportunistic infection (Table 6) in persons who had no previously known immune deficiency. *Pneumocystis carinii* pneumonia was the index diagnosis in 56%. Most patients presenting with opportunistic infection had been symptomatic 1–12 months with illness of variable severity.[1-3] Symptoms prior to diagnosis in patients with *Pneumocystis* pneumonia diagnosed at UCLA Medical Center included fever (often accompanied by drenching night sweats), malaise, and diarrhea. Weight loss of 10–30 lb (4.5–13.5 kg) was typical in patients who developed *Pneumocystis* pneumonia or other opportunistic infection. Among those followed for ARC, accelerated weight loss and fever were associated with incipient AIDS. Although patients commonly reported anorexia and intermittent diarrheal illness, the degree of weight loss was usually out of proportion to these symptoms.

During the later phase of this febrile prodrome,

TABLE 6. Causes of Fever in Patients with AIDS

Pneumocystis carinii pneumonia
Cytomegalovirus infection
Mycobacterium avium complex bacteremia
Salmonella bacteremia
HIV infection (probable)
Other occult opportunistic infection
Occult non-Hodgkin lymphoma, Hodgkin disease, or Kaposi
    sarcoma
Drug fever (typically sulfonamides)

culminating in opportunistic infection, lymphadeno-pathy was not a prominent feature. Slight tachypnea on exertion has occurred shortly before overt pneumonia, although lung auscultation may be normal. Common physical findings include forehead and mid-facial seborrheic dermatitis, retinal "cotton-wool" patches,[65–68] patchy oral candidiasis, or hairy leukoplakia.[69]

The etiology of the febrile prodrome may vary, depending on the country of origin and risk group. In our experience with homosexual and bisexual males, it was prodromal to *Pneumocystis* pneumonia in most cases. Other causes of fever included Kaposi sarcoma limited to lymph nodes, non-Hodgkin lymphoma, disseminated mycobacterial infection, CMV infection, and other opportunistic pathogens. The wide spectrum of such pathogens make thorough microbiologic studies mandatory; nevertheless, the high frequency of eventual *Pneumocystis* pneumonia in patients with the febrile prodrome emphasizes the need for aggressive pursuit of this diagnosis.

A marked reduction of percentage and absolute numbers of helper T cells during the febrile prodrome is often clinically useful in increasing suspicion that these fevers are related to an evolving opportunistic infection (i.e., overt AIDS). The finding of 300 helper T cells per mm^3 should hasten medical evaluation.

Abrupt onset of opportunistic infection: While the febrile prodrome is characteristic of AIDS patients presenting with opportunistic infections, there are noteworthy exceptions: some have presented with *Pneumocystis* pneumonia or cryptococcal meningitis who have reported feeling entirely well until several days before the onset of symptoms. The opportunistic infections associated with AIDS should therefore be included in the differential diagnosis of infection, particularly among groups with increased

relative risk. This diagnosis should be considered in the febrile patient with pneumonia and a history suggesting previous exposure to HIV, which would include blood transfusions since 1978 and sexual contact with members of high-risk groups.

Onset with Kaposi sarcoma: Approximately 22% of the first 1000 AIDS cases in the United States presented with Kaposi sarcoma and an additional 6% with both Kaposi sarcoma and *Pneumocystis pneumonia.*[70] Kaposi sarcoma in AIDS has generally occurred among homosexual/bisexual males aged 20–49. The lesions are typically red-violet plaques that become more deeply purple as they mature. The diagnosis is established by punch biopsy with local anesthesia. The surveillance definition of AIDS is met if the patient is less than 60 and has no other condition associated with immune deficiency. At diagnosis, systemic symptoms are absent in most cases. The presence of fever and weight loss at diagnosis of Kaposi sarcoma usually indicates evolving opportunistic infection or, in some cases, concurrent lymphoma.[55,71–73]

5.2. Clinical Approach to Fever in AIDS and in Population Groups at Increased Risk

Fever in all immunocompromised hosts is a major challenge to the clinician. As defined by CDC criteria, fever is characteristic in patients with AIDS. Moreover, it is a feature of evolving AIDS and in some cases, of ARC.

Fever in the Patient with Known AIDS

Several aspects of investigating fever in patients with known AIDS are important. The major challenge is to determine whether the fever stems from the underlying disease state, a documented but inadequately treated opportunistic infection, the onset of a new infection or lymphoma, or a hypersensitivity reaction to medications.

Most infectious complications of AIDS have been accompanied by fever, which should immediately trigger investigations for etiologic clues. Because localizing symptoms are frequently absent, the need for comprehensive clinical and microbiologic studies is greater. Moreover, AIDS patients tend to have concurrent infections, e.g., *Pneumocystis* and CMV pneumonia, with or without atypical mycobacterial bacteremia. On rare occasions, overwhelming bacterial or fungal infection has been observed in the absence of fever.

The development of recurrence of *P. carinii* pneumonia is a common cause of fever among patients in whom a diagnosis of AIDS has already been established by the presence of Kaposi sarcoma or another opportunistic infection (e.g., cryptococcal meningitis). In some instances, fever due to *P. carinii* is accompanied by accelerated weight loss, dry cough, dyspnea at rest or with exertion only, and night sweats.

Although fevers may be sustained, daily spikes are more frequent. Several investigators and a National Institutes of Health (NIH) working group have concluded that flexible bronchoscopy with bronchoalveolar lavage is a highly sensitive means of establishing the diagnosis of *Pneumocystis* infection.[74–79] Occasionally, expectorated or induced sputum samples are positive for *Pneumocystis,* but such identification should only be attempted by experienced observers. Laboratory evaluations can be used to provide a rationale for an urgent diagnostic procedure. Suggestive findings include respiratory distress and infiltrates on chest radiographs. The latter, which are typically diffuse and interstitial, may be localized and alveolar. Arterial blood gases (ABGs) usually reveal hypoxemia with slight reduction in the P_{CO_2} value.[77]

While patients with fever, cough, and dyspnea due to *P. carinii* pneumonia typically have infiltrates and hypoxemia, cases have been reported of patients with both chest radiographs and room air ABGs demonstrating no abnormal findings.[77] Abnormalities of the diffusing capacity[77] and pulmonary gallium scan[75,80] are sensitive indicators of an interstitial process and provide rationale for proceeding to bronchoscopy. If noninvasive studies cannot be performed within 24 hr, it is advisable to proceed directly to an invasive diagnostic procedure or to institute a therapeutic trial of anti-*Pneumocystis* therapy.

Recurrent *P. carinii* pneumonia should be strongly suspected in febrile patients who have recovered from a previous episode. Recrudescent pneumonia was observed in 33–50% of AIDS patients at UCLA prior to the routine use of chronic prophylaxis with trimethoprim–sulfamethoxazole or sulfadoxine–pyrimethamine.[81]

Mycobacterium avium complex is a frequent cause of fevers in AIDS patients.[76,82–84] It manifests as high grade bacteremia detected on mycobacterial blood culture. A firm tender spleen or enlarged liver usually indicates visceral mycobacterial infection. To establish this diagnosis in patients whose blood is culture negative, bone marrow aspirate and culture may be required.

Disseminated CMV infection is a common cause of fever and may be associated with a variety of end-organ lesions, including pneumonitis, retinitis,[65,68] encephalitis, colitis, and adrenalitis.[30,71,85]

Occult neoplasia (usually non-Hodgkin lymphoma) may produce new fevers in AIDS patients. Lymph nodes and bone marrow are typically involved sites, although gastrointestinal (GI) and CNS lymphomas are not uncommon.[55,86] Computed tomography (CT) scan and brain biopsy may be appropriate components of fever evaluation in patients with CNS signs. Gastrointestinal lymphomas in AIDS, usually found in the upper GI tract, may be associated with minimal symptoms. They are readily identified by noninvasive studies.

More in infants and children than in adults with AIDS, bacterial infections with pyogenic organisms and enteric pathogens are common. Pneumococcal and *Salmonella* bacteremias have been prominent.[5,87,88] For these reasons, blood cultures, and in some instances sputum and stool cultures, are appropriate components of fever evaluation.

Fever due to sulfonamide drugs is common in patients with AIDS,[77,88,89] particularly during initial therapy of *Pneumocystis* pneumonia with trimethoprim–sulfamethoxazole. Drug fevers may occur as early as day 4 or as late as day 14. Such fevers tend to be accompanied by diffuse maculopapular skin eruption. Fevers may also be associated with long-term anti-*Pneumocystis* prophylaxis for which trimethoprim–sulfamethoxazole or sulfadoxine–pyrimethamine is usually prescribed. Sulfonamide medications should be discontinued when drug fever is suspected. Pentamidine is recommended instead if the patient has not yet received adequate therapy (14–21 total days) for *P. carinii*. Long-term prophylaxis can be temporarily interrupted in patients in whom suspected drug fever develops, although such patients should also be studied for additional opportunistic infections.

In those with advanced AIDS, how vigorously

should the evaluation of persistent fever be pursued in the absence of localizing signs or symptoms? The central issues are the likelihood of discovering a treatable cause and the morbidity as well as the cost effectiveness of additional procedures. In our experience, fevers in late-stage patients are usually due to *Pneumocystis* pneumonia, disseminated mycobacterial or CMV infection, or occult lymphoma. It seems reasonable to pursue a diagnosis of *Pneumocystis* infection when clinical circumstances are suggestive. In these cases, most will respond favorably to trimethoprim–sulfamethoxazole, with resolution of fever and infiltrates. Blood cultures for bacteria, mycobacteria, and CMV may also reveal the source of fever. Diagnostic studies beyond these simple measures depend on the specific clinical circumstances. It is our experience that further studies infrequently reveal a readily treatable infection or neoplasm.

When the original fevers remain unknown it is often necessary to empirically prescribe antipyretics for patient comfort. Acetaminophen is generally preferred over aspirin because of the possibility of thrombocytopenia in advanced patients. True fever of unknown origin in ARC may respond to indomethocin at a dose of 25 mg three times daily.

6. Laboratory Studies in AIDS and HIV-Related Syndromes

The term AIDS has been used exclusively for cases meeting the surveillance criteria defined by the CDC. The detection of antibody to HIV is in some instances a component of the case definition.[13] Prior to this modification, diagnosis of AIDS was made exclusively on the basis of clinical criteria. Laboratory evaluations of patients with CDC-defined AIDS and those with possible AIDS or other HIV-related syndrome differ and are discussed separately.

The initial laboratory evaluation should be based in part on the medical history and physical findings. A number of baseline laboratory studies are recommended following definitive microbiologic diagnosis of opportunistic infection or biopsy-proven Kaposi sarcoma. Baseline studies permit determination of extent of disease, assessment of progression, and adverse effects of antimicrobial or chemotherapeutic agents. The need for additional studies may be dictated by specific infections and clinical circumstances.

6.1. Routine Diagnostic Studies

Recommended studies include complete blood count (CBC) with differential and platelet count. The absolute lymphocyte count can be calculated by multiplying total WBC number by the percentage lymphocytes on Wright's-stained smear (normal greater than 1500). Additional recommended baseline studies include chest radiography, chemistry panel, and urinalysis.

6.2. Specific Serologic and Immunologic Tests

Immunologic tests and viral serologies have limited clinical value in patients with established AIDS, but the absolute T-helper cell number may have some prognostic significance in AIDS/Kaposi sarcoma[50] (Table 7). This is not the case in the syndrome with opportunistic infection in which these cells are typically virtually absent (e.g., 0–150/mm^3). This test is occasionally of value in confirming the diagnosis in cases of opportunistic infection in which no risk factor can be identified and other disorders remain in the differential diagnosis. The virtual absence of T-helper cells in such cases strongly supports the AIDS diagnosis. Most patients

TABLE 7. Immunologic Abnormalities in AIDS

Characteristic pattern
  Quantitative T-lymphocyte deficiency
    Total T lymphocytopenia
    Selective T4 lymphocytopenia
  Qualitative T-lymphocyte defect
    T4 functional defect
    Selective functional defect T4 subset
  Hyperactivity of B-cell repertoire
    Increased spontaneous immunoglobulin secretion by individual B cells
    Elevated serum immunoglobulin levels

Consistently observed pattern (probably secondary to A)
  Decreased in vitro lymphocyte proliferative responses
    Predominant defect of antigen-specific responses
    Defect of mitogen responses in bulk T-cell cultures
    Defect in allogeneic and autologous mixed-lymphocyte cultures in bulk cultures
  Decreased cytotoxic responses

with CDC-defined AIDS are anergic, and routine skin tests are not recommended.

While increased serum IgG and IgA are characteristic of AIDS, quantitative immunoglobulin determinations have not added clinically useful information. Serum antibody to EBV and CMV is present in most patients but does not provide diagnostic or prognostic information. Likewise, most patients have antibody to HIV, although the titer does not appear to have prognostic value. Certain immunologic abnormalities have no value in clinical decision making. The indiscriminate application of panels of immunologic and serologic tests in CDC-defined AIDS in settings other than clinical trials is neither informative nor cost effective and should be discouraged.

6.3. Cultures

Cultures of blood for bacterial pathogens, mycobacteria, fungi, and CMV may be indicated in patients with fever of unknown origin. Viral culture of oral, genital, or anal ulcers frequently yield Herpes simplex.[3] Disseminated CMV infection is often accompanied by positive urine and semen cultures. All specimens and endoscopic biopsies should be subjected to complete microbiologic evaluation.

6.4. Other Studies

Additional studies are based on specific clinical problems. The role of GI endoscopy and lymph node biopsy procedures for staging of Kaposi sarcoma has not been established. The evaluation of diarrhea should include complete stool microbiologic studies, including examination for cryptosporidia and *Isospora belli*. Persistent headache or abnormal state of consciousness should include CT scans and lumbar puncture to obtain fluid for cryptococcal antigen detection. Bone marrow examination may be indicated when evaluating persistent leukopenia, lymphoma, or mycobacterial infection.

7. Differential Diagnosis

7.1. General

The extension of HIV infection into the general population makes it essential that the diagnosis of AIDS and ARC be considered in all patients with consistent symptomatology. Several examples serve to illustrate this point. A 65-year-old man had fevers and weight loss due to evolving *Pneumocystis* pneumonia rather than to suspected pancreatic carcinoma for which multiple studies had been performed over a 6-month period. The critical historic point was that blood transfusions had been administered during coronary artery bypass surgery 3 years earlier. Similarly, dyspnea and pulmonary infiltrates in a 20-year-old woman were due to *Pneumocystis* pneumonia and not to asthma as was suspected. History obtained from her husband indicated that he had a past history of intravenous drug use in New York. Along the same lines, a detailed history revealed that a 6-month-old infant with oral thrush and lymphadenopathy had been born prematurely and had received four blood transfusions in the neonatal intensive care unit (ICU). Thus, occult risk factors including drug use, transfusion, and homosexual activity must be sought in a thorough yet sensitive way by the physician. The risk factor may be distant, as in the case of the women who have had a bisexual or drug-using sexual partner years earlier.

7.2. Homosexual and Bisexual Males

The differential diagnosis of AIDS and ARC in the known homosexual or bisexual patient is complicated by several issues. Foremost is the high background incidence of infection caused by sexually transmitted pathogens. Numerous signs and symptoms of common sexually transmitted infections also occur in AIDS and ARC. For example, the symptom complex of diarrhea and fever may occur with enteric bacterial infection or herpes simplex proctitis[10] in nonimmunocompromised hosts as well as in patients with AIDS. Similarly, in young adults the symptom complex of fever and lymphadenopathy is a feature of both CMV mononucleosis and ARC. Thus, a broad differential diagnosis including common illnesses as well as AIDS and ARC should be considered in homosexual patients with fever, sweats, diarrhea, lymphadenopathy, new skin lesions, or other complaints. Laboratory studies to search for common syndromes and pathogens should not be overlooked.

The high frequency of HIV exposure among urban homosexuals, an additional complicating factor, ranges from 25% to 60%, depending on the city and sample selection.[90] The presence of antibody to

HIV does not establish that an illness is AIDS related. As with any laboratory test, the result should be interpreted in the context of the history, physical examination, and other laboratory findings. Evolving AIDS or ARC must be considered in the HIV-seropositive patient, especially when alternative explanations are not apparent. Most patients with ARC have serum antibody to HIV, and other etiologies of lymphadenopathy are more likely in seronegative patients. Inasmuch as antibody to HIV may not be detected in patients with late-stage AIDS, the absence of antibody does not exclude the diagnosis in patients who are eveluted late in their disease course.

Clinical manifestations of other illnesses may be modified when they occur in patients with ARC or asymptomatic HIV infection.[58] For example, uncomplicated Herpes zoster may be an indicator of underlying ARC or immunologic abnormality related to HIV. Severe Herpes zoster ophthalmicus has been reported in patients with ARC/PGL.[56] Speculation has centered on a possible relationship between refractory *Entamoeba histolytica* infections and underlying immune deficiency. Other stool pathogens generally considered commensals have been suspected causes of diarrheal illness. Preliminary cases suggest that HIV infection may predispose to unusual manifestations of syphilis, including ocular and CNS disease. In particular, conventional penicillin therapy of earlier stages of syphilis has not prevented progression to CNS disease in HIV-infected individuals. Thus, anyone with simultaneous evidence of syphilis and HIV infection merits both more intensive therapy (including treatment regimens usually reserved for neurosyphilis) and closer clinical follow-up.[90a,b,c] Oral thrush in homosexual patients receiving antibiotics appears in some cases to suggest underlying immune deficiency. In such patients, measurement of absolute numbers of T-lymphocyte populations tions may provide useful clinical information.

7.3. Women

To date the majority (54%) of women with AIDS in the United States have used intravenous drugs, and 11% have a history of sexual contact with a male who had AIDS or who was in a group at risk for AIDS. As HIV infection extends further into the female population, cases associated with this risk factor are expected to increase. Sexual contacts of females include bisexual males, intravenous drug users, Haitians, and hemophiliacs. Blood product transfusion has been implicated in 9% of cases occurring among women, but in 25% of women no known risk factor could be identified. In recent studies in Haiti, antibody to HIV was found in 55% of asymptomatic female sexual partners of patients with AIDS. In Central African countries, heterosexual promiscuity and prostitution appear to be significant risk factors for both AIDS and HIV seropositivity among women.

7.4. Intravenous Drug Users

AIDS and ARC are common among users of intravenous drugs and appear to be increasing among sexual contacts and children of drug users.[91,92] The major predisposing factor for AIDS among intravenous drug users is assumed to be shared needles and subsequent blood-borne transmission. It is widely believed that regional aspects of drug subcultures, such as storefront "shooting galleries" in New York, contribute to increased prevalence of HIV seropositivity and AIDS in drug users.

Together with bacterial endocarditis, abscesses, and other infectious processes, AIDS must be considered in the differential diagnosis of fever in drug users. Indeed, fevers, sweats, and weight loss are features of both AIDS and bacterial endocarditis. Thus, the evaluation requires cardiac valvular studies and blood cultures as well as studies directed toward the diagnosis of evolving *Pneumocystis pneumonia*. *Pneumocystis* infection presenting as a butterfly pattern infiltrate on chest radiographs must be considered in the differential diagnosis of heroin-associated pulmonary edema.

Lymphadenopathy per se has been described in intravenous drug users, and it may bear a clinical resemblance to persistent generalized lymphadenopathy associated with HIV infection. Lymph node biopsy, HIV serologic studies, and quantitative T-cell subset determinations are often useful in discriminating among these diagnostic possibilities.

7.5. Blood Product and Organ Transplant Recipients

AIDS and HIV infection must be included in the differential diagnosis of febrile illnesses in blood product recipients, hemophiliacs, and organ transplant recipients. More than 500 cases of AIDS have been attributed to administration of blood or clotting factor concentrate. Opportunistic infections were the presenting manifestation in the large majority. Exposure to multiple units appeared to increase the risk of AIDS.[28] Eighteen transfusion cases studied by the CDC had received blood from a mean of 15.9 different donors. In blood transfusion recipients, AIDS occurred at a median 24 months after transfusion with a range of 3 months to 8 years.[28] Coronary bypass surgery was the most common surgical procedure associated with this complication. The highest incidence of transfusion-related AIDS has been in the major geographic foci of the epidemic: 60% of transfusion cases were reported from New York, California, New Jersey, and Florida, areas accounting for 83% of the first 1000 AIDS cases.

Illustrative Case 2

A 47-year-old woman presented with a 4-day history of fever, nonproductive cough, and increasing shortness of breath. The patient had been well until 2 years previously, when she suffered an upper GI hemorrhage requiring the transfusion of 12 units of blood. Subsequent evaluation revealed a bleeding duodenal ulcer, ultimately requiring surgical treatment with a pyeloroplasty and vagotomy. Recovery was uncomplicated, and she had remained well until 4 days prior to admission, when increasing respiratory distress was noted. Other members of her family were in good health, and there had been no significant travel history.

Physical examination revealed an acutely dyspneic middle-aged woman with a respiratory rate of 34 breaths/min, an oral temperature of 101.6°F, and a blood pressure of 140/90. The rest of the examination was entirely within normal limits, with the exception of a well-healed abdominal scar.

Laboratory studies included Hct 37, WBC 3800/mm³, with 86% polys, 8% monocytes, 4% lymphocytes, and 2% eosinophils. Chest radiographs revealed a bilateral lower lobe interstitial pneumonitis. Room air ABGs were determined to be Pao₂ 47 mm Hg, Paco₂, 38 mm Hg, and pH 7.48. Fiberoptic bronchoscopy with bronchoalveolar lavage yielded *Pneumocystis carinii*.

Comments. Prior to the occurrence of the AIDS epidemic, previously healthy individuals presenting with acute respiratory failure and a chest radiographic picture of interstitial pneumonia were usually thought to be infected with such infectious agents as influenza, adenovirus, or *Mycoplasma pneumoniae*. This case of transfusion-associated AIDS presenting as acute *P. carinii* pneumonia emphasizes the importance of a complete medical history in leading the clinician to the correct diagnostic procedure, diagnosis, and therapy. Notable in the patient's presentation is the absence of any physical findings except for an increased respiratory rate. This is typical of patients with *Pneumocystis* pneumonia.

It is essential to obtain a complete transfusion history in patients revealing symptoms and signs consistent with HIV-related disease. The introduction in early 1985 of HIV antibody screening of blood products will decrease future cases of AIDS related to transfusion and clotting factors; nevertheless, this measure will not eliminate transfusion as a risk factor. Additional cases are expected to follow from blood transfused during the period 1981–1985, i.e., before routine screening was instituted.

AIDS has also been reported as a complication of renal and bone marrow transplantation.[93,94] This has led to recommendations that all potential organ and tissue donors be screened for evidence of HIV infection.[93] Clearly, AIDS must be considered in the differential diagnosis of fevers and infections in immunocompromised hosts who have received blood products or who have some other recognized risk factor for exposure to HIV.[95]

7.6. Pediatric Age Group

Diagnosis of AIDS in children is complicated by the background congenital disorders of cell-mediated immunity. In addition to the typical infections that occur in adults with AIDS, children have a markedly increased incidence of bacterial infection, resulting from impaired specific antibody responses secondary to the defect in T-helper lymphocytes. Infants with AIDS are usually small for gestational age (SGA). During the first 6 months of life, they fail to thrive and tend to develop chronic diarrhea, lymphadenopathy, hepatosplenomegaly, and recurrent or chronic infections,[92,96,97] including mucocutaneous candidiasis, *Pneumocystis* pneumonia, and *Salmonella* septicemias, as well as a lymphoid interstitial pneumonitis.[98] In contrast to most congenital immune deficiencies, children with AIDS have elevated quantitative immunoglobulin levels.

A detailed history from the parents is essential in the medical evaluation of the child with suspected AIDS or ARC; virtually all have an association with intravenous drug abuse, prostitution, or promiscuity. In most cases, the risk factor was associated with the mother; however, there are instances in which the father was either bisexual or an intravenous drug user. Moreover, in several cases the parents were apparently healthy Haitians. It is believed that premature infants are particularly susceptible to transfusion-related HIV infection. Premature infants are known to be susceptible to severe post-transfusion hepatitis and CMV syndromes.

8. Therapy

8.1. General Approach

The many unknowns and the poor prognosis associated with AIDS often lead to considerable anger and frustration in patients as well as family members. Care of such medically and emotionally complex patients is obviously a challenge for the physician. In our experience, the most satisfactory outcomes have occurred when care has been coordinated by one physician working closely with consultants. The ongoing participation of a generalist in the patient's care provides coordination that becomes increasingly important as the disease advances and as major decisions on life-prolonging measures are considered. Involvement of one coordinating physician also favors a holistic, comprehensive approach to the needs of the patient. Subspecialties in infectious diseases, oncology, and other disciplines can be involved in the context of specific clinical developments.

At the time of diagnosis, the patient experiences profound emotional distress, similar in intensity to that experienced by patients with incurable forms of cancer. Aware of the stigmas associated with the disease, the patient frequently has profound feelings of guilt about responsibility for the illness. The physician should attend to these needs and engage additional psychiatric or psychological consultants to help the patient deal with this disabling, life-threatening illness. Early social services consultation is to be encouraged.

8.2. Management of Infection

As a general rule, opportunistic infections in AIDS patients require longer courses and in some cases indefinite use of antimicrobial agents. For *Pneumocystis* pneumonia, 14–21 days of therapy is recommended when AIDS is the underlying condition compared with the standard 14-day regimen in other patients.[77] Relapse is frequent in those not placed on long-term anti-*Pneumocystis* prophylaxis.[81] Toxoplasmosis of the CNS in AIDS pa-

tients consistently relapses if pyrimethamine and sulfamethoxazole therapy are discontinued.[98,99] Indefinite therapy with multiple-agent regimens usually fails to eradicate disseminated infection with *Mycobacterium avium* complex. Severe ulcerative perioral and perianal herpes simplex infection usually heals after therapy with intravenous acyclovir; however, relapses occur unless the patient is chronically maintained on oral acyclovir.[57] Similarly, preliminary studies with the acyclovir analogue 9-(1,3-dihydroxy-2-propoxymethyl)guanine (DHPG or gancyclovir) indicate its efficacy in stabilizing lesions of CMV retinitis, although recrudescence tends to occur when the drug is stopped.[100] Intravenous immunoglobulin may be useful in infants and in children with AIDS or ARC and in those with frequent or recurrent infection.

8.3. Presentation and Management of Common Opportunistic Infections

For a summary of this subject see Table 8.

8.3.1. *Pneumocystis carinii* Pneumonia

Pneumocystis pneumonia has been the presenting opportunistic infection in 51% of all AIDS cases in the United States. Most of these patients have presented with fever, nonproductive cough, and dyspnea. Antecedent weight loss and thrush are common. Chest radiographic findings range from entirely normal to diffuse interstitial and alveolar infiltrates, frequently with a perihilar distribution. Additional findings that may be useful in increasing the diagnostic index of suspicion are arterial hypoxemia[79] and uptake over the lungs on gallium scan.[75,80] Flexible bronchoscopy with bronchoalveolar lavage is a sensitive method for establishing the diagnosis.[76] *Pneumocystis* can occasionally be found in the expectorated sputum of heavily infected patients. Rarely, repeat bronchoscopy with lavage and transbronchial biopsy or open-lung biopsy is required for diagnosis.

When *Pneumocystis* infection is strongly suspected, prompt pulmonary consultation and bronchoscopy should be obtained; there is no reason to delay antibiotics if AIDS and *Pneumocystis* are suspected. Cysts typically persist in bronchoalveolar lavage washings for as long as 3 weeks after suc-

TABLE 8. Most Common Etiologic Agents of Infections in AIDS Patients

Microorganism	Common locations	Clinical manifestations
Protozoa		
Pneumocystis carinii	Lungs	Pneumonia
Cryptosporidium	Intestine	Diarrhea, cholecystitis
Toxoplasma gondii	Brain	Encephalitis
Entamoeba histolytica	Intestine	Enterocolitis
Giardia lamblia	Intestine	Diarrhea
Fungi		
Candida species	Oropharynx, esophagus	Thrush, esophagus
Cryptococcus neoformans	Brain, lung, lymph nodes, bone marrow, blood, urine	Meningitis, pneumonia
Mycobacteria		
Mycobacterium avium-intracellulare	Lymph nodes, bone marrow, liver, spleen, blood, urine, lungs, skin	Lymphadenitis, hepatosplenomegaly, pancytopenia, pneumonia
Viruses		
Cytomegalovirus	Lungs, adrenals, eyes, brain, intestine, blood, liver, seminal vesicles	Pneumonia, retinitis, encephalitis, hepatitis, esophagitis, enterocolitis, adrenal insufficiency
Epstein-Barr virus	Blood	EBV-positive Burkitt lymphoma
Herpes simplex virus	Mucocutaneous	Ulcerative mucocutaneous lesions
Herpes zoster	Cutaneous	Shingles (dermatomal zoster)
Poxvirus	Mucocutaneous	Molluscum contagiosum
Polymavirus	Brain	Progressive multifocal leukoencephalopathy

cessful treatment.[101] Thus, in cases in which bronchoscopy cannot be promptly obtained, empiric therapy can be instituted and bronchoscopy performed 24–48 hr later if the patient's condition permits.

High-dose intravenous trimethoprim–sulfamethoxazole for 14–21 days is recommended as initial therapy for proven *Pneumocystis*, except for patients with a history of hypersensitivity to sulfonamides. In such patients, therapy with pentamidine isethiocyanate (4 mg/kg per day) by the intramuscular route or slow intravenous infusion is recommended.

The dose of trimethoprim–sulfamethoxazole established in studies of other immunocompromised hosts is calculated according to the trimethoprim component at 15–20 mg trimethoprim per kg body weight per day in three divided doses.[102–104] A 70-kg patient given 20 mg/kg per day will receive 1400 mg trimethoprim or approximately 18 ampules per day (80 mg trimethoprim per ampule). Anecdotal information suggests that concurrent administration of folinic acid (leucovorin) may decrease TMP-SMZ-associated myelosuppression, but this is unproven. Leucovorin may be administered intravenously (3 mg/day) or by tablet (5 mg).

Trimethoprim–sulfamethoxazole therapy of *Pneumocystis* infection in AIDS has an 80% overall response rate.[77] Approximately 20% of patients treated initially with this agent have continued fever and deterioration of gas exchange. In such patients, therapy is often changed to pentamidine between day 4–7 of therapy, depending on clinical circumstances. In these cases, a complete 14–21-day course of pentamidine is recommended. Clinical and animal experience with *Pneumocystis* infection does not support the concurrent use of trimethoprim–sulfamethoxazole and pentamidine.

Numerous investigators have pointed to the high incidence of adverse reactions to sulfonamides in AIDS patients. These include myelosuppression, cutaneous eruptions, and drug fevers—frequently necessitating discontinuation of sulfonamide therapy[83,97,110] and a crossover to pentamidine. Leukopenia in the range of 1500–2000/mm^3 frequently occurs in AIDS patients receiving trimethoprim–sulfamethoxazole. In my experience, the course can usually be completed without sequelae of long-term marrow suppression or infection due to neutropenia.

AIDS patients with *Pneumocystis* infection requiring intubation and mechanical ventilation have an overall poor prognosis.[77] In a series from six U.S. medical centers, only 12 of 101 patients requiring controlled ventilation survived to hospital discharge. Despite this discouraging experience to date, intubation is a reasonable approach, particularly during the first few days of therapy in a patient with newly diagnosed AIDS. The criteria for intubation are similar to those employed for other causes of respiratory failure. Worsening of gas exchange with declining arterial oxygen tension below 50 mm Hg or extreme tachypnea with fatigue are indications for controlled ventilation. Anecdotal experience suggests that in some patients gas exchange may worsen acutely following bronchoscopy with alveolar lavage. In such instances, close observation is warranted in order to decide on possible intubation.

The need for long-term prophylaxis in AIDS patients after recovery from *Pneumocystis* infection remains controversial. A high recurrence rate has been documented in several series of AIDS patients with *P. carinii* pneumonia.[81] The rate of relapse was 33–50% in those followed at the UCLA Medical Center before the routine use of long-term prophylaxis. Prior to AIDS, long-term prophylaxis had been recommended for immunocompromised patients when the probability of recurrent *Pneumocystis* was higher than 10% (see Chapter 10).

In patients without a history of sulfonamide hypersensitivity, long-term prophylaxis is instituted immediately after adequate therapy for the first episode, using either oral trimethoprim–sulfamethoxazole at a dose of one double-strength tablet twice daily or pyrimethamine–sulfadoxine (Fansidar) administered as one tablet weekly. The sulfonamide component in Fansidar has a half-life of approximately 160 hr. The use of trimethoprim–sulfamethoxazole prophylaxis is based on studies in pediatric leukemia; the use of Fansidar is based on growing experience in AIDS.[81] Not a single case of well-documented relapse has occurred when continu-

ing prophylaxis with trimethoprim–sulfamethoxazole has been administered in AIDS patients who have *Pneumocystis* infection. Chronic trimethoprim–sulfamethoxazole therapy has been accompanied by GI intolerance, skin rashes, and leukopenia. While controlled studies have not yet been done, Fansidar prophylaxis appears to be rarely associated with recrudescence of *P. carinii*. The CDC has received reports of Stevens-Johnson-like syndrome in AIDS patients with previous sulfonamide hypersensitivity given Fansidar for *Pneumocystis* prophylaxis.[105] We have found that Fansidar could be given without adverse reaction to patients who had previous cutaneous reactions to high-dose trimethoprim–sulfamethoxazole. Nevertheless, it is best to be cautious in view of the high incidence of adverse reactions to sulfonamide in AIDS patients and wait 2–3 weeks after the last administration of trimethoprim–sulfamethoxazole.

Because of the side effects of each of these therapeutic regimens in the treatment and prophylaxis of *Pneumocystis* infection in AIDS patients, other alternatives are being sought. At present, the most promising appears to be the aerosolized administration of pentamidine, which controls the infection but without significant toxicity because of low blood levels.[105a]

8.3.2. Oral and Esophageal Candidiasis

Candida infections of the mouth and esophagus are common in AIDS patients. Deep organ involvement or fungemia has been rare, usually occurring as a complication of indwelling central catheters. Oral candidiasis involving the tongue can generally be distinguished on clinical grounds from a characteristic lingual lesion described as hairy leukoplakia.[69] The latter typically persists despite topical or systemic antifungal therapy, a useful point in differential diagnosis. Minor degrees of oral thrush can be managed effectively with nystatin oral suspension or clotrimazole troches. Patients whose chronic candidiasis is limited to the oropharynx usually respond to ketoconazole at a dose of 200–400 mg/day.

Candida esophagitis may be present in the absence of thrush, and vice versa. Florid cases are apparent on barium swallow; however, with milder degrees of involvement, endoscopy is usually required. Herpes simplex and CMV are less common causes of esophagitis in AIDS patients. In addition, esophageal and gastric Kaposi sarcoma occur often in patients with cutaneous disease; thus, cultures and histology of endoscopic biopsy specimens are important. Some AIDS patients with odynophagia are found to have extensive nonhealing esophageal ulcers for which an infectious or neoplastic etiology is not apparent despite extensive biopsies. Severe *Candida* esophagitis usually requires treatment with amphotericin-B, 0.3–0.5 mg/kg per day. Ketoconazole alone may be effective in milder cases at a dose of 200 mg two or three times daily.

8.3.3. *Mycobacterium avium* Complex Infection

Disseminated *Mycobacterium avium* complex infection is remarkably characteristic in AIDS and contributes to the overall high mortality from infection.[83,106] Systemic infection typically presents with fevers, weight loss, and wasting and is associated with high-grade bacteremia and bone marrow involvement. The diagnosis is generally established from blood or bone marrow cultures.

These organisms are usually resistant to conventional antituberculous drug combinations, and microbiologic cure has not been demonstrated. While drug treatment for disseminated infection probably should be offered, it must be recognized that current regimens have a poor response rate and a high incidence of adverse drug reactions. It is not clear whether therapy is required in AIDS patients in whom atypical mycobacteria are isolated from pulmonary secretions in the absence of symptoms and chest radiographic findings. At the very least, this finding indicates a need for ongoing close surveillance for disseminated infection.

Clofazimine, an agent used in leprosy, and ansamycin, a derivative of rifampin, have good in vitro activity against *M. avium* complex isolates; however, clinical studies have been less promising. No convincing data are available to indicate efficacy of any one regimen. Reasonable regimens are based on in vitro testing and may include rifampin, ethambutol, ansamcin, clofazimine, and amikacin.[84]

8.3.4. Tuberculosis

Mycobacterium tuberculosis causes pulmonary, extrapulmonary, and disseminated infection, primarily among AIDS patients from such areas as Haiti and South America, where this infection is more prevalent than in the United States.[107,108] Isolates have been sensitive to conventional antituberculous drugs, which are recommended according to standard treatment regimens.

8.3.5. Cryptosporidiosis

Organisms of the Coccidia group, *Cryptosporidium* and *Isospora belli,* have been common causes of profuse watery diarrhea in patients with AIDS.[11,110] The enteritis typically involves both small and large bowel. In the parasitology laboratory, cryptosporidium is diagnosed in stool specimens by acid-fast stains. No specific antimicrobial therapy has been definitively proved effective; however, the agent spiramycin has been reported to give symptomatic relief in some patients; in others, diarrhea has responded to opiates.[111]

8.3.6. Cytomegalovirus

Cytomegalovirus is an important pathogen in most AIDS patients. Retinitis, frequently bilateral, occurs late in the disease course and usually leads to blindness. Pneumonitis with impaired gas exchange is likely to be fatal. In addition, some data indicate that CMV infection concurrent with *Pneumocystis* pneumonia is associated with increased mortality. No curative therapy for disseminated CMV infection or retinitis has been devised. Preliminary studies in AIDS patients demonstrate that DHPG (gancyclovir) treatment may be effective in stabilizing retinal infection and in preventing blindness in some cases. When DHPG therapy is stopped, the disease typically recurs.

8.3.7. Cryptococcal Meningitis

The neurologic manifestations of AIDS are listed in Table 5. *Cryptococcus neoformans* is a common cause of meningitis and fungemia.[86,112] Meningitis may be the initial opportunistic infection, usually presenting with persistent headache, occasionally with associated photophobia and confusion. Fever and nuchal rigidity may be absent. Cranial neuropathies have been observed when the disease is advanced.

Computed tomographic scans are indicated to

exclude mass lesions such as toxoplasmosis, intra-cerebral lymphoma, and progressive multifocal leu-koencephalopathy. Lumbar puncture should be per-formed if the intracranial pressure (ICP) has not been increased. CSF analysis should include routine stud-ies, India ink preparation, cryptococcal antigen, and fungal culture.

The recommended regimen for cryptococcal in-fection includes amphotericin-B plus fluorocytosine (5-FC). Initial therapy consists of a 6-week course of amphotericin-B (0.3 mg/kg per day) and oral fluo-rocytosine (150 mg/kg per day in four oral divided doses).[113] It is important to follow carefully for renal functional impairment due to amphotericin and bone marrow depression secondary to fluorocytosine. Ad-ditional amphotericin to a total dose of 1.5–2.0 g has been recommended. Relapse of cryptococcal disease in AIDS patients frequently occurs, although in some cases cure has been achieved. Remission is marked by a fall in the cryptococcal antigen titer and rever-sion to a culture-negative status in CSF and blood. After therapy, it is advisable to obtain regular cultures and cryptococcal antigen from CSF and blood. In patients with cryptococcal antigen titers greater than 1 : 8, weekly or biweekly amphotericin suppression may be necessary.

8.3.8. Toxoplasmosis of the Central Nervous System

Central nervous system *Toxoplasma gondii* in-fection is manifested by confusion, headache, sei-zure, paresis, or sensory deficit. In some patients, retinopathy has been the major manifestation of this infection.[98,99,114] Ring-enhancing lesions on CT scan may be multiple, suggesting this diagnosis. The basal ganglia and frontal lobes are common sites of involvement; brain biopsy can therefore be useful for diagnosing infectious and neoplastic mass lesions in AIDS patients. In many instances, however, this pro-cedure has not resulted in definitive diagnosis of tox-oplasmosis. Empirical therapy is warranted in se-verely ill patients when CNS toxoplasmosis is suspected or in patients with lesions inaccessible to biopsy.

Illustrative Case 3

A 26-year-old female intravenous drug abuser presented with a 3-day history of increasing fever and confusion. The patient had been ill for the last 6 months with an illness characterized by intermittent fevers, weight loss, and diarrhea. Medical evaluation had revealed *Cryptosporidium* in her stool; she was HIV antibody positive by ELISA testing. Therapy with spiramycin had not al-tered her diarrhea or the presence of *Cryptosporidium* in her stool. She had been relatively stable until 4 days prior to admission, when her family found her in increasing confusion.

Physical examination revealed a thin white woman with a number of needle tracks on both arms. She was disoriented to time, place, and person. Her neck was supple, and there was no focal neurologic abnormalities.

Laboratory data included Hct 32, WBC 2600/mm³, with 90% polys, 4% lymphs, and 6% monocytes. Lumbar puncture revealed an opening pressure of 200 cm H₂O, 25 WBCs (90% lymphs, 10% monocytes), protein 58 mg/dl, and sugar 60 mg/dl. Cryptococcal antigen and cultures were negative. HIV was isolated from the CSF. The CT scan revealed bilateral ring-enhancing lesions in the frontal lobes. Stereotactic biopsy of one of these lesions yielded *Toxoplasma gondii*.

Comment. This AIDS patient presented with CNS infection due to two different pathogens: HIV and *Toxoplasma gondii* after a 6-month illness consistent with ARC. The range of CNS pathogens present in AIDS patients is very different from that seen in the normal host and includes CNS lymphoma as well as the microbial pathogens outlined in Table 5.

Standard therapy includes oral pyrimethamine, 75 mg the first day, followed by 25 mg/day and sulfadiazine, 4 g/day, in four divided doses orally or parenterally for a period of 4–6 weeks in non-compromised hosts. A short course of dex-amethasone may rapidly decrease cerebral edema. In AIDS patients, CNS toxoplasmosis typically recurs within weeks after therapy. It is therefore recom-mended that therapy be continued for at least several months and usually as tolerated for the lifetime of the patient.

8.3.9. Severe Ulcerative Herpes Simplex

Chronic oral or anal ulcers often progressing to form deep and extensive lesions are frequent findings in AIDS patients, particularly homosexual males.[3,10] Herpes proctitis has occurred in some. Intravenous acyclovir administered at a dose of 2.5 mg/kg every 8 hr for 7–10 days has been effective in managing these frequently painful lesions.[6] Recurrence is the rule, however, within weeks of discontinuing therapy. Our experience indicates that recurrence can be pre-vented by continuous therapy with oral acyclovir in divided doses of 600–2000 mg/day.

8.4. Immunotherapy and Antiretroviral Therapy

Effective therapy of the underlying immune deficiency in AIDS is a major objective of ongoing research. Before its retroviral etiology was identified, the first therapeutic trials in AIDS employed various biologic response modifiers with known immune-modulating effects and cellular replacement techniques.[115] These had little or no clinical efficacy and had minor effects on immune function. Treatment with α-interferon (IF$_\alpha$) produces tumor shrinkage in 20–30% of patients with Kaposi sarcoma, although this effect does not appear to be immunologically mediated.[116]

Characterization of the biology of HIV has permitted the development of improved rationales for therapy. The enzyme reverse transcriptase, which is unique to retroviruses and is absent in mammalian cells, represents a potential target for antiviral therapy. Several inhibitors of the reverse transcriptases of animal retroviruses (suramin, HPA-23, azidothymidine) appear to be active against HIV. Suramin, a compound used to treat African sleeping sickness and onchocerciasis, inhibits HIV infection of susceptible lymphocytes; however, clinical trials indicate no improvement in AIDS and ARC patients. Preliminary clinical trials of these agents in AIDS and ARC have been terminated due to drug toxicity. Adverse effects include cutaneous eruptions, fever, influenzalike symptoms, proteinuria, and rarely, anaphylactoid shock. HPA-23 (antimonial tungstate) therapy is associated with thrombocytopenia. Early case studies indicate that during treatment with these agents, the virus cannot be grown from lymphocytes; however, virus is again recovered when therapy is discontinued.[116a,b,c]

The first major advance in the chemotherapy of HV infection came in the fall of 1986 with the announcement of preliminary results of a placebo-controlled trial of azidothymidine (AZT).[117] Of more than 300 patients entered into the trial, mortality was significantly reduced, opportunistic infections were fewer, and improvement in T-helper lymphocyte concentrations were noted in AZT recipients. The results were apparent in patients with prior *Pneumocystis* infection, and the drug was made available in the United States to patients meeting this eligibility criterion. Obviously, further studies are needed, such as in patients with Kaposi sarcoma and ARC. AZT is not innocuous, with toxic effects to bone marrow exacerbating neutropenia and anemia. Recent success with human granulocyte-macrophage colony-stimulating factor in the treatment of leukopenia in patients with AIDS,[117a] suggests that the combination of this substance with AZT could be beneficial.

Enrollment of patients with advanced AIDS in clinical trials makes interpretation of efficacy and toxicity more complex. Those who have the AIDS-related complex or HIV infection with asymptomatic immunologic abnormality may have greater potential for benefit. Quantitative viral detection techniques and T-cell subpopulation studies will probably remain major outcome variables in these trials.

As effective antiviral agents are identified, certain immunomodulators studied early as single agents probably deserve reevaluation. Therapy for AIDS may require combining antiretroviral agents with immunomodulators such as IL-2 or IF$_\alpha$, administered either simultaneously or in sequence. For example, in vitro AZT and IF$_\alpha$ have been shown to be synergistic.[117b] It seems possible that effectively inhibiting HIV replication could improve or stabilize immune function, although the probable cellular integration of provirus in most HIV-seropositive individuals makes the long-term prognosis uncertain. Such patients will undoubtedly have a lifelong risk of adverse sequelae, including AIDS.

9. Hospital Infection Control and Protection of Health Workers

There is no convincing evidence for casual transmission of HIV infection.[118] The evidence for a blood-borne route of transmission raised legitimate concerns about the welfare of health care and laboratory personnel who are at increased risk for occupationally transmitted blood-borne infection, notably hepatitis B. Several case reports indicate the possible association of AIDS with occupational exposure.[119,120] However, preliminary studies among health workers participating in the care of AIDS patients and in processing of laboratory specimens reveal no major increased incidence of HIV antibody above the background for the general population. Nevertheless, continued diligence in following recommended asepsis techniques is indicated as very rare cases of apparent HIV transmission in the hospital and laboratory have been noted.

10. Appendix

The CDC has proposed the following classification system for HIV infection:[121]

Group I. Acute HIV Infection: This mononucleosis-like syndrome, with or without aseptic meningitis, is associated with seroconversion for HIV antibody.

Group II. Asymptomatic HIV Infection: This group shows the absence of any manifestations or history of HIV infection, except for a possible past history of a mononucleosis-like illness.

Group III. Persistent Generalized Lymphadenopathy: There is palpable lymphadenopathy (lymph node enlargement of >1 cm) at two or more extrainguinal sites persisting for greater than 3 months in the absence of a concurrent illness or condition other than HIV infection.

Group IV. Other HIV Disease:

Subgroup A. Constitutional Disease: One or more of the following: fever persisting more than 1 month, involuntary weight loss of greater than 10% of baseline, or diarrhea persisting more than one month with no explanation other than HIV infection

Subgroup B. Neurologic Disease: One or more of the following: dementia, myelopathy, or peripheral neuropathy occurring without explanation other than HIV infection

Subgroup C. Secondary Infectious Diseases: The occurrence of an infectious process associated with defects in cell mediated immunity without a non-HIV infection explanation for such a defect being present, further subdivided into two categories:

Category C-1: Includes patients with symptomatic or invasive disease due to one or more of the 12 specified secondary infectious diseases listed in the CDC surveillance definition of AIDS: *Pneumocystis carinii* pneumonia, chronic cryptosporidiosis, toxoplasmosis, extraintestinal strongyloidiasis, isosporiasis, candidiasis (esophageal, bronchial, or pulmonary), cryptococcosis, histoplasmosis, mycobacterial infection with *M. avium* complex or *M. kansasii,* CMV infection, chronic mucocutaneous or disseminated HSV infection, and progressive multifocal leukoencephalopathy

Category C-2: Includes patients with symptomatic or invasive disease due to one of six other specified secondary infectious diseases: oral hairy leukoplakia, multidermatomal herpes zoster, recurrent *Salmonella* bacteremia, nocardiosis, tuberculosis, or oral candidiasis (thrush)

Subgroup D. Secondary Cancers: The diagnosis of one or more of the types of cancers associated with HIV infection and included as part of the surveillance definition of AIDS: Kaposi sarcoma, non-Hodgkin lymphoma (small noncleaved lymphoma or immunoblastic sarcoma), or primary lymphoma of the brain

Subgroup E. Other Conditions in HIV Infection: The presence of other clinical findings or diseases, such as chronic lymphoid interstitial pneumonitis, not classifiable above, that may be attributed to HIV infection or that may be indicative of a defect in cell-mediated immunity (also included are those patients whose signs or symptoms could be attributed either to HIV infection or to another coexisting disease not classified elsewhere as well as patients with other clinical illnesses for which the course or management may be complicated or altered by HIV infection)

ACKNOWLEDGMENT. This chapter was supported in part by grant AI20672 from the National Institute of Allergy and Infectious Diseases, and by a grant to the UCLA AIDS Center from the University of California Task Force on AIDS.

References

1. Gottlieb MS, Schroff R, Schanker HM, et al: *Pneumocystis carinii* pneumonia and mucosal candidiasis in previously healthy homosexual men: Evidence for a new severe acquired cellular immunodeficiency syndrome. *N Engl J Med* **305**:1425–1431, 1981.
2. Masur H, Michelis MA, Greene JB, et al: An outbreak of community acquired *Pneumocystis carinii* pneumonia: Initial manifestation of cellular immune dysfunction. *N Engl J Med* **305**:1431–1438, 1981.
3. Siegal FP, Lopez C, Hammer GS, et al: Severe acquired immunodeficiency in male homosexuals, manifested by chronic perianal ulcerative herpes simplex lesions. *N Engl J Med* **305**:1439–1444, 1981.
4. Fauci AS, Macher AM, Longo DL, et al: Acquired immunodeficiency syndrome: Epidemiologic, clinical, immu-

nologic, and therapeutic considerations. *Ann Intern Med* **100:**92–106, 1984.

5. Simberkoff MS, El Sadr W, Schiffman G, et al: Streptococcus pneumoniae infections and bacteremia in patients with acquired immune deficiency syndrome *Am Rev Respir Dis* **130:**1174–1176, 1984.

6. Balfour H Jr, Bean B, Laskin O, et al: Acyclovir halts progression of herpes zoster in immunocompromised patients. *N Engl J Med* **308:**1448–1453, 1983.

7. Barre-Sinoussi F, Chermann JC, Rey F, et al: Isolation of T-lymphotropic retrovirus from a patient at risk for acquired immune deficiency syndrome (AIDS). *Science* **220:**868–871, 1983.

8. Rogers MF, Morens DM, Stewart JA, et al: National case-control study of Kaposi's sarcoma and *Pneumocystis carinii* pneumonia in homosexual men. Part 2. Laboratory results. *Ann Intern Med* **99:**151–158, 1983.

9. Centers for Disease Control. Update on acquired immune deficiency syndrome (AIDS)—United States. *MMWR* **31:**507–514, 1982.

9a. WHO: Immunodeficiency. *WHO Technical Report Series* **630:**28–31, 1978.

10. Goddell SE, Quinn TC, Mkritichian E, et al: *Herpes simplex* virus proctitis in homosexual men. *N Engl J Med* **15:**868–871, 1983.

11. DeHovitz JA, Pape JW, Boncy M, et al: Clinical manifestations and therapy of *Isoopora belli* infection in patients with the acquired immunodeficiency syndrome. *N Engl J Med* **315:**87–89, 1986.

12. Gottlieb MS, Wolfe PR, Fahey JL, et al: The syndrome of persistent generalized lymphadenopathy: Experience of 101 patients. In Gupta S (ed): *AIDS-Associated Syndromes.* Plenum, New York, 1985, pp. 85–91.

13. Centers for Disease Control: Revision of the case definition of acquired immunodeficiency syndrome for national reports—United States. *MMWR* **34:**373–375, 1985.

14. Salahuddin SZ, Groopman JE, Markham PD, et al: HTLV-III in symptom-free seronegative persons. *Lancet* **2:**1418–1420, 1984.

15 Sarngadharan MG, Popovic M, Burch L, et al: Antibodies reactive with human T-lymphotropic retroviruses (HTLV-III) in the serum of patients with AIDS *Science* **224:**506–508, 1984.

16. Centers for Disease Control. Update on acquired immune deficiency syndrome (AIDS)—Europe. *MMWR* **34:**585–589, 1985.

17. Clumeck N, Mascart-Lemone F, de Maubeuge J, et al: Acquired immune deficiency syndrome in black Africans *Lancet* **1:**642, 1983.

18. Clumeck N, Sonnet J, Taelman H, et al: Acquired immunodeficiency syndrome in African patients. *N Engl J Med* **310:**492–497, 1984.

19. Van de Perre P, Robert-Guroff M, Clumeck N, et al. Seroepidemiological studies of HTLV-III antibody prevalence among selected groups of heterosexual Africans *International Congress for Infectious Diseases, Cairo, April 1985* (abst).

20. Pape JW, Liautaud B, Thomas F, et al: Characteristics of the acquired immunodeficiency syndrome (AIDS) in Haiti *N Engl J Med* **309:**945–950, 1983.

21. Pitchenik AE, Fischl MA, Dickinson GM, et al· Opportunistic infections and Kaposi's sarcoma among Haitians. Evidence of a new acquired immunodeficiency state. *Ann Intern Med* **98:**277–284, 1983

22. Broder S, Gallo RC: A pathogenic retrovirus (HTLV-III) linked to AIDS. *N Engl J Med* **311:**1292–1297, 1984.

23. Gallo RC, Salahuddin SZ, Popovic M, et al: Frequent detection and isolation of cytopathic retroviruses (HTLV-III) from patients with AIDS and at risk for AIDS. *Science* **224:**500–502, 1984

24. Schroff RW, Gottlieb MS, Prince H, et al. Immunological studies in homosexual men with immunodeficiency and Kaposi's sarcoma. *Clin Immunol Immunopathol* **27:**300–314, 1983.

25. Poiesz BJ, Ruscetti FW, Gazdar AF, et al: Detection and isolation of type C retrovirus particles from fresh and cultured lymphocytes of a patient's cutaneous T-cell lymma. *Proc Natl Acad Sci USA* **77:**7415–7419, 1980.

26. Wong-Staal F, Gallo RC: Human T lymphotropic retroviruses. *Nature (Lond)* **317:**395–403, 1985.

27. Kalyanaraman VS, Sangadharan MG, Robert-Guroff M, et al: A new subtype of human T-cell leukemia virus (HTLV-II) associated with a T-cell variant of hairy cell leukemia. *Science* **218:**517–573, 1982.

28. Curran JW, Lawrence DN, Jaffe H, et al: Acquired immunodeficiency syndrome (AIDS) associated with transfusions. *N Engl J Med* **310:**69–75, 1984.

29. Groopman JE, Mayer KH, Sarngadharan MG, et al: Seroepidemiology of human T-lymphotropic virus type III among homosexual men with the acquired immunodeficiency syndrome or generalized lymphadenopathy and among asymptomatic controls in Boston *Ann Intern Med* **102:**334–337, 1985.

30. Dalgleish AG, Bevereley PC, Clapham PR, et al: The CDC4 (T4) antigen as an essential component of the receptor for the AIDS retrovirus. *Nature (Lond)* **312:**763–767, 1984.

31. Klatzman D, Barre-Sinoussi F, Nugeyre MT, et al: Selective tropism of lymphadenopathy associated virus (LAV) for helper-inducer T lymphocytes. *Science* **225:**59–63, 1984.

32. Klatzmann D, Champagne E, Chameret S, et al: T-lymphocyte T4 molecule behaves as the receptor for human retrovirus LAV. *Nature (Lond)* **312:**763–767, 1984.

33. Lifson JD, Reyes GR, McGrath MS, et al: AIDS retrovirus induced cytopathology: Giant cell formation and involvement of CD4 antigen. *Science* **232:**1123–1127, 1986.

34. Zagury D, Bernard J, Leonard R, et al: Long-term cultures of HTLV-III-infected T cells: A model of cytopathology of T-cell depletion in AIDS. *Science* **231:**850–853, 1986

35. Gartner S, Markovits P, Markovitz DM, et al. The role of mononuclear phagocytes in HTLV-III/LAV infection. *Science* **233:**215–219, 1986.

36. Koenig S, Gendelman HE, Orentein JM, et al: Detection of AIDS virus in macrophages in brain tissue from AIDS patients with encephalopathy *Science* **233:**1089–1093, 1986.

37. Chayt KJ, Harper ME, Marselle LM, et al: Detection of HTLV-III RNA in lungs of patients with AIDS and pulmonary involvement *JAMA* **256:**2356–2359, 1986.

38. Stoler MH, Eskin TA, Benn S, et al. Human T-cell lympho-

tropic virus type III infection of the central nervous system: A preliminary in situ analysis. *JAMA* **256**:2360–2364, 1986

39. Gartner S, Markovits P, Markovitz DM, et al: Virus isolation from and identification of HTLV-III/LAV-producing cells in brain tissue from a patient with AIDS. *JAMA* **256**:2365–2370, 1986.

40. Streiden HZ, Joynt RJ: HTLV-III/LAV and the monocyte/macrophage. *JAMA* **256**:2390–2393, 1986.

41. Arya SK, Chan G, Josephs SJ, et al: Transactivator gene of human T-lymphotropic virus type III. *Science* **229**:69–73, 1985.

42. Sodroski JG, Rosen CA, Haseltine WA: Trans-acting transcriptional activation of the long terminal repeat of human T lymphotropic viruses in infected cell. *Science* **225**:381–385, 1984.

43. Sodroski J, Rosen C, Wong-Staal F, et al: Trans-acting transcriptional regulation of human T-cell leukemia virus type III long terminal repeat. *Science* **227**:171–173, 1985.

44. Gottlieb MS, Groopman JE, Weinstein WM, et al: The acquired immunodeficiency syndrome. *Ann Intern Med* **99**:208–220, 1983.

45. Jaffe HW, Choi K, Thomas PA, et al: National case-control study of Kaposi's sarcoma and *Pneumocystis carinii* pneumonia in homosexual men. Part 1. Epidemiological results. *Ann Intern Med* **99**:145–151, 1983.

46. Fauci AS: Immunologic abnormalities in the acquired immunodeficiency syndrome (AIDS). *Clin Res* **32**:491–499, 1984.

47. Lane HC, Masur H, Edgar LC, et al: Abnormalities of B lymphocyte activation and immunoregulation in patients with the acquired immunodeficiency syndrome. *N Engl J Med* **309**:453–458, 1983.

48. Schupbach J, Halelr O, Bost M, et al: Antibodies to HTLV-III in Swiss patients with AIDS and pre-AIDS and in groups at risk for AIDS. *N Engl J Med* **312**:265–270, 1985.

49. Heagy W, Kelley VE, Strom TB, et al: Decreased expression of human class II antigens on monocytes from patients with acquired immune deficiency syndrome. Increased expression with interferon gamma. *J Clin Invest* **74**:2089–2096, 1984.

50. Taylor J, Afrasiabi R, Fahey JL: A prognostically significant classification of immune changes in AIDS with Kaposi's sarcoma. *Blood* **67**:666–71, 1986.

51. Gottlieb MS, Wolfe PR, Fahey JL, et al: The syndrome of persistent generalized lymphadenopathy: Experience with 101 patients. In *International Conference on the AIDS-Related Complex*. Wiley, New York, 1986.

52. Mathur-Wagh U, Enlow RW, Spigland I, et al: Longitudinal study of persistent generalized lymphadenopathy in homosexual men: Relation to the acquired immune deficiency syndrome. *Lancet* **1**:1033–1038, 1984.

53. Metroka CE, Cunningham-Rundles S, Pollack MS, et al: Generalized lymphadenopathy in homosexual men. *Ann Intern Med* **99**:585–591, 1983.

54. Domingo J, Chin NW: Lymphadenopathy in a heterogeneous population at risk for the acquired immunodeficiency syndrome (AIDS): A morphologic study. *Am J Clin Pathol* **5**:649–654, 1983.

55. Levine AM, Meyer PR, Begandy MK, et al. Development of B-cell lymphoma in homosexual men. *Ann Intern Med* **100**:7–13, 1984.

56. Cole EL, Meisler DM, Calabrese LH, et al: Herpes zoster ophthalmicus and acquired immune deficiency syndrome. *Arch Ophthalmol* **102**:1027–1029, 1984.

57. Glasser JB, Seligman SJ: Acyclovir for immunocompromised patients with herpes zoster. *N Engl J Med* **20**:1254, 1983.

58. Rowland-Payne CM, Farthing C, Byrom N, et al: Shingles in seven homosexuals. *Lancet* **1**:103–104, 1984.

59. Fahey JL, Detels R, Gottlieb MS: An immune cell augmentation (with altered T subset ratio) that is common in healthy homosexual males. *N Engl J Med* **308**:842–843, 1983

60. Smith PD, Ohura K, Masur H, et al: Monocyte function in the acquired immune deficiency syndrome. Defective chemotaxis. *J Clin Invest* **74**:2121–2128, 1984.

61. Fahey JL, Prince H, Weaver M, et al: Quantitative changes in Th or Ts lymphocyte subsets that distinguish AIDS syndromes from other immune subset disorder *Am J Med* **76**:95–100, 1984.

62. Jaffe HW, Feorino PM, Darrow WW, et al. Persistent infection with human T-lymphotropic virus type III/lymphadenopathy-associated virus in apparently healthy homosexual men. *Ann Intern Med* **102**:627–633, 1985.

63. Abrams DI, Lewis BJ, Beckstead JH, et al: Persistent diffuse lymphadenopathy in homosexual men: Endpoint or prodrome? *Ann Intern Med* **100**:801–808, 1984.

64. Wachter RM: The impact of the acquired immunodeficiency syndrome on medical residency training. *N Engl J Med* **314**:177–180, 1983.

65. Holland GS, Gottlieb MS, Yee RD, et al: Ocular disorders associated with a new severe acquired cellular immunodeficiency syndrome. *Am J Ophthalmology* **93**:393–402, 1982.

66. Holland GN, Pepose JS, Pettit TH, et al. Acquired immune deficiency syndrome: Ocular manifestations. *Ophthalmology* **8**:859–873, 1983.

67. Holland G, Gottlieb MS, Foos RL: Retinal cottonwool patches in patients with acquired immunodeficiency syndrome. (Letter.) *N Engl J Med* **307**:1704–1705, 1982.

68. Holland GS, Pepose JS, Pettit TH, et al: Acquired immune deficiency syndrome: Ocular manifestations. *Ophthalmology* **90**:859–873, 1983.

69. Greenspan D, Greenspan J, Connant M, et al: Oral hairy leukoplakia in male homosexuals: Evidence of association with both papillomavirus and herpes group viruses. *Lancet* **2**:831–834, 1984.

70. Jaffe HW, Bregman DJ, Selik RM: Acquired immune deficiency syndrome in the United States. The first 1,000 cases. *J Infect Dis* **2**:339–345, 1983.

71. Macher AM, Reichart CM, Straus SE, et al: Death in the AIDS patient: Role of cytomegalovirus. *N Engl J Med* **3**:1454, 1983.

72. Steinberg JJ, Bridges N, Feiner HD, et al: Small intestinal lymphoma in three patients with acquired immune deficiency syndrome. *Am J Gastroenterol* **80**:21–26, 1985.

73. Zeigler JL, Beckstead JA, Volberding PA, et al: Non-Hodgkin's lymphoma in 90 homosexual men: Relation to generalized lymphadenopathy and the acquired immunodeficiency syndrome. *N Engl J Med* **311**:565–570, 1984.

74. Blumfeld W, Wagar E, Hadley WK: Use of the trans-

bronchial biopsy for diagnosis of opportunistic pulmonary infections in acquired immunodeficiency syndrome (AIDS). *Am J Clin Pathol* **81**:1–4, 1984.

75. Coleman DL, Hattner RS, Luce JM: Correlation between gallium lung scans and fiberoptic bronchoscopy in patients with suspected *Pneumocystis carinii* pneumonia and the acquired immune deficiency syndrome. *Am Rev Respir Dis* **130**:1166–1170, 1984.

76. Coleman DL, Dodek PM, Luce JM, et al: Diagnostic utility of fiberoptic bronchoscopy in patients with *Pneumocystis carinii* pneumonia and the acquired immunodeficiency syndrome *Am Rev Repir Dis* **128**:795–799, 1983.

77. Murray JF, Felton CP, Garay S, et al: Pulmonary complications of a national heart, lung, and blood institute workshop. *N Engl J Med* **310**:1682–1688, 1984.

78. Ognibene FP, Shelhamer J, Gill V, et al: The diagnosis of *Pneumocystis carinii* pneumonia in patients with the acquired immunodeficiency syndrome using subsegmental bronchoalveolar lavage. *Am Rev Respir Dis* **129**:929–932, 1984.

79. Stover DE, White DA, Romano PA: Spectrum of pulmonary diseases associated with the acquired immune deficiency syndrome. *Am J Med* **78**:429–437, 1985.

80. Barron TF, Birnbaum NS, Shane LB, et al. *Pneumocystis carinii* pneumonia studied by gallium-67 scanning. *Radiology* **154**:791–793, 1985.

81. Gottlieb MS, Knight S, Mitsuyasu R, et al: Prophylaxis of *Pneumocystis carinii* pneumonia in AIDS with pyrimethamine-sulfadoxine (Fansidar). *Lancet* **2**:398–399, 1984.

82. Cohen RJ, Samoszuk MK, Busch D, et al: Occult infections with *M. avium intracellulare* in bone marrow biopsy specimens with AIDS. *N Engl J Med* **308**:1475–1476, 1983.

83. Elliot JL, Hoppes WL, Platt MS: The acquired immunodeficiency syndrome and *Mycobacterium avium intracellulare* bacteremia in a patient with hemophilia. *Ann Intern Med* **98**:290–293, 1983.

83a. Zakowski P, Fligiel S, Berlin GW, et al: Disseminated *Mycobacterium avium-intracellulare* infection in homosexual men dying of acquired immunodeficiency. *JAMA* **259**:2980–2982, 1982.

84. Young LS, Inderlied CB, Berlin OG, et al: Mycobacterial infections in AIDS patients, with an emphasis on the *Mycobacterium avium* complex. *Rev Infect Dis* **8**:1024–1033, 1986.

85. Guttman D, Raymond A, Gelb A, et al: Virus-associated colitis in homosexual men: Two case reports. *Am J Gastroenterol* **3**:167–169, 1983.

86. Levy RM, Bredesen DE, Rosenblum ML: Neurological manifestations of the acquired immunodeficiency syndrome (AIDS): Experience at UCSF and review of the literature. *J Neurosurg* **62**:475–495, 1985.

87. Jacobs JL, Gold JW, Murray HW, et al: Salmonella infections in patients with the acquired immune deficiency syndrome. *Ann Intern Med* **102**:186–188, 1985.

88. Read EJ, Orenstein JM, Chorba TL, et al: *Listeria monocytogenes* sepsis and small cell carcinoma of the rectum: An unusual presentation of the acquired immunodeficiency syndrome. *Am J Clin Pathol.* **3**:385–389, 1985.

89. Jaffe HS, Abrams DJ, Ammann AJ, et al: Complications of co-trimoxazole in treatment of AIDS-associated *Pneumocystis carinii* pneumonia in homosexual men. *Lancet* **2**:1109–1111, 1983.

90. Centers for Disease Control: Update on acquired immune deficiency syndrome in the San Francisco Cohort Study, 1978–1985. *MMWR* **34**:573–575, 1985.

90a. Johns DR, Tierney M, Felsenstein D: Alteration in the natural history of neurosyphilis by concurrent infection with the human immunodeficiency virus. *N Engl J Med* **316**:1569–1572, 1987.

90b. Berry CD, Hooton TM, Collier AC, Lukehart SA: Neurologic relapse after benzathine penicillin therapy for secondary syphilis in a patient with HIV infection. *N Engl J Med* **316**:1587–1589, 1987.

90c. Tramont EC: Syphilis in the AIDS era. *N Engl J Med* **316**:1600–1601, 1987.

91. Harris C, Small CB, Klein RS, et al: Immunodeficiency in female sexual partners of men with the acquired immunodeficiency syndrome. *N Engl J Med* **308**:1181–1184, 1983.

92. Oleske J, Minnefore A, Cooper R, et al: Immune deficiency syndrome in children. *JAMA* **249**:2345–2349, 1983.

93. Hasset JM, Zoroulis CG, Greenberg ML, et al: Bone marrow transplantation in AIDS. (Letter.) *N Engl J Med* **309**:665, 1983.

94. L'Age-Stehr J, Schwarz A, Offermann G, et al: HTLV-III infection in kidney transplant recipients. *Lancet* **2**:1361–1363, 1985.

95. Anderson KC, Gorgone BC, Marlink RG, et al: Transfusion acquired human immunodeficiency virus infections among immunocompromised persons. *Ann Intern Med* **105**:519–525, 1986.

96. Amman AJ, Wara DW, Dritz S, et al: Acquired immunodeficiency in an infant: Possible transmission by means of blood products. *Lancet* **1**:956–958, 1983.

97. Scott GB, Buck BE, Letterman JG: Acquired immunodeficiency syndrome in infants. *N Engl J Med* **310**:76–81, 1984.

98. Horowitz SL, Bentson JR, Benson F, et al: CNS toxoplasmosis in acquired immunodeficiency syndrome. *Arch Neurol* **10**:649–652, 1983

99. Wong B, Gold JW, Brown AE, et al: Central nervous system toxoplasmosis in homosexual men and parenteral drug abusers. *Ann Intern Med* **100**:36–42, 1984

100. Stahl-Bayliss CM, Kalman CM, Laskin OL: 9-[2-hydroxy-1(hydroxymethyl)ethoxymethyl]guanine (BW759): Clinical experience in AIDS patients with severe cytomegalovirus infections. In *Twenty-fifth Interscience Conference on Antimicrobial Agents and Chemotherapy (ICAAC), Minneapolis*, 1985 (abst.).

101. Shelhamer JH, Ognibene FP, Macher AM: Persistence of *Pneumocystis carinii* in lung tissue of acquired immunodeficiency syndrome patients treated for pneumocystis pneumonia. *Am Rev Respir Dis* **130**:1161–1165, 1984.

102. Hughes WT, Feldman S, Chaudhary S, et al: Comparison of pentamidine isethionate with trimethoprim sulfamethoxazole in the treatment of *Pneumocystis carinii* pneumonia. *J Pediatr* **92**:285–291, 1978.

103. Sattler F, Remington J. Intravenous trimethoprim sulfamethoxazole therapy for *Pneumocystis carinii* pneumonia. *Am J Med* **70**:1215–1221, 1981.

104. Winston DJ, Lau WK, Gale RP, Young LS: Trimethoprim–sulfamethoxazole for the treatment of *Pneumocystis carinii* pneumonia *Ann Intern Med* **92**:762–769, 1980.

105. Gottlieb MS, Young LS: Adverse reactions to pyrimethamine–sulfadoxine in the context of AIDS. (Letter to the editor.) *Lancet* **1**:1389, 1985.

105a. Montgomery AB, Debs RJ, Luce JM, et al: Aerolized pentamidine as sole therapy for *Pneumocystis carinii* pneumonia in patients with acquired immunodeficiency syndrome. *Lancet* **2**:480–482, 1987.

106. Macher AM, Kovacs JA, Gill V, et al: Bacteremia due to *Mycobacterium avium intracellulare* in the acquired immunodeficiency syndrome. *Ann Intern Med* **99**:782–785, 1983.

107. Pitchenik AE, Fischl MA: Disseminated tuberculosis and the acquired immunodeficiency syndromes. *Ann Intern Med* **97**:112, 1983.

108. Pitchenik AE, Robinson HA: The radiographic appearance of tuberculosis in patients with the acquired immune deficiency syndrome (AIDS) and pre-AIDS. *Am Rev Respir Dis* **131**:393–396, 1985.

109. Forgacs P, Tarshis A, Ma P, et al: Intestinal and bronchial cryptosporidiosis in an immunodeficient homosexual man. *Ann Intern Med* **6**:793–794, 1983.

110. Mitsuyasu R, Groopman JE, Volberding P: Cutaneous reaction to trimethoprim–sulfamethoxazole in patients with AIDS and Kaposi's sarcoma. *N Engl J Med* **308**:1535–1536, 1983.

111. Portnoy D, Whiteside ME, Buckley E, et al: Treatment of intestinal cryptosporidiosis with spiramycin. *Ann Intern Med* **101**:202–204, 1984.

112. Snider WD, Simpson DG, Nielsen S, et al: Neurological complications of acquired immune deficiency syndrome: analysis of 50 patients. *Ann Neurol* **14**:403–418, 1983.

113. Bennett JE, Dismukes WE, Duma RJ: A comparison of amphotericin B alone and combined with flucytosine in the treatment of crytococcal meningitis *N Engl J Med* **301**:126–131, 1979.

114. Alonso, R, Heiman-Patterson T, Mancall EL: Cerebral toxoplasmosis in acquired immune deficiency syndrome *Arch Neurol* **41**:321–323, 1984.

115. Gottlieb MS, Wolfe PR, Mitsuyasu R: Immunotherapy of AIDS in acquired immune deficiency syndrome. In Fauci A, Gallin J (eds): *Advances in Host Defense Mechanisms*. Raven, New York, 1985, pp. 149–170.

116. Krown SE, Real FX, Cunningham-Rundles S, et al: Preliminary observations on the effect of recombinant leukocyte: A interferon in homosexual men with Kaposi's sarcoma. *N Engl J Med* **18**:1071–1076, 1983.

116a. Vogt M, Hirsch MS: Prospects for the prevention and therapy of infections with the human immunodeficiency virus *Rev Infect Dis* **8**:991–1000, 1986.

116b. DeVita VT Jr, Broder S, Fauci AS, et al: Developmental therapeutics and the acquired immunodeficiency syndrome. *Ann Intern Med* **106**:568–581, 1987.

116c. Hirsch MS, Kaplan JC: Treatment of human immunodeficiency virus infections. *Antimicrob Agents Chemother* **31**:839–843, 1987.

117. Barnes DM: Promising results halts trial of anti-AIDS drug. *Science* **234**:15, 1986.

117a. Groopman JE, Mitsuyasu RT, DeLeo MJ, et al: Effect of recombinant human granulocyte-macrophage colony-stimulating factor on myelopoiesis in the acquired immunodeficiency syndrome. *N Engl J Med* **317**:593–598, 1987.

117b. Hartshorn KL, Vogt MW, Chou T.-C., et al: Synergistic inhibition of human immunodeficiency virus in vitro by azidothymidine and recombinant alpha A interferon. *Antimicrob Agents Chemother* **31**:168–172, 1987.

118. Friedland GH, Saltzmann BR, Rogers MF, et al: Lack of transmission of HTLV-III-LAV infection to household contacts of patients with AIDS or AIDS-related complex with oral candidiasis. *N Engl J Med* **314**:334–347, 1986.

119. Centers for Disease Control: Prevention of acquired immune deficiency syndrome (AIDS): Report of interagency recommendations. *MMWR* **32**:101–103, 1983.

120. Centers for Disease Control: An evaluation of the acquired immunodeficiency syndrome (AIDS) reported in health care personnel—United States. *MMWR* **32**:358–360, 1983

121. Centers for Disease Control: Classification system for human T-lymphotropic virus type III/lymphadenopathy associated virus infections. *MMWR* **35**:334, 1986.

16

Infections Complicating Congenital Immunodeficiency Syndromes

HARRY R. HILL

1. Introduction

Nothing is more challenging to the physician than the management of a serious infection in an immunocompromised host. Under such circumstances, the clinician must bring to bear all of his knowledge of microbiology and antimicrobial therapy, but in addition, he must have a firm understanding of the host defense abnormality underlying that individual patient's disease. As indicated by Stollerman in a recent review,[1] we can no longer have a primarily parasite-oriented approach to infectious diseases but must include host factors in the data on which we make potentially life-saving decisions.

Nowhere is this more true than in the management of the patient with a congenital defect in his host-defense mechanisms. Moreover, no clinician (pediatrician, internist, otolaryngologist, surgeon) can afford to ignore this area of medicine, since many such patients are being discovered and are being kept alive and functioning almost normally well into adulthood. It is absolutely essential that the diagnosis of a congenital immunodeficiency disease be made as soon as possible. The reader might ask, "Why?" since there are few definitive procedures for correcting serious defects in the host-defense mechanism. The answer to that question lies in the fact that survival and often the quality of life have improved in almost all instances in which the basic underlying pathophysiology of an immune defect has

been elucidated. A prime example of this is chronic granulomatous disease, once known as fatal granulomatous disease. Since the basic defect in phagocyte intracellular bactericidal activity was discovered in this disease, more appropriate antimicrobial therapy combined with judicious use of surgical drainage have resulted in fewer deaths. Similarly, appropriate use of antibiotics along with γ-globulin or plasma therapy has had an extremely beneficial effect in patients with hypogammaglobulinemia.

A critical factor in the detection of immunodeficient patients is to maintain a high degree of suspicion in order to discover such individuals as early as possible. In one study of patients with acquired common variable hypogammaglobulinemia, a period of approximately 10 years lapsed between onset of recurrent infections and diagnosis of the antibody deficiency.[2] This is unacceptable by present-day standards since simple tests are available in most hospital and commercial laboratories for adequately screening for hypogammaglobulinemia. Although there are several excellent reviews on detecting the immunodeficient patient,[1,3-7] I shall briefly review the factors that should alert the clinician to the possibility of a defect and then discuss the readily available tests that are useful in screening suspected patients.

Deciding which patients are suffering from a host-defense abnormality and which require further investigation is difficult in many instances. A careful history detailing the number, type, and severity of infections is critical. Particular attention should be addressed to determining if the infection and its etiology were documented by culture results, roent-

HARRY R. HILL • Departments of Pediatrics and Pathology, Division of Clinical Immunology and Allergy, University of Utah School of Medicine, Salt Lake City, Utah 84132.

genograms, scans, antibody titer rises, or other means. This is essential since often a diagnosis of pneumonia or blood poisoning is mentioned to the patient by the physician without any documentation being available. A complete family history concentrating on recurrent infections, early deaths, malignancies, and consanguinity may also yield valuable data. A thorough physical examination and appropriate laboratory tests should be performed to rule out physical or anatomic defects that might lead to recurrent infections. Recurrent meningitis because of dermal sinuses or basilar skull fractures and recurrent urinary tract infections secondary to ureteral problems are prime examples of such anatomical abnormalities. I have yet to find a patient with immunodeficiency who has a major problem with recurrent urinary tract infections.

Moreover, one must exclude those patients who are normal but who are exposed in their environment to a number of respiratory illnesses and thus are often ill. It has been shown that preschool and school-aged children may have six and up to 12 respiratory infections per year.[8] If one assumes a 2-week period for each individual infection, including prodrome, disease, and convalescence, then it would not be unusual for a child to be sick 12 (3 months) to 24 weeks (6 months) per year. An adult probably averages two to four respiratory infections per year. These figures should be kept in mind, as they are very useful in explaining recurrent infections to the individual who turns out on testing to have a normal immune system. Again, I would point out that, as in the case of urinary tract infections, I have yet to see pharyngitis, tonsillitis, or colds be a serious problem in any of our true immunodeficient patients.

After determining that a patient's recurrent infections are not the result of anatomical defects or epidemiologic exposure, then it is important to divide the host defense mechanism into its major components and consider the type of infection generally seen with defects in each system. Patients with abnormalities in the thymus-dependent portions of their immune systems tend to have severe or recurrent viral infections caused by varicella–zoster virus (VZV), herpes simplex virus (HSV), cytomegalovirus (CMV), or fungal and yeast infections such as those caused by *Candida albicans*.[9–12] A variety of intracellular bacterial pathogens and *Pneumocystis*

carinii infections also occurs. Abnormalities in T-lymphocyte numbers and function can be screened for fairly simply by employing skin tests for delayed hypersensitivity, lymphocyte mitogenic responses, and enumeration of T cells and T-cell subsets.[13] We currently employ *Candida albicans* antigen (Hollister Stier), streptokinase and streptodornase (SK–SD) (Varidase), and diphtheria–tetanus toxoid. Tritiated thymidine incorporation is used to determine the mitogenic response of lymphocytes exposed to the nonspecific mitogens, phytohemagglutinin or concanavalin A, or to tetanus toxoid, *Candida* antigen, or SK–SD. Sheep erythrocyte-rosetting T lymphocytes are determined by the method of Jondal et al.[13] and usually range from 40 to 70%.

One of the major functions of antibody in the host-defense mechanism is to opsonize or coat bacteria so that phagocytic cells may ingest and kill them. Antibody-deficiency syndromes are often characterized, therefore, by severe and recurrent pyogenic bacterial infections. Almost all such patients have recurrent respiratory infections, which include draining otitis media, mastoiditis, sinusitis, bronchitis, and multiple episodes of pneumonia.[2,14] This often leads to the development of bronchiectasis and chronic respiratory problems.[15] These patients also suffer from chronic diarrhea and may have systemic infections such as sepsis, meningitis, or osteomyelitis.[2,14,15]

The diagnosis of hypogammaglobulinemia is dependent on (1) the history of severe or recurrent bacterial infections, (2) a low level of immunoglobulins, and (3) the inability to make good specific antibodies. Hypogammaglobulinemia is best documented by determining IgG, IgM, and IgA levels by radialimmunodiffusion or nephalometry. These tests are far more sensitive and specific in quantitating immunoglobulins than is protein electrophoresis or immunoelectrophoresis.

The ability of a patient to make good specific antibody can also be assessed fairly easily using common serologic techniques that are available in most hospital or commercial laboratories. Anti-blood group A and B titers, or isohemagglutinins, can be run wherever blood typing is performed. These are predominantly IgM antibodies directed against cross-reacting polysaccharide antigens on bacteria normally present in the gastrointestinal (GI) flora. By 6 months of age, a child should have a titer of 1 : 8 or greater against A or B substance unless the blood type is AB.[6] Other serologic tests that can be used to assess specific antibody production include the anti-streptolysin O, anti-DNAase B, or streptozyme test if a patient has had a past streptococcal infection, or a rubella titer if the patient has already received this vaccine. (Note that immunization with live virus vaccines is not recommended in patients with immune deficiencies including antibody deficiencies since severe reactions may occur.) Alternatively, one can measure influenza titers, febrile agglutinins, or hemagglutinins following immunization with influenza vaccine, typhoid vaccine, or diphtheria–tetanus toxoid. Finally, one can enumerate the number of peripheral blood lymphocytes that have immunoglobulin on their surface or receptors for the third component of complement by erythrocyte antibody complement (EAC) rosettes.

Congenital deficiencies in the complement system are often associated with infections similar to those observed in hypogammaglobulinemia and include respiratory infections, sepsis, and meningitis.[16-23] Commonly available tests for measuring complement activity and levels include radialimmunodiffusion (commercial kits are available for measuring C3, C4, C5, and factor B) and a radial hemolytic assays for determining total hemolytic complement. Through the use of these tests, it is often possible to detect total absence of a single complement component and to define activation of one or more pathways during specific infections or other disease processes.

Infections in patients with phagocyte abnormalities often become manifest as abscesses or cutaneous episodes of cellulitis.[24-32] Staphylococci predominate as the etiologic agent and this is probably because this organism is the most numerous among the skin flora. Streptococci and some gram-negative infections as well as those caused by *Candida albicans* also occur in these patients.[24,26,33] The metabolic activity of phagocytes, which relates to their ability to activate the hexose monophosphate shunt and generate toxic oxygen radicals essential to microbicidal activity, can be assessed with the nitroblue tetrazolium (NBT) dye-reduction test[34,35] or a procedure employing the detection of chemiluminescence.[36,37] In the NBT test, a yellow dye solution is mixed with a drop of blood and often with a substance such as endotoxin that stimulates phagocyte metabolism. After an appropriate interval, a smear is made, and the cells that have activated their hexose monophosphate shunt and developed a black deposit within their cytoplasm are enumerated.[34] Patients with defects in this important microbicidal pathway fail to reduce the dye and therefore do not form black deposits in their cells.

In the chemiluminescence (CL) assay, polymorphonucleocytes (PMNs) are incubated with a phagocytizable particle in a dark-adapted scintillation vial.[36,37] The mixture is placed in a liquid scintillation counter, out of phase, with one photomultiplier tube disconnected, and counted at intervals for 60–90 min. Following particle ingestion, the microbicidal mechanism of both PMNs and monocytes are activated, and excited molecular oxygen species are generated.[38,39] On decaying to the ground state, these emit photons that can be measured as light in the scintillation system. Patients with defects in the generation of these oxygen species either fail to generate or produce lower levels of chemiluminescence than do controls.[40-42] This technique represents a simple and sensitive means for screening for defects in phagocyte oxidative metabolism. Myeloperoxidase deficiency may also be detected using this technique as well as by a simple histochemical stain.[41] All suspected defects in microbicidal activity should be confirmed by more classic phagocytosis and killing assays.[43]

Defects in leukocyte motility are best screened for in vitro using the Boyden chamber or a migration under agarose technique.[44-47] These assays have been found to correlate more closely with clinical abnormalities than do the results of skin window techniques.[48] These are more difficult tests, of course, and are not commonly available except at larger medical centers. One additional laboratory test, the serum level of IgE, may be of value in the diagnosis of a number of patients with the syndrome of hyperimmunoglobulinemia E, recurrent infections, and defective PMN chemotaxis.[24,25] Extremely high levels of IgE are usually present in these patients[24] as well as in the closely related syndrome of Job.[49] Table 1 summarizes the appropriate tests to be employed in the patient suspected of an immune deficiency.

TABLE 1. Immunologic Screening Tests

Portion of the immune system	Tests
Antibody	Quantitative IgG, IgM, IgA
	Isohemagglutinin titers
	Rubella titer, Diphtheria–tetanus titer
	Response to pneumococcal vaccine
	Response to *Hemophilus influenzae* type B vaccine
Complement	Total hemolytic complement
	C3, C4, C5, Factor B
Phagocytes	WBC and differential cell count
	Nitroblue tetrazolium (NBT)
	IgE
Cell-mediated immunity	PMN chemotaxis
	Skin tests (*C. albicans*, diphtheria–tetanus)
	T cells and T-cell subsets
	Mitogen responses

2. Aim of Therapy in Congenital Immunodeficiency Diseases

2.1. Treatment of Life-Threatening Infections

After the diagnosis of immunodeficiency disease is established, what are the therapeutic goals in the management of infections in these patients? These can be grouped as follows: (1) prevention or therapy of potentially life-threatening infections; (2) therapy of less severe acute infections; and (3) management of chronic infection so as to minimize the development of long-term sequelae.

Patients with congenital immune deficiency are often especially prone to develop sudden overwhelming and often fatal infection. In such cases, it is absolutely essential that the clinician have an understanding of the basic underlying defect in the host defense mechanism, the most likely etiologic agents in infection, and the available therapeutic modalities. The following illustrate a few examples.

1. Patients with the Wiskott–Aldrich syndrome are particularly susceptible to the development of serious overwhelming infections with *Pneumococcus, Hemophilus influenzae*, and other encapsulated bacteria because they fail to make good antibodies to polysaccharide antigens.[50,51] A number of individuals with this syndrome have died of such infection. Thus, in an acutely ill patient with this particular immunodeficiency, therapy would logically include the intravenous administration of an antibiotic that would be effective against these organisms and intravenous immunoglobulin in an attempt to supply missing antibodies.

2. Patients with chronic granulomatous disease (CGD) often develop severe pneumonias and other infections caused by staphylococci because their leukocytes fail to kill these organisms following ingestion.[27–30] A CGD patient with severe pneumonia should be treated initially with antimicrobial agents directed against staphylococci and especially ones that are known to penetrate into cells. Thus, nafcillin or methicillin along with agents such as rifampin might be employed for best results.[52,53]

3. Patients with congenital absence of their terminal complement components (C6, C7, C8) often suffer repeated disseminated infections with *Neisseria meningitidis* or *N. gonorrheae*.[20–23] An acutely toxic patient known to have such a defect in his complement system should receive appropriate intravenous antimicrobial therapy for these organisms. Fresh frozen plasma therapy might also conceivably be of value in supplying the missing complement components. No data on the clinical efficacy of such therapy is available, however.

Such dramatic examples point out the need for a thorough knowledge of host-defense abnormalities, likely microbial pathogens, and newer therapeutic modalities in the successful therapy of these life-threatening infections in the congenital immunodeficient syndromes.

2.1.1. Early Diagnosis of Infection

Early diagnosis of infection and correct definition of the etiologic agent are extremely important in managing severe life-threatening infections in immune deficient hosts. Again, a high degree of suspicion must be maintained for infection in these patients. A variety of diagnostic tests may lend additional support in suggesting the presence of infection. These include routine and more specialized cultures such as transtracheal aspirates,[54] lung aspirates,[55,56] or open biopsies[57] in diagnosing pneumonias and cerebrospinal fluid taps or even brain biopsies in central nervous system (CNS) infections.

A variety of scans are now available that have proven useful in defining infections in these patients and include technetium (^{99m}Tc) bone scans, gallium (^{67}Ga) scans, radiolabeled leukocyte scans, and computed tomography (CT). Although a positive result with these latter techniques may be quite helpful, a negative one does not rule out the presence of infection in an immunocompromised host. On several occasions, I have seen osteomyelitis progress significantly in the face of negative bone scans in such patients or abscesses be present without being detected on routine scanning procedures. Again, the most likely problem in these patients is infection, and one should not rule it out on the basis of laboratory tests or radiographs alone.

A number of techniques have recently come into widespread use for the rapid diagnosis of bacterial and other infections by means other than cultures. Microbial antigen detection in the definition of infection has several advantages over more classic microbiologic techniques. These include (1) the rapidity of diagnosis, (2) efficacy even in the face of prior antimicrobial activity, and (3) proof of an etiological relationship, since contamination is seldom a problem in these rapid tests. Counterimmunoelectrophoresis was once of the most widely used techniques.[58–61] In this procedure, negatively charged (predominantly polysaccharide) antigens are drawn by an electrical field toward the anode while less negatively charged hyperimmune antibody is pulled toward the cathode by movement of buffer (endosmosis). This results in the development of a precipitin band within a small reaction area in a short period (30–90 min). This test has been used to detect antigens of many of the pathogens affecting immunodeficient patients including *Hemophilus influenzae*,[62–64] *Streptococcus pneumoniae*,[65–67] *Neisseria meningitidis*,[68,69] *Escherichia coli*,[70] *Pseudomonas aerugginosa*,[71] and groups B[72] and D[73] streptococci. In addition, it can be used to detect viral antigens such as Australia antigen and even mycoplasma.[74,75]

A potentially important new application of this test has been the detection of circulating antigens of *Pneumocystis carinii* in immunosuppressed patients with pneumonia.[76] Hughes and co-workers, using hyperimmune rabbit antiserum, have been able to detect circulating antigens of these organisms in 95% of 20 patients with biopsy-proven disease. However, the test is not specific for pneumocystosis and has been positive in a number of patients with non-*Pneumocystis* pneumonia.[77]

Antigen detection systems such as counterimmunoelectrophoresis, Latex agglutination, staphylococcal coagglutination, and enzyme-linked immunosorbent assay (ELISA) have been shown to be quite promising in defining the etiology of sepsis[58,78,79] meningitis,[57,80–82] pneumonia,[61,83,84] and deep tissue infections[71] in normal hosts. Most of these studies have been carried out in pediatric populations. Improved results have been obtained by examining multiple specimens, including serum, urine, and body fluids such as cerebrospinal (CSF), pleural, or pericardial accumulations.[63,80,81] Many of these antigens are actually filtered out in the urine and can therefore often be detected in an unconcentrated or concentrated urine specimen.[66,80] Moreover, persistence of antigen secretion in the urine has occasionally been associated with persistence of infection in the face of antimicrobial therapy.[66] Unfortunately, these techniques have not been used to examine a large number of immunodeficient patients with infections, so there are no data on its efficacy in these individuals. Excellent results have been obtained in otherwise normal hosts, however. Again, it is important to stress that serum, urine, and the appropriate body fluid should be examined in each instance in order to increase the sensitivity of the procedure. A positive result indicates, in almost all instances, that antigens of that particular organism are present in the fluid and, thus, strongly suggests an etiologic relationship. A few cross-reactions are known such as that between some α-hemolytic streptococci and pneumococci,[85] one between group B meningococcal antiserum and the *Escherichia coli* K1 antigen[70] and one between *E. coli* and *H. influenzae* polyribose phosphate.[83] In practice, however, these do not represent serious problems.

One recent advance in the methodology for antigen detection systems may greatly assist the physician caring for the immunodeficient patient. Several investigators have indicated that examination of sputum is a useful technique for defining the etiology of pneumonia.[83,84,87] Unfortunately, some false-positive results have been noted in patients with chronic bronchitis.[87] Further study may prove this to be a useful diagnostic tool.

The CIE procedure can be reversed to detect specific antibodies against certain bacterial and mycotic pathogens. Such serum antibody determinations have received widespread use in immunocompromised patients with variable degrees of success. The *Candida* precipitin test is probably the most popular of these techniques.[88-90] Remington and co-workers[88] originally reported the detection of serum antibodies against *Candida albicans* in 100% of patients with systemic disease as opposed to 0% in those without disease. Subsequent studies[89] have indicated a higher false-positive rate and suggested that antibody titers might be capable of discriminating between infection and colonization. In a study in immunocompromised patients, we[90] demonstrated that the tests had only 50% sensitivity and 69% specificity. Thus, one has to be extremely careful in interpreting serologic tests in patients who may have impairment of specific antibody production. Counterimmunoelectrophoresis and double immunodiffusion have also been used to detect serum antibodies in patients with invasive staphylococcal disease and endocarditis.[58,91,92] Again, false-positive results represent a problem here.[93]

Other means for microbial antigen detection have been used in immunocompromised and normal hosts. These include latex agglutination[94,95] and staphylococcal coagglutination[96,97] in which antibody is attached to either Latex particles or to staphylococci by protein A–Fc fragment interaction. A Latex agglutination test is available for detecting cryptococcal antigen in CSF, and this is a useful adjunct to the diagnosis of this disease in immunocompromised hosts. Agglutinin tests employing similar reagents to detect bacterial antigens including *H. influenzae*,[95] *N. meningitidis*,[96] *S. pneumoniae*,[97] and group B streptococci[95] have been reported.

Two additional tests for the rapid diagnosis of meningitis that may be of value in the immunodeficient patient should be mentioned. These include the limulus lysate test for gram-negative endotoxin in CSF and CSF lactate levels.[99-101] The limulus lysate test has been reported to give positive results in up to 99% of patients with gram-negative meningitis.[101] The CSF lactate, which increases during bacterial but not viral CNS infection, is generally elevated in almost all patients with culture-proven bacterial meningitis.[101,102] These two tests along with one or more of the antigen-detection techniques will probably result in high yields regarding the diagnosis of a bacterial or even mycotic process in an immunodeficient patient.

In summary then, the key to early diagnosis of infection in the congenitally immunodeficient patient is a high index of suspicion for infection. On the first sign of such a problem, appropriate routine and specialized diagnostic cultures and antibody studies should be obtained. If the illness appears less than immediately life threatening, radiographs and scans may be helpful. If the illness does appear life-threatening, appropriate antimicrobial therapy should be administered immediately and should be based on a clear understanding of the patient's host-defense abnormality and the most likely etiologic agents.

2.1.2. Appropriate Antimicrobial Therapy

Selecting an appropriate antimicrobial agent in the severely ill immunocompromised host is a difficult task. We must often forsake much of what is taught in infectious disease training programs and initiate antimicrobial therapy with the broadest, most potent antimicrobial agents. Thus, initial therapeutic regimens should be designed to quickly stem the progression of infection and prevent a fatal outcome. To illustrate, we were recently challenged by the presentation of one of our Wiskott–Aldrich syndrome patients in the emergency room with a history of sudden onset of fever, chills, and extreme lethargy. On physical examination, he had a fever of 104°F and the usual eczema and petechiae seen in these patients. Knowing that such patients have great difficulty in making antibodies to polysaccharide antigens, we initially suspected infection with *S. pneumoniae*, *H. influenzae*, or *N. meningitidis*, but we could not rule out other organisms such as *E. coli* or *Klebsiella pneumoniae*. Since this was obviously a life-threatening infection, we drew appropriate cultures, did a rapid spinal tap, and began him on penicillin, chloramphenicol, and gentamicin. In this critically ill patient, we believed we were justified in treating all or most of the potential pathogens immediately. The next day, the patient was alert, active and clamoring to go home when a blood culture from the preceding day grew out *S. pneumoniae*. Again, this course of therapy was initiated for a brief period of time to give us time to make a specific diagnosis. As soon as the etiology of his infection was known and its sensitivity to penicillin was determined (pneumococci resistant to penicillin have been described and can, on occasion, be isolated from immune deficient patients who often receive a number of oral antibiotics),[103] the patient was continued only on this drug. Thus, only a very limited course of broad-spectrum antimicrobial therapy was given, which would be highly unlikely to result in abnormal colonization or superinfection. The antimicrobial agents selected for treating life-threatening infections in the immunocompromised host should be chosen based on the patient's host-defense defect and the most likely pathogen involved, as will be discussed later in this chapter. In addition, an attempt should be made to select bactericidal rather than bacteriostatic antibiotics when possible, since the host's immune system may not be capable of microbial killing. Intravenous therapy is indicated for all such serious infections. As pointed out in Chapter 10, a new intravenous form of trimethoprim–sulfamethoxazole is likely to become available, and this agent should be preferentially used in any patients who are not able to accept oral therapy.[104–105]

2.1.3. Immunologic Adjuncts to Therapy

After appropriate cultures and laboratory tests have been obtained and antimicrobial therapy has been instituted in the critically ill congenitally immunodeficient patient, the clinician should consider what he might do to enhance host defenses.

In the antibody-deficient patient, an effort should be directed toward supplying missing antibodies. In the acutely ill individual, this can be done with fresh, frozen plasma, since a large amount of antibody can be given in a relatively short period of time.[106–108] Administration of 10–15 ml/kg plasma results in an immediate increase in immunoglobulin levels of 200 mg/dl for IgG, 30 mg/dl for IgM, and 30 mg/dl for IgA[104] compared with only a 100-mg/dl increase in IgG following 0.6 ml/kg immune serum globulin IM (no significant rises in IgA or IgM are noted after intramuscular gammaglobulin). Moreover, the γ-globulin in plasma rapidly equilibrates with extracellular spaces within 24 hr and has a longer half-life than does that of γ-globulin in the intramuscular preparations.[107] This fact combined with the ability of plasma to raise the levels of IgA and IgM to some degree make it a useful therapeutic tool.

There are several hazards associated with the use of plasma, one being the transmission of hepatitis or HIV virus to the immunodeficient patient. Every effort should be made to ensure that the plasma is Australian-antigen-negative, since rather severe hepatitis and the development of the chronic carrier state for this antigen have been reported in hypogammaglobulinemics.[109,110] One common practice is to plasmapherese a close relative who is unlikely to have hepatitis and use his plasma exclusively on the patient.[106–108] Two or three 250-ml units may be collected at one bleeding and then frozen for later use. Such freezing probably destroys most immunocompetent lymphocytes, but in the patient who also has a T-cell deficiency, it would seem wise to irradiate the plasma before use (3000 rad). Plasma therapy has also been used with some success in Wiskott–Aldrich syndrome patients,[108] in patients with ataxia telangiectasia,[111] and in patients with complement component deficiencies.[106] There are now several γ-globulin preparations modified for intravenous use. These preparations are altered in some way so that they do not contain immunoglobulin aggregates that are capable of activating the complement system. Intramuscular γ-globulin preparations containing aggregates can trigger the complement system if inadvertently injected intravenously and thereby cause anaphylactic-like reactions.[106,112] Such intravenous immunoglobulin preparations have been found to be superior to intramuscular globulin preparations in reducing specific acute illnesses and reducing the number of days that hypogammaglobulinemic individuals required antibiotics.[113] Furthermore, they have also been found to be effective in preventing symptomatic CMV infection following transplantation,[114] and treating chronic echovirus encephalitis.[115]

Additional immediate immunotherapeutic maneuvers that one might employ in the severely infected immunocompromised host include the use of granulocyte transfusions in patients with marked neutropenia or a serious granulocytopathy. Good results have been reported in such patients treated with daily infusions of three to four units of granulocytes by Fudenberg and co-workers.[116] Attempts to correct T-cell abnormalities in the acutely ill patient have not met with much success and are best carried out after infection is brought under control. Efforts at transplantation during such episodes have not often resulted in survival.

2.2. Minimizing the Effects of Less Severe Acute Infections

Immunocompromised patients are seldom entirely free from pyogenic infections. Thus, the antibody-deficient patient often suffers recurrent or chronic episodes of sinusitis, otitis media, mastoiditis, or bronchitis. Patients with absence of C3 or C5 have similar problems, whereas those with phagocyte movement or killing defects suffer recurrent abscesses, episodes of cellulitis, and pneumonias. These recurrent acute infections detract significantly from the patient's quality of life and may evolve into either the severe life-threatening infections discussed above or chronic, indolent infections that have serious sequaelae as discussed in Section 2.3. Every attempt should be made to control these infections by using both antimicrobial therapy and immunologic regimens. In many cases, the etiologic agents may be different from those seen in normal hosts and may have different antibiotic sensitivity patterns, in part because of the chronic use of antimicrobial agents by these patients. These acute infectious processes may be divided as follows.

2.2.1. Respiratory Infections

Acute sinusitis is not uncommon in the patient with deficiency of antibodies, C3, or C5 or with phagocyte dysfunction. This type of infection is characterized by low-grade fever, congestion, postnasal drip, and tenderness over the involved sinus. Such infection is associated in many instances with recurrent otitis media. The organisms involved are often similar to those in the uncompromised host and include *H. influenzae, S. pneumoniae,* and occasionally *S. pyogenes,* or *Neisseria* species. Anaerobes may also be involved in sinusitis.[117] In contrast to normal patients, immune deficient hosts may have organisms such as *S. aureus* or gram-negative bacilli such as *P. aeruginosa* isolated from the middle ear in association with symptoms of otitis media. We have found cultures taken with nasopharyngeal swab to be very useful in selecting antibiotics for these patients. Excellent correlation has been detected in studies comparing the culture results of middle ear aspirates with those of nasopharyngeal cultures.[118] It is surprising how many times immunodeficient patients will yield essentially pure cultures of a pathogen such

as *H. influenzae* or *S. pneumoniae* from nasopharyngeal specimens. In the face of clinically apparent disease, antimicrobial agents should be administered, but in the absence of infection, we have elected to withhold treatment of the carrier state since this would probably only result in replacement of one pathogen by another or in the emergence of antibiotic resistance.

Therapy of sinusitis and otitis media should be initiated with an antibiotic such as ampicillin or amoxacillin, although these agents may not be effective if *Staphylococcus* is involved or if other resistant organisms are present. Nasopharyngeal, sinus, or middle ear fluid cultures should be taken in the immunodeficient patient, and antimicrobial susceptibility patterns determined on significant isolates. This is in contrast to the usual practice in the normal host with acute otitis or sinusitis where such cultures are really not indicated and are not cost effective. Failure to evaluate the immune–deficient host with appropriate cultures and sensitivity determinations often results in significant delay in the initiation of appropriate therapy. Moreover, should infection disseminate and become life threatening, the initial culture and sensitivity results would be of great benefit in selecting appropriate therapy.

Acute bronchitis and pneumonia are also common occurrences in the patient with a congenital defect in the immune system. Low-grade fever, cough, and sputum production with bronchitis are common in antibody and complement deficiencies and may also be seen in T-lymphocyte and phagocyte abnormalities. Typable and nontypable *H. influenzae* are often isolated from sputum specimens in these patients. A host of other organisms may also be involved. A gram stain of expectorated sputum combined with culture results should be the guide to therapy. Initially, a drug such as ampicillin or, in the adult, tetracycline is often helpful in bronchitis. Therapy should be altered when the results of cultures and sensitivities are returned. Cloxacillin, dicloxacillin, or an oral cephalosporin may be used if staphylococci are involved. Antimicrobial therapy for bronchitis is generally limited to 7–10 days.

Recurrent pneumonia is one of the most common problems faced by physicians caring for immunodeficient patients. Pyogenic infections caused by *H. influenzae* and *S. pneumoniae* as well as a host of other pathogens occur in antibody or complement deficiencies. In patients with phagocyte dysfunction, *S. aureus* is more prevalent as an etiologic agent. Sputum or transtracheal cultures should be obtained as well as blood, urine, and pleural fluid when possible for culture and examination for microbial antigens. If the patient appears toxic and if empyema or pneumatocoeles are present, the patient should be hospitalized and treated parenterally. In the less ill patient, we have been successful on numerous occasions with oral therapy combined with chest physical therapy, postural drainage, and close follow-up evaluation. Ampicillin, cloxacillin, or an oral cephalosporin have usually been selected based on the results of cultures and gram stains. Penicillin is the drug of choice for almost all *S. pneumoniae* infections. In the nonhospitalized patient, close follow-up is required, including radiographs to rule out progression, effusion, empyema, or pneumatocoele. If such complications should develop in the face of antimicrobial therapy, the patient should be hospitalized, and additional diagnostic procedures such as transtracheal aspirate or lung biopsy should be carried out in order to document the etiology. Plasma therapy (10–15 ml/kg) or IGIV (100–200 mg/kg) should be administered to antibody-deficient patients in addition to their regular maintenance doses when pneumonia develops.

2.2.2. Gastrointestinal Infections

The respiratory and GI tracts are the prime sites for microbial challenge in the normal and immunodeficient patient. Thus, it is not unusual that these two areas should be the major focus of infection in the compromised individual. Most patients with combined T- and B-cell defects have some degree of diarrhea and malabsorption.[119]

Patients with isolated IgA deficiency or IgA deficiency associated with other immunoglobulin abnormalities often suffer chronic diarrhea because of *Giardia lamblia* infection. This agent is probably the leading cause of infectious diarrhea in immunodeficient patients. Symptoms have their onset within 6–8 days of infection and usually consist of cramping abdominal pain, nausea, diarrhea, and occasionally low-grade fever. The disease may last for weeks or months in the immunodeficient individual. The diagnosis may be established by examining multiple stools for cysts and trophozoites in approximately

50% of patients. More reliable means for establishing the diagnosis consist of examining duodenal or jejunal aspirates or biopsies. Since this disease is so common in our IgA- and combined immunoglobulin-deficient patients, we will often initiate therapy with atabrine or metronidazole after several stools have been collected for examination but before a specific diagnosis has been made. Therapy is continued for 1 week and results in an approximate cure rate of 70%. The symptomatic patient may be retreated with the alternative antimicrobial agent if no response is observed following initial therapy (see Chapter 9).

Bacterial overgrowth in the small intestine has also been suspected as a cause of diarrhea in immunodeficient patients. Good data are not available, however, correlating bacterial counts in the small bowel and symptomatology. On occasion, an immunodeficient patient with marked diarrhea and no specific isolatable pathogen will respond to antimicrobial therapy. A nonabsorbable drug such as neomycin may be employed, or occasionally an absorbable drug such as tetracycline will be of benefit in the older patient. Although the data on such therapy are practically nonexistent, a trial in the patient with marked diarrhea may be indicated after specific pathogens have been ruled out as the etiology.

Plasma infusions have often been found to decrease the severity and frequency of diarrhea in the immunodeficient patient.[106,108,120] The reason for this is unclear, since the IgA in plasma does not appear to cross into the GI tract. Perhaps the plasma contains other factors such as lymphocyte products that are helpful in enhancing local secretory immunity. One or two units of plasma may be given on a biweekly basis in such patients, and this is often followed by dramatic improvement.

2.2.3. Cutaneous Infections

Recurrent cutaneous infections are the hallmark of patients with phagocyte defects.[121] Abscess formation is common in patients with neutrophil and macrophage chemotactic, phagocytic, and killing defects. These may consist of small "pimples," larger boils, or huge abscesses. Interestingly, the patients with the largest abscesses often have phagocyte motility defects leading to their recurrent infections. The reason for this may be related to observations made in animals by Miles and co-workers.[122,123]

This group found that there was a critical 2–4-hr period during which phagocytes must arrive at the site of bacterial invasion if infection is to be contained. If phagocyte accumulation was delayed past this time interval, larger local lesions or systemic infection occurred. Thus, the large abscesses in the patients with chemotactic defects probably result from delayed accumulation of the first wave of phagocytes. This allows further bacterial multiplication with subsequent production of an increased amount of inflammatory mediators via the complement system and other pathways. This added stimulus continues to call in additional cells and results in the large abscesses observed.

Microbicidal defects such as those seen in CGD allow intracellular growth of bacteria, lysis of PMNs and other cells, and release of important inflammatory mediators that also result in accumulations of bacteria, phagocytes, and debris. The abscesses in these patients are often caused by staphylococci but may involve a whole host of organisms.[27] Needle aspiration or open drainage usually yields an etiological agent on which sensitivity testing can be carried out. Many of the patients with CGD have serious problems in wound healing, so that recently we have not recommended incision and drainage except where absolutely necessary. When possible, aspiration with a large-bore needle has been successful in relieving pressure and obtaining an etiologic diagnosis. Therapy is then instituted with an appropriate bactericidal agent. Such medical management of what used to be considered surgical cases has resulted in far less overall morbidity in CGD patients.

Cutaneous and mucocutaneous candidiasis have also been observed in patients with phagocyte abnormalities.[33,124] Some may also have T-lymphocyte problems so that the exact role of each abnormality in the overall clinical picture is unknown. The candidiasis in these patients is usually quite difficult to treat and may require prolonged topical and even systemic therapy for a brief period of time. Nystatin has generally been used in topical therapy, with agents such as amphotericin, 5-fluorocytosine, and miconazole having occasional use in a severely affected patient to decrease the overall numbers of these organisms in lesions. Recently a new antifungal agent, ketoconazole, has been used to treat a variety of fungal infections. Whereas it is quite effective against superficial infections,[125] it has been less suc-

cessful when used against deep infections such as those in bones and joints.[126]

Cellulitis caused by streptococci, staphylococci, and other agents has also occasionally been a problem in patients with phagocyte immune-deficiency diseases.[24,25] These generally require rapid diagnosis based on blood cultures or local needle aspirates of spreading margins and are treated initially with parenteral bactericidal antimicrobial agents.

2.3. Prevention of Chronic Infections and Their Sequelae

2.3.1. Antimicrobial and Other Therapy

A third and perhaps most important objective in the management of the congenital immune deficient patient is to prevent the long-term sequelae of infections. Acute, recurrent, and chronic infections often lead to the development of serious sequelae. Death in the antibody-deficiency syndromes, for instance, is usually the result of respiratory failure secondary to bronchiectasis and recurrent pneumonias. Similar respiratory problems may occur in ataxia telangiectasia and even in diseases associated with phagocyte disorders such as chronic granulomatous disease. On occasion, recurrent staphylococcal pneumonias with pneumotocoele formation and chronic pulmonary fibrosis have resulted in lobectomy and the attending complications. When infection becomes manifested in other lobes, the patient with a history of such surgery is even more compromised. For this reason, such procedures are now discouraged in most centers. Postural drainage and physiotherapy cannot be overstressed in these patients, since adequate removal of plugs, inflammatory cells, and bacterial debris contributes greatly to the prevention of long-term pulmonary complications. All of our patients with pulmonary disease are followed with at least yearly chest roentgenograms and pulmonary function studies. Some chest physicians employ the intermittent use of oral antibiotics (ampicillin or tetracycline) in these patients on a 1-week-on, 1-week-off basis. We do not do this and only employ antibiotics when clinical or radiographic findings point to an increasingly purulent bronchitis or pneumonia.

Additional Therapy. The patient with chronic sinusitis may benefit from drainage procedures such as the Caldwell–Luc procedure, whereas recurrent otitis media patients may benefit from adenoidectomy and insertion of tympanic membrane drainage tubes.

Patients with recurrent abscesses, especially those caused by staphylococci may respond to vigorous washing with an agent containing PhisoHex or Betadine. These preparations tend to dry out the skin, however, and may actually increase abscess formation. In other individuals with severe, essentially incapacitating abscess formation, we have had to resort to chronic long-term antimicrobial prophylaxis. One patient with Job syndrome with severe staphylococcal abscesses was treated for more than 8 years with cloxacillin with an excellent response. As soon as this medication was stopped, abscesses recurred. We do not advocate the indiscriminate use of antibiotic prophylaxis, but in a few instances it can be quite useful. In general, the choice of such therapy should be limited to situations in which (1) one etiologic agent predominates, (2) therapy is not associated with significant toxicities, and (3) resistance is not likely to readily develop. In general, we have tended to use full therapeutic doses rather than the low-dose therapy commonly associated with prophylaxis. Although there are few hard data on this point, we believe that low-dose therapy might favor the selection of resistant organisms.

Trimethoprim–sulfamethoxazole combinations may have several uses in the therapy or prevention of infection in patients with recurrent infections. Such preparations have been used in children with recurrent episodes of otitis media[127] and recurrent urinary tract infections with some success.[128] More recently, Hughes and co-workers[129] showed that 150 mg trimethoprim combined with 750 mg sulfamethoxazole per square meter per day was 100% effective in preventing the development of Pneumocystis carinii pneumonia in immunosuppressed patients. This is an exciting observation, since infection with this agent is a very common complication in immunodeficiency disease. Johnston and co-workers[130] also indicated that sulfonamides may have a beneficial effect in patients with chronic granulomatous disease. This stems from the observation that a number of these patients have had fewer infectious complications while on long-term sulfonamide therapy, and their PMNs have shown slightly better bactericidal activity in the presence of sulfonamides.

2.3.2. Immunotherapy

In the antibody-deficient patient, prevention of chronic infections and sequelae is aided significantly by the use of γ-globulin or plasma therapy. Intramuscular γ-globulin is administered prophylactically in a dose of approximately 0.6 ml/kg every 3 weeks after an initial loading dose of twice that amount. In the larger person, this can result in the requirement for a substantial injection volume (70 kg × 0.6 ml = 42 ml). For this reason, many of the larger patients prefer weekly doses amounting to approximately one-third of the dose; 10 ml/week usually offers adequate protection against pyogenic infections in most patients. We do not routinely check immunoglobulin levels following injection since the level seldom correlates specifically with protection against infection. An attempt is made, however, to adjust the dose according to the patient's symptoms. Approximately 10% of patients will develop reactions following γ-globulin administration. Most will be caused by the inadvertent injection of the material into small veins in the muscle. The aggregates contained within the intramuscular preparation will result in complement activation and an anaphylaxis-like picture. Patients may also develop IgE or IgG antibodies directed against various proteins in the γ-globulin preparations. Patients with total absence of IgA are likely to develop such antibodies to this immunoglobulin that may result in anaphylactoid reactions after intramuscular administration. Such patients may be skin tested for such reactivity using low concentrations of the preparation. Both types of reactions, and especially those caused by aggregates, may be managed subsequently through the use of the plasma therapy mentioned above. This must be administered carefully with emergency equipment readily available in the event that a reaction should occur.

Plasma therapy is also often of benefit in the patient who has hypogammaglobulinemia and who persists with chronic respiratory infections or diarrhea in spite of IM γ-globulin. Chronic use of plasma in these patients has resulted in an improvement in symptomatology and slower progression of developing sequelae in some instances.[108] The new intravenous immunoglobulin preparations have already been discussed. They appear to represent a significant advance in the therapy of patients with antibody deficiency disease. Trials are now under way to assess their role in the therapy of acute infections in otherwise normal individuals who lack antibody to a specific pathogen or in secondary immune deficiencies.

A number of substances derived from human or animal sources or synthesized chemically have been used in attempts to enhance the host defense mechanism of immunodeficient patients. Transfer factor, a small-molecular-weight (<10,000), nonimmunogenic protein derived from human leukocyte lysates has been used with some success to prevent infections in patients with Wiskott–Aldrich syndrome or chronic mucocutaneous candidiasis.[131–133] Unfortunately, results have been quite variable, and the use of this agent has been associated with renal toxicity and the development of hemolytic anemia in a small number of patients.[131]

Thymosin, a partially purified extract of beef thymic tissue, has been reported to increase T-cell numbers in a variety of congenital and acquired immunodeficiency syndromes.[134] Conversion to positive mitogenic responses and mixed leukocyte reactions has followed in vitro incubation with the agent, whereas in vivo therapy has been reported to cause clinical improvement in patients with (1) Nezelof syndrome of cellular immunodeficiency with immunoglobulins, (2) ataxia–telangiectasia, (3) DiGeorge syndrome, and (4) Wiskott–Aldrich syndrome.[135] In general, these studies have involved small numbers of patients, and the results have not always been impressive. Moreover, allergic reactions and hepatitis have occurred during the use of this agent.

Neither transfer factor nor thymosin are widely available in a standardized form. It seems clear that their use at the present time should be restricted to investigational settings, and considerably more experience will be required before their clinical value can be established.

Patients with enzyme defects in their purine metabolic pathways including adenosine deaminase and nucleoside phosphorylase deficiency have a picture similar to that of patients with severe combined immunodeficiency disease, although the sympatomatology may be less severe initially. Polmar and co-workers[136] have treated one such individual with repeated administrations of glycerol-frozen packed human erythrocytes that contain high levels of adenosine deaminase. This has been followed by return of lymphocyte function to normal in vitro and positive skin test reactivity, and the patient has re-

mained well. Similar therapy has been attempted in a patient with nucleoside phosphorylase deficiency with some success.

Bone marrow, fetal thymus, and fetal liver transplant have been used in a variety of immunodeficiency diseases.[137–139] Marrow transplantation between HLA-matched siblings (especially HLA-D matched, mixed lymphocyte culture nonreactive pairs) have been successful in a number of cases of severe combined immunodeficiency disease and in several cases with Wiskott–Aldrich syndrome.[140] Excellent results have been obtained when HLA matched donors have been available. Almost all patients who receive marrow from an individual not matched at the D locus have died of severe graft-versus-host disease and overwhelming infection within the first 1–2 months after transplant. Recent attempts at transplanting mismatched marrow have employed lectin or monoclonal antibody removal of mature T cells from donor marrow. These have met with considerable success. Gram-negative enteric pathogens, viruses, or *Pneumocystis carinii* have usually been the etiologic agents in the severe infections developing in these patients. This had led to attempts aimed at suppressing the gastrointestinal flora of patients after transplantation with a variety of systemic and oral, nonabsorbable antibiotics.[141,142] In addition, laminar flow rooms have been used to manage these susceptible individuals, but without great success.

Fetal thymic and hepatic tissue obtained before immunocompetence has been established have been used in cases of severe combined immunodeficiency disease for which no HLA-D-matched marrow donor has been available. Reconstitution has been successful in several instances but has not usually been of a longlasting nature.[133] Transplantation of fetal thymus or thymic epithelial cells maintained in vitro has been attempted in a variety of immunodeficiency disorders including the DiGeorge syndrome,[143] Nezelof syndrome,[144] chronic mucocutaneous candidiasis,[145] and ataxia–telangiectasia.[144] Transient improvement in skin test reactions and in vitro lymphocyte responses and a decrease in infectious complications have been reported following such therapy, but permanent reconstitution has been rare.

Recently, a number of substances with possible immune-potentiating effects have been investigated in patients with congenital immune deficiencies. Some years ago, we and others[146,147] showed that neutrophil chemotaxis and lysosomal enzyme release were modulated, in part, by cyclic 3',5'-guanosine monophosphate (cGMP) and cyclic 3',5'-adenosine monophosphate (cAMP). Moreover, microtubular polymerization and function appeared to be dependent on the intracellular levels of these cyclic nucleotides. Oliver and Zurier[148] showed that patients with Chediak–Higashi syndrome, who have PMNs filled with large lysozomal granules and that have chemotactic and bactericidal defects, have disordered microtubular function that could be corrected with cGMP or its acetylcholine (ACh). Boxer and co-workers[149] subsequently treated a patient with this disease with ascorbic acid, an agent that has been shown to alter cGMP and cAMP and to alter leukocyte function.[150] Following such treatment, the patient improved clinically and had partial reversal of his in vitro leukocyte function abnormalities. More recently, we have employed moderately high doses of ascorbic acid in several patients with hyperimmunoglobulinemia E, recurrent infections, and defective PMN chemotaxis. We believe, but have not proven, that this syndrome is also the result of an imbalance of cGMP and cAMP resulting from chronic stimulation of the PMN by allergic mediators such as histamine. In several such patients, we have observed rather dramatic results with a marked decrease in infections after in vivo therapy with 1000–2000 mg ascorbic acid per day. In others, no effect has been observed. Thus, as in the other congenital immunodeficiency syndromes that have a variable course, it is extremely difficult to evaluate therapy.

The last agent used for immunopotentiation is levamisole. This agent has been reported to enhance antibody production, increase bloodstream clearance of particles, and enhance monocyte chemotaxis.[151–153] We have shown[154] that the agent alters the levels of cGMP and cAMP within PMNs and markedly enhances the chemotactic response of normal and deficient cells. Preliminary reports[155] have suggested that it may also have an effect in vivo, but, unfortunately, side effects such as agranulocytosis have markedly limited its use.[156]

3. Specific Infections in Immunodeficiency Syndromes

This section reviews the major congenital immunodeficiency syndromes, discusses their major

host-defense abnormalities, and underscores the most common infections that complicate each disorder. The discussion is confined to the most serious and most common etiologic agents in these patients.

3.1. Combined B- and T-Cell Defects

3.1.1. Severe Combined Immunodeficiency Disease

This disease occurs as an X-linked lymphopenic form and as an autosomal-recessive form. The disease is characterized by lymphopenia, a marked decrease in T- and B-cell numbers, low serum immunoglobulins, no antibody responses following immunization, negative skin test reactions, and severe and recurrent infections. Desquamating skin rashes are common and should lead one to suspect immune deficiency if associated with diarrhea, failure to thrive, or pulmonary infiltrates. Most patients become symptomatic within the first few months of life, but a few will do relatively well until 6–9 months of age. Persistent cutaneous *Candida* infection, chronic diarrhea, and failure to thrive should suggest the need for T-cell quantitation or a study of the lymphocyte mitogenic response. Respiratory infection is also very common and may be caused by *Pneumocystis carinii*. A chronic, pertussislike cough is often present and may be associated with tachypnea, retractions, and a markedly decreased arterial P_{O_2} (Pa_{O_2}). When *Pneumocystis* pneumonia is suspected, an open lung biopsy is indicated to confirm the diagnosis since sputum, transtracheal aspirates, or needle aspirates of the lung itself are difficult to obtain in an infant and may lead to false-negative results.[57] It is essential to make an appropriate etiological diagnosis of pneumonia in severe combined immunodeficiency disease (SCID), since other bacterial and viral pathogens may produce very similar findings. To begin treatment without documentation of the etiology usually results in a therapeutic dilemma several days later if the response is less than dramatic. One is then forced to add or subtract antibiotics at random, since routine cultures can no longer be relied on. Therefore, if at all possible, the patient with SCID with severe pneumonia should have an open lung biopsy to define the etiology.

Trimethoprim–sulfamethoxazole is probably the treatment of choice for both children[104] and adults[105] with *Pneumocystis* pneumonia. This combination antibiotic has replaced pentamidine, which had a high reaction rate despite being fairly effective.[105] Hughes and co-workers[104] first reported on the successful therapy of 16 of 20 patients with pneumonia caused by *Pneumocystis*. Subsequently, other investigators have confirmed and extended these results in both children[157] and adults.[105] The recommended dose in children is 20 mg/kg trimethoprim and 100 mg/kg sulfamethoxazole, whereas doses in adults have ranged from 960 to 1200 mg trimethoprim and 4800 to 6000 mg of sulfamethoxazole per day. Survival rates of 80% in children and 83% in adults have been reported in small series compared with an overall reported cure rate of 42% using pentamidine.[158] In general, a response is seen within 2 to 4 days with defervescence of fever if present, lowered respiratory rate, and gradual clearing of the chest radiographs. Therapy is continued for 14–21 days. Pentamidine has been used in common with trimethoprim–sulfamethoxozole in several critically ill patients, but no evidence of a synergistic or additive effect has been observed. Pentamidine preferably should be given intramuscularly and is associated with immediate reactions including hypotension, tachycardia, nausea, and vomiting. In addition, microscopic hematuria, azotemia, granulocytopenia, and hypoglycemia have occurred with its use.

In the patient with severe combined immunodeficiency disease with suspected bacterial pneumonia or sepsis, therapy should initially be broad spectrum and should include an aminoglycoside agent such as gentamicin and ampicillin. Should penicillin-resistant staphylococci subsequently be cultured, then a penicillinase-resistant derivative such as nafcillin or methicillin should be added. In general, the gentamicin should be adequate to cover such organisms initially unless central nervous system infection is present. Later, after the staphylococcal etiology is defined, a combination of nafcillin or methicillin plus the aminoglycoside would be expected to have a synergistic effect against most penicillin-sensitive as well as penicillin-resistant staphylococci.[159]

Systemic candidiasis may also occur in such patients and especially those subjected to hyperalimentation for failure to thrive.[160,161] The presence of one or more positive blood cultures coupled with the presence of *Candida* in the urine or *Candida* lesions in the eye grounds should suggest systemic involvement. The *Candida* precipitin test does not appear to be of value in the very young[162] or in immunocompromised individuals.[90] Therapy should logically consist of low-dose amphotericin therapy with or without flucytosine. This latter agent has the advantage that oral administration results in excellent serum and CSF levels of the drug shortly after therapy is initiated (in contrast to amphotericin).[162] For this reason, I elect to use it in the seriously ill immunodeficient patient, even though a number of *Candida* isolates will be resistant. It should always be combined with amphotericin or other antifungals to prevent the development of resistance. Other agents, miconazole and clotrimazole, have been used with some success in candidiasis in normal individuals and may also be of value in the immune-deficient patient. Ketoconazole also appears to be beneficial.

Disseminated viral infections are also common in patients with severe combined immunodeficiency diseases. Herpes virus, vaccinia, and CMV may produce disseminated disease. Adenine arabinoside in a dose of 15–20 mg/kg per day or Acyclovir may be of value in disseminated herpes virus infection, although few large studies have been carried out in immunodeficient patients. Live virus vaccines should not be given to these individuals as paralytic polio or encephalitis has developed following polio, measles, or mumps vaccines.

Following bone marrow transplant in patients with SCID, graft-versus-host disease often leads to severe infection. Two weeks after transplant, a severe reaction often ensues that is characterized by bloody diarrhea, desquamating skin rash, and abnormal liver function. At this time the patient is most susceptible to overwhelming sepsis and death from enteric organisms, including *E. coli*, *Enterobacter*, *Klebsiella*, and *Pseudomonas aeruginosa*. Broad-spectrum antimicrobial therapy is indicated in such patients when signs of infection develop.

Because of the combined nature of their defect, patients with SCID have a profound defect in antibody production and thus critically need to be supplied with immunoglobulin. γ-Globulin (IM or IV) should routinely be administered (0.6 mg/kg every 3 weeks after a loading dose of twice as much), or plasma therapy may be utilized. This latter therapy or IGIV may prove more useful in the cachectic patient with little muscle mass for intramuscular injections. In addition, it may offer some relief to the patient with severe diarrhea. A parent who is negative for hepatitis antigen would seem to be the most logical donor. Because of the marked propensity of these patients to develop graft-versus-host disease, all blood products should probably be irradiated (3000 rad) prior to administration in order to eliminate immunocompetent lymphocytes.

Permanent reconstitution in SCID is generally attempted after acute infection has been controlled and is best carried out with an HLA-matched sibling bone marrow transplant as indicated earlier.[137] Alternative procedures include fetal liver transplantation with or without fetal thymus transplant.[138-140]

3.1.2. Purine Pathway Enzyme Deficiencies

Patients with defects in their purine metabolic pathways have infections identical to those with SCID described above except they may have later onset and are often somewhat less severe because a degree of immune function remains in some instances.[163-165] The immune deficiency in these patients probably results from the accumulation of substances toxic to the developing immune system because of an enzyme deficiency. Adenosine deaminase and nucleoside phosphorylase deficiencies have both been associated with combined B- and T-cell immunodeficiency or separate B- or T-cell abnormalities.[12] Generally, some immune functions may remain, so that initial symptoms of infection may not appear until 6–12 months of age. Examination of the patients' RBCs for adenosine deaminase or nucleoside phosphorxlase levels is diagnostic, since affected patients' levels are quite low. Serum or urine uric acid concentrations are also quite low because of the purine metabolic block and may be used as a rapid screening test for the disorder.

Therapy for the common infections in these patients would be similar to those reported above for SCID. In addition, these patients may respond with partial immunologic reconstitution to the administration of glycerol-frozen packed erythrocytes containing high levels of the missing enzymes. Immunoglobulin or plasma therapy should also be included when evidence of defective antibody production is present.

3.1.3. Wiskott–Aldrich Syndrome

These patients have as their major host-defense abnormality an inability to make antibody directed at polysaccharide (and to a lesser degree protein) antigens.[50,51] The basic defect is unknown, but many believe it results from abnormal macrophage processing of antigen.[51] Later, these patients seem to lose T-cell function, making this a combined B- and T-cell abnormality. Thrombocytopenia in the 50,000 to 100,000 range often suggests the diagnosis. Infections seldom are a problem until maternal γ-globulin disappears in the infant 4–6 months after delivery. The Wiskott–Aldrich syndrome patient then suffers repeated episodes of otitis media, pneumonia, and sinusitis, mostly caused by *S. pneumoniae* and *H. influenzae*. Polysaccharide-encapsulated enteric organisms such as *E. coli* and *K. pneumoniae* may also be a problem. The most severe infectious problem in the Wiskott–Aldrich patient results from overwhelming sepsis with *S. pneumoniae*. In such individuals, less than 6 hr may elapse between onset of symptoms and death. It is critical that clinicians managing such patients be aware of this and that they inform the patient or the parents of the possible consequences of such infection. Our patients with Wiskott–Aldrich syndrome are cautioned to call us immediately and/or report to an emergency room if they have onset of chills, fever, or other signs of systemic infection. Furthermore, they are instructed to warn the clinician they see of the potential life-threatening nature of their disease. After one such patient died of pneumococcemia on a hurried 4-hr trip in from a rural area, we have started giving large doses of ampicillin or a cephalosporin to such patients to take immediately if they cannot reach a medical facility or physician within an hour. There is no proof that such oral therapy will be beneficial, and it may make subsequent cultures invalid, but the fulminant nature of infection in these patients is the basis for this recommendation. Immediately upon seeing such a patient, I would recommend blood, urine, and CSF cultures followed within minutes by the administration of high intravenous doses of a cephalosporin or ampicillin and chloramphenicol. *Streptococcus pneumoniae* and *H. influenzae* are by far the most likely pathogens so that this combination should cover both ampicillin-sensitive and -resistant strains. Since antibody deficiency is a prime component of this disease as well as shock, I would also give one or two units of fresh-frozen plasma or IGIV to the critically ill Wiskott–Aldrich syndrome patient.

Unfortunately, splenectomy, which greatly aids the thrombocytopenia observed in this disease, may contribute to the incidence of overwhelming infection. Some investigators have been resorting to such therapy in severely symptomatic thrombocytopenia patients, however.[166] These patients have then been placed on oral antibiotic prophylaxis with excellent results.

Less severe acute and chronic infections in Wiskott–Aldrich syndrome patients need to be treated promptly with appropriate antimicrobial therapy to prevent the subsequent development of serious infection and to inhibit the development of local complications such as mastoiditis or osteomyelitis underlying otitis media or sinusitis. I have also seen *S. pneumoniae* meningitis develop in a Wiskott–Aldrich patient in the hospital while undergoing oral therapy for otitis media. These cases serve to point out how serious a problem such infections can be in these individuals and how rapidly they can develop.

Long-term immunotherapy in the Wiskott–Aldrich syndrome cannot be carried out with intramuscular γ-globulin because of bleeding secondary to thrombocytopenia. Moreover, little IgM (which is quite low in these patients) is contained in such preparations. In the severely affected patient with recurrent infections, plasma therapy has been attempted; 10–15 ml/kg every 2–3 weeks may result in a decrease in symptomatic infection.

3.1.4. Ataxia Telangiectasia

These patients develop cerebellar ataxia, telangiectasia (most prominent on the bulbar conjuctiva, nose, ears, and antecubital fossae), and recurrent sinopulmonary infection. Many have depressed skin test reactivity and lymphocyte responses and also may have absent IgA and IgE. chronic sinopulmonary infections with *H. influenzae*, *S. aureus*, and *S. pneumoniae* are common, and bronchiectasis develops in most cases.

Antimicrobial agents should be selected on the basis of nasopharyngeal, tympanocentesis, or sputum cultures and be used on an intermittent rather than continuous basis. Plasma therapy has resulted in beneficial results in several instances.[108,111] Since chronic respiratory infection and failure are often the cause of death in this disease, every emphasis should be made to ensure that adequate pulmonary physiotherapy and postural drainage are accomplished.

3.2. Pure T-Cell Congenital Immunodeficiencies

3.2.1. Cellular Immunodeficiency with Immunoglobulins

Cellular immunodeficiency with immunoglobulins is primarily a T-cell defect, although abnormalities in immunoglobulin synthesis may also occur. These are felt to be secondary to the primary defect in T cells. The disease may be inherited in an autosomal-recessive pattern or may be sporadic and is characterized by failure to develop a thymus. The time of onset of infection varies but is usually between 6 months and 1 year. Recurrent otitis media, monilial diaper rash, and diarrhea are often presenting complaints. Viral infections such as varicella or reactions to live virus vaccines may result in severe disease in these individuals. Gram-negative sepsis with agents such as *E. coli* and *Pseudomonas aeruginosa* or *Pneumocystis pneumonia*[167,168] may result in fatalities. Therapy is similar for these agents to that described for SCID.

As mentioned, these patients may have a deficiency of one or more immunoglobulin classes but, in addition, may fail to make adequate antibodies against T-dependent antigens. For this reason, such patients should receive intramuscular γ-globulin replacement therapy and should receive plasma or IGIV on admission with serious systemic infection.

Thymosin has been used in several patients with this disorder with variable results. One patient was reported to have an increase in T-cell rosettes, positive delayed hypersensitivity skin tests, and a decrease in infectious complications following such therapy.[169] Others have seen little response to this preparation.

3.2.2. DiGeorge Syndrome

This syndrome, which results from abnormal embryologic development of the third and fourth pharyngeal pouches, often results in absence or partial absence of the thymus and a marked deficiency in the T-lymphocyte system. Abnormalities of the aortic arch, the parathyroids, and occasionally the thyroid gland may also occur along with dysmorphic facial features. The diagnosis should be suspected in the presence of seizures, hypocalcemia, and cardiac anomalies in a newborn. Roentgenograms may reveal absence of thymic tissues, and T-cell quantitation will be quite low. Thus, cardiac and parathyroid complications may alert the clinician to the diagnosis before infections occur. Later, chronic mucocutaneous candidiasis, chronic rhinitis, and recurrent pneumonias develop. *Pneumocystis carinii* pulmonary infection is not uncommon. Diarrhea and failure to thrive may also occur. Therapy for these infections is as outlined for SCID.

Although immunoglobulins are usually normal in these patients, there may be some problems in making specific antibodies to T-cell-dependent antigen. Thus, γ-globulin or plasma therapy may be beneficial.

3.2.3. Chronic Mucocutaneous Candidiasis

Chronic mucocutaneous candidiasis probably represents a spectrum of diseases, and, in fact, defective function has been observed at different points in the immune system in different patients. An autosomal recessive pattern has been detected as well as sporadic cases. The disease may also occur in association with multiple endocrine abnormalities including hypoparathyroidism, diabetes mellitus, and Addison disease. Abnormal immune parameters may include (1) decreased skin test and in vitro lymphocyte mitogenic responses to *Candida* and other antigens, (2) a specific defect in skin test and in vitro mitogenic responses to *Candida,* or (3) normal skin test and in vitro mitogenic responses to *Candida* but absent production of migration inhibition factor (MIF) by lymphocytes challenged with *Candida* antigen. We[33] and others[124] have also observed chronic candidiasis in association with both neutrophil and monocyte chemotactic defects.

Infections in these patients are almost entirely limited to candidiasis[12] unless several defects in the immune system are present.[33] Infection is usually confined to the skin and mucous membranes, with systemic involvement being extremely rare. I have seen one case with the granulomatous form of the disease (in which large granulomas develop) in which the patient developed *Candida* endocarditis, and one patient who had associated anorexia nervosa who had a blood culture taken shortly before death that grew *Candida.* Otherwise, *Candida* infection has not been invasive.

Topical therapy with gentian violet, nystatin, or miconazole may be helpful in the patient with limited disease. Applications should be made several times (3–4) daily in a viscous suspension that will hold the antimicrobial agent in contact with the organism for as long as possible. Nystatin suppositories have been most useful in treating both vaginal and oral infections since they are in a viscous, slow-release form. With more severe disease, it is often necessary to use systemic therapy to decrease the overall load of organisms so that immunotherapy or topical antimicrobials may be effective. Amphotericin B, 5-fluorocytosine, and miconazole have been employed with limited success, but it is not clear whether clinical failures have resulted from development of drug resistance that can be documented in vitro. The new antifungal agent ketoconazole appears to be particularly useful in this condition.

Transfer factor as well as thymosin have been reported to cause at least temporary improvement in some patients with chronic mucocutaneous candidiasis[133,135] but cannot be accepted as standard therapy at this time.

3.3. B-Cell Immunodeficiency

Congenital abnormalities of the B-cell system are associated with severe and recurrent infections and may be classified as follows.

3.3.1. Transient Hypogammaglobulinemia of Infancy

A small number of infants have a lag in antibody production that may or may not be associated with some increase in infections.[170] Unfortunately, this condition is grossly overdiagnosed and is often used as the pretext for the inappropriate use of γ-globulin. A study by Buckley and co-workers[170] suggested that most such patients do not have serious bacterial infections and most can make specific antibody when immunized. Such individuals would seldom, therefore, appear to require routine administration of γ-globulin. If the clinician would confine γ-globulin use to those individuals who (1) have IgG levels in the ≤200 mg/dl range, (2) suffer severe and recurrent bacterial infections, and (3) do not produce antibody in response to immunization, then the inappropriate use of this agent would be greatly reduced.

3.3.2. Sex-Linked Hypogammaglobulinemia

This disease, which is X-linked, occurs exclusively in males and is associated with extremely low levels (<100 mg/dl) of IgG, IgM, and IgA, low numbers of B lymphocytes, absent germinal centers in lymph nodes, and a marked decrease in plasma cells. Infections usually begin at 4–6 months of age, when maternal antibody disappears from the infant. Recurrent pyogenic infections including otitis media, sinusitis, conjunctivitis, pneumonia, and sepsis occur and are commonly caused by *S. pneumoniae, H. influenzae, S. aureus, N. meningitidis,* and *P. aeruginosa.*[171,172] Such patients are especially prone to overwhelming infection and usually develop chronic pulmonary disease secondary to recurrent respiratory infections. Initial antimicrobial therapy of the seriously ill patient should be broad spectrum and include an aminoglycoside, a penicillinase-resistant penicillin, and perhaps an agent such as chloramphenicol that would cover ampicillin-resistant *H. influenzae.* Intravenous immunoglobulin (200 mg/kg) or plasma (10–15 ml/kg) should also be administered. More localized acute infections should also be treated promptly. These usually respond to oral therapy with penicillin, ampicillin, cloxacillin, dicloxacillin, or an oral cephalosporin derivative, depending on the results of cultures and sensitivity patterns. Therapy of sinusitis may require 3–4 weeks, whereas otitis will usually respond within 14 days. As described previously, an attempt should be made in immune-deficient patients to determine the etiologic agent and its sensitivity through the use of nasopharyngeal, middle ear fluid, sinus, or sputum cultures.

Prevention of chronic pulmonary disease is dependent on prompt treatment of acute infections as well as attention to pulmonary physiotherapy and drainage. Judicious use of oral antibiotics in treating exacerbations of bronchitis and decreasing purulence in chronic bronchiectasis is also indicated. Oral ampicillin, cephalosporins, or tetracyclines (in the adult) may be utilized.

Although viral infections are not usually a problem in antibody-deficient patients, such patients may develop serious disease from live virus vaccines and also may develop chronic CNS infection with enteroviruses.[173] These may be treated effectively with high-dose intravenous immunoglobulins.

3.3.3. Hypogammaglobulinemia Associated with Hyperimmunoglobulinemia M

This is a sex-linked disorder characterized by normal to increased levels of IgM and IgM-producing B and plasma cells but with low levels of IgG and IgA. The disorder has recently been shown to be due to a primary disfunction of isotype switching.[174] The patients also have neutropenia and thrombocytopenia and may have hemolytic anemias and lymphomas. Antibodies directed against polysaccharide antigens such as isohemagglutinins or opsonins for *S. pneumoniae* and *H. influenzae* are present in serum and are of the IgM variety. Low to absent levels of such antibodies are present in tissue fluids and respiratory and GI secretions, however. These patients, therefore, have respiratory, soft tissue, and GI infections but do not often suffer overwhelming episodes of sepsis. Therapy should be like that described under sex-linked hypogammaglobulinemia (Section 3.3.2) and should include γ-globulin replacement therapy to supply missing IgG antibodies.

3.3.4. Selective IgM Deficiency

This disease is probably of genetic origin, but the exact inheritance pattern has not been elucidated. It is characterized by extremely low levels (<20 mg/dl) of IgM without other detectable abnormalities. Because these patients lack production of IgM antibodies directed against the polysaccharide capsules of many pyogenic bacteria, they tend to have severe systemic infections caused by *S. pneumoniae, H. influenzae,* and *E. coli* as well as other encapsulated pathogens. These often present as sepsis or meningitis and should be treated with broad-spectrum antimicrobial regimens such as gentamicin, ampicillin, and chloramphenicol along with plasma infusions to supply missing IgM. Long-term γ-globulin is not indicated, since commercial preparations contain low levels of this immunoglobulin, and the half-life is quite short.

3.3.5. Selective IgA Deficiency

This immune deficiency is one of the most prevalent abnormalities in the host defense mechanism, occurring in approximately 1 in 700 individuals.[175] These patients usually have absent serum and secretory IgA but normal to only slightly decreased IgA-bearing B cells. There appears to be a terminal block in B-cell differentiation into plasma cells and subsequently a block in actual IgA synthesis. At least one individual has also been described who lacked secretory piece and had undetectable IgA in external secretions but normal serum levels of IgA.[176] Absence of IgA has been found in a number of relatively normal individuals who do not appear to have an increased incidence of infection.[177] Such patients may, however, have an increased incidence of cutaneous, respiratory, and GI allergies, which has led to the speculation that secretory IgA has a major role in preventing absorption of potential allergens. Autoimmune diseases such as rheumatoid arthritis and systemic lupus erythematous (SLE) are also more common in these patients. Other individuals with absent IgA do appear to have recurrent viral and bacterial respiratory infections. These may present as upper respiratory infections, chronic bronchitis leading to bronchiectasis, or pneumonias. Such infections should be treated with antimicrobial agents based on the specific pathogens isolated, and treatment should include strict attention to pulmonary therapy. Allergic therapy for rhinitis or asthma may also greatly benefit certain individuals with IgA deficiency. Plasma has on occasion had a beneficial effect in some of these patients despite the fact that little infused IgA can be demonstrated in external secretions.[178]

Gastrointestinal symptoms are also common in IgA deficiency and often include the development of lymphonodular hyperplasia. Chronic diarrhea secondary to *G. lamblia* is quite common and should be treated.

3.3.6. Common Variable Hypogammaglobulinemia

This immune deficiency is usually classified as acquired; however, studies have indicated a possible genetic basis.[179] This is the most common form of serious immune deficiency that we see. It has its onset several years to several decades after birth and is characterized by a variable incidence of γ-globulin deficiency. Immunoglobulin G is usually low with or without low concentrations of IgM and IgA. Approximately one-third of patients have defective T-cell function, and 25% eventually develop malignancies

including thymomas and lymphoreticular tumors.[2] Respiratory infections including otitis media, sinusitis, bronchitis, and recurrent pneumonias are present in up to 98% of patients.[2] These are usually caused by *H. influenzae, S. pneumonia, S. pyogenes,* and *S. aureus.* Bacteremia and meningitis are less common but do occur. Chronic diarrhea in association with giardiasis occurs in up to one-third of individuals with this syndrome. A number of associated problems such as thyroid abnormalities, achlorhydria, nodular lymphoid hyperplasia, and arthritis are common.

Respiratory infections are managed in a manner similar to that described for sex-linked hypogammaglobulinemia. γ-Globulin replacement therapy is usually beneficial, and plasma may markedly limit chronic diarrhea along with therapy aimed at giardiasis. Pulmonary therapy as well as sinus drainage procedures may be beneficial in preventing long-term sequelae of respiratory infections.

3.4. Complement Component Deficiencies

The complement system represents an important aspect of the humoral portion of the host defense mechanism. Individual components play a major role in bacterial and yeast opsonization (C3b and C5b), viral neutralization (C4b), phagocyte chemotaxis (C3a, C5a, and C567), and lysis of some microorganisms (C6, C7, C8, and C9). Total or partial deficiency of individual components is genetically determined by autosomal inheritance. The homozygous state generally results in serious disease and complete absence of the component, whereas heterozygosity leads to little in the way of symptomatology, but the component is present in approximately one-half the normal concentration.[16-23] Infections in patients with complement deficiencies vary significantly according to the nature of the missing component. The classic complement pathway involving C1, 4, 2, 3, 5, 6, 7, 8, and 9 is triggered predominantly by antigen–antibody complexes. In the absence of antibody, another system, the alternative pathway, which involves properdin, Factor A or C3b, and Factor B or C3 proactivator, is triggered and acts directly on C3 to activate the terminal part of the system. In general, therefore, the classic pathway, which is somewhat more efficient, is important in the immune host, whereas the alternative pathway functions in the individual lacking antibodies. Two of the most important functions of the complement system appear to be to generate chemotactic factors and inflammatory mediators (C3a, C5a, and C567) and to opsonize microorganisms (C3b and C5b).

3.4.1. Early Classic Pathway Component Deficiencies

Deficiencies of Clq, r, s, C2, and C4 do not usually result in an increased incidence of infections, probably because the alternative complement pathway remains intact. Rather these patients suffer from disease that resembles collagen vascular disorders.[180–183] Nephritis is particularly common and may be associated with rashes, Raynaud phenomena, and arthritis. Severe infections occasionally occur, and these may result, in part, from the fact that the alternative pathway is somewhat less efficient than the classic one. Such patients have suffered from meningitis, sepsis, pneumonia, otitis media, paronychia, and sinusitis caused by agents that include *S. aureus*, *S. pneumoniae*, and *Salmonella*. In several cases, there have been underlying conditions that would predispose an individual to infection (including a skull fracture), or the individual suffered only one serious infection. Thus, it is quite difficult to relate unusual or recurrent infections to a deficiency of the early complement components. Of interest is a recent report by Newman et al.[184] in which two patients with C2 deficiency who developed repeated episodes of *S. pneumoniae* sepsis are described. In addition to C2 deficiency, however, both individuals were found to have low levels of Factor B of the alternative complement pathway and deficient functional activity of this pathway. Each of these individuals as well as patients with other early component deficiencies have responded to appropriate antimicrobial therapy without added therapeutic maneuvers.

3.4.2. C3 and C5 Deficiency

As mentioned, C3 and C5 breakdown products play a major role in the host defense mechanism, assisting in immune adherence, opsonization, and chemotaxis and being important as inflammatory mediators. Absence of C3 leads to infections that are

similar to and even more severe than those in patients with hypogammaglobulinemia. Recurrent otitis media, sinusitis, pneumonias, paronychia, and impetigo are common.[17,185] Moreover, sepsis is not uncommon.[17,185] Etiological agents include *S. pneumoniae*, *S. pyogenes*, *Klebsiella*, *N. meningitidis*, *H. influenzae*, and *E. coli*. Of interest is the fact that at least one patient had little response in the way of a leukocytosis despite repeated pyogenic infections. This may be related to the role of C3b breakdown products in releasing bone marrow PMN reserves. In general, these patients have responded well to appropriate antimicrobial agents alone. Initial therapy of the critically ill patient should include agents effective against the organisms listed above. Ampicillin and gentamicin with or without added chloramphenicol for resistant *H. influenzae* would seem appropriate. In the critically ill patient, a unit or two of fresh-frozen plasma might also be of some benefit, especially if shock is present.

Functional deficiency of C5 was initially reported by Miller and associates.[18,186] These infants each had severe seborrheic dermatitis, intractable diarrhea, and recurrent infections with yeast and gram-negative bacilli. All had marked failure to thrive. Normal levels of C5 were detected by immunochemical means in each instance, but the patient's serum did not support phagocytosis of Baker's yeast particles in vitro. Moreover, addition of purified C5 to these sera corrected the defect in opsonization, suggesting that the patient's own C5 was not functionally active. Administration of fresh plasma to these individuals resulted in significant clinical improvement and restoration of opsonic activity in vitro. Thus, this entity became the first complement component deficiency which was found to be at least partially responsive to plasma therapy. Such individuals should be treated, therefore, with appropriate antimicrobial agents or topical antifungal drugs but should also receive a trial of fresh plasma therapy. It should be pointed out that plasma or blood stored at refrigerator temperature for 24 hr or more has little remaining functional C5 and will not correct this abnormality. Miller[187] has subsequently pointed out the similarity between this disease and that described by Leiner[188] and has suggested that these two entities are the same.

Total deficiency of the fifth component of complement has also been described.[19] This patient suffered severe and repeated infections including chronic oral and vaginal candidiasis, infected cutaneous ulcers, subcutaneous abscesses, otitis media, and sepsis. Etiological agents have included staphylococci, *Proteus, Pseudomonas, Enterobacter*, enterococci, and *S. pyogenes*. The patient also had a lupuslike syndrome and Raynaud phenomena. Persistent shedding of cytomegalovirus occurred in her urine. Response to antimicrobial agents was not dramatic, and other therapy was not attempted according to the report. It would seem that appropriate antimicrobial agents combined with fresh plasma therapy might have been of some benefit in this individual and in other patients with this disorder.

3.4.3. C6, C7, and C8 Deficiency

Absence of the sixth, seventh, and eighth components of complement have been reported in man.[20-22] In a recent report, Petersen and co-workers[23] indicated that 13 of 24 patients with absence of one of these components had at least one and usually several episodes of disseminated *Neisseria gonorrheae* or *Neisseria meningitidis* infection. Most had joint or skin lesions associated with dissemination, and few had problems with other infections except for one patient with C6 deficiency who also had four episodes of pneumococcal pneumonia.[20] Associated problems included Raynaud phenomena, sclerodactylia, telangiectasia, ankylosing spondylitis, and SLE. Subsequently, sera from such individuals have been shown to lack bactericidal activity for *Neisseria* species. All patients with disseminated neisserial disease, particularly those with recurrent episodes, should probably be screened for complement component deficiencies using a total hemolytic complement assay. Therapy of the acutely ill patient with such a defect should include high-dose parenteral penicillin, since this would seem to cover most of the pathogens causing serious disease in these individuals.

3.4.4. Alternative Pathway Defects

Absence or deficiency of alternative pathway components may be congenital, developmental, or acquired. Newborn infants, for instance, have low levels of Factor B and impaired nonspecific serum

opsonic activity.[189] This is apparently a developmental problem, since levels subsequently become normal. Patients with the nephrotic syndrome apparently lose Factor B in their urine and, thus, also have defective nonspecific opsonic activity. Congenital deficiency of Factor B has also been described in association with C2 deficiency as mentioned above.[184] Absence of properdin associated with recurrent infections has also been reported.[190] Patients with defects in the alternative complement pathway have in common an unusual incidence of severe and often overwhelming infections. The organisms involved are often polysaccharide-coated ones that can activate the alternative pathway in normal serum and include *S. pneumoniae, Hemophilus influenzae*, and *C. albicans*. The overwhelming nature of the infections in such patients demands that therapy be instituted promptly and be directed toward the organisms mentioned above. A useful adjunct in preventing serious infection might be through the use of vaccines against *S. pneumoniae, H. influenzae*, and *N. meningitidis*.

3.5. Phagocyte Abnormalities

The importance of phagocytes including PMNs, macrophages, and other fixed tissue histiocytes is illustrated best in the individual who has a marked deficiency of these cells. Profound neutropenia with a variety of causes including congenital, autoimmune, toxic, or those associated with malignancy usually result in severe infections and often death. Once the absolute PMN count drops below $500/mm^3$, an increase incidence of infection is observed, and when the level is below $100/mm^3$, one out of four individuals dies of overwhelming infection.[191] Moreover, the infections in these patients are ones not commonly observed in individuals with adequate numbers of phagocytes and include severe gram-negative and gram-positive sepsis, severe pneumonia, perirectal and abdominal abscesses, cutaneous and systemic candidiasis, and *Aspergillus* infection. Many of these patients have normal antibody and complement levels as well as adequate T-cell function but still contract these serious infections, indicating the critical role that phagocytes play in the host defense mechanism against a number of bacterial, fungal, and even viral pathogens.[192,193]

3.5.1. Congenital Neutropenias

Several forms of congenital neutropenia occur which may or may not result in serious infection. These are briefly discussed below.

3.5.1a. Infantile Lethal Agranulocytosis.
this is an autosomal recessive disease associated with a profound neutropenia, eosinophilia, and monocytosis. The bone marrow reveals a striking absence of neutrophilic precursors. Steroids, splenectomy, or other maneuvers have little effect, and the patients suffer severe infections with staphylococci, *E. coli*, *Proteus mirabilis*, *P. aeruginosa*, streptococci, and *Candida* organisms.[194] Despite antibiotic prophylaxis or prompt therapy of individual infectious episodes, death almost always results early in life. It would seem that bone marrow transplantation should be attempted early if an HLA-D-matched marrow donor is available. Knostmann[195] first described these patients in several Swedish families, but similar cases have been described elsewhere.

3.5.1b. Chronic Benign Neutropenia.
This is usually a sporadic disease, but autosomal recessive inheritance has been reported. Unlike the fatal neutropenia described above, these patients have a much milder course.[196] They also have an eosinophilia and often a marked monocytosis, which may help to explain their ability to overcome infections. Bone marrow examination reveals arrest at the myelocyte or metamyelocyte stage. During acute infection, some of these patients appear to be able to mount a neutrophilic response. Infections include cutaneous and deep abscesses caused by staphylococci, streptococci, and gram-negative bacteria, recurrent pneumonias, and mouth ulcerations. Prompt antimicrobial therapy based on the results of aspirate cultures and limited incision and drainage is indicated. In general, these patients do not require therapeutic granulocyte transfusions since they have some neutrophilic response. Moreover, as they grow older, infectious complications become fewer, and most live an essentially normal life span. Initial antimicrobial therapy should include a penicilinase-resistant penicillin and, in life-threatening infections, an aminoglycoside. Oral antimicrobial therapy should be utilized for cutaneous abscesses to prevent dissemination, and limited drainage should be accomplished.

3.5.1c. Neutropenia with Hypogammaglobulinemia with Increased IgM.
As mentioned under antibody-deficiency syndromes, patients with this sex-linked disease have a rather profound neutropenia that contributes to their infectious complications including pneumonias, episodes of sepsis, and occasional cervical adenitis and abscesses. The neutropenia in this disease may be cyclic or constant in nature. Therapy should include IgG replacement but rarely requires white cell transfusion except in the severely ill neutropenic patient.

3.5.2. Chemotactic Defects

A number of individuals suffer severe and repeated infections secondary to phagocyte chemotactic defects. As mentioned, animal studies have shown that a critical 2- to 4-hr period exists during which phagocytes must arrive at the site of microbial invasion if infection is to be suppressed or contained.[122,123] Individuals with chemotactic defects have a variety of infections that are usually confined to the skin, lymph nodes, mucous membranes, and respiratory tract. Staphylococci predominate, probably because they make up a large part of the normal skin flora. Other common pathogens observed in patients with chemotactic defects include streptococci, *Candida albicans*, *E. coli*, and *Trichophyton rubrum*.[24–26,33,124,197] The following disorders are probably congenital and are associated with chemotactic defects and recurrent infections.

3.5.2a. The "Lazy-Leukocyte" Syndrome.
Miller and associates[26] described two patients in 1971 who had gingivitis, recurrent otitis media, rhinitis, and stomatitis. Each was found to have marked neutropenia, but, in addition, PMN random migration and chemotactic function were markedly abnormal. Both patients grew normally, and severe life-threatening infections were not reported. Therapy of such patients would best be directed at the etiological agent involved with oral antibiotics.

3.5.2b. Congenital Ichthyosis.
Subsequently, Miller and co-workers[197] described two kindreds with congenital ichthyosis who suffered chronic, recurrent *Trichophyton rubrum* infections as well as otitis media, recurrent upper respiratory infections, deep abscesses, and generalized impetigo.

Peripheral neutrophil counts were normal as was the random motility of their PMNs. Chemotaxis was markedly depressed, however. Griseofulvin therapy of the dematoses, incision and drainage of abscesses, and oral therapy of otitis media and sinusitis should be reasonably effective in these individuals.

3.5.2c. Hyperimmunoglobulinemia E, Defective Chemotaxis, and Recurrent Infection.

Hill and Quie,[24] Clark and co-workers,[124] and others[33,198,199] have described a whole host of patients with a syndrome of hyperimmunoglobulinemia E, allergic manifestations, recurrent infection, and defective PMN and monocyte chemotaxis. Several aspects of the syndrome including its association with bone disease have recently been reviewed.[200] In at least one report,[33] there appears to be a familial pattern in the inheritance of this syndrome. These patients have usually had severe eczema,[24,33,124,198] although urticaria[201] and allergic rhinitis[202] have also been reported. The infections suffered by these patients vary from multiple superficial cutaneous abscesses to deep-seated abscesses in the buttocks, scalp, or other tissues.[24,33,124,198,201,202] Chronic rhinitis, bronchitis, and otitis media also occur. Furthermore, serious systemic infections such as sepsis and pneumonia have been reported.[201] These are almost always caused by staphylococci, but streptococci and *P. aeruginosa* have also been incriminated on occasion. Chronic cutaneous candidiasis may also be a problem.[33,124] These patients may be related to those described by Buckley and co-workers[203] and are most certainly a variant of Job syndrome described by Davis, Schaller, and Wedgewood.[49] In fact, we studied the original Job syndrome patients, who are red-haired females with severe eczema, hyperimmunoglobulinemia E, and recurrent staphylococcal abscesses, and found them to have a profound defect in chemotactic function. The defect in these patients is not always present and may be related to the release of allergic mediators that can depress PMN chemotaxis.[24,188,201] Of interest are recent[204] findings suggesting that allergen-induced reactions can depress chemotactic function and that several of these patients have high levels of IgE antibody directed against staphylococci, their most prominent pathogen.[205] Thus, in the individual with the appropriate genetic factors, staphylococci may evoke a strong IgE response that, on subsequent challenge, leads to allergic release of mediators, thereby depressing the phagocyte system. Depressed neutrophil chemotaxis has even recently been described in patients with cow's milk or soy protein intolerance.[206] These patients are prone to recurrent respiratory infections.

Therapy of these patients should be undertaken after appropriate cultures are obtained from abscesses, areas of cellulitis, or otitis media. Initial therapy should be directed at staphylococci and streptococci, as these are by far the most common pathogens. In abscesses and localized cellulitis, an oral agent such as cloxacillin usually is sufficient. Limited incision and drainage is often required from which large volumes of purulent material will often be obtained. Healing from such surgical procedures is usually excellent, in contrast to that of the patients with chronic granulomatous disease. Cutaneous *Candida* infection is quite difficult to treat and often requires extremely prolonged therapy with nystatin or clotrimazole. Systemic therapy with coverage aimed predominantly at *S. aureus* is indicated for pneumonia and sepsis in these patients.[201] Nafcillin and gentamicin should be used initially in such patients because of the synergism reported for these agents against both penicillin-sensitive and penicillin-resistant strains.[159] Levamisole is capable of enhancing chemotactic function both in vitro[154] and in vivo[155] in these patients. A recent controlled study with this agent failed, however, to decrease the number of serious infections, even though chemotactic function was increased.[207] More recently, we have observed some response to oral ascorbic acid in several individuals with hyper-IgE and recurrent infections. Following in vitro studies of ours[201] suggesting that histamine H_2-blocking agents might improve chemotaxis in these patients, Mawhinney and associates[208] treated such a patient with 200 mg four times a day of cimetidine. The patient's chemotaxis remained normal throughout the treatment period. Soderberg-Warner et al.[209] recently suggested that trimethoprim–sulfamethoxazole may be useful in preventing infections in these patients.

3.5.2d. Defective Chemotaxis, Neutropenia, and Hyperimmunoglobulinemia A.

Björkstein and Lundmark[210] described four siblings with recurrent bacterial infections, a defect in PMN chemotaxis, neutropenia, eosinophilia, and hyperimmunoglobulinemia A. These patients had recurrent cutaneous abscesses, otitis media, and pneumonia. *Staphylococcus aureus* and *C. albicans* were isolated from cultures and responded to therapy like that described above for the Hyper-IgE syndrome.

3.5.2e. Actin Dysfunction. Boxer and coworkers[211] described an infant with blepharitis, vesicular skin lesions, abscesses, and sepsis with organisms including *S. aureus, C. albicans, S. faecalis,* and *E. coli.* This patient had a profound defect in PMN chemotaxis and phagocytosis and was found to have actin that polymerized poorly after treatment with potassium chloride. The patient eventually received a bone marrow transplant. Subsequent outcome is unknown.

3.5.2f. Monocyte Chemotactic Deficiency. Defective monocyte chemotactic responsiveness has, on occasion, also been observed in the patients with hyperimmunoglobulinemia E. In addition, Snyderman et al.[212] and Gallin[213] have reported patients with chronic mucocutaneous candidiasis who had defective monocyte chemotaxis. In at least one case, transfer factor therapy significantly enhanced function and improved the patient's clinical condition.[213]

3.5.3. Microbicidal Defects

Microbicidal defects in phagocytes also result in serious infections and may lead to rather marked sequelae. The major microbicidal mechanism of the PMN involves the production of toxic oxygen products or radicals including hydrogen peroxide, superoxide, and perhaps singlet oxygen via the hexose monophosphate shunt.[192] Additional factors important in microbicidal activity include the lysosomal enzyme, myeloperoxidase, and a halide.[214] Several defects in this system exist that result in the intracellular survival or even multiplication of bacteria. The specific syndromes associated with microbicidal defects are discussed below.

3.5.3a. Chronic Granulomatous Disease. Chronic granulomatous disease was the first granulocyte defect to be described and have its mechanism elucidated. This disease is usually sex-linked but may occur in autosomal-recessive form or in association with severe G6PD deficiency.[27,215,216]

Following particle uptake, the cells of these patients fail to undergo the respiratory burst, do not activate their hexose monophosphate shunt, and do not produce those toxic oxygen products necessary for microbicidal activity. In the sex-linked form of the disease, this was thought to be caused by the absence of an NADH or NADPH oxidase required to activate the cell. Recent evidence, however, suggests that the abnormality may be due to the absence of cytochrome b that is responsible for electron transfer in the initial stages of the respiratory burst.[206] Glutathione peroxidase deficiency was once believed to be behind the autosomal-recessive form of the disease. It appears that this form may be due to an abnormal, poorly functioning cytochrome b.[217] These patients usually have early onset of recurrent abscesses, especially about the nose and mouth, hepatic abscesses, pneumonias, and osteomyelitis. The organisms involved are either catalase positive or they do not make hydrogen peroxide themselves. *Streptococcus pneumoniae,* group A and D streptococci, and α-streptococci are killed normally by these patients' cells.[218] By contrast, *S. aureus, S. epidermidis, E. coli, Serratia marcescens,* and *C. albicans* are not killed by the PMNs of these patients. *Aspergillus* as well as disseminated bacille Calmette-Guérin (BCG) infection has also been reported in these individuals.[219,220] Fungal infections were found in 20.4 percent of a large series of 245 cases of chronic granulomatous disease.[221] In addition to the infections mentioned, many of these patients have GI symptoms including diarrhea and stomach outlet obstruction because of granulomas. Granulomas also form in the abdomen and urinary tract and can lead to obstruction and additional infectious complications. Infection is usually caused by staphylococci, with *Klebsiella, E. coli, Serratia marcescens, C. albicans, Pseudomonas, Aspergillus, Proteus,* and *Salmonella* also being involved on occasion.

Therapy of these patients can be extremely difficult, since both PMNs and monocytes lack the ability to kill the organisms described. It is essential, whenever possible, to make an etiologic diagnosis by needle aspirate of abscesses, osteomyelitis, liver abscesses, or pneumonias. The use of open biopsies and drainage procedures should be limited because these individuals heal very poorly. I have seen an inguinal incision and drainage site require 6 months to heal even with constant topical care. Moreover, the use of lobectomy in these patients should be greatly discouraged since the patient simply goes on to develop disease in other lobes and then is even more compromised.

Initial antimicrobial therapy in deep-seated bone or tissue infections (sepsis is very rare) should always include a penicillinase-resistant penicillin such as nafcillin. It may be combined with gentamicin for synergism or to cover other enteric gram-negative bacilli. More recently, several investigators have used agents such as rifampin, clindamycin, or chloramphenicol which appear to penetrate WBCs more efficiently.[52,53,222] Such agents have been shown to have better activity in vitro in the presence of PMNs. Therapy must be continued for long periods, especially when incision and drainage are not carried out. After an initial 2–3-week period, oral antimicrobial agents may be substituted for parenteral therapy.

Antimicrobial prophylaxis per se was not recommended in this disease because of the large number of organisms that can be involved and because Candida and other fungal and bacterial pathogens may emerge and cause even more serious infection. Some success has been observed, however, through the use of sulfonamides or trimethoprim–sulfamethoxazole. This agent as well as rifampin and clindamycin are extremely effective in penetrating the cell membrane of PMNs and concentrating within the cell. Chronic use of these agents has been reported to result in some reduction in infectious complications and a slight increase in in vitro PMN bactericidal activity.[130] Granulocyte transfusion therapy has been used on occasion in severe infection, but results, overall, have not been dramatic. In one large study, patients with untreated fungal pneumonia or systemic disease usually succumbed.[221] More than one-half the patients who were treated with appropriate antifungal agents survived, but granulocyte administration had no significant effect.[221] A number of older individuals are now known to have the disease, and it appears that infections become somewhat less severe with age.

3.5.3b. Myeloperoxidase Deficiency.
Hereditary deficiency of the lysosomal enzyme myeloperoxidase has been described in association with Candida infections.[224] In addition, patients with Chediak–Higashi syndrome who have recurrent infections, oculocutaneous albinism, and giant PMN lysosomal granules also have a relative deficiency of myeloperoxidase, since their granules do not readily discharge myeloperoxidase into phagocytic vacuoles. Absence or deficiency of myeloperoxidase results in delayed killing of bacteria and may play a major role in killing yeasts such as Candida albicans. A simple histochemical stain can be used to diagnose this disorder. Infections include those caused by Candida which may be cutaneous or systemic but also may include abscesses caused by S. aureus. Systemic Candida infection should be treated with low-dose amphotericin[225] combined with flucytosine initially, whereas topical therapy with nystatin should control cutaneous infections.

3.5.3c. Down Syndrome.
Patients with Down syndrome may have defective PMN bactericidal activity against Staphylococcus aureus associated with recurrent infections by this agent.[226,227] Nitroblue tetrazolium dye reduction was somewhat less than in controls in these patients, but other metabolic parameters have not been systematically examined. Patients with Down syndrome probably have an increased incidence of staphylococcal abscesses and pneumonia, and this agent should be suspected as the etiological agent in such patients. Therapy with a penicillinase-resistant penicillin should be aggressive. Incision and drainage is often indicated in abscesses.

3.5.4. Neonates with Combined Defects in Chemotaxis and Phagocytosis

Newborn infants have a rather profound defect in PMN and perhaps monocyte chemotactic responsiveness.[228–230] In addition, the PMNs of stressed but not normal neonates also seem to have a defect in oxidative metabolism and intracellular killing.[37,231,232] Thus, the neonate has abnormalities in both major functional activities of the PMN and suffers infections that are compatible with such defects. Cutaneous abscesses caused by S. aureus or gram-negative organisms or cellulitis caused by group A or group B streptococci are not uncommon in such infants. Chronic candidiasis is also quite common and may be related to abnormal PMN function since the T-lymphocyte system is usually normal at this age. Systemic or pulmonary infection with group B streptococci, *E. coli, Klebsiella pneumoniae, S. aureus, H. influenzae, Listeria monocytogenes,* and *S. pneumoniae* may occur and have a very high incidence of morbidity and mortality.[233-238] Such serious infections must be treated early with appropriate antimicrobial therapy which should probably consist of ampicillin or penicillin and an aminoglycoside such as gentamicin. Such a drug combination has synergism against many organisms including group B streptococci and *E. coli,* the most common pathogens isolated. Despite appropriate therapy, however, the mortality rate in neonatal sepsis and meningitis remains quite high. Recently, we have turned to evaluating the results of transfusion of fresh whole blood on mortality in early-onset group B streptococcal sepsis.[239-241] In limited studies, transfusion of relatively large amounts of blood containing antibodies against the infecting organism has dramatically improved survival. Further studies have been carried out in neonatal animals to confirm the efficacy of passive antibody administration in protection and to determine if white cell transfusions will also be of benefit. Experiments indicated that the administration of antibody and functional phagocytes offers significant protection against overwhelming infection in these immune-compromised neonatal animals.[240] These results underscore the importance of the statement attributed to George Bernard Shaw that ''There is at bottom only one genuinely scientific treatment for all diseases and that is to stimulate the phagocyte.''[192] This may be especially true in the congenital immunodeficient patient with infection in whom antimicrobial therapy alone may not suffice.

ACKNOWLEDGMENT. I should like to acknowledge the excellent secretarial assistance of Deborah Camomile.

References

1. Stollerman GH: Immunologic deficiencies in the training of physicians. *J. Chronic Dis* **26**:679–688, 1973.
2. Hermans PE, Diaz-Buxo JA, Stobo JD: Idiopathic late-onset immunoglobulin deficiency, *Am J Med* **61**:221–237, 1976
3. Hill HR: Evaluating the patient with recurrent infections. *South Med J* **70**:230–235, 1977.
4. Hill HR: Laboratory aspects of immune deficiency in children. Pediatr. Clin *North Am* **27**:805–830, 1980.
5. Hill HR: Immunodeficiency diseases. In Stefanini M, Benson ES (eds): *Progress in Clinical Pathology.* Grune & Stratton, New York, 1981, pp. 205–238.
6. Johnston RB Jr, Janeway CA. The child with frequent infections: Diagnostic considerations, *Pediatrics* **43**:596–600, 1969.
7. Johnston RB Jr, Lawton AR III, Cooper MD: Disorders of host defense against infection: Pathophysiologic and diagnostic considerations *Med Clin North Am* **57**:421–440, 1973
8. Dingle JH, Badger GF, Jordan WS Jr: *Illness in the Home.* Cleveland, Press of Case Western Reserve University, 1964.
9. Kretschmer R, Say B, Brown D, et al: Congenital aplasia of the thymus gland (DiGeorge's syndrome). *N Engl J Med* **279**:1295–1301, 1968.
10. Groshong T, Horowitz S, Lovchik J, et al: Chronic cytomegalovirus infection, immunodeficiency, and monoclonal gammopathy-antigen-driven malignancy. *J Pediatr* **88**:217–223, 1976.
11. Lawlor GJ Jr., Ammann AJ, Wright WC Jr., et al. The syndrome of cellular immunodeficiency with immunoglobulins. *J Pediatr* **84**:183–192, 1974.
12. Ammann AJ: T Cell and T–B cell immunodeficiency disorders. In Miller ME (ed): *The Child with Recurrent Infection.* WB Saunders, Philadelphia, 1977, pp. 293–311.
13. Jondal M, Holm G, Wigzell H. Surface markers on human T and B lymphocytes. I. A large population of lymphocytes forming nonimmune rosettes with sheep red blood cells. *J Exp Med* **136**:207–215, 1972.
14. Goldman AS, Goldblum RM: *Primary deficiencies in humoral immunity. In Miller ME (ed). The Child with Recurrent Infection.* WB Saunders, Philadelphia, 1977, pp. 277–291.
15. Hecht F, McCaw BK, Koler RD: Ataxia-telangiectasia-clonal growth of translocation lymphocytes. *N Engl J Med* **289**:286–291, 1973
16. Ballow M, Shira JE, Harden L, et al: Complete absence of the third component of complement in man. *J Clin Invest* **56**:703–710, 1975.
17. Alper CA, Colten HR, Gear JSS, et al: Homozygous human C3 deficiency. *J Clin Invest* **57**:222–229, 1976.
18. Miller ME, Seals J, Kaye R, et al: A familial, plasma-associated defect of phagocytosis: A new cause of recurrent bacterial infections. *Lancet* **2**:60–63, 1968
19. Rosenfeld SI, Baum J, Steigbigel RT, et al: Hereditary deficiency of the fifth component of complement in man *J Clin Invest* **57**:1635–1643, 1976.
20. Leddy JP, Frank MM, Gaitner I, et al: Hereditary deficiency of the sixth component of complement in man. *J Clin Invest* **53**:544–553, 1974.
21. Boyer JT, Gall EP, Norman ME, et al. Hereditary deficiency of the seventh component of complement *J Clin Invest* **56**:905–913, 1975
22. Petersen BH, Graham JA, Brooks GF: Human deficiency of the eighth component of complement. *J Clin Invest* **57**:283–290, 1976
23. Petersen BH, Lee TJ, Snyderman RJ, et al: *Neisseria meningitidis* and *Neisseria gonorrheae* bacteremia associated with C6, C7, or C8 deficiency. *Ann Intern Med* **90**:917–920, 1979

24. Hill HR, Quie PG: Raised serum-IgE levels and defective neutrophil chemotaxis in three children with eczema and recurrent bacterial infections. *Lancet* 1:183–187, 1974.

25. Hill HR, Quie PG: Defective neutrophil chemotaxis associated with hyperimmunoglobulinemia E. In Bellanti JA, Dayton DH (eds): *The Phagocytic Cell in Host Resistance.* Raven, New York, 1975, pp. 249–266.

26. Miller ME, Oski FA, Harris MB: Lazy-leucocyte syndrome. *Lancet* 1:665–669, 1971.

27. Johnston RB Jr, Baehner RL: Chronic granulomatous disease: Correlation between pathogenesis and clinical findings. *Pediatrics* 48:730–739, 1971.

28. Oh MK, Rodey GE, Good RA, et al: Defective candicidal capacity of polymorphonuclear leukocytes in chronic granulomatous disease of childhood. *J Pediatr* 75:300–303, 1969.

29. Curnutte JT, Whitten DM, Babior BM: Defective superoxide production by granulocytes from patients with chronic granulomatous disease. *N Engl J Med* 290:593–596, 1974.

30. Holmes B, Park BH, Malawista SE, et al: Chronic granulomatous disease in females: A deficiency of leukocyte glutathione peroxidase. *N Engl J Med* 283:217–221, 1970.

31. Quie PG, Hill HR: Granulocytopathies. *DM* 1:1–32, 1973.

32. Quie PG: Bactericidal function of human polymorphonuclear leukocytes. *Pediatrics* 50:264–270, 1972.

33. Van Scoy RE, Hill HR, Ritts RE Jr., et al: Familial neutrophil chemotaxis defect, recurrent bacterial infections, mucocutaneous candidiasis and hyperimmunoglobulinemia E. *Ann Intern Med* 82:766–771, 1975.

34. Baehner RL, Nathan DG: Quantitative nitroblue tetrazolium test in chronic granulomatous disease, *N Engl J Med* 278:971–980, 1968.

35. Park BH: The use and limitations of the nitroblue tetrazolium test as a diagnostic aid. *J Pediatr* 78:376–378, 1971.

36. Cheson BD, Christensen RL, Sperling R, et al: The origin of the chemiluminescence of phagocytizing granulocytes. *J Clin Invest* 58:789–796, 1976.

37. Shigeoka AO, Santos JI, Hill HR: Functional analysis of neutrophil granulocytes from healthy, infected and stressed neonates. *J Pediatr* 95:454–469, 1979.

38. Allen RC, Stjernholm RL, Steele RH: Evidence for the generation of an electronic excitation state(s) in human polymorphonuclear leukocytes and its participation in bactericidal activity. *Biochem Biophys Res Commun* 47:679–684, 1972.

39. Allen RC, Yevich SJ, Orth RW, et al: The superoxide anion and singlet molecular oxygen: Their role in the microbicidal activity of the polymorphonuclear leukocyte. *Biochem Biophys Res Commun* 60:909–917, 1974.

40. Stevens P, Winston DJ, Van Dyke K: *In vitro* evaluation of opsonic and cellular granulocyte function by luminol-dependent chemiluminescence: Utility in patients with severe neutropenia and cellular deficiency states. *Infect Immun* 22:41–51, 1978.

41. Rosen H, Klebanoff SJ: Chemiluminescence and superoxide production by myeloperoxidase-deficient leukocytes. *J Clin Invest* 58:50–60, 1976.

42. Shigeoka AO, Hill HR: Recurrent pseudomonas infection

43. associated with neutrophil dysfunction. *Scand J Infect Dis* 10:307–311, 1978.

43. Quie PG, White JG, Holmes B, et al: *In vitro* bactericidal capacity of human polymorphonuclear leukocytes: Diminished activity in chronic granulomatous disease of childhood. *J Clin Invest* 46:668–679, 1967.

44. Ward PA, Cochrane CG, Müller-Eberhard HJ: The role of serum complement in chemotaxis of leukocytes *in vitro*. *J Exp Med* 122:327–346, 1965.

45. Hill HR, Hogan NA, Mitchell TG, et al: Evaluation of a cytocentrifuge method for measuring neutrophil granulocyte chemotaxis. *J Lab Clin Med* 86:703–710, 1975.

46. Cutler JE: A simple *in vitro* method for studies on chemotaxis. *Proc Soc Exp Biol Med* 147:471–474, 1974.

47. Nelson RD, Quie PG, Simmons RL: Chemotaxis under agarose: A new and simple method for measuring chemotaxis and spontaneous migration of human polymorphonuclear leukocytes and monocytes. *J Immunol* 115:1650–1656, 1975.

48. Miller ME: Leukocyte movement—*in vitro* and *in vivo* correlates. *J Pediatr* 83:1104–1106, 1973.

49. Hill HR, Quie PG, Pabst HF, et al: Defect in neutrophil granulocxte chemotaxis in Job's syndrome or recurrent "cold" staphylococcal abscesses. *Lancet* 2:617–619, 1974.

50. Ayoub EM, Dudding BA, Cooper MD: Dichotomy of antibody response to group A streptococcal antigen in Wiskott–Aldrich syndrome. *J Lab Clin Med* 72:971–979, 1968.

51. Blaese, RM, Strober W, Waldmann TA: Immunodeficiency in Wiskott–Aldrich syndrome. *Birth Defects* 11:250–254, 1975.

52. Ezer G, Soothill JF: Intracellular bactericidal effects of rifampin in both normal and chronic granulomatous disease polymorphs. *Arch Dis Child* 49:463–466, 1974.

53. Philippart AI, Colodny AH, Baehner RL: Continuous antibiotic therapy in chronic granulomatous disease: Preliminary communication. *Pediatrics* 50:923–925, 1972.

54. Hahn HH, Beaty HN: Transtracheal aspiration in the evaluation of patients with pneumonia. *Ann Intern Med* 72:183–187, 1970.

55. Hughes JR, Sinha DP, Cooper MR, et al: Lung top in childhood. *Pediatrics* 41:477–484, 1969.

56. Finaldn M: Diagnostic lung puncture. *Pediatrics* 44:471–485, 1969.

57. Wolff LJ, Bartlett MS, Baehner RL, et al: The causes of interstitial pneumonitis in immunocompromised children: An aggressive systematic approach to diagnosis. *Pediatrics* 60:41–49, 1977.

58. Rytel MW: Counterimmunoelectrophoresis in diagnosis of infectious disease. *Hosp Pract* 10:75–82, 1975.

59. Coonrod JD, Rytel MW: Determination of aetiology of bacterial meningitis by counterimmunoelectrophoresis. *Lancet* 1:1154–1157, 1972.

60. Rytel MW: Rapid diagnostic methods in infectious diseases. *Adv Intern Med* 20:37–60, 1975.

61. Hill HR: Rapid detection of specific identification of infections due to group B streptococci by counterimmunoelectrophoresis. In Borodina VM, Meisel MN (eds). *Microbiol 1975 (Vol. 44)* American Society for Microbiology, Washington, DC, 1975, pp. 84–88.

62. Edwards EH, Muehl PM, Peckinpaugh RO: Diagnosis of bacterial meningitis by counterimmunoelectrophoresis. *J Lab Clin Med* **80**:449–454, 1972

63. Smith EWP, Ingram DL: Counterimmunoelectrophoresis in *Hemophilus influenzae* type B epiglottis and pericarditis. *J Pediatr* **86**:571–573, 1975.

64. Ingram DL, Anderson P, Smith DH: Countercurrent immunoelectrophoresis in the diagnosis of systemic diseases caused by *Hemophilus influenzae*, type B. *J Pediatr* **81**:1156–1159, 1972.

65. Coonrod JD, Leach RP: Antigenemia in fulminant pneumococcemia. *Ann Intern Med* **84**:561–563, 1976.

66. Fossieck B Jr, Craig R, Paterson PY: Counterimmunoelectrophoresis for rapid diagnosis of meningitis due to *Diplococcus pneumoniae. J Infect Dis* **127**:106–109, 1973.

67. Coonrod JD, Rytel MW: Detection of type-specific pneumococcal antigens by counterimmunoelectrophoresis. I. Methodology and immunologic properties. *J Lab Clin Med* **81**:770–777, 1973.

68. Ferstenfeld JE, Rytel MW: Fulminating meningococcemia with high serum level of meningococcal capsular antigen. *JAMA* **22**:1301–1302, 1974

69. Greenwood BM, Whittle HC, Dominic-Rajkovic O: Counter-current immunoelectrophoresis in the diagnosis of meningococcal infections. *Lancet* **2**:519–521, 1971.

70. Fallon RJ: *Escherichia coli* K1. *Lancet* **1**:201, 1976.

71. Bartram CE, Crowder JG, Beeler B, et al: Diagnosis of bacterial diseases by detection of serum antigens by counterimmunoelectrophoresis, sensitivity, and specificity of detecting *Pseudomonas* and pneumococcal antigens. *J Lab Clin Med* **83**:591–598, 1974.

72. Hill HR, Riter ME, Menge SK, et al. Rapid identification of group B streptococci by counterimmunoelectrophoresis. *J Clin Microbiol* **1**:188–191, 1975.

73. Portas MR, Hogan NA, Hill HR: Rapid specific identification of group D streptococci by counterimmunoelectrophoresis. *J Lab Clin Med* **88**:339–344, 1976.

74. Wenzel RP, Teates CD, Galapon Q, et al: Acute viral hepatitis in adults: Comparison of the radioimmunoassay and counterimmunoelectrophoresis methods of detecting HBsAg. *JAMA* **232**:366–368, 1975.

75. Cho HJ, Langford EV: Rapid detection of bovine mycoplasma antigens by counterimmunoelectrophoresis. *Appl Microbiol* **28**:897–899, 1974.

76. Pifer LL, Hughes WT, Stagno S, et al: *Pneumocystis carinii* infection: Evidence for high prevalence in normal and immunosuppressed children. *Pediatrics* **61**:35–41, 1978.

77. Myers JD, Pifer LL, Sale GE, et al: Value of *Pneumocystis carinii* antibody and antigen detection for diagnosis of *Pneumocystis carinii* pneumonia after marrow transplantation. *Am Rev Respir Dis* **120**:181–182, 1979.

78. Shackelford PG, Campbell J, Feigin RD: Countercurrent immunoelectrophoresis in the evaluation of childhood infections. *J Pediatr* **85**:478–481, 1974

79. Dorff GJ, Coonrod JD, Rytel MW: Detection by immunoelectrophoresis of antigen in sera of patients with pneumococcal bacteremia. *Lancet* **1**:578–579, 1971.

80. Feigin RD, Wong M, Shackelford PG, et al: Countercurrent immunoelectrophoresis of urine as well as of CSF and blood for diagnosis of bacterial meningitis *J Pediatr* **89**:773–775, 1976.

81. Colding H, Lind I. Counterimmunoelectrophoresis in the diagnosis of bacterial meningitis *J Clin Microbiol* **5**:405–409, 1977

82. Hill HR. Detection of bacterial antigens in meningitis American Society of Clinical Pathology, Check Sample MB 82-3, 1982.

83. El-Refaie M, Dulake C Counter-current immunoelectrophoresis in the diagnosis of pneumococcal chest infections. *J Clin Pathol* **28**:801–806, 1975

84. Michaels RH, Poziviak CS. Countercurrent immunoelectrophoresis for the diagnosis of pneumococcal pneumonia in children. *J Pediatr* **88**:72–74, 1976

85. Sottile MI, Rytel MW. Application of counterimmunoelectrophoresis in the identification of *Streptococcus pneumoniae* in clinical isolates. *J Clin Microbiol* **2**:173–177, 1975.

86. Bradshaw MW, Parke JL, Schneerson R, et al. Bacterial antigens cross-reactive with the capsular polysaccharide of *Haemophilus influenzae* type B *Lancet* **1**:1095–1096, 1971

87. Miller J, Sande MA, Gwaltney JM, et al: Diagnosis of pneumococcal pneumonia by antigen detection in sputum. *J Clin Microbiol* **7**:459–462, 1978

88. Remington JS, Gaines JD, Gilmer MA. Demonstration of *Candida* precipitins in human sera by counterimmunoelectrophoresis. *Lancet* **1**:413–415, 1972.

89. Dee TH, Rytel MW: Clinical applications of counterimmunoelectrophoresis in detection of *Candida* serum precipitins. *J Lab Clin Med* **85**:161–166, 1975

90. Guinan ME, Portas MR, Hill HR: The *Candida* precipitin test in an immunosuppressed population *Cancer* **43**:299–302, 1979.

91. Crowder JG, White A: Teichoic acid antibodies in staphylococcal and nonstaphylococcal endocarditis. *Ann Intern Med* **77**:87–90, 1972.

92. Tuazon CV, Sheagren J: Teichoic acid antibodies in the diagnosis of serious infections with *Staphylococcus aureus. Ann Intern Med* **84**:543–546, 1976.

93. Nagel JG, Tuazon CV, Cardella TA, et al: Teichoic acid serologic diagnosis of staphylococcal endocarditis. *Ann Intern Med* **82**:13–17, 1975.

94. Fisher BD, Armstrong D: Cryptococcal interstitial pneumonia. *N Engl J Med* **297**:1440–1441, 1977.

95. Newman RB, Stevens RW, Goafar HA: Latex agglutination test for the diagnosis of *Hemophilus influenzae* meningitis. *J Lab Clin Med* **76**:107–113, 1970.

96. Zimmerman SE, Smith JW: Identification and grouping of *Neisseria meningitidis* directly on agar plates by coagglutination with specific antibody-coated protein A-containing staphylococci. *J Clin Microbiol* **7**:470–473, 1978.

97. Kaldor J, Asznowicz R, Burst DGP: Latex agglutination in diagnosis of bacterial infections, with special reference to patients with meningitis and septicemia. *Am J Clin Pathol* **68**:284–289, 1977.

98. Edwards MS, Kasper DL, Baker CJ. Rapid diagnosis of type

III group B streptococcal meningitis by latex particle agglutination. *J Pediatr* **95**:202–205, 1979.

99. Nachum R, Lipsey A, Siegel SE: Rapid detection of gram-negative bacterial meningitis by the limulus lysate test. *N Engl J Med* **289**:931–934, 1973.

100. Berman NS, Siegel SE, Nachum P, et al: Cerebrospinal fluid endotoxin concentrations in gram-negative bacterial meningitis. *J Pediatr* **88**:553–556, 1976.

101. McCracken GH Jr: Rapid identification of specific etiology in meningitis. *J Pediatr* **88**:706–708, 1976.

102. Controni G, Rodrigues WJ, Hicks JM, et al: Cerebrospinal fluid lactic acid levels in meningitis. *J Pediatr* **91**:379–384, 1977.

103. Cates KL, Gerrard JM, Giebink GS, et al: A penicillin-resistant pneumococcus. *J Pediatr* **93**:624–626, 1978.

104. Hughes WT, Feldman S, Chaudhary SC, et al: Comparison of pentamidine isethionate and trimethoprim–sulfamethoxazole in the treatment of *Pneumocystis carinii* pneumonia. *J Pediatr* **92**:285–291, 1978.

105. Lau WK, Young LS: Trimethoprim–sulfamethoxazole treatment of *Pneumocystis carinii* pneumonia in adults. *N Engl J Med* **295**:716–718, 1976.

106. Miller ME: Uses and abuses of plasma therapy in the patient with recurrent infections. *J Allergy Clin Immunol* **51**:45–56, 1973.

107. Stiehm ER: Plasma therapy. An alternative to gamma globulin injections in immunodeficiency. *Birth Defects* **11**:343–346, 1975

108. Stiehm ER, Vaerman JP, Fudenberg HH. Plasma infusions in immunologic deficiency states: Metabolic and therapeutic studies. *Blood* **28**:918–937, 1966.

109. Good RA, Page AR: Fatal complications of virus hepatitis in two patients with agammaglobulinemia. *Am J Med* **29**:804–810, 1960.

110. Gelfand SG: Agammaglobulinemia associated with Australia-antigen-positive chronic active hepatitis *Postgrad Med* **55**:263–265, 1974.

111. Ammann AJ, Good RA, Bier D, et al: Long-term plasma infusions in a patient with ataxia–telangiectasia and deficient IgA and IgE. *Pediatrics* **44**:672–676, 1969.

112. Henney CS, Ellis EF: Antibody production to aggregated human αG-globulin in acquired hypogammaglobulinemia. *N Engl J Med* **278**:1144–1146, 1968.

113. Cunningham-Rundles C, Siegel FP, Smithwick EM, et al: Efficacy of intravenous immunoglobulin in primary humoral immunodeficiency disease *Ann Intern Med* **101**:435–439, 1984.

114. Condie RM, O'Reilly RJ: Prevention of cytomegalovirus infection by prophylaxis with an intravenous, hyperimmune, native unmodified cytomegalovirus globulin. *Am J Med* **76**:5134–5141, 1984

115. Mease PJ, Ochs HD, Wedgewood RJ: Successful treatment of echovirus meningoencephalitis and myositis-fasciitis with intravenous immune globulin therapy in a patient with X-linked agammaglobulinemia. *N Engl J Med* **304**:1278–1281, 1981.

116. Fudenberg HH, Spitter LE, Levin AS: Treatment of immune deficiency. *Am J Pathol* **69**:529–535, 1972.

117. Editorial: Chronic sinusitis. *Lancet* **1**:442–443, 1974.

118. Howie VM, Ploussard JH. Simultaneous nasopharyngeal and middle ear exudate cultures in otitis media. *Pediatr Dig* Feb:31–35, 1971.

119. Ament ME: Immunodeficiency syndromes and gastrointestinal disease. *Pediatr Clin North Am* **22**:807–825, 1975.

120. Binder HJ, Reynolds RD: Control of diarrhea in secondary hypogammaglobulinemia by fresh plasma infusions. *N Engl J Med* **277**:802–803, 1967.

121. Hill HR: Clinical disorders of leukocyte function In Snyderman R (ed): *Regul Leukocyte Function: Contemporary Topics in Immunobiology* **14**:345–393, 1984.

122. Miles AA, Miles EM, Burke J: The value and duration of defense reactions of the skin to primary lodgement of bacteria. *Br J Exp Pathol* **38**:79–96, 1957.

123. Miles AA: The acute reaction of injury as an antimicrobial defense. In Thomas L, Uhr JW, Grant L (eds): *International Symposium on Injury, Inflammation and Immunity*. Williams & Wilkins, Baltimore, 1964, pp. 162–182.

124. Clark RA, Root RK, Kimball HR, et al: Defective neutrophil chemotaxis and cellular immunity in a child with recurrent infections. *Ann Intern Med* **78**:515–519, 1973.

125. Horsburgh CR Jr, Kirkpatrick CH: Longterm therapy of chronic mucocutaneous candidiasis with ketoconazole: Experience with twenty-one patients. *Am J Med* **74**:23–29, 1983.

126. Horsburgh CR, Cannody PB, Kirkpatrick CH: Treatment of fungal infections in the bones and joints with ketoconazole. *J Infect Dis* **147**:1054–1069, 1983.

127. Perrin JM, Charney E, MacWhinney JB Jr, et al: Sulfasoxazole as chemoprophylaxis for recurrent otitis media *N Engl J Med* **291**:664–667, 1974.

128. Hardin GM, Ronald AR: A controlled study of antimicrobial prophylaxis of recurrent urinary infections in women. *N Engl J Med* **291**:597–601, 1974.

129. Hughes WT, Kuhn S, Chaudhary S, et al: Successful chemoprophylaxis for *Pneumocystis carinii* pneumonitis. *N Engl J Med* **297**:1419–1426, 1977.

130. Johnston RB Jr., Wilfert CM, Buckley RH, et al. Enhanced bactericidal activity of phagocytes from patients with chronic granulomatous disease in the presence of sulphisoxazole. *Lancet* **1**:824–827, 1975.

131. Ballow M, Dupont B, Good RA: Autoimmune hemolytic anemia in Wiskott–Aldrich syndrome during treatment with transfer factor. *J Pediatr* **83**:772–780, 1973.

132. Wybran J, Levin AS, Spitter LE, et al: Rosette-forming cells, immunologic deficiency diseases and transfer factor. *N Engl J Med* **288**:710–713, 1973.

133. Pabst HF, Swanson R: Successful treatment of candidiasis with transfer factor. *Br Med J* **2**:442–443, 1972

134. Wara DW, Ammann AJ. Activation of T-cell rosettes in immunodeficient patients by thymosin. *Ann NY Acad Sci* **249**:308–314, 1975.

135. Goldstein AL, Cohen GH, Rossio JL, et al: Use of thymosin in the treatment of primary immunodeficiency diseases and cancer. *Med Clin North Am* **60**:591–606, 1976.

136. Polmar SH, Stern RC, Schwartz AL, et al: Enzyme replacement therapy for adenosine deaminase deficiency and severe

combined immunodeficiency. *N Engl J Med* **295:**1337–1343, 1976.

137. Bortin MM, Rimm AA, et al: Severe combined immunodeficiency disease: Characterization of the disease and results of transplantation. *JAMA* **238:**591–600, 1977.

138. Hong R: Thymus transplants: A look to the future. *Birth Defects* **11:**357–360, 1975.

139. Buckley RH, Whisnant JK, Schiff RI, et al: Correction of severe combined immunodeficiency by fetal liver cells. *N Engl J Med* **294:**1076–1081, 1976.

140. Buckley RH: Immunoreconstitution. In Miller ME (ed): *The Child with Recurrent Infection*. WB Saunders, Philadelphia, 1977, pp. 313–328.

141. Thomas FD, Stork R, Clift RA, et al: Bone-marrow transplantation. *N Engl J Med* **292:**832–843, 1975.

142. Levine AS, Siegel SE, Schreiber AD, et al: Protected environments and prophylactic antibodies. *N Engl J Med* **288:**477–483, 1973.

143. Cleveland WW: Immunologic reconstitution in the DiGeorge Syndrome by fetal thymic transplant. *Birth Defects* **11:**352–356, 1975.

144. Ammann AJ, Wara DW, Doyle NE, et al: Thymus transplantation in patients with thymic hypoplasia and abnormal immunoglobulin synthesis. *Transplantation* **20:**457–466, 1975.

145. Kirkpatrick CH, Wells SA, Burdick JF, et al: Effects of fetal thymus transplantation on defective cellular immunity. *Transplantation* **20:**367–369, 1975.

146. Hill HR, Estensen RD, Quie PG, et al: Modulation of human neutrophil chemotactic responses by cyclic 3′5′-guanosine monophosphate and cyclic 3′5′-adenosine monophosphate. *Metabolism* **24:**447–456, 1975.

147. Zurier RB, Weissmann G, Hoffstein S, et al: Mechanism of lysosomal enzyme release from human leukocytes. II. Effects of cAMP and cGMP, autonomic agonists, and agents which affect microtubule function. *J Clin Invest* **53:**297–309, 1974.

148. Oliver JM, Zurier RB: Correction of characteristic abnormalities of microtubule function and granule morphology in Chediak–Higashi syndrome with cholinergic agonists. *J Clin Invest* **57:**1239–1247, 1976.

149. Boyer LA, Watanabe AM, Rister M, et al: Correction of leukocyte function in Chediak–Higashi syndrome by ascorbate. *N Engl J Med* **295:**1041–1045, 1976.

150. Goetzl EJ, Wasserman SI, Gigli I, et al: Enhancement of random migration and chemotactic response of human leukocytes by ascorbic acid. *J Clin Invest* **53:**813–818, 1974.

151. Verhaegen H, DeCree J, Cock WD, et al: Levamisole and the immune response. *N Engl J Med* **289:**1148–1149, 1973.

152. Hoekeke J, Franchi G: Influence of tetramisole and its optical isomers on the mononuclear phagocytic system Effect on carbon clearance in mice. *J Reticuloendothel Soc* **14:**317–323, 1973.

153. Pike MC, Synderman R: Augmentation of human monocyte chemotactic response by levamisole. *Nature (Lond)* **201:**136–137, 1976.

154. Hogan NA, Hill HR: Levamisole enhances PMN chemotaxis and elevates cellular cyclic GMP. *J Infect Dis* **138:**437–444, 1978.

155. Wright DG, Kirkpatrick CH, Gallin JI: Effects of levamisole on normal and abnormal leukocyte locomotion. *J Clin Invest* **59:**941–950, 1977.

156. Rosenthal M, Trabert U, Muller W: Leucocytotoxic effect of levamisole. *Lancet* **1:**369, 1976.

157. Larter WE, John TJ, Sieber OF Jr, et al: Trimethoprim–sulfamethoxazole treatment of *Pneumocystis carinii* pneumonitis. *J Pediatr* **92:**826–828, 1978.

158. Walzer PD, Perl DP, Krogstad PJ, et al: *Pneumocystis carinii* pneumonia in the United States: Epidemiologic, diagnostic, and clinical features. *Ann Intern Med* **80:**83–93, 1974.

159. Watanakunakorn C, Glotzbecker C: Enhancement of the effects of antistaphylococcal antibiotics by aminoglycosides. *Antimicrob Agents Chemother* **6:**802–806, 1974.

160. Curry CR, Quie PG: Fungal septicemia in patients receiving parenteral hyperalimentation. *N Engl J Med* **285:**1221–1225, 1971.

161. Montgomerie JZ, Edwards JE Jr: Association of infection due to *Candida albicans* with intravenous hyperalimentation. *J Infect Dis* **137:**197–201, 1978.

162. Hill HR, Mitchell TG, Matsen JM, et al: Recovery from disseminated candidiasis in a premature neonate. *Pediatrics* **53:**748–752, 1974.

163. Parkman R, Gelfand EW, Rosen FS, et al: Severe combined immunodeficiency and adenosine deaminase deficiency. *N Engl J Med* **292:**714–719, 1975.

164. Stoop JW, Zegers BJM, Hendricks GFM, et al: Purine nucleoside phosphorylase deficiency associated with selective cellular immunodeficiency. *N Engl J Med* **96:**651–655, 1977.

165. Ackeret C, Pluss HJ, Hitzig WH: Hereditary severe combined immunodeficiency and adenosine deaminase deficiency. *Pediatr Res* **10:**67–70, 1976.

166. Lum LG, Tubergen DG, Corasti L, et al: Splenactomy in the management of the thrombocytopenia of the Wiskott–Aldrich Syndrome. *N Engl J Med* **302:**892–896, 1980.

167. Greenberg AH, Ray M, Tsai YT: Thymic alymphoplasia and dysgammaglobulinemia type I. Clinical, immunologic, and pathologic studies of one case. *J Pediatr* **75:**95–103, 1969.

168. Allibone EC, Goldie W, Marmon BP: *Pneumocystis carinii* pneumonia and progressive vaccines in siblings. *Arch Dis Child* **39:**26–34, 1964.

169 Wara DW, Goldstein AL, Doyle NE, et al. Thymosin activity in patients with cellular immunodeficiency. *N Engl J led* **292:**70–74, 1975.

170. Tiller TL Jr, Buckley RN. Transient hypogammaglobulinemia of infancy: Review of the literature, clinical and immunologic features of 11 new cases, and long-term followup. *J Pediatr* **92:**347–353, 1978

171. Bruton OC: Agammaglobulinemia. *Pediatrics* **9:**722–728, 1952.

172. Davis SD. Antibody deficiency diseases. In Stiehm ER, Fulginiti VA (eds): *Immunologic Disorders in Infants and Children*. WB Saunders, Philadelphia, 1973, pp 184–198

173. Wilfert CM, Buckley RH, Mohammakeimar T, et al: Persistent and fatal central-nervous-system echovirus infections in patients with agammaglobulinemia. *N Engl J Med* **26:**1485–1489, 1977

174. Levitt D, Haber P, Rich K, et al: Hyper IgM immunodeficiency. *J Clin Invest* **72**:1650–1657, 1983.

175. Ammann AJ, Hong R: Selective IgA deficiency. In Stiehm ER, Fulginiti VA (eds): *Immunologic Disorders in Infants and Children.* WB Saunders, Philadelphia, 1973, pp. 199–214.

176. Strober W, Krakauer R, Klaeveman HL, et al: Secretory component deficiency: A disorder of the IgA immune system. *N Engl J Med* **294**:351–356, 1976.

177. Ammann AJ, Hong R: Selective IgA deficiency: Presentation of 30 cases and a review of the literature. *Medicine (Baltimore)* **50**:223–236, 1971.

178. South MA, Cooper MD, Wollheim FA, et al: The IgA system. II. The clinical significance of IgA deficiency: Studies in patients with agammaglobulinemia and ataxia–telangiectasia. *Am J Med* **44**:168–178, 1978.

179. Douglas SD, Goldberg LS, Fudenberg HH: Clinical, serologic and leukocyte function studies on patients with idiopathic "acquired" agammaglobulinemia and their families. *Medicine (Baltimore)* **48**:48–53, 1970.

180. Day NK, Geiger H, Stroud R, et al: C1r deficiency: An inborn error associated with cutaneous and renal disease. *J Clin Invest* **51**:1102–1108, 1972.

181. Klemperer MR, Woodworth HC, Rosen FS, et al: Hereditary deficiency of the second component of complement (C'2) in man. *J Clin Invest* **45**:880–890, 1966.

182. Osterland CK, Espinoza L, Parker LP, et al: Inherited C2 deficiency and systemic lupus erythematosus studies on a family. *Ann Intern Med* **82**:323–328, 1975.

183. Gilliland BC, Schaller JG, Leddy JP, et al: Lupus syndrome in a C4-deficient child. *Arthritis Rheum* **18**:401, 1975.

184. Newman SL, Vogler LB, Feigin RD, et al: Recurrent septicemia associated with congenital deficiency of C2 and partial deficiency of factor B and the alternative complement pathway. *N Engl J Med* **299**:290–292, 1978.

185. Alper CA, Colton HR, Rosen FS, et al: Homozygous deficiency of C3 in a patient with repeated infections. *Lancet* **2**:1179–1181, 1972.

186. Miller ME, Nilsson UR: A familial deficiency of the phagocytosis-enhancing activity of serum related to a dysfunction of the fifth component of complement (C5). *N Engl J Med* **282**:354–358, 1970.

187. Miller ME, Kablenzer PG: Leiner's disease and deficiency of C5. *J Pediatr* **80**:879–880, 1972.

188. Leiner C: Uber Erythrodermia desquamativa, eine Eigenartige universelle Dermatose der Brustkinder. *Arch Dermatol Syph* **89**:163, 1908.

189. Hill HR, Hogan NA, Bale JF, et al: Evaluation of nonspecific (alternative pathway) opsonic activity by neutrophil chemiluminescence. *Int Arch Allergy Appl Immunol* **53**:490–497, 1977.

190. Neu RL, Stockman JA III, Spitzer RE, et al: 46,XY/46,XY,21q-Mosaicism in an infant with neutropenia and properdin deficiency. *J Med Genet* **13**:332–334, 1976.

191. Bodey GP, Buckley M, Sathe YS, et al: Quantitative relationships between circulating leucocytes and infection in patients with acute leukemia. *Ann Intern Med* **64**:328–340, 1966.

192. Stossel TP: Phagocytosis. *N Engl J Med* **290**:717–723, 1974

193. Van de Meer JWM, and Van den Brock PJ: Present status of the management of patients with defective phagocyte function. *Rev Infect Dis* **6**:107–121, 1984.

194. Kauder E, Mauer AM: Neutropenias of childhood. *J Pediatr* **69**:147–157, 1966.

195. Kostmann R: Infantile genetic agranulocytosis. *Acta Paediatr* **45**(suppl 105):1–78, 1956.

196. Zuelzer WW, Bajoghli M: Chronic granulocytopenia in childhood. *Blood* **23**:359–374, 1964.

197. Miller ME, Norman ME, Koblenzer PJ, et al: A new familial defect of neutrophil movement. *J Lab Clin Med* **82**:1–8, 1973.

198. Jacobs JC, Norman ME: A familial defect of neutrophil chemotaxis with asthma, eczema, and recurrent skin infections. *Pediatr Res* **11**:732–736, 1977.

199. Dahl MV, Greene WH Jr, Quie PG: Infection, dermatitis, increased IgE, and impaired neutrophil chemotaxis. *Arch Dermatol* **112**:1387–1390, 1976

200. Hill HR: The syndrome of hyperimmunoglobulinemia E and recurrent infections. *Am J Dis Child* **136**:767–771, 1982.

201. Hill HR, Estensen RD, Hogan NA, et al: Severe staphylococcal disease associated with allergic manifestations, hyperimmunoglobulinemia E, and defective neutrophil chemotaxis. *J Lab Clin Med* **88**:796–806, 1976.

202. Hill HR, Williams PB, Krueger GG, et al: Recurrent staphylococcal abscesses associated with defective neutrophil chemotaxis and allergic rhinitis. *Ann Intern Med* **85**:39–43, 1976.

203. Buckley RH, Wray BB, Belmaker EZ: Extreme hyperimmunoglobulinemia E and undue susceptibility to infection. *Pediatrics* **49**:59–69, 1972.

204. Rubin JL, Griffiths RW, Hill HR. Allergen induced depression of neutrophil chemotaxis in allergic individuals. *J Allergy Clin Immunol* **62**:301–308, 1978.

205. Schopfer K, Baerlocher K, Price P, et al: Staphylococcal IgE antibodies, hyperimmunoglobulinemia E and *Staphylococcal aureus* infections. *N Engl J Med* **300**:835–838, 1979.

206. Butler HL, Byrne WJ, Marmer DJ, et al: Depressed nuetrophil chemotaxis in infants with cow's milk and/or soy protein intolerance. *Pediatrics* **67**:264–268, 1981.

207. Donabedian H, Alling DW, Vallin JI: Levamisole is inferior to placebo in the hyperimmunoglobulin E recurrent infection (Job's) syndrome. *N Engl J Med* **307**:290–292, 1982.

208. Mawhinney H, Killen M, Fleming WA, et al: The hyperimmunoglobulinemia E syndrome—A neutrophil chemotactic defect reversible by histamine H2 receptor blockade? *Clin Immunol Immunopathol* **17**:483–491, 1980.

209. Soderberg-Warner M, Rice-Mendoza CA, Mendoza GR, et al: Neutrophil and T lymphocyte characteristics of two patients with the hyper IgE syndrome. *Pediatr Res* **17**:820–824, 1983.

210. Bjorksten B, Lundmark KM: Recurrent bacterial infections in four siblings with neutropenia, eosinophilia, hyperimmunoglobulinemia A, and defective neutrophil chemotaxis. *J Infect Dis* **133**:63–71, 1976.

211. Boxer LA, Hedley-Whyte ET, Stossel TP. Neutrophil actin dysfunction and abnormal neutrophil behavior *N Engl J Med* **291**:1093–1099, 1974

212 Snyderman R, Altman LC, Frankel A, et al. Defective

mononuclear leukocyte chemotaxis: A previously unrecognized immune dysfunction *Ann Intern Med* **78:**509–513, 1973.

213. Gallin JL: Abnormal chemotaxis: Cellular and humoral components. In Bellanti JA, Dayton DH (eds): *The Phagocytic Cell in Host Resistance.* Raven, New York, 1975, pp 227–248.

214. Klebanoff SJ: Myeloperoxidase–halide–hydrogen peroxidase antimicrobial system. *J Bacteriol* **95:**2131–2138, 1968

215. Holmes B, Park BH, Malawista SE, et al: Chronic granulomatous disease in females: A deficiency of leukocyte glutathione peroxidase. *N Engl J Med* **283:**217–221, 1970

216. Gray GR, Klebanoff SJ, Stamatoyannopoulos G, et al: Neutrophil dysfunction, chronic granulomatous disease, and non-spherocytic haemolytic anaemia caused by complete deficiency of glucose-6-phosphate dehydrogenase. *Lancet* **2:**530–534, 1973.

217. Segal AW, Cross AR, Garcia RC, et al: Absence of cytochrome b-245 in chronic granulomatous disease. *N Engl J Med* **308:**245–251, 1983.

218. Kaplan EL, Laxdal T, Quie PG. Studies on polymorphonuclear leukocytes from patients with chronic granulomatous disease of childhood: Bactericidal capacity for streptococci. *Pediatrics* **41:**591–599, 1968.

219. Raubitschak AA, Levin AS, Stites DP, et al: Normal granulocyte infusion therapy for aspergillosis in chronic granulomatous disease. *Pediatrics* **51:**230–233, 1973.

220. Verronen P: Presumed disseminated BCG in a boy with chronic granulomatous disease of childhood. *Acta Pediatr Scand* **63:**627–630, 1974.

221. Cohen MS, Isturiz RE, Malech HL, et al: Fungal infection in chronic granulomatous disease. *Am J Med* **71:**59–66, 1981.

222. Quie PG: Infections due to neutrophil malfunction. *Medicine (Baltimore)* **52:**411–417, 1973

223. Jacobs RF, Wilson CB: Activity of antibiotics in chronic granulomatous disease granulocytes. *Pediatr Res* **17:**916–919, 1983.

224. Salmon SE, Cline MJ, Schultz J, et al: Myeloperoxidase deficiency. *N Engl J Med* **282:**250–253, 1970.

225. Medoff G, Dismicker WE, Meade RH, et al: A new therapeutic approach to *Candida* infections. *Arch Intern Med* **130:**241–249, 1972.

226 Gregory L, Williams R, Thompson E: Leukocyte function in Down's syndrome and acute leukemia *Lancet* **1:**1359–1361, 1977.

227. Rosner F, Kozinn PJ, Jervis GA: Leukocyte function and serum immunoglobulins in Down's syndrome *NY State J Med* **73:**672–675, 1973.

228. Miller ME: Chemotactic function in the human neonate: Humoral and cellular aspects. *Pediatr Res* **5:**587–592, 1971.

229 Klein RB, Fischer TJ, Gard SE, et al: Decreased mononuclear and polymorphonuclear chemotaxis in human newborns, infants, and young children. *Pediatrics* **60:**467–472, 1977.

230. Tono-Oda T, Nakayama M, Uehara H, et al. Characteristics of impaired chemotactic function in cord blood leukocytes. *Pediatr Res* **13:**148–151, 1979.

231. Mills EL, Thompson T, Björksten B, et al. The chemiluminescence response and bactericidal activity of polymorphonuclear neutrophils from newborns and their mothers. *Pediatrics* **63:**429–434, 1979.

232. Wright WC Jr, Ank BJ, Herbert J, et al: Decreased bactericidal activity of leukocytes of stressed newborn infants. *Pediatrics* **56:**579–584, 1975.

233. Hemming VG, McClosky DW, Hill HR: Pneumonia in the neonate associated with group B streptococcal septicemia *Am J Dis Child* **130:**1231–1233, 1976.

234. Headings DL, Overall JC Jr. Outbreak of meningitis in a newborn intensive care unit caused by a single *Escherichia coli* K1 serotype. *J Pediatr* **90:**99–102, 1977.

235 Hill HR, Hunt CE, Matsen JM. Nosocomial colonization with *Klebsiella* type 26 in a neonatal intensive care unit associated with an outbreak of sepsis, meningitis and necrotizing enterocolitis. *J Pediatr* **85:**415–419, 1974.

236 Pickering LK, Simon FA: Reevaluation of neonatal *Hemophilus influenzae* infections. *South Med J* **70:**205–208, 1977.

237. Filice GA, Cantrell HF, Smith AB, et al: *Listeria monocytogenes* infection in neonates: Investigation of an epidemic. *J Infect Dis* **138:**17–23, 1978

238 Bortolussi R, Thompson TR, Ferrieri P: Early-onset pneumococcal sepsis in newborn infants *Pediatrics* **60:**352–355, 1977.

239 Shigeoka AO, Hall RT, Hill HR: Blood-transfusion in group-B streptococcal sepsis. *Lancet* **1:**636–638, 1978

240. Hill HR: Host defenses in the neonate: Prospects for enhancement. *Semin Perinatol* **9:**2–11, 1985.

241. Hill HR: Diagnosis and treatment of sepsis in the neonate. In Root RK, Sande MA (eds). *Septic Shock* Churchill Livingstone, New York, 1985, pp. 219–232.

17

Diagnosis and Management of Infectious Disease Problems in the Child with Malignant Disease

PHILIP A. PIZZO

Among the first questions to be raised in considering the infectious complications that occur in the child with cancer is whether they are different from those found in adults. Are the predominant pathogens, susceptible hosts, patterns of presentation, and response to therapy sufficiently different in children such that age-specific management guidelines are necessary? Does the antigenic naiveté and susceptibility of healthy children to "common" ubiquitous pathogens (e.g., respiratory viruses, herpes viruses, encapsulated bacteria) influence the pattern of infections that occur when a malignancy intercepts the normal process of growth and development? Clearly, infection is a common event during normal childhood, the "average" child experiencing 6–10 febrile illnesses per year. Against this backdrop, an understanding of the types of malignancies that occur during childhood, the modalities used to treat them and their impact on host defenses permits additional insights into the types of infections that might be anticipated. In generating an approach to management, the facts that children may require modifications of the diagnostic techniques used in adults and that therapy must be individualized to the growing child's body weight or surface area are important additional considerations. That the child and adolescent may cooperate with the diagnostic plan or treatment differently from the adult and, importantly, that they may tolerate greater pathogenic burdens as well as therapeutic assaults should also be considered. In this chapter, an attempt is made to highlight some of the features unique to childhood cancers and that may be important to the successful management of the infectious complications associated with them.

1. Cancers of Childhood

There are striking and important differences in the type of malignancies that occur in children as compared with adults.[1,2] For the most part, pediatric cancer can be considered a rare disease. Approximately 6000 new cases of childhood cancer are diagnosed each year in the United States. In spite of this low incidence, cancer is second only to accidents as the leading cause of death in children younger than 15 years of age. Leukemias and lymphomas account for nearly one-half of all pediatric malignancies and are followed by tumors of the central nervous system (CNS) (20%), the sympathetic nervous system, soft tissues, kidney, bone, liver, eye, and germ cells. As a group, pediatric malignancies are characterized by a high growth fraction and a propensity for rapid expansion. In contrast to adults, carcinomas are rare during childhood. Pediatric tumors have unique age

PHILIP A. PIZZO • Pediatric Branch, Clinical Oncology Program, Division of Cancer Treatment, National Cancer Institute, Bethesda, Maryland 20892

TABLE 1. Predominant Pediatric Cancers by Age and Site[a]

Tumors	Newborn (<1 year)	Infancy (1–3 years)	Children (3–11 years)	Adolescents and young adults (12–21 years)
Leukemias	Congenital leukemia AML AMMoL CML (juvenile)	ALL AML CML (juvenile)	ALL AML	AML ALL
Lymphomas	Very rare	Lymphoblastic	Lymphoblastic Undifferentiated	Lymphoblastic Undifferentiated (Burkitt) Hodgkin
Solid tumors				
CNS	Medulloblastoma Ependymoma Astrocytoma Choroid plexus papilloma	Medulloblastoma Ependymoma Astrocytoma Choroid plexus papilloma	Cerebellar astrocytoma Medulloblastoma Astrocytoma Ependymoma Craniopharyngioma	Cerebellar astrocytoma Astrocytoma Craniopharyngioma Medulloblastoma
Head and neck	Retinoblastoma Rhabdomyosarcoma Neuroblastoma PNET	Retinoblastoma Rhabdomyosarcoma Neuroblastoma	Rhabdomyosarcoma Lymphoma	Lymphoma Rhabdomyosarcoma
Thoracic	Neuroblastoma Teratoma	Neuroblastoma Teratoma	Lymphoma Neuroblastoma Rhabdomyosarcoma	Lymphoma Ewing Rhabdomyosarcoma
Abdominal	Neuroblastoma Mesoblastic nephroma Hepatoblastoma Wilms (>6 mo)	Neuroblastoma Wilms Hepatoblastoma Leukemia	Neuroblastoma Wilms Lymphoma Hepatoma	Lymphoma Hepatocellular carcinoma Rhabdomyosarcoma
Gonadal	Yolk sac tumor of testis (endodermal sinus tumor) Teratoma Sarcoma botyroides Neuroblastoma	Rhabdomyosarcoma YST of testis Clear cell sarcoma kidney	Rhabdomyosarcoma	Rhabdomyosarcoma Dysgerminoma Teratocarcinoma, teratoma Embryonal carcinoma of testis Embryonal cell and endodermal sinus tumors of ovary
Exremity	Fibrosarcoma	Fibrosarcoma Rhabdomyosarcoma	Rhabdomyosarcoma Ewing	Osteosarcoma Rhabdomyosarcoma Ewing sarcoma

[a]From Pizzo et al [1]

peaks and some have sex, racial, and geographic predilections. Table 1 lists the predominant pediatric tumors that occur at various stages of development.

In addition to the types of cancers that occur, the second (and perhaps most important) distinctive feature of pediatric oncology has been the enormous therapeutic progress that has been achieved during the last decade. To a large extent, this reflects the general chemosensitivity of childhood neoplasms and the real prospect that cure might be attained with multimodality therapy, particularly combination chemotherapy. Recent analyses confirm that during the last decade, increased numbers (now more than half) of children with cancer are being cured. Thus, a guiding principle in the treatment of pediatric cancers is that no child should be considered to have disease that is so far advanced that treatment for cure could be ruled out.

Since micrometastases are frequent in childhood neoplasms at the time of diagnosis, chemotherapy has become the cornerstone of the therapeutic armamentarium. The drugs used in children are, for the most part, similar to those used in adults. Combination chemotherapy is the rule rather than the exception and, in general, higher dosages of chemotherapeutic agents are employed in children. Outside the newborn period, the tolerance of children to the acute side effects of chemotherapy appears to be greater than that of adults. Thus, many chemotherapeutic regimens in children consist of more intensive and frequent drug administrations, usually with fewer dosage modifications for myelosuppression or infection, than are made in adults. In some childhood cancers, chemotherapy regimens are given over a period of years (frequently 1–3 years), thereby extending the period of risk for immunosuppression and infection.

It has also become increasingly apparent that most pediatric tumors can be divided into "good" and "poor" prognostic categories. While the stage, site, and extent of the cancer have been the traditional methods for classifying patients, additional refinements have been achieved by using tumor histology, immunologic typing, and molecular analysis. Importantly, the identification of risk groups permits therapy to be more appropriately tailored, so that patients likely to do well can receive less intensive (and less toxic) regimens, while the more intensive therapies can be restricted to patients who have a poorer prognosis. This has consequences in planning for the supportive care requirements of children receiving cancer chemotherapy. For example, the risk of developing a fever or infection for good-risk patients (for whom standard dosages of chemotherapy result in periods of neutropenia of less than a week) is generally 0–30%.[3] By contrast, patients undergoing intensive chemotherapy regimens for the treatment of high- (poor) risk malignancies are likely to be rendered neutropenic for 2 or more weeks and have virtually a 100% chance of developing an episode of fever or infection and requiring scrupulous monitoring and care.[4] Indeed, because of the nature of the treatments being given, infection should be considered an expected sequela of the therapy of most childhood cancers.[5,6] Accordingly, skills in the diagnosis and management of these complications are critical for both the oncologist and the infectious disease specialist, particularly if the curative potential of current cancer treatments are to be realized.

2. Interface between Cancer and Infection

Infection and cancer are not infrequently confused before and after the diagnosis of a childhood malignancy. For example, the signs and symptoms heralding the hematopoietic malignancies of childhood frequently include fever and malaise, and the diagnosis of an acute bacterial or viral infection is frequently entertained as the primary cause of the child's symptoms. Similarly, non-Hodgkin lymphoma is not infrequently initially misdiagnosed as infectious mononucleosis, while the lytic bone lesions associated with Ewing sarcoma can be confused with osteomyelitis. Conversely, it should be noted that an infection is occasionally misdiagnosed as a malignancy. For example, histoplasmosis involving the bone marrow has been confused with lymphoma. Acute cryptococcal pneumonia can present in the child with cancer as one or more radiographic nodules and can therefore be misinterpreted as being tumor metastases. It is therefore essential to maintain a heightened index of suspicion; the physician should critically evaluate and obtain appropriate biopsy or aspirate samples for histologic, cytologic, and microbiologic analysis before simply proceeding to treat the patient for an assumed infection or cancer. It is also possible that a malignancy and an infection might have the same etiologic agent. For example, the Epstein-Barr virus (EBV) can cause infectious mononucleosis in normal hosts but in some families may result in a fatal X-linked lymphoproliferative syndrome.[7] Moreover, EBV may be a cofactor, with other infectious agents (e.g., malaria), in the genesis of African Burkitt lymphoma. In light of the recent appreciation that retroviruses can be directly implicated in both malignancy (HTLV-I) and acquired immunodeficiency syndrome (AIDS) and opportunistic infection, the interface among infection, immune deficiency, and malignancy has been more firmly established than ever before.[8]

3. Perturbations of Host Defenses That Contribute to the Risk of Infection in Children with Cancer

While treatment-induced myelosuppression is the single most important and unifying risk factor for both children and adults with cancer, the malignancy itself and the regimens used to treat it may alter other components of the host–defense matrix and, as a consequence, the risk of infection.[9] For example, the child's physical integumentary or mucosal defense barriers can be altered by tumor obstruction (e.g., urinary outlet obstruction secondary to a prostatic rhabdomyosarcoma, defective sinus drainage due to an nasopharyngeal lymphoma) or by the tools for treatment (e.g., indwelling Hickman–Broviac catheters) or the artificial prostheses used in limb-sparing procedures. Moreover, both chemotherapeutic and antimicrobial agents can alter the ease of attachment and the adherence of potential pathogens to mucosal surfaces, thereby facilitating the essential link between colonization and subsequent infection.[10,11]

The cytotoxic chemotherapy used in childhood cancer treatment can adversely affect both B- and T-cell functions, resulting in diminished opsonic activity, inadequate agglutination and lysis of bacteria, and defective neutralization of bacterial toxins. In some children with leukemia, the malignant cells may retain functional (e.g., suppressor) activity and may result in depressed immunoglobulin production.[12] Moreover, we have observed that children with malignancy have lower levels of antibody to the core glycolipid of the Enterobacteriaceae than do normal children and that these antibody levels fall further while patients are receiving cytotoxic chemotherapy.[13,14] In addition, cytotoxic therapy depresses the antibody response of children immunized with viral or bacterial vaccines.

The spleen provides a mechanical filter and an early source of opsonizing antibody. Splenic infiltration is common in childhood leukemias and lymphomas, and the spleen can be a target for infection with both bacteria and fungi (e.g., *Candida*). Splenectomy may sometimes be a component of the diagnostic and therapeutic plan of management (albeit less commonly than in adults), further diminishing the patient's production of antibody, and thus increasing the risk for fulminant infection with encap-sulated bacteria, particularly *Streptococcus pneumoniae*, *Hemophilus influenzae*, and *Neisseria meningitis*. These organisms may also be important in nonsplenectomized children, although it is not clear that their incidence is increased in children with cancer.[15] Of interest, Giebink et al.[16] reported an antibody decline and altered antibody response to pneumococcal vaccine (particularly types 7F, 8, and 19 polysaccharides) in children who were splenectomized because of hereditary spherocytosis or trauma, further emphasizing the role of the spleen in antibody production.

In addition to disease and treatment-related quantitative deficiencies of neutrophils, qualitative abnormalities of phagocyte function can result from cancer and various treatment modalities (e.g., radiation, cytotoxic agents, opiates), further enhancing the risk for developing a potentially life-threatening infection.

Although the balance between the perturbed host defenses and the patient's endogenous and exogenous microbial flora delineates the risk for developing an infection, the degree and duration of neutropenia serves as the common denominator and ultimate equalizer. Thus, children undergoing intensive therapy for solid tumors (with a consequent duration of neutropenia exceeding 2 weeks) have the same risk for developing a serious infection as do patients with hematopoietic malignancies.

4. Fever in Childhood Cancer

Illustrative Case 1

A 15-year-old high school student was in good health until a month prior to hospital admission, when he began to experience pain in his left hip and leg during football practice The pain became increasingly severe during the ensuing weeks and was accompanied by swelling over his left lateral pelvic area, which he attributed to a hit and fall that occurred during the prior week's game. The pain did not improve with rest. During the next 2 weeks, he began experiencing chills and sweats, particularly at night, even though he lacked any symptoms suggestive of an infection. When his parents noted that his oral temperature was 101.8°F (38.8°C), they arranged for him to see his family physician. Examination revealed a firm, warm, and slightly erythematous swelling over the lateral aspect of the left ileum which was tender to palpation. Concerned that he might have an infected hematoma, a cellulitis, or an osteomyelitis, his physician ordered a complete blood count (CBC), erythrocyte sedimentation rate (ESR), blood cultures, and a radiograph of the pelvis Aspiration of the mass was dry, and the Gram stain and cultures were negative Although a malignant process was not suspected initially, the plain radiographs of the pelvis demonstrated extensive destruction of the ileum along with a soft tissue mass. These findings were confirmed on a computed tomograph (CT) scan of the pelvis and a chest radiograph revealed multiple pulmonary nodules. A biopsy of the soft tissue mass confirmed a small round cell tumor, compatible with Ewing sarcoma. No source for fever other than the tumor could be demonstrated. After staging, he was begun on antineoplastic chemotherapy (vincristine, doxyrubicin, and cyclophosphamide), after which his pain improved; the pelvic mass decreased in size, and he defervesced.

Fever has had a long association with malignancy. In the prechemotherapy era, fever was usually attributed to tumor-related necrosis, hemorrhage, or pyrogens.[17] With the advent of chemotherapy, fever in the cancer patient has been more closely linked with infection, especially when the patient is neutropenic. In our prospective review of 1001 episodes of fever in pediatric and young adult patients with cancer at the National Cancer Institute (NCI), the importance of fever was underscored by the fact that nearly one-half of all the patients undergoing cancer treatment we evaluated during the 5-year study period became febrile, frequently necessitating hospitalization for treatment of proven or presumed infectious complications.[18] Approximately 80% of the febrile episodes occurred while patients were granulocytopenic, with polymorphonuclear leukocytes (PMNs) $<500/mm^3$, nearly three-fourths eventually being associated with a clinically or microbiologically defined infection. In contrast, less than 20% of the fevers that occurred in nongranulocytopenic patients could be ascribed to an infectious etiology. In our series, most fevers that occurred in nongranulocytopenic patients took place during the administration of chemotherapy (especially methotrexate, cytosine arabinoside, cyclophosphamide, and actinomycin D). The underlying malignancy itself rarely appeared to be the cause of fever in pediatric patients with leukemias or lymphoma. However, tumor-related fevers occurred more frequently in patients with solid tumors, although this depended on the underlying malignancy (e.g., 14 of 32 patients with Ewing sarcoma had tumor-related fever in contrast to 6 of 47 patients with osteosarcoma or 4 of 24 patients with soft tissue sarcoma), perhaps reflecting the degree of necrosis associated with the malignancy.

5. Primary Causes of Fever and Infection in the Granulocytopenic Child

5.1. Bacteria

When fever occurs in concert with granulocytopenia, or when the granulocyte count is rapidly falling following antecedent chemotherapy, infection must be considered the most likely diagnosis. Of the 793 episodes of fever and granulocytopenia we evaluated, 411 (51.8%) were associated with a defined site of infection at the time of the initial evaluation.[18] While the remaining 382 episodes (48.2%) were initially classified as being unexplained fevers (FUOs), close to one-half of these patients appear to have had occult infections, presumably controlled by the early initiation of empirical antibiotics. Importantly, we observed no difference in the incidence or types of infection that occurred in patients with leukemia, lymphoma, or solid tumors, once they were rendered granulocytopenic. Bloodstream infections, together with infections of the upper and lower respiratory tract, accounted for nearly 65% of these complications. Of note, although the gastrointestinal (GI) tract harbors a multitude of organisms responsible for systemic infection and provides a portal for their potential entry, it served as the primary focus of infection in less than 5% of episodes of fever and granulocytopenia. Similarly, genitourinary tract infections were uncommon (perhaps reflecting the infrequent use of bladder catheters in younger patients), while infections of the CNS were distinctly unusual and were mainly associated with intraventricular shunt contamination or infection. In our analysis, nearly 85% of all initial infectious isolates were bacteria. The pattern of infection was similar in all granulocytopenic patients, regardless of their underlying malignancy. Gram-positive bacteria (particularly *Staphylococcus aureus* and *S. epidermidis*) predominated and accounted for more than one-half of all the bacterial isolates. Of the gram-negative bacteria, *Escherichia coli* and *Klebsiella sp* were most frequent, with *Pseudomonas aeruginosa* being less common. While the specific bacterial isolates responsible for infection in children with cancer appeared to vary from center to center, three factors appear to be shared in common: (1) gram-positive isolates appear to be on the increase, particularly coagulase-negative *Staphylococcus,* most likely as a consequence of the increased utilization of indwelling intravenous catheters; (2) infections due to *P. aeruginosa* appear to be on the decrease, although gram-negative bacilli still remain important causes of infection in children with cancer; and (3) although anaerobes are unusual causes of primary bacteremia in children, they may be important in mixed infections (e.g., perianal cellulitis).

In light of the fact that acute febrile illnesses in young but otherwise healthy children can sometimes be associated with bacteremias, particularly with *S. pneumoniae* or *H. influenzae,* it is surprising that these organisms have not played a more significant role in children with cancer. While pneumococcal or *H. influenza* sepsis certainly can occur in children with cancer, particularly in those who have also been splenectomized, Siber[15] did not observe a significantly increased incidence of infection with these organisms in children with acute leukemia, lymphomas, or solid tumors. Of note, 80% of the pneumococcal bacteremias occurred in association with granulocytopenia.

5.2. Viruses

In otherwise healthy children, viruses account for most acute febrile illnesses and may also account for a number of prolonged unexplained fevers.[19] What role do these viruses play in the primary or secondary infections of children with cancer? As might be anticipated, the frequency of viral isolations depends on the degree to which they are sought. For example, Kosmidis et al.[20] isolated a virus or demonstrated viral serocoversion in 29 of 119 (24%) febrile episodes in children with leukemia. We recently observed that 25% of the throat washings obtained in patients presenting with fever and granulocytopenia were positive by enzyme-linked immunosorbent-assay (ELISA) to common respiratory viruses (15% influenza, 3% adenovirus, 2% parainfluenza).[21] However, patients with positive viral washings could not be distinguished from those with negative washings by their initial presenting symptoms, chest radiograph, fever, or the depth and duration of their granulocytopenia. While these respiratory viruses may have contributed to the patient's fever, the lack of distinguishing clinical features does not clarify the role played by these agents in the genesis of infection or in the management of the fevers which occur in granulocytopenic children.

By contrast, herpes viruses can be significant pathogens for children with cancer. Herpes simplex virus (HSV) can result in serious gingivostomatitis, particularly in patients receiving intensive chemotherapy or undergoing bone marrow transplantation.[22] Of interest, oral or parenteral prophylaxis of high-risk patients with acyclovir appears to reduce the incidence of these infections.[23,24] Cytomegalovirus (CMV) is ubiquitous and can be isolated in the urine or saliva of 27% of children with leukemia.[25] Although CMV can result in extensive organ involvement, its primary target organ is the lung, particularly in patients undergoing allogeneic bone marrow transplantation.[26] CMV is rare in children receiving an autologous bone marrow transplantation, underscoring the importance of graft vs. host disease (GvHD) in the pathogenesis of CMV pneumonitis. To date, the incidence of mortality associated with CMV interstitial pneumonitis in the patient with GvHD has been in excess of 80%.[26-28] Of interest, several recent studies suggest that it may be possible to prevent this infectious complication by passive immunization with hyperimmune CMV antisera or with pooled immunoglobulins.[29,30]

Primary varicella is a major concern for the child with cancer, since the mortality in untreated patients ranges from 7 to 20%, usually because of visceral dissemination to the liver, lung, and CNS.[30] Severe abdominal pain, back pain, or evidence of inappropriate antidiuretic hormone secretion (SIADH) may herald signs of multisystem involvement, indicating the need for prompt therapeutic intervention, usually with acyclovir.[32] An important objective in the care of children with cancer is the prevention of primary varicella. Careful education of the parents, child, and school to avoid exposure to known cases of chickenpox is essential. In order to anticipate and plan for prompt intervention, it is important to know the child's history of varicella (or antibody status) before initiating chemotherapy. If a seronegative child is exposed to varicella, defined by the Centers of Disease Control (CDC) as either a continuous household contact, a playmate contact (generally >1 hr of play indoors), or a hospital contact, varicella–zoster immune globulin (VZIG) should be administered within 96 hr of exposure, preferably sooner.[33] Children who have received ablative therapy regimens associated with bone marrow transplantation should receive VZIG regardless of their prior immune status. Although a preliminary study has suggested that passive immunization with pooled intravenous immunoglobulins may be an alternative to VZIG, definitive data are lacking.[34] Of current interest to the child with cancer is the role of the live-attenuated varicella vaccine. A controlled trial has shown this vaccine to be 100% protective and safe in normal children, and although it is undergoing evaluation in children with leukemia as part of a multiinstitutional study, it remains to be determined how safe this vaccine will be in more intensively immunosuppressed children with cancer and whether antibody titres will remain elevated (and protective) during repetitive and prolonged courses of cytotoxic chemotherapy.[35,36]

5.3. Fungi

In contrast to bacteria and viruses, fungi are infrequently identified when the granulocytopenic child first becomes febrile. With the improved control of bacterial pathogens, however, fungi have emerged as important pathogens, especially in patients with protracted granulocytopenia who have received extended courses of antibiotics. The predominant fungal pathogens are *Candida* (including *Torulopsis*), *Aspergillus,* and less commonly *Cryptococcus* and the Phycomycetes.[37,38] There is considerable institutional variation in the incidence and types of fungal infections that occur. Clusters of *Aspergillis* sinusitis and pneumonitis have been observed, underscoring the importance of environmental exposure (e.g., construction dust, fireproofing material) as well as the critical association between acquisition and colonization in the pathogenesis of infections in the immunocompromised host.[39] An important problem, however, is that even invasive fungal infections remain difficult to diagnose in the granulocytopenic patient, and while colonization can be a helpful indicator, it is far from diagnostic.

Less frequent fungal pathogens in children with cancer include *Trichosporon bigelli, Fusarium solanii,* and *Petryllidium boydii.* Endemic fungi (i.e., *Histoplasma, Coccidioides immitis, Blastomycetes, Cryptococcus*) may be important, depending on the geographic location and exposure of the child.

5.4. Protozoa

Protozoa are infrequent causes of primary fever in children with cancer. Nonetheless, *Pneumocystis carinii* remains an important pathogen, classicially occurring in the child with leukemia who is in remission. It is of interest that the incidence of *P. carinii* pneumonitis is highly variable among different centers and, like *Aspergillus,* clusters of *P. carinii* have been described, suggesting that exogenous exposures, as well as reactivation of latent organisms, may account for some of these infections.[40]

6. Diagnostic Evaluation of the Febrile Child with Cancer

Illustrative Case 2

A 7-year-old child had received actinomycin D and cyclophosphamide a week ago as part of maintenance chemotherapy for a stage II vulvovaginal rhabdomyosarcoma. Even though she had received the same dosage of these drugs twice previously without consequence, this time she felt poorly following her chemotherapy and on the day of admission was noted by her mother to be listless and lethargic. She had no specific complaints and only wished to sleep. Her oral temperature was noted to be 101.5°F (38.6°C). Since both her younger sister and brother had been ill with "colds," her mother's first impression was that her daughter was coming down with a similar illness. However, because she had been instructed to contact her pediatric oncologist for any temperatures above 100.4°F (38°C), she did so and was told to bring her daughter to the hospital immediately for blood counts and evaluation. Since her daughter had had fevers previously, she was a little surprised by the urgency of her summons.

When she arrived at the outpatient clinic, the patient's oral temperature had risen to 102.4°F (39.1°C). Except for lethargy, the physical examination was completely within normal limits. She did not have an indwelling catheter or other foreign body in place. A chest radiograph and urine analysis were both normal, but the patient's total WBC count was 400 per mm³, with an absolute neutrophil count of 121 per mm³. Two sets of blood cultures were obtained, and the patient was admitted to the hospital and was begun on broad-spectrum antibiotic therapy. By the next day, she had become afebrile and was feeling better. Her preantibiotic blood cultures, however, were found to be positive in both sets for *K. pneumoniae.*

The extent and pace of the diagnostic evaluation hinge on whether the child is granulocytopenic (or has a rapidly falling leukocyte count) at the time the fever occurs. In light of the relative infrequency of infection in the nongranulocytopenic patient, the evaluation of these patients should also focus on uncovering noninfectious causes (e.g., drugs, blood products, malignancy) and, in the absence of signs or symptoms pointing to infection, should not be accompanied by immediate empirical antibiotic therapy. An important exception to this is the patient with an indwelling Hickman–Broviac catheter (Fig. 1). We have observed that the incidence of bacteremia is increased nearly 40-fold in nongranulocytopenic patients who have indwelling intravenous catheters. The predominant isolate in such patients is *S. epidermidis*.[41] However, we have also observed a number of nongranulocytopenic children with polymicrobial catheter-associated infections. It is therefore important to obtain blood cultures from both the catheter as well as a peripheral vein when a new fever occurs. It is also important to obtain blood cultures from each of the ports of double or triple lumen catheters, since we have observed some patients in whom only one of the lumens was infected. We currently begin nongranulocytopenic patients who become febrile and who have an indwelling catheter on a combination of vancomycin and gentamicin until the results of the preantibiotic cultures are available (generally 48–72 hr). If the cultures are negative, the antibiotics are discontinued. If the cultures are positive, a full 10–14-day course of antibiotics is given, and the catheter is not removed unless the culture(s) remains positive after 48 hr of antibiotics, or unless they become

positive again after the 10–14-day course of therapy has been completed. It should be noted that if the patient has a double- or triple-lumen catheter, the antibiotics should be delivered through each of the ports, since we have observed treatment failures when this was not done.

Evaluation of the granulocytopenic child in whom a fever develops should focus on uncovering an infectious etiology. Bacteria account for approximately 85% of the new fevers, and since untreated these infections can be rapidly fatal (especially if due to gram-negative bacteria), the guiding principle should be to gather all diagnostic data promptly, followed by initiation of broad-spectrum antimicrobial therapy empirically in order to prevent early morbidity and mortality. Indeed it is of central importance to define and rigidly adhere to established criteria for fever and granulocytopenia that will mandate, without exception, admission to the hospital, immediate evaluation, and the initiation of empiric antibiotic therapy. We define granulocytopenia as fewer than 500 PMNs or bandforms per mm^3, and fever as either a single oral temperature elevation above 101.3°F (38.5°C) or as three oral temperatures above 100.4°F (38°C) during a consecutive 24-hr period. Having identified patients who require hospital admission for empirical antibiotic therapy, the next goal is to attempt to differentiate patients with sites of

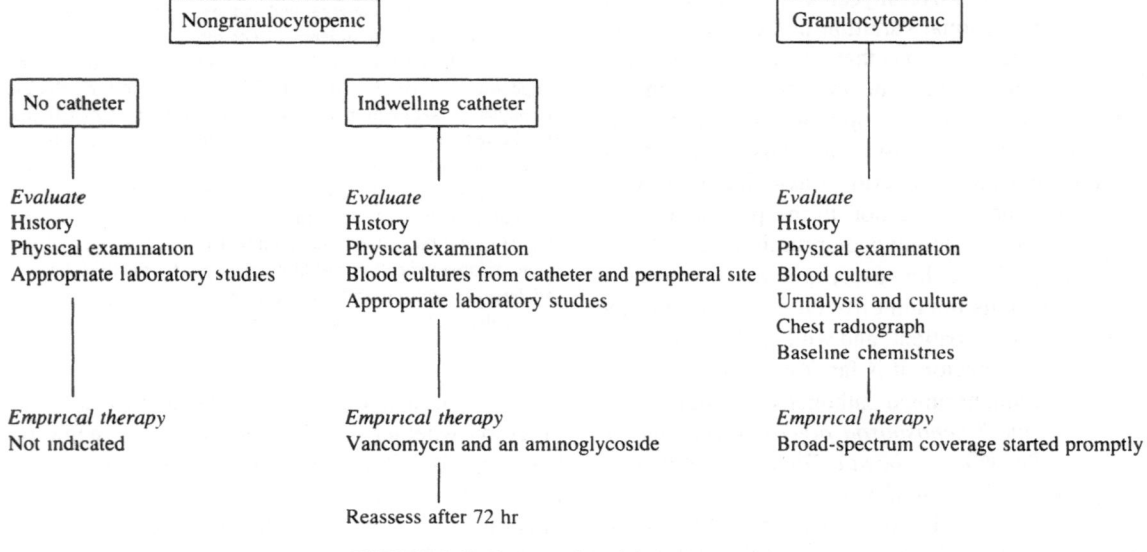

FIGURE 1. Evaluation of the febrile cancer patient

infection that may require additional modifications of therapy. As a guide to initial management, we evaluated 140 consecutive pediatric patients to determine whether any of their presenting signs, symptoms, or pretreatment laboratory findings could be used to differentiate patients who had a bacteremia as the cause of their fever from those whose initial evaluation failed to reveal a clinically or microbiologically defined infectious etiology.[18] However, we were unable to distinguish patients by age; sex; the type, duration, or status of their underlying cancer; the types of therapeutic modalities the patients had received during the prior 6-week period; or the use of invasive diagnostic or therapeutic procedures (e.g., venipuncture, spinal tap, biopsy, surgery) during the week prior to the onset of fever. In this study, we found no difference between bacteremic and nonbacteremic patients in the degree of their presenting neutropenia or lymphopenia. Moreover, physical examination was helpful only if a site of putative infection was discernible. Conversely, the absence of signs or symptoms of infection did not rule out a life-threatening bacteremia (e.g., 55% of patients with a bacteremia had no obvious signs or symptoms of infection). Moreover, some of the classic clinical dictums (e.g., a toxic appearance or a shaking chill) did not correlate reliably with a greater likelihood that a bacteremia would be diagnosed. Thus, the routine clinical and laboratory evaluation may fail to provide data that reliably differentiates patients who might have a serious infection from those in whom an infection process cannot be defined.

Since most infecting organisms arise from the patient's endogenous microbial flora, it is appropriate to question whether surveillance cultures might aid in the clinical management of febrile neutropenic children with cancer. We evaluated the clinical value of serial surveillance cultures of the nose, throat, urine and stool from 271 pediatric patients during 652 episodes of fever and neutropenia.[42] In all, 3470 culture specimens were evaluable. However, the clinical usefulness of these surveillance cultures was limited, since no one particular body site was consistently predictive, and multiple organisms were nearly invariably isolated from the same site, making it difficult to distinguish prospectively the true pathogen(s). Most importantly, these cultures did not alter the initial or the subsequent management of the patients in a manner which would justify their cost effectiveness. Hence, routine surveillance cultures do not appear to be a worthwhile component of the diagnostic repertoire, although selective cultures (e.g., the anterior nares for *Aspergillus*) may be helpful in centers where particular risks from nosocomial infection exist or where monitoring for antimicrobial resistance is being conducted.[43]

If routine physical examination and surveillance cultures are not diagnostically discriminating, are there other tests that can be used to evaluate the child with fever and neutropenia? Although not specifically evaluated in children, transfusion of ^{111}In radiolabeled allogeneic or autologous leukocytes has been investigated in adults to localize occult sites of infections. Although the numbers of neutropenic patients who have been studied are small, the results suggest that this technique may permit the detection of inapparent sites of infection. However, it is unclear whether such findings, in the absence of microbiologic confirmation, contribute to useful changes in patient management. Improvements in culture technique, such as the use of the lysis-centrifugation blood culture methodology (e.g., Dupont Isolator) may increase the yield of certain organisms (e.g., *Candida* sp., *S. epidermidis*) and permits a quantitation of blood culture isolates that may correlate with diagnosis.[44]

In general pediatrics, rapid diagnostic assays, such as ELISA, radioimmunoassay (RIA), counterimmunoelectrophoesis, and Latex particle agglutination) are used to diagnose a variety of common viral and bacterial infections (e.g., *S. pneumoniae, H. influenzae. N. meningiditis*). Unfortunately, these diagnostic techniques have not yet found an application in the rapid detection of the organisms that are of particular concern to the management of the cancer patient (i.e., Enterobacteriaceae, *Candida, Aspergillus*), primarily because they have been associated with an unacceptably high number of false negatives.

Nonspecific correlates of infection have also been used to differentiate between bacterial and viral infection in children. Among these, the C-reactive protein, an acute-phase protein synthesized in the liver in response to infection, may be of help in distinguishing infectious from noninfectious etiologies and may provide a means of assessing the efficacy and response to antimicrobial therapy.[45] This approach requires additional study and confirmation.

What, then, is the appropriate initial evaluation of the child who presents with fever and neutropenia? Since approximately 30–50% of patients will have a focus of infection at the time of their pretreatment evaluation, a careful history and physical examination are clearly important. Moreover, since the patient's signs or symptoms may change over time, it is essential that serial (i.e., at least daily) reevaluation be done, even though the patient may have been placed on empirical antibiotics. While surveillance cultures from asymptomatic body sites are not cost effective in guiding management, at least two sets of preantibiotic blood cultures should be obtained, ideally from separate venipunctures. If the child has an indwelling catheter in place, cultures should be obtained both through the line as well as from a peripheral vein. Also, if the catheter has multiple lumens, each port should be sampled for culture. A pretreatment urinalysis and culture should be obtained, since bacteriuria may occur without pyuria or symptoms when the patient is granulocytopenic. A pretreatment chest radiograph is of help in defining whether an infiltrate is present at the time of presentation as well as serving as a baseline to monitor infiltrate(s) that may appear in association with a rise in the granulocytes or that represent a superinfection. Any accessible lesions suggestive of infection (e.g., cellulitis, skin lesions) should be aspirated or biopsied for microbiologic stains, culture, and histology. Baseline chemistries to monitor organ dysfunction and secondary antibiotic-related toxicity should also be part of the pretreatment evaluation.

7. Is There a Correct Starting Regimen for Granulocytopenic Children Who Become Febrile?

The prompt initiation of empirical broad-spectrum antibiotic therapy to reduce the early morbidity and mortality associated with an untreated infection when the granulocytopenic patient becomes febrile remains as much of a cornerstone of management in the 1980s as it did when it was introduced into clinical practice during the early 1970s. In children, as in adults, combination antibiotic regimens have been the standard of therapy and indeed the only means to provide coverage against the large array of gram-positive and gram-negative bacteria that may be potential pathogens. In addition to the pathogens shared in common with adults (e.g., *S. aureus, S. epidermidis, Streptococcus,* Enterobacteriaceae, *Pseudomonas*), starting regimens in children should also provide coverage for *S. pneumoniae* and *H. influenzae.* In general, effective antibiotic regimens have included a first-generation cephalosporin (e.g., cephalothin, cefazolin) or an antistaphylococcal penicillin (e.g., methicillin, nafcillin, oxacillin), together with either an aminoglycoside (gentamicin, tobramycin, amikacin) and/or an antipseudomonal penicillin (e.g., cabenicillin, ticarcillin, piperacillin). Dosages in children must be based on body weight or surface area; if an aminoglycoside is included in the regimen, serial monitoring of blood levels is an essential aspect of management, both to ensure efficacy as well as to minimize potential nephro- and ototoxicity (Table 2). It should be recognized that to achieve therapeutic levels, the necessary starting dosages for certain drugs (especially aminoglycosides) are higher in children as compared with adults. For example, the starting dosage of gentamicin or tobramycin in the child or adolescent is 6 mg/kg per day compared to 4.5 mg/kg per day in the adult.

A question of current relevance is what impact some of the newer β-lactam antibiotics (e.g., the third generation cephalosporins, the ureido- and piperazine penicillins and the carbapenems) will play in the management of children with granulocytopenia and infection.[46] In their favor is the fact that many of the third-generation cephalosporins (e.g., cefotaxime, ceftizoxime, moxalactam, cefoperazone, ceftazidime) have a very broad spectrum of activity, including the Enterobacteriaceae, *H. influenzae, S. pneumoniae.* Some are also very effective against *P. aeruginosa* (particularly cefoperazone and ceftazidime), while others provide additional coverage against anaerobes (e.g., moxalactam). However, none of the third-generation cephalosporins is as effective against gram-positive bacteria (including *S. aureus*) as are the first-generation cephalosporins, and none is effective against *Enterococcus, Listeria,* or methicillin-resistant *Staphylococcus aureus* (MRSA). By contrast, the third-generation cephalosporins have a longer-serum half-life than other β-lactam antibiotics, they achieve high serum cidal levels against most of the major pathogens and are rela-

TABLE 2. Commonly Used Antimicrobial Agents for Pediatric Cancer Patients

Antibiotic	Trade name	Major indications	Usual daily dosage (IV) (mg/kg)	Daily dosage schedule	Usual maximum dose per day (g)
Penicillins					
Penicillin G	Benzathin Permapen Bicillin	S. penumoniae, S. pyogenes, S. viridens, S. bovis Neisseria, most anaerobes (except B. fragilis)	25–500,000 units/kg	q4h	20
Isoxozyl penicillins					
Methicillin	Staphcillin, Celbenin	S. aureus, Streptococcus	1–300	q4h	12
			1–300	q4h	12
Nafcillin	Unipen		1–300	q4h	12
Oxacillin	Prostaphin, Bactocill				
Aminopenicillin					
Ampicillin	Omipen Principen Polycillin Penbritin	S. fecalis, L. monocytogenes, Hemophilus, E. coli, Salmonella, Proteus	2–400	q4h	12
Carboxypencillins					
Carbenicillin	Pyopen, Geopen	P aeruginosa, Enterobacter, Proteus, Serratia, Acinetobacter, Providentia,	500	q4h	36
Ticarcillin	Ticar	Anaerobes (including some Bacteroides sp., some Clostridium sp., Peptostreptococcus, Fusobacter)	300	q4h	21
Extended-spectrum penicillins					
Mezlocillin	Mezlin	Same as carboxypenicillin plus Klebsiella sp.	300	q4h	21
Piperacillin	Pipercil	Same as mezlocillin plus increased activity against P. aeruginosa	300	q4h	21
Azlocillin	Azlin	Same as piperacillin	300	q4h	21
Cephalosporins					
First generation					
Cephalothin	Keflin	E. coli, Klebsiella, Proteus, Hemophilus, S aureus, S. epidermidis, Streptococcus	170	q4h	12
Cefazolin	Kefzol, Ancef	Similar to cephalothin, more active	50	q6h	2–6

(*continued*)

TABLE 2. (*Continued*)

Antibiotic	Trade name	Major indications	Usual daily dosage (IV) (mg/kg)	Daily dosage schedule	Usual maximum dose per day (g)
		against *Klebsiella*, *E coli*			
Second generation					
Cefamandole	Mandol	More active against *Hemophilus*, *Klebsiella*, *E. coli*, *Enterobacter* sp., *Proteus*, less active against gram-positive cocci	100–200	q4h	6–12
Cefoxitin	Mefoxitin	Same as cephalothin plus *Proteus* sp. and anaerobes (including *B fragilis*)	200	q4h	6–12
Cefuroxime	Zinacef	Similar to cefamandole, Penetrates into CSF	25	q6h	4–5
Third generation					
Cefotaxime	Claforan	Same as cephalothin plus *Enterobacter* sp., indole-positive *Proteus*, *H. influenza*, *Citrobacter* sp., *Serratia* sp., and some *P. aeruginosa* and *Bacteroides* sp	200	q4h	12
Moxalactam	Moxam	Same as cefotaxime but better aneaerobe coverage (including *B fragilis*)	200	q8h	12
Cefoperazone	Cefobid	Same as moxalactam but with better *P aeruginosa* activity	200	q8	12
Ceftizoxime	Cefizox	Same as moxalactam	200	q8	12
Ceftazidime	Fortaz Tazidine Tazicef	Same as cefoperazone but with less anaerobic activity; most active agent against *P. aeruginosa*	100	q8	6
Aminoglycosides					
Gentamicin	Garamycin	*P. aeruginosa*, *Enterobacteriaceae*, *Enterococcus* (with ampicillin)	3–6	q6-q8	

TABLE 2. (*Continued*)

Antibiotic	Trade name	Major indications	Usual daily dosage (IV) (mg/kg)	Daily dosage schedule	Usual maximum dose per day (g)
Tobramycin	Nebicin	Similar to gentamicin (except not as active against *Enterococcus* with ampicillin) Most active for *P. aeruginosa*	3–6	q6-q8h	
Amikacin	Amikin	*Serratia, Proteus, Pseudomonas, Enterobacteriaceae, Providentia*	15	q8–12h	
Miscellaneous					
Chloramphenicol	Chloromycetin	*Hemophilus, B. fragilis, S pneumoniae, Neisseria, Salmonella, Klebsiella*, most anerobes, *Rickettsia*	50–100	q6h	3–6
Erythromycin	Ilotycin gluceptate	*Legionella, Mycoplasma*	30–50	q6h	6
Clindamycin	Cleocin	*B. fragilis, Clostridium, S. pneumoniae, S. viridens, S pyrogenes, S. aureus*	30	q6h	2400
Vancomycin	Vancocin	*C. difficile, S. aureus, S epidermidis, S. fecalis*, multiply resistant *Corynebacterium, S. bovis*	25–40	q8–12h	3
Trimethoprim–sulfamethoxazole (1 : 5 ratio)	Bactrim Septra	*P. carinii, S. aureus, S. pneumonia, S pyogenes, Salmonella, Serratia, Hemophilus, Neisseria*	10–20 as trimethoprim	q8–12h	960 as trimethoprim
Antiparasitic agents					
Pentamidine	Lomidine	*P carinii*	4 (IM)	Once/day q12h	3
Thiabendazole	Mintezol	*Stongyloides*, visceral larva migrans	50		
Antifungal agents					
Amphotericin B	Fungizone	*Candida, Aspergillus, Zygomycetes, Torulopsis, Cryp-*	0 5–1.0	Once/day	

(*continued*)

TABLE 2. (*Continued*)

Antibiotic	Trade name	Major indications	Usual daily dosage (IV) (mg/kg)	Daily dosage schedule	Usual maximum dose per day (g)
		tococcus, Histo-plasma			
5-Fluorocytosine	Flucytosine, Anco-bon	*Cryptococcus, Can-dida, Torulopsis, Chromomycosis*	50–150	q6h	
Clotrimazole	Lotrimin	*Candida* sp., derma-tophytes	50 mg (troches)		
Miconazole	Monistat	*Candida* sp., *Asper-gillus* sp., *Zygo-mycetes, Torulopsis, Cryp-tococcus, Pseudal-lescheria, Blastomyces, Coc-cidioids, Histo-plasma, Paracoccidiodes, Sporothrix*	7–13	q8h	
Ketoconazole	Nizoral	Similar to miconazole	5–10 mg/kg/day (PO)	qd	
Antiviral agents					
Adenosine ara-binoside (ara-a)	Vidarabine	H. simplex, vari-cella–zoster	10–15 mg/kg/day	12-hr infusion	
Acycloguanosine	Acyclovir	H. simplex, vari-cella–zoster	750 mg/m²/day (H. simplex) 1500 mg/m²/day (VZV)	q8h	
Interferons (IF$_\alpha$, IF$_\beta$, IF$_\gamma$)		H simplex	1×10^4 5×10^5 units/kg/day	qid	

tively free of toxicity. In addition, they have good tissue penetration, particularly into the CNS, thereby offering some unique advantages over earlier antibiotics. If, for example, these drugs could be used alone in empirical therapy and still provide effective coverage along with reduced cost and toxicity, they would clearly have an important place in the management of cancer patients.

During the past several years, the third-generation cephalosporins have been studied in both children and adults with fever, granulocytopenia, and/or infection. Investigators have used third-generation cephalosporins together with either an aminoglycoside, an extended-spectrum penicillin (i.e., a double β-lactam combination), or vancomycin. These regimens have been clearly efficacious, although not necessarily more so than standard (and probably less expensive) regimens. Of particular interest, however, is that at least 13 studies have explored the use of third-generation cephalosporins as monotherapy for the empiric management of fever and neutropenia.[46] Most of these studies have been done in adults, although children have been included in some of the trials. Many of these trials have serious deficiencies, and while some have tested inappropriate antibiotics and/or have used questionable control groups, it is notable that 9 of these 13 studies have found that the monotherapy was comparable in efficacy to combination antibiotic regimens.

To test the role of single-drug therapy, five-hundred-and-fifty episodes (half being children) of fever were randomly assigned to either standard combination therapy, consisting of cephalothin, gentamicin, carbenicillin (KGC), or monotherapy with ceftazidime.[47] Both children and adults have been entered into this trial, the patients ranging in age from 1 to 74 years. Several points have emerged from this ongoing trial. First, there has been no difference between the combination (KGC) or the monotherapy group in its efficacy in the early empiric management (i.e., from the time of presentation through 72 hr, at which point the results of the preantibiotic cultures and evaluation are available). Second, patients whose preantibiotic evaluation revealed a defined site of infection or who remained granulocytopenic for a week or more frequently required, over time, the addition of other antibiotics or antifungal agents to their antimicrobial regimen. However, the need for the modification of therapy, predominantly for the addition of a specific antianaerobic agent (e.g., clindamycin), vancomycin, and/or an antifungal agent (e.g., amphotericin B), were comparable for patients who were started on either combination or single drug therapy. Third, for patients whose initial evaluation did not reveal a clinically or microbiologically defined site of infection (i.e., unexplained fever), particularly when the duration of neutropenia was short (i.e., 1 week or less), successful treatment could be accomplished in the vast majority without the need to add to or modify the initial antimicrobial regimen. This is important, since in our study (and in others), 50–70% of all patients who present with an episode of fever and neutropenia will fall into this unexplained fever category. Thus, most patients presenting with fever and neutropenia might be safely treated with a single drug (assuming that the "right drug" was available), thus simplifying their management and reducing the cost of their care.

Thus, it does appear that some of the new β-lactam antibiotics may well have a role in the treatment of both children and adults with fever and neutropenia. From the current data, however, it would seem that the unique advantage of selected third-generation cephalosporins or carbapenems is their potential use as a single agent. By contrast, the combination of a third-generation cephalosporin with an extended-spectrum penicillin or with an aminoglycoside, although effective, is not clearly more efficacious than less expensive antibiotic combinations. Similarly, the combination of a third-generation cephalosporin with vancomycin, while also effective, may be unnecessary for most patients and certainly is a more costly regimen. Thus, it might be appropriate to begin with an effective, but single, broad-spectrum antibiotic with the expectation that in some patients, particularly those who remain granulocytopenic for protracted periods, additions or modifications of therapy might be necessary.

8. When Is It Appropriate to Modify the Initial Empirical Antibiotic Regimen?

The neutropenic cancer patient is best considered to be in a state of dynamic instability. As the period of neutropenia continues, particularly for patients already receiving antibiotics, the risk of second infections or superinfections increases. Accordingly, the persistence of fever or the onset of a new fever or sites of infection after the initiation of an empirical antibiotic regimen may mean that a second infectious process has emerged. We have observed that the incidence of such complications correlates with the duration of the patient's neutropenia. For example, we reviewed 590 episodes of fever and neutropenia presenting during 1979–1984. The initial evaluation in each of these 590 episodes failed to reveal a clinically or microbiologically defined focus of infection (i.e., FUOs), and the goal of management was simply to support the patient empirically until the neutropenia resolved. The risk period for such patients can be subdivided into low, (meaning that the patient was neutropenic for 1 week or less) or high (meaning that the duration of neutropenia exceeded 1 week and in some cases 2 weeks). We observed that 331 (56%) of the FUO episodes fell into the low-risk groups and that additions or modifications of the primary antibiotic regimen were rarely necessary (<4% of cases). However, as the duration of neutropenia lengthened, so did the need for modifications of the patient's

TABLE 3. Modifications of Therapy

Clinical event	Possible modifications of therapy
Breakthrough bacteremia	If gram-positive isolate (e.g., *S. epidermidis*), add vancomycin If gram-negative isolate (i.e., presumably resistant), switch to new regimen
Catheter-associated infection	Add vancomycin (as well as gram-negative coverage if not already being given)
Severe oral mucositis or necrotizing gingivitis	Add specific antianaerobic agent (e.g., clindamycin or metronidazole)
Esophagitis	Trial of oral clotrimazole, ketoconazole, or IV amphotericin B
Pneumonitis Diffuse or interstitial	Trial of trimethoprim–sulfamethoxazole and erythromycin (plus broad-spectrum antibiotics if the patient is granulocytopenic)
New infiltrate in a granulocytopenic patient also receiving antibiotics	If granulocyte count is rising, watch and wait If granulocyte count is not recovering, biopsy to establish diagnosis, if biopsy cannot be done, add amphotericin B empirically
Perianal tenderness	If patient is already receiving broad-spectrum antibiotics, add a specific antianaerobic agent If patient is not on antibiotics, begin broad-spectrum therapy with anaerobic coverage
Persistent fever and neutropenia	Continue antibiotics and after 1 week of persistent fever and neutropenia; add systemic antifungal therapy empirically

initial empirical regimen. For example, 19% of the 166 FUO episodes remaining neutropenic for 1–2 weeks required some modification of their antimicrobial regimen, while 65% of those who were neutropenic for 2 or more weeks needed such a modification. However, the fact that greater than 97% of these patients survived, regardless of the duration of

neutropenia or the number of the therapeutic modification required, suggests that an aggressive and flexible management plan is essential in patients with protracted periods of neutropenia. Table 3 illustrates examples of how therapeutic additions or modifications might be integrated into the management plan. The rationale or data to support some of these modifications are considered in greater detail.

9. If a Microbial Isolate Is Identified and the Antibiotic Sensitivities Are Known, Should the Antibiotic Spectrum Be Narrowed?

Illustrative Case 3

A 10-year-old child with acute myelogenous leukemia (AML) became febrile and neutropenic 10 days following his second induction cycle of daunomycin and cytosine arabinoside. He was readmitted to the hospital, where a physical examination was unrevealing and a chest radiograph was unremarkable Nonetheless, because he met the criteria for fever (see Section 6) he was begun on empirical broad-spectrum antibiotics with cephalothin, gentamicin, and carbenicillin. Two days later, his preantibiotic blood cultures were found to be growing *S. aureus* in two separate sets. He had defervesced after beginning antibiotics, and all the blood cultures obtained since then were negative. He was feeling well and had an unremarkable cardiac and musculoskeletal examination. It was therefore elected to narrow the spectrum of his antibiotics to intravenous oxacillin. On this regimen, the patient continued to do well until 4 days later, when he became febrile again, 103.3°F (39 6°C). The physical examination was still unremarkable and the patient did not note any specific complaints. He was, however, still profoundly neutropenic (total granulocyte count was less than 100 per mm³). He had two sets of blood cultures obtained, a urinalysis, and a chest radiograph. Because of his new fever in concert with continued neutropenia, the antibiotic regimen was broadened by the addition of an aminoglycoside and antipseudomonal penicillin. By the next day, the patient was again afebrile, and blood cultures prior to the change in antibiotics were found to be positive for *E. coli*. He remained on broad-spectrum therapy for an additional 14 days, at which time his granulocytopenia also resolved.

In a previous retrospective study, we evaluated 78 neutropenic pediatric patients who had a gram-positive bacteremia (predominantly *S. aureus*) and who were treated with either a narrow-spectrum antibiotic (e.g., oxacillin, nafcillin) or a broad-spectrum combination of antibiotics.[48] Patients who were neutropenic for less than 1 week (i.e., low-risk) did well regardless of whether their antibiotic spectrum was narrowed or remained broad. However, if the patient remained neutropenic beyond 1 week (i.e., high-risk), second infections were observed in 47% of the patients whose antibiotic spectrum had been narrowed. Since these second infections were all due to gram-negative bacteria, we had concluded that the continuation of broad-spectrum antibiotics in patients with prolonged neutropenia might be providing a systemic prophylaxis in addition to effective therapy for the primary infection. However, because this study was retrospective, we sought to confirm these results in a prospective randomized trial.[49] In the prospective study, patients with a documented infection have been randomized to receive either pathogen-specific or broad-spectrum therapy once their antibiotic sensitivities were available. Of 46 evaluable episodes, new fevers or second infections were observed in 11 of 20 (55%) of the episodes randomized to pathogen-specific therapy compared with 12 of 25 (40%) of those randomized to continue broad-spectrum antibiotics. There was no difference in mortality, although a greater percentage of patients randomized to pathogen-specific therapy (45%) required a modification of their antimicrobial regimen compared with patients randomized to continue receiving broad-spectrum antibiotics (27%). Thus, it seems reasonable to narrow the antibiotic spectrum, as long as the potential need for additional therapy is recognized and the patient is monitored appropriately.

10. If the Patient Has a Bacteremia and Also Has an Indwelling Catheter, Are Additional Modifications of Therapy Necessary?

Illustrative Case 4

An 11-year-old youngster was receiving an adjuvant chemotherapy regimen for osteosarcoma that required frequent intravenous treatment. Because venous access was a problem, a double-lumen Hickman catheter had been placed 2 months earlier. Both the patient and her mother did the daily care procedures in a meticulous manner. On the day of admission, the patient had suddenly became febrile to 102.4°F (39.1°C) orally along with a chill. She was taken to the outpatient clinic, where her physical examination was unremarkable. In particular, the exit site and subcutaneous tunnel of the Hickman catheter were nontender and without erythema or induration. A chest radiograph was also within normal limits and her WBC count was 6700/mm³, with 68%

PMNs. Blood cultures were obtained from both ports of the Hickman catheter and from a peripheral vein. Even though she was non-neutropenic, because of her new fever and the fact that she had a Hickman catheter, it was elected to admit her to the hospital and begin her on parenteral vancomycin and gentamicin. The next day, the blood cultures from the red port was growing a gram-positive coccus (later identified as a *S. epidermidis*) as well as a lactose-fermenting gram-negative rod (subsequently identified as an *E. coli*). The blood culture drawn from a peripheral vein was also growing these same two organisms, although in a lower colony count. The other (i.e., brown Hickman port) cultures, however, were negative. Although the preliminary sensitivities suggested that the organisms were sensitive to these antibiotics, the patient remained febrile, and blood culture obtained after 24 hr of antibiotics revealed that the red port was still positive for the same two organisms, although the cultures obtained from a peripheral vein had become negative. While a decision to remove the Hickman catheter was seriously entertained, it was determined that the antibiotics had only been delivered to the brown (i.e., the uninfected port) and not into the red port. It was elected to continue with a trial of antibiotics, assured that they were rotated to both catheter lumens. Within 1 day of this change, the patient defervesced and all subsequent blood cultures remained negative. She completed a 14-day course of therapy without further consequence and did not have the Hickman catheter removed.

Indwelling right atrial (Hickman–Broviac) catheters, initially designed for home parenteral nutrition, are being used increasingly to provide venous access for the delivery of chemotherapy to children with cancer. Double- and triple-lumen catheters also permit repeated blood sampling and can even provide a means of intensive monitoring of patients. Conversely, these foreign bodies provide a nidus for local infection and a portal for systemic invasion. While initial reports suggested that the incidence of catheter-related bacteremia was low, more recent observations suggest that there is a significant risk for both infectious and noninfectious complications with these catheters. The reasons for these variable rates of complications (3–60%) may relate to differences in techniques of catheter insertion, care, and maintenance.[50] Differences in patient populations, their therapy, degree of catheter use, and the definition of catheter-related infection also influence the appreciation of these complications. These complications must nonetheless be balanced against the considerable advantages offered by these catheters. A question of practical importance is whether the catheter needs to be removed if positive blood cultures are obtained. While the classic principles of infectious disease support the importance of removing a potentially infected foreign body, this is not a simple matter for the neutropenic (and frequently thrombocytopenic) pediatric cancer patient (Fig. 2).

We evaluated our experience in pediatric patients with catheter-associated bacteremia (defined as two or more positive blood cultures obtained from two or more separate sites at two separate times). Positive cultures were usually obtained from both the catheter as well as a peripheral vein as part of the evaluation of a new fever. Of 51 catheters in 43 patients, 39% were associated with an episode of bacteremia; of these, 60% occurred while the patient was granulocytopenic. Gram-positive organisms (especially *S. epidermidis*) were most common, particularly in nongranulocytopenic patients.[50] To assess the impact of indwelling catheters on the incidence of bacteremia, we compared the frequency of bacteremias in patients with and without catheters, both during the study period as well as during the 2-year

period prior to our routine insertion of Silastic catheters. In granulocytopenic patients who had been febrile, the incidence was fourfold higher than in patients without catheters; in nongranulocytopenic patients with indwelling catheters, the incidence was 40-fold higher than for comparable patients without catheters. Thus, there is no doubt that a catheter places the patient at heightened risk of developing a bacteremia, regardless of whether patients becomes granulocytopenic. The consequences of these bacteremias and their ease of management are therefore crucial. Overall, we have observed that more than 90% of these bacteremias can be treated without the need for catheter removal. Similar results have been reported by Abrahm et al.[51] in a prospective study of patients with Silastic catheters. However, the need for caution still exists, since long-term experience with these catheters is still relatively brief. During

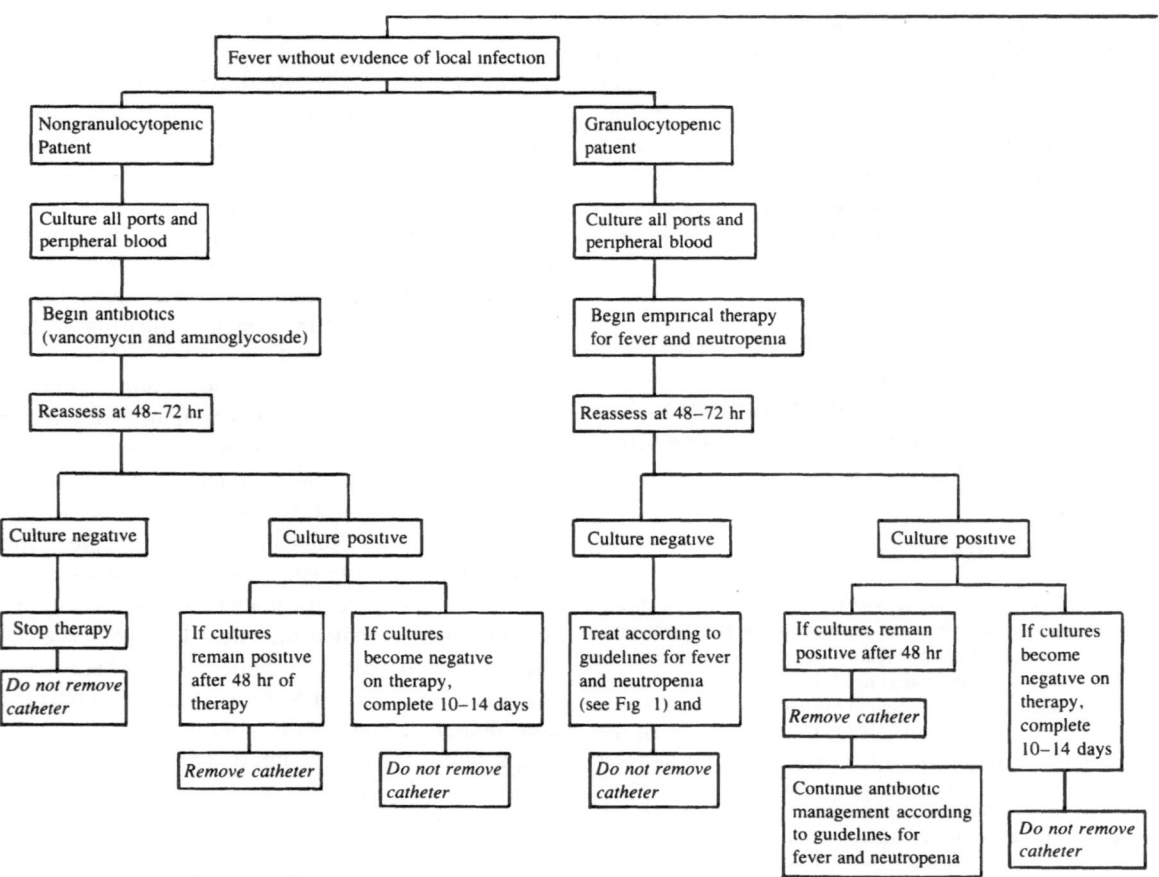

FIGURE 2. Management of patients with indwelling catheter.

1985, with more than 150 catheter placements at the NCI, we have observed a patient with endocarditis due to *Candida* sp. and another in whom osteomyelitis developed due to *S. aureus* bacteremia. While most patients responded to parenteral antibiotics (generally with vancomycin), we have recently observed two bacteremic patients with penicillin sensitive *Bacillus* sp. whose infections could not be cleared until their catheters were removed.[52] Similarly, patients with significant exit site or subcutaneous tunnel inflammation require catheter removal to erradicate their infection. This probably also applies to patients with fungemia. We also have noted that colonization (or infection) can be restricted to only one of the lumens in patients with double- or triple-lumen catheters. This is important, since we have noted treatment failure unless the antibiotic delivery was rotated to include each of the lumen ports.

Subcutaneously implantable catheters are also being introduced into the clinic. To date, experience with these devices is still too early to permit an assessment of their utility or complications. We are comparing their risks and benefits to those of Hickman–Broviac catheters in a prospective clinical trial.

11. Do the Principles Gleaned from the Management of Intravascular Catheters Apply to Other Types of Foreign Bodies?

In addition to indwelling intravenous access devices, other types of foreign bodies may also be implanted as part of the management of the child with cancer. For example, limb-sparing operations or in-

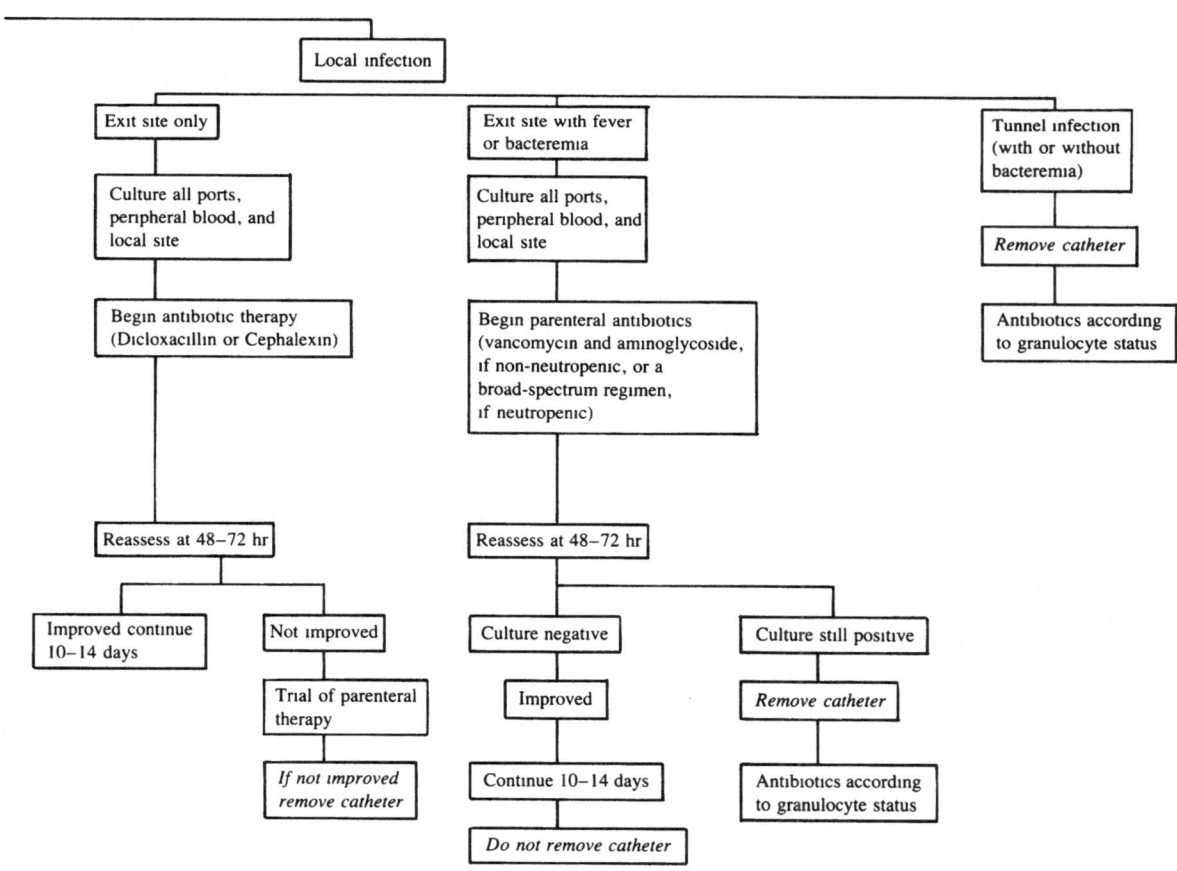

FIGURE 2. (*Continued*)

tramedullary rods are being used in the multimodality plan for patients with osteosarcoma. While these devices do offer some preservation of function, they may become a nidus for infection, particularly if they become seeded during an episode of bacteremia (e.g., secondary to adjuvant chemotherapy-induced myelosuppression). Unfortunately, there is a paucity of data regarding the management of these devices in the pediatric cancer patient. Because of the increased risk of bacteremia associated with Hickman–Broviac catheters, we have not permitted these catheters to be placed in patients who have had limb-sparing hardware implanted, with the hope that this would decrease the risk for seeding and infection. We have nonetheless encountered several patients in whom bacteremias still occurred and in whom evidence of infection went on to develop around the prosthesis. Clearly, the question in such patients focuses on whether the foreign body needs to be removed in order to control or clear the infection. Although anecdotal, we have observed that it may be possible to treat patients with an extended course of antibiotics (i.e., 6 weeks), without removing the foreign body. These observations clearly require confirmation, but they also suggest that aggressive antibiotic therapy may avoid the need for surgery.

Another type of foreign body used in pediatric cancer patients is the intraventricular Ommaya reservoir. These reservoirs are important in the management of patients with leukemic or carcinomatous meningitis. It is well recognized that intraventricular shunt infections occur in 15–27% of patients with hydrocephalus and that these infections may carry a mortality of 17–40%.[53] It is commonly assumed that these shunts must be removed in order to clear the infection. However, few data exist regarding the management of Ommaya reservoir infections in cancer patients, and it is unclear whether the guidelines generated for patients with hydrocephalus are applicable to patients with cancer.

To understand the infectious complications associated with such reservoirs, we reviewed our 10-year experience with 61 children who had intraventricular reservoirs placed for chemotherapy delivery.[54] The average age of these children was 9¼ years, and the reservoirs were in place for a median of 36 weeks (range 3 days to 416 weeks) and had been punctured 29.5 times (range 1–155). In spite of their frequent use and their lengthy periods of placement,

approximately three-fourths of patients never had a reservoir-associated infectious complication. Moreover, unlike the 40% mortality associated with shunt infection in patients with hydrocephalus, none of the patients we studied died of a reservoir-associated infection. Moreover, the incidence of infection was considerably lower than that noted when Ommaya reservoirs were used for the installation of amphotericin B in patients with fungal meningitis.[55] Furthermore, unlike the patients with hydrocephalus in whom S. epidermidis appears to be the most frequent isolate, P. acnes was the most common organism found in patients with Ommaya reservoir-related infections. We observed three types of clinical problems associated with these reservoirs: (1) patients who had symptoms of meningitis (particularly fever, headaches, nausea, vomiting, lethergy, and meningismus) and whose CSF revealed a pleocytosis and whose CSF cultures were positive; (2) those in whom CSF cultures (obtained during routine CSF-cytology sampling) were found to be culture positive even though the patient was completely asymptomatic; and (3) albeit rare, a small number of patients developed evidence cellulitis around the catheter insertion site. Within each of these settings, the question arises as to when therapy is required and whether the reservoir should be removed if a microbial isolate is obtained.

From our study, it appears that if the isolate is obtained in a patient who is symptomatic, a trial of parenteral or intraventricular antibiotics should be given. The choice of antibiotics depends on the isolate and may include vancomycin, rifampin, and/or a third-generation cephalosporin. Only if the antibiotic treatment turns out to be unsuccessful in clearing the CSF is removal of the reservoir a necessary consideration. By contrast, if an isolate is obtained but the patient is completely asymptomatic, it does not appear that immediate antibiotic intervention is necessary. However, these latter patients should be followed closely, since we have observed that two of five such patients eventually went on to develop symptomatic meningitis with the same organism (P. acnes in both cases) that had been found when the patient was asymptomatic.

The risk of infection should therefore not be considered a serious deterrent from using an intraventricular reservoir in the child with cancer (if there is a likely benefit from one); the isolation of an organism per se from an Ommaya reservoir should not be considered a criterion for removal of the reservoir.

12. What Is the Role of Invasive Diagnostic Procedures in the Evaluation and Management of the Febrile Child with Cancer?

If there is an accessible site of infection (e.g., a skin lesion), an aspirate or biopsy is indicated for microscopic examination and culture. The problem is complicated, however, when the putative site of infection is not accessible without an invasive procedure. For example, when a pulmonary infiltrate is detected, the question arises of whether the risk of the procedure justifies its use, or whether simply an empirical approach to therapy should be used. Central to this question is whether the diagnostic procedure will provide sufficient material to guide management. Alternatively, if patients are treated empirically, what is the likelihood that the drugs selected will be successful? If not, will valuable time be lost in treating the patient? A clinical setting in which this dilemma is frequently debated occurs in the patient with a diffuse pulmonary infiltrate. If the patient is non-granulocytopenic, *Pneumocystis carinii* is the most likely pathogen, particularly if the patient has received steroids. Thus, empirical therapy with trimethoprim–sulfamethoxazole may be quite successful. If the patient is neutropenic and/or has been on other antibiotics, other etiologies also need to be considered and the empirical regimen may need to include broad-spectrum antibiotics or even an antifungal agent. The balance between the potential side effects of polypharmacy must then be weighted against the risks from an invasive diagnostic procedure. This is further complicated by the slow response time (e.g., approximately 3–4 days for *P. carinii* pneumonia), making rapid changes in therapy difficult. With trimethoprim–sulfamethoxazole, a 60–80% response can be expected. Failure to improve (continued fever, depressed Po_2, progressive infiltrates), after 4 days of therapy serves as an indication to modify therapy, usually with the addition of pentamidine isothionate. However, if a histologic diagnosis is sought, not all procedures (e.g., transtracheal aspirate, transbronchial biopsy or aspirate,

open lung biopsy) are of comparable diagnostic accuracy. Burt et al.[56] examined each of 17 patients having an open-lung biopsy for the diagnosis of a diffuse interstitial infiltrate with a transthoracic needle aspirate as well as a transbronchial brush and biopsy. The patients in this study thus served as their own controls. A diagnosis was established from only 30% of the aspirates and from 59% of the transbronchial biopsy samples, compared with 94% of the open-lung biopsies (OLB). Although this trial evaluated a relatively small number of patients, it suggests that the OLB may be the procedure of choice. An open lung biopsy provides the soundest guidance for patient management, especially if the patient is neutropenic and requires multiple antimicrobial agents.

In order to assess the risks and benefits of empirical therapy versus an early diagnostic procedure more carefully, we have been conducting a clinical trial that directly addresses this problem.[57,58] Patients in whom a diffuse pulmonary infiltrate developed have been randomly assigned to undergo either an immediate OLB with therapy then dictated according to the results of the procedure, or to receive an initial trial of empirical antibiotics. Use of the empirical antibiotics depended on whether the patient was granulocytopenic or was receiving antibiotics when the infiltrate appeared. Patients randomly assigned to receive empirical antibiotics who were either stable or improved after a 4-day trial of therapy then received a standard course of therapy. However, patients who failed to improve after a 4-day trial of empirical therapy underwent an OLB. Twenty-two non-neutropenic pediatric and adult cancer patients have been evaluated to date. The median room air Po_2 in 21 hypoxic patients was 55 mm Hg. Eight of 10 patients randomized to empirical therapy improved after 4 days. Both patients who failed to improve and who then underwent OLB on day 4 turned out to have *P. carinii* pneumonia; one subsequently improved while the second succumbed to hemorrhage. The time to clinical resolution in the nine surviving patients receiving empirical therapy was 14 days. Of the 12 patients randomized to immediate OLB, five had PCP, while seven had nonspecific pneumonitis. Three deaths appeared to be related to OLB. Although there were no significant differences in mortality between the two groups ($p = 0.54$), there was substantially greater morbidity among patients randomized to immediate OLB. These data suggest that initial empirical therapy for nongranulocytopenic cancer patients with diffuse pneumonitis may be as efficacious as immediate OLB and may be associated with decreased morbidity (Fig. 3). However, it must be underscored that it is not established that these data can be applied to patients who are granulocytopenic.

Illustrative Case 5

A 4-year-old child with acute lymphoblastic leukemia was started on empirical broad-spectrum antibiotics when she was febrile and neutropenic following a course of consolidation chemotherapy. Prior to starting antibiotics, the child's physical examination, blood cultures, and chest radiograph were all negative. She had defervesced within 3 days after starting antibiotics and appeared to be doing nicely. By the eighth hospital day, however, she began having an intermittent hacking cough (but without sputum production); a chest radiograph obtained at that time revealed a patchy right lower lobe infiltrate. In spite of her cough, she was afebrile and was feeling generally well. Blood cultures were obtained, as was a cryptococcal antigen; both were negative. Since her WBC count during the previous 3 days was rising, it was elected to watch her expectantly and not to perform an invasive diagnostic procedure at that time. She remained afebrile, and over the next 2 days her cough improved and her WBC count returned to normal. In concert with her granulocyte recovery, the pulmonary infiltrate at first became slightly worsened and then began to improve. The patient was treated for a full 14-day course of therapy for an assumed bacterial pneumonitis that had only become clinically definable when her inflammatory potential normalized.

Another similar management dilemma arises when a new pulmonary infiltrate develops in a gran-

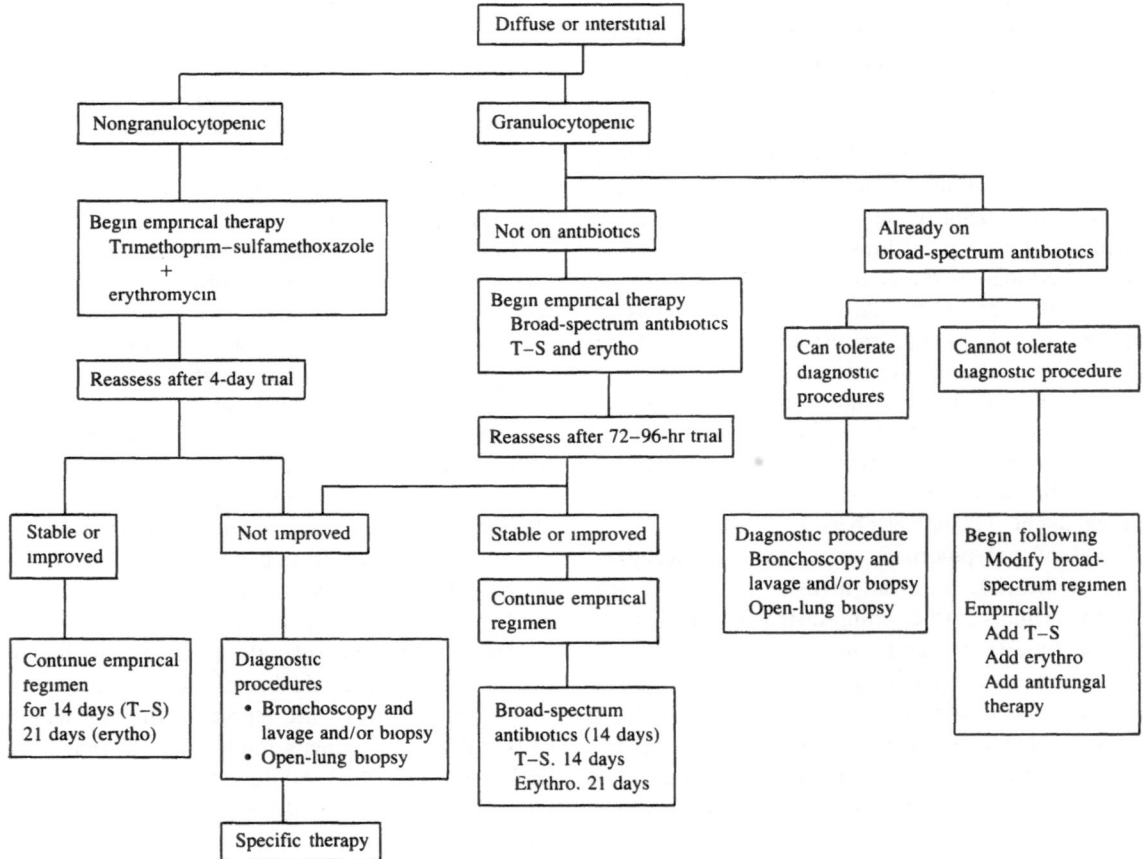

FIGURE 3. Pulmonary infiltrate. T–S, trimethoprim–sulfamethoxadole; erythro, erythromycin.

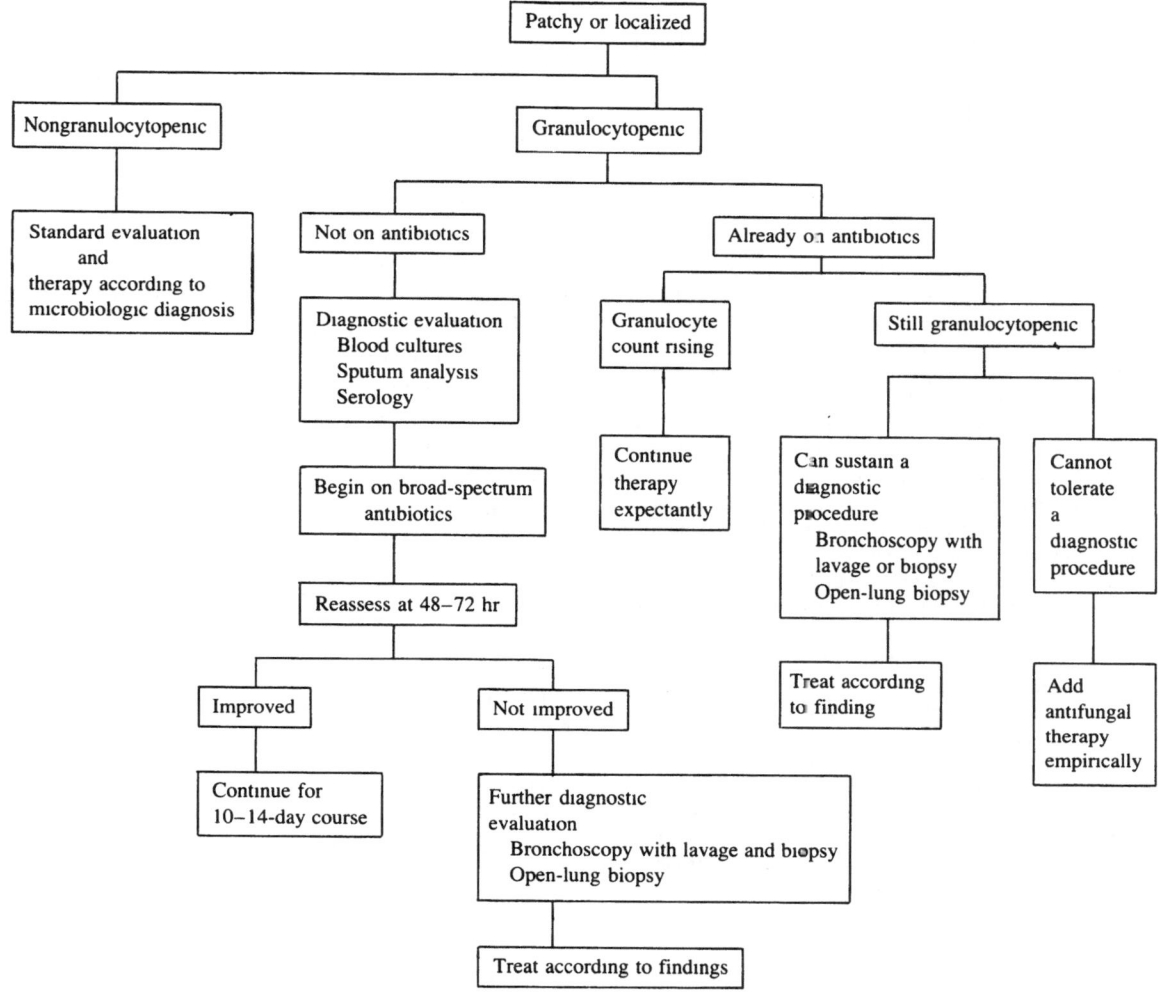

FIGURE 4. Pulmonary infiltrate.

ulocytopenic patient who is already receiving broad-spectrum antibiotic therapy. We recently reviewed our experience with 34 such pediatric patients and observed that they could be divided into two groups: patients in whom a new infiltrate developed while the granulocyte count was rising and patients whose new infiltrate appeared while they remained granulocytopenic.[59] The main question for patients recovering from granulocytopenia is whether a new infiltrate simply reflects the lighting-up of a previously inapparent site of infection or whether it is a new infection. We observed that patients in whom

infiltrates developed in conjunction with bone marrow recovery did well without the need for therapeutic modifications. By contrast, patients in whom a new and progressive infiltrate developed during antibiotic therapy and granulocytopenia were likely to have a fungal pneumonia. Ideally, an OLB should be performed in these patients, in order to establish the diagnosis and guide the duration of therapy. If a biopsy cannot be performed, amphotericin B should be instituted empirically, since we observed a survival advantage for patients who received early empirical antifungal therapy (Fig. 4).

13. Are There Situations in Which Surgery Should Be Incorporated into the Management Plan, Even If the Patient Is Profoundly Granulocytopenic?

Illustrative Case 6

A 15-year-old boy with a T-cell leukemia developed fever and neutropenia and was admitted to the hospital and begun on broad-spectrum antibiotics (cephalothin, gentamicin, and carbenicillin). His preantibiotic examination was remarkable for severe oral mucosal lesions, presumably secondary to the high-dose methotrexate he had received days earlier. He was afebrile by the second day of antibiotics and all the preantibiotic cultures were negative. On the third hospital day, however, he again developed fever, this time with the sudden onset of right lower quadrant abdominal tenderness along with spasm and mild rebound. An abdominal radiograph was remarkable for an ileus, but ultrasound failed to reveal any mass or fluid collection. Clindamycin was added to the antibiotic regimen. Over the next 12 hr, the abdominal pain, spasm, and rebound tenderness worsened. It was assumed that the patient had an acute abdomen due either to an appendicitis or a cecitis (i.e., infiltration of the cell wall with gram-negative bacteria, resulting in a necrotic bowel syndrome). In view of the patient's progressive symptoms, surgical exploration was considered necessary, even though the patient was both neutropenic and thrombocytopenic. In preparation for surgery, the patient received transfusions to maintain his platelet count above 50,000 per mm³. At surgery, the cecum was found to be boggy and necrotic and was resected with an end-to-end anastomasis. Antibiotics were continued, and over the 3 next days the patient improved. Examination of the resected cecum showed the infiltration with gram-negative bacilli, cultures of which grew *P. aeruginosa*.

Because of granulocytopenia and thrombocytopenia, there is frequently a reluctance to consider a surgical procedure in the child with cancer. While this dilemma is understandable, there are times when surgery is a critical part of the therapeutic regimen and when delays in its implementation may result in fatality. In their review of acute abdomens presenting in 26 children with cancer, Schaller and Schaller[59] noted that the most frequent problems included acute massive GI hemorrhage (10 patients), biliary tract disease (four patients), and typhlitis, also referred to as cecitis (three patients). In our experience at the NCI, acute appendicitis is the most frequent abdominal crisis, with typhlitis second. While these processes can sometimes be treated without surgery, it is not uncommon for the signs and symptoms of right lower quadrant pain and rebound tenderness to develop while the child is already receiving broad-spectrum antibiotic therapy. In such situations, the natural history of these lesions is progression to peritonitis, irreversible shock, and disseminated intravascular coagulopathy (DIC), unless the necrotic portion of the cecum is surgically resected.[60] Thus, our approach to children in whom acute abdominal symptoms develop, particularly if they are granulocytopenic and are already receiving broad-spectrum antibiotics, is to monitor them closely. If there is evidence of rebound tenderness, massive GI hemorrhage, or localizing findings, we proceed to a surgical procedure.

It is also important to reassess the role that surgery has been assumed to play in the management of certain infection in cancer patients. Perianal cellulitis serves as an example. Early reports of perianal cellulitis in neutropenic patients cited significant surgical complications (e.g., hemorrhage, spreading infection), leading to the recommendation that surgery should be avoided in these patients.[61] Recently, however, Barnes et al.[62] reported an increased survival in a group of 16 patients with acute leukemia when surgical drainage of the perianal cellulitis was done early. However, the infections described in this series were very severe, characterized by extensive soft tissue destruction. In our experience, most anorectal infections are not as severe as those described by Barnes et al.,[62] leading to the speculation that the close surveillance and repeated physical examination by these authors may have actually increased the severity of the infection in some of those patients. We recently reviewed our experience with 57 episodes of anorectal infections in 44 pediatric and adult cancer patients.[63] Cultures obtained at the time of surgical drainage or by needle aspiration of the wound revealed multiple organisms in 26 of 29 instances, with anaerobic organisms being the most common isolates. The anorectal infection resolved in 28 of 51 treatment courses (55%) when antibiotics were the only treatment given. However, if the antibiotic regimen included both an aminoglycoside and a specific antianaerobic antibiotic (e.g., clindamycin, metronidazole), resolution occurred in 15 of 17 (88%) cases. At the same time, the infection was controlled or resolved completely in 19 of 26 (73%) of cases treated with surgery and antibiotics. These results suggest that early management of perianal cellulitis with antibiotics, using both a broad-spectrum antibiotic and a specific antianaerobic agent may avoid the need for surgery. However, surgery should be performed if there is obvious fluctuance, if there is definable tissue necrosis or if there is progression of the infection either locally or with continued sepsis after a 48-hr trial of antibiotics.

14. How Long Should Antibiotic Therapy Be Continued, And How Should It Be Modified When the Clinical and Microbiologic Evaluation Has Failed to Reveal an Infectious Etiology for Fever?

The appropriate duration of antimicrobial therapy is problematic when the febrile and granulocytopenic patient's initial evaluation has failed to reveal an infectious etiology. Patients with fever of unexplained origin (FUO) can be divided into low-risk and high risk groups. Low-risk FUO patients resolve their granulocytopenia within 1 week of start-

ing antibiotics and do well when their antibiotics are continued simply until the time of recovery of their granulocyte count to above 500 per mm[3].[18]

The major dilemma pertains to the high-risk FUO patients, who remain neutropenic for more than 1 week. We have addressed the management of these patients in a series of prospective clinical studies, stratifying them according to whether they had defervesced after the initiation of broad-spectrum therapy or whether they remained persistently febrile in spite of empirical antibiotics[64,65] (Fig. 5). Within 3 days of stopping antibiotics on day 7 in patients who had defervesced on therapy but who still remained afebrile, 41% again became febrile; the isolate(s) obtained when these patients became febrile again were sensitive to the antibiotics which had been discontinued. By contrast, no subsequent infections were observed in the patients who simply continued on antibiotics. However, these data did not define whether antibiotics should be continued until the final resolutions of neutropenia or whether a defined

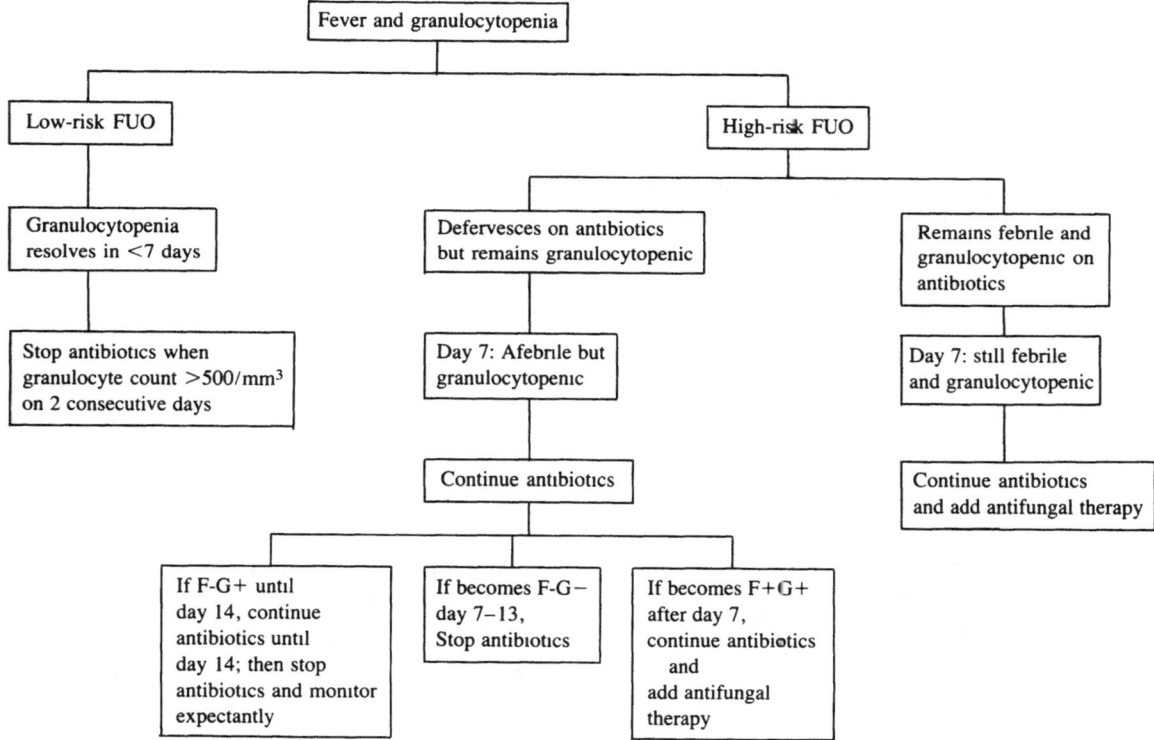

FIGURE 5. Management of granulocytopenic children with fever of unexplained origin (FUO)

but limited course of antibiotic therapy, as if the patient had an occult site of infection, might suffice. Therefore, in an ongoing study, we have tried to further evaluate the appropriate duration of antibiotic therapy by continuing antibiotics for afebrile-but-persistently granulocytopenic FUO patients for a full 14-day treatment course (as if they had an occult infectious etiology for their fever) and then randomizing them to either stop antibiotics or to continue treatment until the resolution of the granulocytopenia. We have observed that after day 14, approximately one-third of the patients either stopping or continuing antibiotic therapy will become febrile again; since patients randomized to discontinue antibiotics responded to the reinstitution of therapy when a new fever developed, it seems reasonable simply to continue FUO patients on a standard 14-day treatment course if they remain granulocytopenic and then to stop the antibiotics, recognizing that approximately 30% of the patients will require further intervention.

The situation is more complicated for patients who remain persistently febrile and granulocytopenic in spite of antibiotic therapy. In a randomized clinical trial, we observed that 56% of the FUO patients who had remained febrile even after receiving empirical antibiotics developed complications within 3 days of stopping therapy. Of these, 38% became hypotensive once antibiotic therapy was stopped. However, simply continuing antibiotics alone in FUO patients with persistent fever and granulocytopenia was not satisfactory, since 31% of these patients eventually developed invasive fungal infections. It is not possible to determine whether these fungal invasions were the cause of the patient's persistent fever or a consequence of their continued antibiotics and prolonged granulocytopenia. However, patients with persistent fever and granulocytopenia appeared to do best when their antibiotics were continued and amphotericin B was added empirically. The efficacy of this approach, however, may depend on the patient population and the predominant fungal pathogens. For example, centers with a high incidence of *Aspergillus* are likely to be less successful, even when amphotericin B is begun early, than are institutions where *Candida* predominates.

While approximately 50% of the patients with prolonged granulocytopenia appeared to benefit from continuing antibiotics, it is important to remember that the remaining patients did well even when antibiotics were stopped. This has led some investigators to suggest that stopping antibiotic treatment may be appropriate, provided that the patient can be closely monitored and the antibiotics promptly reinstituted if the patient becomes febrile again or shows clinical deterioration. However, reliable end points for reinstituting therapy are vague, and because the condition of these patients can sometimes deteriorate quite rapidly, it may be more prudent to continue antibiotics, especially in the persistently febrile and granulocytopenic patient. While this approach certainly results in the overtreatment of some patients, it lessens the possibility that the highest-risk patients will be further compromised.

15. Summary

Although infections continue to remain a major problem in pediatric cancer treatment, it seems clear that infection-related morbidity and mortality can be reduced by aggressive adherence to treatment principles unique to the neutropenic cancer patient. These center around a recognition of the patient at highest risk of infection and incorporate the prompt initiation of broad-spectrum antibiotic therapy when the granulocytopenic child becomes febrile, together with the appropriate additions or modifications of the antimicrobial regimen in patients who remain persistently granulocytopenic or febrile.

References

1. Pizzo PA, Miser J, Cassady JR, et al: Solid tumors of childhood. In DeVita VT Jr, Hellman S, Rosenberg SA (eds): *Cancer: Principles and Practice of Oncology.* ed. 2. Lippincott, Philadelphia, 1985, pp. 1511–1589.

2. Poplack DG, Cassady JR, Pizzo PA: Leukemias and lymphomas. In DeVita VT Jr, Hellman S, Rosenberg SA (eds): *Cancer: Principles and Practice of Oncology.* ed. 2 Lippincott, Philadelphia, 1985, pp. 1591–1622

3. Pizzo PA, Robichaud KJ, Edward BK, et al: Oral antibiotic prophylaxis in cancer patients: A double-blind randomized placebo controlled trial. *J Pediatr* **102**:125–133, 1983.

4. Pizzo PA, Commers JR, Cotton DJ, et al: Approaching the controversies in the antibacterial management of cancer patients. *Am J Med* **76**:436–449, 1984.

5. Pizzo PA: Infectious complications in the child with cancer. I. Pathophysiology of the compromised host and the initial eval-

uation and management of the febrile cancer patient. *J Pediatr* **98**:341–354, 1981.

6. Pizzo PA: Infectious complications in the child with cancer. II. Management of specific infectious organisms. *J Pediatr* **98**:513–523, 1981.

7. Purtillo DT, DeFlorio D Jr, Holt LM, et al: Phenotypic expression of an X-linked lymphoproliferative syndrome. *N Engl J Med* **297**:1077–1981, 1977.

8. Gallo RC, Salahuddin SZ, Popovic M, et al: Frequent detection and isolation of cytopathic retroviruses from patients with AIDS and at risk for AIDS. *Science* **224**:500–503, 1984.

9. Pizzo PA, Young RC: Infections in the cancer patients. In DeVita VT Jr, Hellman S, Rosenberg SD (eds): *Cancer: Principles and Practice of Oncology.* Lippincott, Philadelphia, 1985, pp. 1963–1998.

10. Beachey EH: Bacterial adherence: Adhesin–receptor interactions mediating the attachment of bacteria to mucosal surfaces. *J Infect Dis* **143**:325–345, 1981.

11. Johanson WG, Pierce AK, Sanford JP: Changing pharyngeal flora of hospitalized patients: Emergence of gram-negative bacilli. *N Engl J Med* **281**:1137–1140, 1969.

12. Broder S, Waldman TA: The suppressor-cell network in cancer. *N Engl J Med* **299**:1281–1335, 1978.

13. Peter G, Pizzo PA, Robichaud KR, et al: Possible protective effect of circulating antibodies to the shared glycolipid of enterobacteriaceae in children with malignancy. *Pediatr Res* **13**:466 (abstr.), 1979.

14. Pizzo PA and Young LS: Limitations of antimicrobial therapy. Looking at both sides of the coin. *Am J Med* **76**:101–110, 1984.

15. Siber GR: Bacteremias due to *Hemophilus influenzae* and *Streptococcus* pneumoniae. Their occurrence and course in children with cancer. *Am J Dis Child* **134**:668–672, 1980.

16. Giebink GS, Le CT, Schiffman G: Decline of serum antibody in splenectomized children after vaccination with pneumococcal capsular polysaccharides. *J Pediatr* **105**:576–582, 1984.

17. Browder AA, Hoff JA, Petersdorf RG: The significance of fever in neoplastic disease. *Ann Intern Med* **55**:932–942, 1961.

18. Pizzo PA, Robichaud KJ, Wesley R, et al: Fever in the pediatric and young adult patient with cancer. A prospective study of 1001 episodes. *Medicine (Baltimore)* **61**:153–165, 1982.

19. Pizzo PA, Lovejoy FH Jr, Smith D: Prolonged fever in children. Review of 100 cases. *Pediatrics* **55**:468–473, 1975.

20. Kosmidis HV, Lusher JM, Shope TC, et al. Infections in leukemic children: A prospective analysis. *J Pediatr* **96**:814–819, 1980.

21. Cotton DJ, Yolken RH, Hiemenz JW, et al: Role of respiratory viruses in the etiology of fever occurring during chemotherapy-induced granulocytopenia. *Pediatr Res* **18**:272A, 1984.

22. Whitley R, Barton N, Collins E, et al: Mucocutaneous herpes simplex infections in immunocompromised patients: A model for evaluation of topical antiviral agents. *Am J Med* **73**:236–249, 1982.

23. Wade JC, Newton B, McLaren C, et al: Intravenous acyclovir to treat mucocutaneous herpes simplex virus infections after marrow transplantation: A double blind trial. *Ann Intern Med* **96**:265–269, 1982.

24. Saral R, Ambinder RF, Burns WH, et al: Acyclovir prophylaxis against herpes simplex virus infections in patients with leukemia. A randomized, double blind, placebo-controlled study. *Ann Intern Med* **99**:773–776, 1983.

25. Henson D, Siegel SE, Fuccillo DA, et al: Cytomegalovirus infection during acute childhood leukemia. *J Infect Dis* **126**:469–481, 1972

26. Neiman PE, Reeves W, Ray G, et al: A prospective analysis of interstitial pneumonia and opportunistic viral infection among recipients of allogeneic bone marrow grafts. *J Infect Dis* **136**:754–767, 1977.

27. Hirsch MS and Schooley RT: Treatment of herpes virus infections. *N Engl J Med* **309**:963–970; 1034–1039, 1983

28. Meyers JD, McGuffin RW, Bryson YG, et al: Treatment of cytomegalovirus pneumonia after marrow transplant with combined vidarabine and human leukocyte interferon. *J Infect Dis* **146**:80–84, 1982.

29. Winston DJ, Pollard RB, Ho WG, et al: Cytomegalovirus immune plasma in bone marrow transplant recipients. *Ann Intern Med* **97**:11–18, 1982.

30. Meyers JD, Leszczynski J, Zaia JA, et al: Prevention of cytomegalovirus infection by cytomegalovirus immune globulin after marrow transplantation. *Ann Intern Med* **98**:442–446, 1983.

31. Gershon AA, Steinberg S, Brunnell PA. Zoster immune globulin. A further assessment. *N Engl J Med* **290**:243–245, 1975.

32. Morgan ET, Smalley LA: Varicella in immunocompromised children. Incidence of abdominal pain and organ involvement. *Am J Dis Child* **137**:883–885, 1983.

33. Recommendations of the Immunization Practices Advisory Committee: Varicella–zoster immune globulin for the prevention of chicken pox. *Ann Intern Med* **100**:859–865, 1984.

34. Paryani SG, Arvin AM, Koropchak CM, et al: Comparison of varicella zoster antibody titres in patients given intravenous immune serum globulin or varicella zoster immune globulin. *J Pediatr* **105**:200–205, 1984.

35. Weibel RE, Neff BJ, Duter BJ, et al: Live attenuated varicella virus vaccine. Efficacy trial in healthy children. *N Engl J Med* **310**:1409–1415, 1984.

36. Brunell PA, Shehab Z, Geiser C, et al: Administration of live varicella vaccine to children with leukemia. *Lancet* **2**:1069–1973, 1982.

37. Maksymiuk AW, Thongprasert S, Hopfer R, et al: Systemic candidiasis in cancer patients. *Am J Med* **77**:20–27, 1984.

38. Berkow RL, Weisman SJ, Provisor AJ, et al: Invasive aspergillosis of paranasal tissues in children with malignancies. *J Pediatr* **103**:49–53, 1983.

39. Aisner J, Schimpff SC, Bennett JE, et al: *Aspergillus* infection in cancer patients. Association with fireproofing materials in new hospitals. *JAMA* **235**:411–412, 1976.

40. Ruebush TK, Weinstein RA, Baehner RL, et al: An outbreak of *Pneumocystis* pneumonia in children with acute lymphocytic leukemia. *Am J Dis Child* **132**:143–148, 1978.

41. Hiemenz J, Skelton J, Pizzo PA: Perspective on the management of catheter related infections in cancer patients. *Pediatr Infect Dis* **5**:6–11, 1986.

42. Kramer BK, Pizzo PA, Robichaud DJ, et al: Role of serial

microbiological surveillance and clinical evaluation in the management of cancer patients with fever and granulocytopenia. *Am J Med* **72:**561–568, 1982.

43. Aisner J, Murrillo J, Schimpff SC, et al: Invasive aspergillus in acute leukemia: Correlation with nose cultures and antibiotic use. *Ann Intern Med* **90:**4–9, 1979.

44. Gill VJ, Zierdt CH, Wu JC, et al. Comparison of lysis-filtration and conventional bottles for blood cultures. *J Clin Microbiol* **20:**927–937, 1984.

45. Peltola H, Saarinen U, Siimes M: C-reactive protein in rapid diagnosis and follow up of bacterial septicemia in children with leukemia. *Pediatr Infect Dis* **2:**370–373, 1983

46. Pizzo PA, Thaler M, Hathorn J, et al: The new β-lactam antibiotics in the granulocytopenic patient. New options and new questions. *Am J Med* **79:**75–82, 1985.

47. Pizzo PA, Hathorn J, Hiemenz J, et al. A randomized trial comparing ceftazidime with combination antibiotic therapy in cancer patients with fever and neutropenia. *N Engl J Med* **315:**552–558, 1986.

48. Pizzo PA, Ladisch SL, Robichaud K: Treatment of gram-positive septicemia in cancer patients. *Cancer* **45:**206–207, 1980.

49. Cotton D, Marshall D, Gress J, et al: Pathogen specific vs broad-spectrum antibiotics for granulocytopenic cancer patients with proven infection. Interscience Conference on Antimicrobial Agent Chemotherapy, 1984, p. 188.

50. Hiemenz J, Skelton J, Pizzo PA: Management of Hickman–Broviac catheters in immunocompromised hosts. *Pediatr Infect Disease* **5:**6–11, 1986.

51. Abraham J, Mullen JL, Jacobson N, et al: Continuous central venous access in patients with acute leukemia. *Cancer Treatm Rep* **63:**2099–2100, 1979.

52. Cotton DJ, Gill V, Hiemenz J, et al: Bacillus bacteremia in an immunocompromised patient population. clinical features, therapeutic interventions and relationship to chronic intravascular catheters. *J Clin Microbial* **25:**672–674. 1987

53. Schoenbaum SC, Gardener P, Shillito J: Infections of cerebrospinal fluid shunts: Epidemiology, clinical manifestations and therapy *J Infect Dis* **131:**543–552, 1975.

54 Browne MJ, Perek D, Dinndorf PA, et al: Infectious complications of intraventricular reservoirs in cancer patients. *Pediatr Intel Dis* **6:**182–189, 1987

55. Diamond RO, Bennett JE: A subcutaneous reservoir for intrathecal therapy of fungal meningitis. *N Engl J Med* **288:**186–188, 1973.

56. Burt ME, Flye MW, Webber BL, et al: Prospective evaluation of aspiration needle, cutting needle, transbronchial and open lung biopsy in patients with pulmonary infiltrates. *Ann Thorac Surg* **32:**146–153, 1981.

57. Potter D, Pass HI, Brower S, et al: Prospective randomized study of open lung biopsy versus empiric antibiotic therapy for acute pneumonitis in non-neutropenic cancer patients. *Ann Thorac Surg* **40:**422–428, 1985.

58. Commers JR, Robichaud KJ, Pizzo PA. New pulmonary infiltrates in granulocytopenic patients being treated with antibiotics. *Pediatr Infect Dis* **3:**423–428, 1984.

59. Schaller RT Jr, Schaller JF: The acute abdomen in the immunologically compromised child *J Pediatr Surg* **18:**937–944, 1983.

60. Varki AP, Armitage JO, Feagler JP. Typhlitis in acute leukemia. *Cancer* **43:**695–697, 1979.

61. Sehder M, Dowling M Jr, Seal S, et al: Perianal and anorectal complications in leukemia *Cancer* **31:**149–152, 1973.

62. Barnes S, Sattler F, Ballard J: Perirectal infections in acute leukemia: Improved survival after incision and debridement. *Ann Intern Med* **100:**515–518, 1984.

63. Glenn J, Cotton D, Wesley R, Pizzo PA: Anorectal infection in patients with malignant diseases. *Rev Infect Dis* (in press).

64. Pizzo PA, Robichaud KJ, Gill FA, et al: Duration of empiric antibiotic therapy in granulocytopenic cancer patients *Am J Med* **67:**194–200, 1979.

65. Pizzo PA, Robichaud KJ, Gill FA, et al: Empiric antibiotic and antifungal therapy for cancer patients with prolonged fever and granulocytopenia. *Am J Med* **72:**101–110, 1982

18

Management of Infections in Leukemia and Lymphoma

LOWELL S. YOUNG

1. Introduction

Much of the useful clinical information—as well as persisting controversies surrounding the management of infectious problems in the immunocompromised host—has come from studies of patients with leukemias and lymphomas. That these diseases should be the object of great interest is not difficult to fathom: they are rapidly or ultimately fatal if untreated, the magnitude of treatment with cytotoxic and immunosuppressive agents has few parallels in the therapy of any human illness (probably exceeded only by bone marrow transplantation, which is most often employed for leukemia), and the infectious problems are acute, life threatening, and sometimes highly unusual. Infectious problems developing in other types of immunocompromised patients often result from utilization of the same medications and therapeutic strategies initially attempted in patients with hematologic malignancies. At many medical centers, individuals with acute leukemia have the most severe impairment of host-defense mechanisms and represent the prime example of the immunocompromised host.

It has been gratifying that there has been substantial progress in effectively treating several major types of leukemias and lymphomas to the extent that "cure" can be an accurate and honest assessment of some treatment results. This success has been achieved with more intensive chemotherapy and radiation, better supportive care, and improved management of infectious complications. The nature of infectious complications · has changed somewhat since reviews of a decade or more ago, but the infection risk has not. Some infectious complications have become remarkably more amenable to therapy, like *E. coli* sepsis and pneumocystosis. Effective immunoprophylaxis has become available for chickenpox, and chemoprophylaxis for *P. carinii* infections. On the other hand, a more ominous development has been the emergence of opportunistic fungal infections that are exceedingly difficult to diagnose and treat. Obviously, nature abhors an "ecologic vacuum," and the upsurge in fungal infections is probably a manifestation of better control of bacterial septicemias. Long periods of neutropenia, improved treatment of bacterial pathogens, coupled with failure to achieve substantial improvement in underlying disease are the major prelude to fungal superinfection. In spite of this trend, clinicians need to be alert to the fact that some rather common infectious problems can still come back to haunt the patient with acute leukemia or lymphoma who has experienced "successful" treatment of his underlying disease. Probably the best example of this phenomenon is the problem of pneumococcal sepsis in splenectomized patients with Hodgkin disease[1] or well-engrafted recipients of bone marrow transplants.[2]

Not to be ignored at present is the potential posttransfusion acquired immunodeficiency syndrome (AIDS) in a patient with a hematologic malignancy. These patients receive an enormous number of blood

LOWELL S. YOUNG • Kuzell Institute for Arthritis and Infectious Disease, Division of Infectious Diseases, Pacific Presbyterian Medical Center, San Francisco, California 94115 products and the possibility of AIDS must be considered in any febrile, deteriorating patient who has been transfused since 1978 in the United States, Western Europe, or Africa.

2. Host Defenses against Infection in Leukemias and Lymphomas

There are several well-known shibboleths about the nature of the impairment in host defenses in leukemias and lymphomas and how specific defects relate to the incidence and type of complicating infections.[3] Nevertheless, it would be wise to accept all of these traditional associations with some caution. The "classic" concept is that acute leukemia is associated with a paucity of normally functioning neutrophils, a granulocyte killing defect associated with cellular immaturity, or both, whereas patients with lymphomas have abnormalities in cell-mediated defense mechanisms ("delayed" hypersensitivity). Thus, leukemics experience pyogenic infections (staphylococcal, streptococcal, gram-negative), whereas victims of lymphomas experience infections by agents against which delayed hypersensitivity mechanisms are thought to be important (tuberculosis, fungal diseases). Finally, diseases in which humoral immunity is impaired either through hypogammaglobulinemia (chronic lymphatic leukemia) or the production of an abnormal immunoglobulin (multiple myeloma or macroglobulinemia) would be characterized by a defect in opsonizing or microbicidal antibodies. If levels of opsonizing antibodies are depressed, the net result is impaired granulocyte function, and an increased susceptibility to acute bacterial infections similar to that seen with the acute leukemias is observed.

One of the major problems, however, in attempting to relate types of opportunistic infection to underlying disease involves the major effect of treatment (chemotherapy and radiation being the major factors) on the incidence and nature of infectious complications. Except for those physicians who are caring for patients at the very inception of therapy, it will be rare for a clinician to face an "unmodified" patient. In our experience, the classic association of infections caused by encapsulated bacteria (pneumococci and to a lesser extent *Hemophilus influ-*

enzae) has been observed in untreated patients with multiple myeloma or chronic lymphatic leukemia. These diseases—if unmodified by therapeutic intervention—may show the "classic" associations. If, however, pharmacologic agents with effects on cell-mediated immune function such as the corticosteroids are used to treat these same diseases, the likelihood of infections by fungal organisms, agents such as *L. monocytogenes,* and pneumocystosis will be greatly increased. Likewise, when intensive cytotoxic treatment that depresses the total circulating neutrophil count is given to patients with non-Hodgkin lymphomas and multiple myelomas, we have seen overwhelming gram-negative and opportunistic fungal infections analogous to what has been regularly encountered in patients being treated for acute leukemia. Some antineoplastic agents may actually have antimicrobial effects, and these may be additional factors selecting for the types of organisms that cause infectious complications.[4,5]

In aplastic anemia, the patterns of infection are virtually identical to those observed in acute leukemia. Patients with acute leukemias and the aplastic anemias usually have decreased numbers of normally functioning neutrophils, but it is interesting that within the group of patients with aplasia that we have followed, there appear to be at least two subpopulations: a group with fulminant disease who experience rapid decline of circulating neutrophils to negligible levels and a second group that has more indolent disease and in whom circulating neutrophil counts of 200 to 600/mm³ persist. Clearly, those in the first group are likely to die within weeks to months unless they spontaneously recover hematopoietic function or receive a bone marrow transplant. In contrast, those patients with higher, stable residual white counts may have a life-span of many years. The numbers of neutrophils that are circulating in that latter group of patients give an important clue to what is actually required by the host for adequate defense against pyogenic and gram-negative infections.

No clinician needs to be reminded of the crucial role of neutrophils in the defense against bacterial and fungal infections. In acute leukemia, the paucity of acute neutrophils is clearly related to this susceptibility, and a sharp increase in the incidence of opportunistic infection has been observed with levels

<500/mm^3.[6] Clearly, factors such as the ability of the bone marrow to compensate in times of acute infection and the ability of circulating phagocytic cells to migrate into infected tissues may be of greater importance than the absolute circulating neutrophil count per se. In addition, as we have pointed out earlier in Chapter 4, it may be hazardous to equate risk of infection with only the absolute concentration of circulating neutrophils and not the trend in these levels. For instance, patients now treated with some of the modern aggressive antileukemic protocols will often experience a rapid plummeting of their granulocyte counts such that these levels will halve on each successive day of cytotoxic treatment. Even though patients may have a circulating level of 2000 neutrophils/mm^3 that appear morphologically normal, the production of neutrophils has been virtually halted; such patients with rapidly plummeting neutrophil counts are highly susceptible to acute bacterial infections.

A more interesting issue involves defective functional capacity of phagocytic cells in leukemic patients whose peripheral blood counts may not be at a "neutropenic" level. Recently developed techniques for evaluating microbicidal function of individual leukocytes in mixed populations[8-10] suggest that morphologically mature neutrophils of some patients with acute myelogenous leukemia have impaired ability to kill certain species of fungi and bacteria. The usual presumption has been that cells of the neutrophil series more immature than the metamyelocyte do not phagocytize and kill normally. However, it appears that some leukemic patients who are in hematologic remission or who have mixed populations of normal and leukemic cells in the peripheral blood have phagocytes that are morphologically normal but are functionally abnormal. The abnormality of impaired intracellular killing may not be present in the neutrophils alone but may be present in the mononuclear phagocytes as well. Thus, intracellular bacteria then may find a "sanctuary" from the bactericidal action of systemically administered antimicrobial agents, and this could explain, in part, the persistence of bacterial infection in patients receiving antibiotics. Again, there are many problems in the interpretation of these data including the effect of the underlying disease (in this case acute leukemia) and the added effect of chemotherapy. The

cause of the defective microbicidal activity has not been determined with certainty, but there is concomitant evidence that some of these morphologically normal cells have low levels of lysozyme.[10]

From a clinical view, the adult patient with myelogenous leukemia experiences a marked reduction in the likelihood of infection with the achievement of remission and the repopulation of bone marrow and peripheral blood with morphologically normal cells. Where intensification of remission therapy ("consolidation") has been particularly aggressive, as in some of the protocols for acute leukemia of childhood, the incidence of infection may be high even in remission.[11] The risk of pneumocystosis in patients who have received high-dose steroids during remission underscores this observation. In addition, it has been demonstrated that children with acute lymphatic leukemia undergoing craniospinal irradiation may have defective leukocyte microbicidal[12] function. These observations thus link an increased clinical incidence of infectious complications with a demonstrable abnormality in phagocyte function.[12]

It is widely held that thymus-derived lymphocyte (T-cell)-mediated immune functions are important defenses against a variety of fungal diseases. On the other hand, one of the more significant findings during much of the last decade is the rather striking increase in opportunistic fungal diseases, particularly candidiasis, aspergillosis, and mucormycosis, in the neutropenic acute leukemic population.[13-15] The most plausible explanation for this trend is that intensive multiple-agent treatment protocols given for acute leukemia do more than depress granulocyte precursors and have significant effects on cell-mediated immune function. It also seems likely that neutrophils are important for host defenses against organisms such as *Aspergillus* and *Candida*, something that is suggested by some recent studies[13,16] and the relative paucity of cases of systemic candidiasis and aspergillosis in patients with AIDS. (See Chapter 15.)

In general, humoral immunity as measured by antibody responses and complement levels seems to be relatively well preserved in the acute stages of therapy for acute lymphatic leukemia or acute myelogenous leukemia. Immunization with antigens such as *Pseudomonas aeruginosa* lipopolysaccharides results in brisk type-specific antibody response early in the course of both types of leukemia.[17] A functional assay of circulating antibodies against *P. aeruginosa*, the opsonophagocytosis test, showed no difference between normal serum and serum from children initially treated for acute lymphatic leukemia.[18] However, with resumption of intensive chemotherapy for relapsed leukemia, humoral levels of antibodies as measured by passive hemagglutination and by opsonophagocytosis against *P. aeruginosa* declined. This finding suggests that antibody-synthesizing capacity decreases as the underlying disease progresses and/or as more intensive chemotherapy is given in an attempt to induce remission. Opsonic deficiencies, therefore, parallel levels of circulating neutrophils,[17,19] a finding that may be critical for interpretation of the efficacy of transfused granulocytes (see Section 10).

The effect of antineoplastic chemotherapy in enhancing susceptibility to infection can neither be overlooked nor easily estimated. In addition to their quantitative effects on circulating neutrophils and lymphocytes, large doses of corticosteroids and vinca alkaloids such as vincristine and vinblastine affect bactericidal or locomotive function of phagocytes.[20] Even antibiotics of the polyene class or sulfonamides have been shown, in doses commonly used, to depress neutrophil function.[21,22] The use of pharmacological agents alone or in combination can compound an underlying intrinsic defect in host defenses, and such defects may persist for years.[23]

Patients with advanced Hodgkin disease occasionally exhibit the following immunologic abnormalities: (1) reduced response to a variety of antigens that induce delayed hypersensitivity reactions, (2) delayed homograft rejection, and (3) increased susceptibility to infections caused by varicella–zoster virus (VZV), granulomatous infections such as tuberculosis, and *Listeria monocytogenes*.[24] The blastogenic response of peripheral blood lymphocytes from patients with active Hodgkin disease is reduced on exposure to common antigens used in testing such as phytohemagglutinin. Contrary to widespread impression, delayed hypersensitivity responses as evaluated by a battery of skin tests employed in untreated patients in all stages of disease are normally present[25]: only 11.7% of more than 100 patients in one series were anergic to a battery of six skin-test antigens. No patient with stage I disease was anergic, and the incidence of complete anergy increased to 27% of patients with stage IV disease. Skin-test reactivity was found to correlate with the absence of systemic symptoms of disease as well as histologic type but was not a useful prognostic sign. The mean absolute lymphocyte count was inversely proportional to skin-test reactivity and declined in most advanced stages of disease. Thus, patients found to have stage I Hodgkin disease demonstrated skin test reactivity similar to normal controls, and in all stages of disease, skin test reactivity correlated with absence of symptoms. It was the conclusion of Young et al. that anergy, when it exists, is a result of disease progression and not the cause of the disease.[25] These authors also acknowledge that the prognostic value of the skin test as a measure of cellular immune function may be obscured by successful chemotherapeutic and radiotherapeutic intervention. King et al. have pointed out that patients successfully treated for lymphomas usually are not anergic when treated with ''recall'' antigens. By contrast, most are unable to develop delayed cutaneous hypersensitivity to neoantigens.[23]

There are conflicting data on abnormalities in polymorphonuclear leukocyte, monocyte, and macrophage function in patients with lymphomas. Steigbigel et al. studied patients with Hodgkin disease and other lymphomas in all stages of disease prior to staging laparotomy.[26] These patients were untreated, and none had evidence of active infection. Neutrophil function, serum opsonic activity, and monocyte-derived macrophage phagocytosis and killing were all within normal limits. During the course of in vitro experiments with macrophages incubated with *L. monocytogenes*, these investigators obtained a larger recovery of *L. monocytogenes* from supernatant fluids after macrophage cell lysis. However, these results could not be interpreted as solely reflecting a defect in intracellular killing, since both these workers and others[27] found that macrophages or reticuloendothelial cells from Hodgkin disease patients are more rapidly phagocytic than normal macrophages or reticuloendothelial cells. Furthermore, differences in macrophage function tests between cells from Hodgkin disease patients and normals were observed during the early incubation period (1–2 hr), but later (3–6 hr) there was no significant difference between the two groups. These results suggest that either macrophages from patients with Hodgkin disease are more avidly phagocytic than those of normal subjects or that macrophages from patients with the disease kill intracellular organisms such as *Listeria* more slowly following ingestion.

Although the studies of Steigbigel et al. failed to clarify an immunologic defect in these untreated patients with Hodgkin disease, others[23] have reported that patients receiving chemotherapy or radiation demonstrate impaired monocyte function. The possibility remains that those individuals who actually develop evidence of infection (as opposed to the uninfected patients with Hodgkin disease who were studied by Steigbigel) might manifest defects in intracellular killing, particularly against pathogens such as *Listeria,* mycobacteria, *Nocardia,* or *Salmonella.* Alternatively, some authors propose that defects are present in patients other than those having a nodular sclerosing histological pattern (which was the principal type that Steigbigel et al. studied) or that the defect in cell-mediated immune function lies not with the phagocytic cell but perhaps in the capacity to activate macrophages and to engage in the process of chemotaxis.[26] The latter function has been found to be abnormal in patients with Hodgkin disease because of the presence of a chemotactic factor inhibitor.[28] Thus, although the efferent loop, i.e., postphagocytic killing, may be normal, afferent processes in this immunologic "arc" may be impaired in Hodgkin disease. In vitro tests of bactericidal capacity involve direct mixing of microbes and cells (which may be activated in the process of harvesting or cultivation), whereas a chemotactic factor inhibitor may impair in vivo activation of the locomotion of cells that possess microbicidal activity (i.e., monocytes and neutrophils).

Earlier studies of the primary and secondary antibody response in patients with Hodgkin disease showed these to be unimpaired.[29] It has been stated that serum immunoglobulin levels are generally normal at the inception of treatment.[24] A recent study has reevaluated this concept in the light of more intensive combined treatment modalities that include radiotherapy, chemotherapy, and splenectomy.[30] The clinical observation of increased numbers of infections due to pneumococci and *Hemophilus influenzae* in patients receiving combined radiotherapy and chemotherapy where single treatment modalities reduced antibody titers insignificantly suggests a problem with humoral immunity. Although splenectomy had no effect on antibody titers, splenectomy potentiated the reduction of IgM levels by chemotherapy. However, IgG and IgA levels and alternate-pathway complement activation were either normal or elevated. These authors concluded that aggressive treatment with chemotherapy and radiation therapy impairs humoral defenses against encapsulated microorganisms and thus magnifies the risk of postsplenectomy septicemia in patients with Hodgkin disease. Thus, they concluded that treatment rather than the initial severity of disease is the major determinant responsible for depressed antibody levels. They have called attention to the irony that cure of Hodgkin disease in certain patients by the combination of splenectomy and intensive chemotherapy has transformed a cellular immune defect in the underlying disorder to a life-threatening deficiency in humoral immunity.[30]

3. The Role of Infection in Mortality from Leukemia and Lymphoma

There is no disputing the widely held view that infection plays the major role in the mortality associated with leukemias and some lymphomas. Although this information emanates from the major cancer treatment centers and therefore represents a population in which particularly vigorous chemotherapeutic, radiotherapeutic, and supportive measures have been given, it would be surprising if the role of infection was significantly different in patients with leukemia and lymphoma who received no treatment for their underlying disease. Table 1 is a summary of some of the major series reporting primary causes of death in acute leukemia or hematological malignancy. Five of the series concentrate exclusively on acute leukemia, and one of these four exclusively on childhood leukemia (primarily of the lymphatic type). Of the series summarized by Levine et al. from the National Cancer Institute, a total of 450 patients had hematological malignancies, of which the majority were cases of acute leukemia and malignant lymphomas.[34]

Although the series summarized on Table 1 are by no means comprehensive, they do point towards some interesting trends observed over the past 25 years. Perhaps the most meaningful juxtaposition is the report of Hersh et al. published in 1965, which summarizes the experience between 1954 and 1963

TABLE 1. Primary Causes of Death in Acute Leukemia or Hematologic Malignancy

Investigators	Site	Years	Population	Number of patients	Infection (%)	Hemorrhage (%)	Both (%)	Others (%)
Hersh et al.[31]	NCI	1954–1963	Acute leukemia	366	37.7	20.5	31.7	—
Viola[32]	Yale	1951–1966	Acute leukemia	78	40	33	7	20
Hughes[33]	St. Jude's	1962–1969	Cute childhood leukemia	199	45	—	33[a]	22
Levine et al.[34]	NCI	1965–1971	Hematological malignancy	450	69	11	10	10
Chang et al.[35]	M.D. Anderson	1966–1972	Adult acute leukemia	315	66	15	9	10
Feld and Bodey[38]	M.D. Anderson	1966–1973	Malignant lymphoma	206	51	9	—	40[b]
Estey[38a]	M.D. Anderson	1973–1979	Acute leukemia	123	49	11	20	20

[a]Infection and hemorrhage pooled together
[b]Organ failure and electrolyte imbalance, 23%, neoplasia, 11%, infarction, 6%

at the National Cancer Institute.[31] The period analyzed by Hersh contrasts significantly with the experience reported by Levine et al. from the same institution for the period between 1965 and 1971.[34] Whereas infection accounted for 38% of the primary causes of death in acute leukemia between 1954 and 1963, it had increased to 69% in the latter series from the same institution. One of the major differences between the two series was the decline in percentage of deaths primarily associated with hemorrhage. It is particularly impressive, however, that hemorrhage as the major co-primary cause of death declined at the National Cancer Institute from 31.7% in the 1954–1963 observation period to only 10% in the series reported by Levine and colleagues.[34] The report of Viola et al. from Yale University School of Medicine encompassed the years 1951–1966, for the most part a period during which several modern techniques for control of bleeding were not available; hence, the largest proportion of cases with acute leukemia died from hemorrhage alone.[32] Difficulty must be acknowledged, however, in distinguishing between the roles of infection and hemorrhage as causes of mortality because a number of infectious processes can trigger disseminated intravascular coagulation, and, conversely, a site where bleeding has occurred can become a focus for infection.

The problem in distinguishing between hemorrhage alone and infection plus hemorrhage is emphasized by the experience reported by Hughes at St. Jude's Children's Cancer Research Hospital where the results showed that infection was usually accompanied by hemorrhage, and together they accounted

for 33% of all deaths in this pediatric population.[33] Unquestionably, more effective control of bleeding complications with platelet transfusions and plasma factors seems responsible for the decline in the role of hemorrhage and the relative increase in the proportion of cases where infection has been the major cause of death. Of the more recently analyzed series,[34–37] infection alone appears to account for almost 70% of deaths from acute leukemia. Hemorrhage and infection together represent another 10% of cases, so that it seems reasonable to attribute some 75–80% of deaths in acute leukemia to infection-related causes.

Relatively less information is available on the role of infection in mortality from malignant lymphoma. Casazza reviewed the experience at the National Cancer Institute between 1953 and 1964 and reported that 99 of 134 patients who died had infections demonstrable at autopsy.[36] However, 124 of these 139 patients were believed to have died primarily of the disseminated neoplasm, albeit with serious associated microbial infection. Only two patients in the survey died with infection while the neoplastic disease was apparently in remission. These authors attributed only 10% of deaths in patients with Hodgkin disease and mycoses fungoides primarily to infectious causes. They concluded that even fewer patients, less than 4% with lymphocytic lymphoma and no patients with histiocytic lymphoma, died primarily of infection but rather had a refractory neoplasm as the cause of death.

A larger, more recent study has summarized the experience from the M.D. Anderson Hospital between 1966 and 1973 and is based on 206 patients with malignant lymphomas who had complete postmortem examinations.[38] The most common cause of death was thought to be infection, which accounted for 51% of the overall mortality. Death was thought to result from ''organ failure'' (hepatic and renal) in 25% of patients, hemorrhage in 9%, disseminated neoplastic disease in 8%, infarction of tissue in 6%, a second neoplasm in 3%, and electrolyte abnormalities in 1%. Finally, the experience in the treatment of 300 patients with Hodgkin disease has recently been reported from Stanford University Medical Center by Notter et al.[39] Although the overall mortality in a series of 300 patients was relatively low (19%), histological evidence of Hodgkin disease was present at death in more than two-thirds of patients who came to autopsy, and infection contributed to death in half of all autopsied patients. It was believed that few of these deaths were related to infection in the absence of active neoplasia.

4. Problems with the Interpretation of Fever and Infection Incidence Data in Neutropenic States

There are several major problems that must be acknowledged in any analytic approach to the scope of the infection problem in patients with leukemias and lymphomas: in recognition of these problems, the information summarized in the preceding and ensuing two sections should be accepted in only the broadest of terms, with stress placed on general relationships rather than the precision and accuracy of the information reported.

1. The limitations of extrapolating from autopsy data should be abundantly clear because infections present at autopsy and/or identified as the cause of death may have little relationship to a febrile episode experienced several weeks before. In many referral centers the overall rates at which autopsies have been performed (percentage of total deaths) has been on the decline.

2. Multiple agents may be recovered from blood or histologic material obtained at biopsy or autopsy, and the relative importance of each isolate may be difficult to ascertain.

3. Tumor may coexist with infection, and the causes of death may be multiple, including persistent neoplasm.

4. Different criteria have been used for defining neutropenic states, and most of the lymphomas have been reclassified. Therefore, some series cannot be directly compared.

5. Antibiotic usage has changed over the last 25 years with the introduction of newer systemic agents and the increasing tendency to use prophylactic systemic and oral nonabsorbable antibiotics. This may influence the recovery of pathogens from certain sites and could be responsible for a decreasing ability to establish a link between fever and documented infection in recent studies.

6. Varying criteria have been employed for defining infection. Some studies have included a category such as ''infection caused by unknown organisms,''[40] and others have employed a criterion in which the response to chemotherapy or antimicrobials is used to imply documented infection. One of the more frustrating aspects of dealing with neutropenic patients is that a significant number may have an infected local site such as soft tissue or lung,[41] but the precise cause of the infectious process is never identified. This lack of verification often results from the inability to undertake diagnostic studies or from concurrent antimicrobial therapy at the time that diagnostic attempts are made. Still, in the analysis of such events, it would seem more appropriate to distinguish microbiologically proven infections from febrile episodes whose microbial etiology was not documented.

7. The source of bacteremias in some immunosuppressed patients is never found.[3,42] This may be because of failure to culture the GI tract and distinguish normal flora and potential pathogens such as *P. aeruginosa*. As more careful surveillance studies have been carried out, the role of the GI tract as a source of many septicemias has been firmly established[43] (see Chapter 2).

8. Many studies analyzing the total incidence of fever and infection in neoplastic states fail to take into account the stage of the underly-

ing disease and whether patients are in a pretreatment, posttreatment, or consolidation phase. This factor may be critically related to the incidence and type of infecting agent. For instance, pneumocystosis in children is usually a disease of the remission phase. When it occurs in adults with lymphomas, the underlying disease is most often not under chemotherapeutic control.

5. Causes of Fever in Leukemia and Lymphoma

It is well recognized that fever can be a manifestation of underlying neoplastic disease, and this is particularly true of patients with leukemia and lymphoma. On the other hand, as emphasized in Chapter 4, the appearance of fever necessitates a thorough search for an infectious cause. How often this proves to be rewarding has varied over the last two decades, as shown in the experience of several centers. Table 2 is an attempt to summarize a number of studies primarily carried out in patients with acute leukemia but including some patients with lymphoma. Emphasis is placed on the type of neoplasm, the number of febrile episodes, and the proportion with documented infection vs unexplained fever. Several of these studies are particularly meritorious in that they represent a homogeneous population followed with the same chemotherapeutic protocol; other studies, such as our own, merely represent compilation of underlying diseases, number of episodes for which these patients were followed, and the proportion that turned out to have microbiologically documented infection. Although generalizations are perilous, it can be seen from the studies summarized in Table 2 that up to 70% of febrile episodes in patients with leukemia and lymphoma have been associated with a documented infection. In approximately 10% of patients, another cause such as a transfusion reaction or a drug allergy has been implicated, and the remainder have unexplained fever. On the other hand, some of the more recent studies show a decline in the incidence of documented infection to a range where it is less than 20%[51,52] Factors that may be responsible for this trend are the increasing tendency to use prophylactic nonabsorbable or systemic antibiotics to prevent infection in neutropenic subjects and the aggressive use of empirical antimicrobial therapy given at the very onset of fever in patients with falling neutrophil counts.[52]

The cause of unexplained fever is often the subject of spirited bedside debate. One of the most remarkable findings in our reported experience is that patients who had fever and undocumented infection still responded to a systemic regimen of aggressive antimicrobial therapy in approximately the same proportion as patients who had documented bacterial infection, almost exactly 75%.[50] Defervescence in response to antibiotic treatment even when infection is undocumented in neutropenic subjects is hardly a new observation; for instance, Silver et al., surveying their experience in the National Cancer Institute

TABLE 2. Documentation of Infection in the Febrile Neutropenic Patient[a]

Investigators	Year	Disease	Total number of episodes per total patients	Documented infection (%)	Other cause (%)	Unexplained fever (%)
Silver et al.[44]	1955–1956	AcLK	92/36	48	16	36
Raab et al.[45]	1960[b]	AcLK	149/55	68	6	26
Boggs and Fred[46]	1960[b]	LK, lym	162/97	40	6	54
Bodey et al.[47]	1966–1972	AcLK	1894/494	64	1	35
Goodall and Vosti[48]	1971–1972	AcLK	45/24	24	—	76
Burke et al.[42]	1965–1973	AcLK	180/104	66	8	26
Atkinson et al.[49]	1974[b]	AcLK, aplasia	100/56	62	6	32
Young[50]	1974–1976	AcLK, aplasia	353/198	33	—	67
Wade et al.[51]	1981[b]	AcLK	121/92	18	—	82
Pizzo et al.[52]	1986[b]	AcLK, ST	612/318	28	—	72

[a]AcLK, acute leukemia, Lym, lymphoma, ST, solid tumor
[b]Year published

between 1955 and 1956, reported that 14 of 33 patients with "fever of undetermined origin" responded to systemic antimicrobial therapy.[44] The systemic therapy in that series was often a tetracycline. The authors concede the possibility that antecedent use of penicillin might have been responsible for drug fever in a few cases. On the other hand, all the patients who responded to tetracycline were subsequently rechallenged with a penicillin, and none had recurrent fever, suggesting that the initial febrile elevation while the patient was receiving penicillin was not caused by drug allergy.

For those patients who defervesce after initiation of systemic antimicrobial therapy, the best explanation appears to be effective treatment of a localized infection that has not yet "spilled over" into the bloodstream so that the infecting organism is not recovered from blood cultures or other readily accessible sites. Support for this concept comes from several sources. (1) Those fevers of undetermined origin that persist for several weeks on antibiotics eventually terminate in a serious microbial infection.[44,48] Whether these processes were originally caused by the organism subsequently isolated from blood remains unresolved. Goodall and Vosti noted that roughly one-half of patients who were granulocytopenic from leukemia therapy and had no cause discovered prior to the start of antibiotics subsequently developed an infection that they interpreted as a superinfection.[48] Clearly, however, the possibility that an initially localized process that then spread and was responsible for "breakthrough" sepsis could not be excluded in their series. (2) Surveillance cultures reveal GI colonization by organisms such as *P. aeruginosa* and *Klebsiella* species that are not part of the normal bowel flora. They may be eliminated by systemic antibiotic therapy or oral antimicrobials (aminoglycosides and polymyxins) concurrent with defervescence. (3) We have carried out several studies with paired patient sera and antigens of *P. aeruginosa* and *Enterobacteriaceae* and demonstrated seroconversion after defervescence and achievement of remission (unpublished data).

Illustrative Case 1

A 36-year-old Hispanic man had newly diagnosed acute myelocytic leukemia. He was admitted to the hospital for intensive induction chemotherapy with a combination of thioguanine, cytosine arabinoside, and daunorubicin. He had been treated by his own physician for symptoms of respiratory infection, cough, and easy bruisability. An antimicrobial, ampicillin, had been one of the agents used. Following hospitalization and initiation of treatment, his white count rapidly plummetted to less than 100 mature granulocytes/mm³, and he developed fever to 104 9°F (40.5°C). A chest radiograph revealed right lower lung field consolidation (Fig. 1), and despite a platelet count of only 30,000/mm³, a transtracheal aspirate was performed. Gram stains of the transtracheal aspirate revealed few neutrophils but moderate numbers of gram-negative bacilli. Aerobic cultures of the aspirate revealed pure growth of *Pseudomonas aeruginosa*. Six sets of blood cultures taken at the time of temperature elevation eventually showed no growth. Immediately after the transtracheal aspirate, he was started on amikacin and carbenicillin, and the patient gradually defervesced over the ensuing 3 days. Eventually he achieved a hematologic remission and was discharged from the hospital.

Comment. *Pseudomonas aeruginosa* bacteremia, in our experience, has been one of the most common causes of gram-negative sepsis in the neutropenic subject (see below). However, variations in institutional incidence do occur, and it is our impression that the problem of *Pseudomonas* is most common when very intense cytotoxic regimens are used. Of great interest in this case was that multiple blood cultures drawn when the patient was febrile failed to grow *Pseudomonas aeruginosa*, yet transtracheal aspiration revealed abundant growth of *Pseudomonas* organisms. This case underscores our belief that many patients have localized infections caused by *P. aeruginosa* that have not yet "spilled over" into the bloodstream at the time the patient suddenly develops fever and symptoms of sepsis. The nonbacteremic *Pseudomonas* pneumonia in this case was probably caused by aspiration. Prompt treatment prevented dissemination of disease, and better control of opportunistic infection may have provided the basis for early achievement of remission. Had tracheal aspiration not been performed, this case would be yet another febrile episode in a neutropenic leukemic, attributed to an infectious process, but of undetermined etiology. In reality, the decision to proceed with transtracheal aspiration was made in ignorance of the platelet count. We do not recommend performing transtracheal aspirates with platelet counts less than 40,000/mm³. In this case, the decision to proceed with transtracheal aspiration was probably ill conceived, yet gave information that was highly valuable in the management of the patient. Since platelet transfusions are now readily available, they would have been warranted in this case prior to the procedure.

Febrile episodes are the rule rather than the exception in patients being intensely treated for leukemia and lymphoma. Silver et al. observed that only two patients of a total of 36 remained afebrile throughout the course of their induction therapy for acute leukemia.[44] Most patients experience more than one episode of fever during the course of induction attempts. In the study of Boggs and Frei, children with acute leukemia experienced 4.6 febrile episodes per 100 days of hospitalization; the figure was

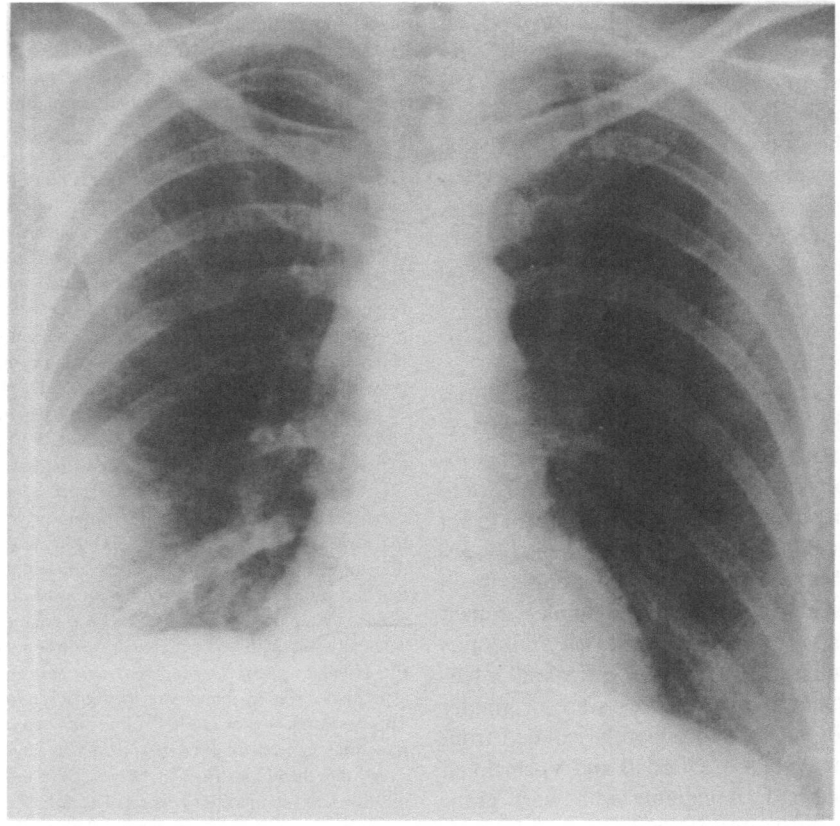

FIGURE 1. PA view of chest in Illustrative Case 1, a febrile neutropenic patient with acute myelocytic leukemia who developed right lower lobe consolidation. All blood cultures were negative, but a transtracheal aspirate grew a pure culture of *Pseudomonas aeruginosa*.

slightly lower, 3.9 episodes per 100 days, in adult patients with acute leukemia, and the latter figure was twice as great for patients with lymphomas.[46] Understandably, most episodes of fever occur while the diseases are in relapse and/or are being intensely treated. In one study, only four of 100 febrile episodes occurred while the underlying neoplastic disease was in remission.[49] All these febrile patients were adults with acute lymphoblastic leukemia immediately prior to or during radiation directed at the central nervous system. In our experience, fevers occurring during hematological remission often suggest allergy or a persistent viral disease such as hepatitis or cytomegalovirus infection.

Although the studies summarized in Table 2 are useful in giving a broad view of the likelihood of infection in febrile conditions, it should be recognized that one of the problems with such data is often

a lack of a clear-cut relationship to the clinical stage of underlying disease. Stated in another way, the likelihood of serious infection will differ if the patient is presenting for initial chemotherapy, is at the beginning of a consolidation cycle, or has developed the severe complications of cytotoxic treatment. Thus. Burke et al. at the Johns Hopkins Hospital noted that almost three-quarters of their patients with acute myelocytic leukemia had fever on presentation, but of these, only 15% had severe infection, and 43% had infected local sites.[42] As chemotherapy was given. fully 90% of patients developed a life-threatening infection. In the latter study, several different antileukemic regimens were used. By contrast, Goodall and Vosti at Stanford University Hospital reported a series of 24 patients who were all treated in the same manner for their acute leukemia.[48] They reported that fever on admission to the hospital prior to the induction of chemotherapy usually resulted from an identifiable cause, but this observation differs somewhat from the Johns Hopkins experience where 40% of patients did not have a documented infection on presentation. During the initiation of chemotherapy, Goodall and Vosti noted fevers in approximately a third of patients, but most of these were short-lived, and some resolved without antimicrobial therapy. As patients became granulocytopenic secondary to treatment, either a cause of fever was found or superinfection subsequently developed. Unfortunately, some infections were not recognized until autopsy. The latter fact illustrates a common dilemma for those investigators attempting to analyze the nature of infection in neutropenic cancer patients—namely, whether autopsy or terminally documented infection can be etiologically linked to earlier febrile episode(s).

6. Site of Involvement and the Nature of the Microbial Pathogen(s)

Information published on the nature of fatal infection—the major site of involvement and the relative proportion of bacterial, fungal, and viral etiologies—is somewhat similar for hematological malignancies. Table 3 summarizes four studies, one from the National Cancer Institute (patients with "hematologic malignancy" included those with acute leukemias and lymphomas), and the experience from three studies reported from the treatment of acute leukemia and malignant lymphoma at the M.D. Anderson Hospital. Only two major sites of involvement are listed, systemic infection and respiratory

infections. Obviously, systemic infections must start in some localized area. As pointed out by Burke et al., the most common primary site of acute leukemia infection is the perirectal/genital area, followed by the urinary tract, skin, and only then the lung.[42] In Burke's studies as well as others, approximately 20% of patients had an unknown source of systemic infection. It seems likely that if such patients were systematically studied with surveillance cultures, suggestive evidence for a source in and around the gastrointestinal tract would be found (see Chapter 2).

From the segregation of pneumonia from systemic infections in Table 3 (a respiratory source excludes those patients whose systemic infections might have originated in the lung), the conclusion is inescapable: bacteria are the most common cause of both systemic infections and pneumonia, and non-pulmonary bacterial infections outnumber bacterial respiratory infections. The table does not, however, reflect the current view that the relative proportion of disseminated fungal infections noted at autopsy is increasing. Up to as many as one-half of patients with leukemias and lymphomas autopsied in four series had disseminated fungal disease.[13–15,37,53] Thus, it appears that Table 3 may underestimate the prevalence of fungal disease at autopsy. The most recent study from the M.D. Anderson hospital found that fungal infection was found in 18% of autopsied patients and an additional 18% had both bacterial and fungal infection present at autopsy.[37] Under the category of "other" types of fatal infection are such entities as *Pneumocystis carinii* pneumonia, toxoplasmosis, and several viral diseases. The relatively small proportion of viral isolations may also be a reflection of less adequate techniques for identification of such agents.

TABLE 3. Types of Fatal Infection in Hematologic Malignancies[a]

Investigators	Year	Patients	N	Systemic infection			Pneumonia			Other
				Bacterial (%)	Fungal (%)	B & F[b] (%)	Bacterial (%)	Fungal (%)	B & F[b] (%)	
Levine et al.[34]	1965–1971	Hematologic malignancy	354	37	13	3	19	12	3	13
Chang et al.[35]	1966–1972	Acute leukemia	234	56	10	6	11	3	—	12
Feld and Bodey[38]	1966–1973	Malignant lymphoma	104	44	4	—	36	2	—	13
Estey[38a]	1973–1979	Acute leukemia	90	34	15	11	—	c	—	—

[a]Indicates percentage of total in each series with type of fatal infection
[b]B & F, bacterial plus fungal
[c]No discrete subdivisions between organisms causing systemic infection and pneumonia

TABLE 4. Organisms Implicated in Fatal Septicemic Infections[a]

Organism	Hersh et al [31]		Chang et al [35] 1966–1972	Levine et al [34] 1965–1971[c]	Hughes[33] 1962–1969[d]
	1954–1959	1960–1963			
Pseudomonas aeruginosa	24 6	34 4	18 1	16	36.7
Escherichia coli	21.6	12 8	18 8	—	19.3
Klebsiella pneumoniae	6 7	12.8	18.7	34	5.1
Other bacilli	—	—	18 8	—	9.0
Streptococcus aureus	23.9	4 8	2 0	NA	11 0
Fungi	8.2	23.8	NA	13	33 5
Multiple organisms	NA	NA	22%	3	1 2
Total number on which calculation based	366		149	462	155

[a]Expressed as percentage of total
[b]NA, not available
[c]Patients had negative blood cultures in remainder of infectious deaths
[d]Total exceeds 100%
[e]This figure includes *E coli*, *K pneumoniae*, and other bacilli

With respect to the etiology of fatal septicemic infection in acute adult and pediatric leukemias, Table 4 summarizes the causative organisms expressed as a percent of the total. Two of these reviews, that of Hersh et al.[31] and Levine et al.,[34] come from the National Cancer Institute and highlight the similarities and differences observed during three periods, 1954–1959, 1960–1963, and 1965–1971. Although there are some major differences in the way some of these data are tallied, such as the handling of polymicrobial sepsis, all of these studies emphasize the important role that gram-negative rods and particularly *P. aeruginosa* play in fatal infections. The most dramatic decrease in fatal infections caused by a single organism is nicely detailed in the experience of Hersh et al.[31] Almost 24% of fatal septicemias between 1954 and 1959 were caused by *S. aureus*, whereas the prevalence declined to less than 5% in the ensuing 4-year period. The experience of Chang et al. shows an even lower proportion of staphylococcal infections that end with a fatal outcome.[35] Autopsy data are potentially misleading because they may summarize only those infections that have a terminal outcome and might not reflect an actually greater incidence of a specific infection that was more amenable to successful therapy. In the case of staphylococcal sepsis, however, Goodall and Vosti noted no cases of staphylococcal infection and a predominance of systemic gram-negative bacillary and fungal infections in their cases.[48] Similarly, in our series of bacteremias complicating acute leukemia and aplastic anemia therapy, we observed only six cases of staphylococcal sepsis in comparison to 49 cases of gram-negative septicemia.[50] Perhaps most remarkably, there were no deaths associated with *S. aureus* bacteremia, whereas 30% of the gram-negative bacteremias were associated with a fatal outcome.

Many recent reviews have emphasized resurgence of gram-positive coccal infection in neutropenic subjects[54,55] with the widespread use of indwelling vascular catheters of the Hickman, Broviac, Porta Cath, or similar type. *S. epidermidis* has become one of the most common cases of bacteremia in neutropenic cancer patients. Enterococcal infections also appear to have increased, perhaps because of increased use of cepholosporins. On the other hand, these bacteremic infections are infrequently of a rapidly fatal nature. In some cases, it is the indolent course of the infection that has led clinicians to doubt the validity of an initial blood culture report and delay onset of therapy. It has been our experience that catheter-associated bacteremia caused by *S. epidermidis* can be treated after the results of the cultures are known, and these infections are not fulminant. However, some *S. aureus* infections are now due to methicillin-resistant strains,[55] and aggressive treatment of these complications is still strongly recommended.

Summaries of fatal infection in neutropenic pa-

TABLE 5. Fatal *P. aeruginosa* Bacteremia by Neoplasm[a]

Neoplasm	Number of deaths	All gram-negative bacteremia		*P aeruginosa*	
		N	Percent	N	Percent fatal bacteremias
Leukemia					
Acute myelo/monocytic	19	12	63	10	84
Acute lymphatic	8	4	50	2	50
Chronic myelocytic	12	2	16	2	100
Chronic lymphatic/lymphocytic lymphoma	37	15	40	11	73
Lymphoma					
Hodgkin	56	6	11	3	50
Non-Hodgkin	32	5	16	2	40
Solid tumors	289	7	3	2	28

[a]Modified after Armstrong et al [3]

tients could be misleading if no attempt is made to consider the association between underlying diseases and specific pathogens. Although *P. aeruginosa* is a leading cause of mortality in the data summarized in Table 4, an even more striking means for demonstrating the role played by this pathogen in leukemias and lymphomas is demonstrated in Table 5. Although compiled 15 years ago, this table summarizes fatal gram-negative bacteremias by neoplastic disease at one institution.[31] More than 60% of acute myelo/monocytic leukemias were associated with a fatal gram-negative bacteremia, and of these fatal septicemias, 84% were caused by *P. aeruginosa*. The incidence of gram-negative septicemia was relatively low for Hodgkin disease and non-Hodgkin lymphomas, 11% and 16% respectively, but of those fatal bacteremic infections that did occur, 50% and 40%, respectively, of the entire total were caused by *P. aeruginosa*.

Studies of all bacteremias complicating leukemia, not necessarily only those with a fatal outcome, show a relative similarity in the proportion of types of infecting pathogens. Thus, Bodey et al. reported that systemic infection and pneumonia together accounted for 69% of total episodes of documented infection in leukemics, and the great majority of infecting pathogens were gram-negative bacilli.[47] In their survey of all septicemias, Bodey and colleagues reported a finding similar to our own: namely, a relative decline in *E. coli* infections and an increase

in the proportion of infections caused by *Klebsiella, Enterobacter,* and *Serratia* species. Currently, the relative frequency of *Klebsiella* isolated from bacteremic infections in neutropenic leukemics is as great as *P. aeruginosa*.

In addition to gram-negative bacterial agents commonly isolated from blood cultures, several studies of infection in cancer patients show an association between a specific pathogen and a neoplastic disorder. Such tallies of isolates by underlying diseases have been particularly interesting, as shown in Table 6. For instance, listeriosis has traditionally been associated with Hodgkin disease and lymphomas; indeed, at the one institution from which these data are summarized (Memorial Sloan-Kettering Cancer Center), there were 18 cases of listeriosis in lymphoma patients as contrasted to three cases in patients with acute leukemias.[56] Similarly, there were ten cases of nocardiosis in patients with lymphomas as opposed to two in acute leukemia, 24 cases of cryptococcosis in lymphoma patients as opposed to one with acute leukemia, and seven cases of toxoplasmosis in lymphoma patients versus none with leukemia. The large number of cases of *Bacteroides* infection associated with solid tumors is probably the reflection of infectious complications following gastrointestinal surgery, and a large number of "other tumors" associated with tuberculosis were pulmonary in origin.

We believe that the associations shown in Table

TABLE 6. Relative Frequency of Some Opportunistic Pathogens by Neoplastic Disease[a]

Organism	Acute leukemia	Hodgkin disease	Non-Hodgkin lymphoma	Other tumors
Bacteriodes sp.	4	4	2	41
C. neoformans	1	14	10	3
L. monocytogenes	3	12	6	3
M. tuberculosis	1	4	4	72
N. asteroides	2	5	5	7
P. aeruginosa	11	1	14	20
Streptococcus				
Group A sp	5	5	5	30
pneumoniae	8	6	8	25
T. gondii	0	6	1	3

[a]"Numerator" data only (Memorial Hospital) From Armstrong [56]

6 are valid and consistent with our experience. On the other hand, such information, which might be designated "numerator data" because it refers only to numbers of cases rather than to precise relative incidence, must be qualified in the light of the different frequencies with which the underlying diseases occur. During the period when the information summarized in Table 6 was obtained, the estimated annual incidence of solid tumors in the United States was more than 300 times that of acute leukemia; Hodgkin disease and non-Hodgkin lymphomas were perhaps 20 times more common than acute leukemia.[57] If we were to take these factors into consideration and the disease prevalence data at this particular institution were the same as for the United States as a whole, the classic concept that cryptococcosis, listeriosis, tuberculosis, nocardiosis, and toxoplasmosis are more common in Hodgkin disease and the lymphomas than in acute leukemia would not hold true.

Clearly we are not justified in extrapolating from national incidence data to the experience at a single referral institution. Other investigators have also questioned the "classic associations between underlying disorder and specific opportunistic infection.[58] In future studies it would obviously be desirable to have specific institutional data on the numbers of cases of underlying disease that it treats that can then be used as the appropriate "denominator" figure for calculating relative incidence of infectious complications. Where such information is available, some interesting associations have become apparent: when cases of cryptococcal infection at Memorial

Sloan-Kettering Cancer Center were factored for numbers of patients with an underlying disease admitted during the study period (to determine a case rate per 1000 cases of neoplasm), it was found that the disease most commonly associated with cryptococcosis was chronic lymphatic leukemia.[59] The incidence was 24.3 cases per thousand in contrast to Hodgkin disease with an incidence of 13.3 cases per thousand. Chronic myelogenous leukemia, interestingly, had a case incidence of 10.9 per thousand. These rates for the lymphomas and leukemias were dramatically higher than the incidence of cryptococcosis complicating carcinoma of the breast, where 0.159 cases per thousand were observed.

TABLE 7. Prevalence of Tuberculosis by Neoplastic Disease[a]

Neoplasm	TB case/10,000
Leukemia	
Acute myelocytic	28
Acute lymphatic	37
Lymphoma	
Hodgkin disease	96
Non-Hodgkin	83
Carcinomas	
Lung	92
Stomach	55
Head and neck	51
Colon	6
Bladder	4

[a]Modified from Kaplan et al [60]

TABLE 8. Underlying Diseases in Opportunistic Fungal Infections

Disease	Histoplasmosis[61-63]	Cryptococcosis[59]	Coccidioidomycosis[64]
Hodgkin disease	18	19	6
Chronic lymphatic leukemia	12	5	—
Acute lymphatic leukemia	10	1	—
Other leukemias	6	2	—
Non-Hodgkin lymphoma	4	9	2
Systemic lupus erythematosus	6	—	—
Renal transplant	7	—	1
Other	3	5	4
Total	66	41	13

Applying the same analytic epidemiologic technique to tuberculosis as they did to cryptococcosis, Kaplan et al.[60] confirmed the classic association between Hodgkin disease and tuberculosis. As shown in Table 7, the tuberculosis case rate for patients with Hodgkin disease was the highest for any neoplasm, 96/10,000 cases, which was followed by carcinoma of the lung (92/10,000), and non-Hodgkin lymphoma (83/10,000). The association with cancer of the lung has triggered speculation about etiologic links between the two entities as well as suggesting the possible mechanism that a growing carcinoma might lead to breakdown of calcified foci of tuberculous infection. Despite the convincingly supported data shown in Table 7, it is our impression that the incidence of tuberculous disease in immunosuppressed patients is declining, paralleling the U.S. decline in clinical disease and a reduction in the "reservoir" of tuberculin-positive individuals in the population.

Consistent with the widely accepted view that Hodgkin disease is associated with a T-lymphocyte-mediated defect and increased susceptibility to fungal infection, "numerator" data on the incidence of some of the important opportunistic fungal pathogens are summarized in Table 8. Hodgkin disease has been the most common neoplasm associated with histoplasmosis, cryptococcosis, and coccidioidomycosis (see also Table 4 in Chapter 11 concerning toxoplasmosis). In contrast to the association with Hodgkin disease, the numbers of cases of these fungal infections in acute leukemias has been small. If present trends continue, it is likely that there will be a strong association between Kaposi's Sarcoma seen as part of the AIDS syndrome and opportunistic mycotic infections caused by cryptococci, *C. immitis*, and *H. capsulatum*. This emphasizes the importance of T-lymphocyte mediated defenses against these fungal pathogens.

Just as the incidence and the type of infection complicating acute leukemia is dependent on the treatment status and stage of the disease, a similar conclusion can be drawn about the lymphomas. The older report of Casazza et al.[36] emphasized that the great majority of serious infections occurred during the advanced stages of the lymphomas. This conclusion has been reaffirmed by more recent reviews. Generally, low fatality rates are associated with infections occurring during the early stages of disease,[38,39] but in patients who are unresponsive to further antineoplastic chemotherapy, infection is the primary cause of death. Not surprisingly, a variety of bacterial, viral, and fungal processes occur preterminally. In the experience of Feld and Bodey, there was not much difference between the Hodgkin and the non-Hodgkin lymphoma in the incidence of septicemias and pneumonias.[38] There were, however, larger numbers of urinary tract infections in patients with non-Hodgkin lymphomas, and this may have been related to a higher incidence of genitourinary tract obstruction by tumor.

Another area where there appears to be some difference between Hodgkin and non-Hodgkin lymphomas is in the incidence and type of involvement with herpes zoster. Patients vigorously treated with combination chemotherapy and/or radiation therapy for Hodgkin disease have an incidence of herpes zoster that ranges between 19% and 34.5%.[65-69] This incidence is significantly higher for patients with Hodgkin disease than for non-Hodgkin lymphoma by a factor of 3:1.[38] The highest risk (56%) was found in children who received both combination chemotherapy plus extensive radiotherapy, but splenectomy did not increase the risk of this viral infection.[69] Most patients developed zoster within a year of initiating chemotherapy and/or radiation therapy, and zoster was most frequently associated with a previously irradiated dermatome.[66] The incidence of dissemination of infection has been quoted as approximately 25%,[68,69] but the definition of dissemination has been quite variable. It is common to see vesicular lesions outside of the primary dermatome without evidence of visceral involvement, and Feldman and co-workers cite an incidence of 50% for this phenomenon, which they term "skin generalization."[66] In general, the mortality from herpes zoster has been low,[66–69] but disseminated disease that includes pneumonic involvement has a mortality that in our experience exceeds 75% and has been reported as high as 100%.[66] With the ready availability of acylovir, however, one would expect the incidence of *H. zoster* dissemination to decline and for the case fatality ratio to fall as well.

The advent of more intensive chemotherapy for non-Hodgkin lymphoma has made the infectious complications more similar to leukemia. In one series, 83% of documented infections were due to gram-negative bacilli and staphylococci, with *P. aeruginosa* the major cause of bacteremia and pneumonia.[70] Of 125 patients reviewed, mycobacterial, listerial, nocardial, *P. carinii,* and cryptococcal infections were rare or did not occur at all.

Relatively few modern reports have summarized infection hazards in patients with multiple myeloma. Shaikh and associates reviewed 46 patients with myeloma and found that gram negative bacilli were the predominant pathogens.[71] This contrasts with earlier studies indicating that *S. pneumoniae* is characteristically associated with this neoplastic disease.[72]

One review of Hodgkin disease and the non-Hodgkin lymphomas calls attention to a disturbing number of fatalities resulting from infections that were not associated with presence of neoplasm at autopsy.[37] Often, these were cases in which consolidation chemotherapy or intense chemotherapy was given in an attempt to eradicate the underlying tumor. As deaths have occurred in these groups because of supervening infection, this serves as a reminder that individuals who may have no evidence of tumor involvement can still die from septic processes or septic complications as a result of intensive chemotherapy aimed at eradicating the underlying disease.

Finally, the problem of pneumococcal sepsis in patients who are surgically splenectomized or functionally so (after radiation) should also be placed in the following perspective: even before splenectomy was a routine component of Hodgkin disease management, cases of overwhelming pneumococcal sepsis were observed in patients with leukemias, lymphomas, and solid tumors.[56] As shown in Table 6, the greatest number of cases in that series occurred in patients with solid tumors rather than lymphomas and acute leukemias, If, however, one "factors" for known differences in disease incidence, the risk is still considerable in those patients having a primary defect in neutrophil-mediated host defenses. The incidence of postsplenectomy pneumococcal sepsis appears to be particularly significant in the pediatric age population.[1] One of the most interesting observations has been the poor antibody response[73,74] to the pneumococcal type VI (VIA, VIB, in Danish system, and 6 and 26 in the American system) antigens. Even before the recent licensure of pneumococcal vaccines, type VI pneumococci were the largest single cause of such bacteremia in hematological malignancy.[75] This suggests that the pneumococcal infection risk in an era when splenectomy is commonly performed is but a continuation of an established trend. Type VI organisms are the most commonly isolated in pneumococcal infections complicating bone marrow transplantation which may be regarded as creating a "functionally asplenic" state.[2] The major threat that organisms of the type VI serotype(s) pose is probably related to their poor immunogenicity even in normal subjects[74]; susceptibility to infections by agents with this antigenic composition seems to be increased in immunocompromised subjects.

7. Synthesis

Primarily from information obtained from retrospective or autopsy reviews, clinical trials of antimicrobial therapy, and epidemiologic studies in neutropenic patients, the following "synthesis" is offered as a summary of the changing nature of the problem of fever and infection in the patient with leukemia or lymphoma.

In the neutropenic patient who has never received chemotherapy, approximately one-half of patients present with fever (i.e., at time of diagnosis); of these, one-third are found to have a localized bacterial infection. These localized infections are caused by staphylococci, streptococci, and the more antibiotic-susceptible gram-negative rods including *E. coli*. In patients with lymphomas, tuberculosis and cryptococcosis are perhaps the only pathogens unequivocally associated with untreated underlying disease. The remaining two-thirds of febrile patients on presentation have fevers caused by their neoplasms or quite localized infections in and around the gastrointestinal tract that infrequently spill over and cause detectable bacteremia. If patients are given oral antibiotics such as ampicillin, cephalosporins, or tetracyclines prior to chemotherapy, they are predisposed to GI colonization by the more antibiotic-resistant gram-negative rods such as *P. aeruginosa* and *Klebsiella* species and fungi such as *Candida* and *Torulopsis* species. However, severity of underlying disease alone in the absence of a selection pressure from antimicrobials can result in colonization of the host by these more drug-resistant organisms.

After antineoplastic treatment has been initiated, fevers secondary to drugs, transfusion reactions, and possibly tumor necrosis enter into the differential diagnosis. Perhaps one-third of these fevers are associated with bacterial infection, but infection should be assumed to be the cause of the temperature elevation and antimicrobials promptly started if the patient is markedly neutropenic (neutrophil count < 500/mm^3) or the white count is rapidly falling. During first and second induction attempts, documented infections still are caused by more sensitive organisms such as staphylococci and *E. coli,* but as repeated courses of antibiotics are given, the likelihood progressively increases that the patient will be colonized and infected by fungi such as *Candida* and resistant gram-negative bacilli. Many leukemics and lymphoma patients defervesce on empirical antimicrobial treatment during chemotherapy before evidence of remission is achieved. It is likely that the majority of persistent fevers will eventually prove to have a bacterial cause if the patient is left untreated, although the simultaneous contribution of the tumor to febrile symptoms cannot be excluded. Some of the fevers that persist in the face of antimicrobials may be caused by undiagnosed viral infection. Aggressive use of systemic antimicrobial agents probably terminates localized bacterial infection—low-grade infections originating around the GI tract and possibly associated with anaerobes—in a large number of patients without documented bacteremia. This accounts for the common observation that patients will improve on empirical antimicrobial therapy without documented infection. Furthermore, new approaches to preventing infection such as use of oral antimicrobial agents to suppress the fecal flora may contribute to culture negativity. Irrespective of the cause of fever, most patients become afebrile with achievement of remission or rise in normal neutrophil count. The exceptions to this probably include chronic viral infections caused by herpes and hepatitis viruses.

It is a great oversimplification to regard infection problems in the various leukemias and lymphomas as similar. Considerably more progress has been made in acute lymphocytic leukemia of childhood and Hodgkin disease than in acute nonlymphocytic leukemia in the adult. At one time steroids were commonly used to treat myelocytic leukemia but probably predisposed to more infection (compared to regimens not incorporating steroids), have little effect against the leukemia, and now are infrequently used.[41] This may be a factor in the improving outlook for infection control accompanying use of some of the recent myelocytic leukemia protocols.[68] On the other hand, steroids have a well-accepted antitumor effect in lymphocytic leukemias and lymphomas, so by helping to ameliorate the underlying disease, they reduce the overall infection risk. Still, there are infections that occur in patients with lymphoma and lymphatic leukemia that seem related to depressed cell-mediated immunity, and these infections may occur during the remission phase of the disease because of use of consolidation or maintenance chemotherapy. The best example of such an infection is *Pneumocystis carinii* pneumonia.

If relapse occurs or remission is not achieved, and the patient continues to be treated to the point of neutropenia, the risk of fatal septicemia caused by *P. aeruginosa* or the opportunistic fungi increases. Opportunistic fungal infections have two primary pathways: the gastrointestinal route for *Candida* species and the airborne pneumonic route for aspergillosis and the zygomycosis. This suggests some epidemiologic approaches aimed at control. Nonetheless, the pressing need is for diagnostic methods that will distinguish GI colonization by *Candida* from early systemic invasion. At autopsy, most leukemics and the majority of patients with lymphomas have evidence for infection. Nonetheless, it could be misleading to equate what is found at autopsy with infectious processes or febrile episodes that were evident weeks before death.

Illustrative Case 2

A 36-year-old white woman had a history of stage IVB Hodgkin disease initially diagnosed 8 years prior to admission. After successful treatment with four cycles of MOPP therapy, she was disease-free for almost 7 years but was eventually readmitted to the hospital with increasing fatigue, easy bruisability, and a white count that showed an acute myelocytic leukemia. She noted daily temperature elevations of 102.2°F (39°C). Physical examination revealed a chronically ill patient with slight lymphadenopathy and hepatomegaly. Peripheral blood showed large numbers of blasts, and she was begun on a 7-day course of thioguanine, cytosine arabinoside, and daunorubicin. Shortly thereafter, she became febrile to 102.9°F (39.4°C) and was started on an aminoglycoside and an antipseudomonal penicillin. After 4 days of therapy, she gradually defervesced but was found on chest radiography to have persistent interstitial markings and a left lower lobe infiltrate. Because of the isolation of *Candida* species from stool and urine, she was started on systemic amphotericin B with therapy increased to a total daily dose of 40 mg/day. After 2 weeks of amphotericin, marked febrility returned, a right middle lobe infiltrate developed, and amphotericin B was held because of an increase in serum creatinine. Over the ensuing 4 days, chest radiographs demonstrated both right middle and left lower lobe infiltrates that both contained cavities (Fig. 2A). Fiberoptic bronchoscopy was performed, and brushings revealed multiple

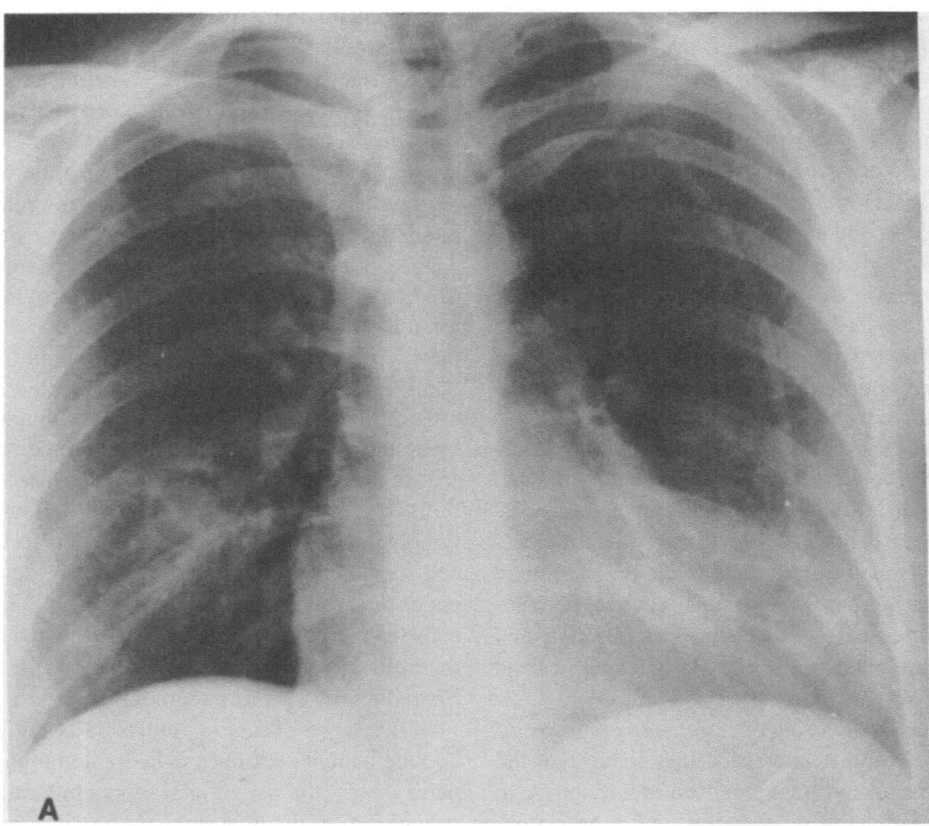

FIGURE 2. (A) Chest radiograph of patient with acute myelocytic leukemia (developing after successful treatment of Hodgkin disease) who developed cavitating infiltrates in the right middle and left lower lobes after prolonged antibacterial therapy. Although this pattern is most commonly seen with *Aspergillus* lung infections, *Petriellidium boydii* was grown from transbronchial biopsies. (B) Multiple infiltrates, many of them cavitating, developed in this young leukemic male with *S. aureus* bacteremia. The prognosis in this infection is far better than with cavitary fungal disease in patients with hematologic malignancies.

branching septate hyphae suggestive of *Aspergillus* species. Systemic antibacterial agents were continued, amphotericin was reinstituted, and a week later *Petriellidium boydii* was grown from the bronchial washings. At this point, miconazole 400 mg q6h was started. The patient developed a pruritic maculopapular rash over her entire body. Both miconazole and amphotericin were held. At this point, the patient experienced daily intermittent fevers as high as 104°F (40°C), confusion, and disorientation, and amphotericin B was resumed after a 4-day hiatus. Progressive consolidation in both lung fields occurred. The patient developed progressive hypoxia and myoclonic seizures and expired almost 2 months after her initial final hospitalization. Autopsy revealed presence of *Petriellidium boydii* in both consolidated lungs.

Comment. This patient was aggressively treated with antibacterial and antifungal chemotherapy for fever, although no bacterial cause of infection was documented. Because of concern that she might have underlying systemic candidiasis, a diagnosis suggested by positive stool and urine cultures, she was started on amphotericin B. Eventually she developed bilateral cavitary pneumonia secondary to *Petriellidium boydii*. This fungus can be mistaken for *Aspergillus* species and causes a similar pathological picture of vascular invasion and infarction of tissue. It is on the latter basis that cavitation occurs, similar to that observed with pulmonary aspergillosis and phycomycosis (mucormycosis).[14,15] Unfortunately, *P. boydii* is usually resistant to amphotericin B but may be inhibited in vitro by miconazole. In this case, therapy with amphotericin and miconazole was ineffective, but the major determining factor underlying the progression of fatal outcome in this disease was a refractory leukemia that developed following successful treatment of Hodgkin disease. Nonetheless, the specific type of superinfection appears to reflect the gradual selecting out of more resistant opportunistic pathogens if the basic disease does not remit. In this case, aggressive diagnostic measures were successful in establishing the diagnosis weeks before death, but death could not be forestalled because of poor status of host defenses. Autopsy revealed disseminated petriellidiosis.

In contrast to the radiographs from this unfortunate case, Fig. 2B shows the chest films from a young leukemic male who developed overwhelming *S. aureus* septicemia (8/8 positive blood cultures), a shocklike clinical picture, and cutaneous dissemination of staphylococcal lesions. Multiple areas of consolidation in the lung also progressed to cavitation, as shown in the film. None-

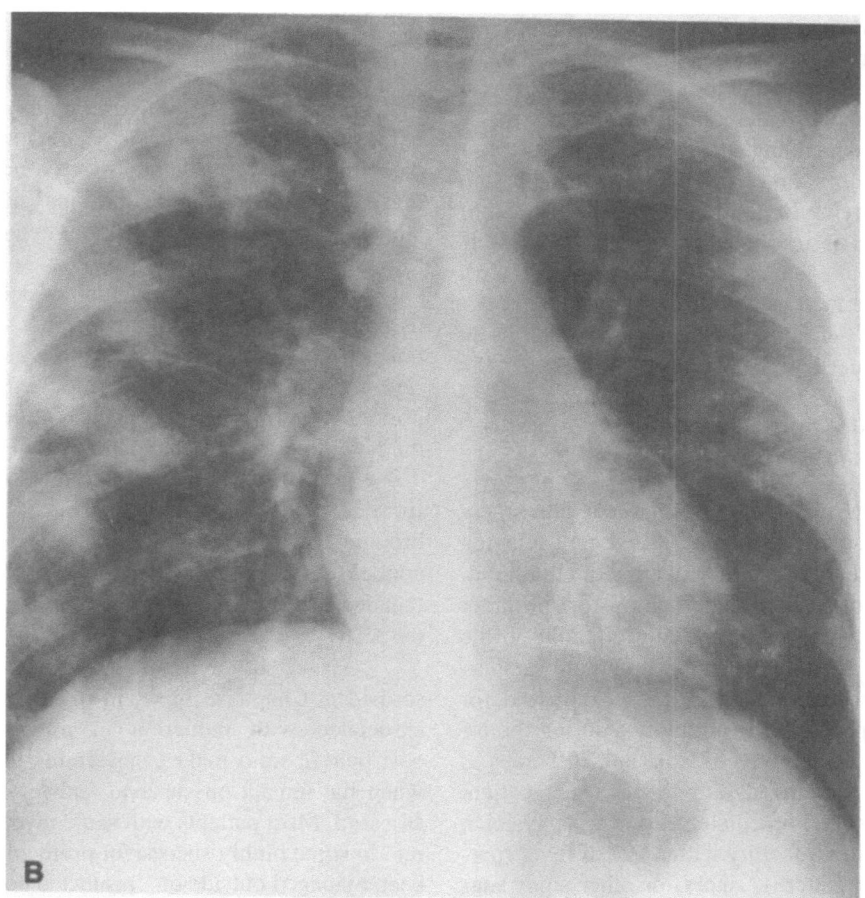

FIGURE 2. (*Continued*)

theless, fluids and antibiotic therapy—oxacillin in doses used for endocarditis—resulted in complete clinical cure and almost complete resolution of lung abnormalities prior to achievement of hematologic remission. Indeed, the patient most likely had right-sided staphylococcal endocarditis as the source for septic emboli to both lung fields. This case illustrates the much better prognosis for treatment of systemic staphylococcal infections in acute leukemic patients, particularly when their disease is newly diagnosed. Staphylococci and filamentous fungi can both cause acute cavitary disease in the lung, but the prognosis with the former infection is usually much better than with the latter.

8. Summary of Recommended Therapeutic Strategies

Other sections of this book, particularly Chapters 3, 4, and 11, have extensively covered the problems of infection risk, approaches to diagnosis, antimicrobial treatment, and supportive care of the neutropenic patient. It would be surprising if there were exact agreement on all approaches, but the degree of concordance among authorities on major issues is remarkable. The recommendations of major centers dealing with these neutropenic patients is likely to vary depending on specific protocols, epidemiologic factors, and local experience. Although there is a gratifying trend to undertake controlled or comparative trials in order to derive more credible and widely applicable guidelines for management, many recommendations still reflect personal experience. It is with that acknowledgment that the following recommendations are made.

8.1. Different Approaches to Leukemia and Lymphoma

There now appears to be markedly divergent infection risk among leukemia (all types) occurring in the adult, acute lymphatic leukemia of childhood, and Hodgkin disease. Chemotherapy for the latter two groups of disorders is initially effective in the great majority of subjects and is commonly undertaken on an outpatient basis. We see no need for special diets, prophylactic antibiotics during the induction phase, or any type of isolation. If therapy is given to nonhospitalized individuals, each patient should be alerted to immediately report to a physician or emergency room facility with onset of fever (particularly a new pattern), rigors, or other signs suggesting infection.

Similar recommendations would apply to most patients with non-Hodgkin lymphoma treated outside of the hospital. However, individuals with refractory lymphomatous disease receiving intensive cytotoxic treatment may be viewed as similar to acute leukemia. Patients with aplastic anemia (e.g., being treated with high-dose steroid or antithymocyte globulin), multiple myeloma receiving intensive cytotoxic therapy, and chronic myelogenous and lymphatic leukemia in an accelerated disease phase (blast crisis) should probably also be treated like acute leukemic patients.

8.2. Environmental Considerations

Patients whose neutrophil counts are likely to plummet to $500/mm^3$ or lower should be placed in a single room and managed with strict handwashing precautions. Numbers of visitors should be held at a minimum. "Reverse isolation" in the traditional sense appears valueless.[76] Masks should be worn by any personnel having upper respiratory infection. Since respiratory infections are often communicable before symptoms appear, it is no major inconvenience to have all personnel wear a nonsterile-type mask on entering the room. This may have an important effect in reminding all persons entering the room to wash their hands.

Sterile bedsheets are not necessary. Recommended technique for bathing includes sponge baths, but if a tub bath is desired, the tub should be first rigorously cleaned and then filled with the hottest possible water from the tap. This is allowed to cool to the level tolerated by the bather.

Fresh fruits and vegetables should be excluded from the diet, and none of these materials or flowers brought into a patient's room. All foods should be cooked and rewarmed before serving. Recommended dietary guidelines are summarized in Chapter 3.

"Protected environments" in the sense described in Chapter 3 have, in most instances, been associated with reduction in infection, but the cost/benefit ratio makes these units hard to justify when the impact on survival and remission rate is assessed. Most patients with acute myelocytic leukemia in some highly successful protocol studies have been managed outside of "protected environments" without laminar air flow, and the remission rate for initial induction attempts has exceeded 80%.[78] Such a rate of success is equal to or better than those of centers using protected environments as an adjunct to leukemia treatment.[79] There is good evidence that the incidence of infection is related to the type of leukemia protocol, i.e., some protocols may be associated with a higher rate of infection than others independent of the use of protected environments.[80] We do acknowledge that protected environments employing the laminar air flow principle should have an impact in reducing true airborne infections. In fact, we are not aware of any case of aspergillosis or mucormycosis developing in a patient managed in a laminar air flow room. Interestingly, attempts to reduce air-borne fungal spores by air-filtration techniques other than incorporating laminar airflow principles also seem to be successful in reducing *Aspergillus* infection.[81]

8.3. Prophylactic Antibiotics

The work of several investigators (summarized in Chapter 3) points towards an effect of oral nonabsorbable antibiotics in reducing infection and permitting more successful leukemia induction attempts. These regimens have usually included an aminoglycoside, vancomycin, and nystatin. There are two major problems with this approach. First, unpalatability of the oral medications added to the extremely "toxic" clinical condition of some patients are two factors contributing to a situation in which patients most at risk will not or cannot take these medications. Thus, those patients most likely to take these medications tend to be less ill, and those who are dropouts (and sometimes excluded by the analysis) are sicker and at greater risk. A special effort has to be made to give patients these regimens, and they are quite expensive. Second, use of gentamicin as a component of the topical regimen may select for resistant strains of *Pseudomonas* and other gram-negative bacilli.

For the past decade, we have used the combination of vancomycin (100 mg q8h), nystatin (400,000 units q4–6h), and colistin or polymyxin B (100 mg q8h) in an attempt to suppress the GI flora. The effect of these efforts has been equivocal at best. The nystatin has had limited impact on fungal colonization, and the vancomycin is the most unpalatable component of this "cocktail." Our regimen differs

from that of Schimpff et al.[82] by the substitution of polymyxin B or colistin for gentamicin. Many investigators have sought an alternative to oral nonabsorbed agents and trimethoprim/sulfamethoxazole has been the compound most extensively evaluated. There are now more than a dozen controlled studies in which trimethoprim–sulfamethoxazole has been used in an attempt to prevent bacterial infection in neutropenic patients.[83] Nonetheless, there are still major reservations to be expressed about this prophylactic approach, which is also reviewed in Chapter 2. Despite the fact that most studies suggest benefit from prophylaxis, the use of trimethoprim–sulfamethoxazole has been reported to be relatively ineffective in some large studies,[84] to be without benefit during consolidation courses of leukemia treatment,[85] to be associated with more prolonged neutropenia in comparison with nalidixic acid[86] and to be associated with emergence of resistance in gram-negative bacilli.[87,88] The fact that trimethoprim–sulfamethoxazole lacks activity against *P. aeruginosa* is another major drawback. An important placebo-controlled study by Pizzo and colleagues at the National Cancer Institute demonstrated that if one corrected for compliance only those patients who were highly compliant with trimethoprim–sulfamethoxazole prophylaxis experienced a significant reduction in documented infections and fever.[89] Perhaps equally important, however, was the observation that even patients who took placebo and were highly compliant experienced a significant reduction in infection. This finding strongly suggests that the nature of the compliant patient per se appears to be associated with a significant reduction in documented bacterial infection.

A comprehensive review of the efficacy of prophylaxis with trimethoprim–sulfamethoxazole suggest that overall the benefit from this approach may depend on local epidemiologic circumstances.[90] In settings in which gram-negative enteric bacteria are very susceptible to this agent, the prophylactic use of trimethoprim–sulfamethoxazole may be effective in reducing infections due to *E. coli, Klebsiella, Proteus, Enterobacter,* and *Serratia* sp. While bacterial infections may be reduced, those that still do occur are more likely to be antibiotic resistant (including resistant to trimethoprim–sulfamethoxazole). Pizzo and associates at the National Cancer Institute have suggested that patients taking prophylactic regimens with trimethoprim–sulfamethoxazole had a significant increase in side effects (skin sensitivity, GI upset) and that these patients experienced significantly more fevers of undetermined origin (FUOs).[89] In a recent editorial, the subject of antibacterial prophylaxis of infection in the neutropenic patients was extensively reviewed.[90] Some of the issues mentioned earlier—that prophylactic antibiotics that suppress the gut flora may merely substitute FUO for documented infections are reviewed, along with proposed criteria for better studies of prophylactic drug efficacy. A desirable prophylactic regimen should reduce the incidence of documented infection as well as the overall incidence of fever and avoid the need for systemic antibiotic therapy. The ultimate benefits of prophylaxis would be reduced numbers of infections, delay in time to onset of fever if it is to occur, and reduced overall use of systemic antibiotics. In addition, a desirable prophylactic regimen should be inexpensive, have a rapid effect, and have few side effects.

We believe that none of the current prophylactic regimens can be routinely recommended. There soon will be a number of studies using the newer fluorinated quinolones as prophylactic agents. Their broad-spectrum includes *P. aeruginosa*[91] as well as *Staphylococcus,* and the early reports are encouraging. Experience is limited, however, in terms of long term use and repetitive use in compromised hosts. The antibacterial spectrum of the quinolones includes many gram-negative and -positive pathogens and *Legionella pneumophila.* There is some evidence that oral erythromycin constitutes effective prophylaxis against Legionnaire's disease, although a published study did not include patients with hematologic malignancy.[92]

Nystatin is not a very effective prophylactic agent against mucosal candidasis in the markedly neutropenic patient, although many failures may be attributed to poor patient compliance rather than to lack of intrinsic activity. Prophylactic amphotericin B taken orally (not a compound licensed in the United States, but can be prepared by a pharmacy) is preferred by some specialists. Topical imidazoles such as clotrimazole have been licensed for prophylaxis of oral thrush and may be quite effective, although prevention of deep-seated systemic or esophageal disease has not been well documented. Similarly, a paucity of studies demonstrate that ketoconazole is effective in the prophylaxis of systemic candidiasis.[93] Ketoconazole does appear to be useful for the treatment of thrush but has neither activity against *Aspergillus* species nor proven prophylactic effect against any deep mycotic pathogen.

For patients with acute childhood leukemia, trimethoprim–sulfamethoxazole is virtually 100% effective in preventing pneumocystosis and has an impressive impact on other childhood-type bacterial infections.[94] Most of these infections occur during remission. Despite the proven efficacy of anti-*Pneumocystis* prophylaxis, we would suggest its use only in populations experiencing a relatively high incidence of *Pneumocystis* infections (more than 5% of patients per year for each diagnostic category). Patients who have had a proven episode of *P. carinii* pneumonia may be given either continuous or intermittent prophylaxis (160–240 mg q12h of trimethoprim) for the total duration of chemotherapy.[95] It is only effective as prophylaxis while it is being administered and does not appear to eradicate the carriage of the parasite.

8.4. Systemic Antimicrobial Agents

The approach to fever and suspected sepsis outlined in Chapter 4 is most directly applicable to the neutropenic patient with leukemia and lymphoma. We would reiterate the following points.

1. In view of our concern about *P. aeruginosa,* we prefer to begin empirical therapy with an aminoglycoside and an antipseudomonal β-lactam compound (penicillin, cephalosporin, and carbapenem). Combination therapy as an initial approach is still to be preferred. We are less concerned about staphylococci and believe there is no advantage to using a third agent such as a vancomycin unless there are specific indications.

2. Prompt initiation of therapy is justified for fever and other clinical signs of infection (tachypnea, hypotension, increased fluid requirements) when the neutrophil count is less than 500/mm³, and proper caution should be exercised in stopping treatment when the patient remains neutropenic in that

range and is colonized by gram-negative organisms such as *P. aeruginosa* or *K. pneumoniae*. It is in such patients that we and others have observed a fulminant "rebound" bacteremia.

3. Major concern should always be exercised about the risk of opportunistic mycotic infection in the patient not responding to treatment with antibacterial agents (see Chapter 4). The febrile, neutropenic patient who develops pulmonary infiltrates while receiving broad-spectrum antibacterial agents most likely has a fungal superinfection and should be started on amphotericin B. The indications for empirical use of amphotericin in the absence of pulmonary infiltrates are not well established, but we would strongly consider empirical amphotericin B in persistently febrile patients (on antibacterial agents) who have (a) symptoms of esophagitis, (b) recovery of *Candida* species in large numbers from the stool, or (c) candiduria without indwelling urinary catheter. (See Chapter 18.)

4. Trimethoprim–sulfamethoxazole is an effective agent for the treatment of *P. carinii* infections and is quite active against many *Enterobacteriaceae* that are aminoglycoside resistant. We would consider using this fixed combination agent with an aminoglycoside as an alternative to cephalosporins in patients with *Proteus* and *Klebsiella* infections and as an alternate to mezlocillin, piperacillin, or azlocillin in patients with *Enterobacter* and *Serratia* infections.

5. Anaerobic pathogens play only a small role in systemic (bacteremic) infections complicating lymphoma and leukemia.[19] They are important in infections of the head and neck area and in acute intraabdominal processes secondary to perforation or obstruction and cellulitis/abscesses around the lower GI tract. Metronidazole, antipseudomonal penicillins and cefoxitin are active against most invasive anaerobic pathogens, including *Bacteroides fragilis*. If patients are receiving broad-spectrum penicillins and aminoglycosides, the addition of chloramphenicol, metronidazole, or clindamycin is

not likely to have an impact on persistent fever.

9. Approach to the Splenectomized Patient

Splenectomized patients, or patients who are functionally asplenic, are candidates for pneumococcal vaccine, but the efficacy of this approach seems limited. An alternative approach is prophylactic oral or parenteral penicillin G (or erythromycin if penicillin allergy is present). However attractive the latter approaches may be, there is no convincing proof of efficacy. Since pneumococcal infections (and *H. influenzae* infections as well) may present with devastating swiftness, we believe that patients should be carefully counseled (1) to seek immediate medical attention with onset of fever accompanied by the first chill, and (2) to carry amoxycillin/clavulanate (Augmentin) and take no less than 1 g PO at onset of upper respiratory infection or chills. The dangers of this latter recommendation are obvious, and there are no studies to prove its value. However, it can be argued that the most likely pathogens in the nonneutropenic outpatient are likely to be susceptible. An alternative agent would be trimethoprim/sulfamethoxazole. Antibiotic suppression of growth in cultures taken subsequent to self-administration of antibiotics may occur, but the most likely pathogens still will be "covered" by this approach.

Illustrative Case 3

A 22-year-old woman was brought to the emergency room with a 6-hr history of fever and shaking chills. The patient had been entirely well until 2 years previously, when she presented with weight loss and night sweats, and mediastinal adenopathy was noted on chest radiography. Diagnostic evaluation revealed Hodgkin disease, nodular sclerosis type, Stage IV-B after staging laparotomy, splenectomy, and liver and bone marrow biopsy. She was treated with total lymph node irradiation followed by six courses of MOPP therapy with an excellent clinical response. No further therapy had been given over the last 6 months, during which time she was asymptomatic and without evidence of overt Hodgkin disease

She remained well until she awoke at 4:00 AM on the day of admission with shaking chills and fever to 103°F (39.4°C). The patient took two aspirin tablets and returned to sleep until she awoke at 7:00 AM complaining of chills, fever, and a moderately severe bifrontal headache. She was noted to be quite lethargic by her parents and was brought to the hospital after the temperature was found to be 102°F (38.9°C) and she had vomited twice

On reaching the hospital at 10:00 AM, she was a confused, sleepy but arousable woman with a temperature of 96°F (35 6°C), pulse of 120, and blood pressure of 50 by palpation. She appeared acutely ill and dehydrated. Her skin was cold and clammy. There were no petechiae or ecchymoses. Her neck was supple without clear evidence of pain on movement. Kernig and Brudzinski signs were absent. The pharynx was somewhat injected. The chest, cardiac, and abdominal examinations were negative except for the well-healed laparotomy scar. Neurologic examination other than the altered state of consciousness was normal.

Initial laboratory data revealed Hct 36, WBC 5,300/mm³ (with 45% polys, 11% bands, 36% lymphs, 4% monocytes). Chest radiographs and KUB were within normal limits. Lumbar puncture revealed an opening pressure of 90, no cells, a CSF protein of 30 mg/dl and CSF sugar of 68 mg/dl. A few pleomorphic gram-negative bacilli were thought to be seen on gram stain of the CSF

Within 30 min of reaching the hospital, the patient received 3 g ampicillin, 3 g nafcillin, and 100 mg gentamicin, as well as 1000 mg methylprednisolone IV. Three liters of normal saline and albumisol were rapidly infused, and dopamine was begun. Despite these measures and a full attempt at cardiopulmonary resuscitation, the patient succumbed 2 hr after reaching the hospital. Both sets of blood cultures and the CSF drawn on admission subsequently grew out *Hemophilus influenzae* type B Postmortem examination revealed very early meningitis, no pneumonia, and no evidence of Hodgkin disease.

Comment. This tragic case illustrates that all-too-common occurrence of effective therapy of the underlying neoplasm but with fatal outcome because of opportunistic infection. Splenectomy and intensive chemo- and radiotherapy probably resulted in marked impairment of host defenses against encapsulated bacteria such as the pneumococcus and, in this case, *H. influenzae* type B Although the therapy could have been initiated some 15–30 min earlier, when the patient first reached the hospital, without taking the time for the usual extensive evaluation, it is unlikely that at that point such therapy would have been successful. Several important lessons are underlined here.

1. Since there is no effective immunization program to prevent such occurrences, the emphasis at this time must be to initiate earlier therapy. The point to begin therapy is with the first shaking chill. Therefore, our patients who are splenectomized for any reason, but most particularly our patients with Hodgkin disease who are splenectomized and undergo chemo- and radiotherapy, are told to start treatment at home at appearance of first chill; they should then contact their doctor or proceed quickly to the hospital. These patients should have antibiotic at home to be used for this purpose. We would recommend initiating therapy with trimethoprim–sulfamethoxazole or the fixed combination of amoxicillin–clavulanate.
2. Speed is of the essence in dealing with this problem—not only speed in initiating therapy at home, but also on reaching the hospital. House officers manning the Emergency Ward must be taught that, in dealing with these patients, a prolonged diagnostic evaluation with delay in initiating therapy is unaccept-

able. Intravenous antibiotics should be initiated within 10 min of these patients reaching the hospital
3. The clinicians should not expect to see established pneumonia or sinusitis or severe pharyngitis at the portal of entry in patients such as this. Bacteremia occurs early in the course of such infection, usually without evidence of established organ invasion that could be ascertained by physical examination or radiography. Therefore, the possibility of bacteremia must be thoroughly investigated and therapy instituted in this clinical setting even without definite evidence of specific organ invasion
4. Better methods of preventing this problem are badly needed.

10. Neutrophil Transfusions in the Treatment and Prophylaxis of Infection

The primacy of phagocytic leukocytes, either those circulating in the blood or those fixed within the reticuloendothelial system in the defense of the host against bacterial infection has never been seriously questioned since the work of Metchinikoff at the turn of the century. More than 50 years ago, neutrophils were injected intramuscularly into neutropenic patients in the hope that their breakdown products would stimulate endogenous neutrophil production.[96] Almost three decades ago, experimental studies in lethally radiated dogs demonstrated that neutrophils harvested by relatively primitive transfusion techniques would circulate and migrate into inflammatory exudates.[97] A realistic dating of neutrophil transfusion therapy in man however goes back only to the mid-1960s when it became possible to harvest granulocytes by a continuous-flow centrifugation technique. In the earlier studies, patients with high circulating white counts secondary to chronic myelogenous leukemia were sought as leukocyte donors, but there always has been a paucity of such patients. Continuous-flow centrifugation techniques required heparinization of the patient. Newer methods have included the harvesting of cells by a discontinuous-flow centrifugation method (which obviates heparinization) and filtration leukopheresis, whereby leukocytes in whole blood are collected by reversible adhesion of cells to nylon wool fibers. Following collection by filtration leukopheresis, cells are eluted and transfused. There may be some functional differences between cells collected by the various techniques, and readers are referred to more technically oriented publications or recent review articles[98–100] for further information about the technical, qualitative, and quantitative aspects of leukocyte collection.

From a simplistic point of view, the half-life of the leukocyte in the circulation, the so-called circulating pool, is approximately 7 hr. In order to raise the circulating neutrophil count from zero to a normal range in an average-size hypothetical 70-kg adult, it would require 10×10^9 or roughly 10 billion cells.[101] It is now within the capability of the aforementioned granulocyte transfusion techniques to approach just this type of theoretical replacement, and the quantitative aspects of replacement would be even more impressive in smaller-sized subjects (i.e., children). On the other hand, careful leukokinetic studies in infected dogs reveal one aspect of the granulocyte transfusion problem that can easily be overlooked, namely, that a normal infected animal has the capacity to augment endogenous granulocyte production by 10–20-fold in the face of infection.[102] Presumably, the same "augmentation" process will occur in normal humans who develop bacterial infection. Thus, the major issue surrounding use of granulocyte transfusions in man is whether the amount that can be replaced by current technology is adequate to cope with the anticipated needs of the subject. The latter involves perhaps a tenfold increment in daily granulocyte production, and it is currently not feasible to deliver such a number of granulocytes. It can be argued that the normal white count is hardly a realistic goal in neutropenic patients who may have infection, because some aplastic individuals remain stable and uninfected with quite low levels of circulating granulocytes ($300+$ cells/mm^3). Indeed, it may not be necessary to replace total daily production in order to tip the balance of defenses in favor of the host.

In the past decade, a series of randomized controlled trials of granulocyte transfusion therapy have appeared, and these are summarized in Table 9. Prior to the publication of these six studies, another study by Fortuny et al. showed no difference between controls and transfused recipients. Unfortunately, the design was not random, as the control group consisted of patients who were too far from the university center to be managed with granulocyte transfusions.[103] Nonetheless, it is remarkable that the response rate in patients treated with aggressive antibacterial therapy was not significantly different from that in those who received that same antimicrobial

TABLE 9. Granulocyte Transfusion Studies: Responses in Randomized Studies in Humans

Investigators	Transfused	Control	Comment[a]
Higby et al.[105]	15/17	5/19	SD fever and survival to day 20 Age differences Four transfusions given
Herzig et al.[106]	13/16	5/14	Median age 16 years (ALL mainly) Meningococcemia in one case Three control patients died >45 days
Alavi et al.[107]	11/14	10/19	NSD by day 21 *Ps.* sepsis 4 in controls, 0 in transfused patients
Vogler and Winton[108]	10/17	3/13	Six "partial responses" in Rx *Candida* and herpes in controls
EORTC[109]	11/16	18/23	Similar pattern in bacteremic patients
Winston et al.[110]	34/47	30/48	One-half of persistently neutropenic patients survive gram-negative septicemia irrespective of transfusions

[a]Rx, treatment group, C, control group, NSD, no significant difference, SD, significant difference, ALL, acute lymphoblastic leukemia

regimen plus therapeutic granulocyte transfusions. One recent study found that, contrary to prior reports, up to 60% of neutropenic patients will recover from gram-negative septicemia without marrow recovery[104] but with appropriate antimicrobial therapy.

Most of the studies summarized in Table 9 that employed simultaneously randomized controls had relatively few patients. The most impressive study from the viewpoint of study design is that of Herzig et al. who treated only patients with documented gram-negative rod septicemia at the National Cancer Institute.[106] This study demonstrated significantly increased survival in recipients of granulocyte transfusions. It is noteworthy, however, that most patients had childhood leukemia (i.e., smaller mass relative to dose of transfused cells), more patients who were transfused had E. coli infections in contrast to the control group, three late deaths (greater than 40 days postbacteremia) were attributed to death from gram-negative septicemia, and a bacteremic infection caused by a meningococcus was judged as successfully treated with granulocytes. Patients were eligible for this study if they had neutrophil counts in the range of 500–1000/mm^3, but it is apparent to us that prognosis is quite different in patients with circulating neutrophils in the 500–1000/mm^3 range than in those who have less than 500 neutrophils/mm^3. There were few Pseudomonas infections in the Herzig study in contrast to the study of Alavi et al.[107] The latter had four patients in the control group with Pseudomonas septicemia, and all died. Herzig and colleagues concluded that no patients recovered without having marrow recovery or granulocyte transfusion. Nonetheless, it is now quite clear from the studies of Love et al.[104] that marrow recovery is not a prerequisite for recovery from infection (i.e., antimicrobial treatment alone may suffice). The two most recent published controlled studies[109,110] show no benefit from use of therapeutic granulocytes in gram negative bacillemia or in febrile neutropenic patients when appropriate antimicrobial therapy was given. The studies of Alavi et al. and Vogler and Winton[108] were discouraging in that, despite some temporary prolongation in life, the survival of transfused versus control patients was not significantly different after 3 weeks. Thus, it appears that granulocyte transfusions for documented infection are somewhat like an iron lung—possibly life-sustaining while the patient is receiving them, but prognosis is dependent on the recovery of the patient's own hematopoietic function.

Considerable confusion has arisen from studies such as those reported by Higby et al.[105] (listed in Table 9) because of poor definition of infection, lack of information on response of specific infections to granulocyte transfusions, and the inclusion of fever without documented bacterial cause as an entity appearing to respond to granulocyte transfusions. By contrast, there is evidence that granulocyte transfusions actually increase the likelihood of febrility because white cells contain endogenous pyrogen.[109] The majority of therapeutic transfusion studies suggest that granulocytes should not be given to patients who are febrile with undocumented infection.

Since most patients with systemic gram-negative bacillary infections will survive on antibacterial therapy alone, the major issue is to identify whether there are any patients who are likely to benefit from granulocyte transfusions. It seems logical that infected individuals with transient drug-induced types of neutropenia (no neoplastic disorder) are logical candidates for granulocyte transfusion. Furthermore, since the hope of inducing remission in leukemia is greatest during the first few induction attempts, therapeutic granulocyte transfusions would appear to be justified in those patients who are severely neutropenic at the time of bacteremia, are failing to improve at 72 hr on appropriate antimicrobial agents, and whose bone marrow is aplastic. The latter group still has a fair chance at achieving hematological remission. Granulocyte transfusions appear to offer little hope to those patients who are refractory to leukemic therapy or to treatment of the underlying condition responsible for neutropenia. The cost of such transfusions, individually in the range of $600–$1000 a day in the 1980s, is large when one considers that at least daily transfusions are required and it may take weeks for bone marrow recovery to occur.

In summary, we advocate reserving granulocyte transfusions for patients with potentially reversible bone marrow diseases who are failing on appropriate two drug combination antibacterial therapy for documented gram-negative bacteremia. Controlled studies now suggest that the area of most concentrated study should be on patients with Pseudomonas infections. Our experience has been that patients with non-*Pseudomonas* infections treated aggressively with antibacterial agents respond just as well as those given the same antibiotic regimen plus granulocytes. Where a difference may possibly exist is for those bacteremic and pulmonary infections caused by *P. aeruginosa*. Patients responding poorly to granulocytes have, in our experience, low circulating levels of opsonins against the host's own infecting strains. This suggests a need for augmentation of both specific antibody and phagocytic cells, and supplementation of the latter alone may not be adequate. For established fungal diseases such as disseminated *Aspergillus* and candidiasis, there are no human studies to support the therapeutic role of granulocytes.

Another logical although not innocuous application of granulocyte transfusion technology has been towards prophylactic use. Theoretically, exogenously supplied granulocytes might be most effective in the prevention of infection, where fewer numbers of cells might be required than to combat an already well-established process. In human subjects, two studies have indicated a reduction in infections,[111,112] whereas three results have been negative.[113–115] The best designed of these studies, a controlled trial reported by Clift et al. with appropriate HLA matching of donors and recipients, still showed that reduction in infection incidence was not paralleled by increased survival.[111] The issue of HLA matching has also been a source of controversy. Higher posttransfusion increments of neutrophils seem related to histocompatibility between donors and recipients. On the other hand, it has not been clearly shown that magnitude of increments or histocompatibility is related to the efficacy of the transfused cells.

The published report of Clift et al. is flawed by a lack of a precise definition of a prophylactic transfusion.[111] More than 40% of their patients given so-called "prophylactic granulocytes" were actually receiving broad-spectrum systemic antibacterial treatment at a time when such granulocyte transfusions were started. Another study carried out at UCLA in afebrile bone marrow transplant recipients who were not receiving antibiotics on admission to study showed no conclusive trend towards efficacy of prophylactic transfusions.[113]

In addition to concerns about efficacy, new information has appeared about the potential hazards of prophylactic granulocyte transfusions. Leukocytes bear a significant number of surface antigens including HLA antigens. Schiffer et al. demonstrated an impressive increase in transfusion reactions when non-HLA-matched granulocytes were given to patients in a prophylactic study; the study was ended because of a significant 70% incidence of transfusion reactions.[114] The possibility is very real that exposure to HLA or other antigens on random white cells might thereby jeopardize the efficacy of platelet transfusions.

An equally great problem is the possibility that prophylactic granulocyte transfusions might be associated with increased risk of leukoagglutinin reactions in the lung or actual increased transfusion-associated viral infection. Effective serological screening techniques now have significantly reduced the incidence of hepatitis B. It has become well established that cytomegalovirus (CMV) is associated with the buffy coat of human leukocytes, and in a large study of dialysis patients, it was shown that a significantly lower incidence of CMV infections resulted from restriction of blood products to leukocyte-poor components.[116] In our study of prophylactic transfusions, we have observed that such granulocyte transfusions are associated with an increased risk of cytomegalovirus infection.[113] In bone marrow transplant recipients, CMV-associated interstitial pneumonitis is now the major cause of posttransplant mortality.

At present, therefore, there appears to be little justification for the prophylactic use of granulocyte transfusions in recipients of marrow transplants or patients with acute leukemia[112]; the risk of complications, including fever and lung infiltrates, is unacceptably high[112] without demonstrated effect on patient survival and success of chemotherapy. Prophylactic granulocyte transfusions are sensitizing, may jeopardize the effectiveness of subsequent platelet transfusions, are associated with a high incidence of transfusion reactions, and appear associated with an increased incidence of CMV infection. If it were possible to (1) avoid sensitization, (2) establish a pool of CMV-negative leukocyte donors, and (3) employ effective anti-CMV immunoprophylaxis or chemoprophylaxis, then the issue of prophylactic transfusions might be justifiably reopened in clinical situations in which there is high risk of acute bacterial infections and the cost of transfusions can be kept low.

11. Immunoprophylaxis and Immunotherapy of Infection

There are some well-established indications for immunoprophylaxis of infection in the immunocompromised host, and these should not be overlooked. In addition, there are areas where licensed vaccines are available, such as pneumococcal vaccine, but doubts persist about their efficacy. Finally, there are several areas of current investigation that involve immunoprophylaxis or immunotherapy of opportunistic infection. There is hope that some of these approaches will bear fruit in the near future.

11.1. Childhood Immunizations

It would be most unfortunate to overlook routine childhood immunizations with antigens such as diphtheria–pertussis–tetanus (DPT) toxoid. On the other hand, live-virus immunizations should be strictly avoided. Killed polio vaccine (Salk type) should be routinely used and is safe.

11.2. Passive Antibody

Postexposure immune serum globulin is recommended for hepatitis and for measles following exposure if the patient lacks a history of disease or immunization. Zoster immunoglobulin (but not regular immunoglobulin) can be used for patients without a history of chickenpox within 72 hr of exposure to varicella–zoster infection. It may be preferable, however, to wait to see whether varicella–zoster infection does develop, in which case the patient can be very effectively treated with acylovir (10 mg/kg every 8 hr IV). Regular pooled γ-globulin routinely given to leukemic patients has been of no effect in reducing the incidence of any infection.[117] Several studies have suggested that plasma or immunoglobulin with high titers of antibody against CMV might reduce the serious complications of interstitial pneumonitis following marrow transplantation. However, a recent study has indicated that CMV immunoglobulin is not beneficial when given to CMV-seronegative marrow recipients, provided that these patients have been given CMV seronegative blood products.[119]

11.3. Influenza Immunization

The Advisory Committee on Immunization Practices of the USPHS continues to recommend influenza immunization for high-risk groups. Influenza vaccines are generally safe because they are killed virus antigens, and most vaccine strains engender antibody responses in cancer patients. However, administration of multiple doses may be necessary for patients receiving immunosuppressive therapy. Aside from antibody responses, there is a paucity of data that influenza immunization reduces active disease or its complications. Problems associated with influenza infection have been infrequent in our patients over the last few years, but this may be because of a generally low incidence of disease in the community. Although we have not routinely immunized our patients with leukemia and lymphomas against influenza, we have no objections to carrying this out on a routine basis.

Despite its longstanding availability for the chemoprophylaxis of influenza, use of amantidine has never been very popular. Modest but consistent efficacy has been demonstrated in controlled studies, and we would consider its use in unimmunized, immunosuppressed patients during outbreaks of influenza A.[119]

11.4. Pneumococcal Immunization

The humoral antibody response to pneumococcal immunization in patients with lymphomas and myeloma has been disappointing.[120] In addition, a number of cases of infection are caused by serotypes that are not incorporated in the vaccine. Patients with Hodgkin disease previously treated with radiation or chemotherapy have particularly impaired antibody responses, whereas patients with untreated disease respond in a manner analogous to controls. Intensity of treatment rather than splenectomy is directly related to blunted antibody responses, and the impairment may persist for years. Some patients, such as with chronic myelocytic leukemia do show better antibody responses if immunized prior to splenectomy rather than afterward.[119] Patients with Hodgkin disease should not be given pneumococcal vaccine during active antineoplastic treatment; it is not certain whether an improved serologic response may result from multiple-dose immunization and delayed therapy of the neoplastic disorder. Those patients in whom a delay in initiating treatment might be considered are likely to have less serious disease (i.e., stages I or II). Since there is no evidence that pneumococcal immunization is effective even in patients with Hodgkin disease who respond well in terms of a humoral antibody response (splenectomy per se might still be the crucial compromising factor), we would not delay treatment of the tumor in symptomatic patients with progressive disease in the hope of obtaining maximum benefit from pneumococcal immunization.

It may be argued that pneumococcal immunization has little or no "downside risks." Even if the calculated efficacy is extremely modest, the use of a relatively inexpensive vaccine may be moderately beneficial to the host. Thus, in concordance with overall guidelines issued by the U.S. Public Health Service Advisory Committee on Immunization Practices, pneumococcal immunization may be viewed as a prudent move backed by epidemiologic principles but for which confirmatory studies (by randomized trials) are lacking.

Several experimental approaches to the prevention or treatment of gram-negative bacillary infections have been described. At present, they are not of established value, yet interest in these approaches runs high. They have obvious appeal because they attempt to augment host defenses rather than eradicate or suppress microbes by pharmacologic means (with all of the possible problems associated with this strategy). There are ample precedents in normal hosts for prevention of bacterial diseases by both active or passive immunization and for treatment of established disease with antiserum. Prior to the introduction of antimicrobial agents, serotherapy was widely used to treat pneumococcal and meningococcal infections as well as "toxic" disorders such as tetanus. We should recognize, however, that there are major obstacles to immunologic approaches aimed at prevention and treatment of gram-negative infections. These problems may be summarized by stating the following questions:

1. What are the antigens that can engender protection?

2. What is the mechanism of this protection?
3. Can comprehensive immunizing preparations be developed?
4. Will the host respond to immunization, i.e., active immunization?
5. If the host is immunologically unresponsive or poorly responsive, will it be better to give passive immunoprophylaxis or therapy?
6. With respect to pulmonary infections, what is the relative importance of "local" immunity as opposed to the systemic immune response?

The answers to these questions are briefly reviewed here, but for more detailed discussion the reader is referred to other publications.[120,121]

Active immunization of human subjects has been accomplished mainly by use of a heptavalent *Pseudomonas aeruginosa* lipopolysaccharide vaccine (Table 10). The immunogen is essentially a set of seven cell wall endotoxins prepared by standard chemical extraction techniques. In cancer patients, the largest *Pseudomonas* vaccine trial carried out in a single center employed the heptavalent lipopolysaccharide antigen and found limited protection against *P. aeruginosa* infection.[17] However, it is important to note that this study, more than a decade old, demonstrated no protection against bacteremic infection. Although 67% of subjects with acute leukemia and Hodgkin disease were found to develop augmented circulating antibody titers against one or more lipopolysaccharide antigens, these elevated titers were short-lived. The immunogenicity of this vaccine in acute leukemics differed in that newly diagnosed cases were usually found to respond with antibody increments as opposed to those individuals who are relatively refractory to antileukemic therapy after multiple relapses of their underlying disease. Progression of underlying disease was associated with low anti-pseudomonal antibody titers and persistent neutropenia. Failures in immunization in that controlled study were related to both low levels of type-specific opsonins and neutropenia. Studies in two other groups of cancer patients involved far fewer patients and were not adequate to assess vaccine efficacy.[125,127]

Of considerable interest was the report of Polk et al. describing the effectiveness of the heptavalent lipopolysaccharide vaccine in preventing *Pseudomo-*

TABLE 10. Summary of Active Immunization with *P. aeruginosa* Vaccines

Study (reference)	Vaccine	Design[a]	Number of subjects		Results
			Vaccinees	Controls	
Feller and Pierson[122]	Whole cell	H B	100	41	Decreased sepsis and deaths
Sachs[123]	Whole cell	N B	39	—	Decreased sepsis and deaths
Alexander et al.[124]	Parke–Davis	H B	96	75	Decreased sepsis and deaths
Young et al.[17]	Parke–Davis	R CA ICU	176	185	Decreased deaths but not sepsis in neutropenic patients
Haghbin et al.[125]	Parke–Davis	R CA	28	30	No differences
Polk et al.[126]	Parke–Davis	R ICU	48	51	Decreased deaths but not sepsis
Pennington et al.[127]	Parke–Davis	R CA	22	20	No differences
Wasserman et al.[128]	Whole cell	H B	287	59	Decreased deaths and sepsis
Jones et al.[129]	Burroughs–Wellcome	A B	18	20	Decreased deaths and sepsis

[a]Abbreviations H, historical controls; N, no controls, R, randomized controls, A, alternate cases, B, with burns, CA, with neoplasms, ICU, intensive care unit

nas respiratory infection in an intensive care unit setting.[126] Studies carried out in burn units[124] with this (Parke–Davis) or other whole cell vaccines[107,122,123,128] suggested protection but did not employ simultaneously randomized controls. Recently, a cell wall extract *Pseudomonas* vaccine was developed by Miler and others using a new process.[130] In burned patients, the results from a field trial in India seemed particularly encouraging; however, much of the protection seemed "nonspecific" in that non-*Pseudomonas* infections also appeared to decline. The use of this vaccine has not been extended to neutropenic cancer patients.

The experience to date suggests that the most expeditious approach in immunocompromised hosts might be to give passive antibody, but there are a number of poorly explored issues relating to quantity of antibody, mode of delivery, and duration of protection. Only one small study has been reported of the use of *P. aeruginosa* immunoglobulin (IgG) to treat *Pseudomonas* infection, and the results of this uncontrolled study are difficult to assess.[131] Even if it were possible to give large quantities of antibody (e.g., by one of the new techniques for intravenous infusion of IgG), this approach alone might not be successful in the neutropenic patient. Mounting evidence from animal studies suggests that protection will be best achieved by giving both granulocyte transfusions and passive antibody.[132] Several preparations of immunoglobulins (IgG) modified for intravenous use are now in clinical evaluation. These preparations contain significantly enriched quantities of antibodies

against gram-negative bacilli, including *P. aeruginosa*.

A multiplicity of immunizing antigens may be required to obtain type-specific protection against clinically significant gram-negative bacilli. An alternate approach is to engender antibody against a common component of the cell walls of these organisms. Studies from several laboratories have identified important immunochemical similarities between lipopolysaccharide (endotoxin) antigens of the family *Enterobacteriaceae*. The inner core regions of endotoxins from *E. coli*, *Proteus*, *Klebsiella*, *Serratia*, *Salmonella*, and so forth are structurally similar. Antibodies directed against "core" antigens prepared from "rough" mutants such as *Salmonella minnesota* R595 (a so-called "Re" mutant) appear to have broad cross-protective activity.[120,133] Anticore antibodies raised in rabbits have given passive protection in mice against a heterologous challenge by *E. coli*, *Klebsiella*, and *Serratia*.

Antibodies directed against the core region of enteric bacteria appear to have a neutralizing or binding effect on lipid A, the toxic portion of bacterial endotoxin.[120] Furthermore, these core antibodies may bind to endotoxin derived from enteric bacteria and *P. aeruginosa*. Ziegler and co-workers have demonstrated that antiserum raised against the J-5 mutant of *E. coli* 0111 (a so-called Rc mutant) offers protection against enteric bacteria and *P. aeruginosa* strains.[134] Active immunization, passive immunization, and serotherapy with antiendotoxin core antibodies appears to be a versatile approach, but type-specific antibodies (against the serotype 0 antigens of bacilli) seem more protective. Encouraging studies in animals led Ziegler and colleagues to initiate an important clinical trial in which hyperimmune plasma was prepared in normal healthy volunteers immunized with a whole-cell vaccine made from the J-5 mutant of *E. coli* 0111. Almost 200 patients with documented gram-negative rod bacteremia were entered into a double-blind clinical trial; the control infusion was preimmunization plasma from the same healthy volunteers.[135] Overall, there was a significant reduction in mortality (38% versus 24% and an impressive ability of J-5 antiserum to reverse profound septic bacterial shock (as defined by systolic blood pressure of <90 mm Hg ≥6 hr). Many of the gram-negative bacteremias treated in this study were due to *P. aeruginosa*. Unfortunately, these investigators were unable to define a protective level of serum antibodies against the J-5 antigen and they could not relate antibody titers in recipients to the clinical response. Unquestionably, this has been one of the most important studies of the adjunctive serotherapy of gram-negative infections ever attempted. It has spurred the development of a number of products that might be more widely available. Several commercial manufacturers have produced hyperimmune plasma or serum fractions that are augmented in type-specific and core antibodies to endotoxin. An equally interesting possibility has been made possible through the advent of the monoclonal antibody (hybridoma) technology. This approach has revolutionized modern immunology because of the ability to produce large quantities of antibodies of predetermined specificity, purity, and consistency from so-called "immortalized" cells derived from the fusion of antibody producing B cells and myeloma cells. Hybridomas are already an important source of either animal (murine) or human antibodies against antigens such as the J-5 antigen of enteric bacteria.[120,136] Indeed, such antibodies have already been produced and have shown varying degrees of protective activity in animal studies. Human clinical trials with such materials are already under way.

Whatever the source of antibodies for prophylaxis or therapy (human or murine, type specific or cross reactive) we should not underemphasize the need for large controlled studies of efficacy, because it is obvious that intervention with antiserum will be only one variable affecting the outcome. In therapeutic studies, it will not be possible to withhold antimicrobial treatment, but double-blind trials evaluating the adjunctive effects of antiserum seem quite feasible. In view of the persistently high mortality from gram-negative bacillary infections in patients with leukemia and lymphoma, this is a goal worth pursuing.

References

1. Chilcote RR, Baehner RL, Hammond D, et al: Septicemia and meningitis in children splenectomized for Hodgkin's disease. *N Engl J Med* **295**:798–800, 1976.
2. Winston DJ, Wang DC, Feig SA, et al: Pneumococcal infections after human bone marrow transplantation. *Ann Intern Med* **91**:835–841, 1979.
3. Armstrong D, Young LS, Meyer RD, et al: Infectious complications of neoplastic disease. *Med Clin North Am* **55**:729–745, 1971.
4. Goldschmidt MC, Bodey GP: The effect of chemotherapy upon microorganisms isolated from cancer patients. *Antimicrob Agents Chemother* **1**:348–353, 1972.
5. Schabel FM, Pittillo RF: Screening for and biological characterizations of anti-tumor agents using microorganisms. *Adv Appl Microbiol* **3**:223–256, 1961.
6. Miller SP, Shanbrom E: Infectious syndromes of leukemia and lymphomas. *Am J Med Sci* **246**:420–428, 1963.
7. Cline MJ: Acute myelocytic leukemia. In Cline MJ (ed): *The White Cell.* Harvard University Press, Cambridge, 1976, pp. 203–224.
8. Cline MJ: Defective mononuclear phagocyte function in myelomonocytic leukemia and in some patients with lymphomas. *J Clin Invest* **52**:2815–2819, 1973.
9. Cline MJ: A test of individual phagocyte function in a mixed population of leukocytes. Identifications of a neutrophil abnormality in acute myelocytic leukemia. *J Lab Clin Med* **81**:311–315, 1973.
10. Lehrer RI, Cline MJ: Leukocyte candidacidal activity and resistance to systemic candidiasis in patients with cancer. *Cancer* **27**:1211–1217, 1972.
11. Hughes WT, Feldman S, Aur RJA, et al: Intensity of immunosuppressive therapy and the incidence of *Pneumocystis carinii* pneumonitis. *Cancer* **36**:2004–2009, 1975.
12 Baehner RL, Neiburger RG, Johnson DE, et al: Transient bactericidal defect of peripheral blood phagocytes from children with acute lymphoblastic leukemia receiving craniospinal irradiation. *N Engl J Med* **289**:1209–1213, 1973.
13. Edwards JE, Lehrer RI, Stiehm ER, et al: Severe candidal infections. *Ann Intern Med* **89**:91–106, 1978.
14. Meyer RD, Young LS, Armstrong D: Aspergillosis complicating neoplastic disease. *Am J Med* **54**:6–15, 1973.
15. Meyer RD, Rosen P, Armstrong D: Phycomycosis complicating leukemia and lymphoma. *Ann Intern Med* **77**:871–879, 1972.
16. Epstein SM, Verney E, Miale TD, et al: Studies on the pathogenesis of experimental pulmonary aspergillosis. *Am J Pathol* **51**:769–777, 1967.

17 Young LS, Meyer RD, Armstrong D. *Pseudomonas aeruginosa* vaccine in cancer patients *Ann Intern Med* **79:**518–527, 1973

18. Wollman MW, Young LS, Haghbin M, et al: Anti-*Pseudomonas* heat-stable opsonins in acute lymphoblastic leukemia of childhood. *J Pediatr* **86:**376–381, 1975

19. Young LS, Martin WJ, Meyer RD, et al: Gram-negative rod bacteremia. Microbiologic, immunologic and therapeutic considerations. *Ann Intern Med* **86:**456–471, 1977.

20. Forsgren A, Schmeling D, Banck G Effect of antibiotics on chemotaxis of human polymorphonuclear leukocytes in vitro *Infection* 6(suppl):S102–S106, 1978.

21. Bjorksten B, Ray C, Quie PG. Inhibition of human neutrophil chemotaxis and chemiluminescence by amphotericin B. *Infect Immun* **14:**315–317, 1976.

22. Lehrer RI. Inhibition by sulfonamides of the candidacidal activity of human neutrophils. *J Clin Invest* **50:**2498–2505, 1971.

23 King GW, Yanes B, Hurtubise PE, et al. Immune function of successfully treated lymphoma patients. *J Clin Invest* **57:**1451–1460, 1976.

24. Cline IJ: Lymphocytic lymphoma Hodgkin's disease, and other chronic lymphoproliferative disorders. In Cline MJ (ed): *The White Cell.* Harvard University Press, Cambridge, 1975, pp 425–456.

25 Young RC, Corder MP, Haynes HA, et al: Delayed hypersensitivity in Hodgkin's disease. *Am J Med* **56:**63–72, 1972

26. Steigbigel RT, Lambert LH, Remington J: Polymorphonuclear leukocyte, monocyte, and macrophage bactericidal function in patients with Hodgkin's disease *J Lab Clin Med* **88:**54–62, 1976.

27 Sheagren JN, Block JB, Wolff SM: Reticuloendothelial system phagocytic function in patients with Hodgkin's disease *J Clin Invest* **46:**855–862, 1967

28 Ward PA, Berenberg JL. Defective regulation of inflammatory mediators in Hodgkin's disease *N Engl J Med* **290:**76–80, 1974

29 Brown RS, Haynes HA, Foley HT, et al: Hodgkin's disease: Immunologic, clinical, and histologic features in 50 untreated patients. *Ann Intern Med* **67:**291–300, 1967.

30 Weitzman SA, Aisenberg AC, Siber GR, et al: Impaired humoral immunity in treated Hodgkin's disease *N Engl J Med* **297:**245–248, 1977

31. Hersh EM, Bodey GP, Nies BA: Cause of death in acute leukemia *JAMA* **193:**105–109, 1965.

32. Viola MV: Acute leukemia and infection. *JAMA* **201:**923–928, 1967.

33 Hughes WT: Fatal infections in childhood leukemia *Am J Dis Child* **122:**283–287, 1971

34. Levine AS, Schimpff SC, Graw RG Jr, et al: Hematologic malignancies and other marrow failure states. Progress in the management of complicating infections. *Semin Hematol* **11:**141–202, 1974.

35 Chang H-Y, Rodriguez V, Narboni G, et al Causes of death in adults with acute leukemia. *Medicine (Baltimore)* **55:**259–268, 1976

36 Casazza AR, Duvall CP, Carbone PP Summary of infectious complications occurring in patients with Hodgkin's disease *Cancer Res* **26:**1290–1296, 1966

37 Coker DD, Morris DM, Coleman JJ, et al. Infection among 210 patients with surgically staged Hodgkin's disease *Am J Med* **97:**109–115, 1983

38. Feld R, Bodey GP Infections in patients with malignant lymphoma treated with combination chemotherapy. *Cancer* **39:**1018–1025, 1977

38a Estey EH, Keating MJ, McCredie KB, et al. Causes of initial remission induction failure in acute myelogenous leukemia *Blood* **60:**309–315, 1982

39 Notter D, Grossman P, Rosenberg SA, et al. Infections in patients with Hodgkin's disease *Rev Infect Dis* **2:**761–800, 1980.

40 Bodey GP, Rodriguez V, Valdivieso M, et al: Amikacin for treatment of infections in patients with malignant disease *J Infect Dis* **134**(suppl).S421–S427, 1976.

41. Valdivieso M, Gil-Extremera B, Zornoza J, et al Gram-negative bacillary pneumonia in the compromised host *Medicine (Baltimore)* **56:**241–254, 1977.

42. Burke PJ, Braine HG, Rathbun HK, et al: The clinical significance and management of fever in acute myelocytic leukemia *Johns Hopkins Med J* **139:**1–12, 1976

43 Young LS: Nosocomial infection in the immunocompromised adult *Am J Med* **70:**398–404, 1981

44. Silver RT, Utz JP, Frei E, et al. Fever, infection and host resistance in acute leukemia *Am J Med* **24:**25–39, 1958.

45 Raab SO, Hoeprich PD, Wintrobe MM, et al. The clinical significance of fever in acute leukemia *Blood* **16:**1609–1628, 1960

46. Boggs DR, Frei E III: Clinical studies of fever and infection in cancer. *Cancer* **13:**1240–1253, 1960

47 Bodey GP, Rodriguez V, Chang H-Y, et al: Fever and infection in leukemia patients. *Cancer* **41:**1610–1622, 1978.

48. Goodall PT, Vosti KL. Fever in acute myelogenous leukemia. *Arch Intern Med* **135:**1197–1203, 1975.

49 Atkinson K, Kay HEM, McElwain TJ: Fever in the neutropenic patient. *Br Med J* **3:**160–161, 1974.

50 Young LS Amikacin. Experience in a comparative clinical trial with gentamicin in leukopenic subjects In Luthy R, Siegenthaler W (eds). *Current Chemotherapy.* American Society for Microbiology, Washington, DC, 1978, pp. 246–248.

51. Wade JC, Schimpff SC, Newman KA, et al. Piperacillin or ticarcillan plus amikacin A double-blind prospective comparison of empiric antibiotic therapy in febrile granulocytopenic cancer patients *Am J Med* **71:**983–989, 1981

52 Pizzo PA, Hathorn JW, Hiemenz J, et al: A randomized trial comparing ceftazidime alone with combination therapy in cancer patients with fever and neutropenia *N Engl J Med* **315:**552–558, 1986

53. Krick JA, Remington JS: Opportunistic invasive fungal infections in patients with leukemia and lymphoma *Clin Haematol* **5:**249–310, 1976

54. Wade JC, Schimpff SC, Newman KA, et al: Staphylococcus epidermidis: An increasing cause of infection in patients with granulocytopenia *Ann Intern Med* **97:**503–508, 1982

55 Carney DN, Fossieck BE, Parker RH, et al: Bacteremia due to *Staphylococcus aureus* in patients with cancer: Report on 45 cases in adults and review of the literature *Rev Infect Dis* **4:**1–27, 1982

56 Armstrong D: Infectious complications of lymphosarcoma In Molander DW (ed): *Lymphoproliferative Diseases.* Charles C Thomas, Springfield, Illinois, 1975, pp. 94–109

57 Walzer PD, Perl DP, Krogstad DJ, et al: *Pneumocystis carinii* pneumonia in the United States: Epidemiologic, diagnostic, and clinical features. In *Symposium on Pneumocystis Carinii Infection* NCI Monograph 43 National Cancer Institute, Bethesda, Maryland, 1976, pp. 55–63

58 Cohen J, Pinching AJ, Rees AJ, Peters DK: Infections and immunosuppression. A study of infective complications of 75 patients with immunologically mediated disease. *Q J Med* **51**:1–15, 1982

59 Kaplan MH, Rosen PP, Armstrong D. Cryptococcosis in a cancer hospital. *Cancer* **39**:2265–2274, 1977

60. Kaplan MH, Armstrong D, Rosen P: Tuberculosis complicating neoplastic disease. A review of 201 cases *Cancer* **33**:850–858, 1974.

61. Kauffman CA, Israel KS, Smith JW, et al: Histoplasmosis in immunosuppressed patients *Am J Med* **64**:923–932, 1978.

62 Davies SF, Khan M, Sarosi GA: Disseminated histoplasmosis in immunologically suppressed patients. Occurrence in a nonendemic area. *Am J Med* **64**:94–99, 1978

63. Cox F, Hughes WT. Disseminated histoplasmosis and childhood leukemia. *Cancer* **33**:1127–1134, 1974

64. Deresinski SC, Stevens DA: Coccidioidomycosis in compromised hosts. *Medicine (Baltimore)* **54**:377–395, 1974.

65. Wilson JF, Marsa GW, Johnson RE: Herpes zoster in Hodgkin's disease. Clinical, histologic, and immunologic correlations. *Cancer* **29**:461–465, 1972.

66. Feldman S, Hughes WT, Kim HY. Herpes zoster in children with cancer. *Am J Dis Child* **126**:178–184, 1973.

67. Schimpff SC, O'Connel MJ, Green WH, et al. Infections in 92 splenectomized patients with Hodgkin's disease. *Am J Med* **59**:695–701, 1975.

68. Sokal JE, Firat D: Varicella zoster infection in Hodgkin's disease. Clinical and epidemiological aspects. *Am J Med* **39**:452–463, 1965.

69. Reboul F, Donaldson SS, Kaplan HS: Herpes zoster and varicella infections in children with Hodgkin's disease *Cancer* **41**:95–99, 1978.

70. Bishop JF, Schimpff SC, Diggs CH. et al: Infections during intensive chemotherapy for non-Hodgkin's lymphoma. *Ann Intern Med* **95**:549–555, 1981

71. Shaikh BS, Lombard RM, Appelbaum PC, et al· Changing patterns of infections in patients with multiple myeloma. *Oncology* **39**:78–82, 1982.

72. Twomey JJ: Infections complicating multiple myeloma and chronic lymphocyte leukemia. *Arch Intern Med* **132**:562–565, 1973.

73 Levine AM, Overturf GD, Field RF, et al. Use and efficacy of pneumococcal vaccine in patients with Hodgkin's disease. *Blood* **54**:1171–1175, 1979

74 Weibel RE, Villa PP, McLean AA, et al. Studies in human subjects of polyvalent pneumococcal vaccines. *Proc Soc Exp Biol Med* **156**:144–148, 1977

75 Folland D, Armstrong D, Seides S, et al. Pneumococcal bacteremia in patients with neoplastic disease *Cancer* **33**:845–849, 1974.

76 Nauseef WM, Maki DG: A study of the value of simple protective isolation in patients with granulocytopenia. *N Engl J Med* **304**:448–453, 1981

77. Pizzo PA, Levine AS: The utility of protected environment regimens for the compromised host. a critical assessment. *Prog Hematol* **10**:311–332, 1977.

78. Gale RP, Cline MJ: High remission induction rate in acute myeloid leukaemia. *Lancet* **1**:497–500, 1977.

79. Rodriguez V, Bodey GP, Freireich EJ, et al. Randomized trial of protected environment—prophylactic antibiotics in 145 adults with acute leukemia *Medicine (Baltimore)* **57**:253–266, 1978.

80. Berdischewsky M, Young LS: Infectious complications of neoplastic disorders and their management. In Franklin EC (ed): *Current Topics in Immunology.* Elsevier North-Holland, New York, 1979, pp. 307–338.

81. Rhame FS, Streifel AJ, Kersey JH Jr, et al: Extrinsic risk factors for pneumonia in the patient at high risk of infection. *Am J Med* **76**(5A):42–52, 1984.

82. Schimpff SC, Greene WH, Young VM, et al. Infection prevention in acute nonlymphocytic leukemia. Laminar air flow room reverse isolation with oral, nonabsorbable antibiotic prophylaxis. *Ann Intern Med* **82**:351–358, 1975.

83. Young LS: Trimethoprim–sulfamethoxazole and bacterial infections during leukemia therapy. *Ann Intern Med* **95**:508–509, 1981.

84. EORTC Antimicrobial Therapy Project Group: Trimethoprim–sulfamethoxazole in the prevention of infection in neutropenic patients *J Infect Dis* **150**:372–379, 1984.

85. Weiser B, Lange M, Fialk MA, et al: Prophylactic trimethoprim–sulfamethoxazole during consolidation chemotherapy for acute leukemia. A controlled trial *Ann Intern Med* **95**:436–438, 1981

86. Wade JC, DeJongh CA, Newman KA, et al: A comparison of trimethoprim–sulfamethoxazole to nalidixic acid: Selective decontamination as infection prophylaxis during granulocytopenia. *J Infect Dis* **147**:624–634, 1983.

87 Dekker AW, Rozenberg-Arska M, Sixma JJ, et al. Prevention of infection with trimethoprim–sulfamethoxazole plus amphotericin-B in patients with acute non-lymphocytic leukemia. *Ann Intern Med* **95**:555–559, 1981

88. Wells EL, Podzorski RP, Rhame F, et al: Incidence of trimethoprim sulfamethoxazole resistant enterobacteriaceae among transplant recipients. *J Infect Dis* **150**:699–706, 1984.

89. Pizzo PA, Robichand KJ, Edwards B, et al: Oral antibiotic prophylaxis in cancer patients: A double blind, randomized placebo controlled trial. *J Pediatr* **102**:125–133, 1983

90 Young LS: Antimicrobial prophylaxis against infection in neutropenic patients. *J Infect Dis* **147**:611–614, 1983.

91. Scully BE, Parry MF, Neu H, et al. Oral ciprofloxacin therapy of infections due to Pseudomonas aeruginosa. *Lancet* **1**:819–822, 1986

92 Vereerstraeten P, Stolean JC, Shoutens E, et al. Erythromycin prophylaxis for Legionnaire's disease in immunosuppressed patients in a contaminated hospital environment *Transplantation* **41**:52–54, 1986.

93. Young LS: Double Beta-lactam therapy in the immunocompromised host. *J Antimicrob Chemother* **16**:4–6, 1985

94. Hughes WT: Pneumocystis carinii pneumonia. *N Engl J Med* **297:**1381–1383, 1977.

95. Hughes WT, Rivera GK, Schell MJ, et al: Successful intermittent chemophrophylaxis for *Pneumocystis carinii* pneumonitis. *New Eng J Med* **316:**1627–1632, 1987.

96. Strumia MM: The effect of leukocytic cream injections in the treatment of the neutropenias. *Am J Med Sci* **187:**527–544, 1934.

97. Brecker G, Wilbur KM, Cronkhite EP: Transfusion of separated leukocytes into irradiated dogs with aplastic marrows. *Proc Soc Exp Biol Med* **84:**54–56, 1953.

98. Goldman JM, Lowenthal RM (eds): *Leukocytes. Separation, Collection and Transfusion.* Academic, New York, 1979.

99. Greenwald TJ, Jamieson GA (eds): *The Granulocyte. Function and Clinical Utilization.* Liss, New York, 1977.

100. Aisner J, Schiffer CA, Wiernik PH: Granulocyte transfusions: Evaluation of factors influencing results and a comparison of filtration and intermittent centrifugation leukopheresis. *Br J Haematol* **38:**121–129, 1978.

101. Boggs DR: Transfusion of neutrophils as prevention or treatment of infection in patients with neutropenia. *N Engl J Med* **290:**1055–1062, 1974.

102. Boggs DR: Neutrophils in the blood bank. *N Engl J Med* **296:**748–750, 1979.

103. Fortuny IE, Bloomfield CD, Hadlock DC, et al: Granulocyte transfusion: A controlled study in patients with acute nonlymphocytic leukemia. *Transfusion* **15:**548–558, 1975

104. Love LJ, Schimpff SC, Schiffer CA, et al: Improved prognosis of granulocytopenic patients with gram-negative rod bacteremia. *Am J Med* **68:**643–648, 1980.

105. Higby DJ, Yates JW, Henderson ES: Filtration leukapheresis for granulocyte transfusion therapy. *N Engl J Med* **292:**761–766, 1975.

106. Herzig RH, Herzig GP, Graw RG Jr, et al: Successful granulocyte transfusion therapy for gram-negative septicemia. *N Engl J Med* **296:**701–705, 1977.

107. Alavi JB, Root RK, Djerassi I, et al: A randomized clinical trial of granulocyte transfusions for infection in acute leukemia. *N Engl J Med* **296:**706–711, 1977.

108. Vogler WR, Winton EF: A controlled study of the efficacy of granulocyte transfusions in patients with neutropenia. *Am J Med* **63:**548–555, 1977.

109. EORTC Antimicrobial Therapy Project Group: Early granulocyte transfusions for high risk febrile neutropenic patients. *Swiss Med J* **113**(suppl 14):46–48, 1983.

110. Winston DJ, Ho WG, Gale RP: Therapeutic granulocyte transfusions for documented infections. A controlled trial in 95 infectious granulocytopenic episodes. *Ann Intern Med* **97:**509–515, 1982.

111. Clift RA, Sanders JE, Thomas ED, et al: Granulocyte transfusions for the prevention of infection in patients receiving bone marrow transplants. *N Engl J Med* **298:**1052–1057, 1978.

112. Strauss RG, Connett JE, Gale RP, et al: Controlled trial of prophylactic granulocyte transfusions during initial induction chemotherapy for acute myelogenous leukemia. *N Engl J Med* **305:**598–603, 1981.

113. Winston DJ, Ho WG, Young LS, et al. Prophylactic granulocyte transfusions during human bone marrow transplantation. *Am J Med* **68:**893–897, 1980.

114. Schiffer CA, Aisner J, Daly PA, et al: Alloimmunization following prophylactic granulocyte transfusion. *Blood* **54:**766–774, 1979.

115. Ford JM, Culen MH: Prophylactic granulocyte transfusions. *Exp Hematol* **5**(suppl):65–73, 1977.

116. Tolkoff-Rubin NE, Rubin RH, Keller EE, et al: Cytomegalovirus infection in dialysis patients and personnel. *Ann Intern Med* **89:**625–628, 1978

117. Bodey GP, Nies BA, Mohberg NR, et al: Use of gammaglobulins in infection in acute leukemia patients. *JAMA* **190:**1099–1102, 1964

118. Bowden RA, Sayers M, Flournoy N, et al: Cytomegalovirus immune globulin and seronegative blood products to prevent primary cytomegalovirus infection after marrow transplantation. *N Engl J Med* **314:**1006–1010, 1986.

119. Delker LL, Moser RH, Nelson JD, et al: Amantidine: Does it have a role in the prevention and treatment of influenza? *Ann Intern Med* **92:**256–258, 1980.

120. Young LS: Immunoprophylaxis and serotherapy of bacterial infections. *Am J Med* **76:**664–671, 1984.

121. Young LS: Gram-negative sepsis. In Mandell G, Douglas JG, Bennett JE (eds): *Principles and Practice of Infectious Diseases.* 2nd Ed. Wiley, New York, 1985, pp. 452–475.

122. Feller I, Pierson C: *Pseudomonas* vaccine and hyperimmune plasma for burned patients. *Arch Surg* **97:**225–229, 1968.

123. Sachs A: Active immunoprophylaxis in burns with a new multivalent vaccine. *Lancet* **2:**959–961, 1970.

124. Alexander JW, Fisher MW, MacMillan BG: Immunological control of *Pseudomonas* infection in burn patients: A clinical evaluation. *Arch Surg* **102:**31–35, 1971

125. Haghbin M, Armstrong D, Murphy ML: Controlled prospective trial of *P. aeruginosa* vaccine in children with acute leukemia. *Cancer* **32:**761–766, 1973.

126. Polk, HC Jr, Borden S, Aldrete JA. Prevention of *Pseudomonas* respiratory infection in a surgical intensive care unit. *Ann Surg* **177:**607–615, 1973.

127. Pennington JE, Reynolds HY, Wood RE, et al: Use of a *Pseudomonas aeruginosa* vaccine in patients with acute leukemia and cystic fibrosis. *Am J Med* **58:**629–636, 1975.

128. Wasserman P, Schlotterer M, Paul P, et al: Systemic utilization of an anti-*Pseudomonas aeruginosa* vaccine in a severe burn unit. *Scand J Plast Reconstr Surg* **13:**81–94, 1979.

129. Jones RJ, Jupta JL, Roe EA: Controlled trials of a polyvalent *Pseudomonas* vaccine in burns, *Lancet* **2:**977–983, 1979.

130. Miler JM, Spilsbury JF, Jones RJ, et al. A new polyvalent *Pseudomonas* vaccine. *J Med Microbiol* **10:**19–27, 1977.

131. Jones CE, Alexander JW, Fisher MW. Clinical evaluation of *Pseudomonas* hyperimmune globulin *J Surg Res* **14:**87–96, 1973.

132. Harvath L, Andersen BR, Zander AR, et al. Combined preimmunization and granulocyte transfusion therapy for treatment of *Pseudomonas* septicemia in neutropenic dogs. *J Lab Clin Med* **87:**840–847, 1976.

133. Young LS, Stevens P, Ingram J: Functional role of antibody against "core" glycolipid of *Enterobacteriaceae. J Clin Invest* **56:**850–861, 1975

134. Ziegler EJ, McCutchan JA, Douglas H, et al: Prevention of lethal *Pseudomonas* bacteremia with epimerase deficient *E. coli* antiserum. *Trans Assoc Am Physicians* **88:**101–105, 1975.

135. Ziegler EJ, McCutchan JA, Fierer et al: Successful treatment of gram-negative bacteremia and shock with human anti-serum to a UDP-Gal epimerase deficient *Escherichia coli. N Engl J Med* **307:**1225–1230, 1982.

136. Teng NNH, Kaplan HS, Hebert JM, et al: Protection against gram-negative bacteremia and endotoxemia with human monoclonal IgM antibodies. *Proc Natl Acad Sci USA* **82:**1790–1794, 1985.

19

Evaluation and Management of Infections in Patients with Collagen Vascular Disease

DONALD G. PAYAN

1. Introduction

The clinical outcome of patients with the various manifestations of collagen vascular disease (CVD) has significantly improved over the past two decades with the increased use of diuretics, cytotoxic agents, dialysis, transplantation, and the judicious use of corticosteroids and other antiinflammatory agents directed at altering or delaying end-organ damage by the underlying immunopathologic process.[1-4] A more rigorous definition of the various CVD clinical syndromes and a greater sophistication in the serologic, radiologic, and pathologic diagnostic methods have meant that patients with these diseases are now coming to clinical attention earlier in the course of their illness. Consequently, the physician is now encountering a greater number of clinical problems over a longer time span for each individual patient, rather than just the well-known complications of their end-stage disease. Despite the beneficial aspects of the newer therapeutic interventions to improve the clinical outcome of patients with CVD, the incidence of infection as a cause of both morbidity and mortality in these patients has not changed significantly over the past 30 years.[1-19] A number of factors discussed in this chapter most likely contribute to the persistence of infectious complications in these patients. These include underlying host-defense ab-

DONALD G. PAYAN • Divisions of Allergy–Immunology and Infectious Diseases, University of California, San Francisco, California 94143.

normalities not significantly altered by therapeutic interventions, prolonged therapy with corticosteroids, and alkylating agents that further suppress an already abnormal immune response, and an increased frequency of hospitalizations with more aggressive medical and surgical interventions, thereby increasing the risk of nosocomial infectious complications.

The management of infections in the two most prevalent collagen vascular diseases—systemic lupus erythematosus (SLE) and rheumatoid arthritis (RA)—are the principal focus of this chapter. Both SLE and RA are characterized by the fact that they are chronic inflammatory multisystem diseases of unknown etiology, with clinical features common to all the collagen vascular disorders.[4,20,21] SLE and RA, which may begin as early as the second decade of life, exhibit diverse clinical and laboratory manifestations and courses characterized by their unpredictability and by periods of remission and relapse.[20,21] The similarity between the symptoms of infection in a patient with either SLE or RA and those due to a flare of the underlying disease pose a significant challenge to the physician.

2. Novel Features of Host–Microorganism Interactions in CVD

The importance of infections in the management of the patient with CVD is underscored by the fact

TABLE 1. Interactions between Infections and Collagen Vascular Activity[a]

1. Clinical symptoms of infection may be indistinguishable from those of CVD (see Table 2).
2. Infection may increase or precipitate CVD activity.
3. Antibiotic therapy for infection may exacerbate CVD activity (penicillins, sulfonamides).
4. Side effects of therapy for infection and CVD may be similar (i.e., diarrhea secondary to gold therapy or antibiotics).
5. Immunosuppressive therapy for CVD may lead to increased susceptibility to infection (see Table 7).
6. Infection increases morbidity and mortality in patients with CVD (see Tables 3 and 4).

[a]CVD, collagen vascular disease

that the symptoms of the host's response to the microorganisms and the therapy of a particular infection may mimic, alter, or exacerbate the underlying immunologic disease (Table 1). The principal clinical manifestations of both SLE and RA are listed in Table 2 along with examples of those infectious disease categories that commonly cause similar symptoms. The musculoskeletal manifestations of SLE present at some time during the clinical course in as many as 90% of patients[20] may be similar to the arthralgias that are common in patients with infectious endocarditis, disseminated gonoccocemia, rubella, and the prodrome of viral hepatitis.[22-25] As in SLE, major joint swelling, bone destruction, and flexion deformities are uncommon with these infections, and the arthralgias and arthritis are usually transient clinical manifestations of the infectious process. Similarly, the one or two tender, swollen, and

TABLE 2. Examples of Clinical Symptoms of Systemic Lupus Erythematosus and Rheumatoid Arthritis Compared with Infectious Diseases[a]

	SLE	RA	Infectious disease[b]
Weight loss	+	+	Chronic infection (e.g., SBE, TB)
Fever	+	+	Most infections
Arthralgia, arthritis	+	+	Septic joint (e.g., bacterial, fungal), disseminated gonococcemia, viral infection
Skin rash	+	+	Bacterial (e.g., erysipelas, rose spots), fungal, treponemal (secondary syphilis), viral
Renal involvement (nephritis)	+	−	Emboli in infectious endocarditis, glomerulonephritis (post-streptococcal, S. epidermidis)
Gastrointestinal (anorexia, nausea, and vomiting)	+	−	Viral hepatitis, bacterial toxins (Staph. sp), bacterial diarrhea (Shigella sp.), antibiotic therapy, pseudomembranous colitis (C. difficile), parasites (Giardia, Amoeba)
Pulmonary (pleurisy, effusions, pneumonia)	+	+	Bacterial, fungal, tuberculous, viral, and parasitic infections
Cardiac (murmurs, pericarditis)	+	+	Bacterial, fungal, tuberculous, viral, and parasitic infections
Lymphadenopathy	+	+	Bacterial, fungal, tuberculous, viral, and parasitic infections
Hepatosplenomegaly	+	+	Bacterial, fungal, tuberculous, viral, and parasitic infections
Central nervous system abnormalities	+	+	Bacterial, fungal, tuberculous, viral, and parasitic infections

[a]Adapted from Schur.[28]
[b]SBE, subacute bacterial endocarditis, TB, tuberculosis

warm joints characteristic of an acute flare of RA may be indistinguishable from the septic joint, and only analysis and culture of the joint fluid permit distinction between the two processes.[21] Nowhere are the differences between the manifestations of an acute flare of a CVD and those of an infectious process more difficult to resolve than when they involve the pulmonary, cardiac, and central nervous system (CNS). As discussed in the clinical cases, pulmonary symptoms of SLE such as pleurisy, pneumonia, and effusions present in as many as 50% of patients,[20] may mimic most infectious processes involving the lungs. When, on occasion, pneumonias caused by organisms such as *Streptococcus pneumoniae,* the group A streptococcus, *Mycoplasma pneumoniae,* and *Mycobacteria* sp., are associated with scant sputum production, they may exhibit clinical characteristics similar to those of an SLE flare involving the lung. Moreover, in the setting of immunosuppressive therapy with corticosteroids or cyclophosphamide, when infections with *Aspergillus* sp. and *Nocardia* sp. are more prevalent,[3] the hemoptysis and pleuritic chest pain caused by these infections may be identical with the symptoms of SLE–pneumonitis. Cardiac manifestations present in 46% of patients with SLE[20] and in 1–2% of patients with RA[21] and that may be heralded by the onset of a new murmur, pericardial friction rub, or conduction abnormality are findings common to all forms of infectious endocarditis (IE). Consequently, only careful serial bedside examinations for the stigmata of IE in addition to blood cultures will help distinguish between Libman-Sacks endocarditis and IE. A third of patients with SLE and a rare patient with RA, will demonstrate neurologic manifestations such as seizures, behavioral disturbances, cranial nerve abnormalities, and a number of other clinical changes consistent with meningeal and cerebral inflammation.[20,21,26,27] A detailed analysis of the cerebrospinal fluid (CSF) will most often permit exclusion of an infectious etiology as the cause of the observed clinical findings. However, infections such as meningeal tuberculosis and viral encephalitis, for example, which can be characterized by an abnormal mental status, focal neurologic findings, computed tomographic (CT) changes consistent with cerebral infarcts due to vasculitis, and negative routine CSF cultures, may be indistinguishable from a patient with a flare of SLE complicated by neurologic manifestations in addition to steroid-induced psychosis. This not infrequent clinical dilemma can occasionally be resolved by pathologic examination of an appropriate biopsy specimen for infectious organisms and a therapeutic trial with antituberculous or antiviral chemotherapy.

Issues involving the relationship between infections that cause increases in CVD activity, the role of antibiotic therapy in precipitating exacerbations of SLE, and whether immunosuppressive therapy predisposes patients with CVD to specific infections are presented as part of the case discussions.

3. Morbidity and Mortality Caused by Infection in Patients with CVD

Infection is a major cause of morbidity among patients with SLE and RA (Table 3). In the series of 70 patients with SLE presenting in the first two decades of life reported by Platt et al.,[7] 55 episodes of infection were documented, with the skin being the principal site of infection. Urowitz et al.[14] described 81 patients with SLE in whom there were 28 instances of proven infection. Eighteen of these were minor, such as cutaneous or urinary tract infections (UTI) requiring only outpatient orally administered antibiotic therapy.[14] In the study by Carpenter et al.,[1] infections complicated the course in 21 patients with SLE, with UTIs affecting 67% of patients, including multiple UTIs in one-half of these. In the 110 patients with SLE reported by Lee et al.,[19] 45 infections were documented in 29 patients. Nine of these patients had multiple infections during the 5-year period of the study. Ten percent had major infections requiring parenteral antibiotics, with pneumonia being the most frequent, and 20% had minor infections, with the most common being UTI and skin infections. In the prospective study of 223 patients with SLE by Ginzler et al.,[12] infection was the major problem leading to hospital admission 100 times, or 29% of all but obstetric hospitalizations among patients in their series. As shown in Table 3, the incidence of infection may vary widely from study to study (26–78%) with the most frequent minor infections involving the skin and urinary tract and major infections most commonly causing pneumonia.

The principal infectious complication causing significant morbidity in patients with RA has been their propensity to develop septic arthritis. The eight

TABLE 3. Infection as a Cause of Morbidity in Systemic Lupus Erythematosus and Rheumatoid Arthritis[a]

Series	Period	Number of patients	Number with infection		Number of infections	Principal site of infection
			N	Percent		
Systemic lupus erythematosus						
Platt et al.[7]	1958–1981	70	55	78		Skin (45%)
Carpenter and Sturgill[1]	1958–1965	40	21	53		Urinary tract (67%)
Urowitz et al [14]	1970–1975	81	21	26	28	Pneumonia/sepsis
Lee et al.[19]	1970–1975	110	29	26	45	Pneumonia (18%), skin (30%)
Ginzler et al [12]	1966–1976	223	150	67	384	Urinary tract (20%) Pneumonia (11%)
Staples et al.[15]	1960–1969	23	13	57	25	Urinary tract (28%)
Rheumatoid arthritis						
Huskisson and Hart[30]		12			24	Tissue abscesses (58%)
Mitchell et al.[29]	1964–1974	2500	8	1		Septic arthritis (100%)

[a]Adapted from Perez and Goldstein [3]

patients with RA in the study by Mitchell et al.[29] all developed indolent septic arthritis frequently after concurrent skin infections. Other studies in patients with RA have documented increased morbidity from recurrent soft tissue abscesses[30] and respiratory infections.[31]

In patients with SLE, infectious complications have been major contributors to the increased mortality of that disease (Table 4). Clinical studies conducted during the preantibiotic era[32,33] found that 30–40% of deaths were caused by infections, with a significant number due to *S. pneumoniae* bronchopneumonia. As described by Dubois[34] and others,[35] bronchopneumonia and pneumonitis continued to be the principal infectious disease complication leading to death in patients with SLE during 1950–1973, despite the introduction of antimicrobial chemotherapy and the improved survival due to advances in the management of CNS damage and uremia. During that period, infections as the cause of death remained unchanged at 5–14% of patients with SLE, whereas uremia declined from 26% to 14%, and death due to CNS damage declined from 26% to 8%. The recent studies of Urowitz et al.[14] and Ginzler et al.[12] underscore the fact that infection contributes to mortality principally during the early phases of SLE. Of the six patients who died in Urowitz's study within the first year after diagnosis, five died from sepsis, whereas in all five of the late deaths, none was attributable to infection, but rather to myocardial infarction. Factors

associated with early death from infection were active lupus nephritis and large doses of corticosteroids. A similar pattern was observed by Ginzler et al.[12] in the 30 patients in their study who died from infection. A majority had their fatal infection early in their clinical course, frequently associated with active lupus nephritis, especially when manifested by red blood cells (RBCs) or cellular casts in the urine sediment.[12] The most recently reported data by Platt et al.[7] and Rosner et al.[8] confirm these earlier observations. Of the 11 deaths in Platt's report caused by infection, five died within one year of diagnosis and two of these patients had diffuse proliferative lupus nephritis. The early deaths from infection were also seen by Rosner and co-workers, however, nearly half of their patients who died primarily of infection did not have active SLE at the time of death, a finding opposite those in earlier series. Nevertheless, in SLE the number of deaths overall due to infection range widely between 3% and 80% and are caused principally by pneumonia (Table 4). The contributions of underlying host-defense abnormalities and immunosuppressive therapy to the increased morbidity and mortality due to infections in SLE are discussed in Section 4.

Infection has also played a major role in the mortality of patients with RA (Table 4). The recent studies by Vanderbroucke et al.[16] and Prior et al.[18] demonstrate that infections were a significant cause of death in RA patients who were hospitalized more

TABLE 4. Infection as a Cause of Death in Systemic Lupus Erythematosus and Rheumatoid Arthritis[a]

Series	Period	Number of deaths	Deaths due to infection		Principal site or type of infection	Time of fatal[b] infection relative to duration of CVD	
			N	Percent		Early in disease (%)	Late in disease (%)
Systemic lupus erythematosus							
Klemperer et al [32]	1930–1941	20	8	40	Pneumonia	—	—
Ropes[33]	1932–1944	—	—	27	—	[c]	—
	1945–1963	5	3	60	—	[c]	—
Harvey et al.[35]	1940–1954	38	1	3	Pneumonia	—	—
Dubois and Tuffanelli[2], Dubois et al.[34]	1950–1955	57	9	16	Pneumonia	—	—
	1956–1962	100	12	12	Pneumonia	—	—
	1963–1973	92	17	18	Pneumonia	—	—
Carpenter and Sturgill[1]	1958–1965	8	4	50	Pneumonia	60	40
Platt et al [7]	1958–1981	11	9	81	Pneumonia/sepsis	55	45
Hashimoto and Shiokawa[37]	1955–1968	17	6	36	—	—	—
	1969–1971	16	4	20	—	—	—
	1971–1976	7	1	14	—	—	—
Estes and Christian[36]	1963–1971	53	10	18	Pneumonia	—	—
Rosner et al.[8]	1965–1978	222	74	30	Sepsis/pneumoia	78	22
Ginzler et al.[12]	1966–1976	55	30	60	Pneumonia	[c]	—
Lee et al.[19]	1970–1975	13	4	30	Pneumonia/sepsis	100	—
Urowitz et al.[14]	1970–1975	11	5	45	Sepsis	100	—
Rheumatoid arthritis							
Vandenbroucke et al [16]	1954–1981	165	4	2	Sepsis	—	[c]
Allebeck[38]	1971–1978	473	5	1	—	—	[c]
Prior et al.[18]	1964–1978	199	4	2	—	25	75
Koota et al.[39]	1959–1976	176	23	13	Pneumonia	—	—

[a]Adapted from Perez and Goldstein [3]
[b]CVD, collagen vascular disease Early in disease within first 2 years of coming to clinical attention Late in disease more than 2 years of clinical follow-up
[c]Present

than 5 years after the onset of their disease. In contrast to SLE, infections in patients with RA occur late in the course of the disease. Furthermore, as in patients with SLE, pneumonia and urogenital sepsis were the principal infectious complications leading to death, findings which are even more striking when autopsy series are examined.[38–41]

4. Host Abnormalities as Potential Contributing Factors to Infections in Patients with CVD

A detailed discussion of abnormal host defenses in CVD is beyond the scope of this chapter, and can be found in several recent scholarly references.[3,42–44] However, a number of both humoral and cellular immune abnormalities have been described in patients with SLE and RA that may predispose them to infectious complications and these will be described within the context of this chapter (Table 5).

The biologic activities of the various components of complement that contribute to the maintenance of normal host defenses include lysis of bacteria (C5, C6, C7, C8, C9), stimulating chemotaxis of phagocytic leukocytes (C5a, C567), opsonization of bacteria (C3b), oxidative metabolism (C3b, C5a), and degranulation of leukocytes (C3b, C5a).[3,45,46] In both SLE[47] and RA,[48] reduction of serum C4 due to increased consumption has been observed con-

TABLE 5. Immunologic Abnormalities in Systemic Lupus Erythematosus and Rheumatoid Arthritis

	SLE	RA
Complement	Decreased levels of C4, C1q, C3, C9, and factor B due to increased consumption and turnover Inherited abnormalities of factors (C1, C4, C2) Decreased heat-labile opsonic capacity for *E. coli* and *S. aureus*	Increased catabolism of C4
Antibodies	± altered antibody response to bacterial antigens Hypergammaglobulinemia	Increased antibody production to native type II collagen
PMN leukocytes	Decreased complement-derived chemotactic activity in endotoxin-activated serum Decreased chemotactic response to ascorbic acid Presence of inhibitor of C5-derived chemotactic activity Decreased phagocytic activity Decreased oxidative metabolism	Altered chemotaxis and phagocytosis
Lymphocytes	Deficient autologous MLR (active SLE) Lymphopenia (decreased number and function of suppressor/cytotoxic T lymphocytes) B-lymphocyte hyperreactivity (polyclonal) Increased T lymphocytes with Ia antigen Decreased NK cell activity (hyporesponsive to interferon) Increased number of antilymphocyte antibodies	Decreased T-lymphocyte production of γ-interferon Increased mononuclear leukocyte activation in synovial tissue Increased T-lymphocyte sensitivity to type II and III collagen Decreased NK cell activity

sistently, in addition to occasionally depressed serum levels of C1q,[49] C3,[49] C9,[59] and factor B,[48,51] all of which lead to decreased serum levels of total hemolytic complement.[52,53] These deficiencies of C3, and other early components of the classic pathway have been associated with an increased incidence of infections with encapsulated bacteria such as *N. meningitidis, S. pneumoniae,* or *H. influenzae.*[54] Systemic infections caused by either *N. meningitidis* or *N. gonorrhea,* however, are more typical of late complement component deficiencies.[54] Other complement abnormalities observed in SLE that may predispose to infection include inherited isolated defi-

ciencies of selected complement components[54] and, in certain patients, decreased heat-labile opsonic capacity for *Escherichia coli* and *Staphylococcus aureus.*[55]

Abnormal immunoglobulin homeostasis has been reported in patients with both SLE[56-58] and RA.[44] Although some studies have detected an abnormally increased antibody response to bacterial antigens in patients with SLE,[59] others have not,[60] suggesting that whatever regulatory defect is present is probably multifactorial in origin. The hyperreactivity of the immune system observed in many patients with SLE[19,36,42] may be manifested by hypergammaglobulinemia principally of the IgG and IgA isotypes.[50] In addition, numerous antibodies directed against the surface antigens of a number of different leukocytes have also been detected in patients with SLE.[61,62] Although it is difficult to assess the role of the hypergammaglobulinemia of SLE in predisposing these patients to infection, it is possible that the antileukocyte antibodies may significantly alter the host's response during periods of increased disease activity.[63]

Altered chemotaxis of polymorphonuclear (PMN) leukocytes has been observed in patients with CVD. In SLE, a number of abnormalities of PMN leukocyte chemotaxis have been detected, including reduced complement-derived chemotactic activity in endotoxin-activated serum,[64] altered responses to ascorbic acid,[65] and the presence of an inhibitor of the chemotactic peptide C5a.[3,66] Of interest is that patients with the heat-stable inhibitor of C5a had a greater number of infectious episodes than did patients without the inhibitor.[67] Other defects of PMN leukocyte function in SLE include defective opsonization,[68] and impaired oxidative metabolism leading to decreased production of hydrogen peroxide and superoxide anion,[69] factors essential to cellular microbicidal activity.[70]

The role of cellular-mediated immunity directed by activated lymphocytes and macrophages in combating infections caused by intracellular organisms (viruses, *Listeria*, *Mycobacteria* sp.) and opportunistic bacteria has been extensively documented.[71] In SLE and to a lesser degree in RA, a multiplicity of abnormalities in cellular immunity have been described (Table 5). To what extent these lymphocyte abnormalities directly contribute to infectious complications in patients with SLE and RA is difficult to establish.

In patients with SLE, conflicting results have been reported on the degree to which delayed hypersensitivity responses to *Candida*, PPD, and other antigens are depressed.[72,73] However, what is clear is that when patients are immunized with specific antigens during periods of SLE activity, they fail to become sensitized.[74] In addition, a number of specific lymphocyte abnormalities have been reported in SLE, which include a deficient autologous mixed lymphocyte response (MLR) during periods of disease activity,[75] a decrease in T-suppressor-cytotoxic lymphocytes,[76] altered B-lymphocyte responses to

pokeweed mitogen,[77] inability of T lymphocytes to generate suppressive signals that turn off B-lymphocyte function,[78] and deficient natural killer (NK) cell function.[79] Parallel abnormalities in cell-mediated immunity have been described in patients with RA, including decreased T-lymphocyte production of γ-interferon (IF$_\gamma$),[80] increased T-lymphocyte sensitivity to type II and III collagen,[81] and decreased NK cell activity.[82] The exacerbations and remissions of SLE and RA over time that have been shown to alter different aspects of immunologic function, most likely predispose the host to varying types of infections depending on which part of the host's response is most severely affected at any one moment by the underlying disease activity. In addition, many of the drugs used to treat RA and SLE can perturb the immune system, altering the host's response even further.

5. Role of Immunosuppressive Therapy in Predisposing Patients with CVD to Infections

The wide use of immunosuppressive therapy in the management of SLE and RA over the past two decades has led to a greater appreciation of the significant interactions between corticosteroids, cytotoxic agents, and gold compounds with various elements of the immune response. Many studies, the results of which are summarized in Table 6, have now established both in vitro and in vivo the extensive degree to which the above classes of drugs inhibit host defenses. In general, glucocorticoids have a greater effect on leukocyte traffic within the circulation and sites of soft tissue inflammation than on their function, and more effect on cellular than humoral processes.[83,84] The ability of glucocorticoids to inhibit recruitment of PMN leukocytes and monocyte–macrophages at sites of inflammation is probably their single most important antiinflammatory effect.[83] Other functions such as lymphokine-mediated recruitment,[85] delayed-type hypersensitivity responses,[86] antigen processing,[88] monocyte bactericidal activity,[89] lymphocyte proliferation,[90] and NK cell activity,[91] are altered by corticosteroid therapy. As will be discussed below, it is not surprising that in addition to the underlying immune alterations that are part of the CVD complex, corticosteroid ther-

TABLE 6. Effects of Immunosuppressive Therapy on the Immune Response of Patients with Collagen Vascular Disease[a-c]

Effect	Corticosteroids	Cyclophosphamide	Azathioprine	Gold
Lymphocytes				
Lymphocytopenia	+[85]	+[99]	+[102]	
Suppression of DTH	+[86]	+[100]	+[103]	
Suppression of proliferation	+[90]	+[100]	±[104]	+[111]
Lysis of activated cells	+[85]			
Decreased cellular recruitment by lymphokines	+[85]			
Inhibition of suppressor T-cell function		+[101]		
Monocyte/macrophage				
Monocytopenia	+[85]			
Inhibition of accumulation at inflammatory site (MIF antagonism)	+[87]		+[105]	+[110]
Altered bactericidal activity	+[89]	+[100]		
PMN leukocyte				
No significant change in function	±[83]			
Accelerated release from bone marrow	+[92]			
Increase in antibody-dependent cellular cytotoxicity	+[83]			
Neutropenia		+[98]		
Altered phagocytic activity				+[110]
Immunoglobulins/mediators				
Inhibition of antibody production	±[93]	+[97]	+[106]	
Inactivation of complement system	+[94]			+[107]
Decreased synthesis of PG and LTs	+[95,96]			+[109]
Potentiation of catecholamine action	+[83]			
Inhibition of lysozomal enzymes				+[108]

[a] Adapted from Parillo and Fauci [83]
[b] Superscript numbers are references
[c] DTH, delayed-type hypersensitivity, MIF, migration inhibition factor, PG, prostaglandins, LT, leukotrienes

apy further inhibits responses that enable the host to combat common pathogenic gram-positive cocci, gram-negative enteric bacilli and intracellular organisms.[3]

Cytotoxic agents such as cyclophosphamide and azathioprine exhibit many of the same alterations of leukocyte function as glucocorticoids. However, the major differences include a more profound inhibition of B-lymphocyte function resulting in significant suppression of immunoglobulin levels in patients on chronic therapy,[97] and marrow suppression resulting principally in neutropenia.[98] The mechanisms in which gold compounds alter host defenses are still controversial. Gold compounds have been shown to inactivate complement,[107] and a number of lysosomal enzymes,[108] in addition to other leukocyte functions (Table 6).

The question as to whether immunosuppressive therapy acting by the above described mechanisms increases the incidence of infection in patients with CVD, is an extremely complex one. This complexity is multifactorial and is caused by the poorly understood interrelationships between a number of interacting elements, including level and extent of disease activity, length of time disease has been present, and degree of immunosuppression secondary to therapy in addition to that already caused by the underlying illness. A number of studies have attempted to examine the various factors associated with infectious complications in patients with CVD and whether they contribute to the commonly held clinical impression that these patients do have an increased incidence of infection as compared with a similar cohort of non-CVD patients.[3] The first study to carefully examine which factors were associated with an increased incidence of infection in patients with CVD was by Staples et al.[15] Their report described 23 patients with SLE, 20 with RA, and 11 with the nephrotic syndrome (NPS), hospitalized at the National Institutes of Health during 1960–1969. The number of infections in each group per 100 days of hospitalization (infection rate, IR) was almost ten times greater in the SLE cohort (1.22) than in the RA (0.0), NPS (0.23), and RA + NPS (0.16) groups, respectively. Of the total of 30 infections that they observed, only 15% occurred during periods of antibiotic therapy or neutropenia. The only other factors associated with disseminated and deep tissue infections was daily prednisone therapy in excess of 20 mg and significant azotemia (BUN >60 mg%). In addition, the IR in SLE was noted to increase with increasing steroid dose from a rate of 0.43 on no steroids to 1.63 on >50 mg prednisone per day. They were able to conclude that patients with SLE on no or low doses of steroids were susceptible to infections as compared with RA and NPS patients and that corticosteroid therapy further increased the risk with increasing dosage. Moreover, azotemia, but not proteinuria or active urine sediment, increased the risk of infection still further. The studies by Urowitz et al.[14] and Lee et al.[19] also noted the association of major infections with corticosteroid therapy and active renal disease. In particular, the former study also showed that the greatest number of fatal infections occurred within one year after diagnosis of CVD had been made, and that these patients had active SLE involving three or more organ systems, including positive renal biopsies for SLE nephritis. These results further underscore the association of increased rate of infection during periods of CVD disease activity, when in vitro studies have demonstrated the greatest degree of functional PMN leukocyte and lymphocyte abnormalities. The association of azathioprine with an increased incidence of infections was noted by Lee et al.[19]; however, in a subsequent study by Ginzler et al.,[12] azathioprine was only associated with an increased incidence of herpes zoster in patients with SLE. Ginzler et al.[12] further noted that with increasing prednisone doses, the rate of bacterial infections and opportunistic infections increased from 10.3/100 patient years of follow-up to 87/100 patient years, and from 0.8/100 patient years to 42/100 patient years, respectively.

The most recent study to examine the question of infection and immunosuppressive therapy in pa-

TABLE 7. Factors Associated with Increased Susceptibility to Infection in Patients with Systemic Lupus Erythematosus and Rheumatoid Arthritis[a]

Late in the course of RA disease activity[114]

First 2 years after diagnosis of SLE (early in the course of disease activity)[14]

Increase in disease severity (increase in manifestations of disease/patient)[14]

Azotemia (BUN >60 mg%)[15]

Active SLE nephritis (RBCs, cellular casts in sediment, positive kidney biopsy for SLE nephritis)[14]

Vascular lesions consistent with sclerosis[113]

Corticosteroid dose >20 mg prednisone/day[15]

Azathioprine therapy (herpes zoster infections only)[12]

Cyclophosphamide therapy (only in the presence of neutropenia)[112]

[a]Superscript numbers are references

tients with CVD, described 22 patients with antiglomerular basement membrane antibody disease (GBM), 19 with SLE, 18 with Wegener's granulomatosis (WG), and 16 with other forms of systemic vasculitis (SV).[112] The 75 patients had a total of 277 infections, with the IR being significantly lower in patients with SV and higher in those with SLE, when compared to the group as a whole. Of importance was that the mean time from the onset of immunosuppression to the first infection for the entire group was 12.7 days but in the SLE group was significantly shorter at 7.8 days ($p < 0.05$). Once again, the association of increased risk of infection with worsening renal failure and corticosteroid therapy was noted. The results of all the above studies therefore support the conclusion that immunosuppressive therapy predisposes patients with CVD to infectious complications. However, it is only one of several important interrelated factors, which include level of disease activity, and time of onset of disease manifestation (Table 7).

6. Spectrum of Infection in Patients with CVD

In most clinical studies over the past decade, bacteria have accounted for the majority of infections in patients with CVD (Table 8). In the recent series by Cohen et al.,[112] clinically significant bacterial

TABLE 8. Types of Infections in Patients with Systemic Lupus Erythematosus and Rheumatoid Arthritis[a]

Infection	Number of patients	SLE/RA[b]	Infection	Number of patients	SLE/RA[b]
Pneumonia		SLE = RA	Skin infections/cellulitis		SLE = RA
S. pneumoniae	5		Varicella zoster	21	
S. pyogenes	2		S aureus	15	
S. aureus	2		S. pyogenes	1	
H. influenzae	2		E. coli	1	
Gram-negative rods (not specified)	35		C. albicans	1	
			Total	39	
Klebsiella sp.	4		Urinary tract infections		SLE = RA
P. mirabilis	1		E. coli	18	
Enterobacter cloacae	1		Klebsiella sp.	1	
M. tuberculosis	7		Enterococcus	2	
Aspergillus sp.	5		Proteus sp.	2	
C. albicans	1		Total	23	
Aspergillus sp., C. albicans	1		Pyelonephritis/perinephric abscess		SLE = RA
Cytomegalovirus	5		E. coli	2	
P. carinii	5		Klebsiella sp.	1	
Total	76		Total	3	
Bacteremia		SLE > RA	Pharyngitis/thrush		SLE > RA
S. pneumoniae	2		C. albicans	24	
S. pyogenes	4		Peritonitis/intraabdominal abscess		SLE > RA
S. aureus	5		P. aeruginosa	1	
E. coli	3		Klebsiella sp.	1	
P. mirabilis	2		Retroperitoneal tuberculosis	1	
S. enteriditis	1		Total	3	
Acinetobacter	1		Soft tissue abscesses		RA > SLE
B. fragilis	1		S aureus	2	
S. typhimurium	1		S pneumoniae	2	
C. albicans	1		C. albicans	1	
C. neoformans	1		Total	5	
Total	22		Prosthetic joint infection		RA > SLE
Meningitis		SLE > RA	Staphylococcus sp.	22	
N. meningitidis	3		S pyogenes	5	
E. coli	1		Diphtheroids	2	
Klebsiella sp.	1		S pneumoniae	1	
Aspergillus sp.	1		Gram-negative bacilli	6	
C. neoformans	2		Anaerobes	3	
Total	8		Mixed infections	14	
			Total	53	

[a]Summarized from Refs 3, 7–9, 12, 14–17, and 19
[b]Comparative frequencies

infections were responsible for 73% of the 277 infections observed in their 75 patients with immunologically mediated disease. Gram-negative enteric bacilli comprised 68% of the bacterial infections in their patients with SLE, whereas in that same group viral, fungal, and *M. tuberculosis* and *P. carinii* accounted for 7%, 15%, and 4% of infections, respectively. In this study, the 15% incidence of fungal infections in patients with SLE was significantly ($p <$ 0.05) greater as compared with the other patients studied which included patients with SV, WG, and GBM disease. The principal sites of infection were the urinary tract, lungs, and blood, with ear, nose, and throat (ENT) infections also being present. UTIs were the most frequent infections in patients with SLE, with *Klebsiella* sp. and *E. coli* the most common isolates. Pneumonias were the second most frequent infection, with gram-negative enteric bacilli again the most common isolates (40%). In addition, pneumonias exhibited the highest mortality, being responsible for 70% of the deaths, with *Aspergillus fumigatus* responsible for 4 of the 5 fatal fungal pneumonias, and cytomegalovirus (CMV) complicating 30% of the fatal pneumonias. Other organisms responsible for fatal pneumonias included *M. tuberculosis*, *P. carinii*, and *Pseudomonas* sp. Of the SLE patients who developed septicemia (5 of 19), only 1 died of *Cryptococcus neoformans* fungemia, whereas the other four with septicemia caused by *S. aureus* (2), *Acinetobacter* (one), and *Salmonella enteritidis* (one), respectively, survived. Furthermore, this study points out the important fact that half of the patients with serious opportunistic infections also became infected with another serious opportunist pathogen, often simultaneously. For example, one patient had a *C. albicans* fungemia rapidly followed by CMV pneumonia, while in another case both *Aspergillus* sp. and *P. carinii* were found in a bronchial biopsy specimen. This type of complication, not unique to immunosuppressed SLE patients, has been observed in renal transplant patients (see Chapter 21) and more recently in those with the acquired immunodeficiency syndrome (see Chapter 15).

The pattern of infections in patients with SLE in the first two decades of life is slightly different from those described above.[7] Infections of the skin (31% with varicella-zoster virus, 13% with *Staphylococcus* sp.) accounted for 44% of all infections, and septicemia with or without endocarditis caused by *Staph.* sp., *S. pneumoniae*, gram-negative bacilli, and *C. albicans* another 20%. The study by Ginzler et al.[12] made the additional observation that in this population, oral thrush was the leading type of opportunistic infection, with pneumonia due to CMV, *P. carinii*, and *Aspergillus* sp. the second most common opportunistic infection. Furthermore, it was noted that a significant number of patients with deep fungal infections had received prior antibiotic therapy for gram-negative sepsis.[12] This study and those by Lee

et al.[19] and by Staples et al.[15] also confirmed that the urinary tract, the lungs, and the skin are the major sites of infection in patients with SLE, with gram-positive cocci and gram-negative enteric bacilli the most frequently isolated organisms. These studies all suggest a progression toward increasing microbial pathogenicity, depending on the level of CVD activity. Patients with inactive SLE have mainly a higher incidence of gram-positive bacterial infections. In the setting of active SLE, however, which involves two or more organ systems, the infections are more aggressive and are caused mainly by gram-negative enteric organisms. In active SLE, when the degree of immunosuppression is furthered by corticosteroid or cyclophosphamide therapy, infections with opportunistic pathogens such as *Aspergillus* sp., *Nocardia* sp., and *Cryptococcus neoformans* become more prevalent.

The types of infections seen in patients with RA are similar, although less frequent, than in patients with SLE. Nevertheless, a number of important differences emerge from several studies over the past 10 years. Whereas, in SLE the majority of infectious complications occur early in the course of the disease, in patients with RA, the greatest number of infections occur late in their clinical course.[114] Moreover, although infections of the urinary tract, lungs, and skin are still significant in number, septic arthritis,[29] relatively silent and localized tissue abscesses,[30] and infected hip, knee, and elbow arthroplasties are the infectious complications with the greatest clinical impact.[11]

In the eight cases of septic arthritis reported by Mitchell et al.,[29] the principal organism was *S. aureus*. Other reports, however, describe many additional organisms implicated in joint infections in this patient population, including *S. pneumoniae*, *H. influenzae*, *Pasteurella multocida*, *Candida* sp., and *Mycobacteria* sp.[22] An increased incidence of severe soft tissue infections in RA patients has also been noted. One report[30] describes 24 episodes of infection in 12 patients with longstanding RA. Extremity abscesses in association with superficial skin infections (5), Intraabdominal abscess (ovarian, 1; gallbladder, 1; pelvic, 1; perinephric, 4), empyema (5), and pneumonia with abscess formation (3), were caused mainly by *S. aureus*, enteric gram-negative bacilli, and *S. pneumoniae*. The gram-positive organisms principally caused the extremity and pulmonary infections, with the gram-negative ones causing the intraabdominal and pelvic infections.

Patients with RA frequently undergo total joint arthroplasty (TJA) in order to relieve symptoms of pain and improve function of severely damaged joints. Although a detailed discussion of the extensive orthopedic literature surrounding the issue of which factors influence the incidence of infections in this setting is beyond the scope of this chapter, several important points should be made. The overall infection rate for all TJA in most series is approximately 1–2%, with the risk in RA patients two to three times that of the osteoarthritic.[115] The operated joint with the highest incidence of infection is the knee, being ten times more frequently infected than the hip and almost twice more often than the elbow. Of interest is that most infections occur within 2 years of surgery, and furthermore, infections occurring during the first year usually result from perioperative complications, but after 3 years there is an increased likelihood that an infected joint may be seeded hematogenously from a distant site. Early TJA infections are caused principally by *Staph.* sp., with late infections exhibiting an increased percentage of gram-negative enteric bacilli, *Pseudomonas* sp., and mixed infections with gram-positive cocci and gram-negative bacilli.

7. Unique Clinical Features of Infection in Patients with CVD

As described in the first part of this chapter, the manifestations of an infectious process in patients with SLE, more often than those with RA, may be identical to a flare of the underlying immunologic illness. Consequently, differentiating between infection and active SLE or RA is a critical aspect of acute medical management in these patients. Relatively few studies, however, have focused exclusively on those clinical features which could be helpful in the early identification of infection in patients with either SLE or RA. The study by Stahl et al.[116] has been particularly useful in helping the physician analyze the etiology of febrile episodes in this population because fever is such a common occurrence in patients with SLE.[4] Their study showed that in 160 patients with SLE who had 63 febrile episodes, the primary cause of febrile episodes was active SLE

TABLE 9. Clinical and Laboratory Features Suggestive of Infection in Patients with Systemic Lupus Erythematosus and Rheumatoid Arthritis

	SLE	RA
Atypical flare	+	+
Shaking chill	+	+
Normalization of previously low WBC count	+	+
Leukocytosis (WBC 12,000/mm³)	+	+
Neutrophilia	+	+
Normal DNA binding (in the absence of SLE flare)	+	−
Active urinary sediment (in the presence of SLE flare)	+	−

alone in 60%, infections in 23% and a variety of miscellaneous causes in 17% of their patients. Of the 19 febrile episodes associated with the infections, bacteremia, which had the highest mortality rate (33%), was the most common single cause of fever (48%), with localized bacterial infections (abscesses and pneumonia) causing 31%. The most important point, however, was that the only clinical feature that was helpful in discriminating infectious from noninfectious febrile episodes, were shaking chills (27% in noninfected versus 68% in infected patients, $p < 0.001$) (Table 9). In patients who had active SLE, the laboratory features that were most helpful in identifying an infectious cause of fever were leukocytosis (WBC count greater than 12,000 mm³), neutrophilia, and an active urinary sediment. When the group as a whole was examined (active plus inactive SLE), normal DNA binding was observed more frequently in infectious than in noninfectious febrile episodes.

Other general clinical features which should alert the physician to an infection in a patient with SLE or RA is a change in the usual pattern associated with a flare of the disease. Manifestations of disease activity in an individual patient will frequently appear as a predictable constellation of signs and symptoms, particularly when the flare occurs in temporal association with efforts to reduce corticosteroid or cytotoxic therapy.[4] Symptoms of pneumonitis and pleurisy, arthritis and skin rashes, or meningitis, will recur repeatedly in patients with SLE on tapering of their prednisone dose. The sudden onset of SLE-like symptoms involving a previously silent organ system should lead to a diligent search for an infectious etiology, particularly in the absence of CVD activity in other systems. Thus, the diagnosis of new onset of arthritis, pleurisy, or fever secondary to SLE should be a diagnosis of exclusion reached only after an evaluation for infection is unrevealing.[116]

8. Clinical Examples of Infection and Their Management

A number of chapters in this book discuss in depth the management of infections in patients with different degrees of immunosuppression in association with an underlying disease process. The clinical approach to complications such as neutropenia, gram-negative sepsis, and pulmonary infiltrates for example, is very similar in practical terms whether the patient has SLE or has had a kideny transplant. However, the unique features of patients with CVD are that the immunologic diseases may mimic an infectious process, that antibiotic therapy can precipitate a flare of CVD activity, and that therapies to suppress CVD activity may cause symptoms indistinguishable from those of an infection. Consequently, the clinical cases below will focus principally on the possible approaches to these particular clinical dilemmas.

8.1. Altered Mental Status in a Patient with SLE

Since the diagnosis of CNS involvement in SLE in any of its forms is largely one of exclusion, it is necessary to rule out other treatable causes of such symptoms or signs.

Illustrative Case 1

A 24-year-old black woman with a 6-year history of SLE was transferred to our hospital for evaluation of possible viral encephalitis because of progressive impairment of memory and unusual behavior over a 4-day period. Six years prior to this admission, the patient had presented with fever to 100 4°F (38°C), arthralgias, and pleuritic chest pain. Evaluation at that time had revealed a normal physical examination except for a friction rub under the right subscapular area. Her laboratory data had revealed a mild normochromic normocytic anemia, a white blood cell (WBC) count of 4500/mm³, an erythrocyte sedimentation rate (ESR) of 80 mm/hr, a positive antinuclear antibody (ANA) test, and a normal urinalysis A presumptive diagnosis of SLE had been made and she

was begun on 60 mg prednisone/day, with prompt resolution of her symptoms During the ensuring 6-year period, numerous attempts to decrease her daily dose of prednisone below 20 mg had resulted in flares of her original symptoms On two of these occasions, when the level of prednisone therapy was increased, she had exhibited a transient period of agitated behavior interpreted as steroid-induced psychosis following unrevealing evaluations for meningitis or SLE as etiologic possibilities. Ten days prior to the present admission, the patient's family stated that she had been suffering from the flu, following a weekend camping trip near a lake, and had complained of a sore throat, a nonproductive cough, fever to 38°C, myalgias, and a mild frontal headache On advice from her family physician, she took acetominophen and increased her prednisone to 60 mg/day (previous evaluation had revealed her to have no significant adrenal reserves under stress conditions). Forty-eight hr later, her family noticed that she displayed increased irritability and had several verbal altercations with her siblings The day before transfer to the hospital, she was examined in an outlying emergency room because of altered personality and further emotional outbursts. She had a normal neurologic examination and computed tomographic (CT) examination of the head, the lumbar puncture was normal, except for CSF showing 20 lymphocytes/mm³. An infectious disease consultation raised the possibility of viral encephalitis as a possible etiology, and the patient was transferred for further evaluation and therapy Examination on admission revealed a cushingoid woman with periods of somnolence alternating with agitation. She was afebrile, and had a normal cardiopulmonary examination Except for her altered mental status, her neurologic examination was normal A chest radiograph was normal A repeat CT examination of the head was normal Lumbar puncture revealed a CSF glucose of 60 mg%, a protein of 100 mg%, and 80 lymphocytes/mm³ India ink, Gram stain, and smears of the CSF for acid-fast organisms were all negative However, her CSF revealed the presence of cryptococcal polysaccharide capsular antigen, and a diagnosis of cryptococcal meningitis was made. CSF cultures subsequently grew *C neoformans* She was treated with the combination of amphotericin B 0.3 mg/kg body weight per day IV and flucytosine 37 5 mg/kg body weight every 6 hr PO for 6 weeks Her neurologic abnormalities resolved, and a lumbar puncture 2 weeks after discontinuation of therapy was normal and failed to grow *C neoformans*

Comment. The dilemma facing the physicians who first saw this patient was to differentiate between infectious meningitis, steroid-induced psychosis, and CNS manifestations of SLE. The fact that the patient's mental status had worsened in association with increasing her prednisone, a pattern that had been previously observed, added to the initial diagnostic difficulties. Nevertheless, several important points can be made to facilitate the management of this case. Although CNS manifestations of SLE can be the sole manifestation of a disease flare,[117] they usually occur when disease activity is manifested in other organs [117–119] Except for her mild flulike symptoms, this patient did not exhibit any of her usual manifestations of active SLE Furthermore, her usual symptoms always had responded to increased prednisone therapy and in this situation had in fact been associated with further clinical deterioration. In several series reporting patients with CNS–SLE, none of the neurologic features appears in the absence of other features of SLE.[118,120] Laboratory abnormalities such as hypoglycorrhacia can very rarely be caused by SLE, but usually only when transverse myelitis is present [121] In addition, CSF pleocytosis may also occur in the setting of CNS–SLE in up to one-third of patients, but usually consists of only a few cells [118,120] Consequently, in this type of case a search for an infectious etiology is imperative, particularly because the symptoms of cryptococcal meningitis may be similar to those of CNS–SLE.[122] As with this patient, more than one lumbar puncture may have to be performed, since the findings of elevated CSF protein and minimal or no lymphocytosis may be the only findings in both early cryptococcal meningitis and CNS–SLE.[122] In a number of series examining deep fungal infections in SLE, the correct diagnosis of cryptococcal meningitis was made in only 36% of patients antemortum.[123] The combination therapy she received with amphotericin B and flucytosine has been effective in erradicating CNS cryptococcal infections.[124] In patients with SLE, however, azotemia is more likely to develop despite the lowered dose of amphotericin B, causing flucytosine levels to rise. Consequently, renal function and flucytosine levels should be carefully monitored in order to avoid the GI and marrow toxicities of this drug. Despite the success of this therapy, mortality due to CNS cryptococcal infection is still approximately 30%, with nearly one-half the patients cured exhibiting residual neurologic abnormalities, and hydrocephalus an occasional late complication even when the infection has been irradicated.[125]

8.2. Pleuritic Chest Pain and Fever in a Patient with SLE

Patients with SLE may develop parenchymal lung disease in addition to pleural and pericardial involvement. In most situations, however, cardiac failure, pulmonary emboli, uremia, and infections play a more important role. A careful and thorough evaluation should provide the basis for a choice between antibiotics and antiinflammatory agents.

Illustrative Case 2

A 37-year-old white woman with a 2-year history of SLE was admitted to the hospital for evaluation of pleuritic chest pain and fever. The patient had presented to her family physician 2 years earlier with pleuritic chest pain, tachypnea, mild hypoxia, arthralgias, and a malar rash. Her initial laboratory examination revealed a normal WBC count, an ESR of 110 mm/hr, an elevated ANA, and a chest radiograph with bilateral alveolar infiltrates She was diagnosed as having SLE following extensive evaluation, including bronchoscopy with transbronchial biopsy that revealed only acute alveolitis on pathologic examination. Her pulmonary symptoms and chest radiographic abnormalities resolved with the use of oral corticosteroids. Even with the judicious use of corticosteroids and the subsequent addition of cyclophosphamide therapy, she had developed the nephrotic syndrome over the 2-year period, and at the time of this admission her degree of azotemia had progressed to the extent that she was being considered for dialysis. Despite her disease, she had remained physically active and had recently

helped her family build an extension to their home. The admission physical examination revealed a visibly tachypneic, cushingoid-appearing white woman, complaining of right-sided pleuritic chest pain. Her temperature was 102.2°F (39°C) and her respiratory rate 24/min. She had dullness to percussion over the right posterior chest with an audible friction rub. Except for mild pitting edema of her lower extremities, the remainder of the physical examination was normal. Her laboratory data revealed a WBC count of 13,000/mm^3, an ESR of 60 mm/hr, a urinalysis with 2+ protein, and a chest radiograph with an area of consolidation in the apical segment of the right lower lobe (Fig 1) Arterial blood gas (ABG) measurements showed her to have a Pao_2 of 74 mm Hg, $Paco_2$ of 25 mm Hg, and pH of 7.48 while breathing room air On further questioning, the patient described several days of a nonproductive cough, intermittent fever to 100.4°F (38°C), and the sudden onset of pleuritic chest pain the day before admission.

Repeated attempts to obtain a sputum sample for examination, including a transtracheal aspirate, were unrewarding. The patient was begun on nafcillin 8 g/day in addition to gentamicin 3 mg/kg per day IV. On her second hospital day, she complained of increasing pleuritic chest pain and had several episodes of a small amount of hemoptysis. Pulmonary arteriography was performed and revealed no changes consistent with pulmonary emboli. Bronchoscopic examination with transbronchial biopsy was performed on the third hospital day because of further clinical deterioration characterized by increasing shortness of breath, and decreasing arterial oxygen content to a Pao_2 of 54 mm Hg on breathing room air. Pathologic examination of the lung biopsy specimen revealed areas of hemorrhagic infarction with abundant hyphal forms growing in blood vessels. The patient's previous antibiotics were discontinued, and she was begun on amphotericin B 0.5 mg/kg per day IV. Aspergillus sp. subsequently were identified in cultures of the biopsy specimen. On the fifth hospital day, the patient suddenly became cyanotic, hypotensive, and unresponsive to stimuli. Resusitation attempts were unsuccessful and she expired Postmortem examination revealed a saddle embolus obstructing the pulmonary artery, and the right lower lobe of the lung with extensive consolidation and hemorrhagic necrosis, with many hyphal forms seen invading the microvasculature.

Comment. Differentiating between SLE pneumonitis, pulmonary emboli, and infectious etiologies to explain this patient's clinical course was the principal difficulty encountered by her physicians Because the patient had previously demonstrated SLE flares that had exhibited a significant pulmonary component, her present tachypnea, nonproductive cough, fever, and hypoxia were all consistent with acute SLE pneumonitis [126] When autopsy series have principally examined the lungs in patients with SLE, those pulmonary manifestations attributed to SLE alone were interstitial fibrosis, vasculitis, and hematoxylin bodies in 100% of cases and interstitial pneumonitis and pleuritis in 73% and 61%, respectively.[127] Chest radiographs are usually characterized by unilateral or bilateral alveolar infiltrates with or without effusions [128,129] It is important to remember however, that pulmonary infections are still the most frequent causes of infiltrates in patients with SLE.[126–131] One feature that may help the physician distinguish between infection and SLE pneumonitis, is that the latter has a predilection for the lung bases [126] In addition, when pulmonary hemorrhage is present in SLE, there are usually bilateral radiographic abnormalities, again usually more pronounced in the

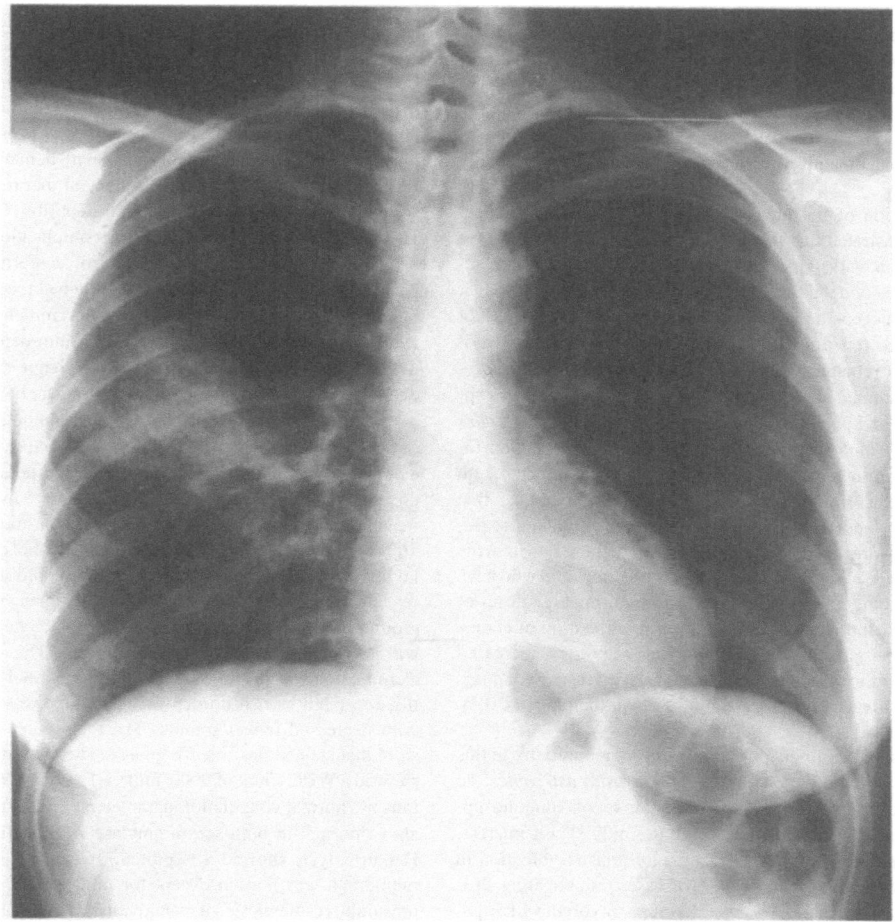

FIGURE 1. Admission chest radiograph for Illustrative Case 2. This 37-year-old patient with SLE presented with pleuritic chest pain, a nonproductive cough, and an audible friction rub over the right posterior chest. The posterior apical (PA) chest radiograph demonstrates a right lower lobe (apical segment) pneumonia

lower lung fields, with pathologic examination revealing a significant number of patients with immune complex deposition in the alveolar septa and bronchioles.[132] In a number of cases of SLE–pneumonitis, once an infectious etiology has been ruled out, there has been prompt clinical response to corticosteroid and immunosuppressive therapy.[126]

The single most important action that will help the physician manage this type of case in an optimal manner, when no sputum can be obtained initially for microbiologic examination and culture, is a lung biopsy. It should be performed as early in the clinical course as possible to obtain material for culture and pathologic examination. Delays to evaluate the results of empirical therapy frequently lead to further clinical deterioration, and should be avoided. Because in autopsy reports of SLE patients bronchopneumonia is present in one-half of cases and is the most common pulmonary finding,[127] every effort should be made to identify an

infectious etiology. Most of these pneumonias are bacterial in origin, but tuberculosis and fungal infections are also common causes. The conspicuous absence of sputum in this case makes a search for tuberculosis and fungal infection particularly urgent.

Tuberculosis (TB) in association with SLE usually presents as fever, cough, hemoptysis, dyspnea, and weight loss, symptoms that frequently initially are attributed to SLE itself.[133] As with most infectious complications of SLE, nearly two-thirds who develop TB will do so within the first 2 years of having had the diagnosis of SLE.[133] Frequently two or more organ systems have manifestations of SLE disease activity at the time TB is detected. Consequently, there usually is an average delay of one to three months in establishing the diagnosis, particularly when extrapulmonary manifestations are present. Therefore, in a patient with SLE, unexplained pulmonary infiltrates, lymphadenopathy, pleural effusion, or ascites should be evaluated aggressively for active TB and not be attributed to the underlying immunologic disease Because in most studies severity of SLE and corticosteroid dosage correlate positively with severity of TB and mortality, an individual patient with a course strongly compatible with TB, in whom a tissue diagnosis of TB has been unobtainable, a judicious trial of antimycobacterial drug therapy is probably indicated [134]

Examination of the lung biopsy specimen and subsequent cultures demonstrated that this patient had developed an invasive fungal infection with *Aspergillus flavus* In one series that reviewed 33 cases of deep fungal infection in association with SLE, most patients had candidiasis (14 of 33), either disseminated (8 of 14) or localized (pneumonitis, peritonitis, or esophagitis) (6 of 14) [123] Of the remaining patients, 10 had infection with *Cryptococcus* (disseminated and meningitis), four with *Aspergillus* sp (disseminated and pneumonitis), and two each with *Coccidioides immitis* and *Histoplasma capsulatum* It was not uncommon for fungus infection to supervene in an area previously infected with bacteria. It is clear from published reports and our experience, that despite the high mortality of invasive pulmonary fungal disease, the patients that are the most likely to survive are those in whom the diagnosis is made early in the course of the infection, and who have few if any ongoing manifestations of SLE requiring high doses of corticosteroids. Intravenous amphotericin B is the drug of choice for invasive aspergillosis The likelihood of a response is increased by its administration early in the course of the disease, with doses being rapidly advanced to therapeutic levels in the range of 0.5–0.6 mg/kg per day

An additional etiologic possibility considered initially in this case was that of an infection caused by *Nocardia asteroides,* an organism frequently complicating the course of immunosuppressed patients on high doses of corticosteroids.[135] Of interest, however, is that norcardiosis is a distinctly unusual infection in women with SLE, with almost 90% of cases complicating SLE being reported in men.[136] In several studies involving SLE patients, lung involvement by Nocardia presented not infrequently as a pulmonary cavity in women, and pneumonia involving the upper and middle lobes in men [136] Most of these patients are almost always on high doses of corticosteroids The striking association of nocardiosis and male patients with SLE seen in the literature suggests that either genetic host factors or hormonal milieu, or both, may contribute significantly to the pathogenesis of this infection.[136]

8.3. Abdominal Pain in a Patient with SLE

Thirty-five to 40% of patients with SLE develop signs or symptoms of GI involvement at some point during the course of their illness, and nearly 20% of these patients complain of abdominal pain at some point. Because of the pleomorphic nature of the symptoms and signs of acute abdominal pain in SLE, it may be impossible to distinguish infectious peritonitis from the abdominal syndromes associated with mesenteric vasculitis.

Illustrative Case 3

The patient was a 31-year-old black woman with a 10-year history of SLE, transferred to our hospital for management of her abdominal pain The diagnosis of SLE had been made 10 years previously when the patient presented with hematuria, arthralgias, fever, and weight loss A renal biopsy at that time had been described as being consistent with SLE nephritis Over the ensuing 10 years, she experienced numerous complications as a result of her SLE, including several episodes of cerebritis, myocarditis, pericarditis, pleuritis, and azotemia She had received continuous therapy with corticosteroids and intermittent therapy with cyclophosphamide, complicated by insulin-dependent diabetes mellitus and several episodes of hemorrhagic cystitis She had been hospitalized for 2 months prior to transfer because of abdominal pain, pleuritis, and pericarditis Radiologic evaluation at the outlying hospital had revealed a normal biliary tree, but a CT examination of the abdomen had raised the possibility of a pancreatic pseudocyst She had been treated with high doses of corticosteroids with no significant relief and on transfer was taking 160 mg/day prednisone She denied any alcohol consumption and no use of thiazide diuretics The admission physical examination revealed a distressed cushingoid black woman, vomiting coffee-ground material Her temperature was 37°C, her blood pressure was $140/100$ mm Hg and her pulse 126/min. The cardiopulmonary examination was positive for a pleuropericardial friction rub over the upper left sternal border Her abdomen was diffusely tender with decreased bowel sounds The rectal examination revealed stool that stained positive for guaiac The laboratory examination showed a WBC count of 9900/mm^3, a Hct of 34.9%, an ESR of 56 mm/hr, normal coagulation parameters, and a fivefold elevation above normal in both serum amylase and alkaline phosphatase Her urinalysis showed 1+ protein and no cells, and the chest radiograph was normal except for mild cardiac enlargement A presumptive diagnosis of pancreatitis complicated by upper GI tract bleeding was made and the patient was placed on antacid therapy by mouth and on intravenous fluids

Initial attempts over the first few days of hospitalization to reduce her dose of prednisone resulted in increased pleuritic chest pain. Further evaluation with a CT examination of the abdomen revealed "fluid collections within the abdomen suggestive of pancreatic pseudocysts," and endoscopy revealed gastritis Because of persistent abdominal pain, paracentesis was performed that revealed yellowish fluid containing 3400 PMN leukocyte/mm^3 and an elevated amylase level Although the Gram stain was negative for organisms, she was begun on antibiotic therapy intravenously as treatment for possible spontaneous bacterial peritonitis. Eight days after admission, she developed sudden left-sided weakness and blurring of vision. CT examination of the head was normal, as was the laboratory evaluation of her CSF. The following morning, because of severe and sudden dyspnea, she was transferred to intensive care, with chest radiography revealing diffuse bilateral interstitial changes consistent with pulmonary edema Because of her deteriorating level of oxygenation, she was intubated. All attempts to identify an infectious etiology for the pulmonary infiltrates were negative, and a presumptive diagnosis of adult respiratory distress syndrome (ARDS) was made Several hours later she complained of severe abdominal pain, became hypotensive and despite resuscitation attempts, expired. Post mortem examination revealed fulminant pancreatitis with extensive fat necorsis and pseudocyst formation, complicated by ARDS and a large acute myocardial infarct In addition, there were focal infarcts in her spinal cord with small vessel thrombosis, and ulceration of the large bowel

Comment. The principal problem that significantly complicated this patient's management among the many other complex and interrelated clinical issues involving this case, was the etiology of her abdominal pain Abdominal pain has long been recognized as a prominent and the most frequent GI manifestation of SLE and other vasculitides such as periarteritis nodosa (PAN)[137] and may have many potential causes such as peritonitis, bowel ulceration and perforation, hemorrhage, and motility disturbances.[138] In a recent series of 140 patients with SLE in whom 11% developed disease-related signs and symptoms of acute surgical abdomen, one-third of this group had nausea, vomiting, diarrhea, and melena, as did our patient.[139] Fever and tachycardia were universally present, and 75% had rebound abdominal tenderness, with hypoactive bowel sounds In those that underwent laparotomy, more than half had intestinal perforations Other causes of pain that needed to be considered in this case were peritonitis and pancreatitis

Acute necrotizing pancreatitis was noted in 4 of 14 SLE patients with severe abdominal pain in Pollack's study [140] The important points from this and other reviews are that (1) there is little correlation between amylase levels and duration or dosage of corticosteroid therapy in those patients who develop pancreatitis,[141] and (2) diagnosis of an acute surgical abdomen due to SLE could be made with increased confidence only when the patient had concomitant disease activity in other organs. Zizic et al [139] pointed out that the index of suspicion should be particularly high in those patients who have evidence of peripheral vasculitis, neurologic involvement, thrombocytopenia, or rheumatoid factor positivity, all of which occur significantly more often in those SLE patients with abdominal crises. In the study by Reynolds et al.,[141] which examined 53 SLE patients with abdominal pain, 49% had hyperamylasemia, with only 20% of these caused by extrapancreatic causes. As was described in other studies,[129] 80% of these patients with pancreatitis and hyperamylasemia manifested SLE activity in more than four organ systems In contrast with our patient, complications such as ARDS, shock, and hemorrhage were not observed in this series Moreover, recovery usually occurred despite continued steroid therapy Gram-positive bacterial spontaneous peritonitis in association with SLE has been reported [142] In SLE patients, this complication has arisen in the setting of marked proteinuria and hypoalbuminemia, although ascites has usually not been demonstrable The symptoms, as in the case of acute pancreatitis, are not distinctive, with abdominal pain, diffuse tenderness, and guarding present in most cases. In the cases reported by Lipsky et al ,[142] all the patients were bacteremic and had abdominal paracentesis revealing the causative organism

In managing these patients, it is important not to delay therapy until all the classic signs of an acute abdomen develop, since they may occur late, if not at all, and be masked by the antiinflammatory properties of corticosteroids Consequently, early analysis of peritoneal fluid for Gram stain and culture to exclude bacterial peritonitis, the judicious use of antibiotics, and prompt laparotomy

when clinical symptoms and signs progress despite medical therapy are all indicated

8.4. Painful Knee in a Patient with Rheumatoid Arthritis

The early identification and treatment of an infectious etiology of a painful knee in a patient with RA will lead to a significant improvement in morbidity.

Illustrative Case 4

A 76-year-old white woman with a long history of seropositive RA was admitted for evaluation of a swollen, painful left knee Over the previous 35 years, she had developed numerous flares of RA involving both her knees and ankle, and had undergone an uncomplicated left knee synovectomy 10 years earlier. Over the preceding 4 months she had experienced periodic painful swelling of her left knee, and on several occasions small amounts of cloudy fluid had been aspirated with Gram stain and routine bacteriologic cultures being negative Intraarticular corticosteroids had been administered with temporary relief of her symptoms She denied any systemic symptoms such as fever or weight loss The physical examination was characterized by the stigmata of longstanding RA involving both her knees and ankles, with her left knee being warm, mildly erythematous, tender to palpation, and demonstrating decreased arc of flexion Radiographs of the left knee showed increased bony and joint destruction, which had progressed over the preceding year. Aspiration of the left knee revealed cloudy fluid with 50,000 PMN leukocytes/mm³, a negative Gram stain but positive Ziel–Nielsen stain for acid-fast bacilli Cultures subsequently yielded *Mycobacterium kansasii*. Surgical exploration of the knee found caseating granulomata with bony and joint destruction and a florid synovitis. On the basis of the diagnosis of tuberculous arthritis, the knee was debrided and an arthrodesis performed. The patient received isoniazid and rifampin therapy for 6 months with resolution of the knee pain and no further radiologic progression

Comment. Patients with chronic RA have a propensity to develop superimposed joint infections This susceptibility to infection is further increased in the presence of Felty syndrome, severe longstanding disease, and immunosuppressive therapy.[143] Moreover, such patients have been shown to be at risk for opportunistic infections with organisms of low virulence, such as *M tuberculosis* and *M kansasii* [144]

The clinical management of cases such as this is always complicated by the difficulty in diagnosing an infectious process in joints of immunocompromised patients who have an underlying chronic inflammatory process Frequently, these joints either fail to show a local articular response to infection such as heat and tenderness or have such frequent rheumatoid flares that no distinguishing features of the suppurative process are detectable

Tuberculous infection of the joints in this population is almost always a combination of osteomyelitis and arthritis, may be a consequence of remote infection, and is frequently monoarticular, with the weight-bearing joints the most commonly affected. *M kansasii* has been reported to cause suppurative arthritis in a number of patients with RA.[145] Distinguishing features have included frequent involvement of the tendon sheaths of the hand and wrist, with common involvement of small bones and joints of the hands.[146] Consequently, the granulomatous process often simulates RA. As in our patient, the earliest clinical manifestation may be pain, which can precede other signs or inflammation by weeks or even months. Joint fluid aspirates in this population should always be carefully examined for an infectious etiology. A sample that is cloudy, with variable viscosity, >10,000 PMN leukocytes/mm^3 and a low to normal sugar, should not only be Gram stained for bacteria, but a Ziehl–Neelsen stain for acid-fast organisms should be done. Definitive diagnosis almost always requires a biopsy, which should be done as soon as the suspicion of tuberculous joint infection is raised. Early chemotherapeutic intervention frequently is curative, with arthrodesis necessary only for control of pain as well as joint stability.[115]

Although the insidious onset of a suppurative process with an organism of low virulence may present a difficult clinical problem, a far more common complication in RA is septic arthritis caused by organisms such as *Staph. aureus*.[22] Mortality in patients with RA for this complication may be high, occurring in approximately 30% of patients. Moreover, the prognosis is largely determined by the speed of initiating antibiotic therapy, with patients who are untreated for a week or more having a much worse prognosis. Not infrequently, the joint infection will be temporally and anatomically close to an infected skin ulcer.[2,29] Therefore, it is important to vigorously treat skin infections in patients with RA, in the same way that an infected lesion would be treated in a patient with diabetes mellitus.

There are a number of significant clinical differences and similarities between our patient with RA and the septic arthritis in patients with SLE. In patients with SLE, septic arthritis also commonly involves the large weight-bearing joints, with the knee being the most frequent. Characteristically, the septic arthritis is monarticular, accompanied by pain, swelling, and erythema.[147] The onset is usually acute, with systemic symptoms such as fever and chills present in 60% of cases. The most significant difference between SLE and RA, however, is that in SLE a wide variety of bacterial organisms may cause septic arthritis.[147] *Neisseria gonorrheae*, *Staphylococcus* sp., gram-negative enteric bacilli, *Hemophilus influenzae*, and *Salmonella* sp. are reported far more frequently in SLE than is RA, where 70–80% of the cases of septic arthritis caused by *S aureus* The management of these cases should be similar to those already described, with prompt joint fluid analysis and culture, synovial tissue biopsy for definitive diagnosis in the more indolent cases, and early antibiotic treatment to prevent further tissue destruction.

9. Conclusions

The management of infections in the immunosuppressed patient with CVD shares many features in common with those in other immunosuppressed groups. Neutropenia and other side effects of cytotoxic therapy, nosocomial infections such as line sepsis, and the complications of corticosteroid therapy are among the many common issues throughout this book. The most distinctive feature, however, that makes infection in the SLE or RA patient difficult to assess is the fact that the manifestation of an infectious process in these patients may be identical to specific aspects of the underlying disease activity. Moreover, infection may not only mimic a flare of SLE or RA but also precipitate one, causing further diagnostic difficulties. In addition, complications of antibiotic and cytotoxic therapy may be indistinguishable from one another, or from the protean manifestations of the immunologic disease.

Patients with SLE are most likely to develop an infection within the first 2 years after diagnosis. These patients have a greater incidence of gram-positive bacterial infections when compared to other patients with immunologically mediated disease. As the level of disease activity increases and immunosuppressive therapy is instituted, infections with enteric gram-negative bacilli and opportunistic pathogens become more frequent. The major causes of morbidity and mortality continue to be pneumonia and sepsis, with minor infections principally involving the skin and urinary tract. By contrast, patients with RA are more likely to develop an infection late in the course of their disease, usually involving the weight-bearing joints. In these patients, joint infections with bacteria commonly causing skin infections, such as *Staph.* sp., are more frequent. In RA patients, when gram-negative organisms are involved, it is principally in the setting of hematogenous spread from the urinary tract.

Atypical flares of disease in the absence of clinical involvement of other organ systems should always raise the possibility that the etiology is an infectious process. Prompt and persistent attempt to obtain a biopsy specimen from the involved area for microbiological analysis is the single most important step in managing infections in these patients. Attempts to evaluate empiric therapy frequently lead to significant delays in the diagnosis, and a far worse prognosis overall. When the appropriate cultures have been obtained, early judicious use of antibiotic therapy most often results in a positive clinical outcome.

ACKNOWLEDGMENT. The author would like to thank Dr. Edward J. Goetzl for his careful reading of the manuscript and for his many helpful suggestions.

References

1. Carpenter RC, Sturgill BC: The course of systemic lupus erythematosus. *J Chronic Dis* **19**:117–131, 1966.
2. Dubois EL, Tuffanelli DL. Clinical manifestations of systemic lupus erythematosus: Computer analysis of the 520 cases. *JAMA* **190**:112–119, 1964.
3. Perez HD, Goldstein IM· Infection and host defenses in systemic lupus erythematosus. In Franklin EC (ed): *Clinical Immunology Update*. Elsevier, New York, 1979, pp 133–159.
4. Steinberg AD: Management of systemic lupus erythematosus In Kelley WN, Harris ED, Ruddy S, Sledge CB (eds). *Textbook of Rheumatology*. WB Saunders, Philadelphia, 1985, pp. 1098–1115.
5. Coplon NS, Diskin CJ, Petersen SJ, et al. The long-term clinical course of systemic lupus erythematosus in end-stage renal disease. *N Engl J Med* **308**:186–190, 1983.
6. Cohen J, Pinching AJ: Infection and immunosuppression. A study of the infective complications of 75 patients with immunologically-mediated disease. *Q J Med* **51**:1–15, 1982
7. Platt JL, Burke, BA, Fish AJ, et al Systemic lupus erythematosus in the first two decades of life. *Am J Kidney Dis* **2**(suppl 1):212–222, 1982.
8. Rosner S, Ginzler EM, Diamond HS, et al: A multicenter study of outcome in systemic lupus erythematosus. II. Causes of death. *Arthritis Rheum* **6**:612–617, 1982.
9. Kiernan M, Bresnihan B: Clinical features and outcome of infection in systemic lupus erythematosus. *Ir J Med Sci* **152**:382–386, 1983.
10. Wallace DJ, Podell TE, Weiner JM, et al. Lupus nephritis Experience with 230 patients in a private practice from 1950 to 1980. *Am J Med* **72**:209–220, 1982.
11. Hashimoto H, Shiokawa Y: Changing pattern of clinical features and prognosis in systemic lupus erythematosus. *Scand J Rheumatol* **7**:219–224, 1978.
12. Ginzler E, Diamond H, Kaplan D, et al: Computer analysis of factors influencing frequency of infection in systemic lupus erythematosus. *Arthritis Rheum* **21**:37–44, 1978.
13. Fish AJ, Blau EB, Westerberg NG, et al. Systemic lupus erythematosus within the first two decades of life *Am J Med* **62**:99–117, 1977
14. Urowitz MB, Bookman AA, Koehler BE, et al: The biomodal mortality pattern of systemic lupus erythematosus *Am J Med* **60**:221–225, 1976.
15. Staples PG, Gerding DN, Decker JL, et al: Incidence of infection in systemic lupus erythematosus. *Arthritis Rheum* **17**:1–10, 1974.
16. Vandenbroucke JP, Hazevoet HM, Cats A: Survival and cause of death in rheumatoid arthritis: A 25-year prospective followup. *J Rheumatol* **11**:158–161, 1984.
17. Hollingsworth JW, Saykaly RJ· Systemic complications of rheumatoid arthritis. *Med Clin North Am* **61**:217–228, 1977.
18. Prior P, Symmons DP, Scott DL, et al Cause of death in rheumatoid arthritis. *Br J Rheumatol* **23**:92–99, 1984.
19. Lee P, Urowitz MB, Bookman AAM, et al: Systemic lupus erythematosus. A review of 110 cases with reference to nephritis, the nervous system, infections, aseptic necrosis and prognosis. *Q J Med* **181**:1–32, 1977.
20. Rothfield N. Clinical features of systemic lupus erythematosus. In Kelly WN, Harris ED, Ruddy S, Sledge CB (eds): *Textbook of Rheumatology*. WB Saunders, Philadelphia, 1985, pp. 1070–1907.
21. Harris ED Jr. Rheumatoid arthritis. The clinical spectrum. In Kelly WN, Harris ED, Ruddy S, Sledge CB (eds): *Textbook of Rheumatology* WB Saunders, Philadelphia, 1985, pp 915–950.
22. Myers AR: Septic arthritis caused by bacteria. In Kelly WN, Harris ED, Ruddy S, Sledge CB (eds): *Textbook of Rheumatology* WB Saunders, Philadelphia, 1985, pp 1507–1527.
23. Schnitzer TJ. Viral arthritis In Kelly WN, Harris ED, Ruddy S, Sledge CB (eds): *Textbook of Rheumatology* WB Saunders, Philadelphia, 1985, pp. 1540–1556.
24. Benson CH, Harisdangkul V Disseminated gonococcal infection in systemic lupus erythematosus. (Letter) *J Rheumatol* **10**:668–669, 1983
25. Churchill MA, Geraci JE, Hunder GG: Musculoskeletal manifestations of bacterial endocarditis. *Ann Intern Med* **87**:754–757, 1977.
26. Ellis SG, Verity MA: Central nervous system involvement in systemic lupus erythematosus: A review of neuropathologic findings in 57 cases, 1955–1977 *Sem Arch Rheum* **8**:212–221, 1979
27. Johnson R, Richardson E: The neurological manifestations of systemic lupus erythematosus. *Medicine (Baltimore)* **47**:1399–1402, 1968
28. Schur PH. Systemic lupus erythematosus In Wyngaarden JB, Smith LH Jr (eds): *Cecil Textbook of Medicine*. WB Saunders, Philadelphia, 1982, pp. 1852–1857
29. Mitchell WS, Brooks PM, Stevenson RD, et al. Septic arthritis in patients with rheumatoid disease: A still underdiagnosed complication. *J Rheumatol* **3**:124–133, 1976.
30. Huskisson EC, Hart FD: Severe, unusual, and recurrent infections in rheumatoid arthritis *Ann Rheum Dis* **31**:118–121, 1972.
31. Walker WC: Pulmonary infections and rheumatoid arthritis *Q J Med* **36**:239–251, 1967
32. Klemperer P, Pollack AD, Baehr G. Pathology of disseminated lupus erythematosus. *Arch Pathol Lab Med* **32**:569–631, 1941.
33. Ropes MW. Observations on the natural course of disseminated lupus erythematosus. *Medicine (Baltimore)* **43**:387–391, 1964.
34. Dubois EL, Wierzchowiecki M, Cox MB, et al Duration and death in systemic lupus erythematosus: An analysis of 249 cases. *JAMA* **227**:1399–1402, 1974.
35. Harvey AM, Shulman LE, Tumulty PA, et al: Systemic lupus erythematosus: Review of the literature and clinical

analysis of 138 cases *Medicine (Baltimore)* **33:**291–437, 1954.

36. Estes D, Christian CL The natural history of systemic lupus erythematosus by prospective analysis *Medicine (Baltimore)* **50:**85–95, 1971.

37. Hashimoto H, Shiokawa Y: Changing pattern of clinical features and prognosis in systemic lupus erythematosus *Scand J Rheum* **7:**219–224, 1978

38. Allebeck P: Increased mortality in rheumatoid arthritis *Scand J Rheum* **11:**81–86, 1982.

39. Koota K, Isomaki H, Mutra O: Death rate and causes of death in RA patients during a period of five years. *Scand J Rheum* **6:**241–244, 1977.

40. Mutra O, Koota K, Isomaki H Causes of death in autopsied RA patients. *Scand J Rheum* **5:**239–240, 1976

41. Cosh JA: Survival and death in rheumatoid arthritis *J Rheum* **11:**117–118, 1984.

42. Zvaifler NJ, Woods VL Jr: Etiology and pathogenesis of systemic lupus erythematosus. In Kelley WN, Harris ED, Ruddy S, Sledge CB (eds)· *Textbook of Rheumatology.* WB Saunders, Philadelphia, 1985, pp. 1042–1070

43. Bennett JC: The etiology of rheumatoid arthritis. In Kelley WN, Harris ED, Ruddy S, Sledge CB (eds) *Textbook of Rheumatology* WB Saunders, Philadelphia, 1985, pp. 879–886

44. Harris ED Jr: Pathogenesis of rheumatoid arthritis. In Kelley WN, Harris ED, Ruddy S, Sledge CB (eds): *Textbook of Rheumatology.* WB Saunders, Philadelphia, 1985, pp. 886–915.

45. Johnston RB, Stroud RM. Complement and host defense against infection. *J Pediatr* **90:**169–179, 1977.

46. Muller-Eberhard HJ Complement. *Annu Rev Biochem* **44:**697–724, 1975.

47. Shur PH: Complement in lupus. *Clin Rheum Dis* **1:**519–524, 1975

48. Kaplan RA, Curd JG, DeHeer DH, et al: Metabolism of C4 and factor B in rheumatoid arthritis· relation to rheumatoid factor *Arthritis Rheum* **23:**911–924, 1980

49. Kohler PF, Ten Beusel R. Serial complement component alterations in acute glomerulonephritis and systemic lupus erythematosus. *Clin Exp Immunol* **4:**1091–1202, 1969

50. Jasin HE, Ziff M: Immunoglobulin synthesis by peripheral blood cells in systemic lupus erythematosus *Arthritis Rheum* **18:**219–228, 1975.

51. McLean RH, Michael AF: Properdin and C3 proactivator. Alternate pathway components in human glomerulonephritis. *J Clin Invest* **52:**634–644, 1973.

52. Schur PH, Sandson J: Immunologic factors and clinical activity in systemic lupus erythematosus. *N Engl J Med* **278:**533–535, 1968

53 Ellis HA, Felix-Davies D. Serum complement, rheumatoid factor, and other serum proteins in rheumatoid disease and systemic lupus erythematosus. *Ann Rheum Dis* **18:**215–244, 1959.

54. Ross SC, Densen P: Complement deficiency states and infection: Epidemiology, pathogenesis and consequences of Neisserial and other infections in an immune deficiency. *Medicine (Baltimore)* **63:**243–273, 1984

55. Jazin HE, Orozco JH, Ziff M· Serum heat-labile opsonins in

systemic lupus erythematosus *J Clin Invest* **53:**343–353, 1974.

56 Louie JS, Nies KM, Shoji KT, et al. Clinical and antibody responses after influenza immunization in systemic lupus erythematosus *Ann Intern Med* **88:**790–792, 1978

57 Williams GW, Steinberg AD, Reinertsen JL, et al Influenza immunization in systemic lupus erythematosus *Ann Intern Med* **88:**729–734, 1978

58 Hess EV Influenza immunization in systemic lupus erythematosus Safe, effective? *Ann Intern Med* **88:**833–834, 1978

59. Meiselas LE, Zingale SB, Lee SL, et al Antibody production in rheumatic diseases. The effect of Brucella antigen *J Clin Invest* **40:**1872–1881, 1961

60. Baum J, Ziff M Decreased 19S antibody response to bacterial antigens in systemic lupus erythematosus *J Clin Invest* **48:**758–767, 1969

61 Messner RP, DeHoratius RJ Epidemiology of antilymphocyte antibodies in systemic lupus erythematosus *Arthritis Rheum* **21:**S167–169, 1978

62 Bluestein HG. Autoantibodies to lymphocyte membrane antigens: Pathogenetic implications *Clin Rheum Dis* **4:**643–647, 1978.

63 Winfield JB, Cohen PL, Litvin DA. Antibodies to activated cells and their soluble products in systemic lupus erythematosus. *Arthritis Rheum* **25:**814–819, 1982

64 Clark RA, Kimball HR, Decker JL: Neutrophil chemotaxis in systemic lupus erythematosus *Ann Rheum Dis* **33:**167–172, 1974

65. Goetzl EJ. Defective responsiveness to ascorbic acid of neutrophil random and chemotactic migration in Felty's syndrome and systemic lupus erythematosus *Ann Rheum Dis* **35:**510–515, 1976

66 Perez HD, Lipton M, Goldstein IM. A specific inhibitor of complement (C5)-derived chemotactic activity in serum from patients with systemic lupus erythematosus. *J Clin Invest* **62:**29–38, 1978.

67. Perez HD, Andron RI, Goldstein IM Infection in patients with systemic lupus erythematosus. Association with a serum inhibitor of complement-derived chemotactic activity *Arthritis Rheum* **22:**1326–1333, 1979

68 Brandt L, Hedberg H. Impaired phagocytosis by peripheral blood granulocytes in systemic lupus erythematosus *Scand J Haematol* **6:**348–353, 1969.

69 Wenger ME, Bole GG: Nitroblue tetrazolium dye reduction by peripheral leukocytes from rheumatoid arthritis and systemic lupus erythematosus patients measured by a histochemical and spectrophotometric method *J Lab Clin Med* **82:**513–521, 1973

70. Karnovsky ML The metabolism of leukocytes *Semin Hematol* **5:**156–165, 1968

71 McLeod R, Wing EJ, Remington JS Lymphocytes and macrophages in cell-mediated immunity In Mandell GL, Douglas RG, Bennett JE (eds). *Principles and Practice of Infectious Diseases* Wiley, New York, 1985, pp 72–93

72 Hahn BH, Bagby MK, Osterland CK Abnormalities of delayed hypersensitivity in systemic lupus erythematosus *Am J Med* **55:**25–30, 1973

73. Rosenthal CJ, Franklin DC. Depression of cellular-mediated

immunity in systemic lupus erythematosus *Arthritis Rheum* **18**:208–212, 1975

74 Horowitz DA. Impaired delayed hypersensitivity in systemic lupus erythematosus *Arthritis Rheum* **15**:353–355, 1972

75 Sakane T, Steinberg AD, Green I: Failure of autologous mixed lymphocyte reactions between T and non-T cells in patients with systemic lupus erythematosus *Proc Natl Acad Sci USA* **75**:3464–3467, 1978.

76 Smolen JS, Chused TM, Leiserson WM, et al· Heterogeneity of immunoregulatory T-cell subsets in systemic lupus erythematosus. Correlation with clinical features. *Am J Med* **72**:783–786, 1982.

77 Ginsberg WW, Finkelman FD, Lipsky PE· Circulating and pokeweed mitogen-induced immunoglobulin-secreting cells in systemic lupus erythematosus. *Clin Exp Immunol* **35**:76–80, 1979.

78 Sagawa A, Abdou NI: Suppressor-cell dysfunction in systemic lupus erythematosus. Cells involved and in vitro correction *J Clin Invest* **62**:789–794, 1978.

79 Katz P, Zaytoun AM, Lee JH Jr, et al. Abnormal natural killer cell activity in systemic lupus erythematosus. An intrinsic defect in the lytic event. *J Immunol* **129**:1966–1970, 1982.

80. Hasler F, Bluestein HG, Zvaifler NJ, et al: Analysis of the defects responsible for the impaired regulation of Epstein-Barr virus-induced B cell proliferation by rheumatoid arthritis lymphocytes. I Diminished gamma interferon production in response to autologous stimulation, *J Exp Med* **157**:173–179, 1983

81. Trentham DE, Dynesius RA, Rocklin RE, et al: Cellular sensitivity to collagen in rheumatoid arthritis. *N Engl J Med* **299**:327–331, 1978

82. Dohlong JH, Forre 0, Kvien TK, et al: Natural killer (NK) cell activity of peripheral blood, synovial fluid, and synovial tissue lymphocytes from patients with rheumatoid arthritis *Ann Rheum Dis* **41**:490–494, 1982.

83 Parillo JE, Fauci AS: Mechanisms of glucocorticoid action on immune processes. *Annu Rev Pharmacol Toxicol* **19**:179–191, 1979.

84. Axelrod L: Glucocorticoids. In Kelley WN, Harris ED, Ruddy S, Sledge CB (eds): *Textbook of Rheumatology* WB Saunders, Philadelphia, 1985, pp. 815–832.

85. Fauci AS, Dale DC, Balow JE: Glucocorticosteroid therapy: Mechanisms of action and clinical considerations. *Am Intern Med* **84**:304–315, 1976.

86. Bovornkitti S, Kangsadal P, Sathirpat P, et al: Reversion and reconversion rate of tuberculin skin reactions in correlation with the use of prednisone *Dis Chest* **38**:51–55, 1960.

87. Balow JE, Rosenthal AS. Glucocorticoid suppression of macrophage migration inhibitory factor *J Exp Med* **137**:1031–1042, 1973.

88. DeSousa M, Fachet J: The cellular basis of the mechanism of action of cortisone acetate on contact sensitivity to oxazolone in the mouse, *Clin Exp Immunol* **10**:673–684, 1972

89. Reinehart JJ, Sagone AL, Balcerzak SP: Effects of corticosteroid therapy on human monocyte function. *N Engl J Med* **292**:236–241, 1975

90. Fauci AS, Dale DC. The effect of in vivo hydrocortisone on subpopulations of human lymphocytes *J Clin Invest* **53**:240–246, 1974.

91 Stavy L, Cohen IR, Feldman M The effect of hydrocortisone on lymphocyte-mediated cytolysis *Cell Immunol* **7**:302–312, 1973.

92. Bishop CR, Athens JW, Boggs DR, et al. Leukokinetic studies XIII: A non steady-state kinetic evaluation of the mechanisms of cortisone-induced granulocytosis, *J Clin Invest* **47**:249–261, 1968.

93 Butler WT, Rossen RD· Effects of corticosteroids on immunity in man. I. Decreased serum IgG concentration caused by 3 or 5 days of high doses of methyl prednisolone. *J Clin Invest* **52**:2629–2640, 1973.

94. Atkinson JP, Frank MM: Effects of cortisone therapy on serum complement components *J Immunol* **111**:1061–1066, 1973.

95. Robinson DR, Tashjian AH Jr, Levine L Prostaglandin-stimulated bone resorption by rheumatoid synovia· A possible mechanism for bone destruction in rheumatoid arthritis. *J Clin Invest* **56**:1181–1189, 1975.

96 Samuelsson B: Leukotrienes. Mediators of immediate hypersensitivity reactions and inflammation *Science* **220**:568–572, 1983.

97. Shand FL: The immunopharmacology of cyclophosphamide. *Int J Pharmacol* **1**:165–180, 1979

98. Decker JL. Toxicity of immunosuppressive drugs in man. *Arthritis Rheum* **16**:89–101, 1973.

99. Cupps TR, Edgar LC, Fauci AS Suppression of human B lymphocyte function by cyclophosphamide *J Immunol* **128**:2453–2457, 1982

100. Hurd ER, Giuliano VJ: The effect of cyclophosphamide on B and T lymphocytes in patients with connective tissue diseases *Arthritis Rheum* **18**:67–75, 1975

101 Askenase PW, Hayden BJ, Gershon RK: Augmentation of delayed-type hypersensitivity by doses of cyclophosphamide which do not effect antibody responses *J Exp Med* **141**:697–703, 1975.

102. Yu DT, Clements PJ, Peter JB, et al. Lymphocyte characteristics in rheumatic patients and the effects of azathioprine therapy. *Arthritis Rheum* **17**:37–43, 1974

103 Maibach HI, Epstein WL. Immunologic responses of healthy volunteers receiving azathioprine (Imuran) *Int Arch Allergy* **27**:102–107, 1965

104. Fournier C, Bach MA, Dardenne M, Bach JF. Selective action of azathioprine on T cells *Transplant Proc* **5**:523–527, 1973

105 Gassman AE, vanFurth R: The effects of azathioprine on the kinetics of monocytes and macrophages during the normal steady state and an acute inflammatory reaction. *Blood* **46**:51–59, 1975.

106 Levy J, Barnett EV, MacDonald NS, et al. The effect of azathioprine on gammaglobulin synthesis in man *J Clin Invest* **51**:2233–2238, 1972

107 Schultz DR, Volanakis JE, Arnold PI, et al· Inactivation of C1 in rheumatoid synovial fluid, purified C1 and C1 esterase, by gold compounds *Clin Exp Immunol* **17**:395–401, 1974.

108 Paltemaa S: The inhibition of lysosomal enzymes by gold

salts in human synovial fluid cells. *Acta Rheum Scand* **14:**161–165, 1968.

109. Penneys NS, Ziboh V, Gottlieb NL, et al: Inhibition of prostaglandin synthesis and human epidermal enzymes by aurothiomalate in vitro: Possible actions of gold in pemphigus. *J Invest Dermatol* **63:**356–361, 1974.

110. Jessop JE, Vernon-Roberts B, Harris, J: Effects of gold salts and prednisolone on inflammatory cells. *Ann Rheum Dis* **32:**294–301, 1973.

111. Lies RB, Cardin C, Paulus HE. Inhibition by gold of human lymphocyte stimulation. *Ann Rheum Dis* **36:**216–220, 1977.

112. Cohen J, Pinching AJ, Rees AJ, et al: Infection and immunosuppression. A study of the infective complications of 75 patients with immunologically-mediated disease. *Q J Med* **51:**1–15, 1982.

113. Hashimoto H, Maekawa S, Nasu H, et al: Systemic vascular lesions and prognosis in systemic lupus erythematosus. *Scand J Rheum* **13:**45–55, 1984.

114. Baum J: Infection and rheumatoid arthritis. *Arthritis Rheum* **14:**135–137, 1971.

115. Poss R, Thornhill TS, Ewald FC, et al: Factors influencing the incidence and outcome of infection following total joint arthroplasty. *Clin Orthop* **182:**117–126, 1984.

116. Stahl NI, Klippel JH, Decker JL: Fever in systemic lupus erythematosus. *Am J Med* **67:**935–940, 1979.

117. Siekert RG, Clark EC: Neurologic signs and symptoms as early manifestations of SLE. *Neurology (NY)* **5:**84–88, 1955.

118. Feinglass EJ, Arnett FC, Dorsch CA, et al: Neuropsychiatric manifestations of SLE: diagnosis, clinical spectrum and relationship to other features of the disease. *Medicine (Baltimore)* **55:**323–339, 1976.

119. Reintz E, Hubbard D, Grayzel AI: Central nervous system systemic lupus erythematosus versus central nervous system infection: Low cerebral spinal fluid glucose and pleocytosis in a patient with a prolonged course. *Arthritis Rheum* **25:**583–588, 1982.

120. Gibson T, Myers AR: Nervous system involvement in SLE. *Ann Rheum Dis* **35:**398–406, 1976.

121. Andrianakos AA, Duffy J, Suzuki M, Sharp JT: Transverse myelopathy in SLE. *Ann Intern Med* **83:**616–624, 1975.

122. Collins JV, Tong D, Bucknall RG, et al: Cryptococcal meningitis as a complication of systemic lupus erythematosus treated with systemic corticosteroids. *Postgrad Med J* **48:**52–55, 1972.

123. Sieving RR, Kaufman CA, Watanakunakor C: Deep fungal infection in systemic lupus erythematosus: Three cases reported, literature reviewed. *J Rheumatol* **2:**61–72, 1975.

124. Bennett J, Dismukes W, Duma R, et al: A collaborative trial of flucytosine-amphotericin B and amphotericin B alone in cryptococcal meningitis. *N Engl J Med* **301:**126–130, 1979.

125. Diamond RD, Bennett JE: Prognostic factors in cryptococcal meningitis. A study of 111 cases. *Ann Intern Med* **80:**176–181, 1974.

126. Matthay RA, Schwarz MI, Petty TL, et al: Pulmonary manifestations of systemic lupus erythematosus: Review of twelve cases of acute lupus pneumonitis. *Medicine (Baltimore)* **54:**397–409, 1974.

127. Haupt HM, Moore GW, Hutchins GM: The lung in systemic lupus erythematosus. Analysis of the pathologic changes in 120 patients. *Am J Med* **71:**791–798, 1981.

128. Matthay RA, Schwarz MI, Petty TL: Pleuro-pulmonary manifestations of connective tissue diseases. *Clin Notes Respir Dis* **16:**3–9, 1977.

129. Hunninghake GW, Fauci AS: Pulmonary involvement in the collagen vascular diseases. *Am Rev Respir Dis* **119:**471–503, 1979.

130. Israel HL: The pulmonary manifestations of disseminated lupus erythematosus. *Am J Med Sci* **226:**387–392, 1953.

131. Webb WR, Gamsu G: Cavitary pulmonary nodules with systemic lupus erythematosus: Differential diagnosis. *Am J Radiol* **136:**27–31, 1981.

132. Eagen JW, Memoli VA, Roberts JL: Pulmonary hemorrhage in systemic lupus erythematosus. *Medicine (Baltimore)* **57:**545–560, 1978.

133. Feng PH, Tan TH: Tuberculosis in patients with systemic lupus erythematosus. *Ann Rheum Dis* **41:**11–14, 1982.

134. Millar JW, Horne NW: Tuberculosis in immunosuppressed patients. *Lancet* **1:**1176–1178, 1982.

135. Palmer DL, Harvey RL, Wheeler JK: Diagnostic and therapeutic considerations in Nocardia asteroides infection. *Medicine (Baltimore)* **53:**391–401, 1974.

136. Gorevic PD, Katler EI, Argus B: Pulmonary nocardiosis. Occurrence in men with systemic lupus erythematosus. *Arch Intern Med* **140:**361–364, 1980.

137. O'Neill PB: Gastrointestinal abnormalities in the collagen diseases. *Am J Dig Dis* **6:**1069–1085, 1961.

138. Hoffman BI, Katz WA. The gastrointestinal manifestations of systemic lupus erythematosus: A review of the literature. *Semin Arthritis Rheum* **9:**237–247, 1980.

139. Zizic TM, Classen JN, Stevens MB: Acute abdominal complications of systemic lupus erythematosus and polyarteritis nodosa. *Am J Med* **73:**525–531, 1982.

140 Pollack VE, Grove WJ, Kark RM, et al: Systemic lupus erythematosus simulating acute surgical condition of the abdomen. *N Engl J Med* **259:**258–266, 1958.

141. Reynolds J: Acute pancreatitis in systemic lupus erythematosus: Report of 20 cases and review of the literature. *Medicine (Baltimore)* **61:**25–32, 1982.

142. Lipsky PE, Hardin JA, Schour L, et al: Spontaneous peritonitis and systemic lupus erythematosus. *JAMA* **232:**929–931, 1975.

143. Seinknecht CW, Urowitz MB, Pruzanski W, et al: Felty's syndrome: Clinic and serologic analysis of 34 cases. *Ann Rheum Dis* **36:**500–507, 1977.

144. Ortbals DW, Marr JJ: A comparative study of tuberculosis and other mycobacterial infections and their association with malignancy. *Am Rev Respir Dis* **117:**39–45, 1978

145. DeMerieux PA, Keystone EC, Hutcheon M, et al: Polyarthritis due to *Mycobacterium kansasii* in a patient with rheumatoid arthritis. *Ann Rheum Dis* **39:**90–94, 1980.

146. Hoffman GS, Myers RL, Stark FR, et al. Septic arthritis associated with *Mycobacterium avium:* A case report and literature review. *J Rheum* **5:**199–209, 1978.

147 Quismorio FP, Dubois EL: Septic arthritis in systemic lupus erythematosus. *J Rheum* **2:**73–82, 1975.

20

Infection Complicating Bone Marrow Transplantation

JOEL D. MEYERS and E. DONNALL THOMAS

1. Introduction

Bone marrow transplantation is being used increasingly as therapy for patients with aplastic anemia or acute leukemia who have an identical twin (syngeneic transplant) or an HLA-identical sibling (allogeneic transplant).[1] Survival of 2 years or more after allogeneic transplant has been reported for more than 65% of patients with aplastic anemia[2] and for 60% of patients with acute nonlymphoblastic leukemia in remission.[3] Marrow transplantation for other malignant diseases (e.g., chronic leukemias, lymphomas, solid tumors), for nonmalignant disorders (e.g., sickle cell anemia), and for primary immunodeficiency diseases has been either suggested or carried out,[1,4] as has the use of donors other than matched siblings or identical twins.[5,6] Thus, it is likely that marrow transplant patients will be seen more frequently in medical centers throughout the world in coming years.

Most patients undergoing marrow transplantation have illnesses that are associated with immunologic deficiency. This deficiency is usually compounded by treatment before arrival at the transplant center and compromised further by pretransplant conditioning. For a substantial period of time before and after transplant, these patients resemble patients with severe combined immunodeficiency disease, with the addition of profound granulocytopenia.

A number of conditioning regimens have been used to prepare patients for allogeneic marrow transplant. The basic regimen for patients with aplastic anemia or hematologic malignancy remains high-dose intravenous cyclophosphamide (CY), with the addition of total-body irradiation (TBI) among patients with hematologic malignancy.[1-3] Some centers use other cytotoxic agents instead of or in addition to CY, whereas others replace TBI with such agents as busulfan. Although TBI was originally given in a single exposure, most protocols currently divide TBI into multiple fractions (fractionated TBI). Intravenous methotrexate (MTX) or intravenous or oral cyclosporine (CSP) is given for approximately the first 100 days after transplant to prevent acute graft-versus-host disease (GVHD). Current areas of investigation include pretreatment of the donor's marrow with monoclonal antibodies or lectins to remove T cells in a further effort to prevent acute GVHD. The result is the same for all regimens: patients lose immune reactivity for varying periods after marrow transplant. Recovery is entirely dependent on the replacement of the hematopoietic and immunologic systems with those of donor origin. Until recovery occurs, patients are subject to many of the natural and most of the opportunistic pathogens of humans.

Patients with identical twin donors or those transplanted for other illnesses such as severe combined immunodeficiency diseases have variations on this theme: patients with syngeneic transplants generally do not receive post-transplant MTX, since GVHD cannot occur, whereas patients with severe

JOEL D. MEYERS and E. DONNALL THOMAS • Fred Hutchinson Cancer Research Center; and Department of Medicine, University of Washington School of Medicine, Seattle, Washington 98104.

525

combined immunodeficiency diseases may need no pretransplant conditioning, since their underlying illness is adequately immunosuppressive. Patients with syngeneic transplants have fewer infections than their allogeneic counterparts. In addition, only patients with allogeneic transplants are subject to GVHD, itself immunosuppressive as is its treatment. This discussion will be limited generally to patients with allogeneic transplants, since these patients pose the more difficult infectious disease problems.

2. Recovery of Host Defenses

The most immediate change in host defense and that which primarily determines the early infection experience of marrow transplant patients is the precipitous loss of circulating granulocytes, which also occurs during a time of disruption of many anatomic barriers, such as the oral and gastrointestinal (GI) mucosa. The granulocyte count may be low before transplant, depending on the underlying illness and recent therapy, and most patients reach a nadir in count within the first 2 weeks after transplant[3]— usually a virtual absence of circulating cells. By 20–30 days after transplant, most patients again have 1000 or more circulating granulocytes/mm^3. Rapidity of recovery of circulating granulocytes, at least among patients with leukemia, is not related to the marrow cell dose within one order of magnitude (1×10^8 to 1×10^9 cells/kg body weight).[1,3] Recovery of circulating granulocyte count is more rapid, however, among patients receiving CSP rather than MTX for post-transplant immunosuppression.[7] Although the clinical status of patients improves dramatically with recovery of circulating granulocytes, neutrophil function is not yet entirely normal, and defects in neutrophil chemotaxis in patients with GVHD and/or antithymocyte globulin treatment have been described.[8]

Recovery of lymphocyte-mediated immunity is also delayed.[9] Total lymphocyte count becomes normal by the second month after transplant, and the proportion and absolute number of EAC-rosette-forming cells and surface immunoglobulin-bearing cells (putative B cells) remain normal throughout the posttransplant period. However, the proportion and sometimes the absolute number of T cells may be abnormal for prolonged periods. The number of help-er-inducer cells (those bearing the OKT4 phenotype) is low in virtually all patients regardless of type of transplant or the presence or absence of GVHD and may remain so for several years after transplant.[10] Conversely, the number and proportion of cytotoxic-suppressor cells (those bearing the OKT8 phenotype) return rapidly and may be higher than normal by 3 months after transplant. The ratio of helper to suppressor cells may therefore be abnormal for 1 year or more after transplant. Some lymphocyte functions in vitro, including reactivity in mixed leukocyte culture and in response to mitogens or viral antigens, are depressed for 4–5 months after transplant in all patients, with more prolonged suppression among patients with GVHD. Related responses such as interferon production in vitro and production of and responsiveness to interleukin-2 (IL-2) are similarly depressed.[11,12] By contrast, cytotoxic activity appears soon after transplant, both natural killer (NK) and antibody-dependent cytotoxic activity against nonspecific targets such as K562 tumor cells or antibody-sensitized cells and activity against virus-infected target cells.[13,14] Activity against virus-infected target cells is mediated by both NK and putative cytotoxic T lymphocytes, with recovery of the latter response associated with survival from cytomegalovirus (CMV) infection.[14]

Serum immunoglobulin levels are low or low normal for the first 3 months after grafting.[9] Serum IgA is depressed in most patients for up to 1 year. After an initial fall, both serum IgM and IgG levels actually become higher than normal in patients with GVHD about 3 months after transplant. By contrast, in patients without GVHD, IgM and IgG levels do not reach the normal range until 6 and 8 months after transplant, respectively.

Although some patients are able to respond to active viral infections with apparently normal antibody production—for example, CMV and varicella–zoster virus (VZV) infection—the response of patients to primary and secondary immunization with bacteriophage ϕX174 and keyhole limpet hemocyanin as well as to pneumococcal polysaccharide remains subnormal for 1–2 years after transplant.[9] Response improves with elapsed time after transplant. Complex functions such as the skin-test response to purified protein derivative or to dinitrochlorobenzene sensitization remain absent for 2 or more years after transplant in some patients.

Many of these immunologic functions are more depressed in patients with GVHD.[9] These patients are at risk of additional infections for longer periods than patients without GVHD. Patients transplanted for aplastic anemia seem to have fewer viral infections than those transplanted for acute leukemia. Whether this is related to the underlying illness and its therapy or to the use of TBI for patients with leukemia is not yet clear. Both aplastics and leukemics transplanted in relapse have approximately a 16% mortality from early bacterial and fungal infections.[3,15] The more aggressive preparative regimens seem to be associated with a higher incidence of and mortality from infection.[2,16]

3. Phases of Infection after Marrow Transplantation

From the viewpoint of the infectious disease consultant, the posttransplant course may be divided into three periods that correspond broadly to the pattern of immunologic recovery outlined above. First, the early granulocytopenic period lasts 20–30 days after transplant in most patients and is highlighted by fever and bacterial or fungal infection. Second, between recovery of circulating granulocytes and day 100, viral and protozoan infections become more prominent. A diffuse, apparently noninfectious pneumonia of unknown cause, called "idiopathic" interstitial pneumonia for lack of a better description, also occurs during this interval. Bacterial infections continue to occur, and fungal infections overlap both early phases, especially in the small number of patients with prolonged granulocytopenia because of graft rejection or graft failure. Third, after day 100, the incidence of most infections decreases. Characteristic infections that do occur include VZV infection and bacteremic pneumococcal infection. The risk of infection depends in part on the occurrence of GVHD and in part on concomitant changes in marrow function and immune reactivity secondary to its treatment.

It must be emphasized that individual patients do not always behave quite so predictably, and the consultant's index of suspicion must remain high at all times. In addition, the total experience with infection after marrow transplantation, although increasing, remains limited, and new presentations of old infections and newly recognized infections will cer-

tainly continue to be described. Willingness to entertain new possibilities and the use of aggressive diagnostic and therapeutic techniques are important in the care of these patients.

4. Phase I: Early Infections

4.1. Bacteremia

Nearly all patients develop fever before or shortly after marrow infusion, temporally related to falling granulocyte count. Patients without fever at any time during their course are uncommon. As in other patients with granulocytopenia, fever often indicates infection, and common signs of infection may be lacking in the absence of a normal inflammatory response. Table 1 is a compilation of organisms isolated from blood cultures in three sequential studies of infection after marrow transplant in the Seattle patients. Study design was different in these three studies, and they are combined primarily for illustrative purposes. The average number of positive blood cultures per patient ranged from 0.3 to 2.4. This difference is due in part to differing study criteria and in part to the increasing use of methods for infection prevention in more recent years (see Section 4.7) with a resultant decrease in the incidence of serious bacterial infection. More than one-half of patients have had no positive blood cultures in our most recent experience, and bacterial infection as the cause of death is now unusual except in patients with either prolonged neutropenia or severe acute GVHD. The organisms recovered from positive blood cultures have also changed: Whereas aerobic gram-negative organisms were more common in early years, it is now more common to find gram-positive bacteria (especially coagulase-negative *Staphylococcus*) as the cause of bacteremia. Although the explanations for this shift are not entirely clear, the universal use of long-term indwelling intravenous catheters and the aggressive use of broad-spectrum antibiotics effective against more gram-negative aerobes have been variously implicated.

Bacteremia was temporally associated with the period of profound granulocytopenia in the study of Stamm and Meyers (Fig. 1). However, 26% of isolates occurred more than 50 days after transplant. Many of these were multiple isolates from patients

TABLE 1. Organisms Isolated from Blood Culture after
Marrow Transplantation

Organism	Study		
	Clift et al.[17] (1969–1973)	Stamm and Meyers[23] (1974–1977)	Buckner et al.[30] (1976–1980)
Gram positive			
Staphylococcus			
Coagulase-positive	0	7	2
Coagulase-negative	0	5	25
Streptococcus sp.	4	9	7
Propionibacterium	0	6	9
Cornyebacterium	0	7[b]	5[a]
Other gram-positive	2	16	4
Total	6	50	52
Aerobic gram negative			
Escherichia coli	11	13	11
Klebsiella sp.	4	13	4
Enterobacter sp.	1	6	5
Proteus sp.	1	4	0
Pseudomonas aeruginosa	10	11	3
Pseudomonas sp.	0	19	0
Serratia sp.	0	3	1
Other aerobic gram-negative	2	1	0
Total	29	70	24
Other organisms			
Bacteroides sp.	0	13	3
Candida sp.	6	14	8
Total isolates	41	147	87
Total patients	52	62	283

[a]Includes *Corynebacterium* sp , as described by Stamm et al [23]
[b]Excludes *Corynebacterium* sp , as described by Stamm et al [23]

with prolonged granulocytopenia. Ten of the 18 *Candida* isolates occurred among 84 positive bloods obtained before day 50 (12%), whereas the remaining eight occurred among only 29 isolates after day 50 (28%). This difference is not significant but may suggest that *Candida* infections occur later among patients with prolonged granulocytopenia. Many of these late bacteremias also occur among patients with acute GVHD.

4.2. Bacterial Pneumonia

Bacterial pneumonia, that is the development of new pulmonary infiltrates accompanied by positive blood cultures or the recovery of organisms from transtracheal aspirates, has been uncommon.[16,17] This may be because of the early use of empirical antibiotics in patients who cannot develop the usual signs of pulmonary consolidation because of severe granulocytopenia. Preliminary study of autologous transplants in dogs suggests that pulmonary macrophages recover both quantitatively and functionally soon after transplant.[18] The situation may be different after allogeneic human transplantation in which the alveolar macrophage is derived from marrow stem cells of donor origin.[19] The presence of functioning alveolar macrophages, although protecting against bacterial infection, may in fact have a pathogenetic role in viral infections.[20]

The diagnosis and treatment of early pulmonary infiltrates are approached aggressively (see Chapter 5). Although transtracheal aspiration should be considered in addition to the usual procedures, we have performed very few because of low platelet counts.

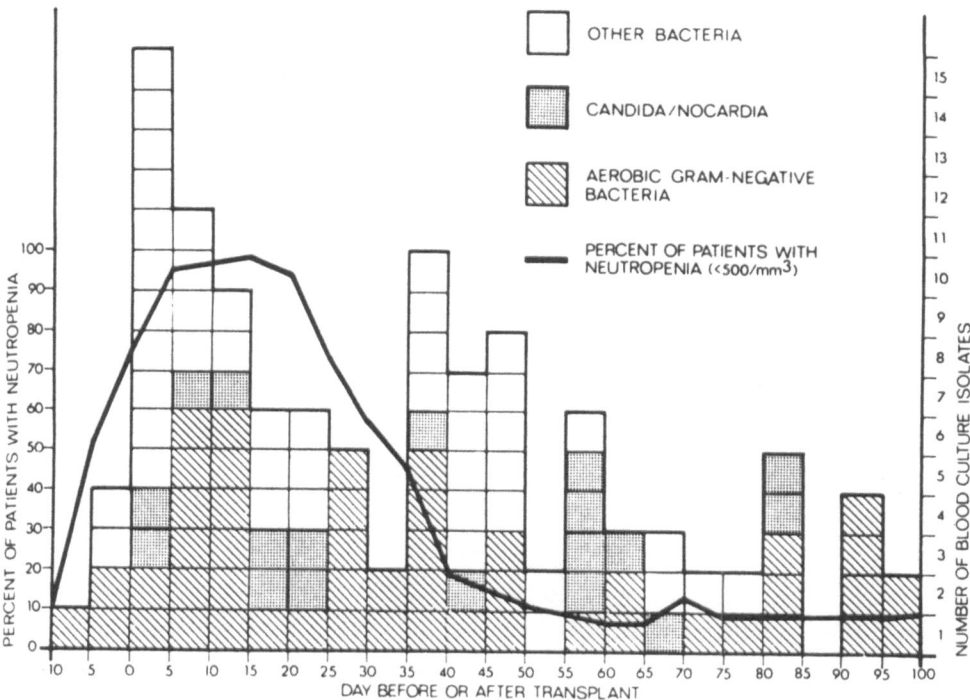

FIGURE 1. Percent of patients with neutropenia (less than 500 neutrophils/mm³) and positive blood cultures, illustrated by day before or after marrow transplant.

These patients usually do not produce adequate sputum, and specimens are often difficult to interpret because of contamination with oropharyngeal flora. If the patient has not improved within 24–48 hr after the initiation of empirical antibiotics (see Section 4.5.1), open lung biopsy is performed. Antifungal treatment is not routinely started in patients with pulmonary infiltrates unless other criteria for the presumptive diagnosis of fungal infection are met (see Section 4.8.1). Some patients cannot be biopsied early in their course because of refractory thrombocytopenia, and of necessity, such patients are maintained on empirical treatment without a specific etiological diagnosis. If the infiltrates remain localized, nonbacterial etiologies are less likely, although localized presentations of both pneumocystis (Fig. 2) and CMV (Figs. 3 and 4) have been observed in our patients and elsewhere.[21,22] If pulmonary infiltrates become diffuse or hypoxia progresses, then empirical anti-*Pneumocystis* treatment is given (see Section 4.5.1).

4.3. Use of Surveillance Cultures

With the exception of patients monitored serially for study of specific infection-control programs, we obtain routine monitoring cultures (nasopharynx, oropharynx, sputum if available, urine, rectum or stool, and multiple skin sites) only at admission and at the onset of fever. By contrast, blood cultures are obtained daily during febrile granulocytopenic periods and when the neutrophil count is less than 200/mm³. Additional cultures from clinically relevant sites including blood are obtained any time the suspicion of infection exists. The use of such "surveillance" cultures may be debated, and these procedures may differ from those described by other marrow transplant groups.[16] It is accepted that granulocytopenic patients usually become infected by resident organisms, either those "endogenous" organisms brought into the hospital with the patient, which include normal flora, or those acquired "exogenously" from the hospital environment and

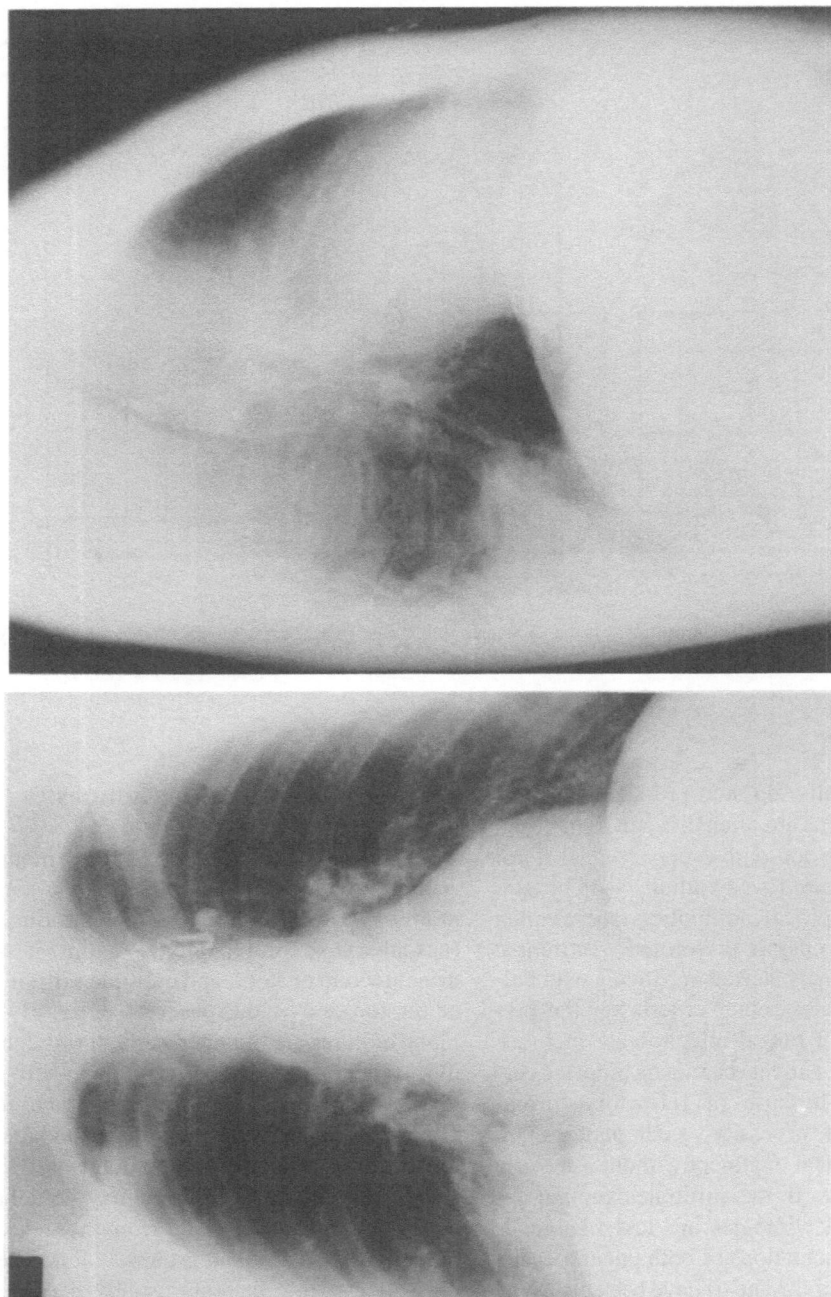

FIGURE 2. Biopsy-proven *Pneumocystis carinii* pneumonia presenting as a segmental infiltrate 62 days after marrow transplant in a 29-year-old man with acute myelocytic leukemia. The patient had received prophylactic oral trimethoprim–sulfamethoxazole for the 2 weeks preceding illness Cultures for *Streptococcus pneumoniae* and *Mycoplasma* serologies were negative

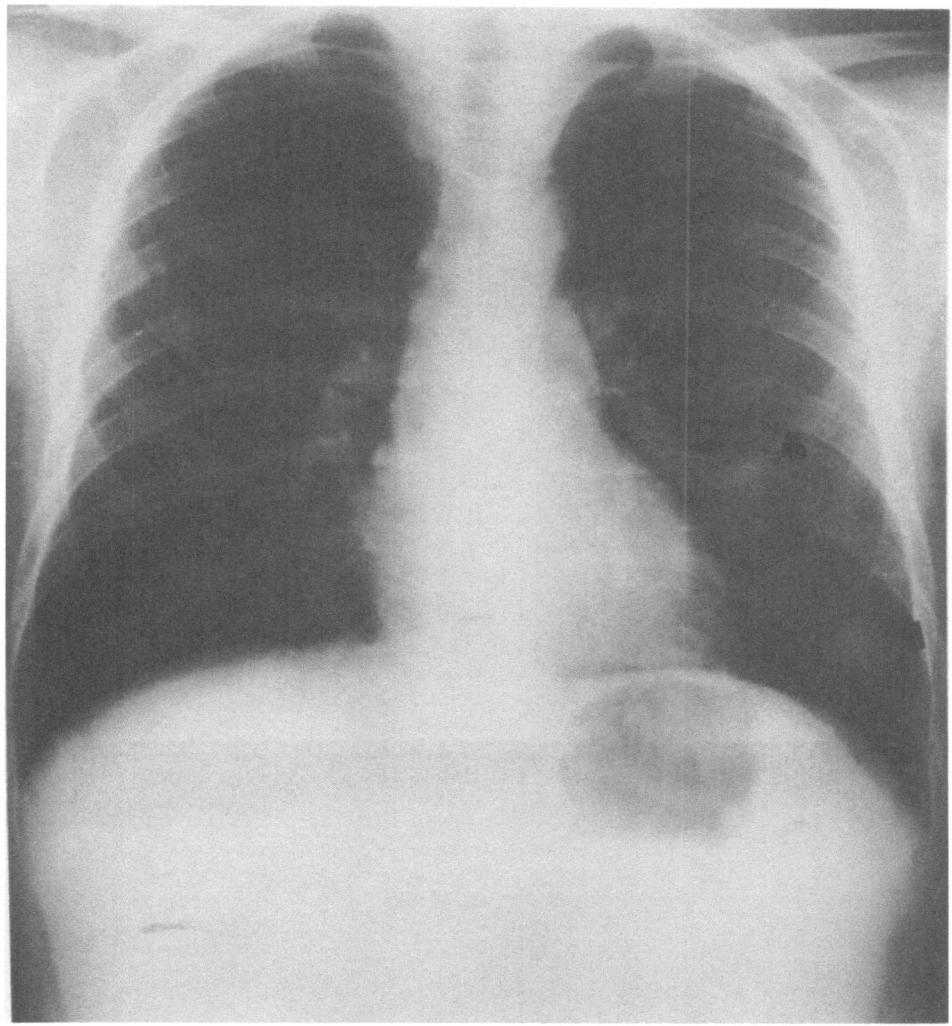

FIGURE 3. "Nodular" cytomegalovirus pneumonia in an 11-year-old boy beginning 70 days after marrow transplant for acute myelocytic leukemia. Two lesions in the left lung are marked by arrows.

which have become part of the patient's flora after admission.

We find surveillance cultures occasionally useful in identifying bacteria that may need additional or alternate antibiotic coverage as part of the empirical regimen (e.g., resistant *Staphylococcus* or *Pseudomonas*) and also in monitoring the unit as a whole for the introduction or persistence of unusual and/or highly resistant organisms (e.g., *Serratia*, corynebacteria[23]). Results of previous surveillance cultures are used at the onset of fever to modify empirical coverage. This has been especially true among patients treated in the protective environment, in whom the recovery of *Staphylococcus aureus, Escherichia coli, Klebsiella pneumoniae,* or *Pseudomonas aeruginosa* from surveillance cultures after entry into the laminar airflow room was predictive of subsequent bacteremic infection, albeit with low positive predictive values.[24] Specific antibiotic policies are reviewed in Section 4.5.

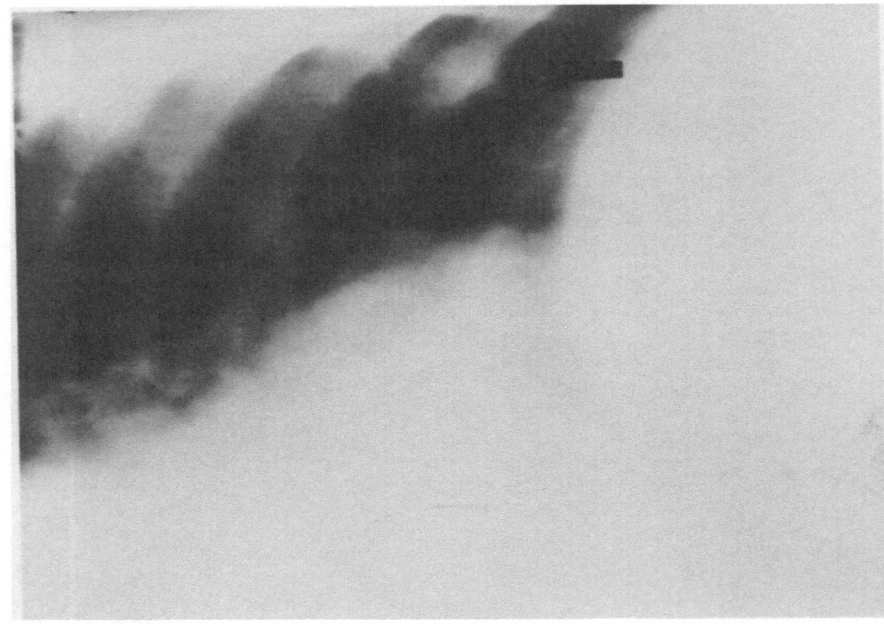

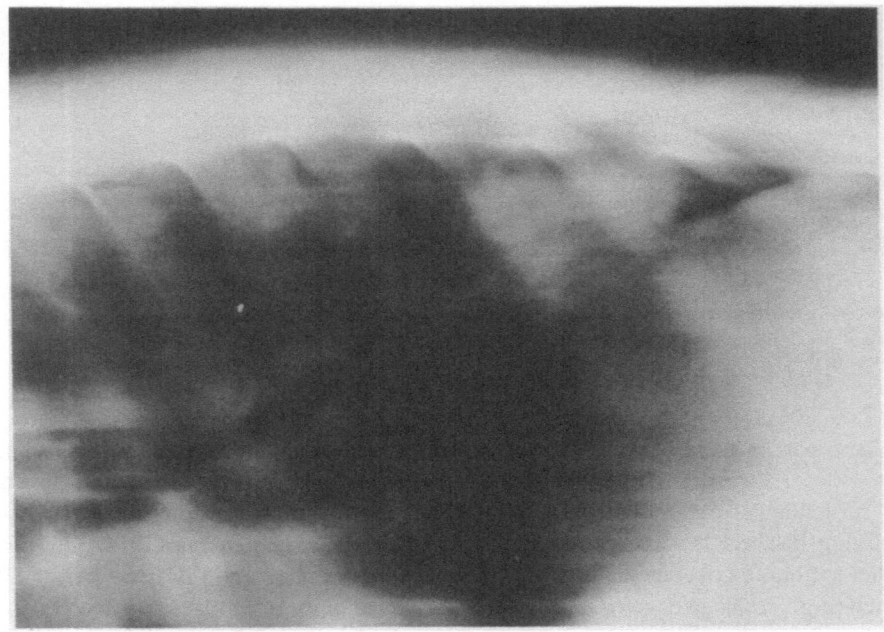

FIGURE 4. Tomograms (posterior–anterior and lateral views) of the left lower lobe lesion in the patient described in Fig. 3.

4.4. Hyperalimentation Lines

Hyperalimentation lines introduced under sterile conditions through a subcutaneous "tunnel" are used in all patients.[25] This eases the problem of venous access for blood samples as well as fluid administration. All blood cultures, unless specified otherwise, are obtained through these central lines. This will occasionally cause uncertainty about the interpretation of a positive blood culture, especially for gram-positive organisms. We regard cultures obtained through these lines as one would regard cultures obtained by usual venipuncture techniques. Simultaneous central and "peripheral" blood cultures have not usually aided in the interpretation of positive blood cultures. These lines have been implicated in both local and bacteremic infections. In our unit, we suggest that lines be changed after two or more positive cultures for fungi or corynebacteria.[23] Bacteremia with other organisms, including *Staphylococcus,* is usually treated with the line left in place unless local signs of hyperalimentation line infection are present; in particular, infection of the subcutaneous tunnel may be difficult to treat without removal of the catheter.

4.5. Antibiotic Treatment

4.5.1. Empirical Antibiotic Coverage

The care of the marrow transplant patient with fever and granulocytopenia is similar to that of other patients with granulocytopenia, and many of the considerations raised in Chapter 4 will apply. The need for careful and frequent physical examinations and for obtaining a full set of cultures processed for bacterial (including anaerobes), fungal, and viral agents before initiating antibiotic treatment will not be further reiterated. Based on the spectrum of bacteria recovered from the blood of marrow transplant patients (Table 1), we have generally used a three-drug empirical regimen consisting of an anti-*Pseudomonas* penicillin, an aminoglycoside, and vancomycin. A third-generation cephalosporin is substituted for the penicillin in patients allergic to penicillin. These antibiotics may be modified further based on the results of surveillance cultures. In recent years, however, we have seen an increase in renal insufficiency due presumably to the concomitant use of CSP and amphotericin among patients already receiving an

aminoglycoside and vancomycin. Therefore, many patients now receive a double β-lactam combination of antibiotics (e.g., an anti-*Pseudomonas* penicillin and a third-generation cephalosporin) for both empirical coverage and treatment of documented infection, with the addition of vancomycin or amphotericin or other antibiotics as the individual situation dictates. The choice of drugs in other centers may depend in part on local usage as well as familiarity with the microbiologic milieu of the particular transplant unit, but in all cases, these drugs should be used in maximum doses for age and weight, and serum levels of aminoglycosides (and other drugs when appropriate) monitored frequently. Peak and trough aminoglycoside levels are measured during the second day of treatment, and these tests are repeated weekly after doses have been adjusted to maintain drug levels in the acceptable range.

4.5.2. Duration of Antibiotic Use and Unresponsive Fever

Various rationales for the use of antibiotics in granulocytopenic patients who do not respond to standard antibiotics after 48–96 hr have been outlined.[26,27] Winston et al.[16] found that bacterial infections were not prominent in marrow transplant patients with such unexplained fever. Nonetheless, the high risk of infection in severely granulocytopenic patients is well known,[28] and studies of the discontinuance of antibiotics in the presence of continued fever and granulocytopenia suggest that bacteremia remains a significant risk.[29] Once empirical antibiotic treatment has been initiated, we continue treatment until the patient recovers 500 circulating neutrophils/mm^3 whether or not fever resolves during treatment. One possible exception to this practice is the patient who is clinically stable and afebrile for at least 1 week with neutrophil counts in excess of 200/mm^3. In such patients, discontinuance of empirical antibiotic coverage can be considered. In patients with demonstrated bacterial infection, duration of therapy is decided according to standard practices after recovery of granulocytes. In patients with unresponsive fever, additional antibiotics are not added to the regimen unless the results of the newly obtained specimens demonstrate a change in flora. The special case of fungal infection and nonbacterial pneumonias will be discussed in Section 4.8.

4.5.3. Prophylactic Antibiotic Use

There are no controlled studies of the use of prophylactic oral antibiotics for marrow transplant patients outside of the protective environment.[30] We do not routinely use oral nonabsorbable antibiotics except for patients in the laminar air flow room, although Winston et al.[16] describe such use for all patients. Although oral nonabsorbable antibiotics and low-bacterial-content food have been associated with a decrease in infection acquisition in adults with acute nonlymphocytic leukemia, poor tolerance of these agents may be associated with increased infection rates.[31] Marrow transplant patients often have difficulty with oral medications because of oral mucosal lesions, and many patients cannot take these antibiotics reliably.[16,30]

The use of TMP–SMX for *Pneumocystis* prophylaxis before transplant is advised. Our regimen consists of the oral administration of TMP–SMX at a dose of 75 mg/m^2 (TMP component) twice daily begun on admission and continued up to 48 hr before transplant. TMP–SMX prophylaxis is resumed later in the post-transplant course (see Section 5.3).

4.6. Therapeutic Granulocyte Transfusions

Some studies suggest that therapeutic granulocyte transfusions are beneficial in the treatment of infection in granulocytopenic patients.[32,33] Whether such studies are definitive is debated.[34] A controlled trial of therapeutic granulocyte transfusions after marrow transplant has not been carried out. We give therapeutic granulocytes from appropriate donors for documented infections when patients have fewer than 200 neutrophils/mm^3 and continue transfusions until the neutrophil count exceeds that level.[35] On occasion, granulocytes are given in seriously ill patients before microbiological documentation of infection. Winston et al.[16] did not find that granulocyte transfusions benefited their patients with either bacterial or fungal sepsis. In general, the use of both therapeutic and prophylactic granulocytes transfusions has decreased, for reasons to discussed in Section 4.7.2.

Illustrative Case 1

A 20-year-old man in second relapse of acute lymphoblastic leukemia was admitted for marrow transplant from his HLA-iden-

tical sister. Pretransplant conditioning included intrathecal methotrexate, 60 mg/kg CY on days −12 and −11, and fractionated TBI (200 rad/day) given daily between days −6 and 0, the day of transplant. Methotrexate was given after transplant. There were fewer than 500 circulating neutrophils/mm^3 on day −10. Temperature reached 39°C on that day, and gentamicin (1.5 mg/kg q8h) and cephazolin (1 g q6h) were started. Fewer than 1% *Pseudomonas aeruginosa* had been found in monitoring stool cultures taken on day −14. The patient became afebrile and remained so until day −6, the first day of irradiation. Temperature reached 40.5°C the following day, and ticarcillin (15 g/day) was added to the regimen. After 1 day of lower temperatures, spiking fevers to 39°C and then 40°C returned. On day −2, three blood cultures were positive for *P. aeruginosa* with sensitivities similar to the earlier stool isolate. Gentamicin was discontinued, and tobramycin at a dose of 1.7 mg/kg, and then 2 mg/kg every 8 hr was substituted. Ticarcillin was increased to 18 g and then 30 g/day. Daily granulocyte transfusions from the patient's mother were started on the day of marrow infusion. Eventually 11 successive blood cultures became positive for *Pseudomonas* between days −2 and +3. Peak serum tobramycin level was only 3.0 μg/ml at a dose of 2.0 mg/kg, and the dose was eventually increased to 2.7 mg/kg given every 6 hr. On day +2, a small perianal ulcer grew *Pseudomonas*. Blood cultures remained negative from day +4 on. Granulocyte transfusions were given from day 0 through day +28. The patient became afebrile on day +29 and circulating neutrophil count reached 500/mm^3 on day 33. Duration of granulocytopenia was 43 days. The perianal lesion never became fluctuant and healed slowly after recovery of granulocytes. Antibiotics were discontinued on day 36, and the patient was discharged on day +40. Renal function remained normal throughout

Comments. This patient developed *Pseudomonas* sepsis from a presumed gastrointestinal (GI) or perianal source. Although *Pseudomonas aeruginosa* with the same drug sensitivities had been isolated from monitoring cultures at the time of admission, treatment of this organism with tobramycin was not initiated at the onset of fever because of the small quantity of *Pseudomonas* (<1%) in the culture. Whether treatment with higher doses of ticarcillin and tobramycin earlier in the course would have prevented the bacteremic infection is conjectural. Although the patient had high fevers and many positive blood cultures, the clinical syndrome of gram-negative sepsis with hypotension and bacteremic skin lesions never developed. Doses of tobramycin higher than expected in conjunction with daily granulocyte transfusions were eventually used in the successful treatment of this patient. Serum levels were crucial in determining the final tobramycin dose. Although high doses of tobramycin were required to achieve acceptable peak levels, renal function remained normal.

4.7. Infection Control Programs

4.7.1. Protective Environment

As in other granulocytopenic patients, an infection control program consisting of skin cleansing, topical and oral nonabsorbable antibiotics, sterile food, and a laminar air flow room for the first 50 days after transplant was successful in preventing serious bacterial infection.[30] The incidence of major local infections and septicemia was decreased as were days of fever, antibiotic usage, and requirement for granulocyte and platelet transfusions. Patients who were better able to tolerate oral antibiotics had a lower infection rate than those who had more difficulty, but the difference was not significant. The incidence of viral infections and nonbacterial pneumonias was unchanged.

A protective environment has theoretical benefits in addition to infection control for marrow transplant patients.[30] Both graft rejection and GVHD may be influenced by reduction in endogenous bacterial flora and infection. Among patients transplanted for aplastic anemia, those treated in the protective environment had significantly less acute GVHD compared with patients not transplanted in the protective environment (some of whom received prophylactic granulocyte transfusions).[36] This effect was also associated with significantly better survival after transplant. Patients with leukemia have not shown such statistically significant benefits, although the incidence of acute GVHD has been lower and survival somewhat better among those transplanted in the protective environment. Patients with leukemia have more difficulty complying with the oral antibiotic regimen due in part to radiation-induced oral mucositis and thus may be less able to benefit from the protective environment compared with patients transplanted for aplastic anemia. Relapse of leukemia is also a major problem in leukemic patients, making any benefit from the protective environment more difficult to demonstrate. Nevertheless, the effect of the protective environment on the incidence and severity of GVHD and on subsequent survival remains of great interest after marrow transplant.

Conversely, the decrease in the rate of serious infection due to bacteria or fungi is less likely to be translated directly into improved survival, in part because death from bacterial or fungal infection is now uncommon after marrow transplant. In similar studies of patients with leukemia, decrease in infection rate did not result in a significant increase in survival.[31,37,38] A cost–benefit analysis of the apparent increased expense of laminar air flow rooms or analogous facilities compared with routine care—and interrelated to survival—is not available. In fact, the protective environment may not be more expensive than conventional ward care when the decrease in supportive care costs is included with the additional

significant short-term benefits of decreased morbidity and increased patient comfort.

However, based on the data described,[30] the protective environment cannot yet be recommended as a necessary adjunct to the care of patients transplanted for leukemia in all centers.

4.7.2. Prophylactic Granulocyte Transfusions

The use of prophylactic granulocyte transfusions was also successful in decreasing bacterial and fungal infection after marrow transplant.[39] This was so only for patients not receiving antibiotics before the initiation of granulocyte transfusions. Granulocytes obtained by both continuous-flow centrifugation and leukofiltration were equally effective, as were granulocytes from HLA-matched and -mismatched donors, although the latter produced more "fevers of unknown origin" in recipients. There were four deaths from bacterial or fungal infection in this study, all among the 40 "control" patients. Overall survival was not significantly different. It was estimated that two of these deaths might have been prevented. Similar preliminary results were reported by Winston et al.[40] among patients not receiving antibiotics at the start of the study.

The use of prophylactic granulocytes is expensive and not widely available, although marrow donors are often willing to make such donations. Indeed, results may be better when single-donor HLA-matched granulocytes such as from the marrow donor are used, with at least a reduction in the incidence of fever seen when HLA-mismatched granulocytes are used. Several problems have been associated with the use of prophylactic granulocyte transfusions, however. The most important of these may be the demonstration that patients seronegative for antibody to CMV before transplant may acquire primary CMV infection from granulocyte transfusions taken from seropositive donors.[41,42] Such patients also have a higher incidence of subsequent CMV pneumonia. Additional problems include clotting of the shunt or other symptoms in the granulocyte donor, and inability to complete the course of prophylaxis because of side effects in the patient or requirement of the donor for platelet (rather than granulocyte) transfusions. One problem that has not been apparent after marrow transplant is a high incidence of pulmonary reactions associated with granulocyte transfusions. The combination of these difficulties has led to a virtual discontinuance of the use of prophylactic granulocyte transfusions in our center, although therapeutic granulocyte transfusions may still be given in appropriate circumstances. One-half of our patients are being treated within the protective environment. For patients not treated in the protective environment, infection control procedures consist of a private room, wearing of surgical masks by all visitors, and careful handwashing for patient contact. Gown-and-glove isolation is used only for specific indications, such as hepatitis or VZV infection. We do not routinely use oral nonabsorbable (or absorbable) antibiotics for patients not in the protective environment.

Illustrative Case 2

This 22-year-old woman with acute myelocytic leukemia in second relapse was admitted for transplant from her HLA-identical brother. During previous chemotherapy she had received granulocyte transfusions from her brother and her father. Pretransplant conditioning consisted of dimethyl busulfan, intrathecal methotrexate, 60 mg/kg of CY given on days −5 and −4, and 1000 rad TBI on day 0. Methotrexate was given after transplant. Circulating neutrophil count fell below 500/mm³ on day +2, and daily prophylactic granulocyte transfusions from the patient's father were started on day +4. Monitoring cultures were unremarkable. On day +4, there was a single temperature elevation to 101.5°F (38.6°C) that resolved. A slow temperature elevation began on day +5, reaching 103.5°F (39.7°C) on day +6, when carbenicillin (24 g/day), gentamicin (1.3 mg/kg q8h), and cephalothin (6 g/day) were started. She had been receiving prophylactic amphotericin (20 mg/day) from day −1 as part of a randomized study. A single blood culture was positive for a corynebacteria sensitive to all antibiotics on day +5; it was considered a skin contaminant. Temperature fell below 100.9°F (38.3°C) until day +11 when fever to 101.8°F (38.8°C) occurred. Repeat cultures and examination were unrevealing. Amphotericin was discontinued because of uncertainty about its role in producing the fever. On day +13, *Pseudomonas aeruginosa*, sensitive by disk testing to gentamicin, was grown from the exit site of the central venous line; blood cultures remained negative. Chest radiographs and renal function were normal. On day +14, hypotension (blood pressure 80/30) and a rise in serum creatinine to 1.7 mg/dl were noted. Arterial blood gases (ABGs) were normal. Blood cultures remained negative. The morning of day +15 the patient had a cardiorespiratory arrest. She was successfully resuscitated. Chest radiography after intubation showed a patchy right lower lobe infiltrate that became bilateral over the next 24 hr. An endotracheal aspirate contained alveolar macrophages but no neutrophils and the next day grew a nearly pure culture of *Pseudomonas maltophilia* sensitive only to sulfonamides and chloramphenicol. Serum creatinine rose progressively to 5.5 mg/dl. Cephalothin was discontinued. Blood pressure was maintained at 80/20, and on day +16 hemodialysis

was started. Ecchymotic skin lesions were noted over the abdomen, and several hemorrhagic papular lesions without central necrosis or pustulation were seen. The decision was made to substitute tobramycin for gentamicin and to add parenteral TMP–SMX in view of the endotracheal isolate. The patient expired later that afternoon. Four blood cultures and an aspirate from a hemorrhagic skin lesion were all subsequently positive for *Pseudomonas aeruginosa*. Minimum inhibitory concentrations of gentamicin and amikacin were 8 µg/ml and of tobramycin 1 µg/ml for this isolate. Postmortem examination showed bilateral bronchopneumonia, hemorrhagic gastritis and enteritis, and acute tubular necrosis. *Pseudomonas aeruginosa* was grown from lung, liver, spleen, kidney, and heart blood.

Comments. This patient died of gram-negative sepsis with hypotension and hemorrhagic skin lesions that developed while receiving prophylactic granulocytes. The responsible organism was first grown from the exit site of the central venous line 3 days before death, but blood cultures were not positive until the day of death. The nearly pure culture of *Pseudomonas maltophilia* from the endotracheal tube was found to be, at most, a colonizer of the upper airway, although it had been presumed to be the cause of her infection. Based on data obtained after death, tobramycin was the preferred drug for treatment of her infection. Prophylactic granulocytes alone were not sufficient in the face of inadequate antibiotic therapy.

4.8. Fungal Infections

Marrow transplant recipients share difficulties in the diagnosis and treatment of fungal infection with other immunosuppressed patients. This topic is last in the discussion of early infections since fungal infection may in fact occur at any time after marrow transplant. Fungal infection is common. M.S. Siegel (unpublished data) reviewed autopsy records of 234 patients transplanted in Seattle between 1969 and 1979. Sixty-four patients (28%) had invasive fungal infections, excluding the skin and GI tract. Incidence was significantly higher among patients transplanted for leukemia (26 of 59, 44%) compared with those transplanted for aplastic anemia (38 of 175, 22%). Approximately two-thirds of these infections were caused by *Candida* sp. (generally *C. albicans*) and the remainder by *Aspergillus* sp., with an occasional infection by other fungi such as *Cryptococcus, Histoplasma,* or *Coccidiomycosis*.

In an earlier study, Martin et al.[43] reviewed 72 patients who received <1 mg/kg total dose of amphotericin B after transplant for risk factors related to invasive fungal infection. Patients with less than 50% of normal marrow cellularity had invasive fungal infection nearly half of the time and significantly more often than those with more than 50%

TABLE 2. Duration of Granulocytopenia and Prevalence of Autopsy-Proven Fungal Infection

	Days of granulocytopenia (<500 neutrophils/mm^3)		
	1–20	21–40	≥41
Total patients	43	22	7
Number with fungal infection	9	9	4
Percent with fungal infection	21%	41%	57%

cellularity ($p = 0.001$). Similarly, there was a direct association between the duration of severe granulocytopenia and incidence of infection (Table 2). This association between circulating granulocyte count and risk of invasive fungal infection presumably explains the higher incidence of fungal infection among patients transplanted for aplastic anemia, in whom prolonged granulocytopenia either before transplant or after graft rejection is more common than among patients transplanted for leukemia.

A smaller group of 42 patients, 21 with invasive infection and 21 without, was compared for prevalence of fungi in monitoring cultures.[43] Four sites were analyzed: sputum, oropharynx, stool, and urine. Only stool colonization was independently associated with proven fungal infection ($p = 0.05$). When all four sites were analyzed together, there was a high incidence of invasive infection among those with three or four sites positive (Table 3). Recovery of fungus from blood cultures was also specific for invasive infection but not very sensitive: 2 of 6 patients with a single positive culture and 10 of 12 with two or more positive blood cultures had invasive infection at autopsy.

These data were collected retrospectively from

TABLE 3. Number of Positive Surveillance Sites and Prevalence of Invasive Fungus Infection

Sites positive for fungus	Autopsy-proven fungus infection	
	Yes	No
3–4	13	3
1–2	6	10
None	2	8

autopsy data and thus should be applied cautiously to the care of living patients. They are consistent with the prospective series of Winston et al.[16] in incidence of fungal infection and association with positive surveillance cultures.

4.8.1. Diagnosis and Treatment of Fungal Infection

In the absence of sensitive, specific, and rapid means for diagnosis of fungal infection, we have utilized the data outlined above in an empirical approach to the treatment of fungal infection after marrow transplant. Granulocytopenic patients who do not become afebrile after 72 hr of empirical antibiotic therapy are treated with amphotericin B if they have two or more surveillance sites positive for fungus (usually *Candida*). Treatment is continued according to the guidelines for empirical antibiotic therapy, namely, amphotericin is continued until the patient becomes afebrile and recovers at least 500 neutrophils/mm^3. If fever continues after recovery of marrow function, amphotericin may be discontinued along with the other antibiotics depending on the individual clinical situation.

When a patient is suspected of having fungal infection, every effort is made to document such infection. Our experience with *Candida* and *Aspergillus* precipitins and a pilot study of the detection of *Candida* antigen in serum by gas–liquid chromatography as described by Miller et al.[44] have been disappointing, and such tests are not obtained routinely. Skin lesions[45] and retinal lesions[46] are searched for, and the former biopsied when present. Other noninvasive tests such as liver scans are obtained when indicated by clinical signs or symptoms but have not been generally useful. Open lung biopsies are obtained whenever possible in patients with pulmonary abnormalities when less invasive procedures fail to yield a diagnosis within 24–48 hr (Fig. 5).

Positive blood cultures for fungi are considered presumptive evidence of fungal infection. We recommend that hyperalimentation lines be changed and antifungal therapy initiated when fungemia occurs. The dose of amphotericin for fungemia and documented fungal infections other than mucocutaneous or esophageal infection is 0.5–1 mg/kg per day if tolerated. Treatment is continued for at least 14 days

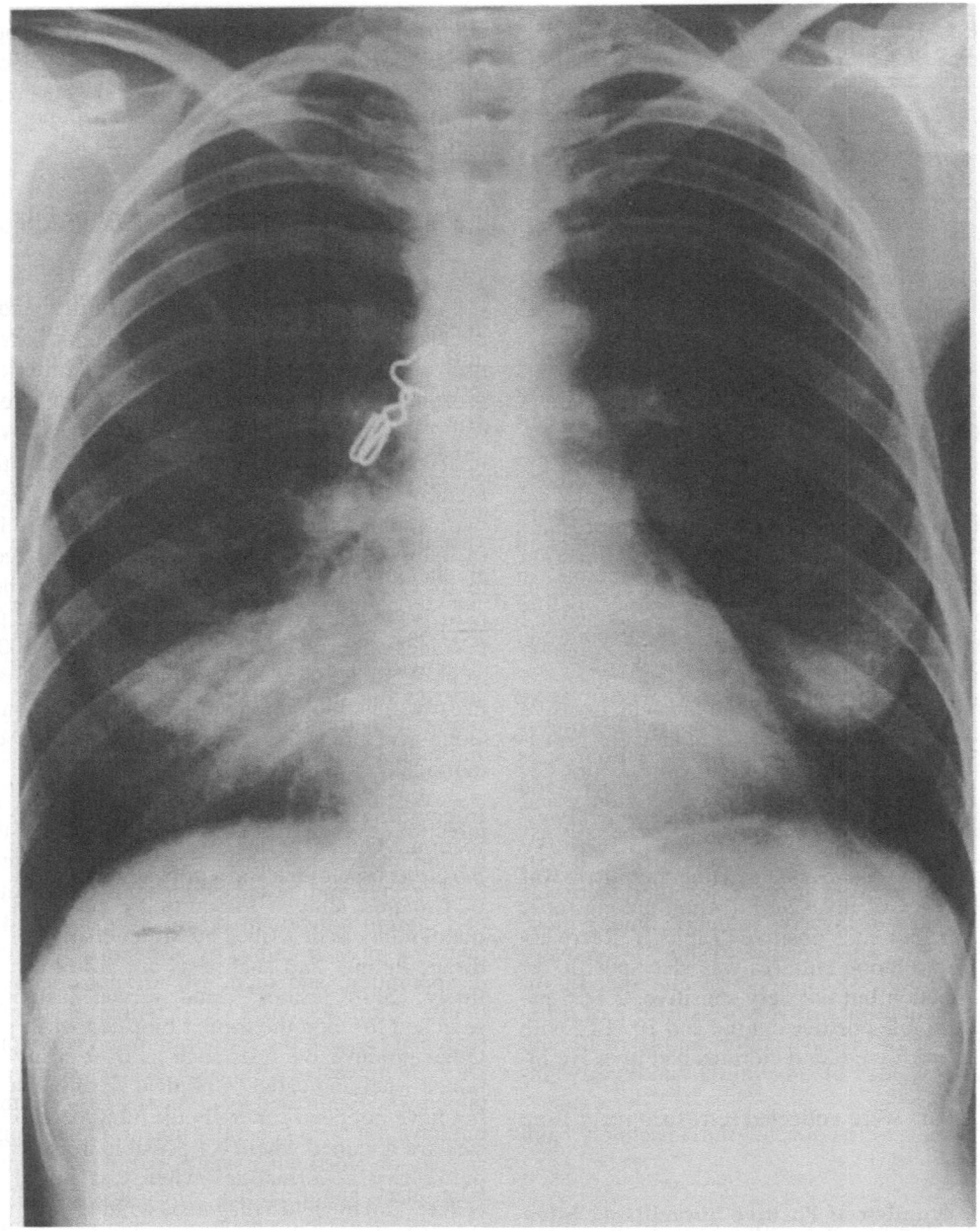

FIGURE 5. *Aspergillus* infection of the right middle lobe proven by open lung biopsy in a 38-year-old woman transplanted for acute nonmyelocytic leukemia in relapse. Involvement of the pericardium was found at the time of biopsy, and at postmortem examination, the anterior descending coronary artery was partially occluded.

after the last positive blood culture for candidemia and for a total of 2–2.5 g for *Aspergillus* or *Cryptococcus* infections. Duration of treatment for other infections (e.g., perineal *Candida* infections) is not standardized. Similarly, varying regimens have been used for oral *Candida* infections or for esophageal candidiasis. In patients with esophageal symptoms suggestive of candidiasis, esophagoscopy is performed whenever possible since it has not been clinically possible to distinguish herpetic from *Can-*

dida infection or from other noninfectious causes of esophagitis such as GVHD. Parenteral amphotericin is used instead of oral agents for all fungal infections including esophagitis during the granulocytopenic period. In some instances, oral nystatin has been used in patients outside of the laminar air flow room to decrease fungal colonization of the oropharynx or GI tract or as adjunctive treatment of *Candida* esophagitis. We recently compared nystatin (3×10^6 units four times daily) with ketoconazole (400 mg/day) for fungal decontamination within the protective environment.[47] Ketoconazole was better tolerated and more effective in reducing *Candida* colonization than nystatin. However, ketoconazole use was associated with a significant increase in detectable colonization with *Torulopsis glabrata,* and there was no difference in the incidence of local or invasive fungal infections in patients in this study. Although ketoconazole may be an acceptable alternative to nystatin in this situation, it cannot yet be generally recommended for fungal prophylaxis, and has been associated with higher cyclosporine levels in one study.[48]

Our experience with the treatment of invasive aspergillosis has been disappointing. Examination of the sinuses is done in all patients with suspected infection. All patients with documented infection are treated with maximum doses of amphotericin, and in a few cases 5-fluorocytosine or rifampin has been added to the regimen. Serum levels of 5-fluorocytosine were kept below 100 μg/ml, and marrow toxicity has not been observed.[49] This drug has not been used otherwise because of marrow toxicity, especially in conjunction with amphotericin. By contrast, local *Aspergillus* infections of tracheostomy or arteriovenous shunt sites or of the maxilla or sinuses have been cured with amphotericin.

Illustrative Case 3

A 49-year-old man with severe aplastic anemia of 3 months' duration was referred for marrow transplantation from his HLA-identical brother. He had been treated with carbenicillin, cephalothin, and gentamicin for recurrent fever for most of the 2 months before transfer. Circulating neutrophil count on admission was 315/mm³, and temperature of 99.9°F (37.7°C). Physical examination was unremarkable, and the chest radiograph was normal. Pretransplant conditioning consisted of 50 mg/kg CY on days −3 and −2, with marrow infusion on day 0; methotrexate was given after transplant The patient also received donor buffy coat on days −4, and +1 through +3. On day −7, the patient's tem-

perature increased to 103.5°F (39 7°C), and carbenicillin (30 g/day), cephalothin (6 g/day), and gentamicin (1.1 mg/kg q8h) were reinstituted. Because of low serum gentamicin levels, the gentamicin dose was raised to 1.4 mg/kg q8h with peak levels of 6.8 μg/ml. Serum creatinine remained normal throughout hospitalization. On day +4, the patient complained of obstruction of the right nasal passage and pressure sensation over the right maxillary sinus. Radiographs showed mucosal thickening of the right maxillary sinus and clouding of several ethmoid air cells but no air–fluid levels. Tomography failed to reveal any bony erosion. However, computed tomography (CT) performed later showed erosion of the medial wall of the maxillary antrum. Examination showed what was initially assumed to be a blood clot attached to the right middle turbinate. Gram stain of a scraping contained hyphal elements with spore formation, and *Aspergillus fumigatus* was grown. Subsequent examination under anesthesia showed that the middle turbinate was, in fact, replaced by a necrotic mass that was partially removed and that grew *Aspergillus*. Fluid recovered from the maxillary sinus during a Caldwell–Luc procedure failed to grow any organisms. Amphotericin treatment was begun on day +6, eventually reaching a dose of 60 mg/day (0.8 mg/kg). Chest radiography on day +8 showed a new lingular infiltrate. By day +13, there were several areas of consolidation seen in the right and left mid-lung fields. Transbronchial biopsy performed on the following day was unrevealing. Open lung biopsy was not performed because of severe hypokalemia caused by combined treatment with carbenicillin and amphotericin. On day +14, 5-fluorocytosine (50 mg/kg per day) was added to the regimen. This was discontinued after 4 days because of slight improvement in the chest radiography and concern about marrow toxicity.

On day +21, the patient's temperature remained below 100.9°F (38.3°C) for the first time since before transplant, and by day +23 he had a circulating neutrophil count in excess of 500/mm³. During this period, the patient began to expectorate clots of fresh blood which he felt originated from the nasopharynx. On the morning of day +25, the patient had a massive nasopharyngeal bleed of at least 2 liters of blood. He aspirated, became apneic, and could not be resuscitated. Postmortem examination revealed mucoid material within the right frontal, ethmoid, and maxillary sinuses, which grew *Aspergillus fumigatus*. No bony or vascular erosion or bleeding site could be identified. Small (0.3–0.8 cm) aspergillomas were found in the apices of both lungs, and a 2-cm cavity in the hilum of the left lung. No fungus was grown from these specimens. There was no involvement of liver or central nervous system.

Comments. This patient had classic sinopulmonary aspergillosis. The improvement during therapy, the return of marrow function, and the absence of viable fungus in the lung suggest that treatment might have been successful had the fatal bleed not occurred. The prolonged course of antibiotic treatment before marrow transplant is a risk factor for the development of aspergillosis. Return of normal marrow function as well as amphotericin therapy may be necessary for recovery from aspergillosis

Illustrative Case 4

A 49-year-old man was referred for marrow transplantation for acute lymphocytic leukemia in relapse. The marrow donor was his brother who was HLA-A and -B identical but not identical at HLA-D. Pretransplant preparation consisted of intrathecal methotrexate, hydroxyurea, CY at a dose of 60 mg/kg on days −10 and −9, and fractionated TBI (200 rad) on days −5 through 0, the day of transplant; methotrexate was given after transplant. Neutrophil count fell below 500/mm³ on day −10. The patient was randomized to treatment in the protective environment where he received oral nonabsorbable antibiotics (vancomycin, polymyxin, tobramycin, nystatin) He was also given oral TMP–SMX prophylaxis during pretransplant conditioning. Fever first occurred on day +1 when the temperature rose to 101.1°F (38.4°C) All monitoring cultures had been unremarkable with the exception of a nasal culture on admission which contained penicillin-sensitive coagulase-positive *Staphylococcus.* Empirical treatment with carbenicillin (30 g/day) and tobramycin (1 mg/kg q8h) was initiated; tobramycin dose was later increased to 1.2 mg/kg. Serum creatinine peaked at 1.7 mg/dl during conditioning but fell to 1.0 mg/100 ml by the beginning of antibiotic treatment. He had had renal failure during previous treatment of gram-negative sepsis. Peak tobramycin levels were between 2.6 and 3.7 μg/ml on this dose. Temperatures as high as 40 7°C occurred over the next 10

days. On day +13, *Candida tropicalis* was found in oropharyngeal cultures, and on day +17, a blood culture drawn on day +15 became positive for the same organism. Amphotericin treatment was instituted, but on day +18 the patient had a cardiorespiratory arrest after receiving 8 mg of amphotericin. Resuscitation was successful, but the patient remained intubated and never again regained consciousness. Serum creatinine peaked at 3.4 mg/dl, and carbenicillin and tobramycin were continued at doses appropriate for his renal function. Amphotericin was discontinued for 1 day but was reinstituted on day +21 after a blood culture from day +19 became positive for *Candida tropicalis.* A total of five additional blood cultures drawn between days +21 and +33 eventually were positive for *Candida tropicalis.* Chest radiography was first noted to be abnormal on day +24 with patchy infiltrates in the left lung (Fig. 6). These infiltrates became bilateral over the next 3 days and progressed slowly thereafter. The patient had intermittent upper gastrointestinal bleeding, but the only additional isolate of *Candida tropicalis* was from an endotracheal aspirate taken on day +37 It was present in small quantities (<1%) and mixed with oral flora and corynebacteria. Temperature fell below 100.9°F (38.3°C) on day +36, and the circulating neutrophil count first

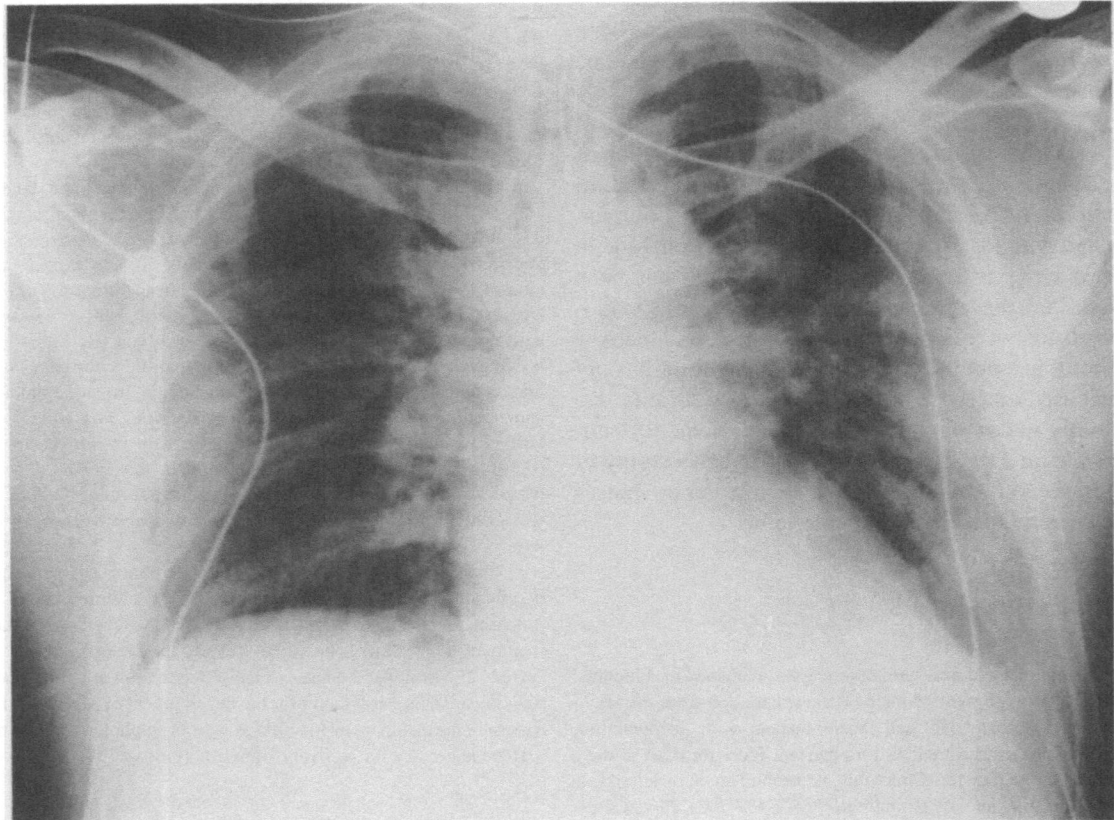

FIGURE 6. Patchy left lung infiltrates in a 49-year-old man transplanted for acute lymphocytic leukemia. Multiple blood cultures were positive for *Candida tropicalis,* and this organism was isolated from numerous organs including the lung at postmortem. Herpes simplex virus was also grown from the lung, although no inclusions were seen.

exceeded 500/mm³ on day +40. Duration of granulocytopenia had been 49 days. Carbenicillin and tobramycin were continued because of the persisting pulmonary infiltrates. On day +47, the neutrophil count again fell below 500/mm³, and fever recurred on day +48.

Gastrointestinal bleeding increased in volume and became nearly constant by day +47. The patient died on day +50 with continued bleeding and hypotension. Postmortem examination showed disseminated candidiasis of lungs, spleen, liver, kidneys, gallbladder, and brain. Severe erosive esophagitis was present, although no *Candida* was found. Herpes simplex virus (HSV) was also grown from both lungs and one kidney, although no inclusions were seen in either lung or esophagus. The patient had multiple oropharyngeal cultures positive for HSV during life.

Comment. This patient had the first positive monitoring culture for *Candida tropicalis* after 23 days of granulocytopenia and 25 days of antibiotics. He had remained afebrile during the first 11 days of granulocytopenia including 7 days of TMP–SMX. It was not possible to decide during life whether the primary source of his candidiasis was GI or from infection of the central venous line. Although no fungus was recovered from stool or postmortem esophageal cultures, neither was there evidence of infection of the venous line at postmortem examination, and the esophagus remains the most likely site of dissemination. Bone marrow cellularity was 40% at postmortem. Evidence of disseminated fungal infection in the face of prolonged granulocytopenia, marrow cellularity less than 50%, and positive blood cultures are consistent with our retrospective analysis of disseminated fungal infection after marrow transplant.[43]

5. Phase II: Infections to Day 100

With the exception of patients who remain granulocytopenic because of graft failure or rejection and who continue to have bacterial (Fig. 1) or fungal (Table 2) infections, the most important infections occurring in the interval between successful engraftment and day 100 are viral or protozoan. Nonbacterial or interstitial pneumonia is the most notorious and overwhelming of these.

5.1. Interstitial Pneumonia

Neither anticipated nor experienced during the early years of marrow transplantation, the striking incidence and mortality of this syndrome became fully apparent in 1976, when fully 60% of all allogeneic transplant recipients developed interstitial pneumonia[50] (Fig. 7). In more recent years, the incidence has averaged 30%, with about one-half of cases diagnosed as CMV pneumonia and one-third as idiopathic interstitial pneumonia (see Section 5.4). The occurrence of interstitial pneumonia is influ-

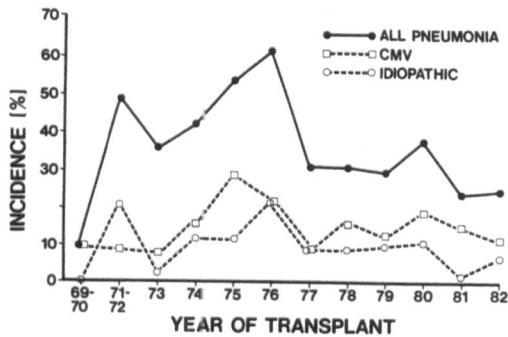

FIGURE 7. Incidence of idiopathic, CMV, and all nonbacterial pneumonias by year of marrow transplant (From Meyers et al.[48])

enced by a number of factors, which vary depending on the etiology of the pneumonia: The risk of CMV pneumonia is increased by any factor that increases the risk of active CMV infection. Thus, patients who are seropositive before transplant have a higher incidence than seronegative patients. Causality of CMV pneumonia is clearly multifactorial, however. For example, patients who receive TBI for conditioning (i.e., leukemics) have a significantly higher incidence of CMV pneumonia than patients who do not receive TBI (i.e., aplastics), and if aplastics are given TBI for conditioning the incidence of CMV pneumonia increases dramatically.[51] By contrast, syngeneic recipients (twins) transplanted for leukemia rarely develop CMV pneumonia even though they also receive TBI.[52] The other major risk factor for CMV pneumonia is the occurrence of acute GVHD.[50,51]

The occurrence of idiopathic interstitial pneumonia is also increased by the use of TBI and is therefore significantly lower among patients transplanted for aplastic anemia. In this case, however, twin recipients transplanted for leukemia develop idiopathic pneumonia at a rate equivalent to allogeneic transplant recipients, a factor suggesting that idiopathic pneumonia is indeed not an infectious process.[51] The use of fractionated rather than single exposure TBI in recent years has been associated with a significant decrease in the risk of idiopathic interstitial pneumonia.[50] The overall significance of interstitial pneumonia is illustrated by the 85% case fatality rate for CMV pneumonia and the 60% case fatality rate for idiopathic pneumonia.

Interstitial pneumonia is a syndrome. The desig-

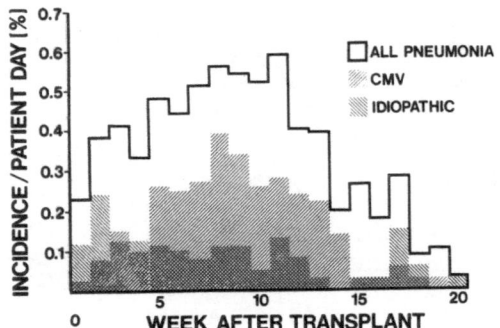

FIGURE 8. Incidence of idiopathic, CMV, and all nonbacterial pneumonias expressed as percentage per patient day for each week after allogeneic marrow transplant. (From Meyers et al [48])

nation interstitial derives from the histologic picture of interstitial inflammation with a mononuclear cell infiltrate.[51] However, many infectious agents produce the radiologic picture of interstitial infiltrates, and *Pneumocystis carinii* is itself predominately an alveolar process,[53] so the radiologic description and clinical designation of this process as interstitial should not narrow the differential diagnosis to the exclusion of bacterial or fungal processes in the investigation of individual patients. The clinical syndrome is not distinctive: although some manifestations may precede others by up to 1 week, patients eventually develop fever, nonproductive or poorly productive cough, tachypnea, dyspnea, and occasionally chest pain. Hypoxia is present. Radiological abnormalities may precede or follow symptoms such as cough or fever, and although infiltrates usually become diffuse, both segmental (Fig. 2) and nodular infiltrates (Figs. 3 and 4) have been observed. The risk period for interstitial pneumonia is highest be-

tween 30 and 90 days after transplant (Fig. 8). Most, but not all, patients have adequate numbers of circulating granulocytes at onset.

The differential diagnosis includes pulmonary damage caused by radiation or cytotoxic chemotherapy, pulmonary hemorrhage or edema, and recurrence of underlying malignancy in addition to infectious agents. We have found that diagnostic procedures short of open lung biopsy are often not sensitive enough to provide a diagnosis in many instances (Table 4).[54] The major exception to this may be bronchoalveolar lavage. Although open biopsy obligates the use of a chest tube, it permits visual inspection of the lung and, therefore, biopsy of obviously involved areas. In addition, bleeding can be controlled under direct visualization in thrombocytopenic patients. We do an open lung biopsy on patients if the platelet level is maintained spontaneously or by transfusion above 50,000/mm^3. Biopsies are done within 24 hr of the clinical diagnosis of interstitial pneumonia whenever possible.

Cytomegalovirus-associated pneumonia (Fig. 9) is defined as pneumonia in which CMV is isolated from lung tissue or typical intranuclear inclusions are identified in the absence of growth of other viral agents. It is the most common form of interstitial pneumonia, occurring in 50% of patients with pneumonia (Table 5). Idiopathic pneumonia, that characterized by similar inflammatory changes without identification of a specific etiologic agent, occurred in one-third of patients, and *Pneumocystis carinii* infection in one-sixth. Herpes simplex virus or adenovirus have been isolated from a small number of patients.[55,56] Only rarely has a patient had a bacterial or fungal process identified, but such diagnoses must be kept in mind.

TABLE 4. Diagnosis of Interstitital Pneumonia after Marrow Transplant by Concurrent Open Lung and Transbronchial Biopsy Procedure[a]

Open lung biopsy		Diagnosis from transbronchial biopsy				
Diagnosis	Number	Idiopathic	Cytomegalovirus	*Pneumocystis*	Bronchiolitis	Nondiagnostic
Idiopathic	9	6	0	0	0	3
Cytomegalovirus	5	2	0	0	0	3
Pneumocystic	5	1	0	3	0	1
Bronchiolitis	1	0	0	0	1	0
Total	20	9	0	3	1	7

[a]Adapted from Peterson et al [54]

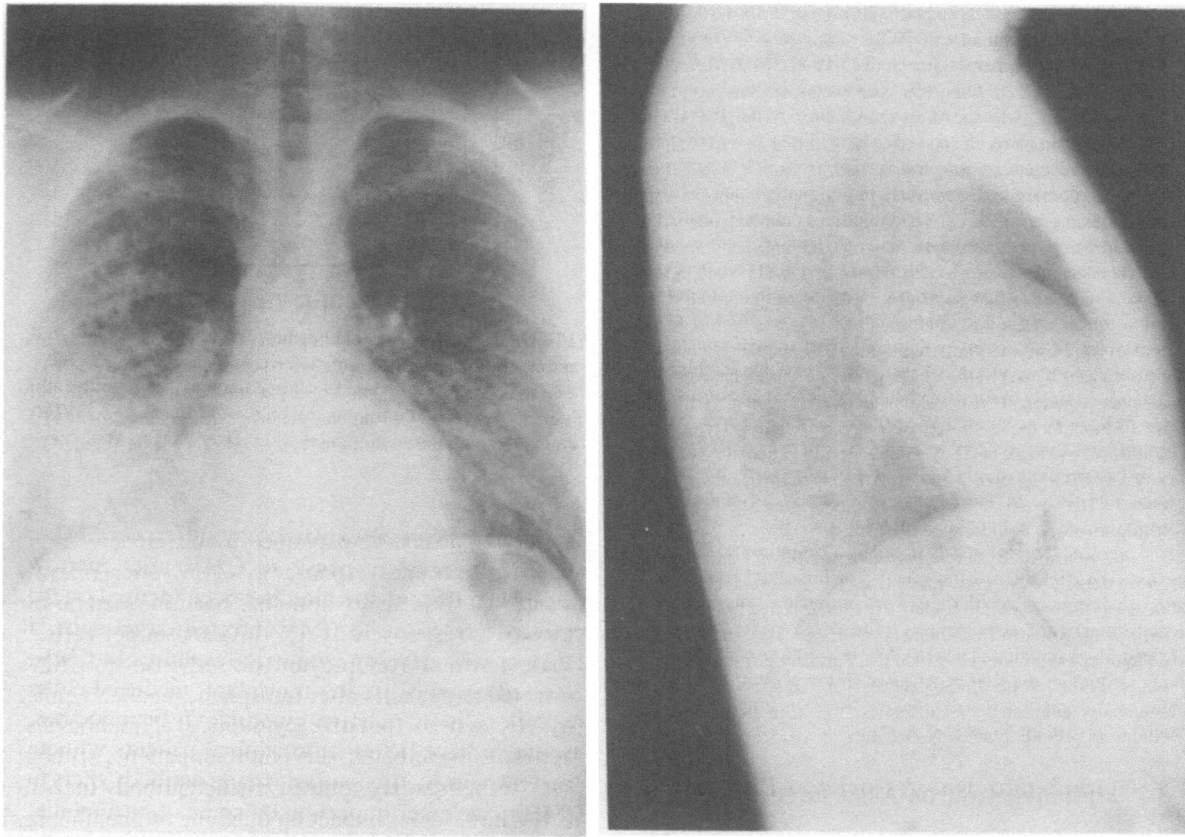

FIGURE 9. Diffuse presentation of cytomegalovirus pneumonia occurring after marrow transplantation.

TABLE 5. Etiology of Interstitial Pneumonia after Allogeneic Marrow Transplantation[a]

Etiology[b]	N	Incidence (%)	Relative incidence[c] (%)
Idiopathic	90	9	32
Cytomegalovirus	147	15	52
Other viruses	25	3	9
Pneumocystis carinii	39	4	14
Total pneumonia[b]	283	30	—
Clinical pneumonia	49	5	—
None	620	65	—

[a]Patients transplanted between 1969 and mid-1982 [50]
[b]Biopsy or autopsy diagnosis only
[c]Incidence among interstitial pneumonias

Illustrative Case 5

A 10-year-old boy was admitted for marrow transplantation from his HLA-identical brother for acute lymphocytic leukemia in relapse. Pretransplant conditioning included intrathecal methotrexate, CY at 60 mg/kg on days −11 and −10, and 200 rad TBI daily on days −6 to 0. Methotrexate was given post-transplant. Neutrophil count remained below 500/mm^3 from day −4 through day +22. The patient was initially treated in the protective environment but was removed on day +19 because of psychological problems. Parenteral antibiotics were given from day −1 through day +29, although the patient became afebrile on day +23. Amphotericin was given for 3 days. Admission CMV titer was 1 : 32. The only infection during the granulocytopenic period was HSV of the left ear and lip. A maculopapular rash of the hands and legs diagnosed as acute GVHD was treated with ATG, with complete resolution. The patient was discharged on day +36, and prophylactic TMP–SMX was started on day +39.

On day +84, he developed a low-grade fever and was found to have mild otitis media and pharyngitis which were treated with an oral cephalosporin. Fever did not improve, and a nonproductive cough developed. Chest radiographs on day +88 showed diffuse infiltrates. White blood cell (WBC) count was 6000/mm³ with 84% lymphocytes. Antibody titer to CMV had risen from 1 : 16 at discharge to 1 : 128. On day +90, hepatosplenomegaly, not previously present, was found on examination. Arterial Po₂ (PaO₂) was 59 mm Hg on room air, and open lung biopsy was performed. This showed discrete granulomas varying from 0.5 to 1.5 cm in diameter, containing predominantly plump macrophages without multinucleated giant cells. The granulomas contained small (1–4 μm) budding yeasts consistent with *Histoplasma capsulatum*, which subsequently grew. This organism was also seen in several sputums and endotracheal aspirates. Amphotericin treatment was initiated immediately, and although there was a period of partial improvement of the chest radiograph, the patient's course was complicated by staphylococcal bacteremia, possible staphylococcal pneumonia, and the development of additional interstitial infiltrates thought to be caused by oxygen toxicity There was no additional evidence of CMV infection. The patient died of respiratory insufficiency on day +143. Autopsy permission was not obtained. The cause of the hepatosplenomegaly, presumed to be histoplasmosis, could not be confirmed.

Comment. This is the only instance of histoplasmosis we have encountered after marrow transplant. The important aspect of this case was the unexpected finding of a disseminated fungal infection in the setting of diffuse pulmonary infiltrates, hypoxia, and a rising CMV titer—a situation in which CMV infection would seem more likely. Although the finding of yeast in the sputum would have eventually suggested the diagnosis, the open lung biopsy was crucial in providing an early diagnosis.

5.2. Cytomegalovirus-Associated Pneumonia

Any factor that increases the incidence of CMV infection increases the risk of CMV pneumonia. Cytomegalovirus infection is more common among patients who are seropositive for antibody before transplant and who have a 75% or greater incidence of virus reactivation compared with seronegative patients in whom primary infection occurs in only one-third. Among seronegative patients the incidence of infection is increased if their marrow donors are seropositive, or if they receive granulocytes from seropositive granulocyte donors.[42] The risk of CMV pneumonia is then superimposed on this risk of CMV infection, and immunologic factors (many undefined) appear to play an important role. Significant risk factors for CMV pneumonia include older patient age, use of conditioning agents in addition to CY for patients with leukemia, and the occurrence of acute GVHD[50] (Fig. 10). Patients with aplastic anemia have a lower incidence of CMV pneumonia unless they receive TBI for conditioning, as do patients with twin donors. It is presumed that many of these

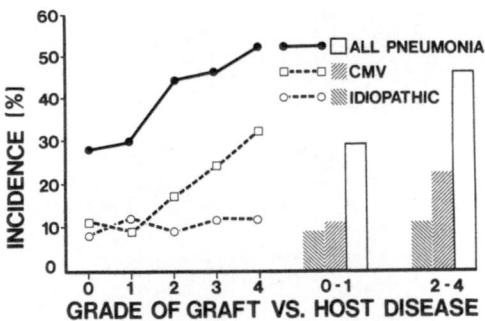

FIGURE 10. Incidence of idiopathic, CMV, and all nonbacterial pneumonias by grade of acute graft-versus-host disease (GVHD). The incidence of CMV and of all pneumonias was significantly higher ($p = 0.00005$) among patients with grades 2–4 GVHD compared with those with grades 0–1. (From Meyers et al.[48])

observations can be explained by differences in the specific immune response to CMV after marrow transplant. Recent attention has been focused on the cytotoxic response to CMV-infected target cells.[14] Patients who develop cytotoxic responses to CMV-infected target cells after transplant, mediated either by NK cells or putative cytotoxic T lymphocytes, appear to have better survival than patients without such responses. By contrast, rising antibody titers to CMV have lesser impact on outcome of pneumonia. Although seroconverters have a slightly longer course and a lower case fatality rate than patients who do not seroconvert, the case fatality rate is still 71% even among seroconverters.

Animal models of many of these risk factors exist and support a number of the clinical and epidemiologic observations. There is insufficient space to review these studies here. However, marrow, renal, and cardiac transplant patients have provided a unique opportunity to investigate the complex biology of this virus in man.

A number of trials of the prevention of primary CMV infection among seronegative marrow transplant patients have been performed. These trials have involved passive immunoprophylaxis using either high-titer plasma,[57] or intramuscular or intravenous CMV immunoglobulins.[58,59] Although study design as well as the prophylactic agent differed between studies, most concluded that passive immunoprophylaxis was effective in preventing either CMV infection[58] or CMV disease (i.e., pneumonia).[57,59] However, a more recent study suggests that passive immunoprophylaxis may not be effective in preventing either CMV infection or disease.[59a] Moreover, use of solely seronegative blood products was highly effective in preventing primary CMV infection in seronegative patients with seronegative marrow donors, although not if the marrow donor was seropositive. The most effective and least expensive means of prevention needs to be determined, and is an issue of some importance in view of both the increasing number of marrow transplant recipients worldwide and the great expense of some of the presently available intravenous globulins. It would appear that prevention of primary CMV infection or CMV disease among seronegative patients should be achievable, particularly with the use of CMV-seronegative blood products.

Prevention of reactivation infection (i.e., infection among patients seropositive before transplant) is more problematic. At least three-fourths of seropositive patients excrete CMV after transplant, and with intensive virologic surveillance this number may approach 100%. Interferon prophylaxis has been effective in reducing the occurrence of CMV disease after renal transplant[60] but has not been effective after marrow transplant in one study.[61] Similarly, the use of vidarabine for prophylaxis was unsuccessful.[62]

Treatment of active CMV infection with available antiviral agents has also been unrewarding. Treatment using vidarabine, acyclovir, and various α-interferons (IF$_\alpha$), both in single agent and combined agent trials, has not reduced the mortality rate of CMV pneumonia.[50] It would appear that both prophylaxis of infection among seropositive patients and treatment of established infection will require development of more effective antiviral agents against CMV. One such agent may be the acyclovir derivative, dihydroxymethylethoxymethylguanine, or ganciclovir, which is 20–50-fold more active against CMV in vitro.[63] This agent shows promise for the treatment of CMV infection, including pneumonia, in immunocompromised hosts, including marrow transplant recipients. Prophylaxis of CMV infection may also be possible, although marrow toxicity observed in initial trials with ganciclovir will obligate careful, controlled trials to determine both safety and efficacy.

Illustrative Case 6

A 20-year-old woman with idiopathic aplastic anemia of 1 month's duration was admitted for marrow transplantation from her HAL-identical sister. The patient's pretransplant CMV titer was <1 : 8, whereas the donor's titer was 1 : 8. Neutrophil count was less than 500/mm³ on the day of admission, and her temperature was 101.8°F (38.8°C). Admitting throat culture contained *Klebsiella* and small quantities of *Candida albicans* (<1%), and both stool and vaginal cultures contained *Klebsiella*. Empirical therapy with carbenicillin (24 g/day), cephalothin (8 g/day), and gentamicin (1.3 mg/kg q8h) was started. Vaginal candidiasis was treated locally with nystatin suppositories. Preparation consisted of CY at 50 mg/kg given on days −5 through −2, with marrow infusion on day 0; methotrexate was given post-transplant. She received unirradiated buffy coat from her marrow donor on days +1 through +5 and prophylactic granulocyte transfusions from her father on days +1 through +12. Carbenicillin was discontinued on day +3 because of pruritic erythematous rash. Admission throat cultures were positive for HSV, and on day +8 the patient developed clinical herpes infection of the buccal mucosa, gingiva, and lips. On day +11 patchy lower lobe consolidation was noted on the chest radiograph. Sputum showed only mixed oral flora without neutrophils. Arterial blood gases showed a fall in Pao₂ from 110 mm Hg (pretransplant) to 62 mm Hg on room air. Over the succeeding 2 days, the patient's clinical condition improved, with progressive clearing of the chest radiograph and increase in arterial oxygenation; biopsy was not done. Improvement was coincident with a rising granulocyte count. By day +13, the circulating neutrophil count was in excess of 500/mm³, and her temperature remained less than 38.3°C after day +16. She was discharged on day +21 on prophylactic TMP–SMX. Antibody titer to CMV was still <1 : 8.

On day +31 the patient was readmitted with temperature to 39.5°C. Physical examination, cultures, and chest radiography were unremarkable, and empirical treatment with cephalothin (4 g/day) and gentamicin (1.3 mg/kg q8h) was initiated. Oral TMP–SMX was continued. Within 24 hr, the patient developed a diffuse, pruritic, maculopapular rash, followed the next day by swelling and discomfort of the wrists and proximal interphalangeal joints of both hands. All antibiotics were stopped. On day +36, she developed a nonproductive cough, although chest radiography remained normal. On day +41, bilateral lower lobe interstitial and alveolar infiltrates were noted on radiography, and Pao₂ on room air was 69 mm Hg. Fever persisted. On the same day, successive transbronchial and open lung biopsies were performed, the latter from the right lower lobe. A single dose of pentamidine isethionate (4 mg/kg) was given on the day of biopsy, and cephalothin and gentamicin were reinstituted. The specimen from the transbronchial biopsy was not interpretable, but the open lung biopsy showed a prominent interstitial inflammatory infiltrate and pulmonary macrophages with intranuclear inclusions suggestive of CMV. *Pneumocystis carinii* was not seen, and pentamidine was discontinued. On day +43 the first of three units of CMV hyperimmune plasma was given. This unit had a CMV CF titer of 1 : 256, and the patient's titer increased to 1 : 32. Pao₂ was 37 mm Hg on 30% inspired oxygen by mask, and a positive-pressure mask with

80% inspired oxygen was used to raise the patient's Pao_2 to 45 mm Hg. A second unit of plasma (titer 1 . 512) was given on day 44. Oxygenation improved with a Pao_2 of 86 mm Hg on inspired oxygen of 50%. The third and last plasma unit (titer 1 : 256) was given on day +46. The patient's titer rose to 1 : 64. The first improvement in chest radiography was seen on day +49, and by the next day Pao_2 was maintained at 75 mm Hg with nasal oxygen alone. Improvement continued, and by day +55, Pao_2 was 75 on room air. Temperature remained less than 101.8°F (38.8°C) from day +59. Antibody titer remained at 1 : 64 until day +64 when it increased to 1 : 128 followed the next week by a further rise to 1 : 256. The patient was discharged on day +64. During this admission, the serum glutamic oxaloacetic transaminase, which was 57 IU/liter on admission, increased to 237 IU/liter, and then fell to 62 IU/liter at discharge. Total bilirubin peaked at 5.0 mg/dl and was normal by discharge. Tissue from the lung biopsy never grew CMV.

Comment. This patient is one of few survivors of CMV pneumonia. Although CMV never grew, the histologic demonstration of intranuclear inclusions in combination with active seroconversion to CMV make another diagnosis unlikely. In particular, failure to grow HSV would be unusual. Although the exact day of active seroconversion cannot be ascertained, the rise in the patient's antibody titer to 1 : 256 2 weeks after the last plasma transfusion suggests that passive immunization may have been superfluous in her treatment. Her serum-sicknesslike symptoms with arthralgias and arthritis may have been caused by CMV infection as well, as might her hepatitis.

It is interesting to speculate about the source of her CMV infection. Her infection was presumed to be primary since she had no detectable antibody before transplant. Her marrow donor was known to be antibody positive. Additional sources include her granulocyte donor and the random-donor platelet transfusions received during the first admission. Unfortunately, CMV titers were not available for these donors.

5.3. *Pneumocystis carinii* Pneumonia

In contrast to CMV pneumonia, *Pneumocystis* infection can be both treated and prevented. Median time of onset of *Pneumocystis* pneumonia is 9 weeks after transplant, similar to that of other nonbacterial pneumonias. The clinical syndrome is indistinguishable both clinically and radiologically from other nonbacterial pneumonias, and unusual radiologic presentations have been observed (Fig. 2). We have not attempted lung aspiration in the diagnosis of *Pneumocystis carinii* infection and have relied on open lung biopsy because of the high incidence of other nonbacterial pneumonias in this population. Serologic techniques including the detection of circulating *Pneumocystis* antigen have not been useful in the diagnosis of *Pneumocystis* infection after marrow transplant.[64] There are as yet no data on the use of bronchopulmonary lavage for the diagnosis of *Pneumocystis* pneumonia after marrow transplant. Although virtually all patients with mixed pneumonias (usually *Pneumocystis* plus CMV) have died, more than one-half of patients treated for pure *Pneumocystis carinii* pneumonia have survived, emphasizing the importance of making the early definitive diagnosis of *Pneumocystis carinii* pneumonia in this population. Treatment is either with pentamidine isethionate or intravenous TMP–SMX, the latter at a dose of 15–20 mg/kg per day (TMP component) given as divided doses either every 6 or 8 hr among patients with normal renal function. TMP–SMX is the current treatment of choice, and all patients treated on this regimen in recent years have survived. We do not use oral TMP–SMX for treatment because of uncertainties about absorption.[65] Treatment with either pentamidine or TMP–SMX is given for 14 days.

Most encouraging has been the ability to prevent *Pneumocystis carinii* infection with oral TMP–SMX. We have observed only one to two cases yearly since instituting routine TMP–SMX prophylaxis. These cases have generally been in patients who have either received no prophylaxis post-transplant because of allergy, or among patients who developed *Pneumocystis* during the granulocytopenic period early after transplant before prophylaxis was reinstituted. However, one case was in a patient who developed a segmental infiltrate 2 weeks after starting TMP–SMX prophylaxis (Fig. 2). We give oral TMP–SMX prophylaxis at the dose of 75 mg/m² (TMP component) twice a day, on two consecutive days of the week. Prophylaxis is started when the patient has 500 circulating neutrophils/mm³ and continues through day 120, encompassing the risk period for *Pneumocystis* pneumonia. Prophylaxis at the same dose given daily may be continued longer among patients with chronic GVHD (see Section 6.2). In addition, TMP–SMX prophylaxis is given daily until 48 hr before transplant in an attempt to prevent the unusual early cases of *Pneumocystis* infection that occur before engraftment (see Section 4.5.3).

Illustrative Case 7

This 29-year-old man was referred in remission for marrow transplantation from his HLA-identical brother for acute myelomonocytic leukemia of 5 months' duration. Pretransplant conditioning included intrathecal methotrexate, CY at a dose of 60 mg/kg on days −5 and −4, and 1000 rad TBI on day 0; methotrexate was given post-transplant. The patient was treated in the protective environment. Neutrophil count fell below 500/mm³ on day +4, and parenteral antibiotics were first given on day +10 for temperature of 103 1°F (39.5°C). On day +11 the patient underwent exploratory laparotomy for severe abdominal pain localized to the area of an old ventral hernia. Operation revealed incarcerated necrotic omentum. With the exception of transient postoperative respiratory distress associated with bibasilar atelectasis and pleural effusions, the remainder of the hospital course was uneventful, and the patient was discharged on day +50 on oral TMP–SMX.

Two days later, he was readmitted with a temperature of 102.9°F (39.4°C), pharyngitis and laryngitis. Examination showed vesicular lesions of the hard and soft palate and posterior pharynx. There were also vesicular lesions of the left fourth and fifth toes. White count was 6200/mm³ with 4340 neutrophils/mm³. Prophylactic TMP–SMX was continued, and ampicillin (4 g/day) and gentamicin (1.3 mg/kg q8h) added. Culture of the oropharynx showed HSV. Culture of the toe lesions showed coagulase-negative *Staphylococcus,* no HSV was recovered. The temperature returned to normal within 36 hr, and the patient was discharged on oral TMP–SMX and dicloxacillin.

Fever to 102.9°F (39 4°C) recurred on day +60 associated with night sweats, fatigue, and mildly productive cough. Chest radiography on day +62 showed a right lower lobe segmental infiltrate (Fig. 2). Temperature at admission was 99.3°F (37.4°C), but rose subsequently to 102.2°F (39°C). Examination showed resolving oral herpes, dullness and rhonchi of the right lower lung, and both crusting and new vesicles of the left fourth toe. PaO₂ on room air was 60 mm Hg. The WBC count was 4450/mm³ with 3650 neutrophils/mm³. Antibody titers to CMV had been negative throughout his hospital course. Sputum contained macrophages and a few neutrophils and grew oral flora. Additional cultures were unremarkable. In spite of the low PaO₂, the clinical impression was that of bacterial pneumonia, and treatment with cephalothin (6 g/day) and gentamicin (1.6 mg/kg q8h) was initiated. Oral TMP–SMX was continued, with the dose increased to 20 mg/kg TMP per day on day +63. Fever persisted, and on day +66 fiberoptic bronchoscopy with transbronchial biopsy was performed as an initial diagnostic procedure. *Pneumocystis carinii* was demonstrated by toluidine blue O staining. Previous sputum examination had been negative for pneumocystis. Treatment was changed from oral TMP–SMX to intramuscular pentamidine isethionate at 4 mg/kg per day and continued for 14 days. Fevers continued throughout pentamidine treatment, and erythromycin was substituted for cephalothin and gentamicin on day +72 because of continued concern about mycoplasma infection. The patient experienced pain from pentamidine injections, and both thighs became erythematous, swollen, and tender. Fever continued until the end of pentamidine treatment. He became afebrile the following day. Cold agglutinin titer in blood taken on day +66 was 1 : 64, and it was 1 : 128 14 days later. However, mycoplasma CF titers were 1 : 8 and <1 : 8 during the same interval.

Comment. This patient had an unusual radiological presentation of *Pneumocystis carinii* pneumonia, perhaps modified by prophylactic TMP–SMX. Although serum levels of TMP to ensure adequate absorption were not measured, the possibility of resistance to TMP–SMX must be considered in this case. Both pneumococcal and mycoplasma infection were considered as etiologies for his segmental infiltrate, but there was no evidence to support either diagnosis. Positive cold agglutinin titers have been observed in *Pneumocystis carinii* infection.[66] Fortunately, bronchoscopic biopsy provided the diagnosis, although we have not found procedures short of open lung biopsy adequate in most cases. It is important to note both the unusual presentation of nonbacterial pneumonia in this patient and to emphasize that tissue examination was needed to establish the diagnosis after the patient failed to respond to 96 hr of empirical antibiotics.

5.4. Idiopathic Interstitial Pneumonia

The most perplexing aspect of the syndrome of interstitial pneumonia has been the inability to identify an infectious agent in one-third of patients with histologically demonstrated pneumonia. Idiopathic pneumonia is otherwise indistinguishable clinically and radiologically from CMV or *Pneumocystis* pneumonia. Time of onset is similar to that of other pneumonias, and the mortality rate is about 60%. Among the etiologies investigated for idiopathic pneumonia have been chlamydia mycoplasma, and BK virus by culture of lung tissue and occasionally oropharynx or nasopharynx, and *Legionella pneumophila* by specific serology.[50,67] None of these studies has been revealing. Although it remains possible that a heretofore unknown infectious agent is responsible for idiopathic pneumonia, the present data suggest instead that it is the result of radiation and chemotherapy toxicity. These data include the lower risk among aplastic anemia patients who do not receive TBI, the lower risk associated with fractionated versus single-exposure TBI as well as the lower risk associated with lower dose rates of radiation, the lack of relationship to acute GVHD, and the equivalent incidence of idiopathic pneumonia among leukemic patients receiving either syngeneic or allogeneic transplants.[50,52] Any procedure that reduces the likelihood of pulmonary toxicity from transplant conditioning (e.g., lung shielding) would therefore be expected to lower the incidence of idiopathic pneumonia.

Specific recommendations about treatment are not possible. Steroids have been tried, but a small randomized trial suggested no benefit. Anti-*Pneumocystis* treatment is started before biopsy in all patients and then discontinued when appropriate after results of the biopsy are known. In patients who cannot be biopsied, treatment for *Pneumocystis carinii* is continued empirically for 14 days.

5.5. Other Manifestations of Cytomegalovirus Infection

More patients develop CMV infection than fatal pneumonia. Seventy-five percent of patients with detectable antibody before transplant have evidence of active infection after transplant if one includes a rise in titer, viral excretion (usually pharyngeal), or CMV pneumonia.[42]

Two nonfatal syndromes commonly attributed to CMV infection are hepatitis and suppression of marrow function. Accurate incidence figures are not available. Patients with significant CMV titer rises frequently have liver abnormalities suggesting hepatocellular dysfunction that cannot be explained fully by GVHD, another hepatic infection, or drug toxicity. Some patients also have unexplained fever and, rarely, arthralgias or even frank arthritis. Clinical symptoms may precede the actual titer rise by several weeks. The usual concepts of primary infection and virus reactivation may not be appropriate in this unusual immunologic situation, and patients with detectable pretransplant antibody may be subject to symptom complexes usually ascribed to primary infection.

The more important manifestation has been the association of CMV infection with depression of marrow function. In some instances, suppression has

been complete, and second grafts have been necessary. Graft rejection has been associated with reactivation of CMV in renal transplant patients[68] as well as in animal models,[69] and whether graft rejection reactivates CMV or CMV infection causes graft rejection is unknown. Twenty-two patients who required marrow boosts or second grafts in 1977–1978 were matched by underlying illness with 44 persons who did not require boosts or regrafts in order to analyze the effect of CMV infection on graft function. These 66 patients were examined for CMV seroconversion and evidence of virus dissemination, including pneumonia. Among patients with CMV infection, 16 of 27 (59%) had a significant fall in leukocyte or platelet count compared with only 14 of 39 (36%) without evidence of CMV infection. This difference is not significant, although it illustrates the relationship described.

Gastrointestinal syndromes have also been of increasing importance. Cytomegalovirus and HSV each caused about one-fourth of endoscopically diagnosed esophagitis in previous years, and CMV will be responsible for an even higher proportion now that HSV infection can be controlled with acyclovir (see Section 5.6).[70] Cytomegalovirus has similarly been implicated as a common cause of nausea and vomiting not due to acute GVHD. Ulceration due to CMV has been identified at all levels of the GI tract from stomach to colon, and fatal colonic hemorrhage due to diffuse colonic involvement has been observed. It should be noted that not all CMV infection, including

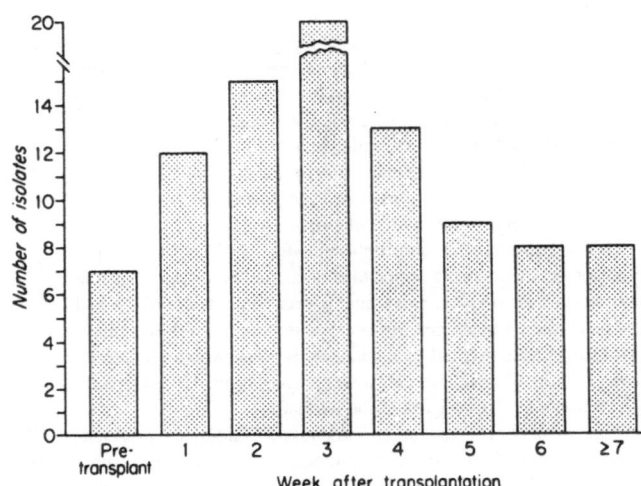

FIGURE 11. Herpes simplex virus isolation by week after transplant from all sites. The 90 patients in the protective environment study are included in this analysis.

locally invasive disease such as esophagitis or enteric ulcers, eventuates in disseminated infection or pneumonia, and most patients recover from CMV infection albeit with sometimes prolonged courses.[70]

5.6. Herpes Simplex Virus Infection

In most patients, HSV infection begins during the granulocytopenic period when it is most difficult to differentiate oral mucosal breakdown (mucositis) from virus infection. Many progress to more typical herpetic lesions involving the lips and nose, although others have HSV recovered from oropharyngeal cultures without such lesions. Eighty percent of seropositive patients excrete HSV, mostly from the oropharynx, at some time during the first 50 days after transplant. By contrast, fewer than 1% of seronegative patients excrete HSV after transplant, and for most purposes (e.g., use of acyclovir prophylaxis) it can be assumed that seronegative patients are not at risk of HSV reactivation. Peak excretion is during weeks 2–3 after transplant (Fig. 11) and only 10% of patients have first excretion detected more than 6 weeks after transplant. Reactivation of HSV clearly increases the severity of oral mucositis (Table 6). Untreated patients heal slowly, beginning with recovery of the granulocyte count, and lesions (and excretion) may recur later after transplant. HSV was a common cause of esophagitis before the availability of acyclovir and has also been recovered from gastric and intestinal ulcers. Patients may develop distant cutaneous lesions, as well as herpes keratitis, through autoinoculation. Cutaneously disseminated HSV infection or encephalitis has been rare, however. Herpetic whitlow has occurred among patient care personnel, and glove isolation should be used for patients with known oral herpes.

One syndrome of note is HSV pneumonia, which has been identified by examination and culture of lung tissue in more than 25 patients.[55] All had either preceding or coincident oral or genital HSV infection, or both. Two modes of pathogenesis were described: contiguous spread from the oropharynx, often in patients intubated for other pulmonary processes, and viremic spread from either oropharyngeal or genital sites of infection. Most patients with contiguous spread had infection with type 1 virus, localized lesions (focal or multifocal) on radiography, and, uncommonly, had spread to other organs. By contrast, patients with viremic spread had infection with either type 1 or type 2 virus, diffuse infiltrates indistinguishable from CMV (and sometimes had co-infections), and, more commonly, spread to other organs including liver and brain. The importance of this syndrome is that it can be diagnosed by commonly available laboratory techniques, and can be treated. Patients with known or suspected oral HSV infection and suspected pulmonary disease should have cultures taken of both oropharyngeal and endotracheal specimens. Since HSV generally grows within a few days, and almost always within 1 week, rapid cultural diagnosis is possible. Specimens, especially those from the tracheobronchial tree or lung, should also be examined by specific immunofluorescence. Treatment with intravenous acyclovir should be effective for HSV pneumonia, although no specific treatment trials have been performed. Seropositive patients should be considered for acyclovir treatment, even in the absence of documented oral HSV infection, if they are to be intubated or otherwise instrumented (e.g., bronchoscopy or endoscopy) to prevent the introduction of HSV to more distant sites.

Systemic acyclovir (intravenous or oral) has been shown to be highly effective in the treatment of established HSV infection after marrow transplant.[71,72] Recommended treatment courses in patients with normal function are 250 mg/m^2 every 8 hr IV or 400 mg PO five times daily; in each case, the course should be a minimum of 7 days. Topically administered acyclovir has also been shown to be effective in the immunocompromised host[73] but is applicable only to patients with solely external lesions. Acyclovir treatment has been associated with

TABLE 6. Severity of Oral Mucositis and Associated Herpes Simplex Virus Excretion

	Clinical severity of mucositis (grade[a])		
	0	1–2	3–4
HSV present	3	15	11
HSV absent	19	29	13
Percentage excreting	14%	34%	46%

[a]Clinical grading system with grade 0 representing no mucositis and grade 4 representing life-threatening mucositis

delay in the specific immune response to HSV after marrow transplant,[74] as well as with the recovery of HSV strains with reduced sensitivity to acyclovir.[75] Neither of these observations should prevent the use of acyclovir for the treatment of active HSV infection after marrow transplant when warranted by the clinical situation.

Because of the predictable timing and high frequency of HSV reactivation among seropositive patients, acyclovir prophylaxis has also been used. Intravenous acyclovir given two or three times daily (250 mg/m^2/dose) and oral acyclovir (400 mg five times daily or 800 mg twice daily) have been shown to be effective, although compliance with oral acyclovir may be a problem early after transplant.[76-78] We use intravenous acyclovir twice daily beginning 1 week before transplant and continuing for 4 weeks after transplant (unless the patient is discharged earlier) to prevent HSV reactivation among seropositive patients. This regimen is 90% effective based on serial virologic surveillance.[78] In some studies, acyclovir prophylaxis has also been associated with more rapid engraftment,[77,78] although this may be apparent only among patients receiving MTX rather than CSP prophylaxis for GVHD.[77] This effect is not mediated by suppression of HSV, and the explanation is unknown.

5.7. Other Protozoan Infections

Toxoplasmosis appears to be rare after transplantation.[79,80] We have observed 10 cases in more than 2000 transplants.[81] Disease has occurred exclusively among patients seropositive before transplant, and thus appears to be due to reactivation of latent infection. Involvement of heart, lung, and brain has been identified at postmortem examination. As in other immunocompromised hosts, serologic studies are usually unrevealing, and biopsy of implicated organs may be needed for diagnosis.[80] We have recovered *Toxoplasma* from blood cultures of three patients with proven disease, and this technique may therefore be considered for diagnosis, although the sensitivity is unknown.[81] Treatment is with pyrimethamine and sulfadiazine and should be continued for 6 months or more.

Cryptosporidiosis also appears to be rare. We have observed one case in our center, the manifestations of which appeared to be less severe than those

reported in patients with acquired immune deficiency syndrome.[82] Although this patient appeared to respond to treatment with spiramycin, this treatment cannot be recommended routinely until additional studies are completed.

6. Phase III: After 100 Days

Infections occurring after 100 days are determined in part by the residual immune deficiency shared by all patients and in part by the additional immunosuppression associated with GVHD and its treatment. The most prominent example of infection determined by the former is VZV infection. A minority of patients with GVHD have an increased incidence of recurrent bacterial infections.

6.1. Varicella–Zoster Virus Infection

Nearly 40% of all marrow transplant patients develop VZV infection. Median time of onset is 5 months after transplant, and most cases occur within the first year (Fig. 12). Of the first 92 patients with VZV infection whom we observed, 77 had herpes zoster, and 15 had varicellalike infection.[83] In some patients, this was undoubtedly true primary infection, whereas others probably had atypical generalized zoster. One-third of patients with untreated herpes zoster had subsequent cutaneous dissemination. The case-fatality rate for untreated varicella is 35%, and for untreated herpes zoster with dissemination is 30%. All deaths have occurred during the first 9 months after transplantation. Other syndromes of importance have included trigeminal zoster with keratitis, post-herpetic neuralgia occurring in 25%, and local scarring or bacterial superinfection in 20%. We have observed second cases of VZV infection in only 3% of patients. The incidence of VZV infection is increased among patients with allogeneic (versus syngeneic) transplants and among those with acute or chronic GVHD. In the subgroup of patients with chronic GVHD, those with demonstrable nonspecific suppressor cells have the highest incidence.[84]

Because of the high mortality rate from VZV infection within the first 9 months after transplant, we recommend treatment of all patients with VZV infection during that interval with acyclovir (500 mg/m^2 every 8 hr). Treatment is continued for 7 days

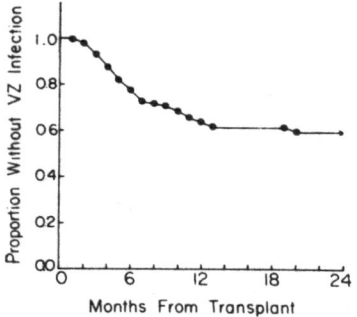

FIGURE 12. Proportion of patients without varicella-zoster virus infection by number of months after transplant. Only patients who survived more than 6 months after marrow transplant are included.

and may be prolonged if patients have persistent new lesion formation. Compared to vidarabine, acyclovir appears to have a more rapid antiviral effect, may have beneficial effects even after cutaneous dissemination has occurred, and is more convenient to use than vidarabine, which requires a 12-hr constant infusion. We have observed relapse of VZV infection within 2 months of acyclovir treatment among six patients, however. No significant toxicity has been observed during that time period among patients with normal renal function treated with either drug for VZV infection at our center. Patients who develop infection more than 9 months after transplant may be treated at the first sign of cutaneous dissemination if they have herpes zoster or at the first sign of visceral spread if they have varicella. Orally administered acyclovir may also have a role in the treatment of VZV infection after marrow transplant, but treatment trials have not yet been reported and it cannot be routinely recommended at this time.

6.2. Late Infections in Patients with Graft-versus-Host Disease

Among 89 patients followed 6 months or longer after transplant, only 30 (34%) remained free of infection.[85] Twenty-five (28%) had three or more infections. Upper respiratory or pulmonary infections were most common. Ten patients had bacterial septicemia. In contrast to the early granulocytopenic period, when gram-negative bacteria were predominant, *Streptococcus pneumoniae* was the most common isolate in proven bacterial infection, followed by *Staphylococcus aureus*. Significant risk factors in the development of these late infections were the occurrence of chronic GVHD and inability

to respond to dinitrochlorobenzene skin sensitization.

The occurrence of pneumococcal bacteremia is especially intriguing. We have observed up to three episodes in a single patient. Whether the same capsular type of *Pneumococcus* was involved is unknown. Males predominate among those with bacteremic pneumococcal infections, both in our experience and that of Winston et al.[86] This male predilection needs to be confirmed by further observation.

The presumed explanation for bacteremic pneumococcal infections is that marrow transplant patients lose and do not subsequently make opsonizing antibody to encapsulated gram-positive organisms, even after recovery from infection. There are several lines of evidence to confirm this. Winston et al.[86] reported that six of seven patients with pneumococcal bacteremia had deficient serum opsonic activity for prototype strain VI compared with normal pooled serum. As reviewed in Section 2, both primary and secondary antibody response to keyhole limpet hemocyanin and bacteriophage ϕX174 are depressed after marrow transplant, although improvement occurs with elapsed time after transplant.[9] This is in contrast to the normal responses seen in most patients recovering from VZV infection and in some patients with CMV infection. Finally, patients respond poorly to immunization with prototype pneumococcal vaccines for the first 1–2 years after transplant, although response again improves with time.[87] In this regard, marrow transplant patients are similar to patients treated for Hodgkin disease.[88] It would seem unlikely that immunization with the available pneumococcal vaccine would provide significant protection for those most in need, patients with chronic

GVHD. As a separate issue, live-virus vaccines in general are considered contraindicated until information about their safety and efficacy after marrow transplant is available.

We continue TMP–SMX prophylaxis in patients with chronic GVHD in the hope of preventing both bacteremic pneumococcal and other infection. Controlled data are not available to evaluate the efficacy of such prophylaxis, but retrospective study of nonrandomized treatment groups indicates that patients with chronic GVHD who receive TMP–SMX prophylaxis have a significantly lower incidence of infection.[89] In prospectively followed patients, the major effect was a decrease in infection due not only to *Streptococcus pneumoniae*, but also to *H. influenzae* and *E. coli*. Unexpectedly, pneumonia due to nonbacterial causes other than *Pneumocystis* was also reduced. TMP–SMX prophylaxis is given twice daily at the dose of 75 mg/m^2 (TMP component) and is continued for as long as patients receive immunosuppressive treatment for chronic GVHD. Oral penicillins have been used among patients who are unable to tolerate TMP–SMX because of rash, GI side effects, or apparent marrow suppression.

Because infection with other organisms including both *Staphylococcus* and gram-negative aerobic bacteria also occurs, empirical antibiotic treatment of marrow transplant patients admitted with clinical sepsis should include broad-spectrum coverage until the identity of the infecting organisms is known. Of interest, apparent recurrences of *Pneumocystis carinii* infection that were clinically unsuspected have been seen in three patients dying with gram-negative sepsis 1–2 years after transplant.

7. Future Considerations

Many issues in the care of the marrow transplant recipient remain unresolved. It has been shown that early bacterial infections can be prevented by the use of the protective environment.[30] This is an expensive procedure and may not be appropriate or cost effective for all patients. Instead, a program of parenteral antibiotics alone or in conjunction with oral antibiotics and sterile food might provide significant protection from early bacterial infection. However, the association between transplantation in the protective environment and improved survival among patients

with aplastic anemia,[36] as well as the possibility that this effect can be extended to patients transplanted for leukemia, is an exciting observation that warrants additional attention.

Problems with early diagnosis and effective treatment of fungal infection are common to all immunosuppressed patients. Our own experience is consistent with others who have found presently available fungal serologies not to be diagnostically useful. Serologic diagnosis will depend on the development of sensitive tests for circulating fungal antigens, since one cannot depend on the ability of immunosuppressed patients to produce antibody. In the absence of such tests, the early empirical use of antifungal drugs must be relied on to decrease the high incidence of fungal infection in patients with prolonged granulocytopenia. An alternative approach is the use of antifungal agents prophylactically.

Opportunistic viral infections are prominent in all transplant populations, and marrow transplant recipients are no exception. The most important viral pathogen remains CMV. Treatment of established infection, and prevention of virus reactivation among seropositive patients, remain elusive goals although the development of newer antiviral agents with improved activity against human CMV suggests that progress may soon be made in this area.[63] Progress has been made in the prevention of primary CMV infection. The sole use of CMV-seronegative blood products for seronegative patients with seronegative marrow donors was highly effective in preventing primary CMV infection, and this approach should be implemented universally for such patients. The role of passive immunoprophylaxis or antiviral prophylaxis among seronegative patients with seropositive marrow donors, and among all seropositive patients, remains to be determined. The ability to both treat and prevent HSV infection with acyclovir and the ability to treat VZV infection are cause for optimism that serious viral infection in the allograft recipient can indeed be controlled. Prophylaxis of VZV infection, in view of the high incidence and defined risk periods, is a future goal that may be achievable either with the long-term use of orally administered antiviral agents such as acyclovir, or through active immunologic manipulations such as the use of live varicella vaccine.[90] Although marrow transplant recipients, like other immunosuppressed patients, are considered at risk of complications from live virus vaccines, varicella vaccine may be a special case. The vaccine virus is sensitive to available antiviral agents, and additional protection to vaccine recipients may be afforded by the use of varicella–zoster immune globulin. Thus it should be possible to use varicella vaccine safely even after marrow transplant, as it is being used among patients with acute lymphocytic leukemia on maintenance chemotherapy. Demonstration of the usefulness of such manipulations to restore specific immunity may subsequently be relevant to CMV[91] and HSV as well, for which investigational vaccines are also under study.

Infections occurring in long-term survivors of marrow transplantation are due both to the persistence of immunologic defects and to the additional effects of chronic GVHD and its treatment. One approach to the prevention of late infections is reconstitution of specific immune responses through the use of antigenic reexposure (i.e., vaccines as just discussed for VZV infection), although the usefulness of nonreplicating agents such as pneumococcal polysaccharide is problematic in view of the poor response to antigens such as bacteriophage φX174 as well as to pneumococcal polysaccharide itself.[87] An alternative approach is nonspecific augmentation of immune responses through the use of immunomodulators such as IF_γ or IL-2. Progress in prevention and treatment of chronic GVHD itself will clearly be needed, as well as a better understanding, and more effective methods, of producing specific immune reconstitution.

ACKNOWLEDGMENTS. The authors thank the physicians, nurses, ward clerks, and technologists of the Seattle Marrow Transplant Team for the care of the patients discussed in this manuscript. Research discussed in this manuscript was supported by grants CA 15704, CA 18029, CA 30924, and CA 26966, awarded by the National Cancer Institute, DHHS. E. Donnall Thomas, M.D., is a recipient of a Research Career Award AI 02425 from the National Institute of Allergy and Infectious Diseases.

References

1. Thomas ED, Storb R, Clift RA, et al: Bone-marrow transplantation N Engl J Med 292:832–843, 895–902, 1975.
2. Storb R, Thomas ED, Buckner CD, et al. Marrow transplantation for aplastic anemia Semin Hematol 21:27–35, 1984.
3. Thomas ED: Current status of bone marrow transplantation. Transplant Proc 17:428–431, 1985.
4. Good RA, Bach FH: Bone marrow and thymus transplants: Cellular engineering to correct primary immunodeficiency. IN Bach FH, Good RA (eds): Clinical Immunobiology Vol. 2. Academic, New York, 1974, pp. 63–114.
5. O'Reilly RJ, Dupont B, Pahwa S, et al: Reconstitution in severe combined immunodeficiency by transplantation of marrow from an unrelated donor. N Engl J Med 297:1311–1318, 1977.
6. Clift RA, Hansen JA, Thomas ED, et al: Marrow transplantation from donors other than HLA identical siblings. Transplantation 28:235–242, 1979.
7. Atkinson K, Biggs JC, Ting A, et al: Cyclosporin A is associated with faster engraftment and less mucositis than methotrexate after allogeneic bone marrow transplantation Br J Haematol 53:265–270, 1983.
8. Clark RA, Johnson FL, Klebanoff SJ, et al: Defective neutrophil chemotaxis in bone marrow transplant patients. J Clin Invest 58:22–31, 1976.
9. Noel DR, Witherspoon RP, Storb R, et al: Does graft-versus-host disease influence the tempo of immunologic recovery after allogeneic human marrow transplantation? An observation on 56 long-term survivors. Blood 51:1087–1105, 1978.
10. Atkinson K, Hansen JA, Storb R, et al: T-cell subpopulations identified by monoclonal antibodies after human marrow transplantation. I. Helper-inducer and cytotoxic-suppressor subsets. Blood 59:1292–1298, 1982.
11. Levin MJ, Parkman R, Oxman MN, et al: Proliferative and interferon responses by peripheral blood mononuclear cells after bone marrow transplantation in humans. Infect Immun 20:678–684, 1978.
12. Azogui O, Gluckman E, Fradeliz D· Inhibition of IL-2 production after human allogeneic bone marrow transplantation. J Immunol 131:1205–1208, 1983.
13. Livnat S, Seigneuret M, Storb R, et al: Analysis of cytotoxic effector cell function in patients with leukemia or aplastic anemia before and after marrow transplantation. J Immunol 124:481–490, 1980.
14. Quinnan GV, Kirmani N, Rook AH, et al: Cytotoxic T cells in cytomegalovirus infection. N Engl J Med 307:6–13, 1982.
15. Storb R, Thomas ED, Weiden PL, et al: One-hundred-ten patients with aplastic anemia (AA) treated by marrow transplantation in Seattle. Transplant Proc 10:135–140, 1978.
16. Winston DJ, Gale RP, Meyer DV, et al: Infectious complications of human bone marrow transplantation. Medicine (Baltimore) 58:1–31, 1979.
17. Clift RA, Buckner CD, Fefer A, et al· Infectious complications of marrow transplantation. Transplant Proc 6:389–393, 1974
18. Springmeyer SC, Altman LC, Hudson LD, et al: The effects of irradiation and autologous bone marrow transplantation on canine bronchoalveolar cell populations. Am Rev Respir Dis 119 (part 2):81, 1979
19. Thomas ED, Ramberg RE, Sale GE, et al: Direct evidence for a bone marrow origin of the alveolar macrophages in man. Science 192:1016–1018, 1976.
20. Brody AR, Craighead JE: Pathogenesis of pulmonary

cytomegalovirus infection in immunosuppressed mice. *J Infect Dis* **129:**677–689, 1974.

21. Cross AS, Steigbigel RT *Pneumocystis carinii* pneumonia presenting as localized nodular densities. *N Engl J Med* **291:**831–832, 1974.

22 Ravin CE, Smith GW, Ahern MJ, et al. Cytomegaloviral infection presenting as a solitary pulmonary nodule. *Chest* **71:**220–222, 1977.

23. Stamm WE, Tompkins LS, Wagner KF, et al. Infection due to *Corynebacterium* species in marrow transplant patients. *Ann Intern Med* **91:**167–173, 1979.

24. Cohen ML, Murphy MT, Counts GW, et al: Prediction by surveillance cultures of bacteremia among neutropenic patients treated in a protective environment. *J Infect Dis* **147:**789–793, 1983.

25. Hickman RO, Buckner CD, Clift RA, et al: A modified right atrial catheter for access to the venous system in marrow transplant recipients. *Surg Gynecol Obstet* **148:**871–875, 1979.

26. Rodriguez V, Burgess M, Bodey GP: Management of fever of unknown origin in patients with neoplasms and neutropenia. *Cancer* **32:**1007–1012, 1973.

27. Schimpff SC, Aisner J: Empiric antibiotic therapy. *Cancer Treatm Rep* **62:**673–680, 1978.

28. Bodey GP, Buckley M, Sathe YS: Quantitative relationships between circulating leukocytes and infection in patients with acute leukemia. *Ann Intern Med* **64:**328–340, 1966.

29. Gill FA, Robinson R, MacIowry JD, et al: The relationship of fever, granulocytopenia and antimicrobial therapy to bacteremia in cancer patients. *Cancer* **39:**1704–1709, 1977.

30. Buckner CD, Clift RA, Sanders JE, et al: Protective environment for marrow transplant recipients. A prospective study. *Ann Intern Med* **89:**893–901, 1978.

31. Schimpff SC, Greene WH, Young VM, et al: Infection prevention in acute nonlymphocytic leukemia. Laminar air flow room reverse isolation with oral, nonabsorbable antibiotic prophylaxis. *Ann Intern Med* **82:**351–358, 1975.

32. Herzig RH, Herzig GP, Graw RG Jr, et al: Successful granulocyte transfusion therapy for gram-negative septicemia. A prospectively randomized controlled study. *N Engl J Med* **296:**701–705, 1977.

33. Alavi JB, Root RK, Djerassi I, et al: A randomized clinical trial of granulocyte transfusions for infection in acute leukemia. *N Engl J Med* **296:**706–711, 1977.

34. Strauss RG: Therapeutic neutrophil transfusions. Are controlled studies no longer appropriate? *Am J Med* **65:**1001–1006, 1978.

35. Clift RA, Buckner CD, Williams B, et al: Granulocyte transfusions in marrow transplant recipients. In Goldman JM, Lowenthal RM (eds). *Leucocytes. Separation, Collection and Transfusion.* Academic, New York, 1975, pp. 340–348.

36. Storb R, Prentice RL, Buckner CD, et al: Graft-versus-host disease and survival in patients with aplastic anemia treated by marrow grafts from HLA-identical siblings. *N Engl J Med* **308:**302–307, 1983.

37. Levine AS, Siegel SE, Schreiber AD, et al: Protected environments and prophylactic antibiotics. A prospective controlled

study of their utility in the therapy of acute leukemia. *N Engl J Med* **288:**477–483, 1973

38. Yates JW, Holland JF: A controlled study of isolation and endogenous microbial suppression in acute myelocytic leukemia patients. *Cancer* **32:**1490–1498, 1973

39. Clift RA, Sanders JE, Thomas ED, et al: Granulocyte transfusions for the prevention of infection in patients receiving bone-marrow transplants. *N Engl J Med* **298:**1052–1057, 1978

40. Winston DJ, Ho W, Gale RP: Granulocyte transfusions for the prevention of infection. *N Engl J Med* **299:**488–489, 1978.

41 Winston DJ, Ho WG, Howell CL, et al. Cytomegalovirus infections associated with leukocyte transfusions. *Ann Intern Med* **93:**671–675, 1980.

42 Hersman J, Meyers JD, Thomas ED et al: The effect of granulocyte transfusions upon the incidence of cytomegalovirus infection after allogeneic marrow transplantation. *Ann Intern Med* **96:**149–152, 1982.

43. Martin DH, Counts GW, Thomas ED: Fungal infections in human bone marrow transplant recipients. In *Seventeenth Interscience Conference on Antimicrobial Agents and Chemotherapy.* American Society for Microbiology, New York, 1977, abstr. 406.

44. Miller GG, Witwer MW, Braude AI, et al: Rapid identification of *Candida albicans* septicemia in man by gas–liquid chromatography. *J Clin Invest* **54:**1235–1240, 1974.

45 Bodey GP, Luna M: Skin lesions associated with disseminated candidiasis *JAMA* **229:**1466–1468, 1974.

46. Fishman LS, Griffin JR, Sapico FL, et al: Hematogenous *Candida* endophthalmitis—A complication of candidemia. *N Engl J Med* **286:**675–681, 1972.

47 Shepp DH, Klosterman A, Siegel MS, et al: Comparative trial of ketoconazole and nystatin for prevention of fungal infection in neutropenic patients treated in the protective environment. *J Infect Dis* **152:**1257–1263, 1985

48. Dieperink H, Moller J: Ketoconazole and cyclosporin. *Lancet* **2:**1217, 1982.

49. Kauffman CA, Frame PT: Bone marrow toxicity associated with 5-fluorocytosine therapy. *Antimicrob Agents Chemother* **11:**244–247, 1977.

50. Meyers JD, Flournoy N, Wade JC, et al: Biology of interstitial pneumonia after marrow transplantation In Gale RP (ed): *Recent Advances in Bone Marrow Transplantation.* Liss, New York, 1983, pp. 405–423.

51. Meyers JD, Flournoy N, Thomas ED: Nonbacterial pneumonia after allogeneic marrow transplantation: A review of ten years' experience *Rev Infect Dis* **4:**1119–1132, 1982.

52. Appelbaum FR, Meyers JD, Fefer A, et al: Nonbacterial nonfungal pneumonia following marrow transplantation in 100 identical twins. *Transplantation* **33:**265–268, 1982.

53. Hughes WT, Price RA, Kim H-K, et al: *Pneumocystis carinii* pneumonitis in children with malignancies. *J Pediatr* **82:**404–415, 1973.

54 Petersen DL, Sale GE, Silvestri RC, et al: Open lung biopsy is superior to transbronchial lung biopsy in immunosuppressed patients with interstitial pneumonia. *Am Rev Respir Dis* **117:**164, 1978.

55. Ramsey PG, Fife KH, Hackman RC, et al: Herpes simplex

virus pneumonia: Clinical, virological and pathological features in 20 patients. *Ann Intern Med* **97**:813–820, 1982.

56. Shields AF, Hackman RC, Fife KH, et al. Adenovirus infections in patients undergoing bone marrow transplantation. *N Engl J Med* **312**:529–533, 1985.

57. Winston DJ, Pollard RB, Ho WG, et al: Cytomegalovirus immune plasma in bone marrow transplant recipients. *Ann Intern Med* **97**:11–18, 1982

58. Meyers JD, Leszczynski J, Zaia JA, et al: Prevention of cytomegalovirus infection by cytomegalovirus immune globulin after marrow transplantation. *Ann Intern Med* **98**:442–446, 1983.

59. O'Reilly RJ, Gold J, Kirkpatrick D, et al: A randomized trial of intravenous hyperimmune globulin for the prevention of cytomegalovirus (CMV) infections following marrow transplantation: Preliminary results. *Transplant Proc* **15**:1405–1411, 1983.

59a. Bowden RA, Sayers M, Flournoy N, et al: Cytomegalovirus immune globulin and seronegative blood products to prevent primary cytomegalovirus infection after marrow transplantation. *N Engl J Med* **314**:1006–1010, 1986

60. Hirsch MS, Schooley RT, Cosimi AB, et al: Effects of interferon-alpha on cytomegalovirus reactivation syndromes in renal-transplant recipients. *N Engl J Med* **308**:1489–1493, 1983.

61. Meyers JD: Prevention and treatment of cytomegalovirus infections with interferons and immune globulins *Infection* **12**(2):143–150, 1984.

62. Kraemer KG, Neiman PE, Reeves WC, et al: Prophylactic adenine arabinoside following marrow transplantation. *Transplant Proc* **10**:237–240, 1978

63. Tyms AS, David JM, Jeffries DJ, et al: BWB759U, an analogue of acyclovir, inhibits human cytomegalovirus in vitro. (Letter.) *Lancet* **2**:924, 1984.

64. Meyers JD, Pifer LL, Sale GE, et al: The value of *Pneumocystis carinii* antibody and antigen detection for the diagnosis of *Pneumocystis carinii* pneumonia after marrow transplantation. *Am Rev Respir Dis* **120**:1283–1287, 1979.

65. Lau WK, Young LS: Trimethoprim–sulfamethoxazole treatment of *Pneumocystis carinii* pneumonia in adults. *N Engl J Med* **295**:716–718, 1976.

66. Rifkind D, Faris TD, Hill RB Jr.. *Pneumocystis carinii* pneumonia Studies on the diagnosis and treatment. *Ann Intern Med* **65**:943–956, 1966.

67. Storch G, Hayes PS, Meyers JD, et al: Legionnaires' disease bacterium: Prevalence of antibody to the organism in patients suspected of having *Pneumocystis carinii* infection. *Am Rev Respir Dis* **121**:483–486, 1980.

68. Simmons RL, Lopez C, Balfour H Jr., et al: Cytomegalovirus: Clinical virological correlations in renal transplant recipients. *Ann Surg* **180**:623–634, 1974.

69. Wu BC, Dowling JN, Armstrong JA, et al: Enhancement of mouse cytomegalovirus infection during host-versus-graft reaction. *Science* **190**:56–58, 1975.

70. McDonald GB, Sharma P, Hackman RC, et al: Esophageal infections in immunosuppressed patients after marrow transplantation. *Gastroenterology* **88**:1111–1117, 1985.

71. Wade JC, Newton B, McLaren C, et al: Intravenous acyclovir

to treat mucocutaneous herpes simplex virus infection after marrow transplantation: A double-blind trial. *Ann Intern Med* **96**:265–269, 1982.

72. Shepp DH, Newton BA, Dandliker PS, et al Oral acyclovir therapy for mucocutaneous herpes simplex virus infection in immunocompromised marrow transplant recipients. *Ann Intern Med* **102**:783–785, 1985

73 Whitley RJ, Levin M, Barton N, et al: Infections caused by herpes simplex virus in the immunocompromised host. Natural history and topical acyclovir therapy. *J Infect Dis* **150**:323–329, 1984.

74. Wade JC, Day LM, Crowley J, et al: Recurrent infection with herpes simplex virus after marrow transplant: Role of the specific immune response and acyclovir treatment. *J Infect Dis* **149**:750–756, 1984.

75 Wade JC, McLaren C, Meyers JD: Frequency and significance of acyclovir-resistant herpes simplex virus isolated from marrow transplant patients receiving multiple courses of treatment with acyclovir. *J Infect Dis* **148**:1077–1082, 1983

76 Saral R, Burns WH, Laskin OL, et al: A randomized, double-blind, controlled trial in bone-marrow-transplant recipients *N Engl J Med* **305**:63–67, 1981.

77. Wade JC, Newton B, Flournoy N, et al· Oral acyclovir for prevention of herpes simplex virus reactivation after marrow transplant. *Ann Intern Med* **100**:823–828, 1984

78. Hann IM, Prentice HG, Blacklock HA, et al: Acyclovir prophylaxis against herpes virus infections in severely immunocompromised patients: Randomised double blind trial. *Br Med J* **287**:384–388, 1983.

79. Emerson RG, Jardine DS, Milvenan ES, et al: Toxoplasmosis: A treatable neurologic disease in the immunologically compromised patient. *Pediatrics* **67**:653–655, 1981.

80. Hirsch R, Burke BA, Kersey JH: Toxoplasmosis in bone marrow transplant recipients. *J Pediatr* **105**:426–428, 1984.

81. Shepp DH, Hackman RC, Conley FK, et al: *Toxoplasma gondii* reactivation identified by detection of parasitemia in tissue culture. *Ann Intern Med* **103**:218–221, 1985.

82. Collier AC, Miller RA, Meyers JD: Cryptosporidiosis after marrow transplant: Person-to-person transmission and treatment with spiramycin. *Ann Intern Med* **101**:205–206, 1984.

83. Atkinson K, Meyers JD, Storb R, et al: Varicella-zoster virus infection after marrow transplantation for aplastic anemia or leukemia *Transplantation* **29**:47–50, 1980.

84. Atkinson K, Farewell V, Storb R, et al: Analysis of late infections after human bone marrow transplantation: Role of genotypic nonidentity between marrow donor and recipient and of nonspecific suppressor cells in patients with chronic graft-versus-host disease. *Blood* **60**:714–720, 1982.

85. Atkinson K, Storb R, Prentice RL, et al: Analysis of late infections in 89 long-term survivors of bone marrow transplantation. *Blood* **53**:720–731, 1979.

86. Winston DJ, Schiffman G, Wang DC, et al. Pneumococcal infections after human bone-marrow transplantation. *Ann Intern Med* **91**:835–841, 1979.

87. Witherspoon RP, Storb R, Ochs HD, et al: Recovery of antibody production in human allogeneic marrow graft recipients: Influence of time posttransplantation, the presence or absence

of chronic graft-versus-host disease, and antithymocyte globulin treatment. *Blood* **58**:360–368, 1981.

88. Siber GR, Weitzman SA, Aisenberg AC, et al: Impaired antibody response to pneumococcal vaccine after treatment for Hodgkin's disease. *N Engl J Med* **299**:442–448, 1978.

89. Sullivan KM, Deeg HJ, Sanders JE, et al: Late complications after marrow transplantation *Semin Hematol* **21**:53–63, 1984.

90. Takahashi M, Otsuka T, Okuno Y, et al: Live vaccine used to prevent the spread of varicella in children in hospital. *Lancet* **2**:1288–1290, 1974.

91. Glazer JP, Friedman HM, Grossman RA, et al: Live cytomegalovirus vaccination of renal transplant candidates. A preliminary trial. *Ann Intern Med* **91**:676–683, 1979.

21

Infection in the Renal and Liver Transplant Patient

ROBERT H. RUBIN

1. Introduction

During the past two decades, remarkable strides have been made in the field of renal transplantation. From a fascinating experiment in human biology, renal transplantation has evolved into a practical therapeutic modality widely applied to the treatment of chronic renal failure. For the first time in history, not only does renal transplantation offer the best chance for rehabilitation of the uremic patient but, in addition, at many centers, it offers at least as good a chance for patient survival as the other widely available treatment modality, chronic hemodialysis. For example, at the Massachusetts General Hospital over the past 3 years, the 1-year patient survival for recipients of kidneys from living related and cadaveric donors has been greater than 95%, with a 1-year graft survival of more than 85%. For patients surviving with a functioning graft at 1 year, the subsequent mortality rate is less than 5% per year. By comparison, the reported patient loss on hemodialysis is 5–10% each year.

This remarkable clinical achievement has been accomplished by the attainment of considerable progress in the five major areas that determine the outcome for a patient receiving a transplant:[1]

1. Optimal tissue typing and matching of donor organ to potential recipient, thus minimizing the incidence and extent of the rejection process
2. Careful procurement and preservation of the donor organ and proper preparation of the recipient
3. Impeccable surgical technique, resulting in a minimum of tissue injury, secure vascular and ureteral anastomoses, and the prevention of fluid collections, be they blood, urine, or lymphatic in origin
4. More precise management of the immunosuppressive regimen; on the one hand, effectively preventing allograft rejection and, on the other, minimizing the global depression of host defenses against infection, the major side effect of the immunosuppressive agents currently available
5. Prompt diagnosis and specific therapy of those infections that do occur

The net result has been better control of rejection and better prevention and treatment of infection—the two major barriers to successful organ transplantation.[1,2] These two are closely related, being essentially mirror images of one another: any intervention that decreases the incidence of infection will permit the safe deployment of more intensive immunosuppressive therapy and thus better management of rejection; and any intervention that decreases the intensity and extent of rejection, thus permitting lesser amounts of immunosuppressive therapy, will be associated with a lower rate of infection. Rejection and infection may be regarded as the two sides of the same problem.

ROBERT H. RUBIN • Infectious Disease and Transplantation Units, Massachusetts General Hospital; and Department of Medicine, Harvard Medical School, Boston, Massachusetts 02114.

It is worth reviewing how far we have come in the past two decades, emphasizing the lessions that have been so painfully learned, in order to present today's infectious disease problems in this patient population in perspective. During the 1960s, not only were surgical techniques, organ procurement and preservation, and tissue typing less advanced than today, but the immunosuppressive therapy was considerably less expert. More than 50% of transplanted patients were dying of infection, with fungal and other opportunistic infections accounting for as many of these deaths as conventional bacterial infections.[3] Rifkind et al.[4] noted that clinical fungal infection occurred with a peak incidence approximately 2–3 months post-transplant, when the average dose of prednisone was 60 mg/day. Bach et al.[5] similarly noted a high incidence of death from fungal infections, particularly *Aspergillus fumigatus,* and related such occurrences to the number of acute rejection episodes that were treated. A typical antirejection program employed at the time was as follows: increasing the prednisone does to 320 mg/day for the first week and then halving the dose weekly until maintenance levels were reached, thus committing the patient to at least four additional weeks of high-dose steroid therapy. The major thrust of modern immunosuppressive therapy has been to devise means of decreasing the dosage of corticosteroids used in clinical transplantation, both for maintenance immunosuppression and for the treatment of acute rejection episodes.[6-8] In addition, a major effort has been mounted to find alternative means of treating and preventing rejection that would be more specific (less globally immunosuppressive) and even more steroid sparing; such efforts to date include polyclonal antilymphocyte sera and globulins,[9-11] monoclonal antibodies specific for particular lymphocytes,[12-14] and total lymph node irradiation.[15-17] In addition, of course, is the clinical revolution associated with the advent of cyclosporine therapy.[18] Table 1 outlines the immunosuppressive regimens currently employed in our transplant program; two crucial points are the markedly lower dose of prednisone employed as standard therapy and the reliance

TABLE 1. Standard Immunosuppressive Therapy Protocols Employed in Adults at the Massachusetts General Hospital

Type of transplant	HLA-identical living related kidney	Other living related and cadaveric donor kidney	Extrarenal allografts and chronic renal rejection
Type of immunosuppression:	Azathioprine[a] + prednisone	Cyclosporine[b] + prednisone	Cyclosporine,[c] azathioprine,[a] and prednisone
Average daily prednisone dose[d]			
Day 0	120	200	200
Day 1	120	160	160
Day 2	120	120	120
Day 3	120	80	80
Day 4	110	40	40
Day 5	100	20	20
Day 6	90	20	20
Day 7	80	20	20
Day 8	70	20	20
Day 9–20	60	20	20
Week 3–7	Reduce by 10 mg q2wk	20	20
Week 8–52	20	15	15
After 1 year	10–15	10–15	10–15

[a]Azathioprine is given at a dose of 5 mg/kg the day prior to transplant, 2–3 mg/kg the day of transplant, and then 1 5–3 mg/kg each day, maintaining the peripheral WBC count in the 4000–10,000/mm^3 range

[b]Cyclosporine therapy is initiated at a dose of 6 mg/kg bid and then is altered to maintain a plasma trough level by radioimmunoassay of 50–150 ng/ml

[c]Cyclosporine therapy is initiated at a dose of 5 mg/kg bid and then is altered to maintain a plasma trough level of 50–100 ng/ml

[d]If acute rejection develops in the face of these programs, the daily prednisone dose is maintained and pulse doses of 500 mg IV methylprednisolone are administered daily for 2–3 days If, at the end of such therapy, rejection is continuing, treatment with a 10-day course of the murine monoclonal antibody OKT3 or equine-derived antithymocyte globulin is initiated. During such therapy, the azathioprine dosage is decreased by 50% and/or cyclosporin is discontinued for 1 week.

on antilymphocyte antibody therapies as the bulwark of antirejection therapy rather than sustained high-dose corticosteroid treatment. Indeed, when such antilymphocyte therapies are employed, other forms of immunosuppression are decreased temporarily in order to avoid the horrendous infectious complications long associated with such treatments. These were particularly common when antilymphocyte antibody therapy was added on top of full-dose azathioprine and prednisone therapy.[11]

Some of the lessons that came out of the early transplant experience that still apply today include the following. First, there is a limit to the amount of corticosteroid a patient will tolerate safely, and it is better to give up on a kidney, return the patient to dialysis, and then retransplant than to continue high-dose steroid therapy with its increased risk of infection in a desperate attempt to salvage the allograft. Second, the addition of cyclosporine and/or azathioprine in moderate doses to the immunosuppressive program allows for the lowering of the steroid dosage, less generalized depression of host defenses, and adequate antirejection effect. Third, in addition to steroid dosage and amounts of other forms of immunosuppressive therapy administered, the other major risk factors predisposing to serious infection are neutropenia, and such metabolic factors as uremia and hyperglycemia.[19]

More recently, a great deal of concern has been paid to the net state of immunosuppression produced in a given patient, whether this state is caused by steroids, azathioprine, viral infection, antithymocyte globulin (ATG), uremia, and/or other factors. For example, we have shown that when ATG is added to a full program of prednisone and azathioprine, there is an increased incidence of cytomegalovirus (CMV) viremia, clinical syndromes caused by the virus, and an attenuation of the beneficial effects of prophylactic interferon against the virus.[20] If, however, the same dose of ATG is combined with an immunosuppressive program in which the prednisone and azathioprine dosage is cut by half, the excess morbidity and potential mortality engendered by this virus are eliminated without decreasing the antirejection effects of the combined program.[21] Such findings should serve as a continued stimulus for the development of more specific immunosuppressive programs that can effectively prevent rejection while decreasing the risk of infection.

Despite the advances in clinical transplantation, infection remains a major problem. More than 80% of renal transplant patients suffer at least one episode of infection in the first year post-transplant,[22] and infection remains the leading cause of death.[23] The challenges to the clinicians responsible for the infectious disease management of renal transplant patients are many[1,24]:

1. The chronic requirement for immunosuppression to prevent allograft rejection will not only increase the incidence and severity of acute infections, but will also result in chronic, progressive disease from microbial agents unlikely to have such effects in immunologically intact individuals. Prime examples of this are the effects of chronic infection with such viruses as cytomegalovirus (CMV), Epstein–Barr virus (EBV), hepatitis B, and papillomaviruses. The combination of chronically impaired host defenses and infection with these agents can lead to progressive eye, liver, and skin disease, and even cancer at a rate and in a form virtually unknown in the normal host.

2. The potential sources of infection for the transplant patient are many, including endogenous organisms, the allograft itself, the environment, and the patients' food and water.

3. The prevention of infection is the primary aim in this patient population, as every episode of clinical infection requiring treatment carries the potential for lethal consequences. In particular, the prevention of opportunistic infection of nosocomial origin and the prevention of infection due to technical error are of greatest importance. Table 2 presents a classification of infections in the organ transplant patient according to the manner in which they are acquired, emphasizing that many of the life-threatening infectious problems are preventable. The major exceptions are those infections acquired in the community or due to transmission and/or reactivation of latent virus by immunosuppressive therapy. The incidence and severity of these infections is directly related to the type and intensity of immunosuppression administered. They are also more difficult to prevent

TABLE 2. Classification of Infections of Major Importance in Organ Transplant Patients

Infections related to technical complications[a]
   Transplantation of a contaminated allograft
   Anastomotic leaks or stenoses
   Wound hematoma
   Intravenous line contamination
   Urinary or biliary catheter contamination
   Iatrogenic damage to the skin
Infections related to excessive nosocomial hazard
   Aspergillus spp.
   Legionella spp.
   Pseudomonas aeruginosa and other gram-negative bacilli
   Nocardia asteroides
Infections related to particular exposures within the community
   Systemic mycotic infections in certain geographic areas
      Histoplasma capsulatum
      Coccidioides immitis
      Blastomyces dermatitidis
   Community-acquired opportunistic infection due to ubiquitous
      saprophytes in the environment[b]
      Cryptococcus neoformans
      Aspergillus spp.
      Nocardia asteroides
      Pneumocystis carinii
   Mycobacterium tuberculosis
   Strongyloides stercoralis
   Respiratory infections circulating in the community
      Influenza
      Streptococcus pneumoniae
   Infections acquired by the ingestion of contaminated food or
      water
      Salmonella spp.
      Listeria monocytogenes
Viral infections of particular importance in the transplant patient
   Herpes group viruses
   Hepatitis viruses
   Papovaviruses
   Human immunodeficiency virus (the causative agent of the
      acquired immunodeficiency syndrome)
   Adenoviruses

[a]All lead to infection with gram-negative bacilli, *Staphylococcus* sp and/or *Candida* sp
[b]The incidence and severity of these infections and, to a lesser extent, the other infections listed are directly related to the net state of immunosuppression present in the particular patient

and treat than other forms of infection, and themselves make a significant contribution to the patient's net state of immunosuppression.

   4. The prompt recognition and aggressive therapy of those infections that do occur is the critical factor in successful treatment of this

patient population. This may be a particularly difficult problem in patients whose inflammatory response may be greatly suppressed by the antiinflammatory effects of the immunosuppressive therapy being administered. This suppressed inflammatory response will often blunt the signs and symptoms of infection, necessitating great skill on the part of the clinician in terms of his ability to interpret the significance of what, in a normal host, might be an innocuous skin lesion or radiographic finding. In this patient population, such lesions might be the first signs of life-threatening infection, and early biopsy may lead to effective therapy.

Although one must recognize the challenges inherent in caring for such chronically immunosuppressed patients, the rewards are great—both for patient and clinician. It is the purpose of this chapter to outline a logical approach to the infectious disease problems of this patient population, based on an analysis of the epidemiologic, clinical, and immunologic events occurring in the individual patient.

2. Timetable of Infection in the Renal Transplant Patient

Different infections occur at different points in the post-transplant period (Fig. 1). For example, although cytomegalovirus infection is the most important single cause of clinical infectious disease syndromes in the period 1–4 months post-transplant, it rarely has clinical effects in the first 20 days. Similarly, cryptococcal disease is unusual earlier than 6 months post-transplant, and clinically significant liver disease from hepatitis B or non-A, non-B hepatitis is usually not manifest for years after transplantation. It is useful to divide the post-transplant period into three phases when evaluating the patient for possible infection[1,24]:

   1. *Infection in the first month post-transplant:* The infectious disease problems in this time period are of three types: (a) infection that was present in the allograft recipient prior to transplant and which continues post-transplant, perhaps exacerbated by post-transplant immunosuppression; the prime concerns here are hepatitis (both B and non-A, non-B), smol-

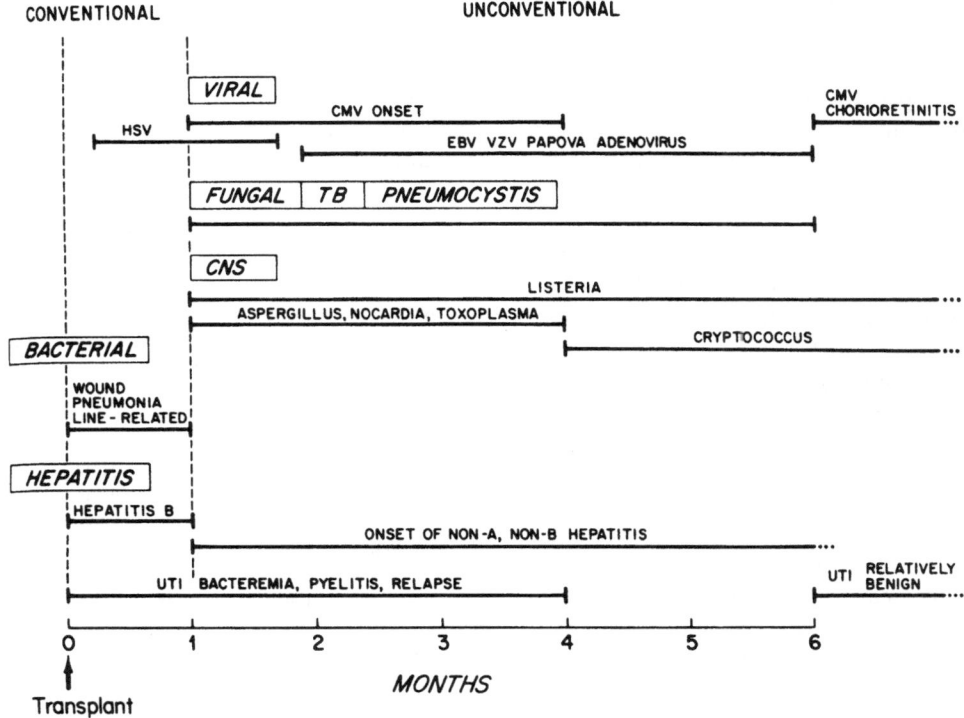

FIGURE 1. Timetable for the occurrence of infection in the renal transplant patient. Exceptions to this timetable should initiate a search for an unusual hazard. CMV, cytomegalovirus; HSV, herpes simplex virus; EBV, Epstein–Barr virus; VZB, varicella–zoster virus; CNS, central nervous system; UTI, urinary tract infection. (Modified from Rubin et al.[1])

dering old bacterial infection, tuberculosis, strongyloidiasis, and the geographically restricted systemic mycoses (blastomycosis, coccidioidomycosis, and histoplasmosis); (b) infection transmitted with a contaminated allograft, with allograft infection either being acquired from the donor (usually) or in the procurement and preservation process prior to the transplant operation; and (c) the routine bacterial infections of the surgical wound, lungs, intravenous lines, and bladder catheters found in nonimmunosuppressed patients undergoing comparable types of surgery. It is these last that are the most important causes of infection in the first month post-transplant.

It is important to emphasize that infection with such opportunistic pathogens as *Aspergillus* sp., *Legionella* sp., and *Nocardia asteroides* is not normally observed the first month post-transplant. The lack of such infections under normal circumstances at a time when the daily dosage of immunosuppressive therapy is at its highest underlines two important

points: the duration of immunosuppression is a more important determinant of the net state of immunosuppression than the particular dose of drug being administered on a given day or over a few days; the cost of excessive immunosuppressive therapy in terms of infection risk will be borne weeks after such therapy is administered rather than immediately, and the physician must guard against a false sense of security engendered by the lack of immediate consequences of high-dose immunosuppressive therapy.

2. Infection 1–6 months post-transplant. Although residual effects of infection acquired earlier may still be noted in this time period, two groups of infections—the second in large measure dependent upon the first—are the major problems in this time period: infection due to a variety of viruses, particularly the herpes group viruses, and most particularly CMV; and infection due to a variety of opportunistic pathogens, such as *Pneumocystis carinii*, the fungi, and *Listeria*. The duration of immunosuppression is now sufficient so that conventional bacterial infection is no longer the major problem, with viral infection now constituting the major hazard. In addition, these viruses, particularly CMV, are themselves immunosuppressing, and it is the subgroup of transplant patients with viral infection that is at major risk of opportunistic infection.

3. *Infection in the late period, more than 6 months post-transplant.* The infectious disease problems of patients with functioning renal allografts (and thus continuing to receive chronic immunosuppressive therapy) in the late period may be divided into three general categories: (1) those with chronic viral infection acquired earlier, and with progressive disease due to the interaction of the chronic viral infection with a chronically immunosuppressed state (the prime examples of this are progressive chorioretinitis due to CMV, progressive liver disease due to hepatitis B or non-A, non-B hepatitis, and hepatocellular carcinoma and B-cell lymphoproliferative disease associated with hepatitis B and EBV, respectively); (2) patients free of chronic viral infection, with good renal function (serum creatinine <2 mg/dl), who are receiving minimal immunosuppressive therapy, and whose infectious disease problems are similar to those in the general community, such as viral upper respiratory infections, trivial urinary tract infections, influenza, and pneumococcal pneumonia; and (3) patients with chronic allograft rejection (serum creatinine >2 mg/dl) who have received too much acute and chronic immunosuppression, who have chronic infection with the immunomodulating viruses, and who are at the greatest risk of life-threatening opportunistic infection with such pathogens as *Pneumocystis carinii, Cryptococcus neoformans, Listeria monocytogenes,* and *Nocardia asteroides.*

The utility of this timetable as the clinician approaches the transplant patient with an infectious disease syndrome such as a pneumonia is twofold: it can be helpful in generating an etiologic differential diagnosis; and it can be extremely helpful as an epidemiologic tool. Our experience has been that whenever exceptions to this timetable occur, it is because an immunosuppressed patient has been subjected to an excessive epidemiologic hazard, usually within the hospital environment. Particularly important in this regard is the occurrence of opportunistic infection in the first month post-transplant. As a general rule, whenever a nosocomial epidemic of *Aspergillus, Legionella, Pseudomonas* or *Nocardia* infection has been observed among renal transplant patients, an early tipoff to the presence of such an epidemic is the occurrence of such cases in the first month post-transplant.

Illustrative Case 1

A 19-year-old white man underwent an uncomplicated renal transplant from a cadaveric donor for end-stage renal disease due to chronic glomerulonephritis. Immunosuppression was accomplished with cyclosporine and prednisone, and by the third transplant day the serum creatinine reached a level of 1 mg/dl, where it remained. Ten days post-transplant, fever, chills, and a nonproductive cough developed. Chest radiography revealed a left lower lobe infiltrate. Transtracheal aspirate was nondiagnostic Therapy was instituted with pipercillin and tobramycin, but over the next 36 hr increasing dyspnea and fever developed. The infiltrate on radiography progressed as well. Because of this, open lung biopsy was carried out which revealed *Legionella pneumophila* Therapy was instituted with 4 g erythromycin intravenously and the patient recovered over a three week period. Epidemiologic investigation instituted on the basis of this one case revealed *L. pneumophila* contaminating a cooling tower that was directly adjacent to the intake duct for the air-conditioning system supplying the transplant unit where this patient was housed. The cooling tower was decontaminated, but not before two other patients developed Legionnaire's disease, with one of these dying despite therapy.

Comment. Prior to this outbreak, none of 350 transplant patients developed Legionnaire's disease; since this outbreak none of 450 transplant patients cared for by this transplant service developed Legionnaire's disease. This small epidemic was due entirely to a new, fortunately temporary, excessive nosocomial hazard. The lessons here are twofold: rapid, specific diagnosis is important (as discussed in Chapter 6), and nosocomial hazards are a constant threat to the immunosuppressed patient. Most importantly, *a single case of infection with an opportunistic pathogen in the first month following renal transplantation constitutes prima facie evidence of a nosocomial epidemic.*[1,24]

3. Infection in the First Month following Renal Transplantation

3.1. Preexisting Infection in the Allograft Recipient

It is axiomatic that a potential renal transplant recipient be rendered free of active infection prior to operation and the initiation of immunosuppressive therapy. The importance of this is underlined by the following catastrophic forms of infection that we have observed in the early post-transplant period when active, although asymptomatic, bacterial infection was not eradicated prior to transplantation: systemic sepsis and deep wound infection with loss of the allograft due to smoldering infection of the native kidneys at the time of transplant; miliary tuberculosis in a patient with unsuspected, active tuberculosis at the time of transplant; and staphylococcal sepsis from a deep abscess that had been present for months at the site of previous surgery. Therefore, a careful evaluation of the urinary tract, lungs, abdomen, and other possible sites of infection, and eradication of such infections (even if ablative surgery is necessary) is obligatory prior to transplant.

Of all the infections that could appear post-transplant, after being asymptomatic pretransplant, one that merits special attention is that due to *Strongyloides stercoralis*. *S. stercoralis* is an intestinal nematode that is endemic in many areas of the world. Even in the United States, it has been found in 36 states.[25,26] The organism has a complex life cycle, the most important aspect of which is an autoinfection component that allows the organism to be maintained in the gastrointestinal (GI) tract of a human host for decades after initial infection was acquired—long after the host has left an endemic area.[25,26] Such individuals may be asymptomatic or have only minor GI complaints. Apparently, tissue invasion is prevented by an intact cell-mediated immune system.[27] Following transplantation, a disastrous hyperinfection syndrome and/or disseminated strongyloidiasis can develop, due to the inhibition of normal cell mediated immune function. The hyperinfection syndrome represents an exaggeration of the normal life cycle of the parasite, with major impact on the GI tract (a severe, ulcerating hemorrhagic enterocolitis) and/or lungs (hemorrhagic pneumonia). Disseminated strongyloidiasis consists of extension of the infection outside its normal domain, with the filariform larvae invading all portions of the body. Both forms of systemic strongyloidiasis in the compromised host are associated with recurrent or persistent gram-negative bacteremia and/or meningitis, despite apparently appropriate therapy, which is primarily due to the adherence of gut bacteria to the external surface of the migrating larvae.[25-36]

Morgan et al.[26] emphasized that although early diagnosis is the key to effective therapy of these po-

tentially devastating infections in the transplant patient, there are a number of barriers to achieving this: the persistence of the organism long after the individual has left endemic areas; eosinophilia, a cardinal sign of parasitic infection, is commonly absent due to exogenous immunosuppression and concomitant systemic bacterial infection; routine stool examination for ova and parasites are negative in more than half of cases and more useful diagnostic tests such as sampling of proximal small bowel contents and sputum cytology are usually not done; symptoms are nonspecific and complicating bacterial infection will frequently obscure the picture.

Therapy of established systemic strongyloidiasis with oral thiabendazole plus systemic antibacterial therapy aimed at the complicating bacteremia or meningitis is possible (see Chapter 10 for details of management), but mortality remains greater than 50%.[26] It is of potential interest that cyclosporine appears to have anti-parasitic properties against *S. stercoralis*.[37] However, it is far better to identify the asymptomatic carrier prior to the transplant, and eradicate infection prior to the initiation of immunosuppressive therapy.[38,39] Since routine stool ova and parasite examinations will diagnose only 27% of asymptomatic carriers,[40] it is recommended that residents or former residents of endemic areas should be screened through examination of Papanicolaou (PAP) stained smears of sputum and duodenal aspirates and of purged stool specimens. Positive individuals should be treated with thiabendazole 25 mg/kg per day twice daily for 3 days and then monitored at 1–2-month intervals for the possible need for retreatment.[26]

Illustrative Case 2

A 14-year-old boy who had immigrated from Cambodia 2 years previously developed end-stage renal disease due to reflux nephropathy. While being maintained on chronic hemodialysis, he underwent bilateral nephrectomies in preparation for transplantation. Pretransplant evaluation also noted a negative tuberculin test, no eosinophilia on peripheral blood smear, and three negative stool examinations for ova and parasites. Three weeks after receiving an HLA-identical kidney from his brother, he presented with fever, rigors, cough productive of bloody sputum, abdominal pain, and bloody diarrhea. Chest radiography revealed bilateral patchy densities consistent with bronchopneumonia. Peripheral white blood cell count was 18,000 with 85% polymorphonuclear leukocytes and 15% band forms. Two blood cultures grew *Escherichia coli* sensitive to all antibiotics, with persistent bacteremia documented despite therapy with high-dose ampicillin and gentamicin. He began complaining of headache 24 hr after admission, and a lumbar puncture revealed an opening pressure of 300 mm H_2O, 400 leukocytes (100% polymorphonuclear leukocytes)/mm³, cerebrospinal fluid (CSF) glucose <20 mg/dl, and protein 110 mg/dl. CSF cultures grew the same antibiotic-sensitive *E. coli*. Despite continued broad-spectrum antibiotics, the patient died 4 days after admission. Postmortem examination revealed systemic strongyloidiasis involving the gastrointestinal tract, brain, heart, lungs, liver, and renal allograft. There was evidence of an extensive hemorrhagic bronchopneumonia and enterocolitis.

Comment. This patient represents a tragic case of disseminated strongyloidiasis that emphasizes several important points. Increasing numbers of such cases are being observed among recent immigrants from Southeast Asia and Central America. They usually present in the first few months post-transplant. Negative routine stool examinations for ova and parasites do not rule out the possibility of this infection, nor does the lack of eosinophilia. The diagnosis of the underlying *S. stercoralis* infection is often obscured by the protean clinical manifestations and the pace of this disseminated syndrome. Treatment of the accompanying bacteremia and bacterial meningitis alone is inadequate if the patient is to be salvaged.

3.2. Infection from the Donor

An important consideration in the choice of a kidney donor for transplantation is to minimize the risk of transmitting infection to a patient who will be immunosuppressed on receipt of the allograft. For example, before an individual may become a living donor, multiple negative urine cultures should be obtained, and the individual should have been free of any systemic infection that could involve the kidney, such as staphylococcal sepsis, for at least 1 year. Even after an extensive evaluation, latent infection may still be transmitted with the donated organ. The best-documented example of this is CMV infection: it has been well established that transplantation of a kidney from a CMV-seropositive donor into a seronegative recipient will frequently result in the development of primary CMV infection in the recipient. In this instance, the virus travels in latent form within the allograft from the seropositive donor and is subsequently reactivated within the recipient by the effects of the rejection process and the immunosuppressive therapy that is administered (see Section 4.1).[41-43] Similarly, hepatitis B can be transmitted with the allograft, with potentially drastic consequences, and all potential donors must be screened for hepatitis B surface antigen (HBsAg). A positive test would rule out such an individual as a donor.[44,45]

Clearly, other viruses can be carried with the graft. The most important new example of this is the transmission of acquired immunodeficiency syndrome (AIDS) from asymptomatic carriers of the human immunodeficiency virus,[46] formerly called human T-cell lymphotrophic virus type III (HTLV-III), lymphadenopathy-associated virus (LAV) immunodeficiency-associated virus (IDAV), or AIDS-associated retrovirus (ARV). Although the experience with AIDS and transplantation is a new one, it is already clear that the epidemiologic characteristics of this virus-initiated condition make it a major potential hazard to clinical transplantation. This transmissible blood-borne infection can also be spread by intimate personal contact. It has a prolonged viremic phase in both symptomatic and asymptomatic individuals. There is a high rate of subclinical, but contagious, infection among individuals of high-risk population groups, with the virus being present in transmissible form in virtually all bodily fluids of such people. Finally, anyone shown to have antibodies to the virus must be considered as harboring transmissible virus.[47-50] Not surprisingly, transmission of AIDS from asymptomatic but infected organ donors to recipients of allografts has now been reported.[47,51-53] In addition, as in other populations, transmission via blood transfusions has occurred to organ and bone marrow transplant recipients.[47,53-55] Accordingly, we have made the following recommendations to prevent exogenous infection of transplant recipients with the human immunodeficiency virus (HIV) (see also Section 4.2.2, for a discussion of AIDS in transplant patients).[47]

First, HIV infection can be transmitted to HIV seronegative individuals via kidney allografts and blood transfusions. Because of the known presence of infectious virus in the blood, tears, cornea, saliva, and semen of antibody-positive individuals, it should be assumed that recipients of liver, bone marrow, heart, pancreas, and corneal transplants, as well as those undergoing artificial insemination are also at risk of acquiring HIV infection from these biologic materials. All possible donors should therefore be screened for the presence of antibody to this virus, with any antibody-positive donor, even if asymptomatic, being regarded as an unacceptable donor.

Second, because currently available antibody tests for rapid screening for HIV antibody have a small but definite false-negative rate, potential donors from one of the population groups at high risk of

HIV infection (homosexual or bisexual males, intravenous drug abusers, hemophiliacs, individuals with a history of being a prisoner in a correctional facility, and, perhaps, immigrants from Central Africa or Haiti) should not be considered potential donors under normal circumstances. Under exceptional circumstances, as when considering a living related donor for a highly sensitized person, an individual from one of the high-risk population groups might be considered a potential donor. In such cases, testing for HIV antibody must be carried out by Western blot analysis as well as by the usual screening enzyme-linked immunosorbent assay (ELISA) technique.

Rarely, dormant fungal or mycobacterial infection that had asymptomatically metastasized to the kidney of the donor during recognized or unrecognized primary infection can be passed to the recipient with potentially catastrophic results. Examples of histoplasmosis[56] and cryptococcosis[57] transmitted in this fashion have been reported. It is thus important in the evaluation of a potential living donor that a complete clinical and epidemiologic history be obtained and, when indicated by such information, that tuberculin testing and fungal serologies be carried out. Although we would not rule out a potential donor on the basis of a positive tuberculin test or a history of residence in a geographic area endemic for histoplasmosis, blastomycosis, or coccidioidomycosis, such information is useful in caring for the recipient posttransplant in terms of the index of suspicion and type of evaluation to which the recipient is subjected for otherwise unexplained febrile illnesses.

Similar considerations apply to the evaluation of potential cadaver donors whenever possible, although by the nature of organ procurement from cadaveric donors, such information is usually much more scanty. Of greater practical significance here is the possibility of transmitting acute bacterial[58-60] and candidal[61] infection from the donor to the recipient. This is particularly true since most potential cadaveric donors will have had intravenous lines, bladder catheters, and/or endotracheal tubes—all potential sources of infection—in place for several days prior to the time of organ donation.

All potential donors with clear-cut systemic infection are eliminated from consideration. In addition, further attempts are made to rule out organ contamination by culturing perfusate and transport media. Indeed, a 4–40% rate of positive cultures has

been documented.[58,59,62-66] Most such positive cultures are with nonvirulent skin flora, and these results have correlated poorly with the occurrence of post-transplant allograft infection. By contrast, the occasional instance in which such surveillance cultures have yielded gram-negative bacilli, particularly *Pseudomonas aeruginosa*, and *Candida, sp.* have been highly correlated with infection involving the vascular anastomoses of the transplant, with the development of mycotic aneurysms and/or vascular disruption with life-threatening hemorrhage.[58,67-70] The importance of gram-negative infection of the perfusate has been emphasized in a dog transplant model.[70] In these studies, the perfusate was purposely contaminated with *Escherichia coli;* the kidney was then transplanted. All recipients died in approximately 4 days from either vascular anastomotic disruption or generalized sepsis.

Unfortunately, negative perfusate cultures and careful clinical evaluation of the donor prior to organ procurement does not preclude the possibility of serious allograft infection. We have reported a case of unsuspected donor *Pseudomonas* sepsis (donor afebrile prior to transplant, but with premortem donor blood cultures becoming positive several days later for the identical *Pseudomonas aeruginosa* strain subsequently isolated from the recipient) causing life-threatening infection in both recipients of kidneys from this single donor.[58] In the second post-transplant week, both kidney allograft recipients required emergency graft nephrectomies because of a massive retroperitoneal bleed. At operation, the arterial anastomosis was completely necrotic and disrupted, and grew the same *Pseudomonas*. Because of this problem of unsuspected cadaver donor bacterial or candidal sepsis, we have adopted the following approach[58]:

1. Careful culturing of the donor (including preterminal blood cultures) and of the perfusates should continue to be carried out, with systemic antimicrobial therapy initiated for positive cultures, utilizing shorter durations of therapy (<7 days) for the nonvirulent organisms and longer durations (>14 days) if the cultures yield gram-negative bacilli, *Staphylococcus aureus,* or *Candida,* sp. Some transplant centers recommend the routine use of 1–2 days of prophylactic antibiotics

for all transplant recipients in order to prevent this complication.[66] However, evidence that this practice would work for such difficult-to-treat organisms as *Pseudomonas* is lacking, and is, in our opinion, doubtful.

2. Van der Vliet et al.[71] and Slapak[72] have suggested, and we agree, that certain potential donors are at particularly high risk for occult sepsis and should not be used. These include victims of drowning (who may be infected with microorganisms found in water), burn victims, and patients who have been maintained on a respirator with indwelling lines and catheters for periods of more than 7 days.

Even these steps will not completely solve the problem of occult sepsis contaminating allografts. The ultimate answer will depend on the development of rapid noncultural diagnostic techniques for detecting microbial antigens or DNA so that potential donors can be rapidly screened for occult sepsis.

3.3. Wound Infection

The most important form of treatable infection in this time period, both in terms of frequency and clinical impact, is wound-related sepsis. The reported incidence of wound infection has varied by as much as 1.8–56%.[73–77] The impact of such infections, particularly when deep in the perinephric space, can be great, with 75% of deep perinephric infections resulting in the need for transplant nephrectomy and with many lives lost because of systemic sepsis originating from this site or from the development of a mycotic aneurysm in the area of the vascular anastomoses.[78,79] That such infections should be common in these patients is no surprise in view of the effects of chronic uremia, possible protein malnutrition, immunosuppressive therapy, and so forth, on wound healing and resistance to infection. However, the experience of the transplant group at the University of Minnesota sheds a different light on the subject. In 439 kidney transplants, the incidence of wound infections was 6.1%. If, however, those secondary to hematoma or urinary fistula are excluded, the incidence of wound infection in the uncomplicated wounds is only 1.6%, with all being superficial infections. If diabetics and retransplanted patients are excluded, the incidence of wound infection was only 0.7%, again, all superficial.[79] By way of comparison, the rate of wound infection for clean general surgical procedures in nonimmunosuppressed patients is reported as 1.8%, for herniorrhaphy 4.7%, and for breast surgery 14.3%.[80] Other transplant groups have noted similarly low rates of wound infection.[81–84]

The unavoidable conclusion is that the most important factor in the prevention of wound sepsis in the transplant patient is the technical quality of the surgery performed. There is probably no other area of general surgery in which anything less than impeccable surgical technique can have such disastrous consequences. The incidence of wound infection is determined by the ability of the surgeon to prevent urine leaks, wound hematomas, and the development of lymphoceles—all of which markedly increase the risk of infection. One additional factor is the avoidance of unnecessary "dirty" surgery at the time of transplant. Fisher et al.[85] documented a high rate of *Bacteroides fragilis* bacteremia when elective appendectomy is performed at the time of transplant. This observation is an extension of two general principles: all active infections must be eradicated prior to transplant, and ill-advised surgery is as bad as a technical error.

Prevention of urinary leaks begins at the time of organ procurement. The primary concern here is to preserve the blood supply of the donor ureter, as ureteral vascular insufficiency resulting in distal ureteral necrosis or fibrosis is a major cause of both urinary extravasation and ureteral obstruction. Damage to this blood supply as a result of stripping of the periureteral adventitial tissue in which the blood vessels run, too extensive dissection of the hilum of the kidney, or the failure to recognize the presence of multiple renal arteries are the major technical errors that must be avoided by the organ procurement surgeon.[8,9] If this is accomplished, attention is then turned to the urinary anastomosis, be it a ureteroneocystostomy or ureteropyelostomy, in which watertight nonobstructing anastomoses are essential. Although a discussion of the surgical details of the urinary anastomosis and the choice between the types is beyond the scope of this chapter, their importance cannot be minimized. In the best hands, urologic complication rates of less than 2% can be obtained.[86–88] By contrast, a review of 1301 renal transplants reported in the literature up to 1973 noted an incidence of urologic complications of 13.3%, with approximately one-third of these patients dying as a result of their urologic complication.[89] Similarly, Myerowitz et al.[90] reported that of 53 episodes of bacteremia in 140 patients, the primary focus was in the urinary tract in 60%, and in more than half of these, the cause was urinary leakage or obstruction. Lobo et al.[91] suggested that the combination of urinary tract infection with renal dysfunction in the peritransplant period also plays an important role in the development of the gram negative sepsis seen at this time; i.e., there is spread of uropathogens from the injured kidney to the perirenal tissues, and that these then interact with the other local factors in the development of deep wound infection.

The second major preventable factor in the development of wound sepsis is the formation of a wound hematoma. Any technical errors resulting in bleeding will be exacerbated by the uremic state and by the heparin employed when post-transplant hemodialysis is required. Wound hemostasis at the time of transplantation must be meticulous.[77,78] As pointed out by Kyriakides et al.[79]

> Particularly in cadaver kidneys, which are usually hastily harvested, attention to hemostasis must be extreme. Small bleeding points in the kidney capsule and around the renal pelvis must be controlled after transplantation. This problem may be complicated, since renal flow to the ischemic kidney may be delayed so that small vascular defects might not be noted.

When bleeding or other complications require reexploration or transplant nephrectomy, the incidence of wound infection rises to approximately 20%.[78,92]

The final technical consideration here is the prevention of lymphoceles. Such collections of lymph in the retroperitoneal wound of the renal transplant patient occur at reported rates of 2–18%[93–95] and may result in mechanical obstruction and/or become secondarily infected. Lymphoceles result when, at the time of transplantation, lymphatic vessels, especially those crossing the iliac arteries, are cut without ligation or lymph nodes are removed for tissue-typing purposes, again without adequate ligation of the lymphatic channels. Lymph collecting in the retroperitoneal space will not be absorbed and must be drained surgically, either externally or into the peritoneal cavity. A clinical clue to the presence of such a lymphocele is the development of unilateral leg edema on the side of the transplant.[78,93–96]

Thus far, the factors leading to the development of wound sepsis have been explored. Next to be considered are the questions of how best to prevent (other than with expert surgery), diagnose, and treat wound infections. In the area of prevention, there is general agreement among most transplant surgeons that local irrigation of the transplant wound with antibacterial solutions such as a bacitracin–neomycin mixture is beneficial, although such practice has never been subjected to a careful randomized study in the transplant setting. Similarly, the use of open drains, such as Penrose drains, is thought to result in more harm than benefit by providing a direct conduit to the perinephric space for microorganisms.[77,78,97] Recently, many groups have been employing closed suction drainage in an effort to obliterate dead space and prevent fluid collections. Our practice has been to place a Jackson-Pratt drain at the time of transplantation and to monitor the daily fluid output, maintaining the drain in place until less than 50 ml/day is being delivered into the system. Usually the drain can be removed in less than 5 days. If copious nonbloody drainage continues for a longer period, either a lymph leak or a urine leak is present. The latter can be ruled out by administering intravenously the dye indigo carmine, which imparts a blue color to the urine, and checking the color of the drainage.

In the past, usefulness of prophylactic, perioperative antibiotics in preventing wound infection has been regarded as unproven. Indeed, at the Massachusetts General Hospital, without using prophylaxis we have had a wound infection rate of less than 0.5% over the past 10 years. Recent data,[82–84,92,97,98] however, would suggest that perioperative antibiotic administration can decrease the rate of wound infection if it is above 4% without such prophylaxis. Such therapy should be aimed at uropathogens and staphylococci. An inexpensive program such as one consisting of cefazolin with or without gentamicin, begun on call to the operating room, and continuing for 24 hr post-transplant, would be a reasonable prophylactic choice. The exact choice of antibiotics should be guided by knowledge of the prevalent bacterial flora causing wound infection at a particular institution and the antibiotic susceptibility patterns of these organisms. Two points should be emphasized regarding such a prophylactic program: (1) no antibiotic prophylaxis program can take the place of technically expert surgery, and (2) such a program is aimed at protecting against wound infection, not later urinary tract infection or other problems. There are better methods for preventing urinary tract infection (see Section 4.3), and prolonging broad-spectrum parenteral antibiotic prophylaxis adds little to the care of transplant patients.

The diagnosis of wound infection requires a high index of suspicion. As detailed in Chapter 23, the immunosuppressive therapy being administered will frequently obscure the usual presenting signs of wound infection. Therefore, any transplant patient with an unexplained fever should be subjected to two procedures: sterile needle aspiration of the wound and either ultrasonographic or computed tomographic (CT) scanning of the deeper operative sites.[93,94,99] Such scans should be directed not only at the pelvis where the transplant was placed but also at nephrectomy and/or splenectomy sites if these procedures were carried out in conjunction with the transplant. Although gallium scans have been recommended for this purpose, in our hands they have not been very useful.

Any collection identified should be promptly drained under broad-spectrum antibiotic coverage. If infection is identified, then appropriate antibiotics are usually continued for 10–14 days or until the patient has been afebrile for 5–7 days. Whenever perinephric infection is identified, the possible need for graft nephrectomy to facilitate drainage and to prevent catastrophic anastomotic leaks should always be kept in mind. If deep sterile collections are found, we once again prefer closed suction drainage to the placement of Penrose drains.

3.4. Other Causes of Infection in the First Month

The major remaining causes of infection in the renal transplant patient during the first month following transplantation are pneumonia, urinary tract infection, and intravenous line-related sepsis. One general principle underlines the occurrence of each of these—the immunosuppressed patient tolerates poorly the presence of foreign bodies that bypass normal local host defenses, i.e., endotracheal tubes, urinary catheters, and plastic intravenous catheters.

These should be used sparingly, removed promptly, and managed with impeccable aseptic technique. In the case of pneumonia, the first concern is prevention with the use of appropriate anesthetic and analgesic management so that the endotracheal tube can be removed in the first 12 hr post-transplant, aspiration is prevented, and chest physical therapy and early patient mobilization are employed to prevent atelectasis. These three factors are the most important elements predisposing to bacterial pneumonia in this setting. Urinary tract infection is discussed in detail in Section 4.3, but suffice it to say here that catheters should be removed promptly postoperatively (usually in less than 2 days if a ureteropyelostomy anastomosis has been performed and in less than 5 days if a ureteroneocystostomy has been carried out). In these time frames, urinary tract infections should not occur while the catheters are still in place and, if they do, prior infection or contamination should be considered.

Plastic catheters for intravenous use are to be discouraged, particularly central venous pressure catheters or Swan Ganz pulmonary artery catheters for hemodynamic monitoring. Unless a major complication occurs in the perioperative period, virtually no suitable candidate for a renal transplant should require this type of monitoring. Although the problem of intravenous line-related sepsis is a general one throughout the hospital, its consequences can be particularly disastrous in these patients. For example, although a transient intravenous line-related *Candida* septicemia is associated with metastatic infection and the need for antifungal therapy in less than 5% of normal individuals, among immunosuppressed patients more than 50% will develop metastatic infections if left untreated.[100] The one exception to the rule concerning avoidance of central lines is if sclerosing substances such as antithymocyte globulin are being administered. Severe phlebitis with a potential for secondary infection will often develop unless this drug is administered into a vessel with a rapid flow rate. Thus, arteriovenous fistulas or subclavian lines are usually employed, taking great care to practice even more careful than usual aseptic technique.

Although we are primarily concerned with infection here, there are other causes of fever in the first month post-transplant. The most important ones are acute rejection, allergic reactions to medications such as antithymocyte globulin, and pulmonary emboli. The approach of the clinician when a renal transplant patient mounts a febrile response is to culture fully; to obtain a chest radiograph, urinalysis, and complete blood count; assess any changes in renal function, blood pressure, weight, and urine output (increasing creatinine, hypertension, weight gain, and falling urine output all being signs of rejection); and to ensure the absence of a superficial or deep wound infection by physical examination, needle aspiration, and ultrasound techniques. The white blood cell (WBC) count and differential are of much less use diagnostically in this patient population, as benign elevations are not uncommon in patients receiving cyclosporine and prednisone therapy, while azathioprine may blunt the WBC response when true infection is present. The question usually is whether or not the WBC is adequate. If the granulocyte count is greater than $1500/mm^3$, then empirical antibiotic therapy is usually not needed (and antibiotics are started for the same indications as in nonimmunosuppressed individuals). If the granulocyte count is less than $1500/mm^3$, empirical therapy with a potentially synergistic antibiotic program of penicillin and/or cephalosporin plus an aminoglycoside, as outlined in Chapter 18, should be instituted immediately.

4. Infection 1–6 Months Post-transplant

Unless technical complications have occurred, the time period 1–6 months post-transplant is the critical period for the transplant patient in terms of the greatest risk of life-threatening infection.

1. Immunosuppression is still at a relatively high level, particularly if significant amounts of antirejection therapy have been required. Although opportunistic infection related to immunosuppressive therapy is rare in the first few weeks of administration,[1] the cumulative effects begin to manifest themselves by the end of the first month of such therapy, and opportunistic infection becomes increasingly common. Despite the fact that humoral immunity, granulocyte function, and reticuloendothelial system function are all somewhat inhibited by current immunosuppressive regimens, the most critical factor here appears to be the level of cell-mediated immunity (CMI) present.

2. Infections occurring during this period are usually more difficult to treat with antimicrobial therapy, since most are caused by viruses, resistant bacterial species, fungi, and protozoan agents.

3. Any technical errors lingering from the perioperative period (e.g., persistent urine leaks or lymphocele formation) will, by definition, be serious. These require the presence of drains, ureteral catheters, nephrostomy tubes, etc., for prolonged periods of time. The longer such foreign bodies are required, the greater the incidence of superinfection, and the more difficult to treat the infection becomes, usually evolving from an antibiotic-sensitive bacterial species to increasingly resistant gram-negative and fungal species. Of all the factors leading to serious infection in this period, however, the most important and pervasive effect appears to be that of CMV.

4.1. Cytomegalovirus Infection in the Renal Transplant Patient

Cytomegalovirus is ubiquitous among renal transplant patients, with 60–96% of patients demonstrating laboratory and/or clinical evidence of the infection in the first year post-transplant.[1,2,41–43,100–104] Virtually all such infections have their onset 1–4 months post-transplant, although a few examples of clinically important infection with onset of disease as late as the second year post-transplant have been reported.[105,106] CMV has three important characteristics, which it shares with other members of the human herpes virus group (HSV, EBV, and VZV) that help explain its importance in clinical transplantation[106–108]:

Latency: Primary infection results in lifelong dormant infection capable of being reactivated by such factors as immunosuppression and allograft rejection at any point in the future.
Cell association: Spread of the virus occurs from cell to cell with direct contact between the cells being important, thus rendering neutralizing antibody inefficient and cell-mediated immunity predominant in controlling the infection.
Oncogenicity: As with all the herpes group viruses, CMV must be considered potentially oncogenic.

Because of these characteristics, CMV is modulated by the two phenomena which are unique to the transplant experience—allograft rejection and a chronic state of immunosuppression. The end result is two effects: CMV, which latently infects much of the normal population, will be reactivated, and the ability of the host to eradicate either reactivated or newly acquired virus is greatly impaired, leading to a state of chronic or prolonged viral infection. The consequences of this are a much broader range of clinical effects than usually associated with infectious processes.[108,109] These clinical effects of CMV in the transplant recipient can be grouped into four distinct categories[106,108]:

1. A variety of clinical infectious disease syndromes produced directly by the virus itself, ranging from prolonged fevers, pneumonia, hepatitis, and colitis acutely to a chronically progressive chorioretinitis.
2. An immunosuppressed state produced by the virus that is over and above that caused by the immunosuppressive drugs being administered, but that contributes significantly to the net immunosuppressed state of the transplant patient and plays an important role in the pathogenesis of opportunistic superinfection due to Pneumocystis carinii, a variety of fungi, and Listeria monocytogenes.
3. A form of allograft dysfunction that appears to be associated with CMV, and apparently has a different pathogenesis, histologic appearance, and clinical course than does classic allograft rejection.
4. Malignancy possibly produced or made possible by the virus.

The first two of these clinical effects of CMV are well established; the last two must be regarded as more controversial than proven at the present time.

4.1.1. Epidemiology of Cytomegalovirus Infection in the Renal Transplant Patient

Until recently, two major epidemiological patterns of CMV infection were recognized among renal transplant patients: primary and reactivation infection.[41-43,101-104,106-109] Now, with the advent of such molecular biologic techniques as DNA restriction enzyme analysis, which permit the exquisite characterization of each isolate of CMV, it has been possible to define a third major pattern, superinfection.[110-112] Each of these carries a different significance for the transplant patient.

Primary CMV disease occurs when the transplant patient has had no pretransplant experience with this virus (and is seronegative for CMV before the transplant), and is infected with virus carried latently in cells from a seropositive, latently infected donor. Some 80–90% of the time, the kidney allograft is the source of such infections. In the remainder, viable leukocyte-containing blood products from seropositive donors are the source of primary infection.[41-43,101-104,106-109] Data generated from a multicenter study of 50 transplant centers in the United States demonstrated the following[113]: Approximately 90% of seronegative recipients who receive kidneys from seropositive cadaveric donors, as opposed to approximately 70% of seronegative recipients of kidneys from seropositive living related donors, seroconvert post-transplant. Presumably, this difference in attack rate is due to the increased level of rejection and added amounts of immunosuppressive therapy associated with the transplantation of cadaveric as opposed to living related donors. In addition, approximately 20% of seronegative patients who received allografts from seronegative donors seroconverted. All these patients had received transfusions of blood products containing viable leukocytes post-transplant. In contrast, among 79 seronegative individuals who received kidneys from seronegative donors and who were not transfused, not a single instance of seroconversion could be demonstrated. Thus, although the latently infected allograft is the major source of primary CMV infection, blood transfusions can also provide a sufficient number of latently infected cells to cause primary infection in the transplant patient. There appears to be no differences in either the incidence of symptomatic disease or the severity of these symptoms whether the source of the primary infection is the allograft or blood transfusions.

The second major epidemiologic pattern of CMV infection post-transplant is that of reactivation disease in which the transplant recipient who has been infected with CMV previously (and is seropositive for CMV before the transplant) reactivates endogenous latent virus. It would appear that essentially every patient who is seropositive pretransplant will show some evidence (serologic and/or virologic) of CMV reactivation or superinfection post-transplant.[41-43,101-104,106-109,114,115]

The newest form of CMV infection recognized is superinfection. The possible occurrence of this phenomenon had been a cause of much speculation for some time, as it had long been recognized that human CMV isolates in nature exhibit considerable genomic and antigenic heterogeneity.[106-109] Studies in other forms of CMV infection, i.e., in congenital CMV (for which detailed analysis of viral isolates from consecutive congenitally infected offspring of the same mother demonstrated on rare occasions superinfection),[116] and the AIDS patient[117] had clearly demonstrated that superinfection could occur. Fryd et al.[118] suggested that such was occurring in renal transplant patients as well, and that superinfection was clinically important because seropositive recipients of kidneys from seropositive donors had a worse outcome than if the kidneys came from seronegative donors. Smiley et al.[119] confirmed this observation. Recent studies by Wertheim et al.,[110] Grundy et al.,[112] and Chou,[111] using DNA restriction enzyme analysis techniques, have now proved this hypothesis to be true. In as many as 50% of renal transplant patients who are seropositive prior to transplant and receive a kidney from a seropositive cadaveric donor, the virus that is activated is of donor rather than endogenous origin. In addition, preliminary data suggest that whereas the patients with superinfection are commonly symptomatic, those with true reactivation infection rarely manifest symptoms.

The demonstration that superinfection occurs commonly has important clinical implications as well as scientific ones. Clearly, it increases the desirability of a CMV seronegative donor. More important are the implications of these observations for vaccine development. If natural infection cannot prevent symptomatic superinfection post-transplant, then a monovalent, attenuated live virus vaccine is unlikely to do so. The ineffectiveness of such a vaccine[120] would therefore be predictable for this reason alone.

The level of CMV infection in the general community has important effects on the occurrence of CMV among transplant patients (In general, in Western Europe and North America, the level of seropositivity by age 2 is 15%, 30% in young adults, and 50–60% over the age of 50, with higher rates among lower socioeconomic groups, male homosexuals, recipients of blood transfusions, and the sexually promiscuous.)[107] First, the incidence of CMV infection and the percentage of cases due to primary infection, superinfection, or reactivation disease will vary from center to center depending on the population being served. Second, the transplant patient who escapes CMV infection in the period 1–4 months post-transplant is still susceptible to acquiring the virus due to contacts within the general community. Thus, we have seen two sexually active transplant patients who developed non-fatal primary CMV infection more than two years post-transplant.[106] In contrast to this means of spread, it should be emphasized that person-to-person spread of CMV among dialysis and transplant unit patients and personnel does not appear to occur.[121]

Although the great majority of transplant patients (>95%) who develop CMV infection post-transplant do so in the time period 1–4 months post-transplant, Linnemann et al.[105] reported two patients who developed fatal CMV infection more than 1 year post-transplant. One patient, a 19-year-old male college student, apparently acquired lethal primary infection in the community. The second case was a 53-year-old man who was seronegative prior to transplant but transiently seroconverted (by complement fixation assay) 6 weeks post-transplant; 16 months post-transplant, he developed lethal disseminated CMV infection, with rising levels of complement-fixing and immunofluorescent IgG and IgM antibodies. This represents either a highly unusual case of late reactivation, or, more likely, superinfection from the general community in an individual with an impaired host response to his first episode of infection.[106]

4.1.2. Factors Influencing Cytomegalovirus Infection in Renal Transplant Patients

The most important exogenous factor influencing the course of CMV infection post-transplant is the kind and intensity of immunosuppression administered. Steroids, by themselves, appear to have minimal effects in terms of reactivating latent CMV.[122] Thus, CMV infection in transplant patients was essentially unknown prior to the addition of such cytotoxic drugs as cyclophosphamide and azathioprine to the antirejection regimen.[106-109] Of all the immunosuppressive agents used in transplant patients, antilymphocyte antibody preparations have the greatest CMV-promoting effect.[123–125] In particular, Cheeseman et al.[123] reported that when antithymocyte globulin is added to conventional azathioprine and prednisone regimens (as has been traditionally the practice), there was a higher rate of viremia and symptomatic disease in the ATG group. In addition, beneficial effects of a prophylactic course of α-interferon (αIF) on CMV infection that could be observed in patients receiving azathioprine and prednisone alone were totally abrogated in patients receiving ATG as well. That this was not just the effect of the ATG was suggested by a subsequent study in which the ATG group was given approximately 50% as much azathioprine and prednisone as the group of patients who only received these latter drugs. In this study there was no difference in either the incidence or clinical impact of CMV between the two groups, suggesting that it is the net immunosuppressive effect or net cytotoxic (? lymphocytotoxic) effect that is important, not just the particular agents that are employed, in determining the effects of CMV on the transplant patient.[126] We have made similar observations in patients treated for rejection with the pan-T-cell monoclonal antibody OKT3. Thus, as noted in Table 1, routine practice should include the decrease or cessation of other immunosuppressive agents, when an antilymphocyte antibody preparation of any kind is used in a transplant patient.

The importance of immunosuppressive therapy in modulating the impact of CMV infection was particularly emphasized in the previously mentioned multicenter seroepidemiologic study (which included more than 1200 patients from 50 transplant centers).[113] The findings in recipients of cadaveric renal allografts were striking: patients at risk of primary CMV treated with conventional immunosuppression (azathioprine and prednisone) had a similar rate of survival with a functioning allograft at 6 months to that of those without experience with CMV. When patients at risk for primary CMV had been treated with ATG or antilymphocyte globulin (ALG) in addition to conventional therapy, there was a significant decrease in the percentage of patients surviving with functioning grafts (53.1% versus 70.8%, $p = 0.05$). By contrast, patients at high risk of reactivation disease had a markedly improved outcome (71% survival with a functioning graft at 6

months versus 61%, $p = 0.003$) if they had received antilymphocyte therapy.

These observations have two important implications.[106] First, for more than a decade, antilymphocyte preparations have been employed as immunosuppressive agents in a variety of trials in human transplantation that have failed to demonstrate consistently increased allograft survival, despite clear-cut results in a variety of animal species. It would appear from this study that a possible explanation for this rests in the fact that different transplant centers have contained different mixtures of patients at risk for primary CMV, reactivation CMV (and superinfection CMV), or no CMV. Administering ATG or ALG uniformly to each of these groups without considering the CMV status would be destined to confuse the issue by mixing patients likely to have benefits from such therapy (those at risk for reactivation disease) with those likely to be harmed by it (those at risk for primary disease). Therefore, if antilymphocyte preparations are to be considered for therapy in a given patient, then knowledge of the donor and recipient's CMV status pretransplant should influence the decision-making.

Second, on a broader scale, such findings suggest that whenever innovative immunosuppression is evaluated, the impact on viral infections in general and CMV in particular are important variables to be considered. It is highly likely that one form of immunosuppression will be better or worse depending upon the patient's CMV (and/or EBV, hepatitis, or human immunodeficiency virus) status. No longer is it sufficient to consider only "immunologic variables" when considering efficacy of an immunosuppressive regimen.[106,113]

Clearly, such an evaluation is necessary when considering the impact of cyclosporine therapy. Bia et al.[127] reported little difference in the occurrence of CMV infection whether conventional immunosuppression or cyclosporin was employed. Weir et al.[128] noted that patients at risk for primary infection who are treated with cyclosporine as their main chronic immunosuppressive agent continue to have considerable morbidity and mortality. By contrast, patients who are antibody positive prior to transplant may have less symptomatic CMV infection if they receive cyclosporine. Although the available data are still incomplete, the following observations would appear to be valid at the present time[127,129,130]:

1. Cyclosporine therapy, with or without low-dose prednisone, is associated with a lower incidence of infection than conventional azathioprine–prednisone therapy, when the conventional therapy group also receives antilymphocyte antibody treatment, either prophylactically or as an acute rejection treatment.
2. Cyclosporine therapy, with or without low-dose prednisone, and conventional azathio-prine–prednisone therapy without anti-lymphocyte antibody treatments are associated with similar rates of infection or perhaps even a slightly higher rate in the cyclosporine patients.
3. *Overall, since cyclosporine use is associated with decreased allograft rejection, and a lesser need for adjunctive antilymphocyte treatment, the use of cyclosporine may be associated with a lower incidence of symptomatic infection for a given rate of allograft survival.* Thus, once again the entire immunosuppressive program, not just one component of it, must be kept in mind.

4.1.3. Infectious Disease Syndromes Produced by Cytomegalovirus

Whatever the category of CMV infection—primary, reactivation, or superinfection—its clinical and virologic manifestations are primarily seen in the time period 1–4 months post-transplant. One measure of the importance of CMV comes from the observation that approximately 50% of transplant patients with fever have evidence for CMV infection, and that CMV itself accounts for more than two-thirds of fevers in this time period.[101–104,125,131–135] Approximately 60–70% of patients at risk of primary CMV infection will develop clinical symptoms related to the infection. Traditionally, it has been stated that 20–25% of individuals who are seropositive prior to transplant will develop clinical symptoms due to CMV.[1,107,107] Recent data generated by Grundy et al.[112] suggest that this can be refined further. In their study, 50% of these patients developed superinfection with a new strain of CMV, with 40% becoming symptomatic; the 50% with reactivation of endogenous virus had a 0% incidence of symptomatic disease. If these observations can be

confirmed, new approaches to CMV infection would be reasonable.

As with most viral infections, CMV usually begins insidiously with constitutional symptoms of anorexia, malaise, and fever, often accompanied by myalgias and arthralgias. In many patients, unexplained fever and constitutional symptoms are all that the virus produces—in fact, prolonged fever is the most common recognizable clinical syndrome produced by CMV (approximately one-third of patients with clinically overt disease).[104] These patients resemble normal hosts with CMV mononucleosis, even to the presence of 5–10% atypical lymphocytes on peripheral blood smear. The major difference lies in the usual absence of splenomegaly and lymphadenopathy in the renal transplant patients. In about one-third of patients who develop fever, a dry nonproductive cough develops within a few days of the onset of the constitutional symptoms. Initially, dyspnea and tachypnea are not noted, but over several days progressive respiratory distress can ensue, although most patients with CMV pneumonia experience little respiratory distress at rest. On physical examination in patients with respiratory symptoms secondary to CMV infection, auscultation of the lungs is usually unrevealing. The best correlate on physical examination with the degree of respiratory embarrassment—hypoxemia on arterial blood gas (ABG) determination and pneumonia on chest radiography—is the respiratory rate.

The radiographic manifestations of CMV pneumonia in the renal transplant patient may take a variety of forms. By far the most common form is a bilateral, symmetrical, peribronchovascular (interstitial) process predominantly affecting the lower lobes.[104] Although a few transplant patients with CMV pneumonia progress to total lung whiteout and respiratory failure,[126] in most individuals the lung involvement is relatively minor and would go unappreciated if a chest radiograph had not been obtained. Less commonly, a focal consolidation more suggestive of bacterial or fungal disease,[104] or even a solitary pulmonary nodule may be caused by CMV.[137] Positive gallium scans of the lungs have been reported in patients with CMV pneumonitis,[138] although in our opinion this adds little to the diagnostic decision-making process. An important point that cannot be overemphasized when considering the rate of progression of pneumonia in renal transplant patients is that CMV causes a subacute process that evolves over several days. In this population of patients, the major differential consideration is to rule out *Pneumocystis carinii* infection, which presents in similar fashion and which is frequently present in addition to CMV. If acute respiratory deterioration over less than 12 hr occurs, superinfection with bacterial or invasive fungal agents should be considered rather than attributing such a deterioration to exacerbation of the CMV infection. A relapsing form of CMV pneumonia has been reported, occurring when immunosuppression is reinstituted after recovery from serious CMV infection.[139]

Hematologic abnormalities are common during the course of CMV infection. For example, small numbers of atypical lymphocytes may be detected on examination of the peripheral blood smear. The most important effects, however, are on the WBC and platelet counts. Leukopenia, often to counts less than 1500/mm^3, and/or thrombocytopenia, usually in the range of 30,000–60,000/mm^3 but sometimes even lower, occur about as frequently as pneumonia in patients receiving conventional immunosuppression, and may have a great clinical impact, the former predisposing to serious superinfection (see Section 4.1.4) and the latter to a major bleeding diasthesis.[41-43,101-104,140] It appears that such profound CMV-induced hematologic abnormalities are much less common in patients receiving cyclosporine-based immunosuppressive therapy.

Abnormal liver function tests are not uncommon in the course of CMV. In fact, the combination of fever, transient elevations in the transaminase level, and decreases in the WBC and platelet counts 1–4 months post-transplant is the classic presenting finding with CMV infection. More sustained and profound alterations in liver function may also be observed, meriting a true diagnosis of hepatitis. Although both acute and chronic hepatitis beginning at this point posttransplant in patients with CMV infection has been attributed to this virus, proof of this theory is lacking. Until the nature of non-A, non-B hepatitis is established, and laboratory tests are available to test for its presence, the contribution of an infection as ubiquitous as CMV to the morbidity and mortality of hepatitis in this setting cannot be determined.[41,42,101-104,135,141]

Simmons and colleagues at the University of Minnesota have emphasized what they have termed the lethal CMV syndrome,[134] which begins with fever and leukopenia, as does the more benign form of the illness, but progresses rapidly to include severe pulmonary and hepatic dysfunction, central nervous system (CNS) abnormalities, GI hemorrhage, and death. Death is usually due to superinfection or bowel hemorrhage. Fortunately, this lethal syndrome is quite uncommon with current immunosuppressive regimens. However, an important additional clinical insight emerged from the study of these patients. When their GI tracts are examined, typical CMV inclusions may be seen at the site of ulceration producing the hemorrhage and the virus can be isolated. The virus appears to be playing an important role in causing the ulceration, hemorrhage, perforation, and, possibly, the development of pneumatosis intestinalis. Although the right colon, particularly at the cecal level, is the usual site for this, such areas as the stomach and proximal small bowel may also be affected. It is now recognized that CMV-associated GI lesions can appear in the absence of other manifestations of CMV disease.[134,142-146]

Less common acute clinical problems in the renal transplant patient have been attributed to acute CMV infection. These include encephalitis,[147] transverse myelitis,[148] and skin ulcerations associated with an apparent cutaneous vasculitis.[149]

An important problem in deciphering the contribution of CMV infection to the causation of a particular clinical syndrome has been the fact that the virus is ubiquitous in this patient population, and large numbers of asymptomatic infections occur. The demonstration of viremia (isolation of virus from buffy coat specimens), as opposed to peripheral excretion in the saliva or the urine or rises in antibody titer, is, when present, highly associated with clinically important infection, both acute and chronic.[123,150,151] The absence of viremia, however, does not rule out the presence of clinically important CMV disease, and better laboratory markers of clinically significant disease are badly needed. Approximately 50% of patients with acute CMV infection will continue to excrete the virus in their saliva and/or urine 2–5 years posttransplant, with approximately 20% continuing thereafter, although clinical effects of such viral excretion are not apparent. By contrast, an occasional patient (probably 1%–5%) will have chronic CMV viremia demonstrable, and this can be correlated with the presence of progressive CMV-induced

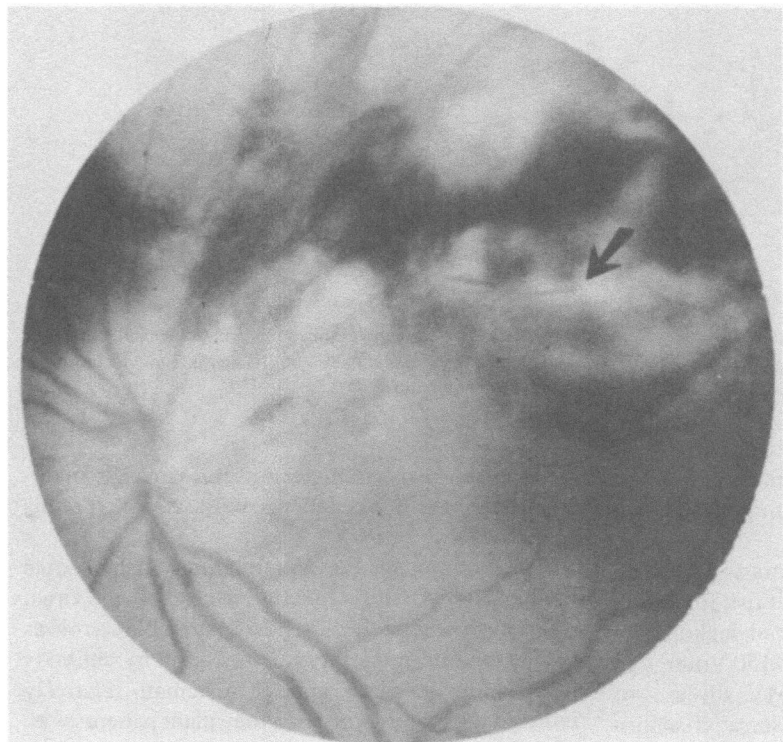

FIGURE 2. Fundoscopic appearance of cytomegalovirus chorioretinitis. Hemorrhagic infarction of retina extends from optic disc along course of superotemporal vessels. Broad expanse of intense white retinal necrosis is largely obscured by extensive hemorrhage. Arteriole coursing through zone of necrosis is attenuated and sheathed (arrow). (From Nicholson [158])

chorioretinitis, apparently in at least 50% of such individuals.[151,152]

Chorioretinitis is the major late manifestation of CMV infection, usually being noted for the first time more than 6 months posttransplant. Although the retinitis may be asymptomatic at the time of discovery, most patients present with complaints of blurred vision, scotoma, and decreased visual acuity. Although symptoms are frequently restricted to one eye initially, progression to bilateral involvement is common. The initial retinal lesion on fundoscopic examination appears as scattered white dots or white granular patches without any characteristic distribution pattern. Irregular sheathing of the adjacent retinal vessels is common. This appearance of a gradually expanding, whitish, necrotic retinitis is thought to be distinctive for CMV in the renal transplant patient (and other chronically immunosuppressed patients). This fundoscopic picture of hypopigmented (white) areas surrounding atrophic retina corresponds to pathological findings in which the retinal pigment epithelium in the involved areas becomes so exten-

sively necrotic that its capacity to proliferate is lost. The white cordlike appearance of the involved retinal arterioles is thought to be secondary to the sloughing of infected endothelial cells from the retinal vessels, which leads to subendothelial hemorrhage and the collection of serofibrinous material in the same area (Figs. 2 and 3). Occasionally, retinal detachment or an anterior uveitis with secondary glaucoma may develop as the retinitis progresses, causing further loss of vision.[152-163]

4.1.4. Superinfection and Depression of Host Defenses Because of Cytomegalovirus

The most important infectious disease effect of CMV infection on the transplant patient is that it predisposes to life-threatening superinfection with a variety of microbial agents. This propensity to superinfection is directly due to the fact that CMV infection, particularly primary infection, has an immunosuppressive effect over and above that produced by the immunosuppressive therapy being administered;

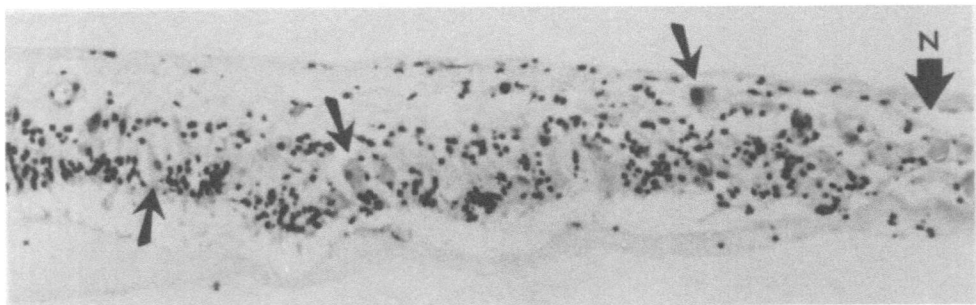

FIGURE 3. Histologic section at margin of retinal necrosis from eye depicted in Fig. 2. Hypertrophied infected cells (smaller arrows) with nuclear and cytoplasmic inclusions are present in region between completely necrotic retinal tissue (N) and that in which normal laminar retinal architecture is preserved. (Hematoxylin and eosin) (× 175) (From Nicholson.[158])

that is, CMV infection is an important contributor to the patient's net state of immunosuppression.[1,2,104,106,108,150,164,165]

The clinical marker that appears to delineate those renal transplant patients most at risk for superinfection appears to be CMV-induced leukopenia. Severe leukopenia (WBC count <1500/mm³) in conjunction with symptomatic CMV disease of greater than 5 days' duration is associated with a greater than 50% mortality caused by superinfection, both of the lung and bloodstream.[104,150] In the lung, *Pneumocystis carinii, Aspergillus fumigatus,* and a variety of gram-negative pathogens are the primary culprits, with a special propensity for concomitant CMV and *Pneumocystis* infection being noted by a number of observers.[164,166] Septicemia with a variety of agents, but most particularly with *Listeria monocytogenes, Candida* sp., and gram-negative organisms, is common in these patients with severe CMV-induced leukopenia. It is of interest that reports of infection in renal transplant patients from centers not actively studying CMV disease have noticed a preponderance of both pneumonia[167] and CNS infection[168–171] in the period 1–4 months posttransplant, suggesting again a major role for this virus in the pathogenesis of serious infection. As with other clinical manifestations of CMV, such events appear to be more common in patients with primary as opposed to reactivation disease (in this context, all patients who are seropositive for CMV prior to transplant are termed reactivation disease, with inadequate information currently available to distinguish between the clinical spectra caused by true reactivation as opposed to superinfection with a new strain of

the virus). Again, viremia is a useful virologic marker to delineate those patients most at risk for this phenomenon.

In addition to the abnormalities in leukocyte number and, possibly, function induced by the virus, a variety of other defects in host defense play a role as well. Humoral immunity, as measured by antibody response to the virus, appears to remain relatively intact in the majority of renal transplant patients with clinical CMV disease[172] except perhaps in those with the rapidly lethal syndrome defined by Simmons et al.[134] One possible detrimental effect of the humoral response to CMV has been suggested by Baldwin et al.,[173–175] who demonstrated that IgM immune complexes appear in renal transplant patients in association with CMV infection, and that these have lymphocytotoxic properties. In addition, some CMV-induced rheumatoid factors may modify the immune response through antiidiotypic activity.[173–175] Cell-mediated immunity, whether measured by skin testing with *Candida,* SKSD, mumps, or intermediate-strength tuberculin recall antigens or by in vitro lymphocyte responsiveness to CMV antigens is markedly impaired.[176,177] It is noteworthy that patients with demonstrable cell-mediated immunity to CMV prior to transplantation, whether naturally induced[177] or vaccine induced,[178] lose this response in the first month posttransplant and may still be unresponsive more than 6 months post-transplant. Morphologic studies on CMV-infected human lung tissue have demonstrated typical CMV inclusion bodies in the endothelial cells, pneumocytes, and alveolar macrophages, with the alveolar macrophages being particularly affected.[179] With the increasing evidence of the importance of alveolar macrophages in protecting the lung against a wide variety of pathogens, it is reasonable to postulate that these abnormal cells in CMV-infected patients would have a decreased ability to prevent bacterial, fungal, or protozoan superinfection.[180] Studies performed in normal hosts with CMV mononucleosis have shown that CMV may be recovered from both mononuclear and polymorphonuclear leukocytes in the peripheral blood, and there is marked hyporeactivity of lymphocytes studied in vitro.[181–185]

The mechanism by which CMV causes depressed cell-mediated immunity has received extensive investigation. At present, it would appear that CMV infection is associated with suppression of both monocyte and NK cell function, and that monocyte-induced suppression of lymphocyte function is the end result.[181–186] A variety of studies, including ones involving bone marrow transplant patients and patients with AIDS, suggest that cellular cytotoxic function, involving NK cells, cytotoxic T lymphocytes, and antibody dependent cytotoxicity are important in the recovery from CMV infection.[186–188]

The most accessible marker of disordered cell-mediated immunity caused by CMV involves the use of techniques (fluorescein-labeled monoclonal antibodies to T-cell surface antigens and flow cytometry) to quantitate the circulating level of so-called immunoregulatory T cells (the helper T cells and the suppressor-cytotoxic T cells). Both in normal individuals[189] and in organ transplant recipients with CMV and/or EBV infection,[190,191] a marked decrease in helper T cells and an increase in suppressor-cytotoxic T cells can be demonstrated. If the normal ratio of T-helper cells to T-suppressor-cytotoxic cells ($T4^+$ as opposed to $T8^+$ cells) is approximately 1.5, CMV-infected transplant patients (and normals with CMV mononucleosis) have ratios of 0.1–0.5, so-called inverted ratios, with clinical recovery being associated with normalization of these ratios. The clinical correlations with these virus-induced inverted ratios are striking[106,190,191]:

1. The great majority of opportunistic infections occur in the subset of renal transplant patients with inverted ratios. Serial measurement of T-cell subsets can therefore be helpful in guiding immunosuppressive therapy: inverted ratios connoting viral infection, an increased risk of invasive superinfection, and a need for decreased immunosuppressive therapy.

2. The rare cases of opportunistic infection that occur in the face of normal T-cell subsets are usually due to an excessive challenge with the invading pathogen. Thus, the few cases of invasive aspergillosis or Legionnaire's disease we have seen in patients with normal T-cell subsets occurred in the setting of a nosocomial epidemic, and was an important clue to the presence of a major environmental hazard.

4.1.5. Allograft Dysfunction Related to Cytomegalovirus Infection

In 1970, Simmons et al.[192] first suggested that CMV infection could in some fashion lead to allograft dysfunction. Since then, a number of studies have failed to settle this issue, with both positive[190,193–200] and negative[42,102,106,107,201] correlations being made. The difficulty in settling this issue has been caused by two problems. First, the ubiquity of CMV infection and the lack of an adequate laboratory marker for distinguishing clinically important CMV infection from the asymptomatic or trivial have greatly handicapped this effort. Second, there has been a problem in most studies with an insufficient number of patients to permit adequate stratification that would control for such variables as type of donor, histocompatibility match, donor and recipient CMV status, and form of immunosuppression administered.

Two separate studies involving large numbers of patients have suggested that CMV does adversely affect allograft function under certain circumstances. A large-scale study from the University of Minnesota involving a large cohort of patients treated at one institution with a uniform immunosuppressive protocol demonstrated that patients with both primary and reactivation CMV infection have a significantly worse outcome in terms of allograft function than do patients without experience with the virus.[118] In the previously described multicenter study,[113] we demonstrated that cadaveric renal allograft recipients treated with antilymphocyte antibodies who were at risk of primary CMV infection had a significantly lower allograft survival rate.

If, then, under intensive immunosuppression, CMV can adversely affect renal allograft function, what is the mechanism? Cameron et al.[202] reported the case of a woman who lost her renal allograft in the setting of systemic CMV infection. Histologic evaluation of the kidney revealed severe tubulointerstitial changes with intranuclear inclusion bodies and intracytoplasmic herpes type viral particles; there was no evidence of rejection. In this case, a reasonable argument could be made that the renal injury was due to a direct cytopathic injury from the virus. However, such cases appear to be vanishingly rare.

The renal lesion that has been the subject of the most discussion[200,201] regarding possible linkage with CMV infection was reported by Richardson et al.[203] In this study, patients were stratified on the basis of the presence or absence of CMV viremia, with renal biopsies obtained at the time of acute functional deterioration of the kidney interpreted without knowledge of their CMV status. The results were striking. Those patients with nonviremic CMV disease and no CMV disease had renal biopsies that revealed the classic tubulointerstitial findings of acute cellular rejection; in contrast, those patients with viremic CMV disease were free of such changes and, instead, had a distinctive glomerular lesion on biopsy characterized by endothelial cell hypertrophy, necrosis, and loss with narrowing or obliteration of capillary lumens and the formation of finely fibrillary material between cells, and mild segmental hypercellularity. Immunofluorescent staining revealed deposits of immunoglobulin and the third component of complement within these glomeruli. Serial serum specimens were available on two patients with this lesion, and these demonstrated by the Raji cell assay circulating immune complexes appearing just before the time of renal deterioration. Patients with this lesion treated with high-dose immunosuppression uniformly lost renal function, whereas the two individuals with this lesion in whom high-dose immunosuppression was discontinued recovered significant function, although chronic glomerulonephritis could be demonstrated in later biopsies. No viral particles were seen by electron microscopy, nor were any viral antigens detectable by immunofluorescent staining with polyclonal anti-CMV antibodies or monoclonal antibodies to CMV early and late antigens. There were minimal findings of interstitial mononuclear infiltrate in these patients, but vascular injury was not uncommon.[203,204]

Since our description of this glomerular lesion,[203] its existence has been confirmed by several groups.[200,201,205] What has been controversial is the issue of whether this lesion is related to CMV infection.[200,201,205] In the original study,[203] CMV viremia was the stratification marker that permitted us to separate out this lesion. Since then, it has become clear in our studies that the glomerular lesion can occur in the absence of demonstrated viremia, but always with some other evidence of CMV infection. Overall, CMV-infected recipients who are viremic have about twice the frequency of glomerulopathy as those who are nonviremic (58% versus 32%). Of 36 biopsies taken for renal allograft dysfunction, the glomerulopathy was observed in 12 of 25 (48%) of those with CMV and 0 of 11 with no virologic or serologic evidence of CMV ($p < 0.005$).[204] In addition, the glomerulopathy is highly associated with the presence of the previously described viral-induced inverted ratio of T-helper/T-suppressor–cytotoxic cells ($T4^+/T8^+$).[190] Other observers, however, have failed to note this same association with CMV infection.[201]

What all observers do agree on is the fact that this glomerular lesion only occurs in renal allografts. Studies in bone marrow transplant patients, AIDS patients, and nonimmunosuppressed individuals with CMV infection who had renal tissue looked at have failed to yield evidence of this lesion.[201,204,206]

Our group has made three additional observations concerning this form of allograft injury since the original description. First, although the absence of classic tubulointerstitial signs of cellular rejection greatly facilitated the original recognition of the glomerular lesion, a number of cases have now been observed in which both the glomerular lesion and interstitial inflammation have been seen.[200,204] Particularly noteworthy are patients in whom both abnormalities are present in the initial biopsy. The patient is then treated with antilymphocyte antibody for rejection, and rebiopsy reveals clearing of the interstitial inflammation but no change or progression in the glomerular lesion.

Second, there is a marked difference in prognosis with antirejection therapy if the patient has or does not have the glomerular lesion on biopsies performed because of decreasing renal function. In patients with a normal T4/T8 ratio and no evidence of the glomerulopathy (and thus allograft dysfunction on the basis of classic rejection), a recovery rate of

95% is noted, whereas patients with these abnormalities have a less than 10% recovery rate.[204,207]

Third, studies of the infiltrating cells present in the glomerulopathy biopsies as opposed to those from patients with tubulointerstitial cellular rejection without the glomerular lesion have been carried out.[208] These studies revealed increased numbers of T cells in the glomeruli of the glomerulopathy cases (11.4 ±2.4 cells/glomerular cross section versus 1.4 ± 1.8, $p < 0.03$); these T cells were virtually all T8 antigen positive; there was an increase in activated mononuclear phagocytes present; and the glomeruli from the glomerulopathy cases stained more intensely for HLA class I antigens than the tubules, in contrast to the typical rejection cases.

There is thus compelling evidence that the glomerulopathy is distinct from classic rejection. It is highly associated with CMV infection, but cases without CMV infection have been described (although the completeness of the virologic workup in at least some of these cases may be questioned). There is no evidence of direct viral injury or immune-complex injury, although CMV infection in general is associated with circulating immune complexes.[174,175,203] How can we put together this information? At present, the leading hypothesis is that this lesion is an indirect result of viral infection and/or other insults. It has been shown that allograft rejection is associated with the upregulation of major histocompatability complex (MHC) antigens on renal allograft cells.[209–212] Several studies have suggested that this upregulation is due to the in situ release of interferon (IF) by a variety of cells, particularly activated T cells.[209–212] CMV infection is associated with the production and release of both IF_γ and IF_α. Recently, von Willebrand and colleagues[199] reported in human renal transplant patients that CMV infection is invariably associated with an upregulation of MHC class II antigen display in the graft, and that in 12 of 14 instances such an increase was associated with evidence of rejection. We would therefore propose that this glomerulopathic lesion represents an unusual form of allograft injury that is due to the interferon-induced upregulation of MHC antigens on glomerular (and, often, arterial endothelium), with alloreactive cytolytic T8$^+$ lymphocytes being the major effectors of the injury. Although local interferon release could be caused by a wide variety of stimuli, in clinical renal transplantation CMV infection is one of the most, if not the most, important

initiating factor in the pathogenesis of this lesion.[204,208]

4.1.6. Effect of Cytomegalovirus Infection in the Occurrence of Malignancy in Transplant Patients

Like other herpes group viruses, CMV must be thought of as a potentially oncogenic agent. Portions of the CMV genome have been shown to be homologous to the *myc* oncogene.[213,214] Not only is the intact virus a transforming agent in certain cell lines (the in vitro correlate of oncogenesis),[107] but also specific cloned CMV DNA fragments are able to transform the NIH 3T3 cell line.[215] In other species, under special conditions, administration of the virus has been associated with the production of malignancy.[107]

What about humans? Rather weak associations between CMV and human colonic carcinoma and prostatic carcinoma have been made, chiefly on the basis of finding CMV DNA in the tumors of some patients with the former and a higher rate of serologic positivity for CMV in the sera of patients with the latter.[107] A better case can be made for a relationship between CMV and Kaposi sarcoma. First, seroepidemiologic studies of African patients with this tumor have reported that nearly 100% of them have antibodies to CMV in their sera, as do 75–100% of European and American patients with Kaposi sarcoma. Secondly, the incidence of Kaposi sarcoma is highest among those two populations of patients with the highest incidence of clinical syndromes due to CMV, patients with AIDS and transplant patients.[106,108] Penn[216] reported that Kaposi sarcoma accounts for 3% of all malignancies among transplant recipients, as opposed to 0.6% in the rest of the population. These tumors usually present in transplant patients approximately 3 years post-transplant.

Finally, more direct studies in which CMV DNA can be found within the nuclei of tumor cells and CMV antigens can be demonstrated with immunofluorescent techniques on the surface of these cells are consistent with the hypothesis that CMV is at least a factor in the pathogenesis of this tumor.[106–108,217] By contrast, biopsies of normal tissue from these patients fail to show evidence of the virus. Thus, CMV is there, but the question remains, which comes first: Does the virus play a causative role or does the tumor develop first and then supply a suitable site for abortive viral growth? The "smoking gun" has not yet been found, and the evidence to choose between these two possibilities is not yet available.[106-108]

4.1.7. Clinical Management of Cytomegalovirus Infection

Efforts to control the effects of CMV infection can be grouped into two categories—the preventive and the therapeutic (Table 3).[218] Within the preventive category, there are three types of strategy: decreasing the risk of virus acquisition and reactivation, specific immunologic manipulation, and antiviral

TABLE 3. Strategies for the Clinical Management of Cytomegalovirus Infection in the Renal Transplant Patient

Strategy	Comment
Preventive	
1. Protective matching of donor and recipient so that an organ from a seropositive donor is not placed in a seronegative recipient	Not indicated for living related donor transplants, of limited applicability to cadaveric donor transplants
2. Appropriate use of blood products from the time of transplant	Viable leukocyte containing blood products from seropositive donors should be avoided
3. Attenuated live CMV vaccine	Of limited, if any, efficacy
4. Passive immunization with hyperimmune anti-CMV antibody preparation	Very promising
5. Prophylactic interferon	Efficacious, but toxicity a concern—cannot be recommended at present
6. Choice of immunosuppressive regimen	Avoid antilymphocyte antibodies in patients at risk for primary disease
Therapeutic	
1. Decrease immunosuppression; in particular, stop cytotoxic drugs and antilymphocyte preparations	Obligatory first step in management
2. Specific antiviral chemotherapy	DHPG, and possibly foscarnet, very promising
3. Passive immune therapy with high titered globulin preparations	Anecdotal efficacy, needs and merits controlled trials

chemotherapy.[106-108,218] The first of these appears to have some applicability at the present time. Thus, blood products used from the time of transplant should either be from CMV seronegative donors or be free of viable leukocytes (frozen washed RBCs are a practical means of accomplishing this[121]). Similarly, in seronegative recipients of kidneys from seropositive donors, antilymphocyte antibody therapy should be avoided.[113] The biggest question is whether protective matching of donor and recipient pairs should be carried out so that an organ from a seropositive donor is never placed in a seronegative recipient. Although eminently reasonable, such a policy would seriously curtail the already in short supply donor pool. Data currently available suggest that the advantages of a living related transplant far outweigh any possible disadvantages from primary CMV,[113] so the only population to which protective matching could be applied would be to patients awaiting cadaveric donor allografts. Even in these patients we would prefer not to decrease the donor pool and instead employ other strategies, i.e., avoid antilymphocyte antibody therapy and use one of the prophylactic therapies.

Two possible immunologic prophylactic interventions against CMV have been evaluated in renal transplant patients: active immunization with an attenuated live CMV vaccine and passive immunization with hyperimmune anti-CMV globulin and serum preparations. There are two major concerns regarding the attenuated vaccine approach: efficacy and possible reversion to virulence of the vaccine strains either causing acute disease or long-term consequences such as oncogenesis. The second series of concerns have not been borne out, but efficacy is a major problem. When the live, attenuated, Towne strain CMV vaccine is given to seronegative dialysis patients prior to transplant an antibody response usually develops, there is no change in T-lymphocyte subsets, and a significant minority of patients do not develop in vitro evidence of cell-mediated immunity to the virus. Even in those patients who develop a cell-mediated immune response prior to transplant, all evidence of this is lost post-transplant.[219-222] When this is coupled with the previously discussed evidence that even natural infection does not confer immunity to superinfection with other strains of CMV, it is then predictable that this vaccine approach would fail, as has been observed.[120] This is not to say that other vaccine approaches might not work or be desirable, rather, it is clear that the task will be difficult and that a simple, monovalent, attenuated vaccine is unlikely to achieve the desired goal.

Much more promising is the use of high-titer hyperimmune anti-CMV globulin preparations of human origin prophylactically. A carefully performed controlled study by Snydman et al.[223,224] and another by Scheuermann et al.[225] suggest this to be the least toxic, potentially effective prophylactic program currently available for preventing clinical CMV disease (although viral excretion appears not to be affected). The fact that the globulin preparations are polyclonal and derived from many donors is at least theoretically appealing, as such a preparation would tend to cover a broader group of naturally occurring viruses than any monovalent vaccine. If the problem of superinfection with CMV continues to emerge, the use of such a globulin preparation in seropositive patients receiving kidneys from seropositive donors would also be of interest.

The final prophylactic strategy is an antiviral one. IF$_\alpha$ of human leukocyte origin has been reported by us[123,226] to be effective in preventing clinical disease in patients at risk for reactivation infection, and may also have decreased the incidence of both opportunistic superinfection and CMV associated glomerulopathy.[226] In these studies, fever and particularly leukopenia were important side effects, but there was no increased evidence of allograft loss. However, more recently, other studies,[227-229] particularly those employing a recombinant alpha interferon preparation, have noted an unacceptably high rate of allograft loss. Although there are differences between interferon of human leukocyte origin and the recombinant preparation (the former is glycosylated and the latter is not), and there were differences in dosage schedules and immunosuppressive regimens among these studies, these reports of increased allograft loss are of great concern. This concern is particularly appropriate, given the present hypothesis regarding interferon's effects on the expression of MHC antigens and the role this plays in allograft injury (see Section 4.1.5). Although IF$_\alpha$ prophylaxis appears to be efficacious in preventing CMV infection, the toxic/therapeutic ratio is too dangerous a one to permit recommending this form of therapy at the present time.

The last consideration in the antiviral prophylaxis category is a theoretical one at the present time, as the appropriate studies have not yet been carried out. For the first time, specific antiviral drug therapy effective against human CMV appears to be on the horizon. Both foscarnet[230] and 9-(1,3,-dihydroxy-2-propoxymethyl)guanine (DHPG, ganciclovir),[231-233] particularly DHPG, have been shown to be useful therapeutically in immunosuppressed patients with CMV disease. It would be appropriate to carry out prophylactic trials with one or more of these agents.

Although CMV, like most other infections in the transplant patient, is better prevented than treated, there is now a rational approach to patients with clinical disease due to this virus. For any patient with clinical CMV disease, the immunosuppression program should immediately be decreased, particularly the cytotoxic therapy, along with the cessation of any ALG, ATG, or OKT3 therapy. Because of the association between CMV and *Pneumocystis carinii* infection, we have chosen to begin trimethoprim–sulfamethoxazole prophylaxis in patients with clinical CMV disease who are not already receiving it. Specific antiviral chemotherapy in the past with adenine arabinoside[234,235] was associated with a high rate of toxicity including a catastrophic neurologic syndrome possibly related to high blood levels in patients with failing kidneys. Acyclovir is without efficacy for human CMV infection, and interferon is unlikely to be effective. Hyperimmune globulin treatment remains to be evaluated in controlled trials. What is new and exciting is the apparent efficacy of DHPG (and perhaps foscarnet) in treating CMV disease. Although virtually all the experience thus far is in AIDS patients, DHPG appears to be of major benefit for CMV chorioretinitis and may be of use in other clinical syndromes.[230-233a] Clearly, there is a new opportunity for optimism in the management of CMV disease in the transplant patient.

Illustrative Case 3

A 64-year-old woman with chronic renal failure secondary to chronic glomerulonephritis had undergone cadaveric renal transplantation 7 weeks previously. Postoperative immunosuppression had included 21 doses of antithymocyte globulin over a 1-month period in addition to conventional doses of prednisone and azathioprine. Renal and bone marrow function on a current regimen of 100 mg azathioprine and 25 mg prednisone per day had remained excellent. Five days previously, BUN was 28, creatinine 1.4, WBC count 5600, and platelet count 160,000. Over the last 2 days prior to admission, the patient had developed fever, malaise, a nonproductive cough, and anorexia.

On physical examination her temperature was 100.6°F (38.1°C), blood pressure 160/100 mm Hg, pulse 85, and respirations 24. She was a slightly cushingoid-appearing woman in no acute distress. Her skin was normal. Examination of the head, eyes, ears, nose, and throat were negative, save for patches of monilia in her pharynx. Chest and cardiac examinations were within normal limits. Abdominal examination revealed a slightly enlarged, minimally tender liver and a swollen, moderately tender renal allograft in the right lower quadrant. The remainder of the physical examination was unremarkable.

Laboratory evaluation revealed a hematocrit (Hct) of 29%, WBC 2900/mm³ (50% polys, 4% bands, 29% lymphs, 4% atypical lymphs, 7% monocytes, 3% basophils, 3% eosinophils), platelet count 64,000/mm³ SGOT was 67, bilirubin 1.4/1.7 mg/dl. BUN was 69 mg/dl, creatinine 2 3 mg/dl. Urinalysis revealed 2+ protein, 20–30 RBCs, and 5–10 WBCs per high-power field. Chest radiography revealed a hazy bilateral lower lobe peribronchovascular (interstitial) infiltrate. Room air ABGs revealed Pao_2 76 mm Hg, $Paco_2$ 31 mm Hg, and pH 7.49. Initial blood, sputum, transtracheal aspirate, and urine cultures for bacteria and fungi were negative. Cytomegalovirus was grown from the transtracheal aspirate, urine, and buffy coat cultures performed on admission (thus establishing viremia), with the cultures turning positive approximately 3 weeks post-inoculation.

Because of a history of sulfonamide allergy, cotrimoxazole prophylaxis was not initiated. Azathioprine was discontinued, and oral mycostatin was begun. Two pulse doses of 1 g IV methylprednisolone were administered in the first 2 days after admission Over the next week, the patient remained febrile with daily temperature spikes to 102°F (38.9°C), and her WBC fell to less than 1200/mm³ and remained there. Her renal function continued to deteriorate, with the serum creatinine reaching 4.7 mg/dl after 1 week. At this point, the patient began to develop severe diarrhea, and her temperature curve became more hectic. Broad-spectrum antimicrobial therapy was begun with vancomycin, ticarcillin, tobramycin, and amphotericin B. Upper and lower GI bleeding began, and she received a total of 6 units of blood Despite these measures, the patient died 48 hr later.

At autopsy, the salient features were as follows: disseminated CMV and *Aspergillus* infections, multiple superficial ulcerations throughout the GI tract, many of which had cells containing the intranuclear inclusions characteristic of CMV infection within the areas of ulceration; and acute glomerulopathy rather than rejection in the kidney. A Raji cell assay drawn on admission was strongly positive for circulating immune complexes. A serum specimen drawn pretransplant revealed antibody to CMV by complement-fixation assay at a titer of 1 : 32, this rose to 1 : 256 at the time of death.

Comment. This case illustrates many of the salient features of severe CMV disease in the renal transplant patient. Viremia was a marker for clinically important infection. The use of antithymocyte globulin in addition to full-dose prednisone and azathioprine therapy probably predisposed to this severe form of

reactivation infection The cause of death here was not a direct result of the CMV infection but was secondary to the superinfection with *Aspergillus fumigatus* that was made possible by the immunosuppressing effect of the virus. Sustained leukopenia was a useful marker of the gravity of host defense suppression that was produced here The cause of the renal dysfunction was glomerulopathy rather than rejection, and this glomerulopathy was probably CMV associated. In retrospect, at the time of admission, in addition to discontinuing the azathioprine, the prednisone dose should have been markedly decreased, and no pulse therapy should have been administered. DHPG therapy would have been appropriate, although it is not yet clear how efficacious it is going to be in this circumstance. It is worth emphasizing that this severe form of infection occurred in a patient who was seropositive for CMV prior to transplant, it is not restricted to patients with primary infection

4.2. Other Viruses

Extensive studies have now been carried out in renal transplant patients to determine the role of most viruses in causing post-transplant morbidity and mortality. At present, it would appear that infection with such agents as rhinoviruses, myxoviruses, paramyxoviruses, rubella, enteroviruses, and arboviruses is not an important problem in transplant recipients. (Similarly, there is currently no evidence of increased incidence or severity of *Mycoplasma* infection in this population.) By contrast, the herpesvirus group (EBV, HSV, and VZV, in addition to CMV), the human immunodeficiency virus (the cause of AIDS), papovaviruses, adenoviruses, and hepatitis viruses (see Section 4.4 for a discussion of liver disease in renal transplant patients) all appear to have a major impact on renal transplant recipients. When one evaluates the impact of these viruses in transplant patients, one needs to consider the same broad range of potential clinical effects previously outlined for CMV: infectious disease syndromes, immunomodulating effects, possible effects on the allograft, and oncogenicity. This last is particularly interesting as the immunosuppressed individual is probably the clearest situation in medicine where viruses appear to play a role in the development of malignancies. Table 4 lists both the most common viral infections seen in transplant patients and the most common malignancies; it is not surprising that in several instances a close association between particular viruses and the development of particular tumors is beginning to emerge. Most of these infections begin 1–6 months post-transplant.[47,107,108,140,236]

TABLE 4. Possible Relationship between Viruses and Malignant Disease in the Renal Transplant Patient

Viruses	Possible virus-associated malignancy
Epstein–Barr virus	B-cell lymphoproliferative disease
Hepatitis B	Hepatocellular carcinoma
Papillomavirus (wart virus)	Sqamous cell carcinoma of the sk.n
Cytomegalovirus	Kaposi sarcoma
Herpes simplex virus	Squamos cell carcinoma of the cervix uteri and/or lips
Human immunodeficiency virus[a]	All of the above
Varicella–zoster virus[b]	?
Polyomaviruses[b]	?
Adenoviruses[b]	?
Non-A, non-B hepatitis[b]	?

[a]This causative agent of AIDS makes possible the occurrence of a wide variety of virus-associated malignancies— particularly the ones listed here There is at present no direct evidence that the human immunodeficiency virus itself is directly oncogenic

[b]These viruses, which are ubiquitous in transplant patients, are not known to be associated with malignancies However, in the case of varicella–zoster virus, the polyomaviruses, and the adenoviruses, the potential for oncogenesis has clearly been demonstrated either in tissue culture or in other species

4.2.1. Herpesvirus Groups Other Than Cytomegalovirus

4.2.1a. Epstein–Barr Virus. EBV may be isolated from the pharyngeal secretions of renal transplant recipients quite commonly, with one-half to two-thirds of such patients excreting the virus posttransplant (as opposed to 15–20% of normal individuals). As is the case for CMV infection, the rate of viral excretion is increased in recipients of cadaveric kidneys as opposed to those receiving kidneys from living related donors, again suggesting that the increased immunosuppression and rejection activity seen in recipients of cadaveric allografts plays an important role in the pathogenesis of EBV infection in this setting.[236–240] Similarly, the administration of ATG in addition to conventional doses of azathioprine and prednisone is associated with an increased rate of viral excretion.[237] Although an occasional patient with primary EBV infection has been reported,[241,242] the great majority of renal transplant patients with evidence of EBV infection have reactivation disease.[101,103,107,108,236–240] Such viral reactivation and excretion may occur without changes in antibody titer. In particular, heterophile antibodies do not appear in renal transplant patients with either viral excretion or rises in specific antibody titer.[103,107,239]

Detailed studies of EBV excretion and specific antibody responses to the virus in renal transplant patients have revealed the following[236–240]: The frequency of EBV excretion rose gradually from a pretransplant baseline of less than 10% to 40–50% by the fifth month. Virtually all adult patients have pretransplant antibody to viral capsid antigen (VCA) and Epstein–Barr virus nuclear antigen (EBNA). Anti-EBNA titers did not change significantly post-transplant. Approximately one-half of patients who received antithymocyte globulin developed fourfold or greater rises in their anti-VCA titers, whereas none of those receiving conventional azathioprine and prednisone immunosuppression developed changes in their titers. Following ATG therapy, antibodies to the restricted (R) component of the early antigen (EA) increased significantly in one-third of individuals, whereas there was no antibody response to the diffuse (D) component of the early antigen. There were no changes in these antibodies in patients receiving conventional immunosuppression.[237]

Primary infection with EBV has been observed occasionally in pediatric transplant recipients, with a range of clinical syndromes observed: asymptomatic disease, a mononucleosis-like syndrome, and a rapidly fatal multiorgan lymphoproliferative disease similar to that seen in boys with the X-linked lymphoproliferative disorder that follows EBV infection.[107,108,241-243] The infectious disease consequences of EBV reactivation probably closely resemble those observed with CMV, although because of the ubiquity of CMV, the contributions of EBV to individual morbidity may be difficult to discern.[108,237,243] It is clear that EBV has immunosuppressive effects similar to those produced by CMV.[108,190,244] Whether EBV infection has any influence on graft function is totally unknown.

Far more important appears to be the contributions of EBV to the development of B-cell lymphoproliferative disease. Approximately 10–15% of the malignancies observed in organ transplant recipients are a form of lymphoma known as immunoblastic sarcoma (formerly called reticulum cell sarcoma). In these individuals, lymphomatous invasion of the central nervous system, nasopharynx, liver, small bowel, heart, and transplanted kidney is commonly observed. EBV-specific antibody titers, immunofluorescent staining of tumors for the presence of EBNA, and DNA hybridization studies all strongly implicate EBV in the pathogenesis of this tumor. These lymphomas can be classified histologically as polymorphic B-cell lymphomas. It is currently believed that these B-cell proliferations evolve from a benign EBV-dependent polyclonal B-cell hyperplasia to a malignant EBV-independent (i.e., elimination of the virus at this stage is without effect) monoclonal B-cell lymphoma.[245-250]

The current hypothesis regarding the pathogenesis of this condition is as follows: In immunologically normal individuals who have had previous infection with EBV (and hence are antibody positive and latently infected with this virus), circulating cytotoxic T-lymphocytes specific for EBV-induced antigens on the surface of infected B-lymphocytes serve as an important surveillance mechanism in preventing the outgrowth of virally induced, transformed cells that are thought to initiate the oncogenic process that ultimately culminates in lymphoproliferative disease. In immunosuppressed patients, this surveillance mechanism is impaired, with the greatest impairment being seen with cyclosporine administration.[251-254] This was dramatically illustrated by Calne's first report of five lymphomas occurring among the first 23 patients treated with cyclosporine.[255] Fortunately, more recent experience with cyclosporine suggests that when lower doses are used and blood levels are closely monitored, there is a relatively low incidence of these tumors. In addition, in the early stages of the tumor, when it is still polyclonal in character, regression occurs when the cyclosporine is discontinued and/or acyclovir (an antiviral drug with activity against EBV) is administered.[248,250,256] However, a recent report[257] of EBV-related B-cell lymphoma developing in a transplant patient treated with relatively low doses of cyclosporine underlines the importance of continuing clinical awareness of this entity.

4.2.1b. Herpes Simplex Virus. HSV is probably second only to CMV among viral agents causing clinical disease in the renal transplant patient. Virtually all the infections caused by the HSV are as a result of reactivation of latent virus. Information currently available would suggest that approximately three-fourths of patients with antibody to HSV pretransplant will excrete the virus in their throat washings, and approximately two-thirds will demonstrate a fourfold or greater increase in their antibody titers. About one-half of the seropositive patients and two-thirds of those who excrete the virus will develop visible mucocutaneous lesions. There appears to be no relationship among the presence, severity, or extent of such lesions and the administration of antithymocyte globulin or the source of the kidney. There is no evidence that HSV infection has an important effect on allograft function.[107,108,140,141,238,258]

By far the most common clinical manifestation of HSV infection in the transplant patient is herpes labialis, usually beginning by the second week posttransplant, peaking in severity by the end of the first month, and then healing over the next 2–6 weeks. Not only are such infections more prolonged than in the normal host, but they are considerably more severe: large, painful, crusted ulcerations that bleed or interfere with normal nutrition and require at least local analgesia. In some individuals, these lesions can interfere sufficiently with the handling of oral secretions to predispose to aspiration. Intraoral and esophageal infection may occur in association with the herpes labialis, particularly if the mucosa has been traumatized by endotracheal or nasogastric tubes. These should be avoided if possible in transplant patients who have active labial or intraoral infection. Both clinically and radiologically, herpetic esophagitis mimics the effects seen with candidal esophagitis. As in normal hosts, virtually all isolates from patients with oral HSV infection are type 1 (HSV-1).[106,108]

Less commonly, anogenital infection may occur, caused predominantly by HSV-2. Stone et al.[259] reported unusually severe anogenital infection in a small group of transplant patients that was characterized by the presence of large, coalescing, ulcerated lesions that presented a difficult diagnostic problem. Routine bacteriologic cultures, biopsy appearance, and Tzanck preparations were of little diagnostic help, although viral cultures of swabs taken of these lesions grew HSV-2 in 18–48 hr. Such lesions may become secondarily infected and act as a portal of entry for a variety of stool flora, resulting in local cellulitis and/or bacteremias, particularly if the patient is leukopenic. We have seen two transplant patients with recurrent zosteriform lesions on the buttocks caused by HSV-2, and chronic chancrelike genital lesions caused by this virus have been reported.[260]

More severe HSV infections in the renal transplant patient are uncommon. In particular, although HSV may act as a secondary pathogen in an intubated patient with severe pneumonia caused by other agents, it is rarely a primary cause of pneumonia. The clinician evaluating a renal transplant patient with pneumonia who grows HSV from sputum or other respiratory samples should never accept this as an adequate explanation for the pneumonitic process that is present.[261] Although several renal transplant patients have been reported with an illness characterized by severe oral lesions followed by high fever, fulminant hepatitis, GI bleeding, and disseminated intravascular coagulation because of HSV,[262–265] this syndrome is exceedingly uncommon in the renal transplant setting. Naraqui et al.[266] reported four cases of HSV viremia in renal transplant patients with severe mucocutaneous infection. We have been unable to demonstrate this in any of our patients,[123] so the incidence of viremia, and therefore the potential for dissemination, remains unclear. We have observed two renal transplant patients with eczema herpeticum (Kaposi varicelliform eruption), a disseminated skin infection with HSV usually developing at sites of previous skin injury. Both patients recovered without visceral dissemination in association with a decrease in the level of immunosuppression. Anora et al.[267] reported an interesting case of a 34-year-old

man in whom fever and then multiple vesicles around the sutures of his transplant incision developed about 2 weeks after receiving a kidney from his brother. HSV-2 was cultured from these vesicles, and an antibody response was documented. It is now apparent that on rare occasions the allograft may convey active HSV infection, which has resulted in disseminated disease in seronegative graft recipients.[267a]

Central nervous system infection by HSV appears to be even less common in the renal transplant patient. Two cases of HSV-2 meningoencephalitis following anogenital infection have been reported, but more typical HSV-1 encephalitis as seen in the normal host has not been observed.[106,108]

Dunn et al.[268] suggested that the combination of HSV and CMV infections in the same individual were associated with a worse clinical outcome than either infection alone. In their experience at the University of Minnesota, concurrent HSV and CMV infection was associated with both increased patient mortality and increased renal allograft loss.

The major advance in the management of HSV infection in transplant patients is the advent of acyclovir. This drug, which has been remarkably free of side effects, is administered intravenously at a dose of 5 mg/kg every 8 hr or at a dose of 200 mg five times per day po (in adults with normal renal function). Such therapy has markedly decreased the morbidity associated with HSV infection in renal transplant recipients. It should be noted that acyclovir therapy may need to be prolonged beyond the usual 5–7 days if acute antirejection treatment is on-going, particularly if such treatment includes an antilymphocyte antibody. An alternative to treatment of overt infection, is the use of acyclovir prophylaxis in seropositive patients (in doses of 200 mg four times per day for the first month post-transplant), which is quite successful in preventing HSV disease.[260,270] Because of the promptness of clinical response to treatment and the difference in cost, we prefer to treat at the first signs of overt disease.

4.2.1c. Varicella–Zoster Virus. Approximately 7–9% of renal transplant patients who remain on immunosuppression will develop clinical zoster post-transplantation. Such infections are uncommon earlier than 2 months and later than 3 years post-transplant, although this latter number may not be completely accurate. Three clinical syndromes are commonly recognized in renal transplant patients as being caused by VZV. One is a typical localized dermatomal zoster resulting from the reactivation of latent virus present in dorsal root ganglia since childhood chickenpox. VZV can be easily isolated from such lesions, and rises in antibody to VZV can be demonstrated in the majority of such individuals. Second, disseminated VZV infection characterized by hemorrhagic pneumonia and skin lesions, encephalitis, disseminated intravascular coagulation (DIC), and hepatitis may be seen in renal transplant patients with primary VZV infection. Third, a syndrome of unilateral pain without skin eruption associated with rises in specific antibody to VZV has been described in renal transplant patients and is presumably also caused by this virus.[108,271,273] In addition, serial studies in renal transplant patients have demonstrated that asymptomatic rises in antibody titer to VZV may occur. This finding has been ascribed to an unstable relationship between virus and host and is cited in support of the argument by Hope-Simpson that subclinical release of virus with resulting antigenic stimulation may maintain immunity to VZV.[272,273]

The important point to be emphasized is that dermatomal VZV infection, which is reactivation infection, rarely if ever disseminates in the renal transplant patient. Therefore, changes in immunosuppressive regimens and specific antiviral chemotherapy are not as pressing clinical needs as they might be in the management of infections by the other herpesviruses in this setting or in the management of patients with malignant disease and VZV infection.[108]

In contrast to the rather benign course of zoster (a reactivation infection) in renal transplant patients, primary varicella infection can be quite virulent. Therefore, particularly in pediatric renal transplant recipients with no history of previous varicella, serious exposure to VZV should be regarded as important and as in indication for immediate zoster immune globulin prophylaxis (see Chapter 3). In patients with primary VZV infection, acyclovir therapy can be life-saving if started early enough.

4.2.2. AIDS: Human Immunodeficiency Virus Infection

The epidemiologic characteristics of the human immunodeficiency virus (HIV) that make the transplant patient so vulnerable to primary infection via the allograft or blood transfusion have already been discussed in Section 3.2, where screening of all potential donors for possible HIV infection was emphasized. In addition to these factors, certain pathogenetic aspects of AIDS render the transplant patient particularly susceptible. HIV has a special tropism for T cells, particularly T cells bearing the T4 antigen, particularly activated T4 cells. With allograft rejection and the other infections occurring in the transplant patient, it is not unreasonable to suggest that transplant patients have more reasons than most patient groups to have a large population of activated T4 cells susceptible to HIV infection. When this is coupled with the exogenous immunosuppressive therapy being administered, and the immunosuppressing effects of such other viruses likely to be present as CMV, EBV, and the hepatitis viruses, it is predictable that AIDS should be a major problem in transplantation.[47-55]

With primary HIV infection, the gamut of clinical events seen in the nonimmunosuppressed host has been observed in transplant patients, including asymptomatic infection, acute mononucleosis syndrome, AIDS-related complex (ARC), full-blown AIDS, and transmission of the virus to a spouse.[47-55] It is clear that primary HIV infection is to be avoided if at all possible.

What is less clear are the consequences of carrying out a transplant in an individual with asymptomatic HIV infection (who is thus seropositive for the virus) prior to transplant. As of 1986, we are aware of three kidney allograft and 15 liver allograft recipients transplanted in the face of pretransplant antibody to HIV. The 6-month patient survival statistics are discouraging; only one of the kidney patients and six of the liver patients has survived for more than 6 months post-transplant. Virtually all the deaths are attributable to infection.[47,53] Because of this initial experience, we have made the following recommendations regarding organ transplantation in asymptomatic carriers of the virus[47]:

1. All potential recipients of organ transplants should be screened for antibody to HIV. All positive individuals should be verified by Western blot analysis, particularly as multiparous women and recipients of past transfusions might have false-positive responses due to the presence of antibodies to histocompatability antigens present on the cell line in which the virus is grown (chiefly DR-4).

2. Although the number of individuals studied thus far is quite small, dialysis rather than transplantation would appear in most such circumstances to offer the best treatment of end-stage renal disease in patients seropositive for HIV.

3. In patients with liver or cardiac failure for whom no potential alternative life support system is as yet available, it may be reasonable to attempt transplantation. However, because of concerns about excess costs and the inappropriate allocation of scarce organs, this should be carried out only at centers with experience both in organ transplantation and AIDS/HIV research.

4. An international registry is needed to serve as a repository of detailed information on the experience with transplantation in persons with HIV infection.

4.2.3. Papovaviruses (Polyomaviruses)

The human papovaviruses BK virus (BKV) and JC virus (JCV) infect most normal individuals during childhood, apparently without demonstrable clinical illness.[274-276] These agents have come under increased scrutiny in recent years for several reasons: (1) immunosuppression results in excretion of these agents in a large number of compromised patients, most particularly renal transplant patients[277-284]; (2) BKV, JCV, and Simian virus 40 (SV40) are closely related both antigenically and structurally[106,107,283,284]; (3) SV40 and JCV have been linked to the development of the devastating neurologic illness progressive multifocal leukoencephalopathy in monkeys and humans, respectively[285,286]; and (4) all three agents are oncogenic outside their normal host.[283,284] This last is of particular concern in the renal transplant patient, who has an incidence of cancer approximately 100 times that of the normal population, particularly reticulum cell sarcomas with an unusual propensity for the CNS and skin cancers.[287,288]

BKV was first isolated by Gardner in 1971 from the urine of a renal transplant patient 3 months posttransplant who presented with a ureteral stricture during an apparent rejection episode.[277] Since then, an additional 12 renal transplant cases with ureteral

strictures and urinary papovavirus excretion have been reported.[277-284] JCV was first isolated from the brain of a 38-year-old man with progressive multifocal leukoencephalopathy[289] and since then has been demonstrated to be the probable agent of this neurological disease which, for practical purposes, only occurs in immunosuppressed patients, including renal transplant recipients.[285,286] Prolonged excretion of both of these agents in the urine of many renal transplant patients has now been clearly documented.[284] BKV can be cultured from the urine in approximately 7% of renal transplant recipients studied longitudinally, with about 20% demonstrating seroconversion. Cytologic methods and electron microscopy have yielded morphologic evidence of papovavirus urinary excretion in a much higher percentage of individuals, but since BKV, JCV, SV40, and perhaps other as yet unnamed papovaviruses are morphologically identical, the meaning of these findings was somewhat unclear.[277-284] For example, in an excellent study using several diagnostic methods, Coleman and colleagues[278] have reported that of 74 renal transplant patients studied, 30% of those tested for papovaviruses by cytology were positive, 16% by electron microscopy, but only 7% were positive for BKV on culture. Once BKV urinary excretion begins, it appears to persist indefinitely.

The answer to these apparently paradoxical differences between morphologic and cultural data may lie in the data reported by Hogan et al.[284] In this study, papovavirus excretion was demonstrated in 20% of patients, with about one-half of these shown to be BKV and one-half JCV by immunofluorescent staining. In addition, 41% of patients showed diagnostic rises in antibody titer to one or both of these agents. Thus, both BKV and JCV may be commonly found in renal transplant patients. Preliminary data would suggest that most JCV infections were primary, whereas BKV infections can result from reactivation or a primary infection with the latter possibly coming with the allograft.[290] This frequent finding of JCV excretion is of particular interest in that several renal transplant patients with progressive multifocal leukoencephalopathy (a progressive demyelinating disease of brain white matter characterized by the development of progressive motor and sensory deficits and death within 3–6 months) have been reported. Papovavirus was demonstrated by electron microscopy in all four, and JCV was isolated from the brain of one of these patients.[107,291]

In the Hogan study,[284] the urinary excretion of

papovaviruses was correlated with the occurrence of ureteral stricture, arterial occlusive disease, and the development of drug-requiring diabetes mellitus. A possible relationship between allograft dysfunction and increases in antibody to BKV was also noted. The correlation with diabetes is particularly interesting in light of the report that two of three patients Cheeseman et al.[283] found excreting BKV developed pancreatitis post-transplant (as compared with only 2 of 38 patients not excreting the virus).

Thus, there are clues that these agents are prevalent and may be linked to clinical disease. The long-term effect of papovavirus excretion in terms of the development of progressive multifocal leukoencephalopathy or malignancy are currently a matter of speculation. Obviously, a great deal remains to be learned in this area. Although clinical management questions cannot yet even be addressed with regard to these agents, it would appear that BKV is resistant to the antiviral effects of interferon.[283]

4.2.4. Adenoviruses

Adenoviruses are a group of DNA viruses commonly causing infection in the normal population, in whom they produce asymptomatic disease or clinical illnesses such as upper and lower respiratory tract infection, conjunctivitis, and hemorrhagic cystitis.[107] It has recently become apparent that this class of virus may have a special relationship with renal transplant recipients. Three patients have now been described with diffuse interstitial pneumonia secondary to adenoviruses previously not recognized (types 34 and 35). Five other renal transplant patients have had adenovirus 35 isolated from their urines. It has been suggested that in at least a few of these cases the virus traveled in latent fashion from the donor within the renal allograft in a manner analogous to that described for CMV.[107,292-296] In addition, several renal transplant patients have had adenovirus type 11 isolated from their urines in the setting of a hemorrhagic cystitis.[296,297]

There are several implications of these findings: (1) hitherto unrecognized adenovirus types are being isolated and should be looked for among immunosuppressed patients, particularly renal transplant patients (the full extent of their clinical impact remains to be established); (2) the major effects of these adenoviruses in renal transplant patients thus far appear to be on the respiratory tract and the bladder; and (3) since adenoviruses in other species have been shown to be oncogenic,[298] the role of these agents, particularly the newly isolated types, needs to be carefully explored in this patient population that has such a high incidence of malignant disease.[107,292-296]

As with several of the other viral agents mentioned in this section, firm guidelines for the clinical management of adenovirus infection in renal transplant patients are not available. Particularly in patients with adenovirus pneumonia, a decrease in the immunosuppressive regimen would appear to be reasonable. Efficacy of antiviral therapy such as interferon and specific antiviral chemotherapeutic agents has not been studied in this clinical context.

4.3. Urinary Tract Infection in the Renal Transplant Patient

The most common form of bacterial infection affecting renal transplant recipients is urinary tract infection (UTI). The incidence of UTI has been reported to vary from 35-79% in different series,[299-305] and, even more importantly, approximately 60% of the bacteremias observed in transplant patients have traditionally taken origin from this site.[90,306] The pathogenesis of such infections is only partially understood. In the earlier days of transplantation, UTI was usually associated with two factors: technical complications associated with the ureteral anastomosis and urinary tract infection present prior to transplantation.[307] Despite recent improvements in surgical techniques and the common practice of pretransplant nephrectomy in patients with past infection in their native urinary tracts, UTI remains a significant cause of renal transplant morbidity. For example at the Massachusetts General Hospital, a retrospective review of 200 consecutive renal transplants performed at this hospital between 1963 and 1976 demonstrated that 41% of the patients developed posttransplant UTIs. The rate of recurrence following conventional antibiotic therapy was 62%, and there was a 12% incidence of gram-negative bacteremia associated with these infections. It was striking that the attack rate of UTI (35-45%) did not change significantly over the past 5 years of review. Particularly during these last 5 years, factors other than technical complications were important, as the urinary tract sepsis could only be ascribed to technical complications in 4% of the cases. In addition, bilateral nephrectomies were performed 6 or more weeks prior to transplant in any patient with a history of urinary tract infection in the previous 6 months; patients with a history of UTI in the more distant past usually underwent bilateral nephrectomies at the time of transplantation. Therefore, other pathogenetic factors had to be responsible for the high incidence of infection.[305]

The two major factors appear to be the postoperative urinary catheter that is routinely used in the peritransplant period and the immunosuppressive therapy that is administered. Now that bladder catheters are routinely removed 1–4 days post-transplant, it is unusual for overt infection to be documented while the catheter is still in place. However, Burleson et al.[308] reported that although culturing the tips of Foley catheters on removal has not been useful in the normal host, it can be useful in the transplant patient. In their study, none of 15 patients with catheter tip cultures negative for urinary pathogens subsequently developed UTI; in contrast, 16 of 24 patients with positive cultures subsequently developed UTIs during the next 2 weeks. None of these 16 had positive urine cultures at the time the catheter was removed. This would lead to three conclusions: (1) despite the brevity of the catheterization procedure, this is the source of many UTIs occurring in the posttransplant period; (2) culturing the catheter tip may be a useful guide to further clinical management; and (3) infection in these patients extends from the catheterized urethral meatus rather than from contaminated urine collection bags.[309,310] Other factors that may play a role in the pathogenesis of UTI in this setting include the type of ureteral anastomosis that is constructed and trauma to the kidney caused by the procurement, perfusion, and implantation procedures as well as rejection. In animal models, the combination of bacteria inoculated into the bladder and trauma to the kidney will result in pyelonephritis, whereas bladder infection without renal trauma results only in a transient cystitis.[311] The role of the ureteral anastomosis is unproven. However, it is not unreasonable to postulate that if the patient's native ureter and bladder are normal (with no reflux present), the construction of a ureterpyelostomy anastomosis is less likely to lead to reflux and the increased opportunity of delivering bladder organisms

to the kidney than is the construction of a new ureterovesical anastomosis in which the possibility of reflux is always present. Mathew et al.[312] reported that not only is ureterovesical reflux common (24%) in patients who have had ureterovesical anastomosis performed, but such reflux was associated with late graft failure, not because of rejection but because of mesangiocapillary glomerulopathy. The pathogenesis of this lesion is unclear, but a reasonable first hypothesis would be to relate it to the combination of reflux nephropathy and UTI in an immunosuppressed host. Once again, it would seem that surgical technique has a major effect on the outcome of an episode of infection.

The impact of UTI in the renal transplant patient lies in two areas: the direct morbidity and mortality from the infection itself, and the possible effects of the infection in the rejection process. In considering these, it is important to delineate when in the post-transplant course the infection is initiated. There is now general agreement that UTI beginning 6 or more months post-transplant is rather benign, can be managed with a conventional 10–14-day course of antibiotics, rarely is associated with a bacteremia or requires hospitalization (unless superimposed on some other urinary tract complication), and has an excellent prognosis.[304,305,313,314] In contrast, UTI presenting in the first 3 months post-transplant is frequently associated with overt pyelonephritis, bacteremia, and a high rate of relapse when treated with a conventional course of antibiotics.[305] Even transient urosepsis in an immunocompromised host can result in metastatic seeding of other body sites.[315] The explanation for this different effect of UTIs occurring at various points in the post-transplant course may lie in the anatomical site of infection. Studies in nonimmunosuppressed patients have shown that kidney infection (symptomatic or asymptomatic) connotes tissue invasion and a propensity to relapse and, in some instances, is associated with the risk of bacteremia; by contrast, bladder infection is a superficial mucosal process that is easily eradicated and rarely associated with bacteremia.[316] It is likely that the reason early UTI is difficult to treat is because of high rates of tissue invasion and that such high rates of tissue invasion are the rule during the early post-transplant period, at a time closely following bladder catheterization, kidney trauma, and the highest doses of immunosuppression employed during the post-transplant course.[305] This information may be immediately translated into a rational program of antimicrobial therapy.

The importance of UTI in the renal transplant population may extend beyond the direct injurious effects of the infection. Experimental studies in animals have shown that both intact Enterobacteriaceae (which account for more than 90% of UTIs in both normal individuals and renal transplant patients) and endotoxin derived from these organisms are nonspecific stimulants of the immune system. In addition, antikidney antibodies have been observed to develop in some animals with clinically infected kidneys.[317] Serum creatinine elevations are frequent in renal transplant patients with evidence of pyelonephritis.[305] Therefore, in addition to the possible role that rejection may play in the invasion of bacteria into an immunologically injured kidney, the converse must be considered, i.e., that the immunostimulatory effects of kidney infection could potentiate the rejection process and lead to long-term loss of allograft function if not appropriately managed. In addition to such effects from gram-negative infection, Byrd et al.[318] suggested a relationship between *Streptococcus faecalis* UTI and graft rejection, possibly because of the triggering of an immune response directed at antigens shared by this organism and certain histocompatibility groups.

A variety of studies carried out in normal individuals have shown that the anatomical site of UTI plays an important role in determining the clinical response to antimicrobial therapy, with kidney infection requiring more intensive therapy than bladder infection. For example, in normal women, antibody-coated bacteria-negative infection is virtually always eliminated with either a single large dose of antibiotic or a conventional 10–14-day course of therapy; by contrast, ACB-positive infection treated with a conventional course of therapy has a 50% relapse rate.[319] This corresponds well with the 62% rate of relapse observed previously in renal transplant patients treated with such conventional antibiotic therapy. Since it appears that normal individuals with kidney infection treated with prolonged courses of antibiotics (6 weeks) are more frequently cured than those treated with conventional courses,[316] we elected to try such prolonged therapy in our ACB-positive patients, reserving conventional 14-day therapy for those with antibody-coated bacteria-negative infec-

tion. The results have been striking: all patients with ACB-negative infection treated conventionally have had their infections eradicated. Of 14 patients with ACB-positive infection treated for 6 weeks, 13 of the 14 (94%) were cured. The one exception, a patient with chronic rejection and poor renal function (serum creatinine of approximately 5 mg/dl), relapsed within 48 hr of discontinuing therapy, with blood and urine cultures positive for the original organism. Since this study was completed, we have treated an additional 19 individuals with early infection (17 of the 19, ACB positive) for 6 weeks with two failures, both with poor renal function (serum creatinine >4.5 mg/dl) and bacteremic relapses within 48 hr of discontinuing therapy. An additional five patients with late infection (four ACB negative, one ACB positive) have been treated with 2-week courses of therapy with 100% success. Therefore, we would make the following recommendations concerning the antibiotic treatment of UTI in the renal transplant patient: (1) unless some test is carried out that proves that a UTI is restricted to the bladder, all UTIs contracted in the first 3 months post-transplant should be treated with an effective antimicrobial agent for 6 weeks; (2) in patients with poor renal function (we have arbitrarily chosen a serum creatinine level of >2.5 mg/dl), that 6 weeks of therapy should be followed by an indefinite course of suppressive therapy. Nitrofurantoin and sulfasoxazole have not worked well for this purpose,[304] and we have had 100% success in five such patients with cotrimoxazole provided the infecting organism is sensitive; (3) in patients with nonbacteremic UTI occurring 4 or more months post-transplant without overt evidence of pyelonephritis, a 2-week course of an effective antimicrobial agent is administered; and (4) prophylactic oral nystatin is administered whenever a broad-spectrum antimicrobial agent is prescribed.[305]

The approach just outlined has been quite successful in preventing relapsing UTI in our renal transplant population. In addition, we[320] have shown, and others[321,322] have confirmed, that UTI can be prevented using trimethoprim–sulfamethoxazole, trimethoprim alone, and, to a lesser degree, sulfonamide prophylaxis. Using one single strength trimethoprim–sulfamethoxazole tablet (containing 80 mg trimethoprim and 400 mg sulfamethoxazole) at bedtime for the first 4–6 months post-transplant (with nystatin administered orally thrice daily at the same time to prevent candidal infection), we now have a UTI incidence of less than 5%. Preliminary results of studies being carried out by us with such quinolone antibiotics as cinoxacin and ciprofloxacin particularly the latter, suggest that these will be effective as well.

Utilizing this regimen, we have essentially eradicated UTI and gram-negative sepsis from our renal transplant population. Side effects have been minimal. Although trimethoprim–sulfamethoxazole-resistant Enterobacteriaceae can be isolated from the feces of these patients, their clinical significance remains to be demonstrated.[323] One possible further benefit of such prophylaxis is on other forms of infection. Although the controlled studies demonstrating efficacy of antibiotic prophylaxis were aimed only at UTI, it is worth noting that both at our center and at the University of Minnesota[321] *Pneumocystis carinii, Listeria monocytogenes,* and nocardial infection have not been observed among recipients of such UTI prophylaxis. At these dosage levels, concerns of potentiating cyclosporine toxicity do not appear to be borne out.[324]

4.4. Liver Disease in the Renal Transplant Patient

Liver function test abnormalities are frequent in renal transplant recipients, with an incidence of 7–67% reported.[325–330] More importantly, the incidence of chronic hepatitis has been estimated to be 6–16%, with considerable morbidity and mortality related to the progressive liver damage.[328–331] In particular, in patients with functioning kidney allografts more than 5 years posttransplant, liver disease (usually with accompanying sepsis) is the leading cause of death.[332,333] The etiology is diverse, probably including both identifiable viral causes of hepatitis (particularly hepatitis B and CMV), as yet undiscovered presumed viral causes of hepatitis (so-called non-A, non-B hepatitis), and toxic causes of hepatitis (particularly azathioprine, cyclosporine, α-methyl-DOPA, and other commonly administered drugs).[325–331]

Most renal transplant patients who develop hepatitis B infection acquire their infection while they are still on hemodialysis prior to transplantation. Hepatitis B is endemic among the staff and patients in many hemodialysis centers, with approximately 70% of infected patients becoming anicteric chronic carriers of the virus (their blood is HBsAg positive) and approximately 85% of the staff being icteric, with acute symptomatic infection.[334] Particularly in transplant programs in which there is a close association between dialysis and transplant patients, with frequent opportunities for contact between the two patient groups, an occasional transplant patient will acquire his hepatitis B infection posttransplant. It is probable that hepatitis B infection may also be transmitted with the allograft if the donor is HBsAg positive at the time or organ procurement. Thus, routine testing for HBsAg should be carried out before accepting a potential donor.[44,45] The suggestion has also been made that the immunosuppressive therapy administered post-transplant can cause reactivation of hepatitis B infection in patients possessing antibody to HBsAg prior to transplant in a manner analogous to that well documented for CMV and shown to occur with hepatitis B in leukemic patients undergoing chemotherapy (see Chapter 12).[335] Other workers[336] have denied this possibility and have suggested that supposed hepatitis B reactivation is artifactual and, rather, what is being observed are fluctuations in the level of viremia above and below that detectable with current techniques for measuring hepatitis B antigenemia.

The impact of hepatitis B on renal transplantation has become much clearer in recent years. First, there can be a major effect on hospital staff—not only those directly involved in the day-to-day care of the patients but also chemistry laboratory employees and cleaning personnel who are at potential risk of coming in contact with the blood of patients with circulating virus.[337] Thus, precautions must be taken to protect hospital employees from contact with this blood. In addition, all individuals involved in the care of these patients or who potentially come into contact with infected blood or secretions should be checked for the presence of antibody to HBsAg. Any seronegative personnel should be encouraged to receive the hepatitis vaccine, with continued monitoring of their HBsAg and HBsAb status post-immunization.

As for the renal transplant patients themselves, there appears to be a major difference between the impact of hepatitis B in the first 6–24 months posttransplant and the impact in the later period. Patients acquiring hepatitis B for the first time in the first 6 months post-transplant appear to do poorly, with a high rate of death from liver failure, and chronic hepatitis developing in the survivors.[338] Fortunately, with routine testing of donors of both blood and organs, such primary infection in renal allograft recipients is unusual. Since available hepatitis vaccines have a low rate of efficacy in both dialysis[339] and renal transplant[349] patients, careful testing of donors to protect the potential recipient is the best way of avoiding this problem.

During the first 6–24 months post-transplant, patients with chronic HBsAg antigenemia prior to transplant continue to have this, only a minority of them (probably less than 15%) developing significant clinical hepatitis, and there is no adverse effect on either graft or patient survival.[338,341–343] Indeed, London et al.[344] suggested that the host response to hepatitis B infection prior to transplant was a useful predictor of transplant graft survival. In this study, those patients able to clear hepatitis B infection and develop antibody to HBsAg while on dialysis had extremely poor graft survival when compared to those with chronic hepatitis B antigenemia or those with no experience with the virus at all. It was concluded that not only do patients who are HBsAg chronic carriers have as good a transplant result over the first 1–2 years post-transplant as noncarriers, but the results of such antigen and antibody testing were useful markers for the immunologic responsiveness of the patient and his ability to tolerate an allograft without major rejection episodes.

However, beginning approximately 1–2 years post-transplant, HBsAg carriers begin to do poorly. An increased patient mortality is observed in these patients because of chronic liver disease, extrahepatic sepsis, hepatocellular carcinoma, and, perhaps, cardiovascular disease.[332,333,345–349] Of these, cirrhosis, hepatocellular carcinoma, and sepsis appear to be the most important adverse effects. It is important to recognize that in these chronically immunosuppressed individuals, liver biopsies and serum liver function tests are poor predictors of the outcome of chronic HBsAg antigenemia.[349,350] For example, Parfrey et al.[349] reported that 5 of 12 patients with an initially benign biopsy (chronic persistent hepatitis or no liver inflammation) eventually developed cirrhosis or chronic active hepatitis. The risk of death from liver-related complications in transplant patients with HBsAg antigenemia was ap-

proximately 5%/year. These results were striking enough that this group[351] has questioned the advisability of transplanting such patients at all. What impact cyclosporine-based immunosuppression protocols will have on this sequence of events remains to be seen.

As early as 1969, it was recognized that progressive liver disease was a major problem in renal transplant patients.[325] Initially, most of the attention was directed at hepatitis B. However, two kinds of observations led to the realization that factors other than hepatitis B were involved. In several renal transplant populations it was noted that the incidence of heptic dysfunction was the same (approximately 15–30%) whether or not the patients had evidence of hepatitis B infection; similarly, even when hepatitis B was not present in a transplant population, the incidence of liver dysfunction did not appear to be much different from that seen in populations with endemic hepatitis B infection. Attention was then shifted to the possibilities of drug-induced toxic hepatitis and to other viral agents.[329,346,352,353]

The therapeutic agent that has received the most attention is azathioprine. Early experience both in man and more intensively in dogs has shown that azathioprine is directly hepatotoxic when administered in a dose of 2–4 mg/kg per day.[354,355] Indeed, there are a number of reports of azathioprine hepatotoxicity beginning 30–900 days post-transplant, with progression in some instances to chronic active hepatitis.[329,356] In recent years, however, during a period of time when the usual dose of azathioprine given to transplant patients is kept under 2 mg/kg per day (usually closer to 1.5 mg/kg per day), documentation of an important role for azathioprine in the causation of clinical liver disease has been lacking.[357,358] In our own experience, we have discontinued azathioprine in 60 patients with liver function test abnormalities and a negative test for HBsAg, with only three of these demonstrating a return of the liver function tests to normal. In two of these patients, the liver function test abnormalities developed within a few weeks of initiating the azathiorpine, resolved within a few weeks of discontinuing the drug, and reappeared quite promptly on rechallenge. In the third, the liver function test abnormalities developed several years after transplantation, resolved on discontinuing azathioprine, and also reappeared on rechallenge. In most patients administered current doses of azathioprine, there is little evidence of direct drug-induced hepatotoxicity that will resolve on cessation of the drug. However, since discontinuing the agent and/or substituting cyclophosphamide is so easy to do, it is worth trying in patients with significant unexplained abnormalities in liver function tests. It should also be noted that cessation of azathioprine therapy several months post-transplant has no impact on the course of hepatitis B infection.[359] Although a similar dose-related hepatotoxicity has been observed with cyclosporine, this appears not to be of major clinical significance at the present time.[360] However, this must be regarded as an open issue at present. Other potentially hepatotoxic agents, such as α-methyl-DOPA, isoniazid, and chlorpromazine, should be sought and eliminated from the patient's therapeutic program in an effort to restore normal liver function.

With there being little evidence now for a toxic hepatitis, other viral causes of hepatitis are being sought. Hepatitis A does not appear to play a significant role here as it does not in virtually all blood-associated cases of hepatitis.[361] Hepatitis A virus appears not to be associated with either a chronic carrier state nor the development of chronic liver disease.[362] Although occasional reports of disseminated herpes simplex virus affecting the liver have appeared, there is no convincing evidence that HSV hepatitis is more than a rare phenomenon. Infections with EBV, VZV, and adenoviruses appear to be equally uncommon causes of significant hepatitis.[358] Less easily evaluated is the possible role of CMV. CMV is ubiquitous among transplant patients; clinical disease in transplant patients is often accompanied by transient abnormalities in liver function tests; and, finally, hepatitis has been commonly demonstrated in other forms of CMV infection seen in nonimmunosuppressed patients, including congenital CMV infection, CMV mononucleosis, and postperfusion CMV infection. However, convincing evidence that CMV plays an important role in the etiology of chronic hepatitis is currently lacking. Although peripheral excretion of CMV for years following transplantation is common, this is by no means proof of progressive CMV hepatic infection. Perhaps the most convincing argument can be made in the rare patient with chronic CMV viremia and hepatitis and in the few patients with characteristic nuclear inclusions and positive cultures on liver bi-

opsy. However, a full understanding of the role of CMV in the pathogenesis of chronic liver disease awaits the development of methods to rule out so-called non-A, non-B hepatitis. It would appear that at present the most important cause of chronic liver disease is non-A, non-B hepatitis, the agent (or agents) responsible for approximately 90% of post-transplant viral hepatitis.[358,363-365]

Non-A, non-B hepatitis in the renal transplant patient closely resembles hepatitis B;[363] blood transfusions are probably the major source of the infection. Once infection occurs, in more than 80% of patients it remains chronic; both liver function tests and liver biopsies are poor predictors of the prognosis for the patient's developing cirrhosis. Unlike hepatitis B, where the virus plays a significant role in the development of hepatocellular carcinoma, there is currently no evidence for oncogenicity of the non-A, non-B hepatitis virus(es); beginning 2 or more years post-transplant, the insidious onset of cirrhosis is a major problem in these patients. Perhaps the most important effect of this form of hepatitis is that it is immunomodulating, an important contributor to the patient's net state of immunosuppression. In the first year postrenal transplantation there is both an increased incidence and mortality of extrahepatic infection among patients with non-A, non-B hepatitis. Conversely, the 1-year kidney allograft survival rate is significantly greater. Any modality that increases the incidence of infections and increases graft survival is by definition immunosuppressing. The increase in septic complications continues into the later period beyond one year as well.[333]

Illustrative Case 4

A 52-year-old woman with end-stage renal disease due to polycystic kidney disease underwent bilateral nephrectomy and cadaveric renal transplantation. Post-transplant, she had no clinical episodes of rejection, and by 1 year post-transplant she had a serum creatinine of 0.7 mg/dl while being immunosuppressed with azathioprine 100 mg/day and prednisone 30 mg every other day. During the first year post-transplant, despite minimal immunosuppression and the absence of CMV infection, she had had bouts of *Listeria* sepsis, invasive pulmonary aspergillosis, and gram-negative sepsis due to a perforated sigmoid diverticulum This last was treated surgically. Her liver function tests, which had been normal prior to transplant, began to show an SGOT level of 75 units/dl (approximately 2.5 times normal), without other abnormalities, by the third month post-transplant

Over the next 5 years, her renal function remained excellent on the same immunosuppressive program. Her SGOT remained elevated at a level of 60–120 units/dl. Percutaneous liver biopsy performed two years post-transplant revealed minimal changes of chronic persistent hepatitis. Substitution of cyclophosphamide for azathioprine had no effect on her SGOT level, and the azathioprine was restarted.

Six years post-transplant, after a 2-month history of progressively increasing abdominal girth and edema, she presented with fever, rigors, and increasing abdominal pain. Physical examination revealed a temperature of 104°F (40°C), blood pressure of 80/60, pulse of 120, and a grossly distended abdomen with ascites and signs of peritonitis. There were large hemorrhoids and the stool was guaiac positive. Pitting edema was present to the knees bilaterally. Laboratory data included Hct 25, WBC count 17,500/mm^3 with 70% polys, 10% bands, 20% lymphocytes; creatinine 1.5 mg/dl, SGOT 220, bilirubin D/T 7.6/8 9 mg/dl, alkaline phosphatase 320 units/dl (2.5 times normal), and alb/glob 2.7/4.8. Abdominal paracentesis and blood cultures grew *E coli* sensitive to all antibiotics. Despite therapy with high dose intravenous ampicillin and gentamicin, the patient died on the second hospital day. At autopsy, far-advanced cirrhosis with esophageal varices and evidence for spontaneous bacterial peritonitis was noted. All tests for hepatitis B virus were negative. The transplanted kidney appeared totally normal grossly and microscopically.

Comment. A tragic case of chronic non-A, non-B hepatitis infection marred the course of an otherwise successful renal transplant. In the first year post-transplant there were three notable events: several episodes of life-threatening extrahepatic infection, no rejection on minimal immunosuppression, and the development of mild elevations of the serum transaminase level. The transaminitis remained constant over the next 6 years and appeared to be of little consequence, particularly in view of the "benign" liver biopsy 2 years post-transplant. She then presented 6 years post-transplant with far-advanced cirrhosis and portal hypertension, and acute, spontaneous bacterial peritonitis that caused her death. This insidious progression of liver disease is occurring increasingly in patients who previously were regarded as asymptomatic, successful renal transplant recipients. Prevention and treatment of this entity is a major challenge in the next few years.

Thus, we have come full circle in 15 years of studying liver disease in renal transplant patients. It still occurs at a high rate with considerable chronic morbidity and some mortality, and it appears to be mediated by a virus that is transmitted through contact with blood and blood products. The discovery of hepatitis B and methods of detecting it provided an explanation for the disease process in some transplant patients. Further understanding awaits the development of techniques for measuring the presence or absence of other hepatitis pathogens. Decisions regarding clinical management likewise await the availability of such techniques.

5. Infection in Renal Transplant Patients More Than 6 Months Post-transplant

One of the measures of the increasing success of renal transplantation in recent years is the fact that investigators are now looking at long-term survival and complications, rather than the 1 year statistics that have been standard for so long. When one considers the infectious diseases present in long-term survivors of successful renal transplantation, three categories of patient can be defined[1,364]:

1. Most patients who are surviving with good renal function (serum creatinine <2 mg/dl), on minimal chronic steroid therapy (<15 mg of prednisone per day or alternate day steroids), no recent acute antirejection therapy, and no evidence of chronic viral infection. Of more than 300 such patients we have followed for periods of up to 10 years, there has only been a single instance of *Listeria* sepsis and one of cryptococcal meningitis. By contrast, there have been 46 instances of UTI that responded to 10 days of therapy, 9 cases of pneumococcal pneumonia, and 14 cases of influenza (most during a communitywide outbreak). These patients, then, are very similar to the general community.
2. A significant minority of patients who have an excessive risk of opportunistic infection. These patients share a similar phenotype—chronic rejection such that the serum creatinine is greater than 2 mg/dl, a daily prednisone dose of ≥20 mg/day, a history of multiple courses of acute antirejection therapy, and a high incidence of chronic infection with such immunosuppressing viruses as CMV and non-A, non-B hepatitis. Among 100 such patients, there have been six cases of *Listeria* sepsis and/or meningitis, nine cases of cryptococcal meningitis, four cases of disseminated nocardial infection, and two cases of invasive aspergillosis. Those patients are thus at high risk of life-threatening infection and would be better served by transplant nephrectomy, cessation of immunosuppression, and return to dialysis.

3. A few patients with the lingering effects of problems acquired earlier. There are three major examples of this: progressive chorioretinitis due to CMV, progressive liver disease due to one of the hepatitis viruses, and viral-associated tumor development (Table 4).

6. Infectious Disease Problems of Particular Importance

6.1. Central Nervous System Infection in the Renal Transplant Patient

Infection of the CNS is a major cause of morbidity and mortality in the renal transplant patient. For example, at the Massachusetts General Hospital over the 10-year period 1969–1979, 21 of 300 individuals undergoing renal transplantation developed significant CNS infection. Although the subject of CNS infection in the immunosuppressed patient is reviewed in more detail in Chapter 7, several points particularly applicable to the renal transplant patient bear emphasis here. Four distinct patterns of infection may be observed in this population: (1) acute to subacute meningitis almost invariably caused by *Listeria monocytogenes*, by far the most frequent cause of bacterial CNS infection in the renal transplant patient; (2) subacute to chronic meningitis, usually caused by *Cryptococcus neoformans*, although uncommonly cases of infection by *Mycobacterium tuberculosis* and *Coccidioides immitis* among individuals acquiring these infections prior to transplant and the initiation of immunosuppressive therapy may be observed; (3) focal brain infection with focal neurologic abnormalities occasionally caused by *Listeria, Toxoplasma gondii*, or *Nocardia asteroides*, but most commonly by *Aspergillus* infection metastatic from a site of active pulmonary infection; and (4) progressive dementia due to progressive multifocal leukoencephalopathy caused by the papovavirus JCV. Together, *Listeria monocytogenes, Cryptococcus neoformans*, and *Aspergillus fumigatus* account for more than three-fourths of the CNS infections occurring in the renal transplant patient. Each of these infections tends to occur at a particular time period post-transplant: the first month post-transplant is relatively free of CNS infections, although a rare patient with listerial or cryptococcal infection has been reported in this period. If one then divided the time intervals into an early period 1–4 months post-transplant (corresponding to a period of maximal immunosuppression from therapy and the effects of CMV infection) and a late period more than 4 months post-transplant (when the effects of CMV have largely abated and the patient is on maintenance immunosuppressive therapy), then the following observations can be made. *Listeria* occurs equally frequently in the early and late period; toxoplasmosis, *Aspergillus fumigatus*, and nocardial infection almost exclusively in the early period; and cryptococcal infection exclusively in the late period (in the Massachusetts General Hospital series, virtually all cases of cryptococcal infection began more than 1 year post-transplant).[170,171]

It is important to emphasize that the presentation of CNS infection in the renal transplant patient may be very different than in the normal host. In particular, the antiinflammatory effects of the immunosuppressive therapy being administered may obscure the signs of meningeal irritation usually associated with meningitis in the normal patient. For example, in the Massachusetts General Hospital experience, only 60% of patients with *Listeria* meningitis had any evidence of meningeal irritation on physical examination, and in many of these the findings were subtle. Mild alterations in the state of consciousness were observed in 70% of patients; however, the most reliable combination of clinical findings for suggesting the possibility of significant CNS infection is the presence of fever and headache. Any renal transplant patient with an unexplained headache, especially if febrile, should undergo careful neurologic examination. If there is no evidence of papilledema or focal neurologic deficit, an immediate lumbar puncture should be carried out. If papilledema or focal deficits are found on neurologic examination, an immediate CT scan should be performed prior to the lumbar puncture. In addition to the usual laboratory evaluations of the cerebrospinal fluid (cell count, protein and sugar determinations, gram stain, acid-fast stain, India ink examination, fungal and bacterial cultures), all such specimens should undergo analysis for cryptococcal antigen. In addition, it is wise to save 2 ml of cerebrospinal fluid (CSF) for any later special studies that may appear indicated.[170,171]

6.1.1. *Listeria monocytogenes* Infection

Listeria monocytogenes is a gram-positive bacillus that can produce a variety of clinical syndromes, but in the immunocompromised patient, the most important are bacteremia alone, meningitis, meningoencephalitis, and cerebritis without concomitant meningitis. In the bacteriology laboratory, this organism may be mistaken for either a diphtheroid or a *Streptococcus* when first isolated from a blood culture bottle. In the setting of an immunosuppressed patient, such initial laboratory reports suggest the possibility of *Listeria* infection, and appropriate therapy should be begun while awaiting definitive diagnosis. All patients with documented *Listeria* bacteremia should undergo lumbar puncture to assess the possibility of CNS seeding. Even if the lumbar puncture is negative, the assumption should be made that subclinical CNS seeding has occurred.[170,171,365–369] Watson et al.[370] reported relapse of listerial infection with cerebritis in patients treated previously with a 10–14-day course of intravenous penicillin for documented bacteremia. Both Watson's group and ours have observed a similar phenomenon in patients treated for 2 weeks for meningitis. Because of this pattern of relapse, we prefer to treat for at least 3 weeks with meningeal doses of antibiotics for documented listerial infection whether or not CNS involvement is initially documented. Choice of therapy remains controversial. In nonallergic patients, penicillin or ampicillin in meningeal doses is the mainstay of therapy. In the renal transplant patient who may have varying degrees of renal dysfunction, we prefer to use ampicillin, because the alternate hepatobiliary route of excretion will prevent toxic accumulation of the drug while allowing full dosages, which will ensure adequate levels, to be administered. In the laboratory, the combination of penicillin or ampicillin and an aminoglycoside leads to synergistic killing of the organism analogous to what is observed with enterococci.[371] Whether this is clinically important is as yet unknown. Our practice is to combine ampicillin in a dose of 2 g IV every 4 hr with gentamicin at full therapeutic doses for the level of renal function present for the first 7–10 days of treatment and then finish the course of therapy with ampicillin alone. In penicillin-allergic patients, optimal therapy is unknown. Although tetracycline, erythromycin, and chloramphenicol have all been suggested as possible alternatives in the penicillin-allergic patient,[372,373] use of these bacteriostatic antibiotics in the treatment of systemic listeriosis has failed in a number of instances.[374,375] In the past, we have preferred to desensitize penicillin-allergic patients with *Listeria* sepsis and/or meningitis and have used this approach successfully in a total of five patients with meningitis.[170] With the clear-cut demonstration that trimethoprim–sulfamethoxazole can be successfully used in the treatment of life-threatening *Listeria* infection,[375,376] we now would regard this as the preferred regimen in pencillin-allergic patients, reserving penicillin desensitization for the patient who cannot tolerate this drug as well.

Illustrative Case 5

A 30-year-old man had undergone transplantation with a kidney from his sister 8 weeks previously. Initial immunosuppression was with azathioprine and prednisone. Approximately 2 weeks post-transplant, an episode of acute rejection was documented and was successfully reversed with a 2-week course of antithymocyte globulin. Six weeks post-transplant, the patient developed fever, mild leukopenia, and mild abnormalities in liver function tests in association with symptoms of malaise and anorexia. These symtpoms resolved in about 1 week. Virologic cultures performed at this time subsequently grew CMV from the urine, buccal swabs, and buffy coat. Over the 4 days prior to admission, the patient had noted fevers with two rigors and progressively increasing headache and photophobia.

On physical examination, the pertinent findings were as follows: temperature 102°F, a nontoxic-appearing male without evidence of meningeal irritation, and a normal neurologic examination. Laboratory evaluation revealed a WBC count of 4200/mm³ (72% polys, 8% bands, 6% monocytes, 14% lymphocytes). Serum creatinine was 2.2 mg/dl and BUN 52 mg/dl. Lumbar puncture revealed an opening pressure of 280 mm H_2O, 160 WBCs (95% polys), CSF 82 mg/dl and sugar 32 mg/dl. Although initial Gram stains of the CSF were negative, the CSF and three sets of blood cultures each grew *Listeria monocytogenes*.

He was treated for 3 weeks, first with 12 g ampicillin per day and 80 mg gentamicin every 12 hr for 1 week and then with ampicillin alone. He was markedly improved within 48 hr of initiation of therapy and was afebrile by the sixth hospital day. By the end of therapy, his serum creatinine level had returned to its baseline of 1.5mg/dl despite the fact that the prednisone dose was tapered from 30 to 15 mg/day and the azathioprine dose from 100 to 50 mg/day during his hospitalization.

Comment. This case illustrates a number of important aspects of *Listeria* infection in the renal transplant patient. Although some renal transplant patients may have an acute course resembling that of conventional bacterial meningitis in the normal host, the majority will have a subacute presentation over 2 or more days. Meningeal findings may be absent, with fever and headache being the only indication for lumbar puncture. CMV infection, by its immunosuppressing effects, may predispose to the development of this infection. There may be a relationship between the development of allograft dysfunction and listerial infection in some patients, since *Listeria monocytogenes* may be shown to have immunostimulatory effects in some settings.[377] At our hospital, in renal transplant patients without UTI and without indwelling intravenous lines, *Listeria* is the most common cause of spontaneous bacteremia, and hence it is not surprising that it is the most common cause of bacterial CNS infection.[1]

6.1.2. *Cryptococcus neoformans* Infection

Cryptococcus neoformans is the single most common cause of CNS infection in the renal transplant patient, occurring almost exclusively in the late post-transplant period. It is the classic cause of subacute to chronic meningitis, often presenting after several weeks of waxing and waning headaches and fever. Approximately one-third of patients will also note coughs related to the primary pulmonary portal of entry of such infection. Indeed, some of these patients will have simultaneous pulmonary and meningeal infection. Any patient with documented pulmonary cryptococcosis should undergo lumbar puncture, for culture and measurement of cryptococcal antigen, as the presence or absence of CNS involvement is a major prognostic indicator in terms of intensity of therapy needed and for predicting ultimate outcome. The other major sites of dissemination include the skin and urinary tract. This last is particularly important to remember in the renal transplant patient, as urologic manipulation of a urinary tract infected with *C. neoformans* can result in further systemic dissemination. Therefore a urine culture for *C. neoformans* is indicated whenever this organism is demonstrated at other bodily sites. Optimal therapy currently includes both amphotericin and 5-fluorocytosine. However, particularly in the renal transplant patient whose renal function may be unstable, great care must be taken to follow 5-fluorocytosine blood levels closely, as toxic levels of this drug may accumulate with potentially disastrous bone marrow suppression resulting. If renal function is unstable, and levels cannot be easily followed, then therapy should be with amphotericin alone. Neither ketoconazole nor miconazole appears to be a satisfactory alternative for meningeal cryptococcal infection.[170,171,378–382]

6.1.3. *Aspergillus fumigatus* Infection

Other than cryptococcal infection, the most common fungal agent affecting the CNS in the renal transplant patient is *Aspergillus fumigatus*. In this setting, *Aspergillus* appears to occur exclusively as a result of metastatic infection from a pulmonary portal of entry. The usual sequence of events begins with a primary viral or bacterial pulmonary infection in a debilitated patient who has responded poorly to therapy, and this is followed by *Aspergillus* superinfection, which metastasizes to the brain via the hematogenous route within days of its invasion of the lung. Alternatively, the normal lung is invaded because of an unusually intense exposure to the organism due to contaminated air, but again with dissemination via the bloodstream to the brain. Such infections are almost uniformly lethal. The best way to deal with *Aspergillus* CNS infection is to prevent it by either preventing the pulmonary infection entirely or by recognizing it early and beginning high-dose amphotericin therapy before hematogenous dissemination has occurred. The approach to *Aspergillus* infection should be very similar to that with cancer of the lung—prevention and/or early diagnosis and aggressive therapy are the only possible means of curing this disease.[170,171]

Other fungal agents and *Nocardia asteroides* may follow a similar pattern, although usually in less lethal fashion and with a greater chance that a single cerebral lesion may be identified and treated. It is our policy that whenever infection with one of the agents that tends to metastasize is identified in the lung or elsewhere (i.e., *Aspergillus fumigatus*, *Nocardia asteroides*, *Phycomycetes*,) a search for metastatic infection, particularly to brain and bone, be carried out with appropriate scanning techniques. As with all serious infections in the renal transplant patient, early diagnosis and aggressive therapy are the only hope for recovery.[170,171,383]

6.2. Bacteremia in the Renal Transplant Patient

Traditionally, the major cause of bacteremia in the renal transplant patient is urinary tract sepsis, both with and without associated surgical complication. An estimated 60–70% of bacteremias in the transplant patient have come from this source.[90,306] With better surgical results and improved methods for treating and preventing urinary tract infections (see Section 4.3), such bacteremias of urinary tract origin are now uncommon. Gram-negative sepsis at present is primarily the result of GI tract complications of transplantation occurring in one of two settings: spontaneously, in a severely leukopenic patient (often due to CMV) in a manner analogous to that seen in leukemic patients (see Chapter 18); and as part of an episode of peritonitis, particularly that occurring as a result of bowel perforation secondary to steroid therapy. As far as this latter is concerned, it is important to emphasize that immunosuppressive therapy will mask the signs of peritonitis in these patients, and although abdominal pain is usually noted, severe peritonitis may be present in the absence of the usual physical signs of an acute abdomen. Any renal transplant patient with apparent sepsis and abdominal symptoms merits an aggressive diagnostic and therapeutic approach as outlined in Chapter 23.

Beginning 1 month post-transplant in renal transplant patients without overt evidence of septic source or without the presence of intravenous lines, *Listeria monocytogenes* is the most frequent cause of bacteremias at many transplant centers. Therefore, when an initial clinical evaluation fails to reveal a source of infection in a patient who appears septic, the empirical antibiotic regimen should include penicillin or ampicillin in order to cover this organism adequately.

An increasingly important cause of bacteremia in the renal transplant patient is nontyphoidal *Salmonellae*. Whereas in the normal host, *Salmonella* gastroenteritis is associated with a risk of bacteremia of less than 5%, in the transplant patient more than 50% of individuals will have bloodstream invasion with this organism. In addition, in the transplant patient metastatic infection as a consequence of such bloodstream invasion is the rule rather than the exception. Seeding of the urinary tract, with positive urine cultures is the rule. The cardiovascular tree, at sites of preexisting atherosclerotic lesions, aneurysms, fistulas, and so forth, is commonly involved. With involvement of the heart and/or vasculature, eradication of infection with antibiotics alone is often not possible. For this reason, prolonged antibiotic therapy is indicated in any transplant patient with documented Salmonella bacteremia or evidence of metastatic seeding.[385–388]

Illustrative Case 6

An 18-year-old boy, 6 months after a successful cadaveric renal transplantation (serum creatinine 1 0 mg/dl on 15 mg prednisone and 100 mg azathioprine/day), entered with a 2-day history of abdominal cramps, diarrhea, fevers to 104°F (40°C), and rigors Cultures of blood, urine, and stool grew *Salmonella typhimurium* sensitive to ampicillin, chloramphenicol, and trimethoprim–sulfamethoxazole. He was treated with intravenous ampicillin 12 g/day for 6 weeks, with defervescence by day 5 of therapy, and clearing of all his cultures (blood and urine by day 3, stool at 6 weeks). Five days after cessation of the antibiotics he reentered the hospital with fever to 103°F (39 4°C) and rigors Blood and urine cultures were again positive for the same *S typhimurium* He received an additional 4 weeks of 12 g/day of intravenous ampicillin, again with prompt defervescence and clearing of his cultures. During the course of this admission, abdominal CT scan, aortography, echocardiography, and an ^{111}In-labeled WBC scan were all carried out, looking for a particular focus of infection. Other than cardiac enlargement consistent with his longstanding hypertension, no abnormalities were detected He was discharged on amoxicillin 500 mg four times a day PO, and remained well on this regimen for 6 months. At this time, the amoxicillin was discontinued. Two weeks later, he returned with a recrudescence of fever, chills, and the same *S. typhimurium* in his blood and urine He again received 4 weeks of intravenous therapy and has been maintained since (2 years) on oral trimethoprim–sulfamethoxazole free of overt signs of infection.

Comment. This represents a typical case of *Salmonella* gastroenteritis and its consequence in a renal transplant patient. Whereas in normal individuals antibiotics are contraindicated in *Salmonella* gastroenteritis, in the transplant patient they are indicated in an effort to prevent bacteremia and its consequences. If bacteremia is documented, we administer a prolonged course of intravenous and then oral therapy (4–6 weeks IV, a minimum of 3–6 months PO) Presumably, the immunosuppression inhibits the functioning of host defenses in the eradication of this intracellular bacterial infection, and the abnormal vascular tree associated with accelerated atherosclerosis and hypertension in the patient with renal disease are responsible for this series of events.

A different kind of problem is present in the renal transplant patient who has undergone a splenectomy as part of the management of his immunosuppressive therapy. There are numerous reports of overwhelming pneumococcal sepsis in these patients,[389–392] and we have observed *Hemophilus influenzae* type B in this same setting.[170] Such observations, which are similar to those being made in lymphoma patients who have undergone splenectomy (see Chapter 18), are not surprising. It would seem reasonable to administer pneumococcal vaccine prior to transplantation (to thereby increase the chances of an appropriate response) to all transplant candidates who are being considered for splenectomy.[393,394] In addition, patients are given a supply of ampicillin, cotrimoxazole, or amoxicillin to keep with them at home and are instructed to begin therapy with this antibiotic with the first onset of shaking chills in association with an upper respiratory infection. Alternatively, others have employed continuous prophylaxis with penicillin or ampicillin. We have favored the former approach to avoid the selection of resistant organisms and to provide adequate coverage of *H. influenzae*. This added approach should help prevent the overwhelming bacteremias that can cause such lethal damage before the patient reaches medical attention.

6.3. Fungal Infection in the Renal Transplant Patient

Fungal infection in the renal transplant patient is of two types: reactivation of latent infection that had been acquired by residence in geographic areas endemic for these agents prior to transplantation, with reactivation and dissemination as a result of the immunosuppressive therapy being administered, and new opportunistic infection acquired posttransplant. In the first category, there are increasing reports of disseminated histoplasmosis,[395–400] coccidioidomycosis,[401–404] blastomycosis,[405,406] and paracoccidioidomycosis[407] in renal transplant patients. The clinical presentation of such infections is various: a subacute respiratory illness, with either local or disseminated interstitial or miliary pattern on radiography; a nonspecific systemic febrile illness of an acute or chronic nature; or an illness in which metastatic aspects of the infection predominate (e.g., skin manifestations in histoplasmosis and blastomycosis or CNS manifestations in coccidioidomycosis). The clinician must be alert to these possibilities. In this age of widespread travel, increasing numbers of cases of disseminated histoplasmosis, coccidioidomycosis, and blastomycosis are being identified at medical centers outside the geographic areas endemic for these infections. Therefore, a careful epidemiologic history is necessary in the evaluation of any immunosuppressed patient with a perplexing infectious disease syndrome. All unexplained skin lesions should be promptly biopsied; bone marrow biopsies should be carried out expeditiously as well as biopsies of other potentially involved areas. Fungal serologies should be checked (see Chapter 8), although the clinician should not delay other diagnostic procedures in patients with compatible clinical presentations and epidemiologic histories.

A more common problem is the acquisition of opportunistic fungal infection posttransplant. Again, two patterns are observed: primary infection, usually of the lungs, occasionally of the nasal sinuses, most commonly by *Cryptococcus neoformans* or *Aspergillus fumigatus;* and sequential and concurrent secondary infection, either of the lungs or via infected intravenous lines, by *Candida albicans, Aspergillus fumigatus,* or *Torulopsis glabrata.* The clinical management of such infections is outlined in Chapters 4 and 8. Two points bear emphasis here. First, metastatic infection is the rule rather than the exception with these agents and the clinically similar *Nocardia asteroides.* Therefore, a search for metastases should be carried out whenever a primary focus of infection is documented (e.g., a lumbar puncture in patients with cryptococcal pulmonary or skin infection, bone and brain scans for patients with *Aspergillus* and *Nocardia* infection). Second, careful surveillance should be maintained for possible clustering of cases of opportunistic fungal infection, particularly *Aspergillus.* Such clustering suggests a major environmental hazard.

6.4. Tuberculosis and Atypical Mycobacterial Infection in the Renal Transplant Patient

One of the more controversial issues in the management of transplant patients is the approach to tuberculosis. The incidence of active tuberculosis in this patient population is approximately 1%, varying from 0.65 to 1.7% in published reports.[408–416] This compares to an overall rate in the United States of approximately 15 per 100,000. Thus, not surprisingly given the depressed cell-mediated immunity characteristic of this population, the incidence of active tuberculosis is many times greater than in the general population. Fortunately, such tuberculosis can be effectively treated, with fatal pulmonary tuberculosis reported in only 4 of 10,000 renal transplant recipients enrolled in the American College of Surgeons Transplant Registry.[408–416]

A variety of forms of tuberculosis have been observed in these patients, from cavitary to miliary disease and from bowel disease to skin disease.[408–416] Particularly noteworthy have been instances in which the graft carried the infection from donor to recipient[417] or when the graft was infected in the recipient as part of hematogenous dissemination of the organisms.[418] An unusually high rate of bone and joint involvement has been reported in transplant patients with tuberculosis.[411,414]

What has been surprising is not that tuberculosis has occurred in these immunocompromised patients, but rather that it has not occurred more frequently. For example, at the Massachusetts General Hospital, we have carried out renal transplantation in more than 300 patients whose pretransplant tuberculin status was known. Of those, 47 were tuberculin positive and did not receive isoniazid prophylaxis either pre- or post-transplant. Only one of these has reactivated his tuberculosis, and this was promptly identified and treated. This is the only case of tuberculosis we have observed over the past 10 years, despite the fact that the tuberculin test may be falsely negative in even well-dialyzed uremic patients.

Why not use isoniazid prophylaxis routinely? The issue of isoniazid prophylaxis is a controversial one. Although the guidelines of the American Lung Association have traditionally recommended 1 year of isoniazid prophylaxis for individuals with positive tuberculin tests who are subjected to a prolonged course of immunosuppressive therapy, we have found such a policy to be nearly impossible to implement in the renal transplant population because of the high incidence of liver function test abnormalities in this setting. We and others[419] have concluded that the risk of isoniazid hepatotoxicity is greater than the benefits of isoniazid prophylaxis in renal transplant patients with positive tuberculin tests as their only manifestation of past experience of tuberculosis. The logic behind this is the low frequency of tuberculosis reactivation in this population coupled with the high frequency of hepatotoxicity. One year of isoniazid prophylaxis is instituted in renal transplant patients who are recent tuberculin converters, in those with a history of untreated or suboptimally treated tuberculosis infection in the past decade, in those with significant abnormalities on chest radiography, or in those who possess other risk factors, such as malnutrition. In our opinion, close surveillance alone is indicated for the most tuberculin-positive transplant recipients.

One other aspect of antituberculosis therapy in the renal transplant patient that bears comment is that antituberculous drugs can have an adverse effect on allograft survival through their effects on steroid metabolism. Rifampin and probably other antitubercular drugs as well cause the induction of hepatic microsomal enzymes that increase the catabolism of steroids. Therefore, a given dose of prednisone will be less effective in a patient receiving such therapy, and rejection may ensue.[420] In addition, rifampin can increase the metabolism of cyclosporine by similar effects on the hepatic cytochrome P450 enzyme system, resulting in severe rejection due to inadvertent underimmunosuppression.

In addition to typical mycobacterial infection, atypical mycobacterial infection has been observed in renal transplant patients. This can be divided into two general categories: pulmonary, skin, and skeletal, and disseminated infection due to *M. kansasii*,[411,414,416,421,422] and skin infection alone with a variety of relatively less virulent mycobacterial species, including *M. marinum*,[423] *M. haemophilum*,[424] and *M. chelonei*.[425]

6.5. Dermatologic Manifestations of Infection in the Renal Transplant Patient

Dermatologic manifestations of infection that are of particular importance in the renal transplant patient may be divided into four categories (see also Chapter 5)[426]:

1. *Infection originating in the skin and typical of that occurring in immunocompetent patients, although with the potential for more serious disease:* The incidence of typical cellulitis due to gram-positive bacteria such as group A streptococci and *S. aureus* is increased in these patients because of the increased fragility of the skin due to chronic corticosteroid therapy. A striking example of this phenomenon is what we have termed transplant elbow, which consists of recurrent staphylococcal or group A streptococcal infection in and about the elbow due to two adverse effects of corticosteroid therapy—the attenuation of the skin integrity, plus a steroid-induced proximal myopathy of the legs, so that patients are unable to rise from a sitting position without pushing off with their elbows and traumatizing them. This provides a portal of entry for the gram-positive pathogens. Therapy requires parenteral antibiotics, frequently surgical excision of the involved olecranon bursa, decrease of steroid dosage, and physical protection to the elbows with basketball elbow guards.

In addition to being alert to an increased propensity to typical infection, the clinician must be aware that the range of microbial invaders may be broader and may include gram-negatives and such fungi as *Cryptococcus neoformans* or *Candida*. Since a cryptococcal cellulitis may be difficult to distinguish from a staphylococcal cellulitis on clinical grounds, an aggressive biopsy approach is indicated, particularly in a patient slow to respond to adequate anti-staphylococcal therapy.

2. *Extensive involvement of the skin with organisms which usually produce localized or trivial infection in immunocompetent individuals:* The two major considerations in this category are viruses and a variety of nonvirulent skin fungi. The major viral skin infections in the renal transplant patients are those due to HSV, VZV (see Section 4.2), and papillomaviruses, i.e., DNA viruses causing human warts.

Because of chronic immunosuppressive therapy, warts are very different in transplant patients than in the normal individual. In the transplant patient warts may be so numerous as to be disfiguring. The incidence and severity of warts in these patients is directly proportional to the intensity of the immunosuppressive therapy, with such therapy apparently reactivating previously acquired latent virus.[238,426–429] The significance of the warts goes beyond the cosmetic, as malignant transformation, particularly in sun-exposed areas, has been well documented. Human papillomavirus DNA has been demonstrated in the skin cancers of these patients,[430,431] and it is likely that such cancers arise as a result of the combined effects of the virus, immunosuppression, and UV irradiation.[432]

Unusually widespread cutaneous infection may be due to nonvirulent fungi in addition to viruses. A variety of fungal species that are ubiquitous in the environment may intermittently colonize and even establish localized superficial skin infection in the normal host, particularly when introduced into areas of injured skin. In the transplant patient, these infections can be extensive, cause disfigurement, and provide a portal of entry for life-threatening superinfection.[426]

3. *Infection originating in the skin caused by opportunistic organisms which rarely produce disease in immunocompetent patients but which may produce localized or disseminated infection in immunocompromised patients:* Examples of localized infection of this type include those caused by the fungus *Paecilomyces*,[433] such atypical mycobacteria as *M. marinum*,[423] and the alga *Protheca wickerhamii*.[434] Of far greater concern are those patients who develop systemic infection following primary skin invasion with *Aspergillus, Candida,* or

Rhyzopus species. The pathogenesis of these cases of disseminated fungal infection taking origin in the skin are distressingly repetitious—trauma to the skin due to maceration by occlusive dressing or tape, followed by invasion of the damaged skin and subsequent systemic dissemination. Others have observed a similar phenomenon in association with the use of Elastoplast tape contaminated with *Rhyzopus* spores.[435,436] Great care must therefore be taken in protecting the skin of these patients.

4. *Disseminated systemic infection metastatic to the skin from a noncutaneous portal of entry:* Cutaneous lesions may be the first clinical sign of disseminated life-threatening infection in the compromised host. Three groups of organisms are responsible for this category of cutaneous infection in the immunocompromised host: (1) *Pseudomonas aeruginosa* and, to a much lesser extent, other bacteria; (2) tuberculosis and the endemic systemic mycoses *Histoplasma capsulatum, Coccidioides immitis,* and *Blastomyces dermatitidis;* and (3) and the opportunistic organisms *Nocardia species, Cryptococcus neoformans, Aspergillus species, Candida species,* and the Mucoraceae.[426] This last category is particularly important in the transplant patient, as some 20–30% of patients with cryptococcal infection will have skin lesions weeks to months prior to the development of CNS disease and 10–15% of patients with disseminated candidal infection will have skin lesions early in their course.[426]

Illustrative Case 7

A 55-year-old black man had undergone cadaveric renal transplantation 14 months previously for chronic renal failure secondary to polycystic disease. Post-transplant immunosuppression was with azathioprine and prednisone. Despite mild chronic rejection, he had maintained a stable serum creatinine of 2.5 mg/dl over the last 6 months on prednisone 20 mg/day and azathioprine 100 mg/day. Four weeks prior to admission, several small papular lesions on an indurated base were noted on both arms but were not further evaluated. Over the last 10 days prior to admission, he had noted a bifrontal headache, first intermittently and then constantly, with increasing severity. Over the last 2 days, nausea and vomiting as well as fever developed, and he sought medical attention

On physical examination the temperature was 100.6°F (38.1°C) and the blood pressure was 150/100. Skin examination revealed four to five nontender papular lesions on the dorsal surfaces of both wrists, with a small area of subcutaneous induration at the base of each papule. Fundoscopic examination revealed papilledema. There were no meningeal signs. Neurologic exam-

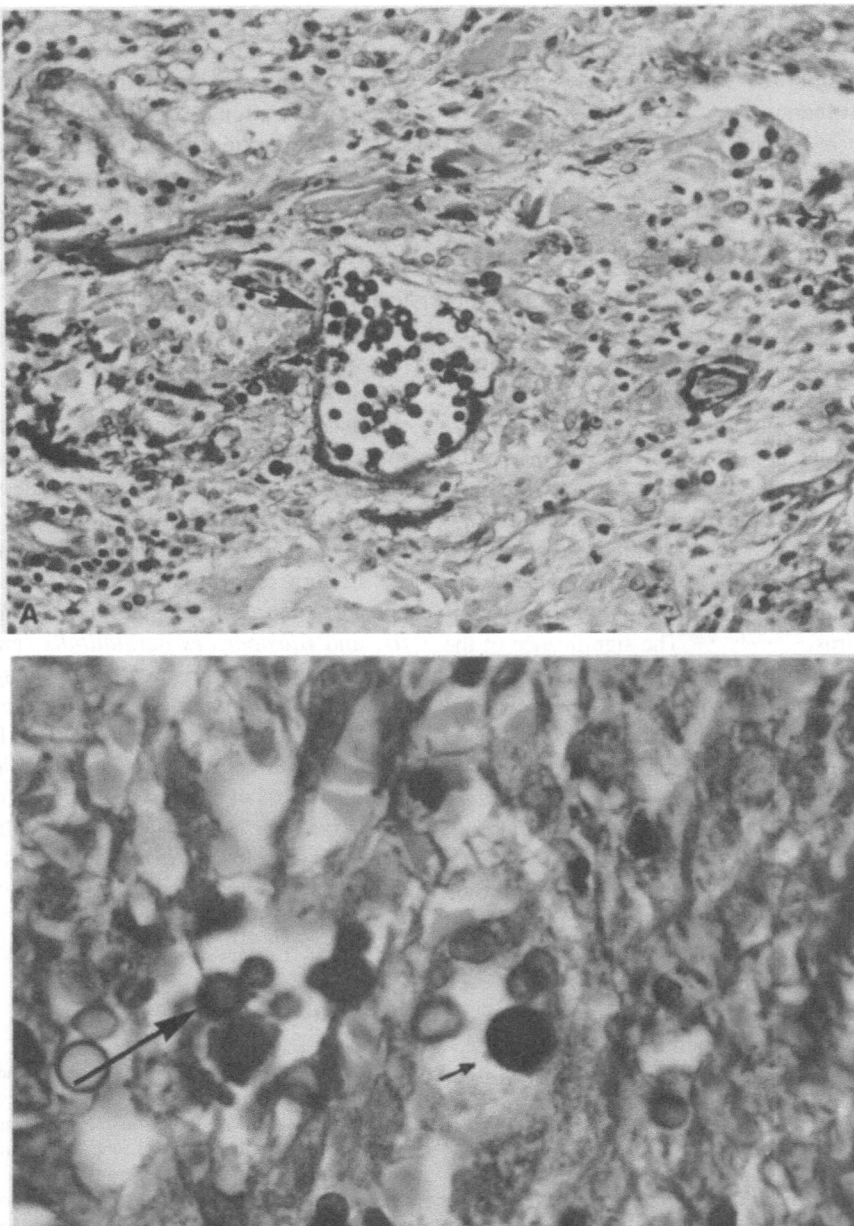

FIGURE 4. Skin biopsy of patient with papular skin lesions caused by disseminated cryptococcal infection (A) In the midst of the dermis were numerous cryptococci present focally as large aggregates (arrow) and singly surrounded by an infiltrate of histiocytes and lymphocytes (Periodic acid-Schiff with diastase) (× 400) (B) Budding forms (small arrow) of *Cryptococcus neoformans* Organisms with well-outlined capsules can be seen as well (large arrow) (Periodic acid-Schiff with diastase) (× 1600)

ination was otherwise unremarkable. A CT scan of the brain was essentially normal, and a lumbar puncture was performed that revealed an opening pressure of 300 mm H_2O, CSF protein 70 mg/dl, sugar 47 mg/dl, 24 WBC (80% lymphocytes), a positive India ink preparation, and a cryptococcal antigen titer of 1 : 128 in the CSF A skin biopsy of the wrist lesions revealed cryptococci in the skin. Both the CSF and skin specimens grew *Cryptococcus neoformans.*

The patient was first treated with amphotericin B and 5-fluorocytosine and then with amphotericin B alone because of 5-fluorocytosine-induced bone marrow toxicity in association with a serum creatinine climbing to 5.2 mg/dl. After a total dose of 2.5 g amphotericin, and with a negative cryptococcal antigen titer in the CSF, therapy was discontinued. Three months later, he presented again with relapsing cryptococcal infection. This time therapy was complicated by progressive renal failure and, despite combined amphotericin B and 5-fluorocytosine therapy, he succumbed to his infection.

Comment. This tragic result might have been avoided if the skin lesions had been biopsied 1 month before the onset of CNS symptoms and the diagnosis and appropriate therapy instituted earlier In contrast to this above case, the patient with the skin biopsy illustrated in Fig. 4 had the biopsy performed within days of the appearance of the lesion, and the diagnosis of cryptococcal infection was made. Lumbar puncture in this second patient was completely negative, and the patient was treated with amphotericin B alone for 6 weeks with complete resolution of his skin lesions. At 48 months follow-up, this patient is free of further clinical cryptococcal infection despite maintenance immunosuppression at a dose of prednisone 15 mg/day and azathioprine 125 mg/day. It is important to emphasize that cutaneous cryptococcal infection practically always signifies systemic dissemination and not just local infection to be treated only with surgical excision. Systemic chemotherapy is always indicated.

Thus, two major principles underline the dermatologic care of the critically ill renal transplant patient: the skin must be protected from injury, and the skin can function as an early warning system of disseminated opportunistic infection at a time when therapy is relatively easy to accomplish. Thus, any unexplained skin lesion merits biopsy for diagnosis, with both cultural and pathologic assessment being necessary[426] (see also Chapter 5).

7. Infection in the Liver Transplant Patient

The advent of cyclosporine immunosuppression, the improvement in surgical techniques for liver procurement and transplantation, and better perioperative patient management have all contributed significantly to the emergence of liver transplantation during the 1980s as an effective therapy for end stage liver disease. Largely through the efforts of Starzl and colleagues, first in Denver and now in Pittsburgh, and of Calne and colleagues in Cambridge, liver transplantation has evolved from a desperate experimental approach to a practical therapeutic option, performed daily at centers throughout the world. In June 1983, a National Institutes of Health Consensus Development Conference concluded that liver transplantation is an appropriate therapeutic approach to patients with end-stage liver disease.[437] Since then, the number of liver transplant centers in the United States has increased from five to more than 30 by 1986, and the liver transplants performed each year have increased during this same period from 170 to more than 600.[438] The current 1-year survival rates approach 70% for adults and 80% for children, with fewer than 5% of these 1-year survivors succumbing over the next four years.[438,439]

This is not to say that liver transplantation teams have solved all their problems, as infection remains a major cause of morbidity and mortality. Although liver, heart, and renal transplant patients all receive similar immunosuppressive regimens (Table 1), the risk of lethal infection in the liver transplant patient is many times greater.[438-443] The difference is clearly related to the technical aspects of liver transplantation, as it has been clear since the first experimental studies of liver transplantation that liver injury is a major factor in the pathogenesis of lethal infection in more than three-fourths of such episodes.[442,444-446] For purposes of this review, it is useful to consider the infectious disease problems of the liver transplant patient in three general categories: those related to events occurring prior to transplant; those occurring in the first month post-transplant; and those occurring in the period beyond 1 month post-transplant.

7.1. Infection Related to Pre-Liver Transplant Events

Important considerations regarding donor and recipient selection to minimize the chances of infection post-transplant are outlined in Sections 3.1 and 3.2. These same points remain relevant in considering donor and recipient for liver transplantation. One additional consideration in liver transplantation, however, is not a factor in renal transplantation. Whereas in renal transplantation, peritoneal or hemodialysis may be employed to support and improve the

TABLE 5. Disease Potentially Treatable by Orthotopic Liver Transplantation[a]

Adults	Children
End-stage cirrhosis due to.	End-stage cirrhosis due to.
Primary biliary cirrhosis	Biliary atresia
Sclerosing cholangitis	Congenital biliary cirrhosis
Autoimmune hepatitis	Congenital hepatic fibrosis
Chronic active hepatitis	Chronic active hepatitis
Non-A, non-B hepatitis[b]	Non-A, non-B hepatitis[b]
Acute overwhelming liver failure due to[a]:	Acute, overwhelming liver failure due to[c].
Toxin exposure	Toxin exposure
Drug reaction	Drug reaction
Hepatitis A	Hepatitis A
Non-A, non-B hepatitis	Non-A, non-B hepatitis
Metabolic disorders	Metabolic disorders
Wilson's disease[c]	α-Antitrypsin deficiency
Protoporphyria	Tyrosinemia
Hemochromatosis	Galactosemia
Type IV hyperlipidemia	Glycogen storage (types I and IV)
Hemophilia (particularly with cirrhosis)	Byler disease
Budd–Chiari syndrome	Sea-blue histiocyte syndrome
Primary hepatocellular carcinoma[b]	

[a]Modified from Busuttil et al [438]
[b]In selected cases in whom disease recurrence is thought to be of low probability
[c]In patients deemed to have irreversible liver damage such that death is highly likely before hepatic regeneration could occur

TABLE 6. Symptoms Suggesting Significant Liver Failure[a]

Progressive jaundice
Diminished hepatic synthetic function
Symptomatic portal hypertension as manifested by either variceal bleeding, increasing ascites, or both
Recurrent or chronic, incapacitating hepatic encephalopathy
Recurrent cholangitis
Progressive weakness and debility

[a]Modified from Busuttil et al [438]
[b]Any patient with two or more of these symptoms should be considered as a possible candidate for liver transplantation

condition of a patient with end-stage renal disease, no such life-support system is available for patients with end-stage liver disease. Liver transplantation is indicated for patients with congenital or acquired non-alcoholic end-stage cirrhosis, a variety of hepatic metabolic defects; certain anatomic disorders, and in selected cases of acute liver failure or primary hepatocellular malignancy (Table 5).[438] This is relatively straightforward. What is much more difficult is assessing the appropriate timing of liver transplantation in these patients. Table 6 outlines the cardinal symptoms of liver failure, and it has been suggested that when two or more of these signs are present in patients with one of the conditions outlined in Table 5, liver transplantation should be considered. On the one hand, too early transplantation, particularly in a patient whose native liver might regenerate (as in certain cases of acute liver failure) is to be avoided. On the other hand, delay can result in catastrophic complications that can have adverse effects on the outcome of liver transplantation. As far as infection is concerned, we have seen three types of complications resulting from delaying too long the performance of liver transplantation:

1. *Aspiration pneumonia:* Because of increasing hepatic encephalopathy, the patient is unable to protect the airway and develops an aspiration pneumonia, often with gram-negative organisms. Such lung injury and infection carries an added risk during the peritransplant period, as progressive superinfection is not infrequent, with death from pulmonary sepsis and respiratory insufficiency developing. Such pneumonias are best prevented. Ideally, transplantation should be carried out before encephalopathy becomes so deep or constant that airway integrity cannot be maintained. In patients (particularly those with acute hepatic failure) in whom this is not possible, early intubation to protect the lungs is indicated. Once such intubation is carried out, if transplantation is to be done, it should be done within 72 hr. After that, the risk of life-threatening pneumonia becomes prohibitive.

2. *Spontaneous bacterial peritonitis:* This is a constant risk in patients with ascites due to end-stage liver disease. Such infections must be completely eradicated before transplantation. A variation on this problem that we have observed is portal venous thrombosis with resulting mesenteric venous compromise, infarction of the bowel, and abscess formation. Although all patients are screened for portal vein patency prior to ac-

ceptance as a liver transplant candidate, we have seen such develop after initially negative studies. The clue to this possibility is recurrent fever and abdominal pain, often without evidence of clear-cut bacterial peritonitis.

3. *Intravenous or intraarterial line-related sepsis:* This becomes an increasing problem as the degree of illness in the patient increases and he requires intensive care prior to transplant.

Because of these concerns and with the increasing success of liver transplantation, we now favor early transplantation for patients with irreversible liver disease, preferably weeks to months before the final downhill spiral occurs. Precise quantitation of the timing of this major moment remains difficult, however, and better guidelines are clearly needed.

Krom[447] suggested one other element in the preparation of patients for liver transplantation. Once a patient is accepted for transplantation, and for the first 21 days post-transplant, selective bowel decontamination is carried out using nonabsorbable antibacterial and antifungal agents. This program, when combined with 2 days of parenteral aminoglycoside and cephalozoin therapy at the time of transplant, has been associated with a very low rate of infection. This stands in direct contrast to a report from Pittsburgh[448] documenting a 44% incidence of fungal infections in their liver transplant patients, with a 16% incidence of fungemia. We use oral nystatin prophylaxis aiming to decrease upper GI tract candidal colonization. With this program, we have had no problems with candidal infection among 30 consecutive liver transplant recipients. Although this issue should be studied with a randomized protocol, the possible benefits of a selective bowel decontamination program aimed particularly at candidal colonization are potentially appealing.

7.2. Infection in the First Month Post-Liver Transplant

As has been noted for the renal transplant patients, infections occurring in the first month post-transplant are largely related to technical aspects of the transplant procedure itself. Because of the technical demands of the liver transplant operation, this is the most critical period in terms of risk from life-threatening infection. In the case of the liver transplant patient, these can be divided into five categories:

1. Infections related to vascular anastomotic problems
2. Infections related to biliary anastomotic problems
3. Wound infections
4. Pulmonary infections
5. Vascular line-related infections

7.2.1. Infections Related to Vascular Anastomotic Problems

Four vascular anastomoses must be accomplished successfully during the course of the liver transplant operation. In order of performance during the operation, these are suprahepatic vena canal anastomosis, infrahepatic vena caval anastomosis, portal vein anastomosis, and reconstruction of the hepatic artery.

Patency of these anastomoses is critical to both graft and patient survival, with portal vein thrombosis or stenosis, hepatic artery thrombosis, and hepatic vein occlusion developing in the first few days post-transplant being well recognized complications.[449,450] Manifestations of these complications include ascites, variceal bleeding, and deterioration in liver function tests and clinical status. Not uncommonly, fever and bacteremia may be the major clues. Sepsis is particularly common following interruption in the hepatic arterial circulation, with secondary infection of hepatic infarcts leading to areas of hepatic gangrene, abscess formation, and fulminant sepsis due to bowel flora or candidal organisms.[438,442,448–450] A more insidious consequence of vascular insufficiency can result when the vascular supply to the liver parenchyma remains intact, but the biliary anastomosis is rendered ischemic. This results in a breakdown of the biliary anastomosis, a bile leak, and secondary infection. Such secondary infection may take the form of deep wound infection, cholangitis, liver abscess, and/or bacteremia, with the microorganisms causing this again derived from the normal flora of the small bowel—streptococci, Enterobacteriaceae, anaerobes, and *Candida* sp. Polymicrobial infection is the rule in these circumstances. This more occult result of vascular insufficiency is totally analogous to the ureteral leaks and stenoses developing after renal transplantation due to vascular insufficiency of the ureter[438,442,448–451] (see Section 3.3).

7.2.2. Infections Related to Biliary Anastomotic Problems

As experience has been gained with liver transplantation, problems with the vascular anastomoses have become less common, particularly in adults, and the fulminant infections related to major ischemic injury have become less common. The biliary anastomosis, however, remains the Achilles heel of liver transplantation. Whenever possible, the anastomosis of choice is a choledochocholedocostomy, which maintains the native sphincter of Oddi intact. When this is not possible for anatomic reasons, as in children with biliary atresia or ducts too small to safely carry out this anastomosis or in adults with sclerosing cholangitis or other abnormalities of the extrahepatic biliary system, a choledochojejunostomy constructed with a Roux-en-Y technique that offers protection against microbial contamination from the gastrointestinal tract can be employed. Although biliary leaks can develop with either anastomosis, obstruction is the major concern with the choledochocholedocostomy procedure, whereas reflux of organisms is the weakness of the choledochojejunostomy anastomosis. In either case, secondary infection is the consequence.[438,442,449–451]

The cardinal rule in the first few weeks following liver transplantation is that any episode of unexplained fever or bacteremia should be regarded as a manifestation of a technical problem involving the vascular tree, the biliary anastomosis, or deep wound infection until proven otherwise. Accordingly, in addition to instituting broad-spectrum antimicrobial therapy aimed at upper small bowel flora (e.g., a second- or third-generation cephalosporin or antipseudomonal penicillin plus aminoglycoside or clindamycin plus aminoglycoside), such diagnostic procedures as abdominal CT scanning and/or ultrasound, cholangiography, and, when appropriate, hepatic angiography must be carried out expeditiously as well. Prompt surgical attack of technical problems under antimicrobial coverage can salvage these patients.[438,442,452]

Colonization of the bile of liver transplant patients with bacteria is the rule rather than the exception, and this can be easily documented by bile cultures in patients with T-tubes left in place to protect the biliary anastomosis. In our hepatic transplantation program, we usually use cefazolin prophylaxis (1 IV every 8 hr beginning on call to the operating room) for 4–5 days postoperatively. This is then followed by oral trimethoprim–sulfamethoxazole (one double-strength tablet orally per day) for 4–6 months. Nystatin or clotrimazole orally is begun preoperatively and continued for 4–6 months postoperatively. With this program, colonization of the biliary tree with *Enterococcus* and/or *Staphylococcus epidermidis* is the rule. Such colonization by itself requires no routine therapy. We have observed, however, that cholangiograms or other manipulations of the biliary tree in the face of such colonization can result in bacteremias. We therefore advocate antimicrobial prophylaxis for 24–48 hr with vancomycin to cover any planned manipulation of the biliary tree. In individuals who develop symptomatic infection with *Enterococcus* or *S. epidermidis* in the absence of manipulation, this should be regarded as an important clue to the presence of a biliary leak or obstruction.

7.2.3. Wound Infections

The incidence of wound infections following surgery in the immunosuppressed host is directly related to the occurrence of technical complications, particularly leaks and hematoma formation (see Section 3.3). By its nature, liver transplantation is particularly likely to be associated with such problems because of (1) the occurrence of bile leaks, and (2) the bleeding problems at the time of surgery. Whenever large volumes of blood are required both intra- and perioperatively (and transfusion requirements of more than 100 units of blood are not uncommon in these patients), intraabdominal hematomas with a risk of secondary infection are important considerations. Adequate drainage, including reexploration when necessary, is essential to prevent such infections from developing. Once again, the technical quality of the surgery and the accomplishment of prompt and complete drainage will be the major factors in limiting the occurrence of serious wound infection. Prophylactic antibiotics are probably useful here, but they are of secondary importance when compared with the technical considerations. Recently, Shaffer et al.[453] reported an unusual form of wound infection in a liver transplant patient—toxic shock syndrome (TSS) stemming from staphylococcal wound infection.

7.2.4. Pulmonary Infections

Postoperative pneumonia has long been recognized as a significant problem after any abdominal operation due to aspiration of pharyngeal flora and postoperative atelectasis. This is a particular problem in the liver transplant patient, as fluid overload, a distended abdomen causing poor respiratory mechanics, and obtundation will frequently necessitate prolonged intubation and mechanical ventilation. In such immunosuppressed patients, intubation beyond 96 hr postoperatively is associated with an increased incidence of pneumonia, often with hospital-acquired antibiotic-resistant gram-negative bacteria. The occurrence of pneumonia is further increased if significant lung injury due to aspiration had occurred preoperatively within 2 weeks of the transplant or if the patient failed an attempt at extubation and had to be reintubated because of respiratory failure. The occurrence of pneumonia can be decreased by aggressive chest physiotherapy to prevent atelectasis and mobilize secretions. In addition, we are impressed that caring for such patients in rooms with HEPA-filtered air (high efficiency particulate air) will also help in the prevention of this complication.

7.2.5. Vascular Line-Related Infections

Any immunocompromised patient is at high risk of systemic sepsis due to contaminated lines. In the renal transplant patient, this is best dealt with by not using central venous lines or Swan Ganz lines in the routine care of such patients. Unfortunately, in the liver transplant patient, fluid management is sufficiently complicated that such invasive monitoring tools are usually required both intra- and perioperatively. However, every effort must be made to discontinue these as quickly as possible. Failing that, new lines inserted through totally new access sites should be carried out at least every 72 hr.

7.3. Infection Beyond 1 Month Post-transplant

Once the patient survives the first month post-transplant, he has survived the most important and most immediately life-threatening infections that threaten his existence. After the first month, the infection problems then can be divided into two general categories: (1) those lingering from an earlier period, and (2) those that are determined by rejection, immunosuppression, and epidemiologic factors and that are virtually identical to those that have been detailed previously in renal transplant patients. In the first category, the major concerns are those related to technical problems associated with the biliary anastomosis. In most instances, these episodes of bacteremia, cholangitis, or intraabdominal abscess are continuations of problems that have already declared themselves but which have not yet been adequately dealt with technically (biliary obstruction, biliary leaks, and intraabdominal collections). In addition, late stenosis of the choledochocholedocostomy anastomosis, with secondary cholangitis, may occur.

For the most part, however, the infectious disease problems are dominated now by the viral infections, particularly CMV, that have received so much attention in renal transplant patients. Three issues regarding CMV in liver transplantation bear particular emphasis here:

1. Because of the lack of a life-sustaining support system akin to dialysis, liver transplant patients regularly receive more immunosuppression than do renal transplant patients. Therefore, it is not surprising that such viral infections as CMV and EBV appear to have, if anything, greater impact on liver transplant patients than on renal transplant patients. Another possible explanation for this is that the potential infecting innoculum in the liver and the blood transfusions is many times greater than in the renal transplant patient. Now that CMV superinfection has clearly been documented in renal transplant recipients (see Section 4.1.1), it is likely that this is playing an important role in liver transplant patients as well. Trials of anti-CMV prophylaxis in liver transplant patients analogous to those carried out in renal transplant patients are badly needed.

2. Episodes of hepatic dysfunction occurring 1–4 months post-transplant may be due to CMV rather than rejection. We have seen several patients in whom the finding of CMV on liver biopsy and subsequent decrease in immunosuppressive therapy resulted in improvement in liver function. Whether DHPG antiviral therapy will be useful in this circumstance as well remains to be determined.

3. There is as yet no information on the possible role of CMV in influencing rejection episodes. With the current emphasis on CMV infection causing upregulation of MHC antigens on transplanted tissue (through the elaboration of interferon by responding cells) leading to rejection (see Section 4.1), this possibility merits investigation.

The major infectious disease area that is poorly understood at present in liver transplantation is the impact of hepatitis viruses post-transplant. Because patients with end-stage liver disease due to hepatitis B infection that is e-antigen-positive have a poor post-transplant course, they are not considered good candidates for liver transplantation at present.[438] Patients who are e-antigen negative but HBsAg positive have been successfully transplanted in terms of 6-month or 1-year survival, but the rate of success is lower than in patients with other forms of liver disease, and it is likely that these patients will develop the same hepatocellular carcinomas and progressive liver disease described in successful renal transplant recipients with chronic hepatitis B infection. We regard infection that is e-antigen negative but HBsAg positive as a strong relative contraindication to liver transplantation. It is hoped that the development of effective antiviral strategies will change this situation in the future.

More problematic is the impact of non-A, non-B hepatitis on liver transplant recipients. This form of hepatitis is associated with an increased risk of extrahepatic infection (it is immunosuppressing), a high rate of chronic infection, and the development of cryptogenic cirrhosis in the renal transplant patient (see Section 4.4). In fact, because of the large amount of blood administered, it is likely that the incidence of non-A, non-B hepatitis in the liver transplant population will be many times greater than in the renal or cardiac transplant populations. Whether patients with end-stage liver disease due to non-A, non-B hepatitis infect their new livers remains to be determined. Much work is necessary to unravel the contributions of this virus (or group of viruses) to liver dysfunction among liver transplant recipients.

8. Summary and Prospects for the Future

In the first edition of this book, several chapters described infectious disease problems of the bone marrow and renal transplant patients. Liver and cardiac transplantation were mentioned only in passing. Because of the great progress made in clinical liver and cardiac transplantation over the past 6 years, both now merit their own extensive review. One may predict that future editions of this treatise will include detailed discussions of pancreatic, lung, bone, and, perhaps, small bowel transplantation. With the development of better immunosuppressive regimens and the increasing skill of the transplant surgeon, success in these newer areas will likely follow the success achieved in renal, bone marrow, cardiac, and liver transplantation thus far. It is incumbent upon all of us involved with the medical side of transplantation to keep pace with our pioneering surgical colleagues to develop better methods for preventing and treating rejection and for preventing, diagnosing, and treating infectious complications of antirejection therapy. The truism that infection and rejection are closely bound together and that progress in one area will affect the other remains as applicable today as it was 20 years ago.

As one approaches both our traditional forms of transplantation and the more experimental areas of transplantation, the following points relevant to infectious disease complications should be kept in mind:

1. Infection may be divided into three general categories: those related to technical complications, those related to epidemiologic exposures, and those due to viruses lurking in the graft recipient or his donor and that are rendered clinically manifest post-transplant. The modulation of these infections is accomplished by the dose, duration, and type of immunosuppressive therapy being administered.

2. There is an expected timetable according to which particular infections occur at particular times in the post-transplant course. Exceptions to this time-

table are usually due to exposure to excessive environmental hazards.

3. The biggest challenge in approaching the infectious disease problems of the transplant patient is the prevention and treatment of those viral diseases that contribute so broadly to the morbidity and mortality still associated with clinical human transplantation. The viruses of greatest importance are the herpes group viruses, the hepatitis viruses, and the human immunodeficiency virus. Each of these can be modulated by immunosuppressive therapy.

4. Because of the impaired inflammatory response of this patient population, signs and symptoms of infection may be greatly muted. Physicians caring for such patients must be alert and aggressive in their approach to "minor" skin lesions or radiographic findings.

5. Although the challenge of caring for these patients is great, the rewards are even greater. We have come a long way in the care of these patients. Continued progress is on the horizon.

References

1. Rubin RH, Wolfson JS, Cosimi AB, et al: Infection in the renal transplant recipient. *Am J Med* **70**:405–411, 1981.
2. Peterson PK, Andersen RC: Infection in renal transplant recipients; current approaches to diagnosis, therapy, and prevention. *Am J Med* **81**(suppl 1A):2–10, 1986.
3. Walker PR, Moorhead JF: Infection in the renal transplant patient. *J R Soc Med* **71**:84–86, 1978.
4. Rifkind D, Marchioro T, Schneck S, et al: Systemic fungal infections complicating renal transplantation and immunosuppressive therapy. *Am J Med* **43**:28–38, 1967.
5. Bach MC, Sahyoun A, Adler JL, et al: Influences of rejection therapy on fungal and nocardial infections in renal-transplant recipients. *Lancet* **1**:180–184, 1973.
6. Vincenti F, Amend W, Feduska NK, et al: Improved outcome following renal transplantation with reduction in the immunosuppression therapy for rejection episodes. *Am J Med* **69**:107–112, 1980.
7. Strom TB: The improving utility of renal transplantation in the management of end-stage renal disease. *Am J Med* **73**:105–124, 1982.
8. Morris PJ, Chan L, French ME, et al: Low dose oral prednisolone in renal transplantation. *Lancet* **1**:525–527, 1982.
9. Howard RJ, Condie RM, Sutherland DER, et al: The use of antilymphoblast globulin in the treatment of renal allograft rejection. *Transplant Proc* **13**:473–474, 1981.
10. Nelson PW, Cosimi AB, Delmonico FL, et al: Antithymocyte globulin as the primary treatment for renal allograft rejection. *Transplantation* **36**:587–589, 1983.
11. Cosimi AB: Antilymphocyte globulin—a final (?) look In

Morris PJ, Tilney NL (eds): *Progress in Transplantation.* Vol 2. Churchill Livingstone, Edinburgh, 1985, pp. 167–188.
12. Cosimi AB, Colvin RB, Burton RC, et al: Use of monoclonal antibodies to T-cell subsets for immunologic monitoring and treatment in recipients of renal allografts. *N Engl J Med* **305**:308–314, 1981.
13. Ortho Multicenter Transplant Study Group: A randomized clinical trial of OKT 3 monoclonal antibody for acute rejection of cadaveric renal transplants. *N Engl J Med* **313**:337–342, 1985.
14. Takahaski H, Okazaki H, Terasaki PI, et al: Reversal of transplant rejection by monoclonal antiblast antibody. *Lancet* **2**:1155–1159, 1983.
15. Najarian JS, Sutherland DER, Ferguson RM, et al: Total lymphoid irradiation and kidney transplantation. A clinical experience. *Transplant Proc* **13**:417–424, 1981.
16. Cortesini R, Molajoni ER, Farmulari A, et al: Total lymphoid irradiation in clinical transplantation: Experience in 28 high risk patients. *Transplant Proc* **17**:1291–1293, 1985.
17. Sampson D, Levin BS, Hoppe RT, et al: Preliminary observations on the use of total lymphoid irradiation, rabbit antithymocyte globulin, and low dose prednisone in human cadaver renal transplantation. *Transplant Proc* **17**:1299–1303, 1985.
18. Stiller CR, Keown PA: Cyclosporine therapy in perspective. In Morris PJ, Tilney NJ (eds): *Progress in Transplantation.* Vol 1. Churchill Livingstone, Edinburgh, 1984, pp. 11–45.
19. Anderson RJ, Schafer LA, Olin DB, et al: Infectious risk factors in the immunosuppressed host. *Am J Med* **54**:453–460, 1973.
20. Cheeseman SH, Rubin RH, Stewart JA, et al: Controlled trial of prophylactic human-leukocyte interferon in renal transplantation; effects on cytomegalovirus and herpes simplex infections. *N Engl J Med* **300**:1345–1349, 1979.
21. Rubin RH, Cosimi AB, Hirsch MS, et al: Effects of antithymocyte globulin on cytomegalovirus infection in renal transplant recipients. *Transplantation* **31**:143–145, 1981.
22. Eickhoff TC, Olin D, Anderson RH, et al: Current problems and approaches to diagnosis of infection in renal transplant recipients. *Transplant Proc* **4**:693–698, 1972
23. Barnes BA, Bergan J, Braun W, et al: The 12th report of the human transplant registry. *JAMA* **233**:787–796, 1975.
24. Auchincloss H Jr, Rubin RH: Clinical management of the critically ill renal transplant patient. In Parillo JE, Masur H (eds): *The Critically Ill Immunosuppressed Patient: Diagnosis and Management.* Aspen, Rockville, MD, 1987, pp. 347–380.
25. Scowden EB, Schaffner W, Stone WJ: Overwhelming strongyloidiasis; an unappreciated opportunistic infection. *Medicine (Baltimore)* **57**:527–544, 1978.
26. Morgan JS, Schaffner W, Stone WJ: Opportunistic strongyloidiasis in renal transplant recipients. *Transplantation* **42**:518–524, 1986.
27. Purtilo DT, Meyers WM, Connor DH: Fatal strongyloidiasis in immunosuppressed patients. *Am J Med* **56**:488–493, 1974.
28. Fogrindes LA, Busato O, Brentano L: Strongyloidiasis: Fa-

tal complication of renal transplantation. *Lancet* 2:439–440, 1971.

29. Scoggin CH, Call NB: Acute respiratory failure due to disseminated strongyloidiasis in a renal transplant recipient *Ann Intern Med* 87:456–458, 1977.

30. Avagnina MA, Elsner B, Iotti RM, et al: Strongyloides stercoralis in Papanicolaou-stained smears of ascitic fluid. *Acta Cytol* 24:36–39, 1980).

31. Venizelos PC, Lopata M, Bardawil WA, et al: Respiratory failure due to *Strongyloides stercoralis* in a patient with a renal transplant. *Chest* 78:104–106, 1980.

32. White JV, Garvey G, Hardy MA: Fatal strongyloidiasis after renal transplantation: A complication of immunosuppression. *Ann Surg* 48:39–41, 1982.

33. Weller IVD, Copland P, Gabriel R: *Strongyloides stercoralis* infection in renal transplant recipients. *Br Med J* 282:524, 1981.

34. Fowler CA, Lindsay I, Lewin J, et al: Recurrent hyperinfestation with *Strongyloides stercoralis* in a renal allograft recipient. *Br Med J* 285:1394, 1982.

35. DeVault GA, Brown ST, Montoya SP, et al: Disseminated strongyloidiasis complicating acute renal allograft rejection Prolonged thiabendazole administration and successful retransplantation. *Transplantation* 34:220–221, 1982.

36. Hirschmann JR, Plorde JJ, Ochi RF: Fever and pulmonary infiltrates in a patient with a renal transplant. *West J Med* 140:914–920, 1984.

37. Schad GA: Cyclosporine may eliminate the threat of overwhelming strongyloidiasis in immunosuppressed patients. *J Infect Dis* 153:178, 1986.

38. Schumaker JD, Band JD, Lensmeyer GL, et al: Thiabendazole treatment of severe strongyloidiasis in a hemodialyzed patient. *Ann Intern Med* 89:644–645, 1978.

39. Leapman SE, Rosenberg JB, Filo RS, et al: *Strongyloides stercoralis* in chronic renal failure: safe therapy with thiabendazole. *South Med J* 73:1400–1402, 1980.

40. Jones CA: Clinical studies in human strongyloidiasis. I. Semeiology Gastroenterol 16:743–746, 1950.

41. Betts RF, Freeman RB, Douglas RH Jr, et al: Transmission of cytomegalovirus infection with renal allograft. *Kidney Int* 8:385–392, 1975.

42. Ho M, Suwansirikul S, Dowling JN, et al: The transplanted kidney as a source of cytomegalovirus infection. *N Engl J Med* 293:1109–1112, 1975

43. Rubin RH, Russell PS, Levin M, et al: Summary of a workshop on cytomegalovirus infections during organ transplantation. *J Infect Dis* 139:728–734, 1979.

44. Wolf JL, Perkins HA, Schreeder MT, et al: The transplanted kidney as a source of hepatitis B infection. *Ann Intern Med* 91:412–413, 1979.

45. Lutwick LI, Sywassink JM, Corry RJ, et al: The transmission of hepatitis B by renal transplantation. *Clin Nephrol* 19:317–319, 1983.

46. Coffin J, Haase A, Levy JA, et al: Human immunodeficiency viruses. *Science* 232:697, 1986.

47. Rubin RH, Jenkins RL, Shaw BW Jr, et al. The acquired immunodeficiency syndrome and transplantation. *Transplantation* 44:1–4, 1987.

48. Gottlieb MS, Groopman JE, Weinstein WM, et al: The acquired immunodeficiency syndrome. *Ann Intern Med* 99:208–220, 1983.

49. Landesman SH, Ginzburg HM, Weiss SH. Special report. The AIDS epidemic. *N Engl J Med* 312:521–526, 1985.

50. Fauci AS, Masur H, Gelman EP, et al: The acquired immunodeficiency syndrome: An update. *Ann Intern Med* 102:800–813, 1985.

51. Prompt CA, Reis MM, Grillo FM, et al: Transmission of AIDS virus at renal transplantation. *Lancet* 2:672, 1985

52. L'Age-Stehr J, Schwarz A, Offermann G, et al: HTLV-III infection in kidney transplant recipients. *Lancet* 2:1361–1362, 1985.

53. Shaffer D, Pearl RH, Jenkins RL, et al: HTLV-III/LAV infection in kidney and liver transplantation. *Transplant Proc* 19:2176–2178, 1987.

54. Anton J, Smith B, Ewenstein B, et al. HTLV-III infection after bone marrow transplantation. *Blood* 67:160–163, 1986.

55. Milgram M, Esquenazi V, Fuller L, et al: Acquired immunodeficiency syndrome in a transplant patient. *Transplant Proc* 17:75–77, 1985.

56. MacLean LD, Dossetor JB, Gault MH, et al: Renal homotransplantation using cadaver donors. *Arch Surg* 91:288–306, 1965.

57 Ooi BS, Chen BTM, Lim CH, et al: Survival of a patient transplanted with a kidney infected with *Cryptococcus neoformans*. *Transplantation* 11:428–429, 1971.

58. Nelson PW, Delmonico FL, Tolkoff-Rubin NE, et al: Unsuspected donor Pseudomonas infection causing arterial disruption after renal transplantation. *Transplantation* 37:313–314, 1984.

59. McCoy GC, Loening S, Braun WE, et al: The fate of cadaver renal allografts contaminated before transplantation. *Transplantation* 20:467–472, 1975.

60. Doig RL, Boyd PJR, Eykyn S: *Staphylococcus aureus* transmitted in transplanted kidneys *Lancet* 2:243–244, 1975.

61. McLeish KR, McMurray SD, Smith EJ, et al: The transmission of *Candida albicans* by cadaveric allografts. *J Urol* 118:513–516, 1977.

62. Anderson CB, Haid SD, Hruska KA, et al: Significance of microbial contamination of stored cadaver kidneys. *Arch Surg* 113:269–271, 1978.

63. Hayry P, Renkonen O-V: Frequency and fate of human renal allografts contaminated prior to transplantation. *Surgery* 85:404–407, 1979.

64 McCoy GC, Loening S, Braun WE, et al: The fate of cadaver renal allografts contaminated before transplantation. *Transplantation* 20:467–472, 1975.

65. Majeski JA, Alexander JW, First MR, et al: Transplantation of microbially contaminated cadaver kidneys. *Arch Surg* 117:221–224, 1982.

66. Spees EK, Light JA, Oakes DD, et al: Experience with cadaver renal allograft contamination before transplantation. *Br J Surg* 69:482–485, 1982.

67. Owens JL, Wilson SE, Maxwell JG, et al: Major arterial hemorrhage after renal transplantation. *Transplantation* 27:285–287, 1979.

68 Fernando ON, Higgins AF, Moorhead JF: Secondary hemorrhage after renal transplantation. *Lancet* 2:368, 1976

69. Vegeto A, Berardinelli L, Storelli G, et al: Spontaneous rupture of the renal atery in kidney transplantation *Transplant Proc* **11**:1276–1279, 1979.

70. Weber TR, Freier DT, Turcotte JF: Transplantation of infected kidneys. *Transplantation* **27**:63–65, 1979

71. Van der Vliet JA, Tidow G, Koostra G, et al: Transplantation of contaminated organs. *Br J Surg* **67**:596–598, 1980.

72. Slapak M: The immediate care of potential donors for organ transplantation. *Anaesthesia* **33**:700–704, 1978.

73. Burgos-Calderon R, Pankey GA, Figueroa JE: Infection in kidney transplantation. *Surgery* **70**:334–340, 1971.

74. Moore TC, Hume DM: The period and nature of hazard in clinical renal transplantation. 1. The hazard to patient survival. *Ann Surg* **183**:266–270, 1976.

75. Schweizer RT, Kountz SL, Belzer FO. Wound complications in recipients of renal transplants. *Ann Surg* **177**:58–62, 1973.

76. Diethelm AG: Surgical management of complications of steroid therapy. *Ann Surg* **185**:251–263, 1977.

77. Muakkassa WF, Goldman MH, Mendez-Picon G, et al: Wound infections in renal transplant patients. *J Urol* **130**:17–19, 1983.

78. Lee HM, Madge GE, Mendez-Picon G, et al: Surgical complications in renal transplant recipients. *Surg Clin North Am* **58**:285–304, 1978.

79. Kyriakides GK, Simmons RL, Najarian JS. Wound infections in renal transplant wounds: Pathogenetic and prognostic factors. *Ann Surg* **186**:770–775, 1975.

80. Brunn JN: Postoperative wound infection. Predisposing factors and the effect of a reduction in the dissemination of staphylococci. *Acta Med Scand* **514**(suppl):3–89, 1970.

81. Belzer F, Salvatierra O, Schwiezer R, et al: Prevention of wound infections by topical antibiotics in high risk patients. *Am J Surg* **126**:180–185, 1973.

82. Tilney NL, Strom TB, Vineyard GC, et al: Factors contributing to the declining mortality rate in renal transplantation. *N Engl J Med* **299**:1321–1325, 1978.

83. Novick AC: The value of intraoperative antibiotics in preventing renal transplant wound infections. *J Urol* **125**:151–152, 1981.

84. Judson RT: Wound infection following renal transplantation. *Aust NZ J Surg* **54**:223–224, 1984.

85. Fisher MC, Baluarte HJ, Long SS: Bacteremia due to Bacteroides fragilis after elective appendectomy in renal transplant recipients. *J Infect Dis* **143**:635–638, 1981.

86. Palmer JM, Chatterjee SN: Urologic complications in renal transplantation. *Surg Clin North Am* **58**:305–319, 1978.

87. Leary FT, Woods JE, DeWeend JH: Urologic problems in renal transplantation. *Arch Surg* **110**:1124–1126, 1975.

88. Salvatierra O, Olcott C, Amend WA, et al: Urologic complications of renal transplantation can be prevented or controlled. *J Urol* **117**:421–424, 1977.

89. Malek GH, Uehling DT, Daouk AA, et al: Urological complications of renal transplantation. *J Urol* **109**:173–176, 1973.

90. Myerowitz RL, Medeiros AAM, O'Brien TF: Bacterial infection in renal homotransplant recipients; a study of fifty three bacteremic episodes. *Am J Med* **53**:308–314, 1972.

91. Lobo PI, Rudolf LE, Krieger JN: Wound infections in renal transplant recipients—A complication of urinary tract infections during allograft malfunction. *Surgery* **92**:491–496, 1982.

92. Kohlberg WI, Tellis VA, Bhat DJ, et al Wound infections after transplant nephrectomy. *Arch Surg* **115**:645–646, 1980.

93. Koehler PR, Kanemoto HH, Maxwell JG: Ultrasonic "B" scanning in the diagnosis of complications in renal transplant patients. *Radiology* **119**:661–664, 1976.

94. Schweizer R, Cho S, Kountz SL, et al: Lymphoceles following renal transplantation. *Arch Surg* **104**:42–45, 1972.

95. Lorimer WS, Glassfor DM, Sarles HE, et al: Lymphocele: A significant complication following renal transplantation. *Lymph* **8**:20–23, 1975.

96. Belzer FO: Technical complications after renal transplantation. In Morris PJ (ed). *Kidney Transplantation. Principles and Practice.* Academic, London, 1979, pp. 267–284

97. Tillegard A: Renal transplant wound infection The value of prophylactic antibiotic treatment *Scand J Urol Nephrol* **18**:215–221, 1984.

98. Townsend TR, Rudolf LE, Westervelt FB Jr, et al: Prophylactic antibiotic therapy with cefamandole and tobramycin for patients undergoing renal transplantation. *Infect Control* **1**:93–96, 1980.

99. Lorber MI, Campbell DA Jr, Konnah JW, et al: Etiology and management of early and late peritransplant infections. *J Urol* **127**:870–872, 1982.

100. Edwards JE Jr, Lehrer RI, Stiehm ER, et al. Severe candidal infections: Clinical perspective, immune defense mechanisms, and current concepts of therapy *Ann Intern Med* **89**:91–106, 1978.

101. Fiala M, Payne JE, Berne TV, et al: Epidemiology of cytomegalovirus infection after transplantation and immunosuppression. *J Infect Dis* **132**:421–433, 1975.

102. Suwansirikul S, Rao N, Dowling JN, et al. Primary and secondary cytomegalovirus infection: Clinical manifestations after renal transplantation. *Arch Intern med* **137**:1026–1029, 1977.

103. Naraqui S, Jackson GG, Jonasson O, et al: Prospective study of prevalence, incidence, and source of herpesvirus infections in patients with renal allografts. *J Infect Dis* **136**:531–540, 1977.

104. Rubin RH, Cosimi AB, Tolkoff-Rubin NE, et al: Infectious disease syndromes attributable to cytomegalovirus and their significance among renal transplant recipients. *Transplantation* **24**:458–464, 1977.

105. Linnemann CC Jr, Dunn CR, First MR, et al: Late onset of fatal cytomegalovirus infection after renal transplantation: Primary or reactivation infection? *Arch Intern Med* **138**:1247–1250, 1978.

106. Rubin RH, Tolkoff-Rubin NE The problem of cytomegalovirus infection in transplantation In Morris PJ, Tilney NL (eds). *Progress in Transplantation.* Vol 1 Churchill Livingstone, Edinburgh, 1984, pp. 89–114.

107. Ho M: *Cytomegalovirus, Biology and Infection.* Plenum, New York, 1982.

108. Rubin RH, Tolkoff-Rubin NE: Viral infection in the renal transplant patient. *Proc Eur Dialysis Transplant Assoc* **19**:513–528, 1982.

109. Ho M: Virus infections after transplantation in man; brief review. *Arch Virol* **55**:1–24, 1977.
110. Wertheim P, Geelen J, van der Nordaa J: Exogenous cytomegalovirus reinfection by renal allograft in seropositive recipients. *Lancet* (In press).
111. Chou S: Acquisition of donor strains of cytomegalovirus by renal-transplant recipients. *N Engl J Med* **314**:1418–1423, 1986.
112. Grundy JE, Super M, Lui S, et al: The source of cytomegalovirus infection in seropositive renal allograft recipients is frequently the donor kidney. *Transplant Proc* **19**:2126–2128, 1987.
113. Rubin RH, Tolkoff-Rubin NE, Oliver D, et al: Multicenter seroepidemiologic study of the impact of cytomegalovirus infection on renal transplantation. *Transplantation* **40**:243–249, 1985.
114. Betts RF, Schmidt SG: Cytolytic IgM antibody to cytomegalovirus in primary cytomegalovirus infection in humans. *J Infect Dis* **143**:821–826, 1981.
115. Betts RF: Cytomegalovirus in transplant patients. *Prog Med Virol* **28**:44–64, 1982.
116. Huang ES, Alford CA, Reynolds DW, et al: Molecular epidemiology of cytomegalovirus infection in women and their infants. *N Engl J Med* **303**:958–962, 1980.
117. Drew WL, Sweet ES, Miner RC, et al: Multiple infections by cytomegalovirus in patients with acquired immunodeficiency syndrome: Documentation by Southern blot hybridization. *J Infect Dis* **150**:952–953, 1984.
118. Fryd DS, Peterson PK, Ferguson RM, et al: Cytomegalovirus as a risk factor in renal transplantation. *Transplantation* **30**:436–439, 1980.
119. Smiley ML, Wlodaver CG, Grossman RA, et al: The role of pretransplant immunity in protection from cytomegalovirus disease following renal transplantation. *Transplantation* **40**:157–161, 1985.
120. Balfour HH Jr, Welo PK, Sachs GW: Cytomegalovirus vaccine trial in 400 renal transplant recipients. *Transplant Proc* **17**:81–83, 1985.
121. Tolkoff-Rubin NE, Rubin RH, Keller EE, et al: Cytomegalovirus infection in dialysis patients and personnel. *Ann Intern Med* **89**:625–628, 1978.
122. Dowling JN, Saslow AR, Armstrong JA, Ho M: Cytomegalovirus infection in patients receiving immunosuppressive therapy for rheumatologic disorders. *J Infect Dis* **133**:399–408, 1976.
123. Cheeseman SH, Rubin RH, Stewart JA, et al: Controlled clinical trial of prophylactic human leukocyte interferon in renal transplantation. Effect on cytomegalovirus and herpes simplex virus infection. *N Engl J Med* **300**:1345–1349, 1979.
124. Pass RF, Reynolds DW, Whelchel JD, et al: Impaired lymphocyte transformation response to cytomegalovirus and phytohemagglutinin in recipients of renal transplants: Association with antithymocyte globulin. *J Infect Dis* **143**:259–265, 1981.
125. Marker SC, Howard RJ, Simmons RL, et al: Cytomegalovirus infection: A quantitative prospective study of 320 consecutive renal transplants. *Surgery* **89**:660–671, 1981.
126. Rubin RH, Cosimi AB, Hirsch MS, et al: Effects of antithymocyte globulin on cytomegalovirus infection in renal transplant recipients *Transplantation* **31**:143–145, 1981.
127. Bia MJ, Andiman W, Gaudio K, et al: Effect of treatment with cyclosporine versus azathioprine on incidence and severity of cytomegalovirus infection posttransplantation. *Transplantation* **40**:610–614, 1985.
128. Weir MR, Irwin BC, Maters AW, et al: Incidence of cytomegalovirus disease in cyclosporine-treated renal transplant recipients based on donor–recipient pre-transplant immunity. *Transplantation* **113**:187–193, 1987.
129. Najarian JS, Fryd DS, Strand M, et al: A single institution, randomized, prospective trial of cyclosporine versus azathioprine - antithymocyte globulin for immunosuppression in renal allograft recipients. *Ann Surg* **201**:142–157, 1985.
130. Tolkoff-Rubin NE, Rubin RH: The impact of cyclosporine therapy on the occurrence of infection in the renal transplant recipient. *Transplant Proc* **18**(suppl 1):168–173, 1986
131. Peterson PK, Balfour HH Jr, Marker SC, et al: Cytomegalovirus disease in renal allograft recipients: A prospective study of the clinical features, risk factors, and impact on renal transplantation. *Medicine (Baltimore)* **59**:283–300, 1980.
132. Peterson PK, Balfour HH Jr, Fryd DS, et al: Fever in renal transplant recipients: Causes, prognostic significance and changing patterns at the University of Minnesota Hospital. *Am J Med* **71**:345–351, 1981
133. Simmons RL, Lopez C, Balfour HH Jr, et al: Cytomegalovirus: Clinical virological correlations in renal transplant recipients. *Ann Surg* **180**:623–634, 1974.
134. Simmons RL, Matas AJ, Rattazzi LC, et al: Clinical characteristics of the lethal cytomegalovirus infection following renal transplantation. *Surgery* **82**:537–546, 1977.
135. Fine RN, Grushkin CM, Malekzadeh M, et al: Cytomegalovirus syndrome following renal transplantation. *Arch Surg* **105**:564–570, 1972.
136. Jeffery JR, Guttmann RD, Becklake MR, et al: Recovery from severe cytomegalovirus pneumonia in a renal transplant patient. *Am Rev Respir Dis* **109**:129–133, 1974.
137. Ravin CE, Smith GW, Ahern MJ, et al: Cytomegaloviral infection presenting as a solitary pulmonary nodule. *Chest* **71**:220–222, 1977.
138. Hamed IA, Wenzl JE, Leonard JC, et al: Pulmonary cytomegalovirus infection: detection by gallium 67 imaging in the transplant patient. *Arch Intern Med* **139**:286–288, 1979.
139. Friedman HM, Grossman RA, Plotkin SA, et al: Relapse of pneumonia caused by cytomegalovirus in two recipients of renal transplants *J Infect Dis* **139**:465–473, 1979.
140. Armstrong JA, Evans AS, Rao N, et al: Viral infections in renal transplant recipients. *Infect Immunol* **14**:970–975, 1976.
141. Luby JP, Brunett W, Hull AR, et al: Relationship between cytomegalovirus and hepatic function abnormalities in the period after renal transplant. *J Infect Dis* **129**: 511–518, 1974.
142. Sutherland DER, Chan FY, Foucar E, et al: The bleeding

cecal ulcer in transplant patients. *Surgery* **86**:386–398, 1980.

143. Ayulo M, Aisner SC, Margolis K, et al: Fatal cytomegalic inclusion disease: Associated skin manifestations in a renal transplant patient. *Arch Dermatol* **113**:1569–1571, 1977.

144. Patel NP, Corry RJ: Cytomegalovirus as a cause of cecal ulcer with massive hemorrhage in a renal transplant recipient. *Am Surg* **46**:260–262, 1980.

145. Franzin G, Muolo A, Griminelli T: Cytomegalovirus inclusions in the gastroduodenal mucosa of patients after renal transplantation *Gut* **22**:698–701, 1981.

146. Van Son WJ, Van der Jagt EJ, Van der Woude FJ, et al: Pneumatosis intestinalis in patients after cadaveric kidney transplantation. Possible relationship with an active cytomegalovirus infection. *Transplantation* **38**:506–510, 1984.

147 Dorfman LJ: Cytomegalovirus encephalitis in adults. *Neurology (NY)* **23**:316–144, 1973.

148. Spitzer PG, Tarsy D, Eliopoulos GM: Acute transverse myelitis during disseminated cytomegalovirus infection in a renal transplant recipient. *Transplantation* (In press).

149. Minars N, Silverman JF, Escobar MR, et al: Fatal cytomegalic inclusion disease; associated skin manifestations in a renal transplant patient; *Arch Dermatol* **113**:1569–1571, 1977.

150. Braun WE, Nankervis G: Cytomegalovirus viremia and bacteremia in renal allograft recipients. *N Engl J Med* **299**:1318–1319, 1978.

151. Cheeseman SH, Stewart JA, Winkle S, et al: Cytomegalovirus excretion 2–14 years after renal transplantation. *Transplant Proc* **11**:71–74, 1979.

152. Fiala M, Chatterjee SN, Carson S, et al: Cytomegalovirus retinitis secondary to chronic viremia in phagocytic leukocytes. *Am J Ophthalmol* **84**:567–573, 1977.

153. Aaberg TM, Cesario TJ, Rytel MW: Correlation of virology and clinical course of cytomegalovirus retinitis. *Am J Ophthalmol* **74**:407–415, 1972.

154. DeVenecia G, ZuRhein GM, Pratt MV, et al: Cytomegalic inclusion retinitis in an adult. *Arch Ophthalmol* **86**:44–57, 1971.

155. Porter R, Crombie AL, Gardner PS, et al: Incidence of ocular complications in patients undergoing renal transplantation. *Br Med J* **3**:133–136, 1972.

156. Wyhinny GJ, Apple DJ, Guastella FR, et al: Adult cytomegalic inclusion retinitis. *Am J Ophthalmol* **76**:773–781, 1973.

157. Astle JN, Ellis PP: Ocular complications in renal transplant patients. *Ann Ophthalmol* **6**:1269–1274, 1974.

158. Nicholson DH: Cytomegalovirus infection of the retina: In PavanLangston D (ed): *Ocular Viral Disease*. Little, Brown, Boston, 1975, pp. 151–162.

159. Murray HW, Knox DL, Green WR, et al: Cytomegalovirus retinitis in adults; a manifestation of disseminated viral infection. *Am J Med* **63**:574–584, 1977.

160. Merritt JC, Callender CO: Adult cytomegalic inclusion retinitis. *Ann Ophthalmol* **10**:1059–1063, 1978.

161. Carson S, Chatterjee SN: Cytomegalovirus retinitis: Two cases occurring after renal transplantation. *Ann Ophthalmol* **10**:275–279, 1978.

162. Broughton WL, Cupples HP, Parver LM: Bilateral retinal detachment following cytomegalovirus retinitis. *Arch Ophthalmol* **96**:618–619, 1978.

163. Moeller MB, Gutman RA, Hamilton JD: Acquired cytomegalovirus retinitis. Four new cases and a review of the literature with implications for management. *Am J Nephrol* **2**:251–255, 1982.

164. Rand KH, Pollard RB, Merigan TC: Increased pulmonary superinfections in cardiac-transplant patients undergoing primary cytomegalovirus infection. *N Engl J Med* **298**:951–953, 1978.

165. Chatterjee SN, Fiala M, Weiner J, et al: Primary cytomegalovirus and opportunistic infections; incidence in renal transplant recipients. *JAMA* **240**:2446–2449, 1978.

166. Rifkind D: *Pneumocystis carinii* pneumonia in renal transplant recipients. *Natl Cancer Inst Monogr* **43**:49–54, 1976.

167. Munda R, Alexander JW, First MR, et al: Pulmonary infections in renal transplant recipients. *Ann Surg* **187**:126–133, 1978.

168. Gantz NM, Myerowitz RL, Medeiros AA, et al: Listeriosis in immunosuppressed patients. A cluster of eight cases. *Am J Med* **58**:637–642, 1975.

169. Schröter GPJ, Weil R III: *Listeria monocytogenes* infection after renal transplantation. *Arch Intern Med* **137**:1395–1399, 1978.

170. Hooper DC, Pruitt AA, Rubin RH: Central nervous system infections in the chronically immunosuppressed. *Medicine (Baltimore)* **61**:166–188, 1982.

171. Rubin RH, Hooper DC: Central nervous system infection in the compromised host. *Med Clin North Am* **69**:281–296, 1985.

172. Rytel MW, Balay J: Cytomegalovirus infection and immunity in renal allograft recipients: Assessment of the competence of humoral immunity. *Infect Immun* **13**:1633–1637, 1976.

173. Baldwin WM III, van Es A, Valentijn RM, et al: Increased IgM and IgM immune complex-like material in the circulation of renal transplant recipients with primary cytomegalovirus infections. *Clin Exp Immunol* **50**:515–524, 1982.

174. Baldwin WM III, Henny FC, Claas FHJ, et al: IgM immune complexes, leucocytotoxins and rheumatoid factors during active cytomegalovirus infection in renal graft recipients treated with azathioprine, cyclosporine A or anti-thymocyte globulin. *Proc Europ Dialysis Transplant Assoc* **22**:655–659, 1985.

175. Baldwin WM III, Claas FHJ, Van Gemert GW, et al: Studies on lymphocytotoxins and rheumatoid factors in renal transplant recipients with cytomegalovirus disease. *Transplant Proc* **17**:616–617, 1985.

176 Rytel MW, Aguilar-Torres FG, Balay J, et al: Assessment of the status of cell-mediated immunity in cytomegalovirus-infected renal allograft recipients. *Infect Immun* **13**:1633–1637, 1976.

177. Linnemann CC Jr, Kauffman CA, First MR, et al: Cellular immune response to cytomegalovirus infection after renal transplantation *Infect Immun* **22**:176–180, 1978.

178. Glazer JP, Friedman HM, Grossman RA, et al: Live

cytomegalovirus vaccination of renal transplant candidates, a preliminary trial *Ann Intern Med* **91**:676–683, 1979.

179. Craighead JE: Cytomegalovirus pulmonary disease. *Pathobiol Annu* **5**:197–220, 1975.

180. Green GM: The J. Burns Amberson Lecture—In defense of the lung *Am Rev Respir Dis* **102**:691–703, 1970.

181. Rinaldo CR Jr, Black PH, Hirsch MS: Interaction of cytomegalovirus with leukocytes from patients with mononucleosis due to cytomegalovirus *J Infect Dis* **136**:667–678, 1977.

182. Levin MJ, Rinaldo CR Jr, Leary PL, et al: Immune response to herpesvirus antigens in adults with acute cytomegaloviral mononucleosis. *J Infect Dis* **140**:851–857, 1979

183. Carney WP, Hirsch MS: Mechanisms of immunosuppression in cytomegalovirus mononucleosis. II. Virus-monocyte interactions. *J Infect Dis* **144**:47–54, 1981.

184 Rinaldo CR Jr, Carney WP, Richter BS, et al: Mechanisms of immunosuppression in cytomegaloviral mononucleosis. *J Infect Dis* **141**:488–495, 1980.

185. Carney WP, Iacoviello V, Hirsch MS: Functional properties of T lymphocytes and their subsets in cytomegalovirus mononucleosis. *J Immunol* **130**:390–393, 1983.

186 Schrier RD, Rice GPA, Oldstone MBA: Suppression of natural killer cell activity and T cell proliferation by fresh isolates of human cytomegalovirus. *J Infect Dis* **153**:1084–1091, 1986.

187. Rook AH, Masur H, Lane HC, et al: Interleukin-2 enhances the depressed natural killer and cytomegalovirus-specific cytotoxic activities of lymphocytes from patients with the acquired immune deficiency syndrome *J Clin Invest* **72**:398–403, 1983.

188. Charpentier B, Espinosa O, Martin B, et al. T cell immunity against cytomegalovirus modifies self-major histocompatability complex antigens in kidney transplant recipients. *Transplant Proc* **17**:161–162, 1985.

189. Carney WP, Rubin RH, Hoffman RA, et al: Analysis of T lymphocyte subsets in cytomegalovirus mononucleosis. *J Immunol* **126**:2114–2116, 1981.

190. Schooley RT, Hirsch MS, Colvin RB, et al: Association of herpes virus infection with T-lymphocyte subset alterations, glomerulopathy, and opportunistic infections after renal transplantation. *N Engl J Med* **308**:307–313, 1983.

191. Dummer JS, Ho M, Rabin BP, et al. The effect of cytomegalovirus and Epstein-Barr virus infection on T-lymphocyte subsets in cardiac transplant patients on cyclosporine. *Transplantation* **38**:433–435, 1984.

192. Simmons RL, Weil R, Tallent MB, et al: Do mild infections trigger the rejection of renal allografts? *Transplant Proc* **2**:419–423, 1970.

193. Balfour HH Jr, Slade MS, Kalis JM, et al: Viral infections in renal transplant donors and their recipients. A prospective study. *Surgery* **81**:487–492, 1977.

194. David DS, Millian SJ, Whitsell JC, et al: Viral syndromes and renal homograft rejection. *Ann Surg* **175**:257–259, 1972.

195. Briggs JD, Timbury MC, Paton AM, et al: Viral infection and renal transplant rejection. *Br Med J* **4**:520–522, 1972.

196. Lopez C, Simmons RL, Mauer SM, et al Association of renal allograft rejection with virus infection. *Am J Med* **56**:280–289, 1974.

197. Betts RF, Freeman RB, Douglas RG Jr, et al: Clinical manifestations of renal allograft derived primary cytomegalovirus infection. *Am J Dis Child* **131**:759–763, 1977.

198. May AG, Betts RF, Freeman RB, et al: An analysis of cytomegalovirus infection and HLA antigen matching on the outcome of renal transplantation *Ann Surg* **187**:110–117, 1978.

199. von Willebrand E, Pettersson E, Ahonen J, et al: CMV infection, class II antigen expression, and human kidney allograft rejection. *Transplantation* **42**:364–367, 1986.

200. Harmon JB, Sibley RK, Peterson P, et al: Cytomegalovirus viremia and renal allograft morphology. Are there distinct pathologic features? *Lab Invest* **46**:35A, 1982.

201. Herrera GA, Alexander RW, Cooly CF, et al: Cytomegalovirus glomerulopathy: A controversial lesion *Kidney Int* **29**:725–733, 1986.

202. Cameron J, Rigby RJ, van Deth AG, et al: Severe tubulointerstitial disease in a renal allograft due to cytomegalovirus infection *Clin Nephrol* **18**:321–325, 1982

203. Richardson WP, Colvin RB, Cheeseman SH, et al: Glomerulopathy associated with cytomegalovirus viremia in renal allografts. *N Engl J Med* **305**:57–63, 1981.

204. Rubin RH, Colvin RB: Cytomegalovirus infection in renal transplantation, clinical importance and control. In Williams GM, Burdick JF, Solez K (eds): *Kidney Transplant Rejection: Diagnosis and Treatment* Dekker, New York, 1986, pp. 283–304.

205. Maryniak R, First RM, Weiss MA. Transplant glomerulopathy: Evolution of morphologically distinct changes. *Kidney Int* **27**:799–806, 1985

206. Pardo V, Aldana M, Colton RM, et al: Glomerular lesions in the acquired immunodeficiency syndrome. *Ann Intern Med* **101**:429–434, 1984.

207. Colvin RB, Cosimi AB, Burton RC, et al: Circulating T-cell subsets in human renal allograft recipients: The OKT4+/OKT8+ cell ratio correlates with reversibility of graft injury and glomerulopathy. *Transplant Proc* **15**:1166–1169, 1983.

208 Tirazon TV, Schneeberger EE, Bhan AK: In situ analysis of mononuclear cells in acute allograft glomerulopathy. *Am J Path* (In press).

209. Skoskiewicz MJ, Colvin RB, Schneeberger EE, Russell PS. Widespread and selective induction of major histocompatibility complex-determined antigens in vivo by gamma interferon. *J Exp Med* **162**:1645–1664, 1985.

210. Pober JS, Collins T, Gimbrone MA Jr, et al: Lymphocytes recognize human vascular endothelial and dermal fibroblast Ia antigens induced by recombinant immune interferon. *Nature (Lond)* **305**:726–729, 1983.

211. Pober JS, Gimbrone MA Jr, Cotran RS, et al: Ia expression by vascular endothelium is inducible by activated T cells and by human gamma interferon *J Exp Med* **157**:1339–1353, 1983.

212. Groenewegen G, Buurman WA, van der Linden CJ: Lymphokine dependence of in vivo expression of MHC class II

antigens by endothelium. *Nature (Lond)* **316**:361–363, 1985.

213. Spector DH, Vacquier JP: Human cytomegalovirus (strain AD 169) contains sequences related to the avian retrovirus oncogene V-myc. *Proc Natl Acad Sci USA* **80**:3889–3893, 1983.

214. Gelmann EP, Clanton DJ, Jariwalla RJ, et al: Characterization and location of myc homologous sequences in human cytomegalovirus DNA. *Proc Natl Acad Sci USA* **80**:5107–5111, 1983.

215. Nelson JA, Fleckenstein B, Galloway DA, et al: Transformation of NIH 3T3 cells with cloned fragments of human cytomegalovirus strain AD 169. *J Virol* **43**:83–91, 1982

216. Penn I: Kaposi's sarcoma in renal transplant recipients. *Transplantation* **27**:8–11, 1979.

217. Drew WL, Conant MA, Miner RC, et al: Cytomegalovirus and Kaposi's sarcoma in young homosexual men. *Lancet* **2**:125–127, 1982.

218. Rubin RH, Russell PS, Levin M, et al: Summary of a workshop on cytomegalovirus infection during organ transplantation. *J Infect Dis* **139**:728–734, 1979.

219. Glazer JP, Friedman HM, Grossman RA, et al: Live cytomegalovirus vaccination of renal transplant candidates, a preliminary trial. cytomegalovirus vaccine. *Ann Intern Med* **91**:676–6683, 1979.

220. Starr SE, Glazer JP, Friedman HM, et al: Specific cellular and humoral immunity after immunization with live Towne strain cytomegalovirus vaccine. *J Infect Dis* **143**:585–589, 1981.

221. Carney WP, Hirsch MS, Iacoviello VR, et al: T-lymphocyte subsets and proliferative responses following immunization with cytomegalovirus vaccine. *J Infect Dis* **143**:958, 1983.

222. Plotkin SA, Smiley ML, Friedman HM, et al: Towne vaccine in the prevention of post-transplant CMV disease. *Lancet* **1**:528–530, 1984.

223. Snydman DR, McIver J, Leszczynski J, et al: A pilot trial of a novel cytomegalovirus immune globulin in renal transplant recipients *Transplantation* **38**:553–557, 1984.

224 Snydman DR, Werner BG, Heinze-Lacey B, et al: Prevention of kidney transplant associated primary cytomegalovirus disease with an intravenous cytomegalovirus immune globulin (CMV Ig-IV). An interim report In *American Society of Transplant Physicians, Fifth Annual Meeting, Chicago, May 1986.*

225. Scheuermann EH, Bechstein PB, Schoeppe W, et al: Cytomegalovirus infections after renal transplantation: Effect of prophylactic hyperimmune globulin. *Proc Eur Dial Transplant Assoc* **22**:630–634, 1985.

226 Hirsch MS, Schooley RT, Cosimi AB, et al. Effects of interferon-alpha on cytomegalovirus reactivation syndrome in renal transplant recipients. *N Engl J Med* **308**:1489–1493, 1983

227. Kramer P, Ten Kate FWJ, Bijnen AB, et al Recombinant leucocyte interferon A induces steroid resistant acute vascular rejection episodes in renal transplant recipients. *Lancet* **1**:989–990, 1984

228 Weimar W, Kramer P, Bijnen AB, et al. The incidence of cytomegalovirus and herpes simplex virus infections in renal allograft recipients treated with high dose of recombinant leucocyte interferon. A controlled study. *Scand J Urol Nephrol* **92**(suppl):37–39, 1985.

229. Kovarik J, Mayer G, Pohanka E, et al. Adverse effects of low dose prophylactic human recombinant leucocyte interferon-alpha treatment in renal transplant recipients—cytomegalovirus infection prophylaxis leads to an increased incidence of irreversible rejections. (In press.)

230. Singer DRJ, Fallon TJ, Schulenburg WE, et al: Cytomegalovirus retinitis in a renal transplant patient with recurrent opportunistic infections: Treatment with foscanet and CMV hyper immune globulin. *Proc Eur Dial Transplant Assoc* **22**:645–650, 1985.

231. Collaborative DHPG Treatment Study Group: Treatment of serious cytomegalovirus infections with 9-(1,3-dihydroxy-2-propoxymethyl)guanine in patients with AIDS and other immunodeficiencies. *N Engl J Med* **314**:801–805, 1986.

233. Shepp DH, Danliker PS, de Miranda P, et al: Activity of 9-[2-hydroxy-1-(hydroxymethyl)ethoxymethyl]guanine in the treament of cytomegalovirus pneumonia. *Ann Intern Med* **103**:368–373, 1985.

233a. Erice A, Jordan C, Chace BA, et al. Ganciclovir treatment and cytomegalovirus disease in transplant recipients and other immuno-suppressed hosts. *JAMA* **257**:3082–3087, 1987.

234. Pollard RB, Egbert PR, Gallagher JG, et al: Cytomegalovirus retinitis in immunosuppressed hosts. I. Natural hsitory and effects of treatment with adenine arabinoside. *Ann Intern Med* **93**:655–664, 1980.

235. Marker SC, Howard RJ, Groth KE, et al: A trial of vidarabine for cytomegalovirus in renal transplant patients. *Arch Intern Med* **140**:1441–1444, 1980.

236. Naraqui S, Jonasson O, Jackson GG, et al: Clinical manifestations of infections with herpesviruses after kidney transplantation: A prospective study of various syndromes. *Ann Surg* **188**:234–239, 1978.

237. Cheeseman SH, Henle W, Rubin RH, et al: Epstein–Barr virus infection in renal transplant recipients. Effects of antithymocyte globulin and interferon. *Ann Intern Med* **193**:39–44, 1970.

238. Spencer ES, Andersen HK: Clinically evident, non-terminal infections with herpesviruses and the wart virus in immunosuppressed renal allograft recipients. *Br Med J* **3**:251–254, 1970.

239. Strauch B, Andrews L, Miller G, et al: Oropharyngeal excretion of Epstein–Barr virus by renal transplant recipients and other patients treated with immunosuppressant drugs *Lancet* **1**:234–237, 1974.

240. Chang RS, Lewis JP, Reynolds RD, et al. Oropharyngeal excretion of Epstein–Barr virus by patients with lymphoproliferative disorders and by recipients of renal homografts. *Ann Intern Med* **88**:34–40, 1978.

241. Rifkind D, Starzl TE, Marchioro TL, et al: Transplantation pneumonia. *JAMA* **189**:808–812, 1964

242. Grose C, Henle W, Horwitz MS: Primary Epstein–Barr virus infection in a renal transplant recipient. *South Med J* **70**:1276–1278, 1977

243. Marker SC, Ascher NL, Kalıs JM, et al: Epstein–Barr virus antibody responses and clinical illness in renal transplant recipients. *Surgery* **85**:433–440, 1979.

244 Junker AK, Ochs HD, Clark EA, et al: Transient immune deficiency in patients with acute Epstein–Barr virus infection. *Clin Immunol Immunopathol* **40**:436–446, 1986.

245. Hanto D, Frizzera G, Purtilo DT, et al: Clinical spectrum of lymphoproliferative disorders in renal transplant recipients and evidence for the role of Epstein–Barr virus. *Cancer Res* **41**:4253–4261, 1981.

246. Frizzera G, Hanto DW, Gajl-Peczalska KJ, et al: Polymorphic diffuse B-cell hyperplasias and lymphomas in renal transplant recipients. *Cancer Res* **41**:4253–4261, 1981

247. Hanto D, Sakamoto K, Purtilo DT, et al: The Epstein–Barr virus in the pathogenesis of posttransplant lymphoproliferative disorders. *Surgery* **90**:204–213, 1981.

248. Hanto D, Frizzera G, Gajl-Peczalska K, et al: Epstein–Barr virus-induced B-cell lymphoma after renal transplantation. *N Engl J Med* **306**:913–918, 1982.

249. Hanto DW, Gajl-Peczalska KJ, Frizzera G, et al: Epstein–Barr virus (EBV) induced polyclonal and monoclonal B-cell lymphoproliferative disease occurring after renal transplantation. Clinical, pathologic, and virologic findings and implications for therapy. *Ann Surg* **198**:356–369, 1983.

250. Hanto DW, Frizzera G, Gajl-Peczalska KJ, et al: Acyclovir therapy of Epstein–Barr virus-induced posttransplant lymphoproliferative diseases. *Transplant Proc* **17**:89–82, 1985.

251. Crawford DH, Swany P, Edwards JMB, et al: Long-term T-cell mediated immunity to Epstein–Barr virus in renal allograft recipients receiving cyclosporin A. *Lancet* **1**:10–12, 1981.

252. Bird AG, McLachlin SM, Britton S: Cyclosporin A promotes spontaneous outgrowth *in vitro* of Epstein–Barr virus-induced B-cell lines. *Nature (Lond)* **289**:300–301, 1981.

253. Crawford DH, Edwards JM, Sweny P, et al: Studies on long-term T-cell-mediated immunity to Epstein–Barr virus in immunosuppressed renal allograft recipients. *Int J Cancer* **28**:705–709, 1981.

254 Yao QY, Rickinson AB, Gastron JS, et al: In vitro analysis of the Epstein-Barr virus: Host balance in long-term renal allograft recipients. *Int J Cancer* **35**:43–49, 1985.

255 Calne RY, Roller K, Thiru S, et al: Cyclosporin A initially as the only immunosuppressant in 34 recipients of cadaveric organs: 32 kidneys, 2 pancreas, and 2 livers. *Lancet* **2**:1033–1036, 1979.

256. Starzl TE, Nalesnik MA, Porter KA, et al: Reversibility of lymphomas and lymphoproliferative lesions developing under cyclosporin-steroid therapy *Lancet* **1**:583–587, 1984.

257. Bia MJ, Flye MW: Immunoblastic lymphoma in a cyclosporine-treated renal transplant recipient. *Transplantation* **39**:673–674, 1985.

258. Korsager B, Spencer ES, Heinrich Mordhorst C, et al: Herpesvirus hominis infections in renal transplant recipients. *Scand J Infect Dis* **7**:11–19, 1975.

259. Stone WJ, Scowden EB, Spannuth CL, et al: A typical herpesvirus hominus type 2 infection in uremic patients receiving immunosuppressive therapy. *Am J Med* **63**:511–516, 1977

260. Burkhart CG: Persistent cutaneous herpes simplex infection. *Int J Dermatol* **20**:552–554, 1981.

261. Ramsey PG, Rubin RH, Tolkoff-Rubin NE, et al: The renal transplant patient with fever and pulmonary infiltrates: Etiology, clinical manifestations, and management. *Medicine (Baltimore)* **59**:206–222, 1980.

262 Anuras S, Summers R: Fulminant herpes simplex hepatitis in an adult: Report of a case in a renal transplant recipient. *Gastroenterology* **70**:425–428, 1976.

263. Holdsworth SR, Atkins RC, Scott DF, et al: Systemic herpes simplex infection with fulminant hepatitis post-transplantation. *Aust NZ J Med* **6**:588–590, 1976.

264. Elliot WC, Houghton DC, Bryant RE, et al: Herpes simplex type 1 hepatitis in renal transplantation. *Arch Intern Med* **140**:1656–1660, 1980.

265. Taylor RJ, Saul SH, Dowling JN, et al: Primary disseminated herpes simplex infection with fulminant hepatitis following renal transplantation *Arch Intern Med* **141**:1519–1521, 1981.

266. Naraqui S, Jackson GG, Jonasson OM: Viremia with herpes simplex type 1 in adults. *Ann Intern Med* **85**:165–169, 1976.

267. Arora KK, Karalakulasingham R, Raff MJ, et al: Cutaneous herpesvirus hominis (type 2) infection after renal transplantation. *JAMA* **230**:1174–1175, 1974

267a. Dummer JS, Armstrong J, Somers J, et al: Transmission of infection with herpes simplex virus by renal transplantation. *J Infect Dis* **55**:202–206, 1987.

268. Dunn DL, Matas AJ, Fryd DS, et al: Association of concurrent herpes simplex virus and cytomegalovirus with detrimental effects after renal transplantation. *Arch Surg* **119**:812–817, 1984

269. Griffin PJA, Colbert JW, Williamson EPM, et al: Oral acyclovir prophylaxis of herpes infection in renal transplant recipients. *Transplant Proc* **17**:84–85, 1985.

270 Pettersson E, Hovi T, Ahonen T, et al: Prophylactic oral acyclovir after renal transplantation. *Transplantation* **39**:279–281, 1985

271. Rifkind D: The activation of varicella-zoster virus infections by immunosuppressive therapy. *J Lab Clin Med* **68**:463–474, 1966.

272. Luby JP, Ramirez-Ronda C, Rinner S, et al: A longitudinal study of varicella-zoster virus infections in renal transplant recipients. *J Infect Dis* **135**:659–663, 1977.

273. Hope-Simpson RE: The nature of herpes zoster: A long-term study and a new hypothesis. *Proc R Soc Med* **58**:9–20, 1965

274. Garner SD: Prevalence in England of antibody to polyomavirus (B.K.). *Br Med J* **1**:77–78, 1973

275 Shah KV, Daniel RW, Warszawski RM: High prevalence of antibodies to BK virus, an SV40-related papovavirus, in residents of Maryland. *J Infect Dis* **128**:784–787, 1973.

276 Brown P, Tsai T, Gajdusek DC: Seroepidemiology of human papovaviruses. Discovery of virgin populations and some unusual patterns of antibody prevalence among remote peoples of the world. *Am J Epidemiol* **102**:331–340, 1975.

277. Gardner SD, Field AM, Coleman DW, et al: New human papovavirus (BK) isolated from urine after renal transplantation. *Lancet* **1**:1253–1257, 1971.

278. Coleman DV, Gardner SD, Field AM: Human polyomavirus

infection in renal allograft recipients. *Br Med J* 3:371–375, 1973.

279. Lecatsas G, Prozesky DW, VanWyk J, et al: Papova virus in urine after renal transplantation. *Nature (Lond)* 241:343–344, 1973.

280. Shah KV, Daniel RW, Ziegel RF, et al: Search for BK and SV40 virus reactivation in renal transplant recipients. *Transplantation* 17:131–134, 1974.

281. Flower AJE, Banatvala JE, Chrystie IL: BK antibody and virus-specific IgM responses in renal transplant recipients, patients with malignant disease, and healthy people. *Br Med J* 2:220–223, 1977.

282. Coleman DV, MacKenzie EED, Gardner SD, et al: Human polyomavirus (BK) infection and ureteric stenosis in renal allograft recipients. *J Clin Pathol* 31:338–347, 1978.

283. Cheeseman SH, Black PH, Rubin RH, et al: Interferon and BK papovavirus—clinical and laboratory studies. *J Infect Dis* 141:159–161, 1980.

284. Hogan TF, Borden EC, McBain JA, et al: Human polyomavirus infections with JC virus and BK virus in renal transplant patients. *Ann Intern Med* 92:373–378, 1980.

285. Narayan O, Penney JB Jr, Johnson RT, et al: Etiology of progressive multifocal leukoencephalopathy. Identification of papovavirus. *N Engl J Med* 289:1278–1282, 1973.

286. Padgett BL, Walker D: New human papovaviruses. In Melnick J (ed): *Progress in Medical Virology.* Karger, Basel, 1976, pp. 1–35.

287. Matas AJ, Hertel BF, Rosai J, et al: Post-transplant malignant lymphoma: Distinctive morphologic features related to its pathogenesis. *Am J Med* 61:716–620, 1976.

288. Sheil AGR: Transplantation and cancer, in Morris PJ (ed): *Kidney Transplantation: Principles and Practice.* Academic, London, 1979, pp. 335–352.

289. Padgett BL, Walker DL, ZuRhein GM, et al: Culturation of papovalike virus from human brain with progressive multifocal leucoencephalopathy. *Lancet* 1:1257–1260, 1971.

290. Andrews C, Shah KV, Rubin R, et al: BK papovavirus infections in renal transplant recipients: Contribution of donor kidneys. *J Infect Dis* 145:276, 1982.

291. ZuRhein GM, Varakis J: Progressive multifocal leukoencephalopathy in a renal allograft recipient. *N Engl J Med* 291:798, 1974.

292. Hierholzer JC, Atuk NO, Gwaltney JM Jr: New human adenovirus isolated from renal transplant recipient: Description and characterization of candidate adenovirus type 34. *J Clin Microbiol* 1:366–376, 1975.

293. Myerowitz RL, Stalder H, Oxman MN, et al: Fatal disseminated adenovirus infection in a renal transplant recipient. *Am J Med* 59:591–598, 1975.

294. Keller EW, Hierholzer JC, Rubin RH, et al: Isolation of adenovirus type 34 from a renal transplant recipient with interstitial pneumonia. *Transplantation* 23:188–191, 1977.

295. Stalder H, Hierholzer JC, Oxman MN. New human adenovirus (candidate adenovirus type 35) causing fatal disseminated infection in a renal transplant recipient. *J Clin Microbiol* 6:257–265, 1977

296. Lecatsas G, Prozesky OW, VanWyk J: Adenovirus type 11 associated with haemorrhagic cystitis after renal transplantation. *S Afr Med J* 48:1932–1935, 1974.

297. Harnett GB, Bucens MR, Clay SJ, et al: Acute haemorrhagic cystitis caused by adenovirus type 11 in a recipient of a transplanted kidney. *Med J Aust* 1:565–567, 1982.

298. Huebner RJ, Rowe WP, Lane WT: Oncogenic effects in hamsters of human adenoviruses types 12 and 18. *Proc Natl Acad Sci USA* 48:2051–2058, 1962.

299. Hinman F Jr, Schmaelzle JF, Belzer FO: Urinary tract infections and renal homotransplantation. II Post-transplantation bacterial invasion. *J Urol* 101:673–679, 1969.

300. Leigh DA: The outcome of urinary tract infections in patients after human cadaveric renal transplantation. *Br J Urol* 101:453–456, 1970.

301. Martin DC: Urinary tract infection in clinical renal transplantation. *Arch Surg* 99:474–476, 1969.

302. Bennett WM, Beck CH Jr, Young HH, et al: Bacteriuria in the first month following renal transplantation. *Arch Surg* 101:453–456, 1970.

303. Prout GR Jr, Hume DM, Lee HM, et al: Some urological aspects of 93 consecutive renal homotransplants in modified recipients. *J Urol* 97:409–425, 1967.

304. Ramsey DE, Finch WT, Birch AG: Urinary tract infections in kidney transplant recipients. *Arch Surg* 114:1022–1025, 1979.

305. Rubin RH, Fang LST, Cosimi AB, et al: Usefulness of the antibody-coated bacteria assay in the management of urinary tract infection in the renal transplant patient. *Transplantation* 27:18–20, 1979.

306. Nielsen HE, Korsager B: Bacteremia after renal transplantation. *Scand J Infect Dis* 9:111–117, 1977.

307. Pearson JC, Amend WJ Jr, Vincenti FG, et al. Post-transplantation pyelonephritis: Factors producing low patient and transplant morbidity. *J Urol* 123:153–156, 1980

308. Burleson RL, Brennan AM, Scruggs BF: Foley catheter tip cultures; a valuable diagnostic aid in the immunosuppressed patient. *Am J Surg* 133:723–725, 1977.

309. Schaeffer AJ: Catheter-associated bacteriuria in patients in reverse isolation. *J Urol* 128:752–754, 1982.

310. Schaeffer AJ, Chmiel J: Urethral meatal colonization in the pathogenesis of catheter-associated bacteriuria. *J Urol* 130:1096–1099, 1983.

311. Heptinstall RH: Experimental pyelonephritis: A comparison of blood-borne and ascending patterns of infection. *J Pathol* 89:71–80, 1965.

312. Mathew TM, Kincaid-Smith P, Vikraman P: Risks of vesicoureteric reflux in the transplanted kidney. *N Engl J Med* 297:414–418, 1977.

313 Murphy JF, McDonald FD, Dawson M, et al: Factors influencing the frequency of infection in renal transplant recipients. *Arch Intern Med* 136:670–677, 1976.

314. Griffin PJA, Salaman JR: Urinary tract infections after renal transplantation: Do they matter? *Br Med J* 1:710–711, 1979

315. Vincenti F, Amend WJ Jr, Feduska NJ, et al: Septic arthritis following renal transplantation. *Nephron* 30:253–256, 1982.

316. Fang LST, Tolkoff-Rubin NE, Rubin RH: Localization and antibiotic management of urinary tract infection. *Annu Rev Med* 30:225–239, 1979

317. Holmgren J, Smith JW: Immunological aspects of urinary tract infections. *Prog Allergy* 18:289–352, 1975.

318. Byrd LH, Tapia L, Cheigh JS, et al: Association between *Streptococcus faecalis* urinary infections and graft rejection in kidney transplantation. *Lancet* 2:1167–1169, 1978

319. Fang LST, Tolkoff-Rubin NE, Rubin RH: Efficacy of single dose and conventional amoxicillin therapy in urinary tract infection localized by the antibody-coated bacteria technique. *N Engl J Med* 298:413–416, 1978.

320. Tolkoff-Rubin NE, Cosimi AB, Russell PS, et al: A controlled study of trimethoprim/sulfamethoxazole prophylaxis of urinary tract infection in renal transplant patients. *Rev Infect Dis* 4:614–618, 1982.

321. Peters C, Peterson P, Marabella P, et al: Continuous sulfa prophylaxis for urinary tract infection in renal transplant recipients. *Am J Surg* 146:589–593, 1983.

322. Fox B, Maki DG, Karreman E, et al: Controlled double-blind study of trimethoprim–sulfamethoxazole (TMP/SMZ) prophylaxis in renal transplantation. I. Efficacy, effects on microflora. Abstract #245. In *Interscience Conference on Antimicrobial Agents and Chemotherapy, Minneapolis, 1985.*

323. Wells CL, Podzorski RP, Peterson PK, et al: Incidence of trimethoprim–sulfamethoxazole-resistant enterobacteriaceae among transplant recipients. *J Infect Dis* 150:699–706, 1984.

324. Maki DG, Fox B, Karreman E, et al: Controlled double-blind study of TMP/SMZ prophylaxis in renal transplantation. II. TMP/SMZ toxicity and interaction with cyclosporine A. Abstract #710. In *Interscience Conference on Antimicrobial Agents and Chemotherapy, Minneapolis, 1985.*

325. Moore TC, Hume DM: The period and nature of hazard in clinical renal transplantation. I. The hazard to patient survival. *Ann Surg* 170:1–11, 1969.

326. Ireland P, Rashid A, von Lichtenberg F, et al: Liver disease in kidney transplant patients receiving azathioprine. *Arch Intern Med* 132:29–37, 1973.

327. Berne TV, Chatterjee SN, Craig JR, et al: Hepatic dysfunction in recipients of renal allografts. *Surg Gynecol Obstet* 141:171–175, 1975.

328. Ware AJ, Luby JP, Eigenbrodt EH, et al: Spectrum of liver disease in renal transplant recipients. *Gastroenterology* 68:755–764, 1975.

329. Mozes MF, Ascher NL, Balfour HH Jr, et al: Jaundice after renal allotransplantation. *Ann Surg* 188:783–790, 1978.

330. Sopko J, Anuras S: Liver disease in renal transplant recipients *Am J Med* 64:139–146, 1978.

331. Anuras S, Piros J, Bonney WW, et al: Liver disease in renal transplant recipients. *Arch Intern Med* 137:42–48, 1977

332. Kirkman RL, Strom TB, Weir MR, et al. Late mortality and morbidity in recipients of long-term renal allografts *Transplantation* 34:347–351, 1982.

333. Weir MR, Kirkman RL, Strom TB, Tilney NL: Liver disease in recipients of long-functioning renal allografts. *Kidney Int* 28:839–844, 1985.

334. Garibaldi RA, Forrest JN, Bryan JA, et al. Hemodialysis-associated hepatitis. *JAMA* 225:384–389, 1973.

335. Nagington J, Cossart YE, Cohen BJ. Reactivation of hepatitis B after transplantation operations. *Lancet* 1:558–560, 1977.

336. Denes AE, Berquist KR, Fields HA, et al. Hepatitis-B reactivation after renal transplantation. *Lancet* 1:1314, 1977.

337. Levy BS, Harris JC, Smith JL, et al. Hepatitis B in ward and clinical employees of a general hospital *Am J Epidemiol* 106:330–335, 1977.

338. Dusheiko G. Song E, Bowyer S, et al: Natural history of hepatitis B virus infection in renal transplant recipients—A fifteen year follow-up *Hepatology* 3:330–336, 1983.

339. Stevens CE, Alter HJ, Taylor PE, et al. Hepatitis B vaccine in patients receiving hemodialysis: Immunogenicity and efficacy. *N Engl J Med* 311:496–500, 1984.

340. Jacobson IM, Jaffers G, Dienstag JL, et al: Immunogenicity of hepatitis B vaccine in renal transplant recipients. *Transplantation* 39:393–395, 1985.

341. Chatterjee SN, Payne JE, Bischel MD, et al Successful renal transplantation in patients positive for hepatitis B antigen *N Engl J Med* 291:62–65, 1974.

342. Fine RN, Malekzadeh MH, Pennisi AJ, et al: HB$_s$ antigenemia in renal allograft recipients. *Ann Intern Med* 185:411–416, 1977

343 Shons AR, Simmons RL, Kjellstrand CM, et al. Renal transplantation in Australia antigenemia. *Am J Surg* 128:699–701, 1974.

344. London WT, Drew JS, Blumberg BS, et al Association of graft survival with host response to hepatitis B infection in patients with kidney transplants. *N Engl J Med* 296:241–244, 1977.

345. Pirson Y, Alexandre GPJ, van Ypersele de Strihou C. Long-term effect of HB$_s$ antigenemia on patient survival after renal transplantation. *N Engl J Med* 296:194–196, 1977.

346. Toussaint C, Dupont E, Vanherweghem JL, et al: Liver disease in patients undergoing hemodialysis and kidney transplantation. *Adv Nephrol* 8:269–294, 1979

347. Hillis WD, Hillis A, Walker WG: Hepatitis B surface antigenemia in renal transplant recipients; increased mortality risk. *JAMA* 242:329–332, 1979

348. Dalgleish AG, Tiller DJ, Horvath J, et al. Hepatocellular carcinoma associated with hepatitis B in a renal graft recipient. *Med J Aust* 2:240–241, 1983

349. Parfrey PS, Forges RD, Hutchinson TA, et al: The clinical and pathological course of hepatitis B liver disease in renal transplant recipients. *Transplantation* 37:461–466, 1984.

350. Parfrey PS, Forbes RDC, Hutchinson TA, et al: The impact of renal transplantation on the course of hepatitis B liver disease. *Transplantation* 39:610–615, 1985.

351. Harnett JD, Parfrey PS, Kennedy M, et al: Is transplantation advisable in hepatitis B positive hemodialysis patients? *Transplantation* (In press).

352. Freiberger Z, Anuras S, Koff RS, et al: Chronic active hepatitis without hepatitis B antigenemia in renal transplant recipients. Report of three cases. *Gastroenterology* 66:1187–1194, 1974.

353. Briggs WA, Lazarus JM, Birtch AG, et al: Hepatitis affecting hemodialysis and transplant patients: Its considerations and consequences. *Ann Intern Med* 132:21–28, 1973.

354. Haxhe JJ, Alexandre GPJ, Kestens PJ: The effect of imuran and azaserine on liver function tests in the dog: Its relation to the detection of graft rejection following liver transplantation. *Arch Int Pharmacodyn Ther* 168:366–372, 1967.

355. Starzl TE, Marchioro TL, Porter KA, et al. Factors determining short and long-term survival after orthotopic liver homotransplantation *Surgery* **58**:131–155, 1965

356 Sparberg M, Simon N, DelGreco F: Intrahepatic cholestasis due to azathioprine. *Gastroenterology* **57**:439–441, 1969.

357 Pirson Y, van Ypersele de Strihou C, Noel H, et al: Liver disease in transplanted patients *Proc Eur Dial Transplant Assoc* **10**:434–445, 1973.

358 Ware AJ, Luby JP, Hollinger B, et al: Etiology of liver disease in renal-transplant patients. *Ann Intern Med* **91**:364–371, 1979.

359 Farge D, Parfrey PS, Forbes RDC, et al Reduction of azathioprine in renal transplant patients with chronic hepatitis. *Transplantation* **41**:55–59, 1986.

360. Stiller CR, Keown PA Cyclosporine therapy in perspective In Morris PJ, Tilney NL (eds) *Progress in Transplantation* Vol 1. Churchill Livingstone, Edinburgh, 1984, pp. 12–45.

361 Szmuness W, Dienstag JC, Purcell RH, et al: Hepatitis type A and hemodialysis. A seroepidemiology study in 15 U.S. centers *Ann Intern Med* **87**:8–12, 1977.

362. Mosley JW: Epidemiology of HAV infection. In Vyas GN, Cohen SN, Schmid R (eds): *Viral Hepatitis A Contemporary Assessment of Etiology, Epidemiology, Pathogenesis, and Prevention.* Franklin Institute Press, Philadelphia, 1978, pp 85–104

363 LaQuaglia MP, Tolkoff-Rubin NE, Dienstag JL, et al: Impact of hepatitis on renal transplantation. *Transplantation* **32**:504–507, 1981.

364. Tolkoff-Rubin NE, Delmonico F, Cosimi AB, et al: Infectious disease problems in long-term survivors of renal transplantation *Transplantation* (In press.)

365. Ascher NL, Simmons RL, Marker S, et al: *Listeria* infection in transplant patients; five cases and a review of the literature. *Arch Surg* **113**:90–94, 1978

366. Schroter GPJ, Weill R III. *Listeria monocytogenes* infection after renal transplantation. *Arch Intern Med* **137**:1395–1399, 1977

367. Niklasson PM, Hambraeus A, Lundgren G, et al. *Listeria* encephalitis in five renal transplant recipients. *Acta Med Scand* **203**:181–185, 1978.

368 Schroter GPJ. *Listeria monocytogenes* and encephalitis. *Arch Intern Med* **138**:198–199, 1978.

369. Tilney NL, Kohler TR, Strom TB: Cerebromeningitis in immunosuppressed recipients of renal allografts. *Ann Surg* **195**:104–109, 1982

370 Watson GW, Fuller TJ, Elms J, et al: *Listeria* cerebritis, relapse of infection in renal transplant patients *Arch Intern Med* **138**:83–87, 1978.

371. Moellering RC Jr, Medoff G, Leech I, et al Antibiotic synergism against *Listeria monocytogenes*. *Antimicrob Agents Chemother* **1**:30–34, 1972

372. Buchner LH, Schneierson SS Clinical and laboratory aspects of *Listeria monocytogenes* infections, with a report of ten cases. *Am J Med* **43**:39–49, 1967

373. Hoeprich PD. Infection due to *Listeria monocytogenes* *Medicine (Baltimore)* **37**:143–160, 1958

374. Ray CG, Wedgewood RJ: Neonatal listeriosis: Six case reports and a review of the literature. *Pediatrics* **34**:378–392, 1964.

375. Scheer MS, Hirschman SZ: Oral and ambulatory therapy of *Listeria* bacteremia and meningitis with trimethoprim–sulfamethoxazole *Mt Sinai J Med* **49**:411–414, 1982

376 Spitzer PG, Hammer SM, Karchmer AW: Treatment of *Listeria monocytogenes* infection with trimethoprim–sulfamethoxazole: Case report and review of the literature. *Rev Infect Dis* **8**:427–430, 1986.

377. Finkelstein FO, Bastl C, Schiff M, et al: *Listeria* sepsis immediately preceding renal transplant rejection. *JAMA* **235**:844–845, 1976

378. Schroter GPJ, Temple DR, Husberg BS, et al: Cryptococcosis after renal transplantation. Report of ten cases *Surgery* **79**:268–277, 1976.

379. Ellner JJ, Bennett JE: Chronic meningitis. *Medicine (Baltimore)* **55**:341–369 1976.

380. Bennett JE, Dismukes WE, Duma RJ, et al: A comparison of amphotericin B alone and combined with flucytosine in the treatment of cryptococcal meningitis. *N Engl J Med* **301**:126–131, 1979.

381. Hellman RN, Hinrichs J, Sicard G, et al: Cryptococcal pyelonephritis and disseminated cryptococcosis in a renal transplant recipient. *Arch Intern Med* **141**:128–130, 1981

382. Plunkett JM, Turner BI, Tallent MB, et al: Cryptococcal septicemia associated with urologic instrumentation in a renal allograft recipient. *J Urol* **125**:241–242, 1981.

383 Morduchowicz G, Shmueli D, Shapira Z, et al: Rhinocerebral mucormycosis in renal transplant recipients. Report of three cases and review of the literature. *Rev Infect Dis* **8**:441–446, 1986

384. Hau T, VanHook EJ, Simmons RL, et al: Prognostic factors of peritoneal infections in transplant patients. *Surgery* **84**:403–416, 1978.

385 Rubin RH, Weinstein L: *Salmonellosis. Microbiologic, Pathologic and Clinical Features* Stratton Intercontinental, New York, 1977.

386. Smith EJ, Milligan SL, Filo RS: Salmonella mycotic aneurysm after renal transplantation. *South Med J* **74**:1399–1401, 1981

387. Berk MR, Meyers AM, Cassal W, et al: Non-typhoid salmonella infections after renal transplantation. A serious clinical problem. *Nephron* **37**:186–189, 1984.

388. Samra Y, Shaked Y, Maier MK: Nontyphoidal salmonellosis in renal transplant recipients Report of five cases and review of the literature. *Rev Infect Dis* **8**:431–440, 1986

389. Schroter GPJ, West JC, Weill R III: Acute bacteremia in asplenic renal transplant patients *JAMA* **237**:2207–2208, 1977.

390 Linnemann CC Jr, First MR: Risk of pneumococcal infections in renal transplant patients *JAMA* **241**:2619–2621, 1979

391 Bourgault AM, Van Scoy RE, Wilkowski CJ, et al: Severe infection due to *Streptococcus pneumoniae* in asplenic renal transplant patients. *Mayo Clin Proc* **54**:123–216, 1979

392. Alexander JW, First MR, Majeski JA, et al: The late adverse effects of splenectomy on patient survival following cadaveric renal transplantation. *Transplantation* **37**:467–470, 1984.

393 Coscio FG, Giebink GS, Le CT, et al. Pneumococcal vac-

cination in patients with chronic renal disease and renal allograft recipients. *Kidney Int* 20:254–258, 1981.

394. Arnold WC, Steele RW, Rastogi SP, et al: Response to pneumococcal vaccine in renal allograft recipients. *Am J Nephrol* 5:30–34, 1985.

395. King RW Jr, Kraikitpanitch S, Lindeman RD: Subcutaneous nodules caused by *Histoplasma capsulatum. Ann Intern Med* 86:586–587, 1977.

396. Kauffman CA, Israel KS, Smith JW, et al: Histoplasmosis in immunosuppressed patients. *Am J Med* 64:923–932, 1978.

397. Davies SF, Khan M, Sarosi GA: Disseminated histoplasmosis in immunologically suppressed patients. *Am J Med* 64:94–100, 1978

398. Davies SF, Sarosi GA, Peterson PK, et al: Disseminated histoplasmosis in renal transplant recipients. *Am J Surg* 137:687–691, 1979.

399. Peterson PK, Dahl MV, Howard RJ, et al: Mucormycosis and cutaneous histoplasmosis in a renal transplant recipient. *Arch Dermatol* 118:275–277, 1982.

400. Wheat LJ, Smith EJ, Sathapatayavongs B, et al: Histoplasmosis in renal allograft recipients. Two large urban outbreaks. *Arch Intern Med* 143:703–707, 1983.

401. Deresinski SC, Stevens DA: Coccidioidomycosis in compromised hosts. *Medicine (Baltimore)* 54:377–395, 1975.

402. Bayer AS, Yoshikawa TT, Galpin JE, et al: Unusual syndromes of coccidioidomycosis: Diagnostic and therapeutic considerations. *Medicine (Baltimore)* 55:131–152, 1976.

403. Schröter GPJ, Bakshandeh K, Husberg BS, et al: Coccidiodomycosis and renal transplantation. *Transplantation* 23:485–489, 1977.

404. Cohen IM, Galgiani JN, Potter D, et al: Coccidiomycosis in renal replacement therapy. *Arch Intern Med* 142:489–494, 1982.

405. Gallis HA, Berman RA, Cate TR, et al: Fungal infection following renal transplantation. *Arch Intern Med* 135:1163–1172, 1975.

406. Butka BJ, Bennett SR, Johnson AC: Disseminated inoculation blastomycosis in a renal transplant recipient. *Am Rev Respir Dis* 130:1180–1183, 1984.

407. Sugar AM, Restrepo A, Stevens DA: Paracoccidioidomycosis of the immunosuppressed host: Report of a case and review of the literature. *Am Rev Respir Dis* 129:340–342, 1984.

408. Rattazzi LC, Simmons RL, Spanos PK, et al: Successful management of miliary tuberculosis after renal transplantation. *Am J Surg* 130:359–361, 1975.

409. Oliver WA: Tuberculosis in renal transplant patients. *Med J Aust* 1:828–829, 1976.

410. Bell TJ, Williams GB: Successful treatment of tuberculosis in renal transplant recipients. *J Soc Med* 71:265–268, 1978.

411. Ascher NL, Simmons RL, Marker S, et al: Tuberculosis joint disease in transplant patients. *Am J Surg* 135:853–856, 1978.

412. Riska H, Kuhlback B: Tuberculosis and kidney transplantation. *Acta Med Scand* 205:637–640, 1979.

413. Vaz AJ: Miliary tuberculosis and the adult respiratory distress syndrome in a renal transplant recipient. *Chest* 75:412, 1979.

414. Lloveras J, Peterson PK, Simmons RL, et al: Mycobacterial infections in renal transplant recipients; seven cases and a review of the literature. *Arch Intern Med* 142:888–892, 1982.

415. Coutts II, Jegarajah S, Starsk JE: Tuberculosis in renal transplant recipients. *Br J Dis Chest* 73:141–148, 1979

416. Spence RK, Dafoe DC, Rabin G, et al: Mycobacterial infections in renal allograft recipients. *Arch Surg* 118:356–359, 1983.

417. Peters TG, Reiter CG, Boswell RL: Transmission of tuberculosis by kidney transplantation. *Transplantation* 38:514–516, 1984.

418. Walker JF, Cronin CJ, O'Neill S, et al: Tuberculosis affecting a cadaveric renal allograft. *Clin Nephrol* 17:262–265, 1982.

419. Thomas PA Jr, Mozes MF, Jonasson O: Hepatic dysfunction during isoniazid chemoprophylaxis in renal allograft recipients. *Arch Surg* 114:597–599, 1979.

420. Buffington GA, Dominguez JH, Piering WF, et al. Interaction of rifampin and glucocorticoids; adverse effect on renal allograft function. *JAMA* 236:1958–1960, 1976.

421. Cruz N, Ramirez-Muxo O, Bermudez RH, et al: Pulmonary infection with *M. kansasii* in a renal transplant patient. *Nephron* 26:187–188, 1980.

422. Bolivar R, Satterwhite TK, Floyd M: Cutaneous lesions due to *Mycobacterium kansasii. Arch Dermatol* 116:207–208, 1980.

423. Gombert ME, Goldstein EJ, Corrado ML, et al: Disseminated *Mycobacterium marinum* infection after renal transplantation. *Ann Intern Med* 94:486–487, 1981

424. Davis BR, Brumbach J, Sanders WJ, et al: Skin lesions caused by *Mycobacterium haemophilum. Ann Intern Med* 97:723–724, 1982.

425. Heironimus JD, Winn RE, Collins CB: Cutaneous nonpulmonary *Mycobacterium chelonei* infection. Successful treatment with sulfonamides in an immunosuppressed patient. *Arch Dermatol* 120:1061–1063, 1984.

426. Wolfson JS, Sober AJ, Rubin RH: Dermatologic manifestations of infections in immunocompromised patients. *Medicine (Baltimore)* 64:115–133, 1985.

427. Koranda FC, Dehmel EM, Kahn G, et al: Cutaneous complications in immunosuppressed renal homograft recipients. *JAMA* 229:419–424, 1974.

428. Mullen DL, Silverberg SG, Penn I, et al: Squamous cell carcinoma of the skin and lip in renal homograft recipients. *JAMA* 229:419–424, 1974.

429. Savin JA, Nobel WC: Immunosuppression and skin infection. *Br J Dermatol* 93:115–118, 1975.

430. Lutzner MA, Gerard O, Dutronquay V, et al: Detection of human papillomavirus type 5 DNA in skin cancers of an immunosuppressed renal allograft recipient. *Lancet* 1:422–424, 1983.

431. Ostrow RS, Bender M, Niimura M, et al: Human papillomavirus DNA in cutaneous primary and metastasized squamous cell carcinomas from patients with epidermodysplasia verruciformis. *Proc Natl Acad Sci USA* 79:1634–1637, 1982.

432. Boyle J, Mackie RM, Briggs JD, et al: Cancer, warts, and sunshine in renal transplant patients. A case-control study. *Lancet* 1:702–705, 1984.

433. Harris LF, Dan BM, Lefkowitz LB Jr, et al: *Paecilomyces* cellulitis in a renal transplant patient: Successful treatment with intravenous miconazole. *South Med J* **72:**897–898, 1979.

434. Dagher FJ, Smith AG, Pankoski D, et al: Skin protothecosis in a patient with a renal allograft. *South Med J* **71:**222–224, 1978.

435. Prystowsky SD, Vogelstein B, Ettinger D, et al: Invasive aspergillosis. *N Engl J Med* **295:**655–658, 1976.

436. Mead JH, Lupton GP, Dillarou CL, et al: Cutaneous *Rhizopus* infection; occurrence as a postoperative complication associated with an elasticized adhesive dressing. *JAMA* **242:**272–274, 1979.

437. Consensus Panel of the Consensus Development Conference on Liver Transplantation. National Institutes of Health Consensus Development Statement: Liver Transplantation—June 20–23, 1983. *Hepatology* **4**(suppl):1075–1105, 1984.

438. Busuttil RW, Goldstein LI, Danovitch G, et al: Liver transplantation today. *Ann Intern Med* **104:**377–389, 1986.

439. Gordon RD, Shaw BW Jr, Iwatsuki S, et al: Indications for liver transplantation in the cyclosporin era. *Semin Dig Dis* (In press.)

440. Fulginiti VA, Scribner R, Groth CG, et al: Infections in recipients of liver homografts *N Engl J Med* **279:**619–626, 1968.

441. Starzl TE, Ishikawa M, Putnam CW, et al: Progress in and deterrents to orthotopic liver transplantation, with special reference to survival, resistance to hyperacute rejection, and biliary duct reconstruction. *Transplant Proc* **6:**129–139, 1974.

442. Schröter GPJ, Hoelscher M, Putnam CW, et al: Infections complicating orthotopic liver transplantation. *Arch Surg* **111:**1337–1347, 1977.

443. Ho M, Wajszczuk CF, Hardy A, et al: Infections in kidney, heart and liver transplant recipients on cyclosporine. *Transplant Proc* **15**(4 suppl 1):2768–2772, 1983.

444. Brettschneider L, Tong JL, Boose DS, et al: Specific bacteriologic problems after orthotopic liver transplantation in dogs and pigs. *Arch Surg* **97:**313–322, 1968.

445. Alican F, Hardy JD: Replantation of the liver. *J Surg Res* **7:**368–382, 1967.

446. Starzl TE, Porter KA, Putnam CW, et al: Orthotopic liver transplantation in 93 patients. *Surg Gynecol Obstet* **142:**487–505, 1976.

447. Krom RAF: Liver transplantation at the Mayo Clinic. *Mayo Clin Proc* **61:**278–282, 1986.

448. Wajszczuk CP, Dummer JS, Ho M, et al: Funal infections in liver transplant recipients. *Transplantation* **40:**347–353, 1985.

449. Calne RY, Williams R: Liver transplantation. *Curr Probl Surg* **16:**1–44, 1979.

450. Starzl TE, Iwatsuki S, Van Thiel DH, et al: Evolution of liver transplantation. *Hepatology* **2:**614–636, 1982.

451. Schröter GPJ, Hoelscher M, Putnam CW, et al: Fungus infections after liver transplantation. *Ann Surg* **186:**115–122, 1977.

452. Starzl TE, Putnam CW, Hansbrough JF, et al: Biliary complications after liver transplantation: With special reference to the biliary cast syndrome and techiques of secondary duct repair. *Surgery* **81:**212–221, 1977.

453. Shaffer D, Jenkins RL, Karchmer AW, et al: Toxic shock syndrome complicating orthotopic liver transplantation—A case report. *Transplantation* **42:**434–436, 1986.

22

Infection in the Cardiac Transplant Patient

LAYNE O. GENTRY and BARRY ZELUFF

1. Introduction

During the two decades since the dramatic report of the first human heart transplant by Barnard[1] in December 1967, cardiac transplantation has evolved into the treatment of choice for patients with end-stage cardiac disease. Largely through the efforts of the cardiac transplant group at the Stanford University Medical Center, cardiac transplantation is now carried out at numerous medical centers throughout the world, offering the patient an 85% chance of surviving 1 year, a 75% chance of surviving 2 years after the procedure, and an excellent chance for full rehabilitation. It should be emphasized that these results are being achieved in patients for whom all other forms of therapy offer a less than 20% 1-year survival.[2-5]

A number of factors have contributed to the increasing success of human cardiac transplantation: careful selection of recipients according to definite criteria (Table 1), improved tissue typing of the donor and recipient, more expert acquisition and transport of the donor heart, advances in the technical aspects of the operative and perioperative management of the cardiac allograft recipient, the routine employment of serial endomyocardial biopsies that allow for the early diagnosis and treatment of rejection, and better programs for achieving and monitoring effective immunosuppression.

Of all these factors, perhaps the most important single advance has been the introduction of cyclosporine as a more effective and selective immunosuppressive agent. As of 1981, using an immunosuppressive program of rabbit antithymocyte globulin (RATG), azathioprine, and prednisone, the Stanford group was achieving a 1-year survival rate of 63%.[6] When cyclosporine was added to this program, an excessive rate of lymphoma was developing.[2,7] However, beginning in 1982, when a program of immunosuppression consisting of just cyclosporine and prednisone (reserving RATG and high-dose steroids for acute rejection episodes) was introduced, the 1-year survival rate of 85% began to be seen.[2,7] This is not to say, however, that factors other than cyclosporine use have not contributed significantly to the increased success of this procedure.[8] Cyclosporine use has been associated with a decrease in the need for acute antirejection therapy (particularly high-dose steroids), a decrease in the incidence of life-threatening infections, and a decrease in the amount of time spent in hospital by patients. The occurrence of lymphoma, renal damage, and hypertension remain as significant problems associated with cyclosporine.[2-10]

Infection, however, remains the most important cause of mortality in cardiac transplant patients. Since the first report of the Stanford group in 1971,[11] it has been clear that the infectious disease complications of the technical and immunosuppressive manipulations required in cardiac transplantation are one of the two major barriers to be overcome if success is to be achieved—rejection being the other.[6,7,11] As is

LAYNE O. GENTRY and BARRY ZELUFF • Infectious Disease Section, St. Luke's Episcopal Hospital, Houston, Texas 77030

TABLE 1. Selection Criteria for Cardiac Transplant Recipients and Donors

Primary selection criteria
 Terminal cardiac disease
 Age under 55
 Noncardiac organ function: normal or reversible dysfunction
 Absence of systemic illness that would limit recovery or
  survival
Absolute contraindications
 Active infection
 Recent pulmonary infarction
 Significant pulmonary vascular resistance
 Psychosis or mental deficiency unrelated to low cardiac output
  or metabolis status
 Drug addiction
Matching requirements with donor
 ABO compatibility
 Absence of donor-specific lymphocyte cytotoxicity
 Appropriate size match
 HLA-A compatibility

discussed more completely in Chapter 21, infection and rejection are closely related phenomena in the transplant patient, the treatment of one often leading to the other. This relationship is particularly important in the cardiac transplant patient, for whom there are currently no practical means of life support off immunosuppressive therapy. Whereas in the renal transplant patient, life-threatening infection is often best managed by discontinuing immunosuppression and returning the patient to dialysis, this option is not available in cardiac transplantation. Thus, it is not surprising that infection has been responsible for 58% of all deaths and 65% of the deaths within 3 months of the cardiac transplant procedure.[6] Overall, bacterial infection is the most common form of clinically important infection observed, with viral, fungal, and protozoan infection also of clinical importance. Gram-negative infection due to the Enterobacteriaceae and *Pseudomonas aeruginosa* are the most common bacterial invaders, with *Staphylococcus aureus* and enterococci also being observed, and being particularly associated with early infection. In recent years, the viral and fungal infections have become more predictable and are usually related to periods of augmented immunosuppressive therapy for acute organ rejection.[2,6,7,9]

Because of the important role of infection in determining the outcome of clinical cardiac transplantation, it is essential to have a logical approach to the prevention, early diagnosis, and effective therapy of these patients' infectious disease problems. The purpose of this chapter is to present such an approach, based upon the published literature and our own experience with 188 patients who have undergone cardiac transplantation over the last 60 months at St. Luke's Episcopal Hospital in Houston.

2. Infection in the First Month Post-transplant

The first few months after transplantation represent the highest risk period for the cardiac transplant patient for life-threatening infection and rejection—this is the time period when immunosuppression is most intense, rejection is most active, and technical interventions in the patient most invasive. In the first month, the infections which are most common are similar to those observed in any postoperative cardiovascular surgical patient—bacteremia, wound, urinary or respiratory tract infection. These are common and are frequently caused by hospital pathogens. Unusual more opportunistic infections, such as those caused by viruses (other than herpes simplex virus), protozoa, or fungi, rarely cause infection during the first month. The one exception to this general rule is the occurrence of opportunistic infection due to *Aspergillus, Nocardia,* or *Legionella* species resulting from excessive contamination of the patient from a nosocomial source. Outbreaks such as that seen with Legionnaires' disease at the Wadsworth VA Hospital[12] can devastate any transplant unit.[7,13] Thus, if infection caused by such opportunistic organisms occurs in cardiac transplant patients within the first few weeks following transplantation, a hospital source for infection must be considered.

Antibiotic prophylaxis in cardiovascular surgery remains controversial, although most cardiac transplantation centers use it. Cephalosporins are commonly used as single agents because they have a broad antibacterial spectrum and a low incidence of toxicity. The specific cephalosporin to be used should be selected on the basis of its efficacy against the common organisms that cause postoperative infections at each center. In our hospital, we have elected to use cefotaxime, because of our early experience with postoperative wound and chest cavity infections caused by *Enterobacter cloacae,* an organism commonly isolated from patients housed in our intensive care areas. Since initiating this prophylactic program, we have successfuly eliminated these infections.

The early removal of all catheters, chest tubes, and invasive monitoring equipment is essential. There must also be meticulous aseptic techniques when dealing with intravenous catheter sites. Antibiotic prophylaxis is continued until these lines are removed. In addition, we have adopted the policy of continuing prophylaxis until the chest tubes are removed, or until there is cultural evidence that suggests that the prophylaxis is no longer effective, and a different agent is indicated.

Wound infections in cardiac transplant patients do not appear to be as frequent a problem as in renal transplant patients, where the incidence has been reported to vary from 1.8 to 56%.[14-17] Although the incidence of wound infection reported has been similar, 3.6–62.5%,[18,19] these are usually related to various catheter sites or vascular cutdown sites and are rarely fatal. Infections related to chest tubes require special attention (see Section 2.3). In our own series of transplant patients, we have seen only one serious wound infection, a midline sternotomy infection with *Staphylococcus aureus*. Sternotomy infections are particularly dangerous, as they may extend into the mediastinum, with life-threatening mediastinitis resulting. Accordingly, sternal wound infections require aggressive attention, with surgical debridement and appropriate systemic antibiotics.[20] It is important to emphasize that because of the suppressed inflammatory response in these patients, the usual physical signs of wound infection may be greatly muted. Therefore, the caring physician must be prepared to do a sterile diagnostic aspiration of the wound in the face of minimal findings.

The organisms associated with wound infections are common hospital pathogens such as *S. aureus, E. cloacae, Serratia marcescens,* and *P. aeruginosa*. These can be easily isolated from wound sites using standard bacteriologic techniques. Although *Staphylococcus epidermidis, Corynebacterium* species, and *Candida* species are rarely associated with wound infections in these patients, they can cause catheter-related infection.

The best method of preventing wound infection is the combination of good surgical technique, meticulous wound and catheter care, and the early removal of all devices which penetrate the all-important skin barrier to infection. Good surgical technique is especially critical when reexploration of the medi-

astinum is undertaken for any reason. Reexploration is most commonly performed for postoperative bleeding, and should be performed in the operating room under strict sterile conditions whenever possible. Emergency life-saving procedures are rarely necessary in the recovery room, and, in our experience, such measures have a significantly increased the incidence of postoperative infectious complications. Rapid removal of chest or mediastinal tubes will decrease the chance of subsequent wound infection. Prolonged intubation of the pleural space leads to an increased incidence of lung infections and empyema, often caused by antibiotic-resistant hospital pathogens. For this reason, we suggest monitoring the bacteriology of these drainage tubes and continuing antibiotic prophylaxis until the chest tubes have been removed.

Once a wound infection has been identified, broad-spectrum antibiotic coverage appropriate for the common hospital pathogens should be instituted after sufficient material has been obtained for Gram stain and culture. The importance of aggressive surgical drainage and/or debridement under the coverage of antibiotics in this situation cannot be overemphasized. In particular, foreign material must be removed from the wound, as it may retard wound healing and interfere with local host defenses, providing a nidus for later recrudescence of the infection. Once the microbial etiology and antimicrobial sensitivity of the infecting organism(s) are known, specific, narrow-spectrum antibiotic therapy should be employed. Although the duration of antibiotic therapy in such patients is controversial, our policy has been to continue therapy for 10–14 days or until the patient has been afebrile for 5–7 days.

2.1. Bacteremia

Bacteremia is the single most important cause of infectious disease morbidity and morality in cardiac transplant patients.[6,7,11] Although such bacteremias may be due to blood stream invasion from other primary sites of infection such as the lungs, surgical wound, or urinary tract, bacteremia from intravenous or intraarterial catheter-related sepsis is far more common.

In most series, gram-negative bacteremia is more common than gram-positive bacteremia.[6,7,11] For example, in a review of 35 cardiac transplant patients treated with cyclosporine and prednisone, there were 10 episodes of bacteremia in eight patients. Of these episodes, seven were caused by gram-negative bacilli and three by gram-positive cocci. Six of the eight patients with bacteremia ultimately died, and four died within a few days of the onset of the bacteremia.[21] In a similar but earlier series of 41 cardiac transplant patients from Stanford, there were 12 episodes of bacteremia in 10 patients, and gram-negative bacteremia also was more common.[18] It is of note that although these two series represent experience over a 12-year period and include two entirely different programs of immunosuppression, the etiology of the bacteremias encountered in both series was similar.

Although bacteremia may occur as a complication of pneumonia, urinary tract or wound infection, most of these are neither predictable nor preventable. By contrast, a common cause of bacteremia, the contaminated intravascular catheter, is both predictable and preventable. Cardiac transplant patients are particularly susceptible to catheter sepsis because they frequently require invasive hemodynamic monitoring equipment after transplantation. The biggest problem appears to be with such central venous catheters as Swan Ganz lines left in place for more than 72 hr. Thus, we urge the removal and/or changing of these lines as soon as possible. Another significant source of bacteremia is the intravascular catheter used for hemodialysis access (acute renal failure requiring temporary dialysis being not uncommon postcardiac transplant). Because these are often placed in the groin, it is virtually impossible to keep them sterile. In addition to gram-negative bacteria, *Candida* species commonly contaminate these catheters, and even transient candidal sepsis in the immunocompromised host can have disastrous consequences. It has been our routine practice to take intermittent surveillance blood cultures through these catheters, especially long-term groin catheters; in addition, all catheter tips are routinely cultured for both bacteria and fungi when removed, with antimicrobial therapy guided in part by the results.

2.2. Urinary Tract Infection

The incidence of urinary tract infection in cardiac transplant patients appears to be approximately 8–12%,[7,18,21] with the risk of acquiring such infections directly proportional to the duration of urinary tract catheterization.[22] The responsible pathogens here are the typical gram-negative uropathogens that invade nonimmunosuppressed patients, with *E. coli* the most common, followed by *Proteus* species and *Pseudomonas aeruginosa*. In addition, *Enterococcus* and *Candida* species are not uncommon uropathogens in this population group. Early removal of the urinary catheter, preferably within 3 days of the transplant, is the best way of preventing urinary tract infection. Treatment of urinary tract infection in female cardiac transplant patients is usually easily accomplished with a conventional 7–14 days course of antimicrobial therapy. In men more prolonged therapy, 4–6 weeks of antibiotics, and even surgery, aimed at removing prostatic foci of infection, may be necessary.[7]

2.3. Pneumonia

The lung has been the most common site for primary infectious complications in cardiac transplant patients.[7,18,19,21,23] Although pneumonia is a problem common to all transplant and immunosuppressed patients, it appears to be a more significant problem in cardiac transplant patients due to the unique relationship of the cardiopulmonary systems. The factors involved with the development of pneumonia are numerous, and include such factors as underlying lung disease, length of intubation, level of immunosuppression, the presence of rejection, and other associated systemic diseases. Gram-negative bacteria are the most common pathogens causing pneumonia in the first month after transplantation, although other pathogens are also seen.

It has been our procedure to obtain routine surveillance cultures of tracheal secretions immediately after surgery and then twice weekly while the patient is intubated. With the onset of clinical and radiographic findings suggestive of pulmonary infection, repeat cultures are done as indicated. It is also our practice to obtain routine cultures of the chest tube drainage at least once before these tubes are removed. Occasionally an early pleural space infection can be detected and with aggressive antibiotic therapy, a subsequent empyema can be avoided. Cultures of the pleural fluid drainage may also provide early clues as to the etiology of pneumonias in patients who are extubated and unable to give good sputum samples.

Chest radiographs are obtained daily at the bedside until the patients are fully ambulatory and then several times per week as indicated. Careful daily review of the sequential radiographs is important to the early detection of pneumonia. Even in cardiac transplant patients, bacterial and fungal pneumonias tend to present as lobar alveolar infiltrates while viruses and *Pneumocystis carinii* are more likely to present as more diffuse interstitial infiltrates. We have found that it is often difficult to detect early pneumonia, especially in the lung bases, on a routine portable film and have found the computed tomography (CT) scan to be much more useful in detecting these basilar pneumonias. This scan is also very good for detecting fluid collections in the pleural space that may represent early empyema. It is also excellent for detecting and localizing small areas of nodular infiltration, and can be used to direct the percutaneous approach for needle biopsy of these suspicious areas. The following case illustrates how the use of the CT scan can be of assistance in detecting pulmonary infection which is not detectable on routine chest radiography.

Illustrative Case 1

LC is a 44-year-old white man who underwent allograft cardiac transplantation on July 4, 1982 for severe ischemic cardiomyopathy. His postoperative immunosuppression included cyclosporine and prednisone. He suffered a right-sided cerebrovascular accident (CVA), with resultant left-sided weakness, after a right-sided cardiac catheterization. During his recovery from the CVA, fever and right upper quadrant pain developed. On physical examination, his temperature was 101°F (38.3°C), the blood pressure was 140/85 mm Hg, pulse 95, and respirations were 30 per minute. He was slightly cushingoid, icteric, and in moderate respiratory distress. The chest examination revealed only coarse rhonchi bilaterally and decreased breath sounds in both bases. The cardiovascular examination revealed only tachypnea. The abdominal examination was positive for a diffuse tenderness with guarding in the right upper quadrant. The neurologic examination revealed left-sided weakness of both upper and lower extremities.

Laboratory evaluation revealed a hematocrit of 35% and WBC count of 18,000/mm (75% polys, 15% bands, 9% lymphs, 1% monos). SGOT was 85, total bilirubin was 3.5, and alkaline phosphatase was 200. Room air arterial blood gases revealed a PaO_2 75 mm Hg, $PaCO_2$ 25, and pH 7.45. Chest radiography revealed a diffuse hazy infiltrate in the right lower lobe with blunting of the right costophrenic angle (see Fig. 1).

A CT scan of the chest and abdomen was performed on August 27, 1982. Cholelithiasis was evident with thickening of the gallbladder wall but no dilatation of the ducts. An abscess involving the right lower lobe of the lung was noted and is seen in Fig 2. The patient had a cholecystectomy and drainage procedure of the right lower lobe abscess. Cultures from both areas grew *E. cloacae*. He was treated with a prolonged course of cefotaxime and the infection resolved.

Once pneumonia is detected or suspected, it is very important to be aggressive in trying to discover the causative pathogens (see Chapter 6). Examination and culture of the sputum are the mainstay of the laboratory evaluation of pneumonia. However, the value of a routine expectorated sputum culture for the diagnosis of pneumonia has been questioned in a normal population[24] and is of even more questionable value in an immunocompromised host. If a patient is intubated and develops a lobar infiltrate, sputum for Gram stain and culture obtained through the endotracheal tube is usually adequate. However, if the infiltrate is interstitial and the patient is severely ill, bronchoscopy is indicated. At bronchoscopy, one should obtain a brushed specimen using a double-sheathed plugged catheter, used for bacterial, viral, and fungal culture; in addition, we take another brushing for cytologic evaluation, plus bronchial washings and transbronchial biopsy. The yield using all these techniques is higher than any one alone.[25] Little is written about the value of bronchoscopy in the diagnosis of pneumonia in cardiac transplant patients. However, one study of renal transplant patients with suspected pneumonia revealed that bronchoscopy could be a useful and accurate tool in the diagnosis of pneumonia.[26] In this study, bronchoscopy was performed for 39 patients with pneumonia, and a specific etiology was detected in 30 (77%). Pathogens detected included cytomegalovirus, Aspergillus, *Chlamydia trachomatis* and various gram-positive and -negative bacteria.

Another technique that is useful in the detection of pneumonia in cardiac transplant patients is the percutaneous biopsy.[27–30] Diagnostic yields have been reported to be 35–76%. Unfortunately, false-negative results have been reported in up to 18% of these patients.[27] In general, attempted biopsy of nodular or localized peripheral lesions has been more rewarding than biopsy of diffuse infiltrates with the percutaneous needle biopsy technique. Organisms recovered include various bacteria, *Aspergillus, Nocardia* and *Legionella* species. Localization of the lesion with a CT scan and either CT scan or fluo-

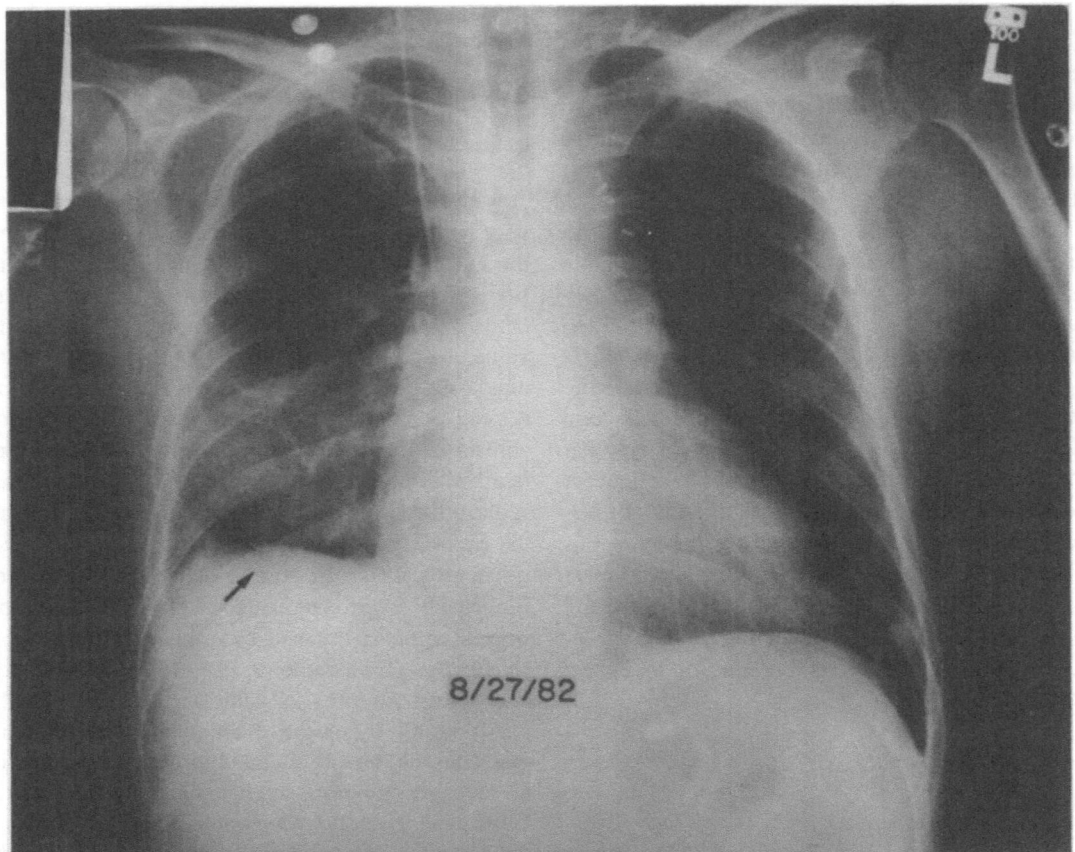

FIGURE 1. PA chest radiograph, patient LC (2/27/82). Note air–fluid level at the tip of the arrows.

roscopic biopsy needle guidance makes this a relatively safe procedure with acceptable complication rates of 5–39%.[27-38]

Open lung biopsy is still the procedure of choice in patients with diffuse interstitial infiltration, who are seriously ill and require respiratory support. In such patients, a rapid diagnosis is essential for proper antibiotic therapy, and we view this as the procedure of choice.

Pneumocystis carinii pneumonia is the most common cause of treatable interstitial pneumonia in the cardiac transplant patient, and can be rapidly fatal if not recognized and treated. The differential diagnosis of interstitial pneumonia includes the viruses cytomegalovirus (CMV) and herpes simplex virus (HSV). In the cardiac transplant patient, as in the renal transplant patient, CMV is virtually not seen until the end of the first month. HSV, although com-

monly isolated from the respiratory secretions, and a frequence cause of orolabial disease, rarely causes primary pneumonia in the cardiac transplant patient. It is usually found in the lungs of patient who have had prolonged endotracheal intubation because of other forms of pulmonary pathology. HSV infection is now treatable with acyclovir. Until recently, the treatment options following the diagnosis of CMV pneumonia were limited to decreasing the level of immunosuppression and supportive care. The acyclovir analogue 9-(1,3-dihydroxy-2-propoxymethyl)guanine (DHPG), appears to be promising in the treatment of human cytomegalovirus infection. Its exact role in heart transplant patients with cytomegalovirus pneumonia, however, remains to be determined.

The use of antibiotics in the management of pneumonia in a cardiac transplant patient in the first

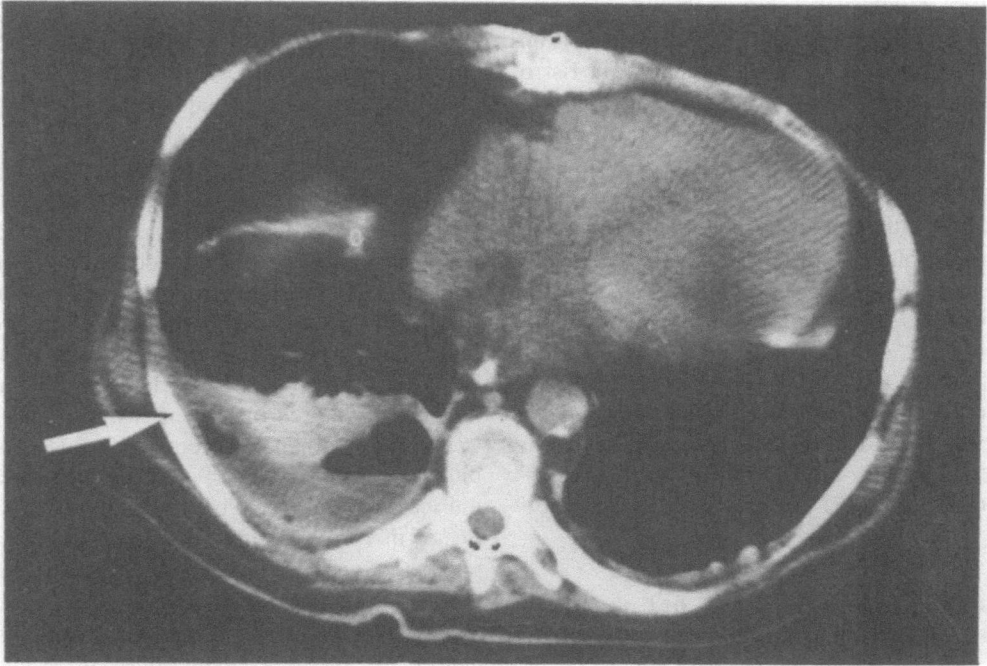

FIGURE 2. Computed tomographic scan view through lower chest, patient LC (same date as Fig 1) Note the dense infiltrate with multiple cavities at the arrow tip.

month is similar to that of any nosocomial pneumonia in a hospitalized patient. In patients with the development of fever, purulent secretions and a new lobar infiltrate, a Gram stain of the sputum may help in selecting the empirical antibiotic therapy. Previous surveillance cultures taken from the endotracheal tube can often be very helpful in this situation; however, colonization of the respiratory tract may change in the hospital, and different pathogens may be causing the pneumonia. Since the pathogens are usually gram negative, we usually begin therapy with either an antipseudomonal penicillin or third-generation cephalosporin plus an aminoglycoside until more specific therapy can be defined by the culture data. Because of the nephrotoxicity associated with both aminoglycosides and cyclosporine, we try to alter our therapy to discontinue the aminoglycosides as soon as possible.

In patients with nodular lung lesions, *Legionella, Nocardia,* and *Aspergillus* species are more common. In these patients, empiric therapy with erythromycin and trimethoprim–sulfamethoxazole is usually started immediately after a definitive

diagnostic attempt has been made. Diffuse interstitial infiltrates are more commonly associated with *P. carinii,* cytomegalovirus, or other viral infections. However, we only have proven chemotherapy for *P. carinii.* Therefore, in this setting, empirical use of trimethoprim–sulfamethoxazole is indicated after tissue has been obtained for special stains. An aggressive diagnostic approach is important in the management of this form of infection in the transplant patient.

3. Infection 1–6 Months Post-Cardiac Transplant

The time period from 1–6 months after transplant can be one of the most critical times for these patients. During this interval, they are at risk for the common hospital-acquired infections. In addition, however, they are at increased risk of opportunistic infections associated with excessive levels of immunosuppression. During this period, the level of immunosuppression is still relatively high because of large doses of both cyclosporine and prednisone, and there is a profound depression of cell-mediated immunity, more so than humoral immunity. The risk of organ rejection also continues to be significantly increased as well. If rejection occurs, increases in the level of immunosuppression, which are necessary to treat rejection, also increase the risk of opportunistic infections.[23] Although the variety of infections that occur in transplant patients seems endless, several are seen more frequently during this period of immunosuppression and appear to be especially related to high-dose corticosteroid therapy and/or antilymphocyte antibody therapy for episodes of rejection. These include CMV, *P. carinii,* and *Legionella pneumoniae,* and disseminated infections with the other members of the herpes virus group: HSV, Epstein–Barr virus (EBV), and varicella–zoster virus (VZV).

3.1. Cytomegalovirus Infection in Cardiac Transplant Recipients

Cytomegalovirus is the single most common cause of morbidity and mortality in cardiac transplant recipients. Active infections occur in 65–93% of individuals post-transplant.[7,21,31–34] The ubiquity of this infection in transplant patients is explained by two important characteristics, which it shares with the other herpes group viruses(HSV, EBV, and VZV). These are latency and high degree of cell association. By latency is meant that although normal individuals who recover from CMV infection no longer have demonstrable, infectious virus, the virus does remain within the host in a dormant state ready to be reactivated under special circumstances. The most important of these special circumstances is the administration of immunosuppressive therapy such as that used in transplantation. Of the immunosuppressive agents, antilymphocyte antibodies have the most CMV-promoting effects, followed by such cytotoxic drugs as azathioprine and cyclophosphamide, cyclosporine, and, least of all, corticosteroids. The sites of CMV latency in man have not been completely defined, but leukocytes and the transplanted allograft itself appear to harbor sufficient virus to transmit CMV from one person to another. Because the virus is so highly cell associated, neutralizing antibody is rendered inefficient as a host defense and cell-mediated immunity is considered

more important. Hence, the impaired cell-mediated immunity of the transplant patient is a major factor in the pathogenesis of these infections.[32,35–37]

Traditionally, two major epidemiologic patterns of CMV infection have been recognized following transplantation: primary infection, in which patients with no prior history of CMV infection and who are seronegative for CMV prior to transplant develop CMV post-transplant; and reactivation infection, in which patients who are seropositive for the virus pre-transplant (and thus harbor dormant virus capable of being reactivated by immunosuppressive therapy) reactivate their own latent infection. Primary infection is usually acquired by one of two routes: from the transplanted organ or from leukocyte-containing blood transfusions.[36–42] Recent studies with murine[43–45] and rat[46] models of CMV have confirmed that the heart in seropositive individuals harbors latent virus that can cause lethal, disseminated primary infection post-transplant. The latent virus appears to be present in intrinsic cardiac tissue rather than in so-called passenger leukocytes.[47]

When considering patients who were seropositive for CMV prior to transplant, it had been assumed that all active CMV infection developing post-transplant was of endogenous origin. However, it has long been recognized that different human CMV strains have a great deal of genomic and antigenic heterogeneity. The biologic significance of this heterogeneity has been unclear, particularly in terms of the possibility of superinfection with a new strain of CMV in a seropositive individual.[37] It has recently been shown using DNA restriction enzyme-analysis techniques that superinfection does occur in renal transplant patients; that is, in approximately 50% of individuals who are seropositive prior to transplant who receive kidneys from seropositive donors, the CMV that develops post-transplant is of donor origin rather than of recipient origin. In addition, superinfected individuals are far more likely to develop symptomatic disease than are patients who reactivate their own endogenous strain.[48,49] This is likely to be true in cardiac transplant patients as well.

In all three types of CMV infection—primary, reactivation, and superinfection—the transplant-associated immunosuppression is sufficient to permit reactivation of latent virus with clinical manifestations. The peak incidence of CMV infection is 1–4 months posttransplant. Unlike most other infections,

CMV has a spectrum of clinical manifestations that exceeds those encountered during the basic disease process caused directly by the virus itself. The spectrum of the clinical manifestations of CMV infection in the cardiac transplant patient can be divided into three categories. The first is the direct infectious disease syndrome caused by the virus itself. Although a significant number of transplant patients have asymptomatic infection, as do normal hosts, the majority of cardiac transplant patients manifest the CMV infection clinically. The second category is a predisposition to superinfection with other pathogens that has been associated with CMV infection. CMV infections appear to cause a depression in host defenses in excess of that produced by the immunosuppressive therapy being administered. Finally, although not well studied in cardiac transplant patients, CMV could play a role in the production of allograft dysfunction (see Chapter 21).

3.2. Infectious Disease Syndromes Produced by Cytomegalovirus

In the normal host, the vast majority of CMV infections are clinically asymptomatic.[50] Although there are asymptomatic infections in transplant patients, clinically apparent disease is much more common. It has been noted that the clinical manifestations of CMV infection can be divided into two groups; one a benign, self-limited mononucleosis-like syndrome and the other a lethal progressive disease with multisystem involvement.[51,52] Patients with primary CMV disease appear to be at greater risk of developing more clinically severe disease than those with reactivation infection.[32,34,36,37,52] In a study that compared the clinical symptoms of primary and secondary CMV infection, it was noted that those patients with primary CMV infection had significantly more fever and hepatic dysfunction than transplant patients with reactivation infection.[35] They also had more pulmonary involvement and leukopenia but the differences were not significantly different statistically.

The clinical manifestations of the mild, self-limited form of CMV disease in transplant patients are much like those of the mononucleosis-like syndrome seen with CMV infection in a normal host. The disease generally beings insidiously with constitutional symptoms such as fever, malaise, my-algias, arthralgias, and anorexia. Fever is the most common clinical manifestation of CMV disease and often presents as the only clinical symptom. As with CMV mononucleosis in the normal host, these patients present with 3–10% atypical lymphocytes in the peripheral blood.[53] Both elevated and depressed total WBC count has been reported with CMV infection.[53] It has been our experience that leukopenia with increased numbers of atypical lymphocytes is much more common as a manifestation of active CMV infection. Other clinical manifestations such as pharyngitis, lymphadenopathy and splenomegaly are uncommon in post-transplant CMV infection.

Pneumonitis is one of the most dreaded complications of CMV infections. CMV pneumonia is one of the most common causes of death in bone marrow transplant recipients (see Chapter 20). It is also a common cause of morbidity and mortality in cardiac transplant patients.[18,21] The typical chest radiograph of CMV pneumonia shows bilateral, symmetric, interstitial infiltrate, primarily involving the lower lobes. CMV involvement of the lungs can be asymptomatic or a total whiteout of the lung with respiratory failure and death. Most patients have the classic chest radiographic changes plus mild hypoxia. Focal lung infiltrate is more suggestive of bacterial or fungal disease but has also been seen with CMV disease. Even solitary nodules have been reported as the presenting sign of CMV pneumonia.[54] The major differential diagnosis in interstitial pneumonia in these patients is between CMV and *P. carinii*. Gallium scanning of the lung is helpful in distinguishing an inflammatory infiltrate from pulmonary edema.[55] However, this will not distinguish between CMV and *Pneumocystis* pneumonia. Clinically, CMV appears to have a more subacute presentation than *Pneumocystis*, but this again is not diagnostic. Bronchoscopy with transbronchial biopsy or open lung biopsy is the only way to reliably distinguish between the two. It is also important to remember that these two infections are often coexistent; thus, it is better to begin empirical treatment for *P. carinii* with trimethoprim–sulfamethoxazole until the distinction is made.[36,37]

Hematologic abnormalities are common with CMV disease in the transplant patient. The presence of atypical lymphocytes is not uncommon and may help in the differential diagnosis of CMV disease. However, leukopenia and thrombocytopenia are also common and usually much more clinically significant. The leukopenia may be profound with counts of less than 1500 cells/mm^3 and may contribute to the increased risk for opportunistic infections. Thrombocytopenia has also been reported and may lead to a significant bleeding diasthesis.[37,53,56]

CMV involvement in the gastrointestinal (GI) tract has become a significant problem in the transplant patient. CMV inclusions have been found in patients with gastric ulcers and various forms of colitis. Bleeding is a major problem associated with these lesions, especially if associated with thrombocytopenia. The histopathologic diagnosis can be made from a biopsy of the affected area. Treatment is difficult, however, because the lesions are usually diffusely spread throughout the GI tract and thus segmental resection of the affected area is not helpful. Until the advent of specific antiviral therapy, management is directed at supportive measures and decreasing the level of immunosuppression.[36,37,57–59]

Abnormal liver function tests due to CMV involvement with the liver are not uncommon in post-transplant infections. Transient elevation of the transaminase levels or alkaline phosphatase are among the typical manifestations of CMV disease. Severe hepatitis has also been reported, and it is impossible to distinguish CMV hepatitis from other causes of viral hepatitis.[60] A problem that has developed with widespread use of cyclosporine is distinguishing between viral hepatitis, in particular CMV, and cyclosporine toxicity. Both can present with elevation of transaminases and alkaline phosphatase. A high bilirubin level with minimal elevation of other enzymes appears more characteristic of cyclosporine toxicity. Again, both problems can be coexistent, with a similar clinical presentation.

Central nervous system signs and symptoms are less common manifestations of CMV infection; however, such involvement may vary from a mild encephalopathy to severe progressive meningoencephalitis indistinguishable from herpes simplex encephalitis. Aseptic meningitis has also been seen with CMV infection. It is important to remember that it is difficult to distinguish the neurologic manifestations of CMV infection from those of other more treatable infections such as herpes simplex or toxoplasmosis. Thus, care must be taken in establishing the correct diagnosis.[62–64]

A late complication of CMV infection is chorioretinitis. This usually occurs later than 6 months post-transplant. Patients may be asymptomatic but often complain of blurred vision or of decreased visual acuity. Scotoma can be detected with visual field testing. The characteristic eye lesion is an expanding whitish, necrotic retinitis on a background of hemorrhagic infarction. The outcome of the retinitis is variable depending on the level of immunosuppression and the control of the underlying CMV infection.[36,37,65–67]

The severe or lethal syndrome associated with CMV infections has the same clinical manifestations as the self-limited form but to a much greater degree. The syndrome usually begins with mild fever and leukopenia and then progresses to prostration, hypotension, and severe respiratory insufficiency. Hepatic failure, GI bleeding and encephalopathy are also common in this severe form of CMV disease. Ultimately, this multisystem failure leads to death. Death is often precipitated by superinfection with bacterial, fungal, or protozoal infection. The host defenses appear to be severely depressed by this overwhelming CMV infection.[68]

3.3. Superinfection Associated with Cytomegalovirus Infection

One of the unique aspects of CMV disease in transplant patients has been the increased incidence of potentially lethal superinfections.[53,56] Cardiac transplant patients have been particularly susceptible to a syndrome characterized by fever, atypical lymphocytes, pneumonia, and pulmonary superinfection.[31,53] Cardiac transplant patients with primary CMV infection are at greater risk of pulmonary superinfection as compared with patients with reactivation disease. In a study of early and late pulmonary infection in cardiac transplant patients with primary and reactivation CMV disease, it was observed that 6 of 12 patients with serologic evidence of primary CMV infection had either bacterial pneumonia or abscess as compared with only 1 of 20 patients who were seropositive prior to infection. This trend continued in later pulmonary infections in patients with primary CMV disease. *P. carinii* pneumonia was specifically more common in patients with primary CMV disease. There did not appear to be any increased rate of fungal or nocardial infections.[31]

This increased propensity for pulmonary superinfections appears to be due to several factors. Severe leukopenia due to CMV infection places patients at greater risk of superinfection. However, other alterations in host defense mechanisms appear to be secondary to CMV infection as well. Humoral immunity appears to be intact in most transplant patients with high levels of circulating antibodies.[69] However in spite of this high level of circulating antibody it does not appear to offer protection against infection.[35,69] Cell-mediated immunity appears to be severely impaired in transplant patients with CMV infection.[32,35,69] Lymphocyte transformation responses were severely diminished to specific CMV antigens in both early and late transplant recipients.[35] Lymphocyte transformation response and interferon production to other herpes viruses were also noted to be depressed in these infected cardiac transplant patients.[32,69] CMV inclusions have been detected in pneumocytes, endothelial cells, and alveolar macrophages.[70] These CMV-infected cells may also have decreased activity, making transplant patients more susceptible to pulmonary superinfections.

Other than leukopenia, the clearest marker of impaired host resistance to superinfection induced by CMV infection has been changes noted in the circulating levels of immunoregulatory T cells. In normal individuals,[71] renal transplant patients,[72] and cardiac transplant patients[73–76] CMV (and/or EBV) infection is associated with a marked decrease in circulating levels of helper-inducer T cells (T4+ cells) and an increase in suppressor-cytotoxic T cells. If the normal ratio of T helper cells to T suppressor-cytotoxic cells is approximately 1.5, CMV-infected transplant patients (and normal persons with CMV mononucleosis) have ratios of 0.1–0.5, so-called inverted ratios. Studies by Schooley et al.[72] in renal transplant patients have shown that the subgroup of transplant patients at highest risk of opportunistic infection are those with virus-induced changes in their T-cell subsets.

3.4. Management of Cytomegalovirus Infection

Because of the great clinical impact of CMV on transplant patients, considerable effort has been devoted to attempts to control this infection. These efforts can be divided into two categories: preventive and therapeutic.[37] Within the preventive category,

other than minimizing the transfusion of CMV seropositive blood and transplantation of organs from seropositive donors into seronegative recipients,[52] three interventions have been systematically evaluated (all in renal transplant recipients): prophylactic monovalent, attenuated CMV vaccine, prophylactic hyperimmune CMV globulin, and prophylactic α-interferon (IF$_\alpha$). Of these, the vaccine appears to be relatively ineffective (not too surprising, given the current evidence of superinfection occurring in the face of even natural infection with a single strain of virus), interferon works but is difficult to use, and the hyperimmune globulin appears quite promising (see Chapter 21). However, before firm recommendations can be made for cardiac transplant patients, trials in this patient population must be carried out.

Therapeutically, until recently, there has been little available for the treatment of acute CMV infection. It is clear that in any patient with significant clinical CMV disease immunosuppressive therapy should immediately be decreased, particularly the cytotoxic drugs, and any antilymphocyte antibody therapy terminated.[37] Initial attempts to use adenine arabinoside in renal transplant patients with serious CMV disease were halted by catastrophic neurologic complications,[77] although Pollard et al.[65] have reported improvement in CMV chorioretinitis in patients treated with 20 mg/kg per day of this drug. In this study, serious hematologic and GI toxicities remained a significant problem. Acyclovir is without significant clinical effect for human CMV infection.[37] However, the advent of DHPG, the acyclovir analogue, has transformed this bleak picture into a more promising one. Initial experiences, primarily in patients with acquired immunodeficiency syndrome (AIDS),[78–80] have been promising, particularly for chorioretinitis. There is also the potential for using this drug prophylactically. It should be stressed, however, that experience with its use in cardiac transplant patients with CMV has been minimal at this point.

3.5. Herpes Group Viruses Other Than Cytomegalovirus

3.5.1. Herpes Simplex

Herpes simplex virus is probably second only to CMV in causing clinical illness in transplant patients.

The problem appears to be due to reactivation of the latent virus rather than acquisition of new virus.[32,41,81,82] The most common clinical manifestation is herpes labialis, usually beginning during the first 3 months post-transplantation. Rand et al.[60] found that cardiac transplant patients had herpes simplex lesions on the lips, nose, face, or oral mucosa. These infections generally began 1.1 months post-transplant and lasted greater than 1 month. In some patients, facial lesions persisted for more than 3 months. They also showed that patients in the first 6 months post-transplant had severely depressed cellular immunity to herpes virus, as demonstrated by lower lymphocyte transformation and interferon production. By contrast, late cardiac transplant patients (defined as more than 6 months post-transplant) had normal lymphocyte respnse to herpes simplex and the same rate of clinical herpes labialis as a control population. Asymptomatic shedding of herpes virus was greater in the late cardiac transplant group than in controls.

Anogenital infections are less common than herpes labialis. They are typically due to HSV-2. The lesions are usually characterized by coalescing, ulcerative lesions in the anogenital area. Biopsy of the lesion or Tzanck smear may be helpful, but culture for HSV is the diagnostic gold standard. Generally, herpes simplex will grow in tissue culture in 48–72 hr. Unfortunately, the diagnosis may be confused due to secondary infection of the lesions. This secondary infection may lead to a localized cellulitis of the surrounding tissue and is frequently infected with bowel flora. Bacteremia has also resulted from severe areas of cellulitis in the perirectal area.[82]

Severe forms of HSV infections, including widely disseminated disease or encephalitis, appear to be unusual in cardiac transplant patients. In several large series, only one death due to herpes simplex infection has been reported.[23] Neurologic complications resulting from HSV infection have also been reviewed.[63] In the first 83 cardiac transplant patients, three had herpes simplex encephalitis and two had evidence of disseminated disease. In another large series,[21] even though 25% of their patients had clinical HSV infections, no cases of either encephalitis or disseminated herpes disease were encountered.

Fortunately, as compared to CMV infections, there is effective antiviral therapy for herpes simplex infections. Both vidarabine and acyclovir have demonstrated efficacy in the management of herpes simplex infections. Vidarabine has been shown to be effective in the treatment of herpes simplex encephalitis using doses of 15 mg/kg per day.[83] It has also been shown to be effective treatment in disseminated disease of neonates.[84] Intravenous acyclovir is only approved for primary or recurrent HSV in the immunocompromised host[85,86] but ongoing trials suggest that this agent has similar if not better efficacy in encephalitis and disseminated disease. Acyclovir definitely appears to have fewer side effects than vidarabine. The availability of an oral as well as an intravenous formulation of acyclovir, together with its essential lack of toxicity in the transplant patient, makes this the drug of choice for treating herpetic infections. Because of its high therapeutic to toxic ratio, it is reasonable to begin therapy at the first signs of infection.

3.5.2. Epstein–Barr Virus

Epstein–Barr virus is commonly isolated from the pharyngeal secretions of transplant patients.[87,88] Up to 87% of the seropositive renal transplant patients excrete EBV at some time in throat washings.[89] EBV reactivation appears to be more common in patients who receive certain immunosuppressants such as antithymocyte globulin or cyclosporine.[90,91]

Even with the high level of viral excretion in transplant patients, clinically apparent infectious disease syndromes are uncommon. Clinically apparent EBV disease has not been reported with cardiac transplant patients and only rarely reported in renal transplant patients.[91,92] In those series, illness associated with EBV was characterized by fever, leukopenia and fleeting pulmonary infiltrates closely resembling CMV infection. No deaths could be directly attributed to EBV infections.

Of greater concern has been the association of EBV and lymphoproliferative diseases in transplant patients. There are recent reports of EBV-associated lymphomas arising in patients with congenital immune disorders[93,94] and after initiation of immunosuppression for organ transplantation.[21,90,95–98] The association of a primary EBV infection and subsequent lymphoma has been very clearly demonstrated in a cardiac transplant patient.[99] A patient previously seronegative for EBV underwent cardiac transplantation and received cyclosporine and prednisone immunosuppression. He subsequently became seropositive for EBV 3–5 months after transplantation. Six months post-transplant he was found to have diffuse histiocytic lymphoma, with 60–70% of the cells staining positively for Epstein–Barr nuclear antigen (EBNA) by immunofluorescent staining. The development of lymphomas in three heart transplant and two heart lung transplant patients has been previously documented.[100] All these patients received cyclosporine and prednisone and some received additional immunosuppression with azathioprine or antithymocyte globulin. Again, the association with EBV infection was definite, and the lymphomas were successfully managed with drastic reduction in the level of immunosuppression. Thus it appears that EBV, not unlike CMV, has effects on transplant patients that are not directly related to clinical infection (see Chapter 21).

3.5.3. Varicella–Zoster Virus

The risk of VZV infection is also increased in transplant patients.[32,69] Clinically apparent disease has been reported in up to 22% in one instance.[101] VZV infections have been reported in both early and late cardiac transplant recipients. As with other herpes virus infections, cell-mediated immunity to VZV appears depressed in cardiac transplant patients as demonstrated by a decreased lymphocyte transformation response to VZV antigen *in vitro*. In contrast to other herpes virus infections, with VZV lymphocyte defects may be detected for more than 1 year. Thus the risk of VZV infections is the same in early and late cardiac transplant recipients.[32,69]

The clinical manifestations of VZV infection in transplant patients is usually one of two presentations. The most common is the typcial skin lesion characterized by a vesicular lesion in a dermatomal distribution. In transplant patients these lesions may be more severe and may persist for longer periods. In one instance, four patients were described who had persistent VZV infection for 5–24 weeks.[101] These lesions resolved only when the level of immunosuppression was significantly decreased. The second and more severe presentation of VZV is the widely disseminated form of VZV infection, which is much less common. However, it has been implicated as a cause of death in a cardiac transplant patient.[32]

As with herpes simplex, there is effective antiviral chemotherapy for VZV infections. Vidarabine appears effectively to halt the dissemination of VZV infection in immunocompromised hosts.[102] Acyclovir has also been demonstrated to halt progression of already disseminated VZV infection.[103] High-dose interferon appeared to decrease the rate of new vesicle formation and visceral complication in VZV infection in cancer patients.[104] As with herpes simplex infections, acyclovir should be considered the drug of choice for VZV infection at the present time. It should be noted that significantly higher dosages of the drug are needed to treat VZV as opposed to herpes simplex virus. Even though most VZV infections appear to be reactivation disease, a small percentage of transplant patients may be susceptible at the time of transplantation. In immunosuppressed patients with negative serology for VZV, varicella–zoster immune globulin (VZIG) passive immunization is indicated for exposure to any form of VZ disease, as primary VZV infection in this setting can be a rapidly lethal process.

4. *Pneumocystis carinii* Infection in Cardiac Transplant Patients

As in other immunosuppressed patients, *P. carinii* pneumonia is common in cardiac transplant patients.[19,21,28] The clinical presentation is similar to that of other immunosuppressed patients, characterized by the progressive development of fever, nonproductive cough and tachypnea. The chest radiograph initially reveals a diffuse interstitial infiltrate that soon progresses to a diffuse alveolar infiltrate with air bronchograms. Severe hypoxia is usually a cardinal sign of the disease. Rarely, atypical presentations may occur, such as solitary lesions, lobar infiltrates, unilateral disease, or even a clear chest radiograph (see Chapter 10).

The diagnosis of *P. carinii* pneumonia can only be made by the demonstration of the organism in the lung tissue or in material obtained from the lung using a methenamine silver stain. Open lung biopsy, transbronchial biopsy, percutaneous lung biopsy, and endobronchial brush technique have all been successful in confirming the diagnosis of *Pneumocystis*.[105–109] It has been our experience that bronchoscopy with bronchial lavage and transbronchial biopsy is the initial procedure of choice. If this is unsuccessful then we proceed to open lung biopsy. Open lung biopsy has been necessary in only two instances in which *Pneumocystis* has been the cause of the lung infiltrates. In patients who are critically ill, open lung biopsy is the procedure of choice (see also Chapter 6).

These aggressive diagnostic techniques are indicated because there is currently no way to diagnose *Pneumocystis* noninvasively. The major differential diagnosis is with CMV pneumonitis. Typically, *Pneumocystis* has a more acute onset than CMV; however, this is not diagnostic. CMV infection can often be coexistent with *P. carinii* pneumonia.[31] Other pulmonary infections which can mimic *Pneumocystis* include those caused by *Legionella, Aspergillus, Nocardia,* and *Candida* species.

In patients presenting with a syndrome compatible with *P. carinii* pneumonia, empirical therapy is necessary because of the potential for rapid progression of the disease. Pentamidine isethionate was the first drug used successfully in the treatment of *P. carinii* pneumonitis.[109] Currently the combination of trimethoprim–sulfamethoxazole is the recommended initial therapy for *Pneumocystis* pneumonia. The fixed combination of trimethoprim–sulfamethoxazole given in high doses (20 mg/kg per day of trimethoprim) has been found to be as effective as pentamidine in a variety of immunosuppressed hosts.[110,111] Although it is not any more effective than pentamidine, it has significantly fewer side effects[109,111] and thus is the suggested initial therapy. Therapy should be continued for a total of 14 days. Patients who do not respond to trimethoprim–sulfamethoxazole therapy should be treated with pentamidine.

5. *Legionella* Infections

Legionella species have become common pathogens in the compromised host and cardiac transplant patients are no exception.[7,112–114] This infection usually presents as a patchy pneumonia with an initial interstitial infiltrate progressing to an alveolar infiltrate. The lesions are usually unilateral but may be bilateral.[113] Nodular infiltrates are also common with *Legionella* infections.[115] Cavitation is unusual but has been reported to occur in 10% of the cases, usually in an immunocompromised host.[112,115]

The culture confirmation of *Legionella* infection can be difficult. Most reports state that expectorated sputum is not helpful in the diagnosis of pulmonary infection.[116] The highest yield for culture-positive *Legionella* infection results from a direct culture of lung tissue.[117] Serologic techniques have also been widely used to diagnose *Legionella* infection. A direct fluorescent antibody (DFA) test can be performed on fresh or formalin-fixed tissue and sputum. This technique is able to detect approximately 60% of the culture positive cases.[118] The most widely used test, however, is the indirect fluorescent antibody test (IFA). A fourfold rise in titer or a single titer of 1 : 256 is considered evidence of recent or active infection. Unfortunately, this test is not generally heplful in the immediate diagnosis of a patient with an infiltrate. Thus, a combination of the techniques using culture, DFA and IFA is often necessary to make the diagnosis of *Legionella* infection (see also Chapter 11).

Again, because culture confirmation of the diagnosis may be delayed, empirical therapy is indicated when *Legionella* infection is suspected. Erythromycin is the antibiotic of choice. In the cardiac transplant patients, intravenous erythromycin should be started in doses of 4–6 g/day. This should be continued for at least 1 week.[119] After completion of intravenous therapy, oral therapy can be started at a dose of 2 g/day and therapy continued for a minimum of 3 weeks. Relapses are common and more prolonged therapy may be necessary for relapses.[113,120] In addition, Naot et al.[122] suggested that the administration of immunosuppressive therapy after a cardiac transplant could result in the reactivation of previously dormant infection in individuals with antibody to *L. pneumophila*. The following illustrative case of *Legionella* pneumonia appropriately treated with erythromycin, but that relapsed as a cavitary lesion, emphasizes the difficulty with this infection in the cardiac transplant patient.

Illustrative Case 2

WC is a 59-year-old white man with a history of ischemic cardiomyopathy who underwent allograft cardiac transplantation on June 6, 1984. His postoperative immunosuppression included prednisone and cyclosporine A. He was discharged home 3 weeks after surgery. In July 1984, he was readmitted with severe herpes simplex stomatitis. He was successfully treated with intravenous acyclovir. He was admitted 1 week later with a complaint of cou-

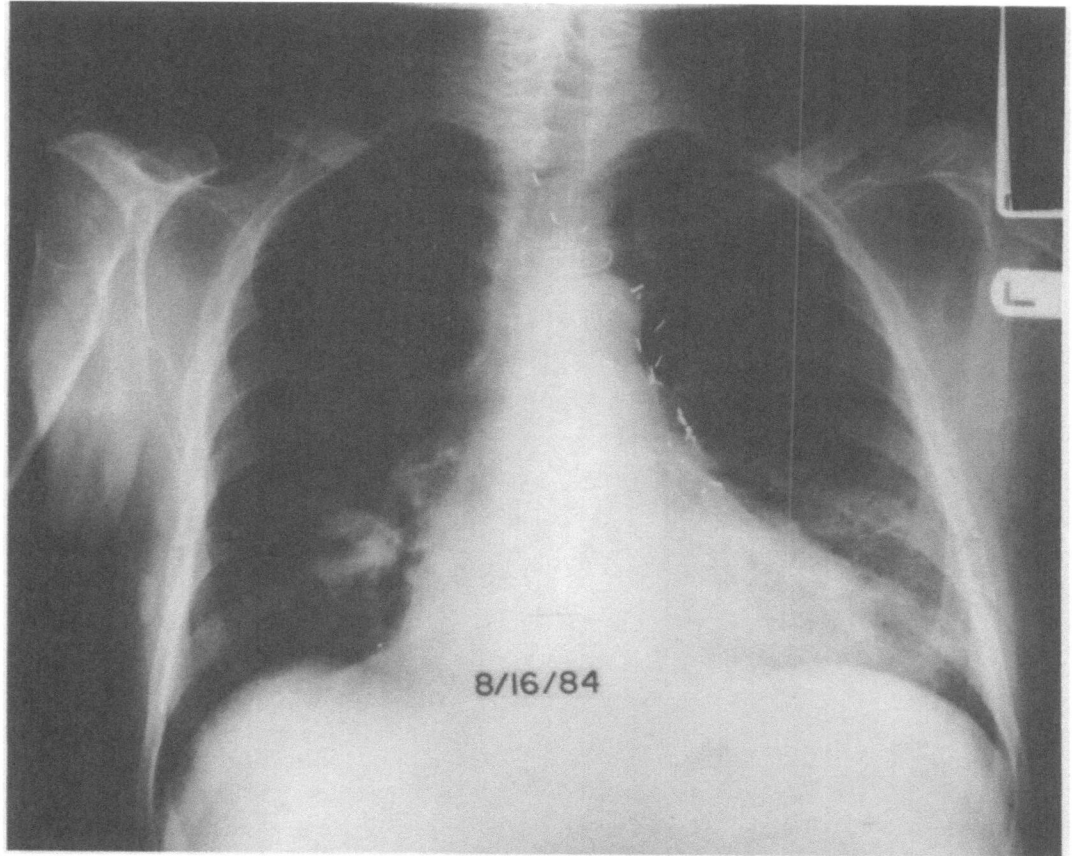

FIGURE 3. PA chest radiograph, patient WC (8/16/84) Note the nodular pulmonary infiltrate with cavitation at the arrow tip

gh, fever, and increasing shortness of breath. A chest radiograph revealed a new right lower lobe infiltrate

He was empirically given piperacillin, erythromycin and trimethoprim–sulfamethoxazole. Initial sputum cultures revealed normal respiratory flora. Because of an increasing infiltrate on chest radiography, a percutaneous aspiration of the right lung infiltrate was performed. Gram-negative organisms were seen in the aspirated material. Cultures subsequently grew a pure culture of *Legionella pneumophila* type I.

The other antibiotics were discontinued and the IV erythromycin was continued. He became afebrile and the infiltrate began to clear. He received a full 14-day course of IV erythromycin and was discharged home with only a small residual right lung infiltrate on chest radiography.

The patient returned for routine follow-up on August 16, 1984 and had no complaints A chest radiograph revealed a right lung nodular density with cavitation, shown in Fig. 3. The patient again had bronchoscopy, from which no positive cultures were obtained. Because of persistent infiltrate, he underwent repeat percutaneous lung aspiration, from which *Legionella pneumophila* type I was grown. The patient received a 2-week course of IV erythromycin followed by a 2-month course of oral erythromycin.

Followup chest radiography done in January 1985 (Fig. 4) revealed complete resolution of the infiltrate

6. Fungal Infections in the Cardiac Transplant Patient

Fungal infections in the cardiac transplant patient may be grouped into two general categories: (1) an occasional patient, like other individuals with impaired host defenses, who has been resident in one of the geographic areas endemic for systemic mycotic infection who develops disseminated coccidioidomycosis, histoplasmosis, or blastomycosis due to the effects of the immunosuppressive therapy administered[121–129]; and (2) the all-too-common patient who develops opportunistic infection with *Candida, Aspergillus, Cryptococcus,* or, rarely, other fungal species.[7,23,130] It is the latter group of infections that

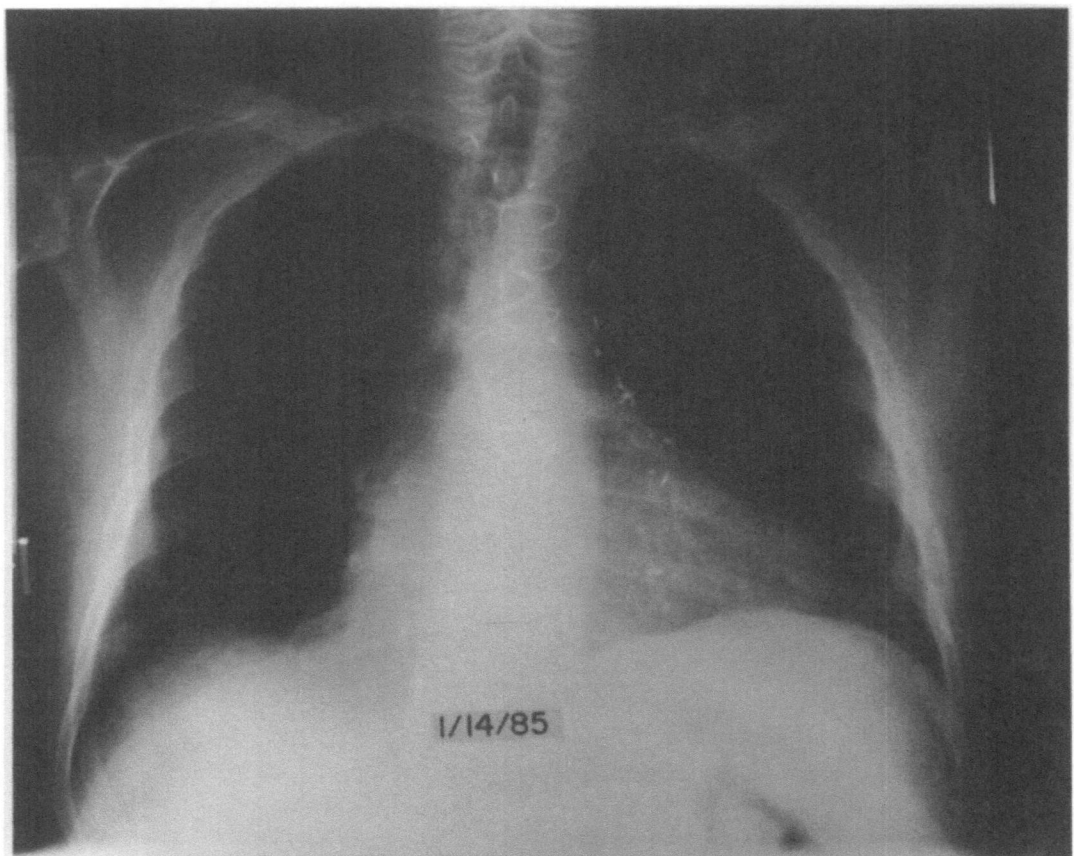

FIGURE 4. PA chest radiograph, patient WC, 5 months later showing complete clearing of infiltrates.

pose the greatest hazard to the transplant patient (see Chapter 8).

6.1. *Aspergillus* Infection in the Cardiac Transplant Patient

Although *Aspergillus* infections have clearly been acquired from a hospital source,[131] the ubiquitous nature of this fungus often makes the actual source of infection impossible to detect. Thirty-nine patients in the Stanford transplant experience have had *Aspergillus* infection, of whom 20 have died.[23] Most patients in this experience had both cavitary and infiltrative lesions in the lung. The usual treatment with amphotericin B has not been uniformly successful, and most patients who are cured of their *Aspergillus* infection have some form of surgically resectable infectious focus. Nine of our 188 patients have had biopsy evidence of disseminated *Aspergillus* infection of the lung and/or other organs. Seven have died and at autopsy had histologic evidence of either local lung infection or disseminated *Aspergillus* infection. We have attributed our two survivors to the use of liposomal amphotericin B. This compound has been used in patients with malignant diseases, particularly acute leukemia; although the results appear to be related to the early diagnosis and early institution of therapy, there have been survivors, including patients with acute leukemia who have survived *Aspergillus* infections which are routinely fatal.[132] The typical progression of *Aspergillus* infection in a severely immunosuppressed cardiac transplant patient despite treatment with liposomal amphotericin B, is presented in the following case report.

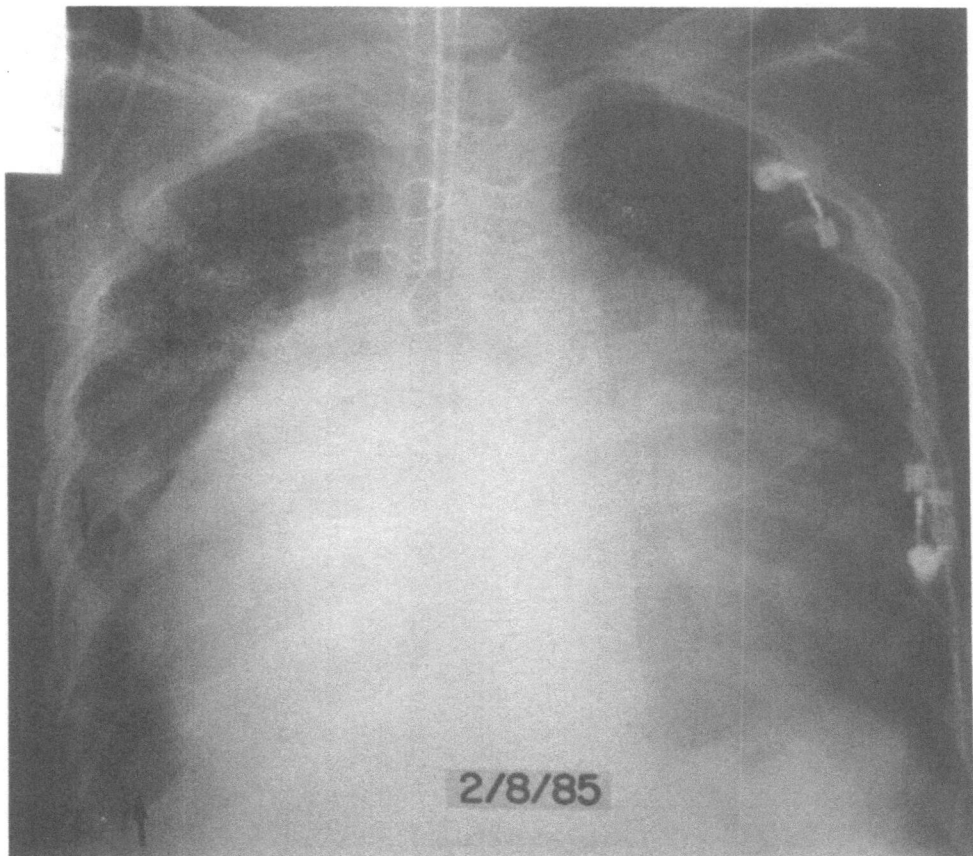

FIGURE 5. PA chest radiograph, patient BD (2/8/85). Note the nodular infiltrate between the two arrows

Illustrative Case 3

BD was a 16-year-old black boy who underwent allograft cardiac transplantation on January 5, 1985 for idiopathic cardiomyopathy His postoperative immunosuppression included prednisone and cyclosporine. His course was complicated by an episode of mediastinal bleeding with subsequent hypotension. Re-exploration of the chest revealed bleeding from the atrial anastomosis site, which was corrected He developed an episode of severe rejection 1 week after surgery. This was treated with cyclosporin, prednisone, and antithymocyte globulin. The patient continued to do poorly, with chronic severe rejection, arrhythmias, hypotension, and renal failure

Four weeks post-transplant, the patient developed a right lung infiltrate (Fig. 5), and sputum cultures grew *E. cloacae* and *Aspergillus* species. A bronchoscopy with transbronchial biopsy revealed invasive *Aspergillus* in the right lung A CT scan of the chest done on February 8, 1985 (Fig. 6) revealed a dense infiltration and cavitation of the right lower lobe

The patient was begun on amphotericin B, but the immunosuppression could not be decreased due to the severe ongoing rejection Because of his failure to respond to amphotericin B as manifested by persistent fever and deteriorating pulmonary status, the patient was placed in an experimental protocol with liposomal amphotericin B In spite of aggressive medical management, the patient continued to deteriorate and died on February 16, 1985 At autopsy he was found to have a massively dilated heart with severe rejection *Aspergillus* was present in both lungs, in the brain, and in an endocardial abscess

6.2. *Candida* Infection in the Cardiac Transplant Patient

Candida infections occur frequently in seriously ill hospitalized patients, as well as in transplantation patients. In a large autopsy series of bone marrow

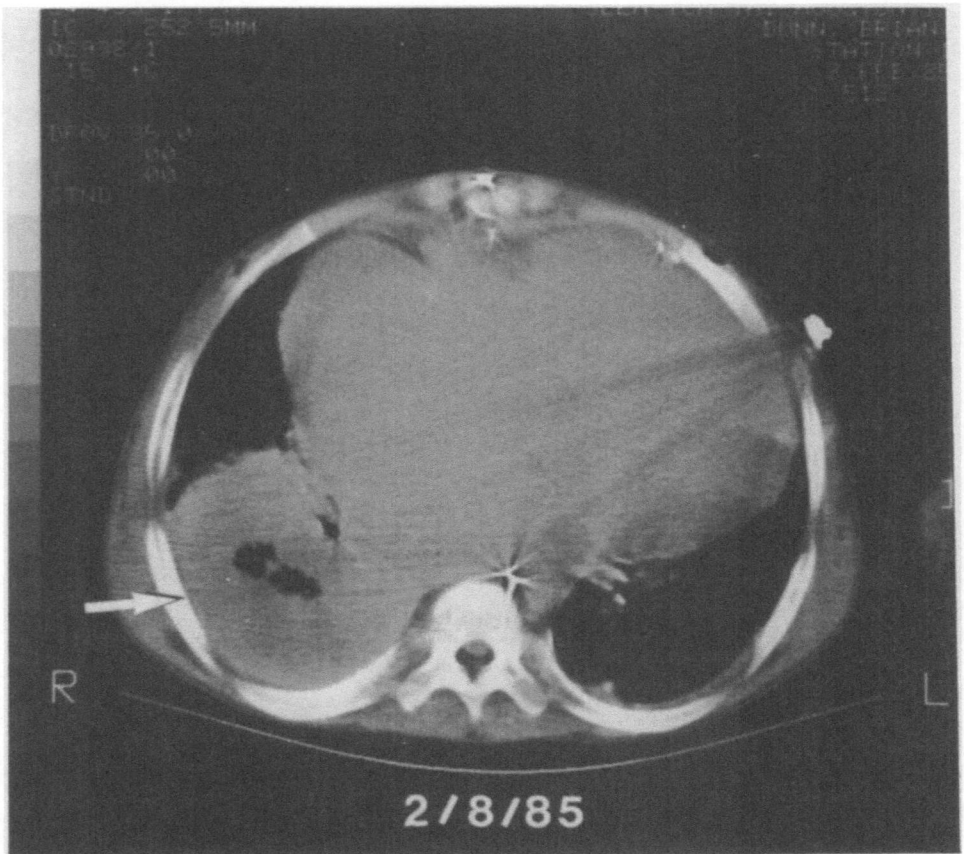

FIGURE 6. Computed tomography scan, patient BD (same date as Fig. 5). Note the dense infiltrate involving right lower lung with multiple cavities

transplantation patients, for example, disseminated candidal infection was the most common fungal infection noted.[133] Indwelling intravenous lines continue to be the most common portal of entry for serious candidal infection. Because the diagnosis of disseminated candidal infection is difficult, maintaining a high index of suspicion and doing frequent cultures from suspicious sites remains the best clinical approach to this problem. Of the 12 patients in the Stanford series who had documented candidal infections, six died of their infection.[23] Most fatal cases go unrecognized until either autopsy or until the morbid condition precludes survival even with appropriate amphotericin B therapy. Three serious candidal infections in our 188 cardiac transplant patients have been successfully treated with 260 mg amphotericin B. We have noted a transient increase

in serum creatinine in both patients after they received this small dose that does not influence renal function in the normal patient. All patients were receiving concurrent cyclosporine therapy, suggesting that amphotericin B and cyclosporine together may be more nephrotoxic.

6.3. *Cryptococcus* Infection in the Cardiac Transplant Patient

Pulmonary infection and meningitis caused by *Cryptococcus neoformans* have been particularly frequent in the renal transplant experience.[120,130,134] In the Stanford series, 10 infections occurred in nine patients, three of whom died despite the institution of appropriate therapy with amphotericin B and 5-fluorocytosine. We have had no cryptococcal infections to date in our transplantation series. Other fungal infections in the Phycomycetes group, which include *Mucor* and *Rhizopus,* have been well documented in all three transplantation groups. As with the case in other immunosuppressed patients, these infections are always serious and frequently fatal.[129,130,135]

7. Nocardial and Mycobacterial Infection in the Transplant Patient

Infection caused by *Nocardia asteroides* in transplantation and other immunosuppressed patients has been the subject of several reviews.[136–139] A complete and thorough analysis of the clinical experience and of the risk factors has been done in the 22 patients in the Stanford series who have had *Nocardia* infections. This analysis confirms that the diagnosis of *Nocardia* infection is extremely difficult, as 40% of the patients had nonspecific or absent symptoms. Pulmonary infection was the primary site of infection in 81% of their patients. However, disseminated infection occurred in 19% and involved multiple organ systems. Cutaneous and soft tissue dissemination is particularly common.[136,137] An association was noted between pulmonary nocardiosis and the subsequent development of atypical mycobacterial infections. An aggressive approach to the diagnosis and the rapid institution of appropriate therapy resulted in no fatalities in that series.[23] *Nocardia* has been associated with bacterial, fungal, viral, and *Pneumocystis* infections. Statistical analysis however, has failed to establish any relationship between the total number, type, or time of infections as related to the subsequent development of nocardial infections. One expection to this however was the association with atypical mycobacteria infections. Eight of the 21 patients who had *Nocardia* infection subsequently developed pulmonary infections with atypical mycobacterial species. Several of these infections were disseminated to other body organs.[140]

Fortunately, prolonged therapy for at least 4–6 months with sulfonamides alone, trimethoprim–sulfamethoxazole, or minocycline is usually associated with a good therapeutic response in heart transplant patients.[136,137,141]

We have experienced four nocardial pulmonary infections in our 188 transplant patients. Three of them have occurred as single infections. However, the following illustrative case occurred concurrently with an invasive *Aspergillus* infection. It is of interest that this patient survived both the nocardial and the *Aspergillus* infections.

Because of careful screening pretransplant and a low rate of active infection in the general community, tuberculosis has not been a major problem in cardiac transplant patients. The occurrence of atypical mycobacterial infection has already been noted. It should be stated, however, that rifampin therapy, presumably by influencing cyclosporine metabolism, can lead to severe rejection.[142]

Illustrative Case 5

DS is a 45-year-old white man who underwent allograft cardiac transplantation on June 13, 1984. His postoperative immunosuppression included prednisone and cyclosporine, and his postoperative course was uncomplicated until June 23, 1984, when he developed fever and had drainage from his chest tube site. Cultures taken from the site grew *E. cloacae* and the patient was treated with piperacillin and tobramycin. In spite of the antibiotics, the patient continued to have fever and drainage from his chest. A CT scan of the chest confirmed a loculated right pleural effusion and lower lobe lung abscess. The patient underwent a right thoracotomy with wedge resection of the right lower lobe and decortication. His IV antibiotic therapy was continued for 2 weeks with clinical improvement, and he was sent home on a 2-week course of trimethoprim–sulfamethoxazole.

On November 3, 1984, he presented with a 3-day history of fever, dyspnea, and a cough productive of a thick brown sputum. He was febrile and had a respiratory rate of 35 per minute. However, the physical examination was remarkable only for diffuse, coarse rhonchi. Laboratory evaluation revealed a Hct of 39% and WBC count of 17,500/mm³ (75% polys, 20% bands, 5% lymphs). Chest radiography (Fig. 7) revealed bilateral nodular infiltrates. Gram stain of the sputum revealed many WBCs, rare epithelial cells, and a mixture of gram-positive cocci, gram negative rods, and a rare gram-positive rod. The patient was begun on IV erythromycin and trimethorpim–sulfamethoxazole. Because of clinical deterioration, he had a percutaneous aspiration of a lung nodule. A Gram stain of the material revealed many branching gram-positive rods which were also weakly acid fast. The sputum and the aspirate subsequently grew *N asteroides* Subsequent cultures were also positive for *Aspergillus* species.

Trimethoprim–sulfamethoxazole was continued, and the erythromycin was discontinued. Because of the positive culture for *Aspergillus* species, the patient reveived 1.5 g liposomal amphotericin B over a 3-week period. Within 5 days, the patient had become afebrile and had some resolution of this infiltrate on chest radiography. The patient also received a 3-week course of parenteral trimethoprim–sulfamethoxazole and was then discharged home to complete a 4-month course of oral therapy with trimethoprim–sulfamethoxazole. A follow-up chest radiograph in January 1985 (Fig. 8) revealed complete clearing of the infiltrates.

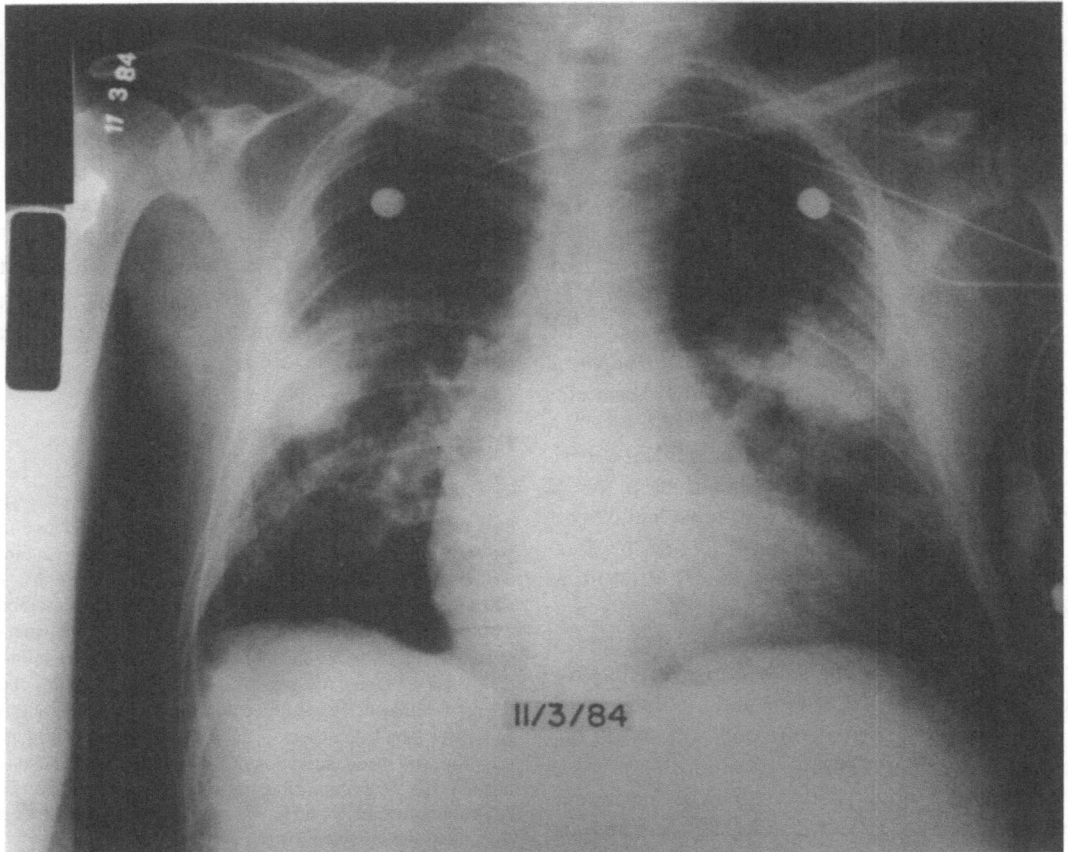

FIGURE 7. PA chest radiograph, patient DS (11/3/84). Note bilateral infiltrates

8. Toxoplasmosis in the Cardiac Transplant Patient

Toxoplasma gondii infection is a major problem in cardiac transplant patients. Myocarditis, disseminated infection, and, particularly, encephalitis have been observed not uncommonly in this patient population. Although reactivation of latent infection with immunosuppressive therapy is possible, in most cases the *T. gondii* is transmitted with the donor heart from seropositive individuals into seronegative recipients.[143–146] In England, it has been estimated that this occurs in 12–17% of cardiac transplants.[136–148] Although not all such individuals will develop clinical toxoplasmosis, the risk in this circumstance appears to approach at least 50%. The Stanford group observed a 10% incidence of clinical toxopolasmosis in their earlier experience with this

agent. Even now, with all their expertise,[7,144,149] there have been 10 cases among their last 290 heart transplants.

As detailed in Chapter 10, the clinical manifestations may be quite nonspecific, resulting in delay in diagnosis. It is important to emphasize that expert review of endomyocardial biopsies taken to assess rejection activity may give the first clue to the presence of active *T. gondii* infection. An important mistake to be avoided is to diagnose rejection and increase the immunosuppressive therapy, when the inflammatory infiltrate is due to the presence of *T. gondii* rather than to rejection activity.[145,150]

Making the diagnosis of toxoplasmosis is quite important, as therapy with pyrimethamine and sulfadiazine is quite effective if instituted early enough. Better yet is prevention. It has been recommended that both donor and recipient be screened serological-

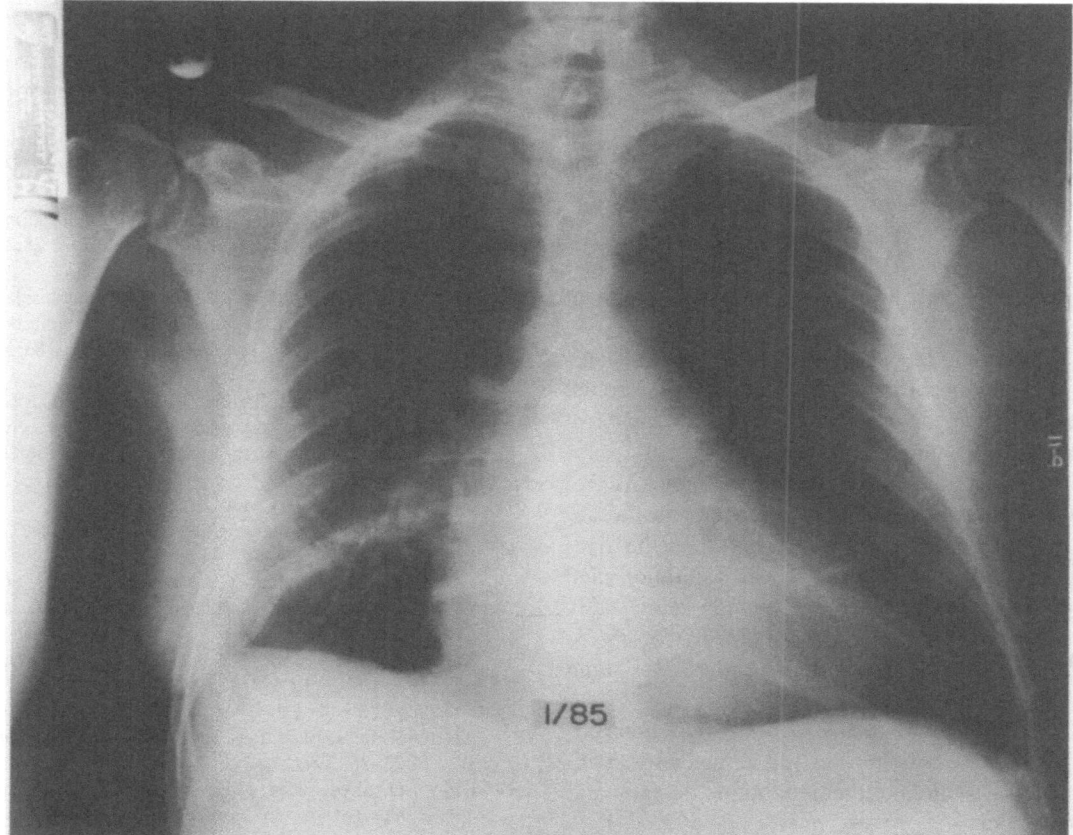

FIGURE 8. PA chest radiograph, patient DS (2 months later). Note the complete clearing of right lung and partial clearing on the left.

ly for *T. gondii*. If the placement of a heart from a seropositive donor into a seronegative recipient cannot be avoided, there is evidence that prophylactic pyrimethamine will prevent the development of clinical disease.[7,147,148]

9. General Surgical Considerations in the Cardiac Transplant Patient

As detailed in Chapters 21 and 23, long-term immunosuppressive therapy, such as that administered to the cardiac transplant patient, is associated with a variety of problems of major interest to the general surgeon. These may be divided into three general categories: surgical correction of problems such as hernias, which are seen in every patient population; surgical problems such as false aneurysms of the femoral artery or repair of a groin lymphocele, that may develop in any patient requiring cardiac bypass for cardiac surgery; and the special emergency intraabdominal problems that develop as a result of the immunosuppressive therapy being administered. This latter category includes perforated or severe gastric and/or duodenal ulcer disease, pancreatitis, acalculous and calculous cholecystitis, and perforating colonic diverticulitis. The details of the diagnosis and management of these problems are discussed in Chapters 21 and 23. It is worth emphasizing here, however, that there must be a high index of suspicion of potential intraabdominal catastrophe in immunosuppressed patients such as these, as their impaired inflammatory response will mask the gravity of the situation, and rapidity of diagnosis and therapy are critical for patient salvage.[151]

10. Special Infectious Disease Problems of Patients Undergoing Heart–Lung Transplants

The availability of cyclosporine as the basis of immunosuppressive programs has made feasible combination heart–lung transplantation. Although the general pattern of infections observed in this patient population has been similar to that seen in patients receiving only hearts, there are some important differences[152,153]:

1. As might be expected, the lung of the heart–lung recipient is particularly vulnerable to microbial invasion. Acute bacterial pneumonia is the most frequent infectious disease problem observed. Because the lower respiratory tract of these patients is frequently colonized with bacterial species in the absence of pulmonary parenchymal invasion, the diagnostic specificity of transtracheal aspiration and bronchoscopy in this patient population is unusually low. There may be a higher incidence of *Pneumocystis carinii* infection among the heart–lung patients.

2. Overall, more than 90% of the infections observed in these patients are life threatening, with more than two-thirds of them involving the lung and thoracic cavity.

3. In long-term survivors of heart–lung transplantation, extensive bronchiolitis obliterans may be observed.[154] This is, presumably, at least in part a result of chronic allograft rejection. In addition, however, there is a possibility that chronic lower respiratory tract infection could be contributory to the pathogenesis of this lesion. Dummer et al.[153] described two patients more than 1 year posttransplant with a clinical syndrome of chronic purulent sputum production, lower respiratory tract colonization with *Pseudomonas aeruginosa,* and symptomatic improvement with intravenous antibiotic therapy. The relative contributions of infection and rejection to the pathogenesis of these conditions remain to be determined.

References

1. Barnard CN: The operation. *South Afr Med J* **41**:1271–1274, 1967.
2. Oyer PE, Stinson EB, Jamieson SW, et al: Cyclosporine in cardiac transplantation· A 2½ year follow-up *Transplant Proc* **15**:2546–2552, 1983.
3. Hardesty RL, Griffith BP, Debsk RF, et al. Experience with cyclosporine in cardiac transplantation. *Transplant Proc* **15**:2553–2558, 1983.
4. Wallwork J, Cory-Pearce R, English TAH: Cyclosporine for cardiac transplantation: U,K trial *Transplant Proc* **15**:2559–2566, 1983
5. Modry DL, Oyer PE, Jamieson SW, et al. Cyclosporine in heart and heart-lung transplantation. *Can J Surg* **28**:274–282, 1985.
6. Pennock JL, Oyer PE, Reitz BA, et al. Cardiac transplantation in perspective for the future. Survival, complications, rehabilitation, and cost *J Thorac Cardiovasc Surg* **83**:168–177, 1982.
7. Hofflin JM, Potasman I, Baldwin JC, et al. Infectious complications in heart transplant recipients receiving cyclosporine and corticosteroids. *Ann Intern Med* **106**:209–216, 1987.
8. Copeland JG, Emery RW, Levinson MM, et al: Cyclosporine. an immunosuppressive panacea? *J Thorac Cardiovasc Surg* **91**:26–39, 1986.
9. Goldman MH, Barnhart G, Mohanakumar T, et al: Cyclosporine in cardiac transplantation *Surg Clin North Am* **65**:637–659, 1985.
10. Kahan BD. Cyclosporine: The agent and its actions *Transplant Proc* **17**(suppl 1):5–19, 1985.
11. Stinson EB, Bieber CP, Griepp RB, et al: Infectious complications after cardiac transplantation in man. *Ann Intern Med* **74**:22–36, 1971
12. Kirby BD, Snyder KM, Meyer RD, et al: Legionnaire's disease: report of sixty-five nosocomially acquired cases and review of the literature. *Medicine (Baltimore)* **59**:188–205, 1980.
13. Fuller J, Levinson MM, Kline JR, et al: Legionnaire's disease after heart transplantation. *Ann Thorac Surg* **39**:308–311, 1985
14. Burgos-Calderon R, Pankey GR, Figueroa JE: Infection in kidney transplantation. *Surgery* **70**:334–340, 1971
15. Moore TC, Hume DM: The period and nature of hazard in clinical renal transplantation: The hazard to patient survival *Ann Surg* **183**:266–270, 1976.
16. Schwiezer RT, Kountz SL, Belzer FO. Wound complications in recipients of renal transplants. *Ann Surg* **177**:58–62, 1973.
17. Diethelm AG: Surgical management of complications of steroid therapy *Ann Surg* **185**:251–263, 1977.
18. Remington JS, Gaines JD, Gripp RB, et al. Further experience with infection after cardiac transplantation. *Transplant Proc* **4**:699–705, 1972.
19. Montgomery JR, Barrett FF, Williams TW: Infectious complications in cardiac transplant patients *Transplant proc* **5**:1239–1243, 1973.
20. Pearl SN, Weiner MA, Dibbell DG. Sternal infection after cardiac transplantation. Successful salvage utilizing a variety of techniques *J Thorac Cardiovasc Surg* **83**:632–634, 1982.
21. Dummer JS, Bahnson HT, Griffith BP, et al: Infections in patients on cyclosporine and prednisone following cardiac

transplantation. *Transplant Proc* **15**(suppl 1, 2):2779–2781, 1983.

22. Kunin CM, McCormack PC: Prevention of catheter-induced urinary tract infections induced by sterile closed drainage *N Engl J Med* **274**:1155–1161, 1966.

23. Copeland DJ, Stinson EB: Human heart transplantation. *Curr Probl Cardiol* **3**:4–51, 1980.

24. Barret-Connor E: The non-value of sputum culture in the diagnosis of pneumococcal pneumonia *Am Rev Respir Dis* **103**:845–849, 1971.

25. Murray JR, Felton CP, Garaz SM: Pulmonary complications of the acquired immunodeficiency syndrome. *N Engl J Med* **310**:1682–1688, 1984.

26. Hedemark LL, Kroneberg RS, Rasp FL: The value of bronchoscopy in establishing the etiology of pneumonia in renal transplant recipients. *Am Rev Respir Tract* **126**:981–985, 1982

27. Palmer DL, Davidson M, Lusk R: Needle aspiration of the lung in complex pneumonia. *Chest* **78**:16–20, 1980.

28. Bandt PD, Blank N, Castellino RA: Needle diagnosis of pneumonitis, value in high risk patients. *JAMA* **220**:1578–1582, 1982.

29. Mammana RB, Peterson EA, Fuller JK, et al: Pulmonary infections in cardiac transplant patients: Modes of diagnosis, complications and effectiveness of therapy *Ann Thorac Surg* **36**:700–705, 1983.

30. Rand KH, Pollard RB, Merigan TC. Increased pulmonary superinfections in cardiac transplant patients undergoing primary cytomegalovirus infection *N Engl J Med* **298**:951–953, 1978

31. Pollard RB, Arvin AM, Gamberg P: Specific cell-mediated immunity and infections with herpes viruses in cardiac transplant recipients. *Am J Med* **73**:679–687, 1982.

33. Adler SP: Transfusion-associated cytomegalovirus infections. *Rev Infect Dis* **5**:977–933, 1983.

34. Dummer JS, White LT, Ho M, et al: Morbidity of cytomegalovirus infection in recipients of heart or heart–lung transplants who received cyclosporine. *J Infect Dis* **152**:1182–1191, 1985.

35. Pollard RB, Rand KH, Merigan TC: Cell-mediated immunity to cytomegalovirus infection in normal subjects and cardiac transplant patients. *J Infect Dis* **137**:541–549, 1978.

36. Ho M. *Cytomegalovirus, Biology and Infection.* Plenum, New York, 1982

37. Rubin RH, Tolkoff-Rubin NE: The problem of cytomegalovirus infection in transplantation. In Morris PJ, Tilney NL (eds): *Progress in Transplantation.* Vol. 1, Churchill Livingstone, Edinburgh, 1984, pp. 89–114.

38. Hersman J, Meyers JD, Thomas ED. The effect of granulocyte transfusions on the incidence of CMV infection after allogenic marrow transplantation. *Ann Intern Med* **96**:149–152, 1982.

39. Fiala M, Payne JE, Berne TV: Epidemiology of CMV infection after transplantation and immunosuppression. *J Infect Dis* **132**:421–433, 1975.

40. Betts RF, Freeman RB, Douglas RH Jr, et al: Transmission of cytomegalovirus infection with the renal allograft. *Kidney Int* **8**:385–392, 1975.

41. Ho M, Suwansirichal S, Dowling JN, et al: The transplanted

kidney as a source of cytomegalovirus infection. *N Engl J Med* **293**:1109–1112, 1975.

42. Preiksaitis JK, Rosno S, Grumet C, et al. Infections due to herpesvirus in cardiac transplant recipients. Role of the donor heart and immunosuppressive therapy. *J Infect Dis* **147**:974–981, 1983.

43. Rubin RH, Wilson EJ, Barrett LV, et al: Primary cytomegalovirus infection following cardiac transplantation in a murine model *Transplantation* **37**:306–310, 1984.

44. Wilson EJ, Medearis DN Jr, Barrett LV, et al. Activation of latent murine cytomegalovirus in cardiac explant and cell cultures. *J Infect Dis* **152**:625–626, 1985.

45. Shanley JD, Billingsley AM, Shelby J, et al: Transfer of immune cytomeglovirus by heart transplantation. *Transplantation* **36**:584–587, 1983.

46. Brunnez JH, Bruggeman CA, Van Boven CPA, et al: Passive transfer of cytomegalovirus by cardiac and renal organ transplants in a rat model. *Transplantation* **41**:605–698, 1986.

47. Wilson EJ, Medearis DN, Barrett LV, et al: The effects of donor pretreatment on the transmission of murine cytomegalovirus with cardiac transplants and explants. *Transplantation* **41**:781–782, 1986.

48. Chou S: Acquisition of donor strains by renal-transplant recipients. *N Engl J Med* **314**:1418–1423, 1986.

49. Grundy JE, Super M, Lui S, et al. The source of cytomegalovirus infection in seropositive renal allograft recipients is frequently the donor kidney. *Transplant Proc* **19**:2126–2128, 1987

50. Kemola E: Cytomegalovirus infection in previously healthy adults *Ann Intern Med* **79**:267–269, 1973

51. Simmons RL, Matas AJ, Rattazzi LC, et al: Clinical characteristics of lethal cytomegalovirus infection following renal transplantation. *Surgery* **82**:537–546, 1977.

52 Rubin RJ, Russell PS, Levin M, et al: Summary of workshop on cytomegalovirus infections during organ transplantation. *J Infect Dis* **139**:728–734, 1979.

53. Rubin RH, Cosimi AB, Tolkoff-Rubin NE, et al: Infectious disease syndromes attributable to cytomegalovirus and their significance among renal transplant patients. *Transplantation* **24**:458–464, 1977.

54. Ravin CE, Smith GW, Ahern MJ, et al: Cytomegaloviral infection presenting as a solitary pulmonary nodule. *Chest* **71**:220–222, 1977.

55. Hamed IA, Wenzl JE, Leonard JC, et al: Pulmonary cytomegalovirus infections: Detection by Gallium 67 imaging in the transplant patient. *Arch Intern Med* **139**:286–288, 1979.

56. Chatterje SN, Fiola M, Weiner J, et al: Primary cytomegalovirus and opportunistic infections: Incidence in renal transplant recipients. *JAMA* **240**:2446–2449, 1978.

57. Goodman ZD, Boitnoot JK, Yardley JH: Perforation of the colon associated with cytomegalovirus infection. *Am J Dig Dis* **24**:376–380, 1979.

58. Goodman MD, Porter DD: Cytomegalovirus vasculitis with fatal colonic hemorrhage. *Arch Pathol Lab Med* **96**:281–284, 1973.

59. Sutherland DER, Chan FY, Foucar E, et al: The bleeding

cecal ulcer in transplant patients. *Surgery* **86**:386–398, 1979.

60. Luby JP, Brunett W, Hull, AR, et al: Relationship between cytomegalovirus and hepatic function abnormalities in the period after renal transplant. *J Infect Dis* **129**:511–518, 1974.

61. Carrafax DM, Archer NL: Cyclosporin immunosuppression. *Clin Pharmacol* **2**:515–524, 1983.

62. Schober R, Herman MM: Neuropathology of cardiac transplantation: Survey of 32 cases. *Lancet* **1**:962–967, 1973.

63. Hotson JR, Pedley TA: The neurological complications of cardiac transplantation. *Brain* **99**:673–694, 1976.

64. Bale JF: Human CMV infection and disorders of the nervous system. *Arch Neurol* **41**:310–320, 1984.

65. Pollard Rb, Egbert PR, Gallagher JG, et al: Cytomegalovirus retinitis in the immunosuppressed host. *Ann Intern Med* **93**:655–664, 1980.

66. Holland GN, Gottlieb MS, Yu RD: Ocular disorders associated with a new acquired cellular immune deficiency syndrome. *Am J Ophthalmol* **93**:393–402, 1982.

67. Murray WH, Known DL, Green WR, et al: Cytomegalovirus retinitis in adults: A manifestation of disseminated viral infection. *Am J Med* **63**:574–584, 1977.

68. Minors N, Silverman JF, Escobar MR, et al. Fatal cytomegalovirus inclusion disease: Associated skin manifestations in a renal transplant patient *Arch Dermatol* **113**:1569–1571, 1977.

69. Rand KH, Rasmussen JE, Pollard RB, et al: Cellular immunity and herpesvirus infections in cardiac transplant patients. *N Engl J Med* **296**:1372–1377, 1977.

70. Craighead JE: Cytomegalovirus pulmonary disease. *Pathol Annu* **5**:197–229, 1975.

71. Carney WP, Rubin RH, Hoffman RA, et al. Analysis of T lymphocyte subsets in cytomegalovirus mononucleosis. *J Immunol* **126**:2114–2116, 1981.

72. Schooley RT, Hirsch MS, Colvin RB, et al: Association of herpes virus infection with T-lymphocyte-subset alterations, glomerulopathy and opportunistic infections after renal transplantation. *N Engl J Med* **308**:307–313, 1983.

73. Dummer JS, Ho M, Rabin B, et al: The effect of cytomegalovirus and Epstein–Barr virus infection on T lymphocyte subsets in cardiac transplant patients on cyclosporine. *Transplantation* **38**:433–435, 1984.

74. Maher P, O'Toole CM, Wreghitt TG, et al. Cytomegalovirus infection in cardiac transplant recipients associated with chronic T cell subset ratio inversion with expansion of a Leu-7+ TS-C+ subset. *Clin Exp Immunol* **62**:515–524, 1985.

75. O'Toole CM, Gray JJ, Maher P, et al: Persistent excretion of cytomegalovirus in heart transplant patients correlates to inversion of the ratio of T Helper/T suppressor-cytotoxic cells. *J Infect Dis* **153**:1160–1162, 1986

76. Wreghitt TG, Hakim M, Gray JJ, et al: A detailed study of CMV infections in the first 136 heart and heart/lung transplant recipients at Papworth Hospital. *Transplant Proc* **(in press.)**

77. Marker SC, Howard RJ, Groth KE, et al: A trial of vidarabine for cytomegalovirus in renal transplant patients *Arch Intern Med* **140**:1441–1444, 1980.

78. Bach MC, Bagwell SP, Knapp NP, et al 9-(1,3-dihydroxy-2-propoxymethyl)guanine for cytomegalvoris infections in patients with the acquired immunodeficiency syndrome. *Ann Intern Med* **103**:381–382, 1985

79 Shepp DH, Dandliker PS, de Miranda P, et al: Activity of 9-[2-hydroxy-1-(hydroxymethyl)ethoxymethyl]guanine in the treatment of cytomegalovirus pneumonia. *Ann Intern Med* **103**:368–373, 1985.

80 Collaborative DHPG Treatment Study Group. Treatment of serious cytomegalovirus infections with 9-(1,3-dihydroxy-2-propoxymethyl)guanine in patients with AIDS and other immunodeficiencies. *N Engl J Med* **314**:801–805, 1986

81. Ho M: Virus infections after transplantation in man, brief review. *Arch Virol* **55**:1–24, 1977.

82 Rubin RH, Tolkoff-Rubin NE. Viral infection in the renal transplant patient. *Proc Eur Dial Transplant Assoc* **19**:513–528, 1982

83. Whitley RJ, Soong S-J, Hirsch MS, et al: Herpes simplex encephalitis: Vidarabine therapy and diagnostic problems. *N Engl J Med* **304**:313–318, 1982.

84. Whitley RJ, Nahmias AJ, Soong S-J, et al Vidarabine therapy of neonatal herpes simplex virus infection *Pediatrics* **66**:495–500, 1980.

85. Mindel A, Adler MW, Sutherland S, et al: Intravenous acyclovir treatment for primary genital herpes. *Lancet* **1**:697–700, 1982.

86. Wade JC, Newton B, McLaren C, et al: Intravenous acyclovir to treat mucocutaneous herpes simplex virus infection after marrow transplantation. *Ann Intern Med* **96**:265–270, 1982

87 Cheeseman SH, Henle W, Rubin RH, et al Epstein–Barr virus infection in renal transplant recipients. Effects of antithymocyte globulin and interferon. *Ann Intern Med* **193**:39–44, 1980.

88. Spencer ES, Andersen HK. Clinically evident, non-terminal infections with herpesvirus and the wart virus in immunosuppressed renal allograft recipients. *Br Med J* **3**:251–254, 1970

89. Change RS, Lewis JP, Reynolds RD, et al: Oropharyngeal exception of Epstein–Barr virus by patients with lymphoproliferative disorders and by recipients of renal allografts. *Ann Intern Med* **88**:34–40, 1980.

90 Nagington J, Graz J: Cyclosporin-A immunosuppression, Epstein–Barr virus antibody and lymphoma *Lancet* **1**:536–537, 1980.

91. Grose C, Henle W, Horwitz MS. Primary Epstein–Barr virus infection in renal transplant recipients. *South Med J* **70**:1276–1278, 1977

92. Marker SC, Ascher NL, Kalis JM, et al· Epstein–Barr virus antibody responses and clinical illness in renal transplant recipients. *Surgery* **85**:433–440, 1979.

93 Purtilo DR: Epstein–Barr virus-induced oncogenesis in immune-deficient individuals. *Lancet* **1**:300–303, 1980.

94. Saemundsen AK, Berkel AL, Henle W, et al: Epstein–Barr virus causing lymphoma in a patient with ataxia–telangectasia. *Br Med J* **282**:425–427, 1981.

95 Hanto SW, Frizzera G, Purtilo DT, et al. Clinical spectrum of lymphoproliferative disorder in renal transplant recipients

and evidence for the role of Epstein–Barr virus. *Cancer Res* **41**:4253–4261, 1981.

96. Hanto DW, Frizzera G, Gajl-Peczalska RJ, et al: Epstein–Barr virus induced B-cell lymphoma after renal transplantation: Acyclovir therapy and transition from polyclonal to monoclonal B-cell transformation *N Engl J Med* **306**:913–918, 1982

97. Thiru S, Calne RY, Nagington J: Lymphoma in renal allograft patients treated with cyclosporin-A as one of the immunosuppressive agents *Transplant Proc* **13**:359–364, 1981.

98. Crawford DH, Thomas JA, Janossy F, et al: Epstein–Barr virus nuclear antigen positive lymphoma after cyclosporine-A treatment in patients with renal allograft. *Lancet* **1**:1355–1256, 1980

99. Dummer JS, Bound LM, Singh G, et al: Epstein–Barr virus-induced lymphoma in a cardiac transplant recipient. *Am J Med* **77**:179–184, 1984

100. Starzl TE, Porter KA, Iwatsuki S, et al: Reversibility of lymphomas and lymphoproliferative lesions developing under cyclosporin-steroid therapy *Lancet* **1**:583–587, 1984

101. Gallagher JG, Merigan TC: Prolonged herpes-zoster infection associated with immunosuppressive therapy. *Ann Intern Med* **91**:842–846, 1979.

102. Whitley RJ, Soong S-J, Dolin R, et al: Early vidarabine therapy to control the complications of herpes zoster in immunosuppressed patients. *N Engl J Med* **307**:971–974, 1982.

103. Balfour HH, Bean B, Laskin O, et al: Acyclovir halts progression of herpes zoster in immunocompromised patients. *N Engl J Med* **308**:1448–1451, 1983

104. Merigan TC, Rand KH, Pollard RB, et al: Human leukocyte interferon for the treatment of herpes zoster in patients with cancer. *N Engl J Med* **298**:981–985, 1978.

105. Rosen PP, Martini N, Armstrong D: *Pneumocystis carinii* pneumonia: diagnosis by lung biopsy. *Am J Med* **8**:794–805, 1975.

106. Hodgkin JE, Anderson HA, Rosenow EC. Diagnosis of *Pneumocystis carinii* pneumonia by transbronchoscopic lung biopsy *Chest* **64**:551–556, 1973.

107. Gentry LO, Ruskin J, Remington JS *Pneumocystis carinii* pneumonia Problems in diagnosis and therapy in 24 cases. *Calif Med* **116**:6–12, 1972

108. Coleman DL, Dodek PM, Luce JM, et al: Diagnostic utility of fiberoptic bronchoscopy in patients with *Pneumocystis carinii* pneumonia and the acquired acquired immune deficiency syndrome *Am Rev Respir Dis* **128**:795–802, 1983

109. Walzer PD, Perl DP, Krogstad DJ, et al. *Pneumocystis carinii* pneumonia in the United States *Ann Intern Med* **80**:83–90, 1974

110. Hughes WT, McNabb PC, Makres TD, et al. Efficacy of trimethoprim and sulfamethoxazole in the prevention and treatment of *Pneumocystis carinii* pneumonia *Antimicrob Agent Chemother* **5**:289–293, 1974

111. Hughes WT, Feldman S, Chaudkary S. Comparison of trimethoprim–sulfamethoxazole and pentamidine in the treatment of *Pneumocystis carinii* pneumonia. *Pediatr Res* **10**:399A–407A, 1976

112. Mayaud C, Carette MF, Dournon E, et al. Clinical features and prognosis of severe pneumonia caused by *Legionella pneumophila*. In Thornsberry C, Balow A, Felley JS, Jakubowski W (eds): *Legionella. Proceedings of the Second International Symposium.* American Society for Microbiology, Washington, DC, 1984, pp. 11–12.

113. Copeland W, Wieden M, Feinberg W, et al. Legionnaires disease following cardiac transplantation. *Chest* **79**:669–671, 1981.

114. Carrington CB: Pathology of Legionnaires' disease. *Ann Intern Med* **90**:496–499, 1979.

115. Beaty HN: Clinical features of Legionellosis. In Thornsberry C, Balows A, Feeley JS, Jakubowski W (eds): *Legionella Proceedings of the Second International Symposium.* American Society for Microbiology, Washington, DC, 1984, pp. 6–10.

116 Broome CV, Chenz WB, Winn WC Jr, et al: Rapid diagnosis of Legionnaires' disease by direct immunofluorescent staining. *Ann Intern Med* **90**:1–4, 1979

117. Edelstein PH, Meyer RD, Feingold SM: Laboratory diagnosis of Legionnaires' disease. *Am Rev Respir Dis* **121**:317–322, 1980.

118. Edelstein PH: Laboratory diagnosis of Legionnaires' disease In Thornsberry C, Balows A, Feeley JC, Jakubowski W (eds): *Legionella: Proceedings of the Second International Symposium.* American Society of Microbiology, Washington, DC 1984, pp. 3–5.

119 Miller AC: Erythromycin in Legionnaires' disease: A reappraisal. *J Antimicrob Chemother* **7**:217–220, 1981.

120. Naot Y, Brown A, Elder EM, et al: IgM and IgG antibody response in two immunosuppressed patients with Legionnaires' disease. Evidence of reactivation of latent infection. *Am J Med* **73**:791–794, 1982.

121. Brewer JH, Parrott CL, Rimland D: Disseminated coccidioidomycosis in a heart transplant recipient. *Sabouraudia* **20**:261–265, 1982

122. King RW Jr, Kraikitpanitch S, Lindeman RD: Subcutaneous nodules caused by *Histoplasma capsulatum. Ann Intern Med* **86**:586–587, 1977.

123. Kauffman CA, Israel KS, Smith JW, et al: Histoplasmosis in immunosuppressed patients. *Am J Med* **64**:923–932, 1978.

124. Davies SF, Khan M, Sarosi GA. Disseminated histoplasmosis in immunologically suppressed patients. *Am J Med* **64**:94–100, 1978.

125. Davies SF, Sarosi GA, Peterson PK, et al: Disseminated histoplasmosis in renal transplant recipients. *Am J Surg* **137**:687–691, 1979.

126. Deresinski SC, Stevens DA: Coccidioidomycosis in compromised hosts. *Medicine (Baltimore)* **54**:377–395, 1975.

127. Bayer AS, Yoshikawa TT, Galpin JE, et al: Unusual syndromes of coccidioidomycosis. Diagnostic and therapeutic considerations. *Medicine (Baltimore)* **55**:131–152, 1976.

128. Schroter GPJ, Bakshandeh K, Husberg BS, et al: Coccidioidomycosis and renal transplantation. *Transplantation* **23**:485–489, 1977.

129 Gallis HA, Berman RA, Cate TR, et al. Fungal infection following renal transplantation. *Arch Intern Med* **135**:1163–1172, 1975.

130. Hooper DL, Pruitt A, Rubin RH: Central nervous system

infections in the chronically immunosuppressed. *Medicine (Baltimore)* **61**:166–188, 1982.

131. Ramsey PG, Rubin RH, Tolkoff-Rubin NE, et al The renal transplant patient with fever and pulmonary infiltrates: Etiology, clinical manifestations, and management *Medicine (Baltimore)* **59**:206–222, 1980.

132. Lopez-Bernstein G, Fainstein V, Hopfer R, et al. Liposomal amphotericin B for the treatment of systemic fungal infections in patients with cancer: A preliminary study. *J Infect Dis* **151**(4):704–710, 1985.

133. Martin DH, Counts GW, Thomas ED: Fungal infections in human bone marrow transplant recipients. Abstract #406. In *Seventeenth Interscience Conference of Antimicrobial Agents and Chemotherapy*. American Society for Microbiology, New York, 1977.

134. Schroter GPJ, Temple DR, Husberg BS, et al: Crypococcosis after renal transplantation: report of ten cases. *Surgery* **79**:268–277, 1976.

135. Mead JH, Lupton GP, Dillarou CL, et al: Cutaneous rhizopus infection: Occurrence as a postoperative complication associated with an elasticized adhesive dressing. *JAMA* **242**:272–274, 1979.

136. Krick JA, Stinson EB, Remington JS: Nocardia infection in heart transplant patients. *Ann Intern Med* **82**:18–26, 1975

137. Simpson GL, Stinson EB, Egger MJ, et al. Nocardial infection in the immunocompromised host: A detailed study in a defined population. *Rev Infect Dis* **3**:492–507, 1981.

138. Palmer DL: Diagnostic and therapeutic considerations in *Nocardia asteroides* infection. *Medicine (Baltimore)* **53**:391–401, 1974

139. Benman BL, Burnside J, Edwards B, et al: *Nocardia* infection in United States, 1972–1974 *J Infect Dis* **134**:286–289, 1976

140. Simpson GL, Raffin TA, Remingston JS: Association of prior nocardiosis and subsequent occurrence of nontuberculous mycobacteriosis in a defined, immunosuppressed population. *J Infect Dis* **146**:211–219, 1982.

141. Petersen EA, Nash ML, Mammana RB, Copeland JG. Minocycline treatment of pulmonary nocardiosis. *JAMA* **250**:930–932, 1983.

142. Modry DL, Stinson EB, Oyer PE, et al: Acute rejection and massive cyclosporine requirements in heart transplant recipients treated with rifampin. *Transplantation* **39**:313–314, 1985.

143. Ryning FW, McLeod R, Maddox JC, et al: Probable transmission of *Toxoplasma gondii* by organ transplantation. *Ann Intern Med* **90**:47–49, 1979

144 Luft BJ, Naot Y, Araujo FG, et al: Primary and reactivated Toxoplasma infection in patients with cardiac transplants *Ann Intern Med* **99**:27–31, 1983

145 Rose AG, Uyus CJ, Novitsky D, et al: Toxoplasmosis of donor and recipient hearts after heterotopic cardiac transplantation. *Arch Pathol Lab Med* **107**:868–873, 1983

146. McGregor CG, Fleck DG, Nagington J, et al: Disseminated toxoplasmosis in cardiac transplantation. *J Clin Pathol* **37**:74–77, 1984.

147. Nagington J, Martin AL· Toxoplasmosis and heart transplantation. *Lancet* **2**:679, 1983

148. Hakim M, Esmore D, Wallwork J, English TAH: Toxoplasmosis in cardiac transplantation *Br Med J* **292**:1108, 1986.

149. Britt RH, Enzmann DR, Remington JS: Intracranial infection in cardiac transplant recipients. *Ann Neurol* **9**:107–119, 1981.

150 Luft BJ, Billingham M, Remington JS. Endomyocardial biopsy in the diagnosis of toxoplasmic myocarditis *Transplant Proc* **18**:1871–1873, 1986.

151. Steed DL, Brown B, Reilly JJ, et al: General surgical complications in heart and heart–lung transplantation *Surgery* **98**:739–745, 1985.

152 Brooks RG, Hofflin JM, Jamieson SW, et al: Infectious complications in heart–lung transplant recipients. *Am J Med* **79**:412–422, 1985.

153. Dummer JS, Montero CG, Griffith BP, et al: Infections in heart-lung transplant recipients. *Transplantation* **41**:725–729, 1986.

154. Yousem SA, Burke CM, Billingham ME. Pathologic pulmonary alterations in long-term human heart–lung transplantation. *Hum Pathol* **16**:911–923, 1985.

23

Surgical Aspects of Infection in the Compromised Host

A. BENEDICT COSIMI

1. Introduction

Steadily increasing numbers of patients with compromised immune responsiveness are being encountered in current surgical practice. The spectrum of these patients (Table 1) ranges from those with severely impaired host resistance, such as acquired immunodeficiency syndrome (AIDS) victims or immunosuppressed transplant recipients, to those with more subtle defects, as occur in diabetics and the elderly. These patients should be expected to respond to inflammation and surgical stress quite differently from normal individuals. Thus, it is not unusual to encounter as great as a 12-fold increase in postoperative sepsis and mortality[1] in patients whose acute condition is complicated by factors that diminish host defense. The surgeon called upon to evaluate a problem requiring possible surgical intervention in such patients must be aware of the special considerations which have been found to greatly influence their prognosis. Successful operative intervention is usually not possible following the solo approach typically employed for acute focal or traumatic conditions. Close collaboration and planning with the internist, infectious disease consultant, and anesthetist are essential. This chapter presents a number of other guidelines found helpful in the diagnostic approach, preoperative preparation, intraoperative techniques, and postoperative management of infection in the compromised host, illustrated by a review of typically encountered cases.

2. Diagnostic Approach

Since impaired immune responsiveness not only provides the soil for atypical infectious conditions but also masks the commonly expected signs and symptoms of the inflammatory process (Table 2), an unusually aggressive diagnostic approach must be pursued in these patients. Their outcome is almost entirely dependent on the rapidity with which the correct diagnosis is established and specific therapy is instituted. In our experience with pulmonary infections in renal transplant recipients, for example, the overall mortality of patients diagnosed in the first 5 days of illness was 21%, as opposed to 65% for those whose diagnosis was not clarified until after 5 days of illness.[2] Similar experience recorded by others has generally led to the impression that pulmonary infection in the immunocompromised patient is the most frequently fatal of the infectious complications. In large part, this reflects the fact that the specific diagnosis is commonly not made until postmortem examination.

2.1. Pneumonia in the Immunocompromised Host

Illustrative Cases 1 and 2

A 42-year-old allograft recipient (Case 1) was admitted with pneumonitis. Following renal transplantation 12 years earlier, he

A. BENEDICT COSIMI • Department of Surgery, Massachusetts General Hospital, Boston, Massachusetts 02114.

TABLE 1. Causes of Impaired Host Resistance

Patient's Underlying Condition
   AIDS
   Neoplasia
   Malnutrition
   Acute stress (burns, trauma)
   Metabolic illness (diabetes, uremia)
   Aging

Iatrogenic
   Antineoplastic chemotherapy
   Immunosuppression (allograft recipients,
      autoimmune disorders)

was initially treated with azathioprine and prednisone. Five years before this admission, cyclophosphamide had been substituted for azathioprine because hepatic dysfunction had developed. The patient remained stable until 1 month before entry, when cough, low-grade fever, and malaise were first noted. Chest radiography showed only linear scarring at the bases. Because of a presumptive diagnosis of viral upper respiratory infection, probably complicating cyclophosphamide-induced fibrosis, azathioprine therapy was reinstituted. When dyspnea continued to worsen, he was referred here for admission. At this time, he appeared acutely ill with fever and severe hypoxemia while breathing room air. Chest radiography showed bilateral hilar infiltrates consistent with fluid overload. Intensive diuresis only marginally improved the respiratory function. Smears and cultures remained nondiagnostic. On the second hospital day, open lung biopsy established the diagnosis of *Pneumocystis carinii* pneumonia, which, despite appropriate therapy, led to the patient's demise.

A 60-year-old woman (Case 2) had been treated for 5 months with cyclophosphamide, methotrexate, and 5-fluorouracil (5-Fu) for stage II breast cancer. She was now admitted with fever and respiratory distress of several days' duration. Chest radiography showed a focal consolidation in the right lung. When the transtracheal sputum aspirate yielded *Streptococcus pneumoniae*, ampicillin and gentamicin therapy were begun. Successive radiographs showed progressive involvement of both lung fields. Further sputum cultures were not helpful. Despite the addition of

TABLE 2. Impaired Host Resistance: Consequences Affecting Surgical Management

Ineffective inflammatory reaction
Unusual presentation of common conditions
Unusual infectious problems
Increased tissue fragility
Impaired wound healing
Side effects of drug therapy for underlying condition (e.g., leukopenia, hyperglycemia)

erythromycin and trimethoprim–sulfamethoxazole her symptoms worsened, requiring tracheal intubation for assisted ventilation. An open lung biopsy then revealed drug-induced pneumonitis with no evidence of significant infection. Following the addition of steroid therapy, the patient's condition rapidly improved, and she was discharged on a different adjuvant chemotherapy regimen for her breast cancer.

Comment. These cases emphasize the nature of the challenge the physician faces when assessing pulmonary infiltrates in an immunosuppressed patient. The differential diagnosis must include not only the usual bacterial or viral pathogens but also noninfectious causes, such as drug-induced pneumonitis[3] or pulmonary emboli[4] and, most importantly, invasion by opportunistic agents such as *Pneumocystis*, *Nocardia*, and *Legionella*. The role of the surgeon in this assessment is to provide, as efficiently and safely as possible, appropriate secretions or tissues for study. Although empirical therapy is often begun immediately in these critically ill patients, one must simultaneously proceed to establish the definitive diagnosis before, as in Case 1, the potentially treatable process has become irreversible. Our first approach is transtracheal aspiration since expectorated specimens almost invariably are nondiagnostic. If aspiration is unproductive, a number of invasive techniques, including aspiration lung biopsy, bronchoscopy with brushing or transbronchial biopsy, and thoracoscopic or open lung biopsy, are available. We favor early open lung biopsy, since the ample tissue obtained almost always provides the diagnosis, whereas the "less invasive" procedures not infrequently result in disappointing delays because an inadequate specimen was taken. Although some investigators continue to question the impact of lung biopsy in the management of these patients,[5] many have concluded it is essential for early specific treatment.[6-8] We have found that the procedure can be accomplished with relatively few complications using a limited intercostal incision through which the involved lung tissue can be identified. The most obviously abnormal area is isolated using noncrushing clamps. After the wedge biopsy is obtained, the incised lung can be oversewn while the clamps maintain complete control of bleeding and air leakage. Despite postoperative mechanical ventilation, bronchopleural fistula formation has not been a problem. Similar results can also be achieved using the automatic stapler for lung repair.

2.2. Colonic Complications of the Immunosuppressed State

Illustrative Case 3

A 61-year-old man was treated with azathioprine and prednisone after receiving a renal allograft from his daughter. With the onset of acute rejection 9 days after transplantation, the steroid dosage was sharply increased, and local graft irradiation was instituted. Renal function gradually improved, and tapering of the steroid dosage was begun. Six weeks after the transplant, the patient was discharged to a neighboring state with normal renal function while receiving azathioprine 125 mg/day and prednisone 40 mg/day. One week later, he complained of lower abdominal discomfort. He was evaluated at his community hospital, where a temperature of 101°F (38°C) was noted and the abdomen was described as slightly distended with moderate direct and rebound tenderness. Laboratory evaluation revealed a white blood cell (WBC) count of 11,500/mm³, hematocrit (Hct) of 33%, and no abnoramlities of hepatic or renal function. Surgical consultation recommended abdominal radiographs. Since these were normal and the patient had remained clinically stable, admission and simple observation were advised. During the succeeding hours, the patient complained of increasing abdominal distention and discomfort. By 12 hr after admission, he had developed oliguria, hypotension, and restlessness consistent with gram-negative septicemia. When emergency laparotomy was finally performed, diffuse fecal peritonitis secondary to perforated sigmoid diverticulitis was found. Despite resection of the involved bowel with construction of an end-colostomy, extensive irrigation and drainage of the abdomen, and intensive postoperative supportive measures, the patient expired 48 hr later.

Illustrative Case 4

A 58-year-old woman with severe asthma and coronary artery disease reported the development of diarrhea over a 3–4-hr interval followed by lower abdominal discomfort precipitating, in addition, typical angina symptoms She had been treated intermittently with steroids over the past year for her asthma and currently was receiving prednisone 40 mg/day. Evaluation revealed her to be afebrile, in moderate distress from the angina, but otherwise stable except for definite lower abdominal direct and rebound tenderness. Hematologic and serum chemistry studies revealed only mild leukocytosis. Plain radiographs and ultrasound examination of the abdomen were not remarkable. Paracentesis produced several milliliters of thin, yellow fluid containing sheets of neutrophils on microscopic examination.

Emergency laparotomy confirmed the preoperative diagnosis of perforated sigmoid colon which was treated by resection and end-sigmoid colostomy. Postoperatively, the patient recovered without incident. The colostomy was successfully closed as a subsequent procedure.

Comment. Since the possible occult sites of acute inflammatory processes in the abdomen or retroperitoneum are numerous, accurate evaluation in this situation is perplexing Furthermore, because of the host's impaired response, typical findings of pain, abdominal tenderness and muscle splinting may be deceptively mild In these compromised patients, active bowel sounds with continuing bowel movements are not unusual, despite extensive peritoneal soilage. The impairment of the inflammatory response, unfortunately, also results in an inability to wall off the pathologic process so that irreversible disseminated sepsis may develop during even brief periods of hopeful observation. Most reports of colonic perforation in steroid-treated or uremic patients emphasize the paucity of symptoms, signs, and laboratory evidence of visceral perforation, leading to fatal delays in treatment or to incorrect preoperative diagnosis in almost all cases [9,10] This complication has been reported so frequently that some authorities suggest that there is a direct adverse effect of steroids on normal colon Certainly, inhibition of the normal inflammatory response, antifibroblastic activity, and atrophy of lymphoid elements of the bowel wall could interfere with normal barriers to invasive infection by intraluminal bacteria Thus, perforation may occur whether the colon was previously diseased or not and, indeed, has been documented in apparently normal areas of the bowel.[11] This, plus the inability to adequately localize the process, results in extensive contamination. Early clinical recognition of this problem, therefore, is essential, and perforation of the colon should always be a prime suspect in any steroid-treated patient with fever and abdominal symptoms. Paracentesis has been particularly helpful in this diagnosis, often yielding purulent fluid despite absence of free air on plain radiographs. If the diagnosis remains in doubt, contrast radiographic studies of the gastrointestinal (GI) tract should not be delayed despite fear of peritoneal soilage In general, a water-soluble contrast agent is preferred, but establishment of the diagnosis of perforated colon with barium enema has been reported without the serious complication of barium peritonitis In fact, the unusual occurrence of free flow of barium into the peritoneal cavity even in the presence of perforated bowel has been documented,[12] although this must remain a concern in these fragile patients who are unable to wall off perforations adequately.

Another bowel complication being encountered with increasing frequency in the immunosuppressed patient is intestinal infarction and perforation unrelated to major vascular occlusion.

Illustrative Case 5

A 57-year-old man received a cadaver-donor renal allograft in the right iliac fossa, after which he was treated with azathioprine, prednisone, and antithymocyte globulin. He was continued on hemodialysis during a period of resolving acute tubular necrosis but otherwise remained stable until the eighth posttransplant day when guaiac-positive stools were noted Left-sided abdominal pain and tenderness and passage of small amounts of grossly bloody stool occurred 24 hr later. Plain radiographs of the abdomen were unremarkable. Sigmoidoscopy revealed pale rectal mucosa up to 18 cm, where the mucosa became edematous, bloody, and ulcerated, and beyond which passage of the sigmoidoscope was impossible. Biopsy revealed only severe inflammation. Barium enema revealed an area of narrowing in the distal sigmoid colon with irregularity and probable shallow ulcerations without perforation. Because of the increasing tenderness and development of hyperkalemia, exploratory laparotomy was performed. The left colon was severely ischemic with multiple areas of infarction despite pulsatile mesenteric vessels along the entire segment of involved bowel. A left colectomy with end-transverse colostomy and a distal mucous fistula were performed Pathology of the resected specimen revealed prominent edema of all layers of the bowel with a diffuse, inflammatory infiltrate, extensive mucosal loss, and several areas of full-thickness infarction.

Postoperatively, the patient's immunosuppressive therapy was discontinued He did well initially, although hyperkalemia necessitated daily hemodialysis Renal scan showed good perfusion but poor function of the allograft. Several days after surgery, while being dialyzed, the patient developed ventricular tachycardia progressing to cardiac standstill from which he could not be resuscitated

Comment. Bowel infarction and perforation in the immunosuppressed host may occur without major vessel obstruction. Various etiological mechanisms have been suggested including steroid-induced vasculitis or connective tissue alterations which reduce mucosal resistance to bacteria.[13] Similar lesions, however, have been described in leukemic patients receiving chemotherapy, not including steroids,[14] as well as in trauma victims who have suffered periods of hypotension.[15]

Undoubtedly, numerous factors, including host immunoincompetence, postoperative blood volume changes, hypotension, marginally adequate blood supply secondary to atherosclerotic disease, uremia, and possibly the use of ion-exchange resin enemas for hyperkalemia,[16] are operative with differing degrees of importance in any individual. The common denominator in all reports, however, is that delay in establishing the diagnosis in the compromised host almost invariably leads to a fatal outcome. In some patients, the acute symptomatology was preceded by reasonably prolonged periods of vague abdominal distress, malaise, and low-grade fevers. The surgeon should proceed with evaluation on the premise that colon pathology is presumed present unless proved otherwise in immunosuppressed individuals. Confirmatory signs, such as guaiac-positive or bloody stool, demand immediate sigmoidoscopic examination which may reveal pale or cyanotic mucosa or areas of edema and ulceration. Barium enema in the early, less severe stages may show only "thumbprinting" secondary to hemorrhage into the bowel wall. This may progress to narrowing of the lumen and pseudopolypoid filling defects, indicating mucosal necrosis, and finally to perforation as total bowel wall infarction ensues. Obviously, hope of salvaging these patients is dependent on definitive surgical therapy during the early, more difficult to diagnose stages.

2.3. Occult Intraabdominal Sources of Fever and Infection

In patients with occult fever but no incidence of an acute intraabdominal catastrophe, the search for a surgically drainable collection often requires more sophisticated studies.

Illustrative Case 6

An 18-year-old patient with end-stage renal disease was being supported with hemodialysis while awaiting renal transplantation when he began having intermittent fevers in the range of 100.4–101.2°F (38°–29°C). Five years earlier, he had undergone a right nephrectomy after several unsuccessful attempts to reconstruct a congenitally deformed drainage system. Renal function of the successfully reconstructed left kidney provided a marginal creatinine clearance, adequate to delay the need for dialysis during the succeeding 4½ years. With the onset of the febrile course, there was occasional right-sided abdominal distress but no significant GI symptoms. Barium enema and ultrasonography suggested a mass effect in the right lower quadrant. The patient was taken to surgery with a preoperative diagnosis of periappendiceal abscess. At laparotomy, a walled-off 200-ml collection of thick, white, purulent fluid that subsequently cultured *Staphlococcus aureus* was drained from the retroperitoneal site of the previous nephrectomy. A normal intraperitoneal appendix was removed as well. The postoperative and subsequent postransplant course was benign

Comment. Noninvasive contrast studies, ultrasonography, and computerized body tomography (CT) are frequently required in the preoperative assessment of immunocompromised hosts with occult fevers. Scanning with radioactive isotopes may be helpful in defining abscesses of the upper abdomen as perfusion defects or "cold areas" on simultaneous liver–lung or liver–spleen studies. For the remainder of the abdomen, some authorities have recommended the use of ^{67}Ga citrate scanning, but this has not proved useful in our experience. Most current reports favor ultrasound or CT-guided percutaneous aspiration of collections as more helpful.[17] Ultimately, however, exploratory laparotomy may be required as the definitive diagnostic maneuver.

Previous, apparently healed incisions should always be regarded with a high index of suspicion in an immunosuppressed patient. Hidden infections may be demonstrated months or even years after apparent uncomplicated healing. Needle aspiration or ultrasonography of any area of tenderness, erythema, or questionable fluctuance is often successful in revealing unbelievably extensive underlying collections

Obviously, an awareness of the likelihood of certain specific infectious complications will also aid in the surgical evaluation. As noted, wound infections and colonic complications are seen regularly in the immunocompromised host. Another common but frequently overlooked condition is the occult perianal abscess which should always be carefully sought—particularly in neutropenic patients.

Interestingly, appendicitis seems to be nearer the opposite extreme of frequency in immunosuppressed hosts except perhaps for children receiving chemotherapy for leukemia. In that group, abdominal pain and fever are usually considered sufficient findings to justify immediate laparotomy and appendectomy. In contrast, appendicitis is a rather unusual complication in transplant recipients, possibly as a result of lymphoid atrophy in the bowel wall making obstruction and inflammation of the appendix unlikely.

Acute pancreatitis, although its etiology remains obscure, unfortunately is not unusual in immunosuppressed patients.

Illustrative Case 7

The patient had received a renal allograft 4 months previously. Excellent allograft function had been maintained with an immunosuppressive regimen including cyclosporine (500 mg/day)

and prednisone (15 mg/day) The patient was admitted with complaints of adbominal pain, "bloating", and fever. He was found to have a serum amylase level of 350 Russel units ($N = 4-25$). With intravenous alimentation and conservative therapy, the symptoms resolved but the amylase level fell only to the 60–70 range. Ultrasound and CT studies identified no abscess cavities but suggested persistent edema of the tail of the pancreas. With each attempt to resume oral alimentation, recurrent pain and low-grade fever developed. Exploratory laparotomy revealed an edematous pancreas with multiple abscesses in the tail. Distal pancreatectomy provided complete relief of symptoms.

Four months later, the patient returned with similar findings while being maintained on cyclosporine and prednisone. Ultimately, subtotal pancreatectomy was performed, again revealing multiple small abscesses in the gland. Following this, he has remained asymptomatic for 1 year.

Comment. In one autopsy study of 54 steroid-treated patients, acute focal pancreatitis was found in 28.5% of the subjects as compared with 3 7% of matched but non-steroid-treated controls.[18] In allograft recipients, the incidence of clinically significant pancreatitis has been reported to be as high as 6%.[19] The mechanism whereby steroids could produce pancreatitis may be ductal ectasia and epithelial metaplasia, which favor obstruction. Perhaps of more significance is the fact that many of these patients have coincident severe infection, often of viral etiology. This may be the important underlying factor, with even direct viral infection of the pancreas being a possibility. Azathioprine has also been implicated as an etiologic agent for pancreatitis,[20] indicating the probable multifactorial origin. The mortality in these patients can be as high as 70%. The major factors responsible for this high mortality are the considerable delay in establishing the diagnosis and the unusually high incidence of postpancreatitis complications such as pseudocyst and abscess formation. In this case, the multiple pancreatic abscesses remained undetected for some time despite numerous radiographic studies Fortunately, the process remained localized (presumably the consequence of the much lower dosages of steroids currently used for allograft recipients) and could be managed by resection on both occasions.

As in colonic perforation, the surgeon is therefore presented with the demanding role of providing early clinical recognition of the condition followed by direction of the necessarily aggressive management, which includes nasogastric suction; fluid, electrolyte, and caloric replacement, and further steroid reduction. Most importantly, prompt detection and appropriate, possibly repeated, drainage of developing collections is essential.

3. Preoperative Preparation

Once the need for surgery in an immunoincompetent patient has been established, the degree to which preoperative preparation can be extended is determined primarily by the nature and urgency of the surgical indication. Usual preoperative resuscitative measures including volume replacement, institution of antibiotic therapy, and correction of electrolyte imbalances, follow the same guidelines employed for any acute surgical state. If the surgical indication is less urgent, a preoperative attempt to begin restoration of immunocompetence toward normal may also be possible. Withdrawal of cytotoxic chemotherapy or high-dosage steroids will permit some recovery of depressed bone marrow and host-defense function and should reduce the risks of superinfection in the postoperative period. In addition, certain conditions unique to these patients must be considered.

3.1. Infection and Adrenal Insufficiency

Illustrative Case 8

A 27-year-old woman had been treated for several years with various immunosuppressive regimens, including steroids, cyclophosphamide, and azathioprine for an ill-defined vasculitis characterized by diabetes, blindness, and impaired renal function Because of the need for frequent venipunctures and hemodialysis, a saphenous vein-to-femoral artery A/V fistula had been constructed for vascular access 6 months previously. The current admission followed the development of fever, chills, and pain in the area of the A–V fistula. On examination, she was found to be obtunded but arousable, temperature was 104.9°F (40.5°C); and blood pressure, which was typically elevated, was found to be 9%o. The soft tissues around the A–V fistula were erythematous and edematous, with a 3×5 cm tender fluctuant mass beneath the site of a recent venipuncture. The patient was begun on antibiotics and intravenous volume replacement. Under local anesthesia, the fluctuant mass was drained of 75 ml purulent fluid containing numerous neutrophils and gram-negative bacteria Despite these measures, she remained obtunded, febrile, and hypotensive, requiring vasopressor and massive fluid support. The diagnosis of relative adrenal insufficiency was eventually suggested. Increased doses of steroids were administered, resulting in satisfactory stabilization of the vital signs, defervescence, and improved mental function. The patient was continued on intravenous antibiotics and local wound care. Over the succeeding 2 weeks, there was complete resolution of the local infection, and the patient was discharged for continuing outpatient hemodialysis

Comment. Of the many side effects of steroid therapy (Table 3), one of the unique conditions to keep in mind is the likelihood of occult adrenal insufficiency during periods of acute stress.[21] In fact, if the patient has received pharmacologic doses of steroids at any time within the previous 6-month period, it should be assumed acute adrenal failure will occur in the face of severe stress. A hypotensive febrile crisis often associated with a variety of central nervous system (CNS) symptoms ranging from obtundation to mania may be rapidly reversed by administration of a single intravenous hydrocortisone bolus. However, the surgeon should avoid this crisis by advising preoperative and intraoperative steroid (hydrocortisone, 50–100 mg) supplementation, with maintenance doses continuing into the postoperative period. A typical schedule might be hydrocortisone, 100 mg every 8h the day of surgery, 50

TABLE 3. Major Side Effects and Complications of Steroid Therapy

Side effects	Complications
Decreased phagocytosis	
Hyperglycemia	Susceptibility to infection
Decreased inflammatory response	Poor wound healing
Lymphopenia	
Capillary fragility	Breakdown of normal barriers
Dermatologic changes	Poor healing
Decreased musocal resistance	Peptic ulceration
? Local vasculitis	Pancreatitis
	Colonic ulceration
Catabolic effects	Myopathy
? Local vasculitis	Osteoporosis
Occult adrenal insufficiency	Hypotension, fever

mg every 8h the following day, and 25 mg every 8h the third day. By this time, resumption of the preoperative maintenance dosage should be adequate, provided continuing severe stress is not present.

3.2. Infection and Ketoacidosis

In addition to the acute infection, the immunocompromised patient's underlying condition must also be considered and appropriately managed.

Illustrative Case 9

A 59-year-old diabetic patient had undergone successful renal transplantation for end-stage diabetic nephropathy, 3 years previously He was admitted at the present time with fever and shaking chills of 2 days' duration and abdominal pain and vomiting for one day. Prior to these symptoms, he had been in good health with normal renal function while receiving maintenance dosages of cyclosporine and prednisone.

On examination, he was found to be severely ill with a temperature of 103°F (39.5°C), pulse rate of 133 beats/min, respiratory rate of 30 respirations/min, and blood pressure of 85/60. The renal allograft was not enlarged but was slightly tender and the abdomen was moderately distended with direct and rebound tenderness, particularly in the epigastrium. Bowel sounds were hypoactive The hematocrit was 43%, and the WBC 17,600/mm^3 Urinalysis revealed many white and red cells and gram-negative bacteria Significant chemical abnormalities included a blood sugar of 595 mg/dl and CO_2 content of 14 mEq/liter. Abdominal and chest radiographs revealed only a distended stomach without evidence of free air

The admitting diagnosis was gram-negative septicemia with consequent diabetic ketoacidosis Although the ultrasound showed no stones, the source of infection was presumed to be acute, possibly gangrenous, cholecystitis. Urinary tract infection was also diagnosed. In preparation for proposed emergency laparotomy, intravenous antibiotics, rehydration, and insulin therapy were instituted. As the dehydration and ketoacidosis were corrected, the abdominal symptoms and signs rapidly resolved, and the patient's vital signs stabilized Surgery was therefore deferred. Subsequent workup of the biliary tree revealed a normally functioning gallbladder without stones.

Comment. Diabetics may present with ketoacidosis in conjunction with a condition requiring surgery, in which case surgery must be delayed while vigorous treatment with insulin and intravenous fluids is initiated. It is important to recognize, however, that diabetic ketoacidosis itself may mimic an acute abdominal emergency In this situation, treatment of the ketoacidosis will result in resolution of the symptoms and signs originally thought to require urgent surgical intervention.[22] In the case reported above, the urinary tract infection apparently precipitated the ketoacidosis and the abdominal symptoms. On the other hand, the surgeon must not fall into the trap of ascribing all acute abdominal symptoms in diabetics to the pseudoperitonitis of ketoacidosis. During the few hours required to begin correcting the ketoacidosis with vigorous insulin and fluid therapy, the significance of the abdominal symptoms will usually become clarified.

3.3. Infection and Malnutrition

Another factor, the importance of which is only recently receiving significant appreciation, is the role that malnutrition plays in the increased morbidity and mortality of surgical patients.

Illustrative Case 10

A 27-year-old man was evaluated for complaints of crampy abdominal pain and bloody diarrhea Barium enema was consistent with the diagnosis of regional enteritis of the distal ileum. Despite intensive medical therapy, intermittent fever, anorexia, and chronic diarrhea persisted over the succeeding 4-month period The patient's weight fell from 165 to 130 lb (75 to 59 kg). Hospital admission was eventually required when increasing colicky pain, abdominal distention, and vomiting suggested partial bowel obstruction. Examination revealed a chronically ill young man who had a normal temperature and blood pressure The abdomen was modestly distended with hyperactive, high-pitched bowel sounds in rushes, resulting in frequent watery stools. Significant laboratory studies revealed Hct 32%, WBC count 13,000/mm^3, and serum albumin 2 6 g/dl Barium enema with reflux into the terminal ileum revealed marked thickening and irregularity of the bowel wall and a narrowed lumen with several enteroenteric fistulas Following resolution of the vomiting with nasogastric suction and intravenous fluids over the first 4 days, the patient was taken to surgery, for resection of all grossly diseased bowel, including the distal ileum and right colon Over the subsequent 3 months, the patient was explored three times for subphrenic and pelvic abscesses and attempted closure of multiple enterocutaneous fistulas. Despite the initiation of intravenous hyperalimentation, his weight continued to fall, to 105 lb (47.7 kg) Renal failure developed, prompting his transfer here for hemodialysis. At the time of admission, he was obtunded and wasted with a temperature of 102.5°F (39°C) and persistent anemia, hypoalbuminemia, and uremia. The partially disrupted abdominal incision was grossly purulent with evident tracking of the purulence into the perineum. Several persistent enterocutaneous fistulas were present.

During the subsequent 3-week hospitalization, the patient was treated with blood products, total parenteral nutrition, various antibiotics, multiple drainage procedures of abdominal and subcutaneous abscesses, suction drainage of the fistulas, and hemodialysis. Despite these measures, he had repeated positive blood cultures for gram-negative organisms, showed little eivdence of wound healing, and finally expired 4 months after the initial surgical procedure.

Comment Inflammatory bowel disease of the transmural type is frequently associated with partial bowel obstruction, fistulas, intraabdominal abscess, and malabsorption. These patients are markedly malnourished, protein and electrolyte depleted, and severely catabolic. Immunocompetence measurements reveal most to be either anergic or severely compromised. Numerous reports indicate a markedly increased likelihood of postoperative sepsis and death in patients with a preoperative weight loss of more than 20%.[23,24] In this setting, preoperative hyperalimentation may be a valuable tool. Improvement in various immune parameters after nutritional repletion in malnourished animals and patients has been described [25] In patients with inflammatory bowel disease, remission of acute symptoms may be achieved, and, even if only partial resolution occurs, the patient has become an improved operative candidate with nutritional deficiencies partially corrected.[26] In fact, the prevalence of some degree of malnutrition, when defined by certain metabolic parameters, has been reported to be as high as 50% in hospitalized patients.[27] Thus, there has been generated a substantial clinical opinion that hyperalimentation might be beneficial for most patients prior to surgery. Objective data that such support can provide decreased operative morbidity when administered fairly regularly to surgical candidates remains to be generated. Nevertheless, the well-documented evidence of poor anastomotic healing in protein-depleted experimental subjects and a number of clinical studies[25] have established the applicability of hyperalimnetation for the management of specific conditions such as enterocutaneous fistulas,[28] acute renal failure,[29] and burns,[30] in addition to inflammatory bowel disease More widespread experience with the use of specific nutritional markers such as weight loss/time and serum protein, albumin, and transferrin levels or the newer measures of immunocompetence[31−33] should help clarify whether other patients at high risk of surgical complications can be prospectively identified and benefited by preoperative nutritional supplementation or immunomodulation. Currently, one may assume that significant malnutrition exists in any patient who presents with derangements such as weight loss of greater than 0.2% per day or 10% of normal, serum albumin of less than 3 0 g/dl, serum transferrin level of less than 200 mg/dl, or inability to respond to common delayed hypersensitivity skin tests. This type of patient should be considered a candidate for preoperative hyperalimentation if time allows. With

selective use of such preoperative therapy, it is hoped that most of the disastrous complications illustrated by this case can be avoided.

3.4. Preoperative Antibiotics

Preoperative administration of antibiotics to the compromised host may have therapeutic and prophylactic goals. Certainly, when a specific infectious process is suspected or has already been identified, or when a contaminated procedure such as bowel resection is planned, appropriate antibiotic coverage should be recommended. The importance of prophylactic antibiotics for "clean" surgical procedures in the compromised host, on the other hand, remains more controversial. Some transplant groups strongly recommend pre- and intraoperative broad-spectrum antibiotic coverage particularly for diabetic patients, and view this therapy as a major reason for the reduced risk of mortality for these patients.[34] Our own experience without routine antibiotic coverage, however, has indicated an extremely low rate of infection of the primary transplant wound or following other uncontaminated procedures in these patients. Thus, prophylactic antibiotics have not been recommended for fear of selecting out resistant, more highly virulent, bacterial flora. The validity of either of these recommendations remains to be established in controlled studies of immunosuppressed patients.

In some compromised patients, the status of the natural bacterial flora may suggest the need for prophylactic antibiotics. For example, in a retrospective study of infection in cancer patients undergoing major surgical procedures, nasal cultures were performed preoperatively to determine the infectious carrier status.[35] Of the subsequent staphylococcal infections observed, 80% occurred in patients carrying the organisms preoperatively. The investigators then evaluated the value of administering antibiotics postoperatively. They observed a 14% infection rate in the treated group in contrast to a 54.3% rate in the placebo group. Later studies using antibiotics both pre- and postoperatively showed a decreased incidence of infection to 8.9%.[36] Based on such results, many surgeons advise the use of prophylactic antibiotics in all patients undergoing major surgical resections for malignancy. Specific recommendations obviously vary, but the antibiotic chosen is usually one with broad-spectrum coverage with particular consideration of the potential pathogens (e.g., oral, respiratory, enteric) expected to be encountered. The type of procedure to be undertaken is also an important determinant. For example, the indications are clearly greater for a major orthopaedic or vascular procedure than for simple excisions or node dissections.

It has generally been accepted that there is a limited time period during which it is possible to augment the host's antibacterial mechanisms with antibiotics and that this period lasts only a few hours beginning at the time of bacterial contamination[37] Thus, if they are to be used, it is essential that prophylactic antibiotics be administered preoperatively and continued intraoperatively. Following surgery, the course of antibiotic administration should be brief lest the host be colonized with resistant organisms.[38]

4. Intraoperative Considerations

4.1. Choice of Anesthesia and Patient-Monitoring Techniques

Selection of anesthetic techniques in these patients is limited primarily by precautions dictated by the underlying disease. For example, in uremics, agents eliminated primarily via renal excretion should be avoided or dosages appropriately decreased. The use of average doses of gallamine triethiodide, for example, in renal transplant recipients results in prolonged paralysis in 20% of patients.[39] We have observed a similar problem following administration of pancuronium bromide, and therefore favor the use of agents such as Atracurium to avoid protracted neuromuscular blockade.[40] This complication can be particularly serious because of the increased risk of pulmonary infection in immunosuppressed patients when prolonged endotracheal intubation is maintained. One important goal of anesthesia management, therefore, is to provide for return of adequate spontaneous respiratory activity and early postoperative extubation. In fact, in some circumstances, even brief intubation can prove unusually hazardous.

Illustrative Case 11

A 34-year-old woman was admitted to the hospital with fever, leukopenia, and thrombocytopenia. She had received a cadaver-

donor kidney 4 months before the present admission Postoperatively, several episodes of acute rejection had required treatment with high dosages of steroids in addition to maintenance azathioprine. Renal function then stabilized with a serum creatinine of 3.0 mg/dl while azathioprine (100 mg/day) and prednisone (30 mg/day) were continued.

Multiple ulcerated lesions developed on the face and lips, a biopsy of which disclosed herpes simplex infection. Local treatment was given, and the prednisone dosage was lowered to 15 mg/day. One week later, the patient noted slowly increasing weight, decreased urine output, tenderness of the allograft, and low-grade fever. She was admitted with a diagnosis of acute allograft rejection.

At the time of admission, the temperature was 101°F (38°C), pulse rate 110/min, and blood pressure 140/100. There were clusters of hemorrhagic, crusting lesions about the nose and upper lip. A few scattered lesions were noted on the forehead and cheeks. Shallow ulcerations were present within the oropharynx. Cardiac examination revealed on S-3 gallop with no murmurs The renal allograft was swollen and tender. Extensive muscle atrophy and 2+ pitting edema of the lower extremities were observed

The urine gave a 4+ test for protein. The Hct was 31%, WBC count 2900/mm³, and the platelet count 78,000/mm³. The serum creatinine was 5.5 mg/dl. Arterial blood gas (ABG) determination with the patient breathing room air revealed a Pao_2 90 mm Hg and pH 7.42. A chest radiograph revealed small bilateral pleural effusions without parenchymal lesions.

Azathioprine was discontinued. Diuretics were administered, and local irradiation of the allograft was begun. During the following week, the serum creatinine continued to rise to 7.0 mg/dl and hemodialysis was instituted in preparation for transplant nephrectomy. During this period, the WBC count remained at 2500–3000/mm³ and the platelet count varied from 75,000 to 100,000/mm³ despite cessation of azathioprine therapy. Following hemodialysis, the chest radiograph revealed clearing of the pleural effusions, and she was taken to the operating room where transplant nephrectomy was performed without incident under general endotracheal anesthesia.

Postoperatively, the patient was maintained on hemodialysis. The steroid dosage was tapered to 15 mg/day over a 72-hr period. A low-grade fever developed with progressive cough and dyspnea. One week after the nephrectomy, chest radiography revealed diffuse hazy opacification throughout both lung fields. A smear of the tracheal secretions disclosed a few polymorphonuclear cells. Cytologic examination disclosed multinucleated cells consistent with herpes infection. The temperature rose each day to a maximum of 101–102°F (38°–39°C). Broad-spectrum antibiotics including cotrimoxazole for possible Pneumocystis infection were added, but progressive hypoxemia developed necessitating nasotracheal intubation and mechanical ventilation. Enteric hyperalimentation was continued via a nasogastric tube. During the following week, gram-negative sepsis developed, and the patient expired. At autopsy, the lungs revealed punctate and confluent areas of a necrotizing bronchopneumonia with the spectrum of nuclear changes in cells characteristic of herpetic infection. Herpetic infection was also found throughout the tracheobronchial tree and larynx, where it produced necrosis and ulceration of the mucosa. No evidence of bacterial pneumonia was noted, and post mortem cultures of the lungs were negative for pathogenic bacteria but did yield HSV Punched-out and confluent herpetic ulcers were also present in the esophagus. There was no other dissemination of herpes infection.

Comment. In a study of herpetic necrotizing tracheobronchitis and bronchopneumonia, it was suggested that this infection was acquired by aspiration, in contrast to the hematogenous spread of disseminated herpes.[41] The common denominator in all cases was the debilitated state of the patients and some form of tracheal trauma, usually intubation. Since herpes simplex has a predilection for traumatized areas, endotracheal intubation should be avoided if at all possible in patients with active infection of the oropharynx. In the present case, for example, regional anesthesia would have been a suitable approach for the transplant nephrectomy and might have avoided the subsequent fatal complication of herpes pneumonitis. It is noteworthy that the esophagus was also involved with active herpes infection after a feeding tube had been present for approximately 1 week, again emphasizing the relationship between mucosal trauma and spread of the ulcerating lesions. Earlier reports of anesthesia techniques for transplantation, in fact, advised regional anesthesia without endotracheal intubation as the approach of choice to avoid pulmonary infection in these immunoincompetent patients. Currently, most groups reserve regional anesthesia for patients whose general condition has not been adequately improved by dialysis or who have already suffered the ravages of immunosuppression, as in this case.

Similar considerations should be observed when placing potentially contaminated percutaneous venous or arterial catheters. Recognition that any indwelling line in these patients can be the source of serious bacteremia should emphasize that their use should never be allowed for only marginal indications, and that they should be removed as soon as clinical conditions permit. With the observation of such possibly obvious precautions, the administration of general or conduction anesthesia to immunocompromised patients can be provided without an unacceptably high incidence of complications.

4.2. Surgical Technique

The surgeon managing these patients must be prepared to constantly reevaluate and modify his usual techniques in order to deal with tissues (Fig. 1) that are weak, hold sutures poorly, and can be expected to require unusually prolonged healing periods.

Illustrative Case 12

A 71-year-old woman with leukemia received 6-thioguanine and cytosine arabinoside treatment for 5 months prior to the present hospital admission which was prompted by the sudden onset of crampy abdominal pain. On admission, her temperature was 104°F (40°C) and blood pressure 90/70. The abdomen was distended and tympanitic, and both direct and rebound tenderness were present. Following institution of antibiotics and rapid rehydration, the patient underwent emergency laparotomy. A volvulus of the distal ileum with dilatation of the proximal bowel was found. A localized

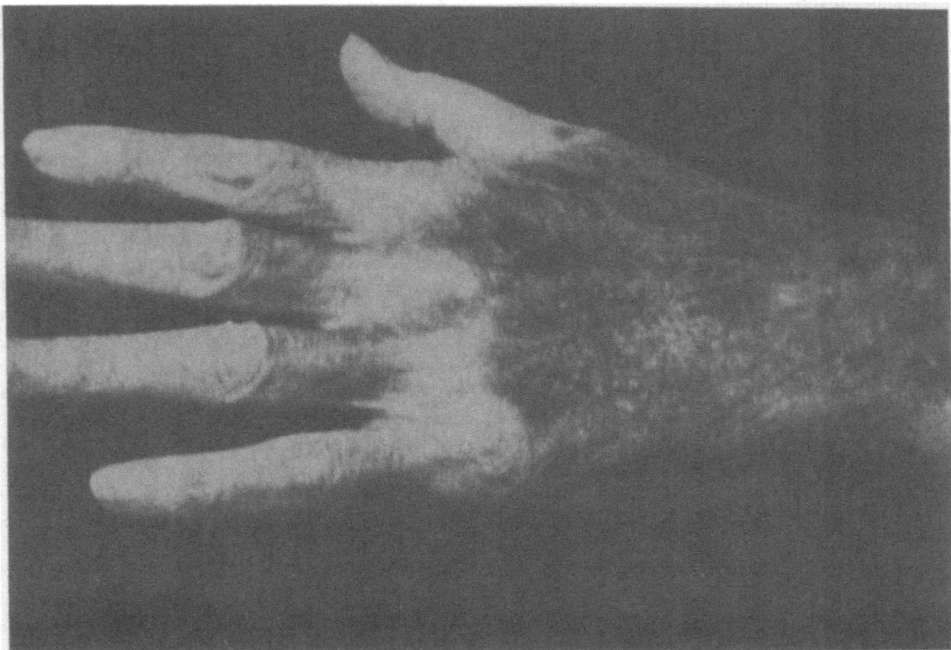

FIGURE 1. Typical thin, friable skin in a steroid-treated patient. Significant injuries after only minor trauma and poor wound healing following surgery can be anticipated.

abscess surrounding a perforation of the antimesenteric border of the ileum was present as well. The volvulus was reduced, and no evidence of nonviable bowel was noted. The edges of the perforation were excised, and the defect was closed in two layers with chromic catgut and silk sutures. Postoperatively, the patient remained febrile with a quiet, distended abdomen until the fifth day, when a fecal fistula was noted at the inferior margin of the abdominal incision. Emergency reoperation revealed dehiscence of the bowel closure with local peritonitis. The involved small bowel segment was resected, and an end-to-end anastomosis constructed. The patient remained stable for several days but then developed fever, hypotension, and blood cultures positive for *Escherichia coli*. Her condition rapidly deteriorated, and she expired shortly thereafter. Postmortem examination revealed dehiscence of the bowel anastomosis and diffuse peritonitis.

Comment. In urgent gastrointestinal tract operations in the compromised host, stomas should be considered in preference to anastomoses more frequently than in the usual surgical subject. Following an emergency bowel resection, the patient's chances of survival are enhanced if ileostomy or colostomy are constructed rather than a primary anastomosis which may result in fatal leakage when replaced into the abdomen. Several months after construction of the stoma, when the patient has recovered from the acute event and host defenses have been at least partially restored, reestablishment of bowel continuity becomes a relatively minor surgical procedure. If sutured bowel must be left in the abdomen, nonabsorbable sutures must be used, and the surgeon should attempt to isolate and reinforce the closure, for example, with omentum, and provide proximal decompression via colostomy, gastrostomy, etc. Similarly, tragic experience has emphasized that local drainage and proximal colonic diversion, which is adequate therapy for perforated diverticulitis in the usual patient, is totally inadequate following sigmoid perforation in the compromised host. In these patients, sepsis continues to spread, despite apparently complete local drainage, because the depressed inflammatory response is unable to provide satisfactory containment. Thus, exteriorization or primary resection of the involved bowel and construction of a descending colostomy and distal mucous fistula is the treatment of choice. With such an approach, one should expect at least a 60–70% salvage rate in these patients for a condition previously found to be almost universally fatal.

Copious intraperitoneal lavage should also be used to reduce the residual contamination and limit the possibility of subsequent abscess formation. Some authors recommend antibiotic or antibacterial irrigations with continuing lavage into the postoperative period,[42] however, saline alone is probably as efficacious and does not expose the patient to any side effects of the irrigation itself. Liberal drainage of all four quadrants and of the subphrenic spaces and pelvic pouch should be considered.

Following abdominal surgery in the immunocompromised host, the surgeon should anticipate the possibility of prolonged periods of gastric dysfunction. Drainage via gastrostomy should therefore usually be employed to avoid the pulmonary and esophageal complications associated with nasogastric tubes. At the same time, consideration should be given to using the small bowel for early resumption of nutritional support. In fact, motility and absorption by the small intestine usually returns within hours of abdominal exploration. Most patients with a reasonable length

of normal small intestine can be given full nutrition via jejunostomy administration of elemental diet beginning in the early postoperative period.[43] The elemental diet is absorbed in the proximal intestine without the need for digestion, thus providing an early return to anabolism without the risks of prolonged hyperalimentation via central venous lines. Because of the poor healing in these patients, special precautions must be taken during placement of cutaneous–enteric tubes. Unless the bowel around the enterostomy is carefully and completely sutured to the anterior abdominal wall, a satisfactory seal of the tract will not develop. Subsequent leakage of enteric contents around the tube and into the peritoneal cavity can be regularly anticipated. Similarly, poor tissue healing should be expected in all incised tissues

Illustrative Case 13

A 10-year-old girl with end-stage liver failure and massive ascites was admitted because of fever and abdominal pain. Following the initial diagnostic impression of acute appendicitis, exploratory laparotomy was performed. Slightly cloudy ascites revealed white blood cells but no organisms on Gram stain. Cultures subsequently yielded *E. coli* The remainder of the examination, including the appendix, revealed no acute inflammatory process. A diagnosis of primarily infected ascites was presumed and continued antibiotic therapy was advised. The wound closure included all layer retention sutures because of the fear of poor healing. Postoperatively, continued ascites leakage around the sutures led to wound disruption, purulent peritonitis, and eventual death

Comment. This patient's history emphasizes two points at which different surgical approaches could have changed her course. The correct diagnosis might have been made if a preoperative paracentesis had been performed. This would have avoided completely the surgical procedure. Once the laparotomy was performed, the possibility of wound complications was correctly recognized, but the inadequate nature of the usual approach taken for this problem is emphasized by the patient's postoperative course.

Because of the expected delayed healing, closure with interrupted nonabsorbable suture material is advisable. We have found fine stainless steel sutures to be particularly appealing, but other synthetic monofilament products are probably equally satisfactory. Silk or cotton sutures are, of course, inadvisable in wounds at high risk of infection. Subcuticular skin closure (Fig. 2) also seems to decrease the incidence of complications since microabscesses, which frequently develop around transcutaneous sutures left in place for more than a few days, are avoided. Similarly, we rigorously avoid the use of all-layer sutures, especially in patients with ascites where direct communication between skin flora and peritoneum can occur along the suture tract because of the host's inability to effectively seal off the sites. The value of topical application of antibacterial solutions into surgical wounds remains controversial. Some reports[44] seem to provide sound evidence that such irrigations lower the frequency of subcutaneous infections, especially in highly contaminated cases. In a nonrandomized series of transplant wounds that required reopening for a variety of indications, the incidence of septic complications was found to be

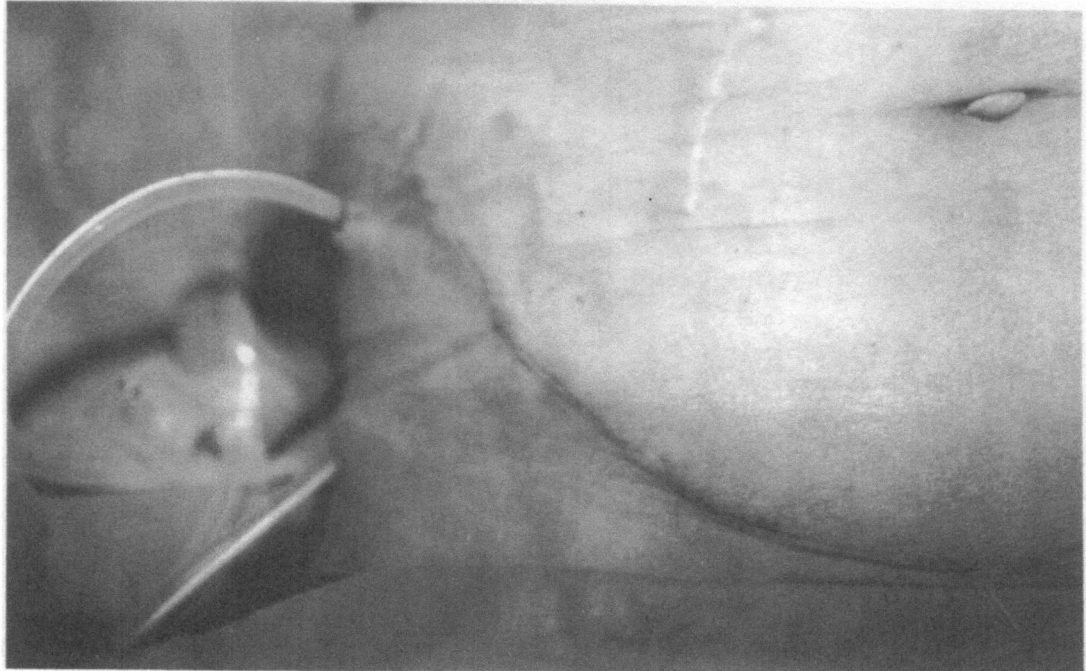

FIGURE 2. Wound closure in renal allograft recipient avoiding the use of transcutaneous sutures. Uncomplicated primary healing regularly results with this approach.

28.6% when no local antibiotics were given but only 4.0% if local antibiotics were used.[45] In our own practice, in which we do not use systemic prophylactic antibiotics but irrigate the transplant wound with local antibiotics, a wound infection rate of approximately 3% has been observed. If the surgical procedure was one of marked contamination, delayed or secondary closure of the skin and subcutaneous tissues is in most instances safer than attempted primary closure.

Recently, a special concern for the surgical team has arisen as the number of patients with AIDS continues to escalate. Surgical intervention for various conditions in these patients is consequently being required with increasing frequency.[46] In addition to the guidelines emphasized for the surgical management of all immunocompromised hosts, the operating team must in these cases, take special precautions to limit their own risk of infection by the AIDS virus. These precautions are quite similar to those employed for patients who are hepatitis B surface antigen Hb_sAg positive and include the wearing of goggles and double gloves and the use of extreme care in the handling and disposal of all sharp instruments and needles.

5. Postoperative Management

As emphasized above, an urgent goal following postanesthesia stabilization of the compromised host is early extubation. In immunosuppressed allograft recipients, we have observed superinfection pneumonitis in 80% of patients who require endotracheal intubation for longer than 72–96 hr. Such experience cautions that the use of even extraordinary techniques should be considered in order to avoid prolonged intubation in these patients.

5.1. Respiratory Management in the Immunocompromised Patient

Illustrative Case 14

A 34-year-old woman was admitted to the hospital with multiple injuries after having been struck by an automobile. She had received a cadaver-donor renal allograft 3 years earlier and had excellent renal function on maintenance dosages of azathioprine and prednisone. At the time of admission, she was alert but in rather severe pain and respiratory distress with obvious paradox-

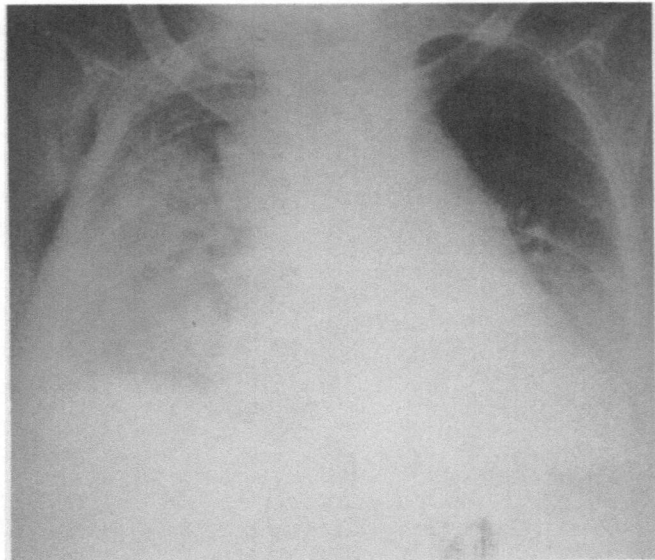

FIGURE 3. Admission chest radiograph demonstrating multiple rib fractures and hemothorax of the right chest resulting in severe respiratory insufficiency.

ical respiratory movement of the right chest. Chest radiographs revealed multiple rib fractures and a right-sided hemothorax (Fig 3), bilateral pubic ramus fractures, and a closed, comminuted fracture of the right tibia. The large flail segment of the right chest necessitated endotracheal intubation with positive-pressure ventilation. Following this procedure and drainage of the hemothorax by tube thoracostomy, the patient's condition stabilized. Continuing evaluation revealed no evidence of significant intracranial or intraabdominal injury. The leg fracture was reduced and externally stabilized under general anesthesia, and the patient was transferred here 24 hours later for further care. At this point, the patient was gratifyingly stable, but it was obvious that the 10–12 day period of internal pneumatic stabilization required to allow satisfactory recovery of chest wall rigidity could result in a fatal superinfection of the underlying contused pulmonary parenchyma. Accordingly, the patient was taken to the operating room where intermedullary wire fixation of ribs 3–10 was performed (Fig. 4). It was possible to extubate the patient 24 hr after this procedure. With aggressive respiratory therapy, she subsequently recovered from these injuries without any serious infectious complications

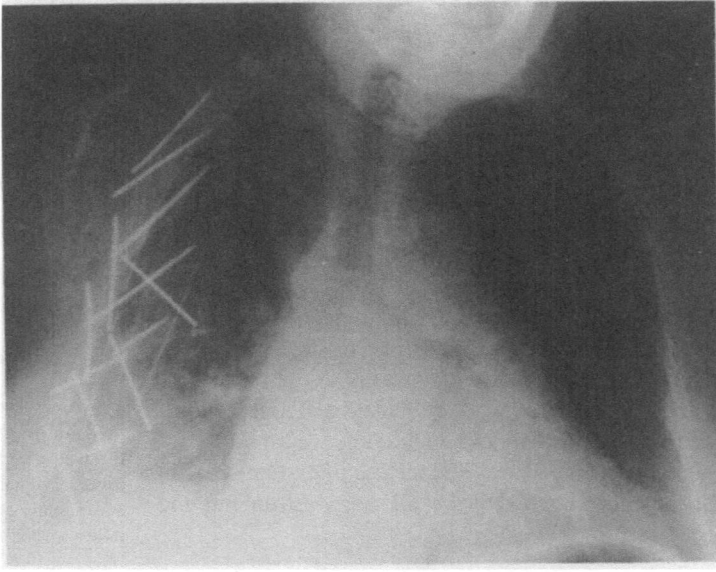

FIGURE 4. Postsurgical radiograph with the large flail segment of the chest wall stabilized by intramedullary pins providing adequate respiratory mechanics without intubation and positive-pressure ventilation.

Comment Traumatic injuries resulting in chest wall instability and diminished ventilation are managed with high degrees of success in healthy individuals by internal pneumatic stabilization with or without tracheostomy. In the compromised host, however, such management would almost surely lead to fatal pulmonary infection even with the availability of excellent respiratory therapy. Thus, as in the diagnostic approach to these patients, the surgeon must sometimes avoid what appears to be conservative techniques in favor of more invasive management, which, however, provides a more rapid resolution of the presenting problem. For similar reasons, the importance of respiratory therapy in the early postoperative period cannot be overemphasized. Moderate areas of atelectasis or pooling of tracheobronchial secretions, which may be inconsequential in lower-risk surgical candidates, can provide the appropriate environment for sepsis in the compromised host. This is all too often followed by pulmonary failure, which is typically the initial event in a cumulative sequence of multiorgan system failure leading to death. Thus, increased attention to positioning, early ambulation, oxygenation and humidification of inspired air, and aggressive respiratory therapy which includes judicious endotracheal suction or even bronchoscopy to clear bronchial plugs is mandatory following extubation.

An important consideration related to endotracheal intubation in immunocompromised patients has been the observation that the naso-tracheal route may favor the development of sinus infection leading to serious complications. Thus, oro-tracheal intubation should usually be employed even when it is anticipated the tube will be in place for a number of days.

5.2. General Postoperative Care in the Immunocompromised Patient

Other postoperative considerations include careful monitoring of wounds for development of collections that may be deceptively asymptomatic. We recommend immediate needle aspiration of any suspicious area of even minimal induration or tenderness. Prompt ultrasound examination of the operative site is also indicated in any patient with signs of occult sepsis. Attempts to accelerate wound healing in these patients with any of the widely studied adjuvant agents (e.g., cartilage, zinc)[47] are probably not warranted. Although the exact value of protein-sparing therapy for correcting surgically induced depression of host resistance continues to be debated,[48] provision of adequate caloric and protein intake to achieve a positive nitrogen balance as early as possible seems appropriate. Similarly, addition of vitamins, particularly A and C, to the chronically malnourished patient cannot be severely criticized.

Severe degrees of anemia should be corrected, with an hematocrit value of 30–33% being the range that appears most appropriate.[49] The usefulness of granulocyte transfusions to prevent gram-negative sepsis in patients with severe neutropenia, although fairly convincingly demonstrated in bone marrow transplant recipients,[50] remains under investigation for other immunocompromised patients. Some studies suggest there may be a place for such therapeutic rather than prophylactic transfusions in the management of severely burned patients,[51] although major questions remain here as well. Vigorous isolation measures, except in patients with marked leukopenia or major burns, are generally not required, although it is clear that significant environmental contamination in the hospital will be first manifested in these patients. Thus, any unusual incidence in the number of infections by organisms such as Aspergillus or Legionella must be immediately investigated and the contaminating source controlled.

5.3. Management of the Burn or Trauma Patient

The syndrome of sepsis and sequential postoperative organ failure may develop in a previously healthy immunocompetent host, particularly in the setting of major trauma such as burns or multiple injuries that produce chronic stress.[52]

Illustrative Case 15

A 9-year-old boy was admitted to the burn unit 9 days after suffering a flaming gasoline injury producing full-thickness burns over 80% of the body surface area. During the period between injury and transfer, the burns had been treated with $AgNO_3$ dressings; but, at the time of admission, early *Pseudomonas* sepsis of the thighs and buttocks was noted. These areas were debrided; the chest and abdomen were primarily excised and covered with autografts from the scalp. The patient was continued on $AgNO_3$ dressings and both enteric and parenteral hyperalimentation while being housed in the protective environment of a bacteria-controlled nursing unit. Initially, the take of the skin grafts was excellent, but by the tenth postgraft day, there was evidence of spread of *Pseudomonas* sepsis and partial graft loss. Multiple procedures of burn excision followed by coverage with allografts and autografts were successful in closing most of the trunk and proximal extremity wounds, but the patient's course was continually complicated by spiking fevers, positive blood cultures, and recurrent pulmonary infiltrates. By the 35th hospital day, GI dysfunction with ileus, distention, and vomiting severely limited oral intake. On the 45th day, the patient developed respiratory insufficiency requiring mechanical ventilation after which he continued to deteriorate metabolically. He eventually died on the 54th day, at which time more than 90% of the burns had been successfully covered with autografts.

Comment. Despite major advances in the immediate resuscitation and surgical management of severe trauma victims, an unacceptably large fraction of these previously healthy, often young patients succumb in the later postoperative period, usually with multiple organ failure. Intensive evaluation of this syndrome indicates that late onset of sepsis enhanced by limitation of protein synthesis is the major underlying etiologic factor.[53] In this patient, the *Pseudomonas* sepsis was already established at the time of admission. Despite institution of intensive efforts to eradicate the infection, it was never possible to regain control. The typical downhill course, inevitably leading to death, ensued even though the burns were nearly covered.

In patients with burns, as with all trauma, the goal must be to convert the open, contaminated wound to a closed, clean wound in the shortest time possible. This is especially important for major burns where continuing immune depression is produced by the wound itself.[54,55] In most cases, repeated skin grafting from uninjured donor areas is an adequate solution to the problem. However, if the area of normal skin available for donor sites is insufficient to provide reasonable prompt skin graft closure, we have again found that a much more aggressive approach is required. Following the serial evaluation of a number of techniques, we initially recommended immediate wound closure with skin allografts, whose survival is prolonged by immunosuppressive agents, as the most useful method of reducing fluid, protein, heat, and energy loss,

controlling infection, and protecting underlying structures.[56] More recently, the use of synthetic "skin" has been even more promising because the need for immunosuppression is avoided.[57,58]

In patients with massive burns, prompt excision and wound closure by a number of successive surgical procedures is begun usually on the first or second day after the burn injury when all available donor sites are harvested to cover a comparable area of excised eschar with autografts. Subsequent procedures consist of excision of eschar and closure with allograft skin or artificial skin. Eventually, the allografts are excised stepwise and replaced with autografts as donor sites regenerate.

All patients are nursed in the protective environment provided by the bacteria-controlled nursing unit until open areas are reduced to less than 5% of the body surface area (Fig. 5). The patient is protected against contact cross-infection by clear plastic access walls and by a system of medical care delivery whereby the nursing and medical personnel do not directly enter the protected environment of the units.

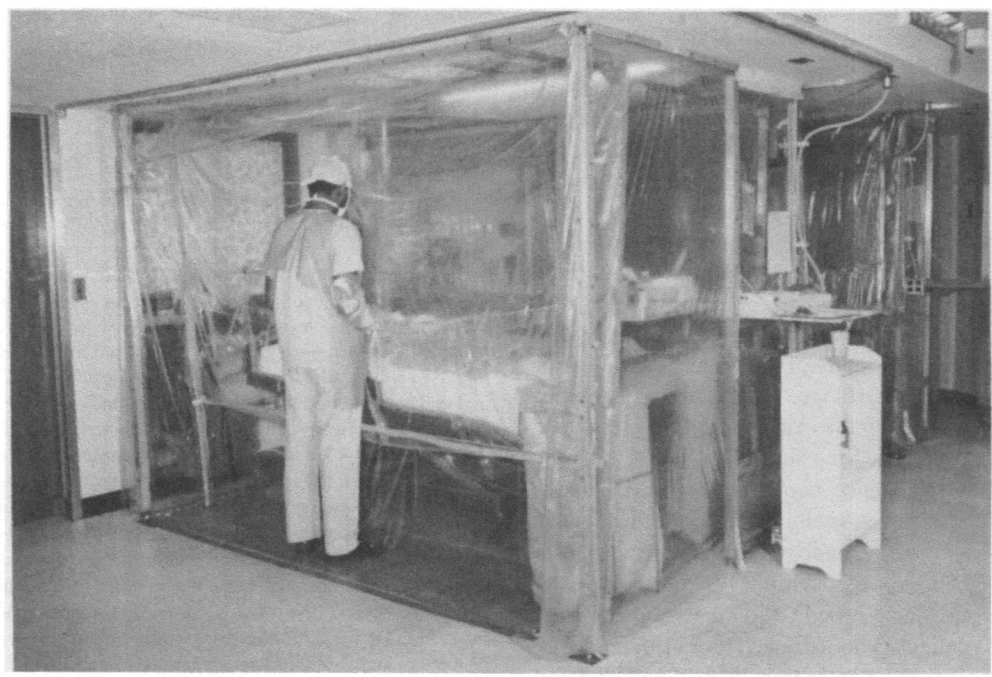

FIGURE 5. Bacteria-controlled nursing unit in which the patient area is provided with a continuous, pistonlike downflow of bacteria-free air at 90°F and 94% relative humidity to protect against energy loss as heat or evaporation as well as air-borne cross-infection. Nursing and medical personnel access is via openings in the plastic walls.

Autoinfection of the burn wound from the patient's respiratory or gastrointestinal tract is reduced by meticulous aseptic precautions and the use of 0.5% aqueous silver nitrate dressings to the burn eschar until excised, to donor sites, and to newly grafted areas of the extremities.

The metabolic balance of these patients is carefully maintained with the goal of daily parenteral and enteric intake of at least 3000 cal/m^2 and 3 g/kg of protein. Malfunction of the gastrointestinal tract taking the form of gastric retention with ileus or diarrhea has been an ominous sign. Its onset usually heralds severe malnutrition and sepsis. Patients who expire usually develop diarrhea followed by persistent ileus and gastric retention that prevents oral alimentation. Surviving patients have occasional limited episodes of ileus, usually following an operative procedure, but gastrointestinal tract dysfunction is not severe enough to interfere with nutrition and body weight is maintained throughout the course of the illness.

A large part of the effective control of bacterial infection demonstrated by these patients must be laid to the beneficial effect of prompt and almost complete wound closure and the maintenance of normal nutrition during periods of maximal stress. The contribution of the protective environment provided by the bacteria-controlled nursing unit is difficult to assess. Cross-infection is rarely seen in this group of highly susceptible patients, however, and late development of bacterial pneumonitis is seen only as a terminal episode in patients who fail to survive. Thus, although a dogmatic statement concerning the exact contribution of a protective environment to the immunosuppressed burn patient cannot be made, the evidence available indicates the contribution is probably significant.

Prior to the addition of immunosuppression to the routine treatment plan, which included prompt excision of dead tissue and immediate wound closure with autografts and allografts, the controlled environment of the bacteria-controlled nursing unit, intensive metabolic alimentation, and topical AgNO$_3$, patients with full-thickness burns of greater than 70% of the body surface suffered 100% mortality. With the addition of immunosuppression, which allowed continued wound closure by the allografts until they were electively replaced with autografts, we found it possible to salvage over half of this group of patients. The latest innovation using synthetic "skin" without

immunosuppression has now simplified the care of these patients further.

Intensive postoperative support including nutritional management is also essential for preventing delayed sepsis and multiple organ failure in other postsurgical patients, in whom it is anticipated that oral alimentation will not be possible within 5–7 days. As noted in Section 3, many malnourished patients can be identified prior to surgery and will have been already begun on a nutritional repletion program that is continued through the postoperative period. In previously healthy patients such as victims of major trauma, however, the extent of the postoperative catabolic response and increasingly negative nitrogen balance may not be appreciated until delayed wound healing, occult fevers, and early hepatic dysfunction become manifest. Unfortunately, at this point, institution of hyperalimentation is often ineffective. Thus, even in these acutely injured patients, it should be anticipated that although the body can initially employ its carbohydrate and fat reserves to meet the increased metabolism and negative caloric balance, these reserves are depleted within a few days of the injury or surgery. Thereafter, protein must be mobilized to provide these needs. Since there are no protein reserves as such, this immediate assault on the functional and structural capacity of the body must be prevented by early enteric or parenteral administration of adequate calories and amino acids.[53]

5.4. Gastrointestinal Bleeding in the Immunocompromised Patient

A particularly difficult postoperative problem is acute upper GI bleeding. The incidence of this life-threatening complication continues to increase, especially as intensive care units (ICUs) managing these patients are more regularly able to resuscitate them with modern technology.[59]

Illustrative Case 16

A 57-year-old woman with severe arthritis requiring steroid therapy was admitted to the hospital with fever and lower abdominal pain. Bowel sounds were present, and the abdomen was nondistended, but lower abdominal direct and rebound tenderness was demonstrable. Urgent laparotomy revealed peritonitis secondary to perforated sigmoid diverticulitis which was managed with resection and end-sigmoid colostomy. A gastrostomy was performed, and extensive peritoneal lavage and drainage were instituted. The wound was managed with delayed primary closure.

The patient initially did well, but on the seventh postoperative day, black, guaiac-positive gastrostomy drainage was noted. This cleared with iced saline lavage. Bright red bleeding developed 24 hr later. Selective angiography showed marked hypervascularity of the gastric mucosa. With vasopressin infusion via the left gastric artery, the bleeding remained controlled for 48 hr. After weaning of the vasopressin infusion, however, active bleeding recurred. Surgery was recommended but the patient and her family adamantly refused. Over the subsequent 7 days, repeated intraarterial vasopressin infusions and embolic occlusion of the left gastric artery only intermittently controlled the slow but persistent bleeding. During this time, multiple blood cultures became positive for Cryptococcus. Culture of the removed angiography catheter similarly was positive for this organism. Despite Amphotericin therapy and broad-spectrum antibiotic coverage, the patient remained febrile and lethargic, eventually developing pneumonia and respiratory failure leading to death.

Illustrative Case 17

An 18-year-old man suffered a severe crushing injury to the abdomen, pelvis, and legs in a jeep accident and required splenectomy, resection of devitalized bowel, and reduction and fixation of multiple fractures. Postoperatively, acute renal failure developed. He remained relatively stable, but intermittent fever occurred usually in association with hemodialysis treatments. On the tenth postinjury day, massive upper GI bleeding occurred. This was only partially controlled with iced saline lavage. Endoscopy revealed several prepyloric bleeding ulcerations. Cimetidine therapy was added, and the bleeding appeared to stop, only to recur 48 hr later. At exploration, a 300-ml foul-smelling hematoma was evacuated from the left subphrenic space. Vagotomy and distal gastrectomy were performed. The patient subsequently recovered without further bleeding or other significant complications.

Comment. Stress ulceration continues to provide a significant surgical challenge. Such ulcers characteristically bleed or perforate during the early postinjury or postoperative period. The incidence is markedly increased when significant complications, particularly sepsis, follow the initial procedure. In fact, the association of systemic or localized infection with acute gastroduodenal ulceration is so constant that a surgical axiom has been coined for these patients. It cautions that in the face of upper gastrointestinal bleeding laparotomy is more urgently indicated for detection of the underlying sepsis than for control of the bleeding site. The occult subphrenic abscess in this case emphasizes this point. Interestingly, this patient also exhibits another diagnostic clue occasionally observed, namely, the febrile episodes associated with hemodialysis. It has been suggested that these may be the result of expansion of the infected collection during the rapid osmotic shifts associated with dialysis.

The pathologic condition of stress ulceration varies from diffuse erosive changes to a single punched-out ulcer with virtually no surrounding re-

action. The progression of mucosal damage is closely related to the duration of sepsis. In patients studied serially, gastroduodenal disease becomes worse as sepsis is prolonged. On the other hand, mucosal lesions show a dramatic improvement when focal infection and septicemia are eradicated.[60] In experimental evaluation of this relationship, Douglass et al.[61] reported that subcutaneous infection with coagulase-positive staphylococci increased the incidence of ulcers in guinea pigs.

Prospective endoscopy performed in high-risk patients has shown frequent acute lesions in spite of clinical silence. Czaja et al.[62] demonstrated gastric erosion in 86% of patients with large burns, LeGall found acute gastric or duodenal lesions in 100% of patients with severe sepsis and positive blood cultures, although many did not have clinical symptoms of macroscopic hemorrhage or digestive perforation.[60]

The mechanism of sepsis-induced gastroduodenal lesion formation is unclear, but it may be favored by ischemia of the mucosa as it is with acute ulcers of other origins. It is possible that a vasoconstrictive process of the gastroduodenal mucosa is associated with the septic focus and is independent of systemic shock. In support of this, endoscopies have shown a pale, ischemic, marbled mucosa that strongly suggests an ischemic etiology.

Medical therapy of stress ulcers is often disappointing. The addition of H_2-receptor antagonists may improve these results, but again, ultimate patient survival can only be achieved if the accompanying sepsis is controlled as well.[63]

The development of bipolar and laser coagulation devices has provided another approach to control for the patient who continues to bleed despite intensive medical therapy.[64] Emergency mesenteric angiography is usually undertaken only after endoscopy has been unsuccessful in identifying or controlling the bleeding site. If a bleeding site is defined by angiography, selective intraarterial infusion with aqueous vasopressin or embolic occlusion is sometimes successful. This is particularly true in patients with the typical gastric mucosal lesions in whom bleeding can usually be controlled following infusion via the left gastric artery.[65] When celiac axis perfusion is required, the bleeding is less well controlled. But again, the ultimate salvage of the patient is dependent on localization and treatment of any septic focus.

In heavily immunosuppressed patients, especially in the presence of leukopenia, we have had little success with long-term angiographic control of gastrointestinal bleeding. An obvious hazard is the development of sepsis from the indwelling catheter as occurred in Illustrative Case 16. Thus, we advise surgical intervention if bleeding is not controlled within 24–48 hr following institution of treatment by selective angiography.

Surgical therapy in these patients also leaves much to be desired. The choice of operation is largely a matter of unsupported preference. Most authorities agree that vagotomy usually should be performed.[66,67] Gastric resection has been advised as well, since the incidence of rebleeding after vagotomy with only gastric drainage is usually higher. Of course, the greater morbidity and mortality following resection must also be taken into consideration. With the addition of postoperative H_2-receptor antagonist therapy, the safer procedure of vagotomy and pyloroplasty appears to be an effective solution.[68]

5.5. Sepsis following Splenectomy

Illustrative Case 18

A 35-year-old man on chronic hemodialysis because of end-stage polycystic kidney disease was admitted to the hospital with fever and hypotension. Two years earlier, he had required left nephrectomy for infection. At that time, splenectomy was also performed because of intraoperative trauma to the spleen. He had been well until 1 week before the present admission when he noted the onset of occasional headaches and malaise. On the day of admission, he had been hiking on the beach, where he felt unusually hot. Swimming precipitated chills and he subsequently noted fever to 103°F (39°C). He was admitted to a local hospital with the possible diagnosis of heatstroke. He was observed there to be intermittently alert with a systolic blood pressure of 70 mm Hg and an oral temperature of 105°F (41°C). Ice packs were applied after which the temperature fell to 103°F (39°C), but the patient became increasingly obtunded and hypotensive. When transferred here, he was found to have generalized petechia and ecchymoses. Despite intravenous pressors, antibiotics, and fluid resuscitation, he died 5 hours after admission. Blood cultures subsequently grew *Streptococcus pneumoniae*.

Comment. The occurrence of fulminant bacterial sepsis in splenectomized patients was first clearly demonstrated by King and Shumacker.[69] For many years, the risk was believed to be limited to infants or young children but subsequent studies have emphasized that splenectomy done at any age and for any reason increases the risks for death due to infection.[70,71] Not surprisingly, the frequency and mortality rate vary with the age and underlying medical condition of the patient. Thus, in patients who underwent splenectomy for trauma, the risk of serious infection is approx-

imately 15%, whereas asplenic patients with thalassemia have a risk of serious infection approaching 25%.[72]

The surgeon's role in the management of this condition should be on several fronts First, it is clear that splenectomy is not always required to achieve hemostasis following splenic disruption. Thus, increasing numbers of reports have emphasized the feasibility of splenic salvage procedures.[73–75] Second, if splenectomy is unavoidable because of exsanguinating hemorrhage or for definitive control of a specific disease process, the patient should be protected as much as possible by polyvalent pneumococcal vaccine and should be appropriately informed of the need for aggressive treatment of all infections. Finally, the surgeon, who may be the first to evaluate these patients in an emergency ward, must keep this possibility in mind lest valuable time be lost, as in the case above, while nonspecific treatment for the fever is being administered.

6. Conclusions

Surgical management of infection in the compromised host requires special considerations related to the diagnosis, preoperative preparation, intraoperative techniques, and postoperative care (Table 4) of these fragile patients. With observation of certain guidelines as outlined here, it is possible to perform even highly complicated procedures with acceptable morbidity and mortality. The surgeon

TABLE 4. Infection in the Immunocompromised Host: Special Surgical Considerations

Aggressive diagnostic approach
  Recognition of impaired signs of inflammation
  Persistent evaluation despite unusual presentation
  Awareness of commonly occurring conditions
Expeditious preoperative preparation
  Systemic antibiotics
  Correction of malnutrition
  Prevention of adrenal insufficiency
  Reduction of immunosuppressive treatment
Special intraoperative attention
  Liberal use of stomas, lavage, drains
  Provision for prolonged gastric drainage and enteric feeding
  Topical antibiotics
  Secure wound closure
  Limit surgical team's exposure to virus (e.g., AIDS)
Careful postoperative management
  Early extubation
  Adequate nutritional support
  Detection of occult septic complications
  Aggressive control of GI bleeding
  Environmental control
  Leukocyte transfusions (selected cases)

should consider appropriately aggressive evaluation and surgical intervention in these patients from the viewpoint that delay in performance of an indicated procedure, far from being the conservative approach, will more likely be the determining factor that prevents the patient's rehabilitation or even precludes survival.

ACKNOWLEDGMENT. This work was supported in part by U.S. Public Health Service grant HL-18646.

References

1. MacLean LD: Host resistance in surgical patients. *J Trauma* **19**:297–304, 1979.
2. Ramsey PG, Rubin RH, Tolkoff-Rubin NE, et al. The renal transplant patient with fever and pulmonary infiltrates: Etiology, clinical manifestations, and management *Medicine (Baltimore)* **59**:206–222, 1980.
3. Ginsberg SJ, Comis RL: The pulmonary toxicity of antineoplastic agents. *Semin Oncol* **9**:34–51, 1982.
4. Fanburg BL, Mark EJ: A 33-year-old woman with a pulmonary nodule two years after renal transplantation. *N Engl J Med* **312**:843–850, 1985.
5. Hiatt JR, Cong H, Mulder DG, et al: The value of open lung biopsy in the immunosuppressed patient. *Surgery* **92**:285–291, 1982.
6. Waltzer WC, Sterioff S, Zincke H, et al: Open-lung biopsy in the renal transplant recipient. *Surgery* **88**:601–610, 1980.
7. Haverkos HW, Dowling JN, Pasculle AW, et al: Diagnosis of pneumonitis in immunocompromised patients by open lung biopsy. *Cancer* **52**:1093–1097, 1983.
8. Jaffe JP, Maki DG: Lung biopsy in immunocompromised patients: One institution's experience and an approach to management of pulmonary disease in the compromised host. *Cancer* **48**:1144–1153, 1981.
9. Warshaw AL, Welch JP, Ottinger LW: Acute perforation of the colon associated with chronic corticosteroid therapy *Am J Surg* **131**:442–446, 1976.
10. ReMine SG, McIlrath DC: Bowel perforation in steroid-treated patients. *Ann Surg* **192**:581–586, 1980.
11. Sterioff S, Orringer MB, Cameron JL. Colon perforations associated with steroid therapy *Surgery* **75**:56–58, 1974.
12. Gardner H, Miller RE: Barium peritonitis. *Am J Surg* **125**:350–352, 1973.
13. Powis SJA, Barnes AD, Dawson-Edwards P, et al Ileocolonic problems after cadaveric renal transplantation. *Br Med J* **1**:99–101, 1972.
14. Koretz MJ, Neifeld JP: Emergency surgical treatment for patients with acute leukemia. *Surg Gynecol Obstet* **161**:149–151, 1985.
15. Flynn TC, Rowlands BJ, Gilliland M, et al: Hypotension-induced post-traumatic necrosis of the right colon. *Am J Surg* **146**:715–718, 1983.
16. Lillemoe KD, Romolo JL, Hamilton SR, et al. Intestinal necrosis due to sodium polystyrene (Kayexalate) in sorbital enemas: Clinical and experimental support for the hypotheis *Surgery* **101**:267–279, 1987.
17. Gerzof SG, Robbins AH, Johnson WC, et al: Percutaneous catheter drainage of abdominal abscesses *N Engl J Med* **305**:653–696, 1981.
18. Carone FA, Liebow AA: Acute pancreatic lesions in patients treated with ACTH and adrenal corticoids *N Engl J Med* **257**:690–697, 1957
19. Renning JA, Warden GD, Stevens LE, et al. Pancreatitis after renal transplantation. *Am J Surg* **123**:293–296, 1972
20. Kawanishi H, Rudolph E, Bull FE: Azathioprine-induced acute pancreatitis. *N Engl J Med* **289**:357, 1973.
21 Hubay CA, Weckesser EC, Levy RP: Occult adrenal insufficiency in surgical patients. *Ann Surg* **181**:325–332, 1975.
22. Steinke J: Management of diabetes mellitus and surgery. *N Engl J Med* **282**:1472–1474, 1970.
23. Mullen JL, Gertner MH, Buzby GP, et al. Implications of malnutrition in the surgical patient *Arch Surg* **114**:121–125, 1979.
24 Christou NV, Meakins JL, MacLean LD The predictive role of delayed hypersensitivity in preoperative patients. *Surg Gynecol Obstet* **152**:297–301, 1981.
25 Powanda MC, Moyer ED: Plasma proteins and wound healing *Surg Gynecol Obstet* **153**:749–755, 1981.
26 Fischer JE, Foster GS, Abel RM, et al: Hyperalimentation as primary therapy for inflammatory bowel disease. *Am J Surg* **125**:165–175, 1973.
27. Bistrian BR, Blackburn GL, Vitale J, et al. Prevalence of malnutrition in general medical patients. *JAMA* **235**:1567–1570, 1976
28. Ota DM, Imbembo AL, Zuidema GD: Total parenteral nutrition *Surgery* **83**:503–520, 1978.
29. Abel RM, Beck CM, Abbott WM, et al Improved survival from acute renal failure after treatment with intravenous essential L-amino acids and glucose. *N Engl J Med* **288**:695–699, 1973.
30. Popp MB, Law EJ, MacMillan BG. Parenteral nutrition in the burned child: A study of twenty-six patients. *Ann Surg* **179**:219–225, 1974
31. Munster AM, Winchurch RA, Keane RM, et al. The "in vitro skin test" A reliable and repeatable assay of immune competence in the surgical patient *Ann Surg* **194**:345–352, 1981
32 Keane RM, Birmingham W, Shatney CM, et al Prediction of sepsis in the multitraumatic patient by assays of lymphocyte responsiveness. *Surg Gynecol Obstet* **156**:163–167, 1983.
33. Hansbrough JF, Bender EM, Zapata-Sirvent R, et al. Altered helper and suppressor lymphocyte populations in surgical patients. *Am J Surg* **148**:303–307, 1984.
34. Tilney NL, Strom TB, Vineyard GC, et al Factors contributing to the declining mortality rate in renal transplantation *N Engl J Med* **299**:1321–1325, 1978.
35 Ketcham AS, Bloch JH, Crawford DT, et al: The role of antibiotic therapy in control of staphylococcal infections following cancer surgery. *Surg Gynecol Obstet* **114**:345–352, 1962
36. Bagley DH, Ketcham AS. Infections and their prevention in surgical cancer patients In Burke JF, Hildick-Smith GY

(eds): *The Infection-Prone Hospital Patient.* Little, Brown, Boston, 1978, pp. 193–208.

37. Burke JF: Host defects caused by surgical operation, in Burke JF, Hildick-Smith GY (eds): *The Infection-Prone Hospital Patient.* Little, Brown, Boston, 1978, pp. 175–181.

38. Boyd RJ, Burke JF, Colton T: A double-blind clinical trial of prophylactic antibiotics in hip fracture patients. *J Bone Joint Surg* **55A:**1251–1258, 1973.

39. Aldrete JA, Daniel W, O'Higgins JW, et al: Analysis of anesthetic-related morbidity in human recipients of renal homografts. *Curr Res* **50:**321–329, 1971.

40. deBros FM, Lai A, Scott R, et al: Pharmacokinetics and pharmacodynamics of Atracurium during isoflurane anesthesia in normal and anephric patients. *Anesth Analg* **65:**743–746, 1986.

41. Nash G: Necrotizing tracheobronchitis and bronchopneumonia consistent with herpetic infection. *Hum Pathol* **3:**283–291, 1972.

42. Stephen M, Loewenthal J: Continuing peritoneal lavage in high-risk peritonitis. *Surgery* **85:**603–606, 1979.

43. Page CP, Ryan JA, Haff RC: Continual catheter administration of an elemental diet. *Surg Gynecol Obstet* **142:**184–188, 1976.

44 Sindelar WF, Mason GR: Irrigation of subcutaneous tissue with povidone–iodine solution for prevention of surgical wound infections. *Surg Gynecol Obstet* **148:**227–231, 1979.

45. Schweizer RT, Kountz SL, Belzer FO: Wound complications in recipients of renal transplants. *Ann Surg* **177:**58–62, 1973.

46 Potter DA, Danforth DN, Macher AM, et al: Evaluation of abdominal pain in the AIDS patient. *Ann Surg* **199:**322–339, 1984

47. Prudden JF, Wolarsky ER, Balassa L: The acceleration of healing. *Surg Gynecol Obstet* **128:**1321–1326, 1969.

48. Christou NV, Superina R, Broadhead M, et al: Postoperative depression of host resistance: Determinants and effect of peripheral protein-sparing therapy. *Surgerx* **92:**786–792, 1982.

49. Czer LSC, Shoemaker WC: Optimal hematocrit value in critically ill postoperative patients *Surg Gynecol Obstet* **147:**363–368, 1978.

50. Clift RA, Sanders JE, Thomas ED, et al. Granulocyte transfusions for prevention of infection in patients receiving bone marrow transplants. *N Engl J Med* **298:**1052–1057, 1978.

51. Workman RD, Faville RJ, Strate RG, et al: Granulocyte transfusions for patients with severe thermal burns. *Transfusion* **18:**142–148, 1978.

52. Saba TM, McCafferty MH, Lanswer ME. Depressed reticuloendothelial function in the surgical patient. *Infect Surg* **2:**124–131, 1983.

53. Border JR, Seibel R, LaDuca J, et al. Trauma and delayed sepsis. In Burke JF, Hildick-Smith GY (eds): *The Infection-Prone Hospital Patient* Little, Brown, Boston, 1978, pp 227–242.

54. McIrvine AJ, O'Mahony JB, Saporoschetz I, et al: Depressed immune response in burn patients. *Ann Surg* **196:**297–304, 1982.

55. Antonacci AC, Reaves LE, Calvano SE, et al: Flow cytometric analysis of lymphocyte subpopulations after thermal injury in human beings. *Surg Gynecol Obstet* **159:**1–8, 1984.

56. Cosimi AB, Burke JF, Russell PS: Transplantation of skin. *Surg Clin North Am* **24:**435–451, 1978.

57. Goodenough RD, Molnar JA, Burke JF: Closure of burn wounds using an artificial skin. *Surg Rounds* **11:**16–22, 1982.

58. Gallico GG, O'Connor NE, Compton CC, et al: Permanent coverage of large burn wounds with autologous cultured human epithelium. *N Engl J Med* **311:**448–467, 1984.

59. Stremple JF, Mori H, Lev R, et al (eds.): The stress ulcer syndrome, in *Current Problems in Surgery.* Vol. 10, no. 4. Year Book Medical, Chicago, 1973, pp. 1–64.

60. LeGall JR, Mignon FC, Rapin M, et al. Acute gastroduodenal lesions related to severe sepsis *Surg Gynecol Obstet* **142:**377–380, 1976.

61. Douglass HO, Falk GA, LeVeen HH: Infection, a cause of acute septic ulceration in hypersecreting animals. *Surgery* **68:**827–830, 1970.

62. Czaja AJ, McAlhany JC, Pruitt BA: Acute gastroduodenal disease after thermal injury; an endoscopic evaluation of incidence and natural history, *N Engl J Med* **291:**925–929, 1974.

63. Martin LF, Max MH. Polk HC: Failure of gastric pH control by antacids or cimetidine in the critically ill: A valid sign of sepsis. *Surgery* **88:**59–68, 1980.

64 Donahue PE, Mobarhan S, Layden TJ, et al: Endoscopic control of upper gastrointestinal hemorrhage with a bipolar coagulation device. *Surg Gynecol Obstet* **159:**113–118, 1984.

65. Nusbaum M, Deren J, Chait A, et al. Angiographic control of bleeding. *Contemp Surg* **23:**79–123, 1983.

66. Drapanas T, Woolverton WC, Reeder JW, et al: Experiences with surgical management of acute gastric mucosal hemorrhage: A unified concept in the pathophysiology. *Ann Surg* **173:**628–640, 1971.

67. Moody FG, Miller TA: Answers to questions on stress ulcer. *Hosp Med* **11:**33–56, 1983.

68. Bubrick MP, Wetherille RE, Onstad GR, et al: Control of acute gastroduodenal hemorrhage with cimetidine. *Surgery* **84:**510–518, 1978.

69. King H, Shumacker HB: Splenic studies. Susceptibility to infection after splenectomy performed in infancy. *Ann Surg* **136:**239–242, 1952.

70. Krivit W, Giebink GS, Leonard A: Overwhelming postsplenectomy infection, *Surg Clin North Am* **59:**223–233, 1979.

71. Malangoni MA, Dillon LD, Klamer TW, et al: Factors influencing the risk of early and late serious infection in adults after splenectomy for trauma. *Surgery* **96:**775–783, 1984.

72. Wilson SA, Johnson WD: Infectious comlicating surgical or functional splenectomy. In Grieco MH (ed). *Infections in the Abnormal Host.* Yorke, New York, 1980, pp 848–865.

73. Barrett J, Sheaff C, Abuabara S, et al. Splenic preservation in adults after blunt and penetrating trauma. *Am J Surg* **145:**313–321, 1983.

74. Tibi P, Ouriel K, Schwartz SI: Splenic injury in the adult: Splenectomy, splenorrhaphy, or nonoperative management. *Contemp Surg* **26:**73–76, 1985.

75 Oakes DD, Charters AC: Changing concepts in the management of splenic trauma *Surg Gynecol Obstet* **153:**181–185, 1981.

Index

Abscess
  brain, nocardiosis and, 246–247
  recurrent, PhisoHex for, 417
Acanthamoeba spp , 309
Acinetobacter spp., CNS infections
    with, 174
Acquired immunodeficiency syndrome
    (AIDS), 3
  and ARC, 381, 386–387
  clinical features of, 388–391
    fever, 389–391
    general, 388–389
  CMV infection in, 358
  CNS infections complicating, 185–
    188
  dermatologic lesions associated with,
    125
  differential diagnosis, 392–394
    in blood product and organ trans-
      plant patients, 393–394
    general, 392
    in homosexual and bisexual males,
      392–393
    in intravenous drug users, 393
    in pediatric age group, 394
    in women, 393
  EBV infection in, 360
  epidemiology
    in Africa and Caribbean, 383–384
    by case definition, 381–382
      in children (provisional), 382
      revisions to, 383
    by surveillance definition, 381–
      382
    in United States and Europe, 382–
      383, 384
  etiologic agents in, 388
  hospital infection control and health
    worker protection, 400
  human T-lymphotropic viruses and,
    376, 381, 384–386
  immunologic abnormalities in, 391
  immunologic features of, 386–387
    ARC, 386–387
    opportunistic infections and/or Ka-
      posi sarcoma, 386
  infectious disease syndromes in, 388
  laboratory studies in, 391
    cultures, 392
    other, 392

Acquired immunodeficiency syndrome
    (AIDS) (*Cont.*)
  laboratory studies in (*Cont.*)
    routine diagnostic, 391
    serologic and immunologic, 391–
      392
  mycobacterial infections in, 237–238
    disseminated *M. avium–intra-*
      cellulare, 238
  P. carinii infection in, 270
    versus non-AIDS patients, differ-
      ences between, 270
  pulmonary infiltrates in, 155–156
  in renal transplant patients, 586–587
  risk groups for, 387–388
  therapy for, 395–400
    general approach, 395
    immunotherapy and antiretroviral,
      400
    infection management, 395–399
  toxoplasmosis in, 288–289
  VZV infection in, 354
Actin dysfunction, in congenital immu-
    nodeficiency syndromes, 430
Acyclovir
  for CMV infection, 357, 359
    following bone marrow transplan-
      tation, 545
  for HSV infection, 351
    following bone marrow transplan-
      tation, 549–550
ADCC. *see* Antibody-dependent cell-
    mediated cytotoxicity
    (ADCC), HSV infection and
3′,5′-Adenosine monophosphate
    (cAMP), as immune-poten-
    tiating substance, 419
Adenoviruses
  case study, 367–368
  cellular immune dysfunction and, 6
  diagnosis, 369
  isolation of, 369
  organ involvement by, 368–369
  in renal transplant patient, 588
Adjuncts, immunologic, to strengthen
    host defense, 413
Adjuvants, immunologic, to strengthen
    host defense, 63
Adrenal insufficiency, surgical con-
    siderations in, 653–654

Adult respiratory distress syndrome
    (ARDS), associated with
    strongyloidiasis, 295
Africa, AIDS incidence in, 383–384
Age, host defense and, 55
Agranulocytosis, infantile lethal, 428
AIDS: *see* Acquired immunodeficiency
    syndrome (AIDS)
AIDS-related complex (ARC), 381,
    386–387
Air. *see also* High-efficiency particulate
    air (HEPA)
  Aspergillus fumigatus in supply,
    132
  microorganisms in, 11–12
  in protective environment: *see* Lami-
    nar airflow rooms
  quality of, 17
Alcoholism, suppressed host-defense
    mechanisms in, 58–59
Allograft, *see also* Renal
    transplantation
  and CMV infection, 577–579
  and preexisting infection in recipient,
    562–564
  transmittal of HIV by, 564–565
Aminoglycosides
  as empirical therapy after bone mar-
    row transplantation, 533
  in fever and septicemia, 100–101
  monitoring, 105
  for systemic therapy, calculation,
    100–101
Amphotericin-B
  for *Candida* infections
    in AIDS patients. 397–398
    as prophylaxis, 26–28
    with Miconazole and Ket-
      oconazole, 29–30
    with fluorocytosine for cryptococcal
      infections in AIDS patients,
      399
Anastomosis, and infection in liver
    transplant patients
  biliary, 606
  vascular, 605–606
Anemia, aplastic. *see* Aplastic anemia
Anesthesia, choice of, 656–657
Angiography, in diagnosis of fever, 90
Antibiotics. *see* Antimicrobial therapy

Antibody
    ability to make, 408–409
    antilymphocyte, immunosuppressive
        effects of, 61
    function in host-defense mechanism,
        408
    in fungal infections, 194–195
    passive, 494
    recovery in bone marrow transplant
        patients, 526
Antibody-dependent cell-mediated
        cytotoxicity (ADCC), HSV
        infection and, 350–351
Antifungal agents, 209–210; see also
        individually named agents
    oral nonabsorbable, 26–30
Antifungal therapy
    agents for, 209–210
        oral nonabsorbable, 26–30
    combined regimens, 211
    empirical, 210–211
    initiation of, 109–111
    granulocyte transfusions, 211–212
    management controversies, 210–212
    optimal dose and duration, 211
    resistant strains, 211
Antigens
    detection systems, in infection diag-
        nosis, 411
    EBV-associated, 361
    in fungal infections, 195
    HBsAg: see HBsAg
Antilymphocyte antibodies, immu-
        nosuppressive effects of, 61
Antimicrobial therapy
    for cardiac transplant patients, 624–
        625
    in childhood cancer, 448–453; see
        also Childhood cancer
        broad- versus narrow-spectrum,
            454–455
        modifications to, 453–454
    in congenital immunodeficiency
        syndromes
        acute infection amelioration, 412–
            413
        chronic infection prevention, 416–
            417
    in documented infection, 107
    in fever and septicemia
        agents used, 100–103
        childhood cancer and: see Child-
            hood cancer, fever in
        continuing versus discontinuing,
            109–111
        monitoring of, 105
        other antibacterial agents used,
            104–105
        recommendation factors, 96–100
        treatment indicators, 95
    following bone marrow
        transplantation
        duration, unresponsive fever and,
            533

Antimicrobial therapy (Cont.)
    following bone marrow
        transplantation (Cont)
        empirical coverage, 533
        prophylactic, 534
    immunosuppressive effects of, 61
    initial versus empirical, 95
    for legionellosis, 318
    for leukemia and lymphoma patients
        prophylactic, 487–488
        systemic, 488–489
    microbial flora shifts and, 9–10
    microbial suppression with, 13–14
    for nocardiosis, 247
    preoperative, 655–656
    and underlying disease, 107
        microbial infection versus fever,
            96
        relationship to outcome, 96
    in undocumented infection, 107–109
Antipseudomonal penicillins, in fever
        and septicemia, 101
Antiretroviral therapy, for AIDS pa-
        tients, 400
Antistaphylococcal therapy, for fever
        and septicemia, 103
Antituberculous agents, for mycobac-
        terial infections
        combined regimens, 242
        first-line, 240–241
        second-line, 241–242
        third-line, 242
Aplastic anemia
        bone marrow transplantation for, 525
        infection patterns in, 468
ARC: see AIDS-related complex (ARC)
ARDS: see Adult respiratory distress
        syndrome (ARDS), associated
        with strongyloidiasis
Aspergillosis
    with Aspergillus spp., 199–200
    case study, 121, 122
    chemoprophylaxis for, 208
    other forms, 201–203
    pulmonary, 200–201
Aspergillus spp.
    in aspergillosis, 199–200
    in bone marrow transplant patients,
        536
        treatment of, 537–541
    in cardiac transplant patients, 638–
        639
    CNS infections with, 178–179
    in renal transplant patients, 597
    fumigatus
        in air supply, 132
        cerebral lesions caused by, 202
        in renal transplant patients, 597
        and transplanted organ rejection,
            558
    granulocytopenia and, 6
        and fever in child, 445
    laminar airflow rooms and, 14
    skin infections with, 121

Aspiration pneumonia, as pre-liver
        transplant infection, 604
Asymptomatic lymphadenitis, 287
Atabrine: see Quinacrine hydrochloride,
        for giardiasis
Ataxia telangiectasia, in immunodefi-
        ciency syndromes, 422
Australia antigen. see HBsAg
Azathioprine, for cardiac transplant pa-
        tients, 623
Aztreonam, recommended dosage and
        properties of, 102–103

B-cell
    immunodeficiency, in congenital im-
        munodeficiency syndromes,
        422–425
    and T-cell defects combined, in im-
        munodeficiency syndromes,
        419–422
Babesiosis, 275–276
    clinical features, 276–277
    laboratory diagnosis, 277–278
    treatment for, 278–279
Babesis spp., 275–276
    divergens, 276
    microti, 277
    versus Plasmodium spp., 276–288
Bacillus Calmette–Guerin (BCG), 222
    vaccine, 236–237
Bacillus spp., CNS infections with, 168
Bacteremia
    in cardiac transplant patients, 625–
        626
    in childhood cancer, 455–457
    defined, 76
    fatal P aeruginosa, by neoplasm, 479
    following bone marrow transplanta-
        tion, 527–528, 529
    in renal transplant patient, 597–599
Bacteria-controlled nursing unit: see
        Protective environment
Bacterial pneumonia, following bone
        marrow transplantation, 528–
        529, 530–532
Bacteriophage ΦX174, immunization in
        bone marrow transplant pa-
        tients, 526
Barriers, body: see Body barriers
BCG: see Bacillus Calmette–Guerin
        (BCG)
Berenil. see Diminazene, for babesiosis
β-Lactam agents
    as antimicrobial therapy, 97–99
    recommended dosage and properties
        of, 102
Betadine, for recurrent abscesses, 417
Biliary anastomotic-related infections,
        following liver transplanta-
        tion, 606
Biotechnology, development of, 3–4
BK virus
    morbidity of, 372
    organ involvement by, 368

Bleomycin lung, 144
Blood culture
    in AIDS patients, 392
    in fever diagnosis, 87–88
    organisms isolated from, following
        bone marrow transplantation,
        528
Blood products
    AIDS and ARC differential diagnosis
        in recipients of, 393–394
    immunosuppressive effects of, 61
Bloodstream, particle clearance from,
    50
Blood transfusions
    and acquisition of non-A, non-B hep-
        atitis, 337–338
    AIDS and ARC differential diagnosis
        in recipients of, 393–394
    hazards posed by, 18
    HIV transmittal by, 564–565
    in pulmonary infection epidemiologic
        history, 135–136
BMT: see Bone marrow transplantation
    (BMT)
Body barriers
    breech in
        avoiding, 34
        host-defense and, 7–8
    skin as: see Skin
Body passages, obstruction of
    host-defense and, 7
    relief of, 34
Body temperature, host-defense and,
    55
Bone marrow biopsy, in fever diag-
    nosis, 90
Bone marrow transplantation (BMT)
    allogeneic
        conditioning regimen for, 525
        interstitial pneumonia etiology fol-
            lowing, 543
    CMV infection following, 358
    fever following, 93
    future considerations, 552–553
    in immunodeficient patients, 418
    infection phases after, 527
        I: early, 527–541
        II: to day 100, 541–550
        III: after day 100, 550–552
    and recovery of host defense, 526–
        527
    syngeneic, 525–526
    as therapy for acute leukemia, 56
Bone scans, in fever diagnosis, 90
Bowel, and complications from immu-
    nosuppressive therapy, 650–
    652
Boyden chamber, and leukocyte motili-
    ty screening, 409
Brain abscess, nocardial, case study,
    246–247
Bronchial brushing, in diagnosis of feb-
    rile pneumonitis syndrome,
    152–153

Bronchoalveolar lavage
    in diagnosis of febrile pneumonitis
        syndrome, 153–154
    in diagnosis of P. carinii pneumonia,
        265
Bronchoscopy, fiberoptic, in diagnosis
    of febrile pneumonitis syn-
    drome, 152
Burn patients, postoperative care for,
    661–663

cAMP: see 3',5'-adenosine monophos-
    phate (cAMP)
Cancer, see also Malignancy, in renal
        transplant patients; Oncology
        patients
    in childhood: see Childhood cancer
    febrile pneumonitis syndrome etiol-
        ogy, 133
    nontuberculous infections in patients
        with, 227
    and tuberculosis
        mimicking, 227–228
        patients with, 227
Candida spp. infection
    in AIDS patients, therapy for, 397–
        398
    albicans
        CMV infection and, 358
        and thymus-dependent portions of
            immune systems, 408
        in bone marrow transplant patients,
            536
        treatment of, 537–541
    in candidiasis, 195
    in cardiac transplant patients, 639–640
    CNS infections with, 177–178
    granulocytopenia and, 6
        and fever in child, 445
    prophylactic agents
        amphotericin-B, 27–30
        antifungal, 25
        clotrimazole, 28
        ketoconazole, 28–30
        miconazole, 28–30
        nystatin, 26–27
    skin infections with, 121, 125
    tropicalis, in bone marrow transplan-
        tation patient, case study,
        539–541
Candidiasis
    and Candida organism, 195
    cardiac, 197
    cerebromeningeal, 199
    chemoprophylaxis for prevention of,
        207–208
    chronic mucocutaneous, in congenital
        immunodeficiency syndromes,
        423
    disseminated, 196
    fungemia, 196–197
    gastrointestinal, 197–198
    oral and esophageal, therapy for
        AIDS patients, 397–398

Candidiasis (Cont.)
    osteoarticular, 199
    other forms, 199
    pulmonary, 199
    urinary tract, 198
Capreomycin, for mycobacterial infec-
    tions, 242
Cardiac candidiasis, 197
Cardiac transplantation
    infection following
        in first month, 624–629
        from 1-6 months posttransplant,
            629–635
        fungal, 637–641
        Legionella spp., 636–637
        nocardial and mycobacterial,
            641
        Pneumocystis carinii, 635–636
        toxoplasmosis, 642–643
    with lung, infectious disease prob-
        lems with, 644
    selection criteria for patients and do-
        nors, 624
    success factors in, 623
    surgical considerations for, 643
Caribbean, AIDS incidence in, 383–
    384
Carrier populations, of HBsAg, 328
Catheters
    indwelling, in childhood cancer,
        455–457
    infection associated with, manage-
        ment of, 105–106
    microbial flora shifts and, 10
    tolerance by renal transplant patients,
        568
Cefotaxime
    as antimicrobial therapy, 98–99
    recommended dosage and properties
        of, 102
Ceftazidime, recommended dosage and
    properties of, 101–102
Cell-mediated immunity
    in CVD, 509
    and herpesvirus infections, 347
        T-lymphocyte, 351
    recovery in bone marrow transplant
        patients, 526
    in tuberculosis pathogenesis, 225
Cellular immune dysfunction
    host-defense and, 6–7
    prophylactic therapies for, 31–
        33
Cellular immunity
    activated macrophages, 53
    defective, 53–54
    initiation, 52–53
    T-lymphocytes, 53
Cellular-mediated immunity see Cell-
    mediated immunity
Centers for Disease Control (CDC)
    HIV classification, 400–401
    surveillance criteria for AIDS, 381–
        382

Central nervous system (CNS) infections, *see also* Meningitis; *individual infectious agents*
  with *Acinetobacter* spp., 174
  in AIDS patients, 185–188
  approach to patient with, 184–188
  with *Aspergillus* spp., 178–179
    fumigatus, in renal transplant patient, 597
  with *Bacillus* spp., 168
  bacterial, 166–174
  with *Candida* spp., 177–178
  clinical presentation with, 184–188
  with CMV, 183
  with *Coccidioides immitis*, 176–177
  and Coxsackie virus involvement, 374
  with *Cryptococcus neoformans*, 88, 123–125, 175–177, 204–205
    in renal transplant patient, 597
  with *Enterobacter* spp., 174
  with *Escherichia coli*, 173
  fungal, 174–181
  gram-negative cocci in, 174
  gram-negative rods in, 172–174
  gram-positive cocci in, 170–172
  gram-positive rods in, 166–170
  with *Hemophilus influenzae*, 174
  with *Histoplasma capsulatum*, 177
  with HSV-1 and HSV-2, 182–183
  with *Klebsiella pneumoniae*, 173
  with *Legionella pneumophila*, 307
  with *Listeria monocytogenes*, 166–168
    in renal transplant patient, 595–596
  and measles virus involvement, 375
  microorganisms causing, 166–174
  with *Mucoraceae* spp., 180–181
  with *Mycobacterium* spp., 170
  with *Neisseria meningitidis*, 174
  with *Nocardia asteroides*, 168–170
  organisms causing, 165–166
  with papovaviruses, 183–184
  parasitic, 181–182
  with *Proteus* spp., 173–174
  with *Pseudomonas aeruginosa*, 172–173
  in renal transplant patients, 595–597
  with *Staphylococcus aureus*, 171
  with *Staphylococcus epidermidis*, 171–172
  with *Streptococcus pneumoniae*, 170–171
  with *Strongyloides stercoralis*, 181–182
  therapy for, 169
  with *Toxoplasma gondii*, 181
  viral, 182–184
  with VZV, 183
Cephalosporines
  for cardiac transplant patients, 624–625
  as empirical therapy after bone marrow transplantation, 533

Cephalosporines (*Cont.*)
  in fever and septicemia, 101–103
  third generation, dosage and properties of, 102
Cerebral spinal fluid (CSF)
  examination in CNS infections, 184–185
  lactate levels, in diagnosis of meningitis, 412
Cerebromeningeal candidiasis, 199
CGD: *see* Chronic granulomatous disease (CGD)
cGMP. *see* 3',5'-guanosine monophosphate (cGMP), as immune-potentiating substance
Chediak–Higashi syndrome, 431
Chemiluminescence (CL) assay, in phagocyte metabolism assessment, 409
Chemoprophylaxis
  in aspergillosis prevention, 208
  in candidiasis prevention, 207–208
  for mycobacterial infections, 238–240
Chemotaxis
  defects, in congenital immunodeficiency syndromes, 428–430
    in neonates, 431–432
  of polymorphonuclear (PMN) leukocytes, altered in CVD, 509
Chemotherapy
  antineoplastic
    differential diagnosis for fever following, 483
    and infection susceptibility, 470
  for childhood cancers, 442
  granulocytopenia following, 5–6
  hepatitis in oncology patients receiving
    B, 335–337
    non-A, non-B, 338
  and induction of pulmonary disease, 143
  for mycobacterial infections, 240
  of VZV infections, 356
Chickenpox, 354
Childhood, immunizations in, 494
Childhood cancer
  versus adult cancers, 439–441
  by age and site, 440
  fever in, 442–443; *see also* Fever, in granulocytopenic child
    antimicrobial agents used, 448–453
      broad- versus narrow-spectrum, 454–455
      duration, 463–464
    bacteremia and, 455–457
    diagnostic evaluation, 445
      invasive procedure role in, 459–461
    and foreign body management, 457–459
    indwelling catheters and, 455–457
    modified therapy, 453–454
    surgery as option, 462–463

Childhood cancer (*Cont.*)
  host-defense perturbations and, 442
  and infection interface, 441
  infectious complications in, 439
  prognostic categories, 441
Children, *see also* Infants; Neonates; congenital immunodeficiency syndromes in
  AIDS in
    and ARC differential diagnosis, 394
    case definition, 381, 382
  with cancer. *see* Childhood cancer
  fever in
    for "average" child, 439
    for granulocytopenic child: *see* Fever, in granulocytopenic child
  immunizations for, 494
Chloramphenicol, in treatment of fever and septicemia, 104
Chorioretinitis, CMV infection and, 575–576
Chronic benign neutropenia, 428
Chronic granulomatous disease (CGD)
  in congenital immunodeficiency syndromes, 430–431
  life-threatening infection in, 410
Chronic mucocutaneous candidiasis, in congenital immunodeficiency syndromes, 423
CIE: *see* Counterimmunoelectrophoresis (CIE), for antigen detection
Ciprofloxacin, prophylactic trials with, 24
Cirrhosis, hepatic, suppressed host-defense mechanisms in, 58–59
CL: *see* Chemiluminescence (CL) assay, in phagocyte metabolism assessment
Clindamycin
  for babesiosis, 279
  in toxoplasmosis therapy, 292
  in treatment of fever and septicemia, 104
Clofazimine, and *M avium* complex isolates, 398
Cloroquine, for babesiosis, 278–279
Clotrimazole, prophylaxis of *Candida* infections, 28
CMV: *see* Cytomegalovirus (CMV) infection
Coccidial infections, 292–295
Coccidioides immitis
  cellular immune dysfunction and, 6
  CNS infections with, 176–177
  in coccidioidomycosis, 205
Coccidioidomycosis
  with *Coccidioides immitis*, 205
  other forms, 205–206
  in pneumonia, 205
Coccidiomycosis spp., in bone marrow transplant patients, 536

Colistin, prophlyactic, for leukemia and lymphoma patients, 487
Collagen vascular disease (CVD), 503, see also Rheumatoid arthritis; Systemic lupus erythematosus (SLE)
  host–microorganism interactions in, 503–505
  infection in patients with, 514–515
    management, 520–521
      clinical examples, 515–520
    morbidity and mortality caused by, 505–507
    and other infection interactions, 504
    spectrum, 511–514
Colon, and complications from immunosuppressive therapy, 650–652
Colonization
  gram-negative, respiratory tract and, 132
  pattern of, 41
  resistance to, 10–11, 41
Combined immunodeficiency disease, severe, 419–421
Common variable hypogammaglobulinemia, 425
Complement fixation test, in diagnosis of P. carinii pneumonia, 266
Complement system
  cascade, 43
  component deficiencies
    in congenital immunodeficiency syndromes, 409, 425–426
      alternative pathway, 427
      C3 and C5, 426–427
      C6, C7, and C8, 427
      early classic pathway, 426
      life-threatening infection in, 410
    in CVD, 507–508
  as host-defense mechanism, 43–44
Conditioning regimens, prior to allogeneic bone marrow transplantation, 525
Congenital ichthyosis, 428–429
Congenital immunodeficiency syndromes, 407–409
  B-cell immunodeficiency, 423–425
  combined B- and T-cell defects, 419–422
  complement component deficiencies, 425–427
  phagocyte abnormalities, 427–432
  pure T-cell defects, 422–423
  screening tests in, 410
  therapeutic aim in, 410–419
    chronic infection prevention, 416–419
    cutaneous, 415–416
    gastrointestinal, 415
    in life-threatening infections, 410–413
    respiratory, 414–415

Congenital neutropenias
  chronic benign, 428
  with hypogammaglobulinemia with increased IgM, 428
  infantile lethal agranulocytosis, 428
Congenital toxoplasmosis, 287
Cooked food diet, in infection prevention, 17
Corticosteroids
  as risk factor for Legionella infection, 309
  as support in P. carinii pneumonia, 271
Cosmetics, exogenous organisms in, 12
Cost-effectiveness, in clinical practice, 3
Cough
  in Legionella pneumonia, 310–311
  in Pneumocystis carinii pneumonia, 260
Counterimmunoelectrophoresis (CIE), for antigen detection, 411–412
Coxsackie virus, 373–374
  organ involvement by, 368
Cryptococcal meningitis, in AIDS patients, 398–399
Cryptococcosis
  case study, 124–125
  in CNS, 204–205
  with Cryptococcus neoformans, 204
  other forms, 205
Cryptococcus spp.
  in bone marrow transplant patients, 536
    treatment of, 537–541
  and fever in granulocytopenic child, 445
  neoformans
    in cardiac transplant patients, 640–641
    cellular immune dysfunction and, 6
    CNS infections with, 175–176, 204–205
      in AIDS patients, 187–188, 398–399
    in renal transplant patients, 597
    skin infections with, 123–125
    in renal transplant patients, 601–603
Cryptosporidia spp., 253
  in AIDS patients, therapy for, 398
  cellular immune dysfunction and, 6
  infections involving, 292–295
Cryptosporidiosis
  in AIDS patients, therapy for, 398
  following bone marrow transplantation, 550
CSF: see Cerebral spinal fluid (CSF)
Cultures
  in AIDS patients, 392
  in fever diagnosis, 87–89
  following bone marrow transplantation, organisms isolated, 528
  in fungal infection diagnosis, 194

Cutaneous infections: see Skin infections
CVD: see Collagen vascular disease (CVD)
CY: see Cyclophosphamide (CY), in conditioning regimen prior to bone marrow transplantation
Cyclophosphamide (CY), in conditioning regimen prior to bone marrow transplantation, 525
Cycloserine, for mycobacterial infections, 242
Cyclosporine, in conditioning regimen prior to bone marrow transplantation, 525
Cyclosporins
  A, immunosuppressive effects of, 61
  for cardiac transplant patients, 623
Cytomegalovirus chorioretinitis, 575–576
Cytomegalovirus (CMV) infection
  in AIDS patients
    affecting CNS, 188
    therapy for, 398
  in cardiac transplant patients, 630–631
    and infectious disease syndromes, 631–632
    management, 633
    superinfection and, 632–633
  case study, 356
  cellular immune dysfunction and, 6–7
  of CNS, 183
    in AIDS patients, 188
  diagnosis and therapy, 359
  epidemiology and patterns, 356–358
  in febrile pneumonitis syndrome, 156
  and fever in granulocytopenic child, 444–445
  following bone marrow transplantation
    associated with pneumonia, 531–532, 544–546
    manifestations of, 548–549
    treatment, 545
  in liver transplant patients, 607–608
  pathogenesis, 358–359
  in renal transplant patients, 569–570
    allograft dysfunction, 577–579
    clinical management, 580–582
    epidemiology, 570–571
    factors influencing, 571–573
    and infectious disease syndromes, 573–575
    malignancy occurrence, 579–580
    superinfection and host-defense suppression, 575–577
Cytotoxic chemotherapeutic agents, in pulmonary disease induction, 143
Cytotoxic drugs, immunosuppressive effects of, 60–61

Decontamination, in infection prevention, 17–18
Defense systems, see also Host defense
  cellular, 46–54
  humoral, 42–46
Defervescence, in FUO in leukemia and lymphoma, 474–475
Dental hygiene, microbial suppression, 31
Dermacentor spp., 276
Dermatologic manifestations of infection, in renal transplant patients, 600–603, see also Skin infections
DFA: see Direct fluorescent-antibody (DFA) test, in diagnosis of Legionella pneumonia
DHPG: see 9-1-(1,3-dihydroxy-2-propoxymethyl)guanine (DHPG), for CMV infection
Diabetes mellitus, suppressed host-defense mechanisms in, 57–58
Dialysis, tuberculosis risk in patients, 228–229
Diet, low microbial, 17–18; see also Nutrition
DiGeorge syndrome, 422–423
9-1-(1,3-Dihydroxy-2-propoxymethyl)guanine (DHPG)
  for CMV infection, 359, 398
  retinitis in AIDS patients and, 188
Diminazene, for babesiosis, 279
Direct fluorescent-antibody (DFA) test, in diagnosis of Legionella pneumonia, 316
Dirty linens, shaking of, 17
Disinfectants, in infection prevention, 17
Disseminated candidiasis, 196
Disseminated mycobacterial infection, and hematologic abnormalities, 233–236
Disseminated nontuberculous mycobacteriosis, 235–236
DNA viruses, morbidity due to, 367–373; see also individually named viruses
  adenoviruses, 367–369
  papovaviruses, 369–372
  vaccinia, 372–373
Donor
  heart, selection criteria, 624
  kidney, infection from, 564–566
Down syndrome
  congenital immunodeficiency syndromes and, 431
  HBsAg in, 328
Drug-induced pneumonitis, 141–144
Drug users, intravenous, AIDS and ARC differential diagnosis in, 393
Dual infection, in legionellosis, 315
Dyspnea
  in Legionella pneumonia, 311

Dyspnea (Cont)
  in Pneumocystis carinii pneumonia, 260

EBV: see Epstein–Barr virus (EBV) infection
Echo virus, 373–374
  organ involvement by, 368
Eczema herpeticum, in HSV infection, 349
Education
  for hepatitis prevention, 338–339
  patient, 34
  staff, 34
Eimeria spp., 283, 292
Electron microscopy, of P carinii, 255–257
Empirical therapy
  alteration to, 103–104
    in childhood cancer, 453–454
  antibiotic, following bone marrow transplantation, 533
  antifungal, 109–111, 210–211
  circumstances for, 155
  in CNS infections, 186
  versus initial therapy, 95
  recommendations for, 96–100
Encephalitis
  IF_α as therapy for, 375
  measles virus and, 375
Endocytosis, 47, 49–50
  primary defects, 51–52
Enterobacter spp.
  associated with strongyloidiasis, 295
  cloacae, in cardiac transplant patients, 624, 641
  CNS infections with, 174
Environment
  affecting normal patients, 408
  cofactors in HIV infection, 386
  and Legionella in water supply, 309
  protective: see Protective environment
Eosinophils, kinetics of, 47, 48
Epstein–Barr virus (EBV) infection
  in cardiac transplant patients, 634–635
  case study, 359–360
  cellular immune dysfunction and, 6
  and childhood cancer risk, 441
  diagnosis and therapy, 361–362
  epidemiology and patterns, 360
  pathogenesis, 360–361
  in renal transplant patients, 583–584
Erythrocyte sedimentation rate (ESR), limited usefulness, 91
Erythromycin
  for legionellosis, 318–319
  prophylactic trials with, 23
Escherichia coli
  CNS infections with, 173
  and fever in granulocytopenic child, 443–444
  granulocytopenia and, 6

Esophageal candidiasis, in AIDS patients, therapy for, 397–398
Esophagitis, in HSV infection, 349
ESR: see Erythrocyte sedimentation rate (ESR), limited usefulness
Ethambutol, for mycobacterial infections, 241
Ethionamide, for mycobacterial infections, 242
Europe, AIDS incidence in, 382–383
Exogenous organisms, sources of acquisition, 11–13
Extrapulmonary legionellosis, 307, 313
  infectious, 314
  noninfectious, 313–314
Extrapulmonary tuberculosis, 232
  case study, 232–233

Fansidar: see Sulfonamide
5-FC: see 5-Fluorocytosine (5-FC)
Febrile pneumonitis syndrome; see also Pulmonary infection
  definitive diagnosis, 149–150
    by conventional sputum examination, 150–151
    by immunologic techniques, 150
    by invasive techniques, 152–155
    by transtracheal aspiration, 151–152
  diagnostic possibilities, 133–134
  etiology, 133
  importance of, 131–134
  noninfectious, diagnostic clinical clues, 140
    drug-induced, 141–144
    neoplastic invasion, 144–145
    other causes, 145–147
    radiation, 140–141
  radiologic diagnostic clues, 147–149
  and superinfection, 156–157
Febrile prodrome, as AIDS clinical feature, 388–389
Felty syndrome, suppressed host-defense mechanisms in, 59
Females, AIDS and ARC differential diagnosis in, 393
Fetal liver transplants, in immunodeficient patients, 418
Fever, 75; see also Infection
  in AIDS
    causes of, 389
    clinical approach to, 389–391
  antibody measurements and skin tests, 89
  antistaphylococcal semisynthetic penicillins and, 103
  clinical approach to, 85–87
  in CMV infection, 357
  criteria for, 75
  diagnostic procedures
    invasive, 90–91
    of limited usefulness, 91
    noninvasive, 89–90

Fever (*Cont*)
  in granulocytopenic child; *see also*
    Childhood cancer, fever in
    antimicrobial therapy for
      broad- versus narrow-spectrum,
        454–455
      duration, 463–464
      modifications to, 453–454
      starting regimen, 448–453
    causes of, 443–445
    diagnostic evaluation, 446–447
    management of, 463–464
    surgery as option, 462–463
  in "average" child, 439
  in *Legionella* pneumonia, 311
  in leukemia and lymphoma, *see also*
    Leukemia; Lymphomas
    causes of, 474–477
    incidence data problems, 473–474
  microbial infection versus, 94–95
  and neoplasia, 94
  occult intraabdominal sources of,
    652–653
  pathogenesis of, 76–78
  persistent and/or recurrent, 77–78
    with negative cultures, diagnostic
      considerations, 91–94
  pneumonitis and: *see* Febrile pneu-
    monitis syndrome
  pulmonary infiltrates versus, differ-
    ential diagnosis, 139
  specific laboratory studies, 87
  from sulfonamide drugs, in AIDS pa-
    tients, 390
  suppression of, 106–107
  syndrome-oriented approach to, 78
  of undetermined origin (FUO), 75–
    76, 463–464
    cultures for, 392
    defervescence and, 474–475
    prophylactic granulocyte transfu-
      sions and, 535
Fiberoptic bronchoscopy, in diagnosis
  of febrile pneumonitis syndrome, 152
  combined with other procedures, 153
  complications from, 154
Fibronectin, as host-defense mechanism, 44
Fibrosis, postinfection, with *P. carinii*
  pneumonia, 272–275
Flagy 1: *see* Metronidazole
5-Fluorocytosine (5-FC)
  amphotericin-B with, for cryptococ-
    cal infections in AIDS pa-
    tients, 399
  as antifungal therapy, 209–210
Folinic acid, in toxoplasmosis therapy,
  291
Food
  cooked versus uncooked, 17
  exogenous organisms in, 11
Foreign bodies
  bloodstream clearance, 50

Foreign bodies (*Cont.*)
  management of, 457–459
  tolerance by renal transplant patients,
    568
FRACON: *see* Framycetin, colistin,
  and nystatin (FRACON), prophylactic trials with
Framycetin, colistin, and nystatin
  (FRACON), prophylactic trials with, 23
Fungal infections, *see also individually
  named fungi*
  antibody detection, 194–195
  antifungal therapy, 209–212
  antigen or fungal metabolite detec-
    tion, 195
  in cardiac transplant patients, 637–
    641
  cultures, 194
    in diagnosis of fever, 88–89
  diagnostic approach, 193–195
  as fever cause in granulocytopenic
    child, 445
  following bone marrow transplanta-
    tion, 536–537
    diagnosis and treatment, 537–541
  future perspectives, 212
  histology, 194
  incidence, 193
  opportunistic, underlying diseases in,
    481
  prevention, 207–208
  in renal transplant patients, 599
  of skin, 123–124
  systemic mycotic, 122–123
Fungemia, 196–197
FUO: *see* Fever, of undetermined origin (FUO)
Furazolidone, for giardiasis, 282
Fusarium spp
  infection with, 207
  solanii, and fever in gran-
    ulocytopenic child, 445

Gallium scans, in diagnosis of fever,
  89–90
Gancyclovir: *see* 9-1-(1,3-dihydroxy-2-
  propoxymethyl)guanine
  (DHPG), for CMV infection
Gastroenteritis, from adenovirus infection, 369
Gastrointestinal bleeding, postoperative
  care for, 663–665
Gastrointestinal infections
  from *Candida* spp., 197–198
  in congenital immunodeficiency syn-
    dromes, therapy for, 415
Genetics, host-defense and, 54
Gentamicin, vancomycin, and nystatin
  (GVN) regimen
  infection prevention, 13–14
  and laminar airflow room combined,
    14–15
  microbial flora suppression, 10

Giardia lamblia, in giardiasis, 279–
  282
Giardiasis, 279
  clinical manifestations, 281
  in the compromised host, 281
  diagnosis, 281–282
  epidemiology, 280
  and *Giardia* spp., 279
  pathogenesis, 280–281
  treatment, 282
Glucocorticosteroids, immunosuppressive effects of, 60
Gomori methenamine silver nitrate
  stain, 255
Government, cost-effective medicine
  and, 3
Graft-versus-host disease (GvHD)
  and bone marrow transplantation
    late infections following, 551–552
    prevention, 525–526
  CMV and, in granulocytopenic child,
    444
  fever and, 93
  host-defense recovery in, 527
  and pneumonia incidence, 544
  protective environment and, 535
Granulocytes
  loss in bone marrow transplant pa-
    tients, 526
  neutrophilic, kinetics of, 47
Granulocyte transfusions, 15–16
  as antifungal therapy, 211–212
  following bone marrow
    transplantation
    prophylactic, 535–536
    therapeutic, 534
  human response to, 491–493
  studies, 491–493
  as prophylaxis, 493–494
Granulocytopenia
  bacteremia associated with, following
    bone marrow transplantation,
    527–528
  duration, 25
  and autopsy-proven fungal infec-
    tion in bone marrow trans-
    plantation patients, 537
  host-defense and, 5–6
  microbial suppression in, 18–19
  prophylactic transfusions: *see* Gran-
    ulocyte transfusions
  "standard" reverse isolation, 16
Griseofulvin therapy, 429
3',5'-Guanosine monophosphate
  (cGMP), as immune-potentiating substance, 419
GvHD: *see* Graft-versus-host disease
  (GvHD)
GVN regimen: *see* Gentamicin, vancomycin, and nystatin (GVN)
  regimen

Handwashing, in infection prevention,
  18

HBLV: *see* Human B-lymphotropic virus (HBLV)
HBsAg
findings in oncology patients receiving chemotherapy, 336–337
in hepatitis B virus infection, 326, 327–328
Heart donor, selection criteria, 624
Heart–lung transplants, infectious disease problems with, 644, *see also* Cardiac transplantation
Helminth, cellular immune dysfunction and, 6
Hemodialysis units, hepatitis infection in
HBV, 329–330
non-A, non-B, 330
Hemophilus influenzae
CNS infections with, 174
dual infection with legionellosis, 315
humoral immune dysfunction and, 7
opsonization of, 51
Hemorrhage, versus infection plus hemorrhage, 472
HEPA: *see* High-efficiency particulate air (HEPA)
Hepatic cirrhosis, suppressed host-defense mechanisms in, 58–59
Hepatitis, 327–329
A, incidence of, 325
from adenovirus infection, 368
B
antigens, 326, 327–328; *see also* HBsAg
clinical expression, 326
hazards to medical personnel, 329
in hemodialysis units, 329–330
immune responses, 326–327
immunoprophylaxis for, 339
in oncology patients receiving chemotherapy, 335–337
pathogenesis, immunologic mechanisms in, 326–327
in renal transplant patients, 331–333
categories, 325
in liver transplant patients, 608
non-A, non-B
hazards to medical personnel, 330
in hemodialysis units, 330
in oncology patients, 337–338
pathogenesis, immunologic mechanisms in, 327
in renal transplant patients, 333–335
in organ transplant patients, 330–331
prevention, 338–340
survival rates, in renal transplant patients, 332, 334
Herpes simplex virus (HSV) infection
in AIDS patients, therapy for, 399
in cardiac transplant patients, 633–634
case study, 347

Herpes simplex virus (HSV) infection (*Cont.*)
cellular immune dysfunction and, 6–7
of CNS, 182–183
diagnosis and therapy, 351
epidemiology and patterns, 348–350
and fever in granulocytopenic child, 444–445
following bone marrow transplantation, 550
site isolation, 548
pathogenesis, 350–351
prophylaxis for, 32–33
in renal transplant patients, 347–348, 584–585
sputum cytology, 349
Herpesviruses, 347; *see also individually named viruses*
in cardiac transplant patients, 633–635
in renal transplant patients, 583–588
and thymus-dependent portions of immune systems, 408
High-efficiency particulate air (HEPA), 13
for fungal infection prevention, 208
Histoplasma spp.
in bone marrow transplant patients, 536
capsulatum
cellular immune dysfunction and, 6–7
CNS infections with, 177
in histoplasmosis, 206
skin infections with, 123
Histoplasmosis
disseminated, 206
with *Histoplasma capsulatum*, 206
primary infection, 206
HIV: *see* Human immunodeficiency virus (HIV)
Hodgkin disease
antibody response in, 471
immunologic abnormalities in, 470
microbial pathogens involvement in, 480–482
and VZV infection, 353
Homosexual males, AIDS and ARC differential diagnosis in, 392–393
Host defense, 1
age and, 55
in AIDS patients, 155
antibody function in, 408
body temperature and, 55
in bone marrow transplant patients, recovery of, 526–527
childhood cancer and infection risk, 442
and CMV infection in renal transplant patients, 575–577
congenital defect in, 407–409; *see also* Congenital immunodeficiency syndromes

Host defense (*Cont*)
defects in, 5–8
causes, 650
as contributing factor to infections in CVD, 507–509
surgical management and, 650
in diabetes mellitus, 57–58
disease affecting, 56–60
genetic control of, 54
immunosuppressive agents and, 60–61
mechanisms, 42
cellular, 46–54
humoral, 42–46
mucosal, 41–42
skin, 41
and mycobacterial infection, 223
nutritional status and, 54–55
in *Pneumocystis carinii* pneumonia, 258
predisposition to pulmonary infection and, 139
radiation and, 61–62
strengthening, 62–63
in congenital immunodeficiency syndromes therapy, 413
Host–microorganism interactions, in CVD, 503–505
Host resistance: *see* Host-defense
HSV: *see* Herpes simplex virus (HSV) infection
HTLV: *see* Human T-lymphotropic virus (HTLV)
Human B-lymphotropic virus (HBLV), 362
Human immunodeficiency virus (HIV); *see also* Human T-lymphotropic virus (HTLV)
CDC classification, 400–401
differential diagnosis
in blood product and organ transplant patients, 393–394
general, 392
in homosexual and bisexual males, 392–393
in intravenous drug users, 393
in pediatric age group, 394
in women, 393
environmental cofactors, 386
etiologic in AIDS, 385
versus HTLV-I and HTLV-II, 385
infection model, 385–386
laboratory studies, 391
cultures, 392
other, 392
routine diagnostic, 391
serologic and immunologic, 391–392
mononuclear phagocyte infection by, 385
in renal transplant patients, 586–587
risk groups for, 387–388
transmittal by kidney allograft, 564–565
tropism of, 386

Human T-lymphotropic virus (HTLV)
AIDS and, 376
morbidity from, 376
type I and II, versus HIV, 385
type III, and CNS disease in AIDS
patients, 185–186
Humoral immune dysfunction
host-defense and, 7
prophylactic therapies for, 33–34
Humoral immunity
legionellosis and, 308
leukemia and, 469–470
Hyperalimentation line, following bone
marrow transplantation, 533
Hyperimmunoglobulinemia
in congenital immunodeficiency
syndromes
A, 429–430
E, 429
M, hypogammaglobulinemia associated with, 424
Hypogammaglobulinemia
common variable, 425
diagnostic criteria for, 408
and hyperimmunoglobulinemia M association, 424
neutropenia with, 428
sex-linked, 424
transient, of infancy, 423

Ichthyosis, congenital, 428–429
Idiopathic interstitial pneumonia, in
bone marrow transplant patients, 547–548
IF$_\alpha$: see α-interferon (IF$_\alpha$)
IFA: see Indirect fluorescent-antibody
(IFA) test, in diagnosis of
Legionella pneumonia
IFNs: see Interferons (IFNs), as host
defense mechanisms
Imidazoles, as antifungal therapy, 210
Imipenem, recommended dosage and
properties of, 102–103
Immune dysfunction
CNS infection and, 165–168
host-defense and
cellular, 6–7
humoral, 7
Immune response
cell-mediated, in VZV infections,
355
in chickenpox and zoster, 354
of CVD patients to immunosuppressive therapy, 510
to hepatitis B virus, 326–327
Immune serum globulin (ISG), 355
Immunity, cellular: see Cellular
immunity
Immunization
in childhood, 494
for influenza, 494
pneumococcal, 494–497
response in bone marrow transplant
patients, 526

Immunodeficiency disease, severe combined, (SCID), 419–421
Immunodeficiency syndromes
acquired: see Acquired immunodeficiency syndrome (AIDS)
congenital: see Congenital immunodeficiency syndromes
Immunogenicity, of hepatitis B vaccine, 339–340
Immunoglobulins
abnormal homeostasis in CVD, 508–509
cellular immunodeficiency with, in
congenital immunodeficiency
syndromes, 422
as host-defense mechanism, 45–46
IgA, in congenital immunodeficiency
syndromes, 424–425
IgG, to strengthen host defense, 62–63
IgM
in congenital immunodeficiency
syndromes, 424
for detecting Toxoplasma spp.
antibodies, 290
recovery levels in bone marrow
transplant patients, 526
Immunology, in diagnosis of febrile
pneumonitis syndrome, 150
Immunoprophylaxis, 494–497; see also
Prophylaxis
Immunosuppression
chronic requirements for, 559
in renal and liver transplant patients,
559
Immunosuppressive therapy
in cardiac transplant patients, 623
colonic complications from, 650–652
and predisposition to infection, in
CVD patients, 509–511
standard protocols for adults, 558
and suppressed host-defense mechanisms, 60–61
Immunotherapy, 494–497
for AIDS patients, 400
in congenital immunodeficiency syndromes, 417–419
Indirect fluorescent-antibody (IFA) test,
in diagnosis of Legionella
pneumonia, 316
Indwelling catheters, management of,
455–457
and foreign bodies compared, 457–459
Infantile lethal agranulocytosis, 428
Infants, see also Children
lethal agranulocytosis in, 428
transient hypogammaglobulinemia in,
423
Infection, see also individually named
infectious agents
and cancer interface, 441
catheter-associated, management of,
105–106

Infection (Cont.)
chronic, prevention in congenital immunodeficiency syndromes,
416–419
control in hospitals, 400; see also
Laminar airflow rooms; Prevention techniques; Protective
environment
cutaneous, in congenital immunodeficiency syndromes, 415–416
development probability, 22
disease: see Infectious diseases
documented
antimicrobial therapy duration in,
107
empirical therapy alteration following, 103–104
and underlying disease therapy,
107
dual, in legionellosis, 315
fatal, in hematologic malignancies,
477
gastrointestinal, in congenital immunodeficiency syndromes, 415
health worker protection, 400
immunoprophylaxis and immunotherapy of, 494–497
incidence data problems in leukemia
and lymphoma, 473–474
life-threatening, in congenital immunodeficiency syndromes,
410–413
mimicking neoplasm, 79
occult intraabdominal sources of,
652–653
organism origins, 8–13
acquisition reduction, 17–18
exogenous acquisition, 11–13
microbial flora shifts, 9–11
prevention techniques: see Prevention
techniques
pyogenic, minimizing effects of, 414
and rejection of transplanted organ,
557–560
respiratory, in congenital immunodeficiency syndromes,
414–415
of skin: see Skin infection
suppressed host-defense mechanisms
in, 59–60
surgical considerations: see Surgery
syndromes of: see Infectious disease
syndromes
undocumented, antimicrobial therapy
and, 107–109
Infectious disease syndromes, 78–79
in AIDS, 388
produced by CMV
in cardiac transplant patients, 631–632
in renal transplant patients, 573–575, 576
Infectious diseases
heart–lung transplants and, 644

Infectious diseases (Cont)
  in renal transplant patients
    bacteremia, 597–599
    of CNS, 595–597
    dermatologic manifestations, 600–603
    fungal, 599
    tuberculosis and atypical mycobacterial, 599–600
  and SLE and rheumatoid arthritis, symptoms compared, 504
  syndromes of: see Infectious disease syndromes
Infiltrates, pulmonary: see Pulmonary infiltrates
Inflammation, phagocyte kinetics during, 47
Influenza, immunization against, 494
INH: see Isoniazid (INH)
α-interferon (IF₀)
  for CMV infection, 356, 359
    following bone marrow transplantation, 545
  for measles encephalitis, 375
Interferons (IFNs), as host-defense mechanism, 44–45
Interstitial pneumonia, in bone marrow transplant patients, 541–544
  case study, 543–544
  diagnosis, 542
  etiology, 543
  idiopathic, 547–548
  incidence, 541–542
Intraarterial line-related sepsis
  as pre-liver transplant infection, 605
  renal transplant patients and, 568
Intracellular killing
  defects, 52
  phagocytosis and, 50
Intramedullary rods, management of, 458
Intraoperative considerations
  anesthesia and patient-monitoring, 656–657
  surgical techniques, 657–659
Intravenous drug users, AIDS and ARC differential diagnosis in, 393
Intravenous line-related sepsis
  as pre-liver transplant infection, 605
  renal transplant patients and, 568
Intraventricular Ommaya reservoir, management of, 458
ISG: see Immune serum globulin (ISG)
Isolation, see also Protective environment
  and GVN regimen combined, 14–15
  for infection prevention, 13
  P. carinii pneumonia and, 271–272
  for prevention of fungal infection, 208
  reverse, 13
Isoniazid (INH)
  in management of mycobacterial infections, 240–241

Isoniazid (INH) (Cont.)
  prophylaxis in tuberculosis patients, 228, 238–240
Isospora belli, 253
  in AIDS patients, therapy for, 398
  infections involving, 292–295
Ixodes spp., 276

JC virus
  case study, 369–370
  organ involvement by, 368
  in PML, 370–372
Job syndrome, 429

Kanamycin, for mycobacterial infections, 242
Kaposi sarcoma, in AIDS patients, 156, 386
  onset, 389
  surveillance criteria for, 381–382
Ketoacidosis, infection and, surgical considerations, 654
Ketoconazole, for Candida infections, 28–30
  in AIDS patients, 398
Keyhole limpet hemocyanin, immunization in bone marrow transplant patients, 526
Kidney donor, infection from, 564–566
Klebsiella spp.
  and fever in granulocytopenic child, 443–444
  pneumoniae
    CNS infections with, 173
    dual infection with legionellosis, 315
    granulocytopenia and, 6
    in pulmonary infection epidemiologic history, 138

Lactoferrin, as host-defense mechanism, 42–43
Laminar airflow rooms
  and GVN regimen combined, 14–15
  reverse isolation in, 13
Laparotomy, in diagnosis of fever, 90–91
Latex agglutination, for antigen detection, 411, 412
LAV. see Lymphadenopathy-associated virus (LAV)
"Lazy-leukocyte" syndrome, 428
Legionella pneumonia, see also Legionellosis
  extrapulmonary complications, 307, 313
    infectious, 314
    noninfectious, 313–314
  immunology, 308
  laboratory findings, 311
  pathology and pathogenesis, 307–308
  radiographic findings, 311–313
  signs, 311
  symptoms, 310–311

Legionella spp., see also Legionella pneumonia
  bozemanii, 306
  in cardiac transplant patients, 636–637
  cellular immune dysfunction and, 6
  classification, 305–306
  cultural and biochemical characteristics, 306–307
  infection with: see Legionella pneumonia, Legionellosis
  longbeachae, 306
  micdadei, 305, 306
    nosocomial infection with, 310
    signs and symptoms associated with, 310–311
  morphology, 306
  pneumophila, 305
    nosocomial infection with, 310
    signs and symptoms associated with, 310–311
  recognized species, 306
Legionellosis, see also Legionella pneumonia
  diagnosis
    approach to patient, 316–317
    differential, 314–315
    of dual infection, 315
    specific, 315–316
  ecological considerations, 309
  general considerations, 309
  nosocomial, 309–310
  prevention and control, 319
  treatment
    animal studies and, 317–318
    antimicrobial efficacy, determination of, 318
    course of, 318–319
    recommendations for, 318
    retrospective studies and, 317
Lesions, dermatologic, associated with AIDS, 125
Lethal CMV syndrome, 574
Leukemia
  beneficial effects of hepatitis virus on, 338
  fever in, 474–477
  infections in, 467–468
    host defenses against, 468–471
    immunoprophylaxis and immunotherapy of, 494
    incidence data problems in neutropenic states, 473–474
    mortality from, 471–473
    neutrophil transfusions, 490–494
    and splenectomized patient, 489–490
    summation of problems associated with, 482–486
    therapeutic strategies, 486–489
  and lymphoma, different therapeutic approaches to, 486
  microbial pathogen(s) involvement and nature in, 477–482

Leukemia (*Cont.*)
suppressed host-defense mechanisms in, 56
tuberculosis in, 233–234
Leukoagglutinin reactions, 146–147, 148
Leukocyte motility, defects in, screening for, 409
Leukopenia
in AIDS, 386
in renal transplant patients, 574
Levamisole, as immune-potentiating substance, 419
Life-threatening infection, in congenital immunodeficiency syndromes, 410–413
Limb-sparing, management of, 457–458
Limulus lysate test
for diagnosis of meningitis, 412
limited usefulness of, 91
Limulus polyphemus, 91
Listeria monocytogenes
cellular immune dysfunction and, 6–7
CNS infection with, 166–168
in renal transplant patients, 595–596
Lithium therapy, to strengthen host-defense, 63
Liver disease, in renal transplant patients, 591–594
Liver failure, symptoms suggesting, 604
Liver function tests, abnormal, in renal transplant patients, 574
Liver transplantation
determinants of patient outcome in, 557
diseases potentially treatable by, 604
infection in, 603
in first month post-liver transplant, 605–606
after first month posttransplant, 607–608
pre-liver transplant-related, 603–605
Lung, bleomycin, 144
Lung biopsy, *see also* Open lung biopsy
in diagnosis of febrile pneumonitis syndrome
open, 152, 154
transpleural, 154
in *P. carinii* pneumonia, 264, 265
Lung lavage, as support in *P. carinii* pneumonia, 271
Lung transplantation, heart and, infectious disease problems with, 644
Lymphadenitis, asymptomatic, 287
Lymphadenopathy-associated virus (LAV), 381; *see also* Human immunodeficiency virus (HIV); Human T-lymphotropic virus (HTLV)

Lymphangiography, in diagnosis of fever, 90
Lymphoceles, prevention of, 567
Lymphocyte-mediated immunity, recovery in bone marrow transplant patients, 526
Lymphomas
fever in, 474–477
infections in, 467–468
host-defense against, 468–471
immunoprophylaxis and immunotherapy of, 494–497
incidence data problems, 473–474
mortality from, 471–473
neutrophil transfusions, 490–494
and splenectomized patient, 489–490
summary of problems associated with, 482–486
therapeutic strategies, 486–489
and leukemia, different therapeutic approaches to, 486
microbial pathogen(s) involvement and nature in, 477–482
suppressed host-defense mechanisms in, 56
Lysozyme, as host-defense mechanism, 42–43

Macrophages
activated, 53
lymphoma and, 470–471
T-lymphocyte interaction, 52
and uptake of bacteria, 50
Madomycosis, 244
Malaria, 253
Malignancy, in renal transplant patients
effect of CMV on, 579–580
and virus relationship, 583
Malnutrition, infection and, surgical considerations, 654
Mantoux test, 223
Marrow transplantation: *see* Bone marrow transplantation (BMT)
Measles
morbidity from, 374–375
organ involvement by, 368
Mebendazole, in strongyloidiasis therapy, 297–298
Meningeal tuberculosis: *see* Extrapulmonary tuberculosis
Meningitis, *see also* Central nervous system (CNS) infections
clinical presentation, 185
cryptococcal, in AIDS patients, therapy for, 398–399
diagnostic tests for, 412
organisms causing, 165–168
Meningoencephalitis, organisms causing, 165–168; *see also*

Meningoenchephalitis (*Cont*)
Central nervous system (CNS) infections
Metabolites, in fungal infections, 195
Methotrexate (MTX), in conditioning regimen prior to bone marrow transplantation, 525
Metronidazole
for giardiasis, 282
for *Trichomonas vaginalis* infection, 282
Miconazole, prophylaxis of *Candida* infections, 28–30
Microbes, survival, 11
Microbial antigen detection, 411–412
Microbial flora, shifts in, factors causing, 9–11
Microbial modulation, selective: *see* Selective microbial modulation
Microbicidal defects, in congenital immunodeficiency syndromes, 430–432
Monocyte chemotactic deficiency, in congenital immunodeficiency syndromes, 430
Monocytes, lymphoma and, 470–471
Mononuclear phagocyte system (MPS), 47, 49
Mononuclear phagocytes
defect, CNS infection and, 167
HIV infection of, 385
kinetics of, 47, 49
MPS: *see* Mononuclear phagocyte system (MPS)
MTX: *see* Methotrexate (MTX), in conditioning regimen prior to bone marrow transplantation
Mucoraceae, CNS infections with, 180–181
Mucormycosis
with *Mucoraceae* spp , 203
other forms, 204
pulmonary, 203–204
rhinocerebral, 203
Mucosa, as first line in host defense, 42
Mycobacteria, *see also* Tuberculosis
in AIDS, 237–238
atypical
management of, 242–243
in renal transplant patients, 599–600
in cardiac transplant patients, 641
classification and microbiology, 221–223
clinical features, 229–238
epidemiology, 226–229
host-defense, 223
infection management, 238–243
by ancillary therapeutic modalities, 242
by antituberculous agents, 240–242; *see also* Antituberculous

Mycobacteria (*Cont.*)
  infection management (*Cont.*)
    agents, for mycobacterial in-
      fections; *individually named*
      agents
      of atypical mycobacteria, 242–243
    by chemoprophylaxis, 238–240
    by chemotherapy, 240
    pathogenesis, 224–226
    skin testing for, 223–224
    virulence, 226
Mycobacteriosis, disseminated nontuberculous, 235–236
Mycobacterium spp.
  avium-intracellulare, 222–223
    in AIDS patients, 237–238, 390
      therapy for, 398
    in cancer patients, 227
    cellular immune dysfunction and, 6
    management of, 243
  bovis, 221–222
  chelonei, management of, 243
  CNS infections with, 170
  fortuitum, 222–223
    in cancer patients, 227
    management of, 243
  kansasii, 222
    in cancer patients, 227
    management of, 242–243
  leprae, 222
    rifampin in management of, 241
  mavinum, management of, 242–243
  scrofulaceum, 222
  skin infections with, 120
  tuberculosis, 221–222
    in AIDS patients, therapy for, 398
    antituberculous agents against,
      240–242
    versus atypical mycobacteria, 225–
      226
    cellular immune dysfunction and,
      6–7
  xenopi, in AIDS patients, 237
Myeloperoxidase deficiency
  in congenital immunodeficiency syn-
    dromes, 431
  testing for, 409

Naegleria, 309
Nalidixic acid, prophylactic trials with,
  22
Natural killer (NK) cells, as host-
  defense mechanism, 52
NBT: *see* Nitroblue tetrazolium (NBT)
  dye-reduction test
Needle aspiration, in diagnosis of febrile pneumonitis syndrome,
  153
Neisseria meningitidis, CNS infections
  with, 174
NEOCON: *see* Neomycin, colistin, and
  nystatin (NEOCON)
Neomycin, colistin, and nystatin (NEO-
  CON), prophylactic trials
  with, 21

Neonates, congenital immunodeficiency
  syndromes in, 431–432
Neoplasia
  fever and, 94
  mycobacterial infection and, 226–
    227
Neoplastic disease
  fatal *P aeruginosa* bacteremia by,
    479
  frequency of opportunistic pathogens
    by, 480
  infection mimicking, 79
  prevalence of tuberculosis by, 480
Neoplastic pulmonary invasion,
  144-145, 146
Neutropenia
  after bone marrow transplantation,
    527–528, 529
  in AIDS, 386
  congenital: *see* Congenital
    neutropenias
  with defective chemotaxis and hyper-
    immunoglobulinemia A, 429–
    430
  and fever and infection incidence in
    leukemia and lymphoma,
    473–474
  fever in, infection documentation for,
    474
Neutrophilic granulocytes, kinetics of,
  47
Neutrophils
  acute leukemia and, 468–469
  defect in, CNS infection and, 167
  transfusions, for leukemia and lym-
    phoma patients, 490–494
Nitroblue tetrazolium (NBT) dye-reduction test
  limited usefulness, 91
  phagocyte activity assessment by,
    409
NK: *see* Natural killer (NK) cells, as
  host-defense mechanism
Nocardia spp., 243
  asteroides
    in air samples, 244
    in cardiac transplant patients, 641
    cellular immune dysfunction and,
      6
    clinical importance of, 243
    CNS infections with, 168–170
  brasiliensis, 243, 244
  in cardiac transplant patients, 641
  classification and microbiology, 243–
    244
  clinical features and diagnosis, 244–
    245
    case studies, 245–247
  epidemiology and pathogenesis, 244
  and infection by related organisms,
    247–248
  skin infections with, 123, 125
  therapy, 247
Nocardiosis
  brain abscess, case study, 246–247

Nocardiosis (*Cont*)
  clinical features and diagnosis of,
    244–245
  pulmonary, case study, 245–246
  therapy for, 247
Non-A, non-B hepatitis
  in oncology patients, 337–338
  pathogenesis, 327
Noncytotoxic chemotherapeutic agents.
  in pulmonary disease induc-
    tion, 143
Nonvirulent fungi, skin infection and,
  118–119
Norfloxacin, prophylactic trials with,
  23–24
Nosocomial legionellosis, 309–310
Nutrition
  host-defense and, 54–55
  parenteral, and management of in-
    dwelling catheters, 455–457
Nystatin, prophylactic
  for *Candida* infections, 26–27
  in FRACON regimen, 23
  in GVN regimen: *see* Gentamicin,
    vancomycin, and nystatin
    (GVN) regimen
  for leukemia and lymphoma patients,
    487, 488

Obstruction, of natural body passages,
  7
Occult miliary tuberculosis, 234–235
Ommaya reservoir, management of,
  458
Oncology patients, *see also* Cancer
  hepatitis B in, 335–337
  non-A, non-B hepatitis in, 337–338
Oocysts
  of *Isospora belli*, 293
  of *T. gondii*, 283–284
Open lung biopsy
  in cardiac transplant patients, 628
  in diagnosis of febrile pneumonitis
    syndrome, 152, 154
  in diagnosis of *P. carinii* pneumonia,
    264, 265
Ophthalmic zoster, 352
Opportunistic infections
  AIDS with, 386
    clinical features of, 388–389
    common etiologic agents, 396
  fungal, underlying diseases in, 481
  in transplant populations, 552–553
Opportunistic pathogens, 2–3; *see also*
  Opportunistic infections
  CNS infection from, 165–168
  fever and, 80, 84
  fungal
    infection prevention, 207–208
    and nocardial infections, 123–125
  by neoplastic disease, frequency of,
    480
  in respiratory tract, 132
  skin infections with, 120–121,
    123

Oral candidiasis, in AIDS patients, therapy for, 397–398
Oral mucositis, severity of, 549
Organ transplantation
    AIDS and ARC differential diagnosis in recipients of, 393–394
    determinants of patient outcome, 557
    heart: see Cardiac transplantation
    hepatitis infection in recipients of, 330–331
    in immunodeficient patients, 418
    and infection
        classification, 560
        from donor, 564–566
    kidney: see Renal transplantation
    liver. see Liver transplantation
    lung, heart and, 644
    thymus: see Thymus transplantation
Organisms
    exogenous, sources of acquisition, 11–13
    isolated from blood culture after bone marrow transplantation, 528
Orifice, body, obstruction of, host-defense and, 7
Osteoarticular candidiasis, 199

Paecilomyces, skin infections with, 120
p-aminosalicylic acid (PAS), for myco-bacterial infections, 242
Pancytopenia, tuberculosis in, 233–234
Papillomavirus
    involving skin, 118, 119
    morbidity of, 372
    organ involvement by, 368
Papovaviruses, 369
    BK, 372
    CNS infections with, 183–184
        in AIDS patients, 188
    JC, 369–372
    organ involvement by, 368
    papillomavirus: see Papillomavirus
    in renal transplant patient, 587–588
Paramyxoviruses, morbidity from, 374–375
    measles, 374–375
    organ involvement, 368
    respiratory syncytial virus, 375
Parasites, 253, see also individually named organisms
Parenteral nutrition, and management of indwelling catheters, 455–457
PAS: see p-aminosalicylic acid (PAS), for mycobacterial infections
Passive antibody, 494
Pathogens, see also individually named organisms
    involvement and nature, in leukemia and lymphoma, 477–482
    opportunistic. see Opportunistic pathogens, individually named pathogens
    potential, suppression of, 18–31

Patient-monitoring techniques, choice of, 656–657
Penicillins
    as empirical therapy after bone mar-row transplantation, 533
    in fever and septicemia
        antipseudomonal, 101
        antistaphylococcal semisynthetic, 103
Pentamidine
    for babesiosis, 279
    as therapy for P. carinii pneumonia, 267
        administration and dosage, 267–268
Percutaeous biopsy, in cardiac trans-plant patients, 627–628
Peritonitis, spontaneous bacterial, as pre-liver transplant infection, 604–605
Petryllidium boydii, as cause of fever in granulocytopenic child, 445
Phagocytes, see also Phagocytic cells
    abnormalities, in congenital immu-nodeficiency syndromes, 427
        chemotactic, 428–430
        congenital neutropenic, 428
        microbicidal, 430–431
        in neonates, 431–432
        testing for, 409
    functions
        deficient, 51–52
        other, 50–51
    kinetics during inflammation, 47
    mononuclear: see Mononuclear phagocytes
Phagocytic cells
    development of, 48
    as host-defense mechanism, 47–52
    in leukemics, 469
Phagocytosis, 49–50
    and intracellular killing, 50
    in neonates, 431–432
Phenolic disinfectants, in infection pre-vention, 17
PhisoHex, for recurrent abscesses, 417
Picornaviruses, morbidity from, 373–374
    Coxsackie and ECHO viruses, 373–374
    organ involvement by, 368
    poliomyelitis, 373
Plants, exogenous organisms and, 11
Plasma, as adjunct to antimicrobial therapy, 413
Plasmodium spp., Babesis spp. versus, 276–277
PML· see Progessive multifocal leuk-oencephalopathy (PML), JC virus and
Pneumococcal polysaccharide, immu-nization in bone marrow transplant patients, 526

Pneumococcus spp.
    humoral immune dysfunction and, 7
    vaccine, 33–34
    immunization against, 494–495
Pneumocystis carinii pneumonia, 253
    in AIDS patients, 386, 389–391
        management of, 395–397
        versus non-AIDS patients, differ-ences between, 270
    in cardiac transplant patients, 628–629, 635–636
    clinical features (non-AIDS related), 259–261
    diagnostic approaches, 263–266
    epidemiology and transmission, 258–259
    following bone marrow transplanta-tion, 528, 530, 546–547
    histopathology, 257
    historic perspective, 254
    host-defense mechanisms, 258
    isolation, 271–272
    and Pneumocystis organism, 254–257
    and pneumocystosis in humans and animals, 257–258
    postinfection fibrosis, 272–275
    predisposing factors, 258
    prophylaxis, 271–272, 275
    radiologic features, 251–263
    treatment of, 266–270, 275
        in AIDS patients, 270
        new therapy, 270–271
        and other supportive meaures, 271
Pneumocystis spp.
    in AIDS patients, 389–391
    carinii
        in AIDS patients, 155
        cellular immune dysfunction and, 6–7
        diagnosed by invasive procedures, 153–154
        and fever in granulocytopenic child, 445
        pneumonia: see Pneumocystis carinii pneumonia
        prophylaxis for, 31–32
        and VZV infection, 355
    jirovecii, 254
Pneumocystosis, conditions associated with, 257–258
Pneumonia, see also Pulmonary infection
    from adenovirus infection, 368
    in cardiac transplant patients, 626–629
    CMV, in renal transplant patients, 573–574
    coccidioidomycosis and, 205
    diagnostic approach, 649–650
    following bone marrow transplantation
        bacterial, 528–529, 530–532
        CMV-associated, 531–532, 544–546

Pneumonia (*Cont*)
  interstitial, 541–544
    idiopathic, 547–548
  Pneumocystis carinii, 546–547
  giant cell, measles virus and, 375
  Legionella. see *Legionella*
    pneumonia
  Pneumocystis carinii: see *Pneumocystis carinii* pneumonia
Pneumonitis
  drug-induced, 141–144
  febrile syndrome: see Febrile pneumonitis syndrome
  radiation: see Radiation pneumonitis
Poliomyelitis, 373
  organ involvement by, 368
Polyenes, as antifungal therapy, 209
Polymorphonuclear (PMN) leukocytes
  altered chemotaxis in CVD, 509
  lymphoma and, 470–471
Polymyxin B, prophlyactic, for leukemia and lymphoma patients, 487
Polypharmacy, nonspecific, for *P carinii* pneumonia, 264–265
Postinfection fibrosis, with *P. carinii* pneumonia, 272–275
Postoperative care
  of burn and trauma patients, 661–663
  following splenectomy, 665
  of gastrointestinal bleeding, 663–665
  general, 661
  and respiratory management, 659–661
Postprimary tuberculosis: see Reactivation tuberculosis
PPD: see Purified protein derivative (PPD)
Prednisone, for cardiac transplant patients, 623
Preoperative preparation, 653
  in adrenal insufficiency, 653–654
  in ketoacidosis, 654
  in malnutrition, 654
Prevention techniques
  complex, 13–16
  ineffective, 16
  for leukemia and lymphoma patients, 486–487
  simplified, 16–18
Primary varicella, mortality from, in children, 444
Prodrome, febrile, as AIDS clinical feature, 388–389
Progressive multifocal leukoencephalopathy (PML), JC virus and, 370–372
Prophylaxis, *see also*
    Chemoprophylaxis,
    Immunoprophylaxis
  antimicrobial
    for bone marrow patients, 534
    for leukemia and lymphoma, 487–488

Prophylaxis (*Cont*)
  in cardiac transplant patients, 624–625
  for CMV infection, 359
  fungal, 25, *see also* Antifungal agents
  granulocyte transfusions as, 15–16
    after bone marrow transplantation, 493–494
  hepatitis B vaccine, 339–340
  by immunization, 494–497
  neutrophil transfusions as, 490–494
  for *P. carinii* pneumonia, 271–272
  trimethoprim–sulfamethoxazole trials, 19–24, *see also* Trimethoprim–sulfamethoxazole
  of varicella, with VZIG, 356
Protective environment, *see also* Laminar airflow rooms; Prevention techniques
  for bone marrow transplant patients, 534–535
  for burn or trauma patients, 661–663
  for leukemia and lymphoma patients, 486–487
Proteus spp., CNS infections with, 173–174
Prototheca, skin infections with, 120–121
Protozoa, *see also individually named organisms*
  as cause of fever in granulocytopenic child, 445
  cellular immune dysfunction and, 6
  coccidial, 253
    infections involving, 292–295
  infections from, following bone marrow transplantation, 550
  Legionella growth within, 309
Pseudoallescheria boydii, infection with, 207
Pseudomonas spp
  aeruginosa
    associated with strongyloidiasis, 295
    as cause of fever in granulocytopenic child, 443–444
    CMV infection and, 358
    CNS infections with, 172–173
    fatal bacteremia by neoplasm, 479
    granulocytopenia and, 6
    immunization with, 495–497
    in renal transplant patients, 131–132
    skin infections with, 122
    sepsis, from donor, 565
Pulmonary aspergillosis, 200–201
Pulmonary candidiasis, 199
Pulmonary disease, chemotherapeutic agents inducing, 143
Pulmonary emboli, as cause of fever, 93
Pulmonary infection, *see also* Febrile pneumonitis syndrome; Pneumonia

Pulmonary infection (*Cont*)
  diagnostic clues
    clinical, 138–140
    epidemiologic, 134–138
  in liver transplant patients, 607
  predisposition to, 139
Pulmonary infiltrates
  after bone marrow transplantation, 528–529, 530–532
  in AIDS patients, 155–156
  in febrile child with cancer, 460–461
  versus fever, differential diagnosis, 139
  in *Legionella* pneumonia, 311–313
  in *Pneumocystis carinii* pneumonia, 261–263, 264
Pulmonary invasion, neoplastic, 144–145, 146
Pulmonary mucormycosis, 203–204
Pulmonary nocardiosis, 245–246
Pulmonary tuberculosis, 229
  case study, 231–232
Purified protein derivative (PPD), 223–224
  INH prophylaxis and, 239
Purine pathway enzyme deficiences, in immunodeficiency syndromes, 421
Pyogenic infection
  in leukemics, 468
  minimizing effects of, 414
Pyrazinamide, for mycobacterial infections, 242
Pyrimethamine
  as therapy for *P. carinii* pneumonia, 268
  for toxoplasmosis, 291, 399

Quinacrine hydrochloride, for giardiasis, 282
Quinine, for babesiosis, 279
Quinolones, fluorinated, for leukemia and lymphoma patients, 488

Rabbit antithymocyte globulin (RATG), for cardiac transplant patients, 623
Radiation, *see also* Total-body irradiation (TBI)
  immunosuppressive effects of, 61–62
  as therapy, granulocytopenia following, 5–6
Radiation pneumonitis, 140–141, 142
  radiologic clues in, 149
Radiology
  in diagnosis of febrile pneumonitis syndrome, 147, 149
  radiation pneumonitis and, 149
Rapid methenamine silver stain, 256
RATG: see Rabbit antithymocyte globulin (RATG), for cardiac transplant patients
Reactivation tuberculosis, 226, 230–231
Rejection, and infection, 557–560

Renal failure, chronic
  hemodialysis in, hepatitis B infection
    and, 329–330
  suppressed host-defense mechanisms
    in, 58
Renal transplantation
  determinants of patient outcome in,
    557
  and febrile pneumonitis syndrome
    etiology, 133
  infection following
    adenoviruses, 588
    bacteremia, 597–599
    CMV, 356, 357, 569–582; see
      also Cytomegalovirus (CMV)
      infection
    CNS, 595
      by Aspergillus fumigatus, 597
      by Cryptococcus neoformans,
        597
      by Listeria monocytogenes,
        595–596
    dermatologic manifestations, 600–
      603
    from donor, 564–566
    EBV, 360, 583–584
    fungal, 599
    hepatitis, 331–335
    HIV (AIDS), 586–587
    HSV, 347–348, 584–585
    other causes in first month,
      568
    papovaviruses, 587–588
    preexisting, 562–564
    timetable, 560–562
      in first month, 560–561, 562–
        569
      in 1-6 months posttransplant,
        561–562, 569–594
      more than 6 months post-
        transplant, 562, 594
    tuberculosis and atypical mycobac-
      terial, 228, 599–600
    urinary tract, 588–591
    VZV, 354, 585–586
    from wound, 566–568
  Legionella and, 309
  liver disease and, 591–594
  P. carinii and, 271
  Pseudomonas aeruginosa and, 131–
    132
Reservoir, intraventricular Ommaya,
  management of, 458
Resistant strains, antifungal therapy
  and, 211
Respiratory infections, in congenital
  immunodeficiency syndromes,
  therapy for, 414–415
Respiratory secretions, in diagnosis of
  Legionella pneumonia, 315–
  316
Respiratory syncytial virus (RSV)
  morbidity from, 375
  organ involvement by, 368
Retinitis, in AIDS patients, 188

Retrovirus
  and childhood cancer risk, 441
  defined, 384–385
  human lymphotropic, 384–386; see
    also Human immunodeficien-
    cy virus (HIV); Human
    T-lymphotropic virus (HTLV)
  therapy against, for AIDS patients,
    400
Reverse isolation, 13
  "standard," 16
Rheumatoid arthritis
  immunologic abnormalities in, 508
  and infection
    as cause of death, 507
    as cause of morbidity, 506
    features, 514
    spectrum, 512
    susceptibility to, factors associated
      with, 511
  and infectious diseases, symptoms
    compared, 504
  painful knee in patient with, 519–
    520
  suppressed host-defense mechanisms
    in, 59
Rhinocerebral mucormycosis, 203
Rhizopus, skin infections with, 121
Rifampin
  for legionellosis, 318
  for mycobacterial infections, 241
  in treatment of fever and septicemia,
    105
RNA viruses, morbidity of, see also in-
    dividually named viruses
  human T-lymphotropic viruses, 376
  organ involvement by, 368
  paramyxoviruses, 374–375
  picornaviruses, 373–374
  rotaviruses, 375–376
Rods, intramedullary, management of,
  458
Rotaviruses
  morbidity from, 375–376
  organ involvement by, 368
  therapy for, 376
RSV. see Respiratory syncytial virus
  (RSV)

Salmonella
  in AIDS patients, 390
  cellular immune dysfunction and,
    6
Sarcosporidia spp , 283
Scanning, in infection diagnosis, 411
SCID: see Severe combined immu-
    nodeficiency disease (SCID)
Selective immunoglobulin deficiency,
    in congenital immunodeficien-
    cy syndromes
  IgA, 424–425
  IgM, 424
Selective microbial modulation
  disadvantages of, 24–25
  regimens compared, 21–23

Sepsis
  following splenectomy, 665
  line-related
    as pre-liver transplant infection,
      605
    renal transplant patients and, 568
    Pseudomonas, from donor, 565
    wound-related: see Wound infections
Septic arthritis, 513–514
Septicemia, see also Fever
  antistaphylococcal semisynthetic pen-
    icillins and, 103
  arthritis, 513–514
  defined, 76
  organisms implicated in, 478
Severe combined immunodeficiency
    disease (SCID), 419–421
Sex-linked hypogammaglobulinemia,
    424
SGOT determination, in tuberculous
    patients, 240
SIADH: see Syndrome of inappropriate
    antidiuretic hormone secretion
    (SIADH), in granulocytopenic
    child
Sickle cell anemia, suppressed host-
    defense mechanisms in, 57
Skin
  as barrier to infection, 115–117
  exogenous organisms and, 12
  as first line in host-defense, 41
  microbial suppression, 30–31
  testing, in mycobacterial infection,
    223–224
Skin infections
  associated with AIDS, 125
  conditions for, 115–116
  in congenital immunodeficiency syn-
    dromes, therapy for, 415–416
  corticosteroids and, 116–117
  diagnostic aspects of, 125–126
  localized and disseminated, 116
  nonvirulent fungi, 118–119
  primary
    with common pathogens, 117
    opportunistic, 120–121
  in renal transplant patient, categories
    of, 600–603
  systemic, metastatic to cutaneous and
    subcutaneous sites, 121–125
  types, 117
  viral, 117–118
SLE: see Systemic lupus erythematosus
  (SLE)
Spiramycin, in toxoplasmosis therapy,
    292
Spleen, role in childhood cancers, 442
Splenectomy
  approach to leukemia and lymphoma
    patients following, 489–490
  and bacteremia in renal transplant pa-
    tients, 598–599
  sepsis following, 665
  suppressed host-defense mechanisms
    in, 56–57

Spontaneous bacterial peritonitis, as pre-liver transplant infection, 604–605
Sputum
  cytology in HSV infection, 349
  in diagnosis of febrile pneumonitis syndrome, 150–151
  in diagnosis of *Legionella* pneumonia, 315–316
Staining, and *P. carinii* pneumonia
  diagnosis of, 265–266
  techniques, 255–256
Staphylococcal coagglutination, for antigen detection, 411, 412
Staphylococcus spp.
  aureus
    CNS infections with, 171
    granulocytopenia and, 6
    and fever in child, 443–444
  epidermidis
    CNS infections with, 171–172
    and fever in granulocytopenic child, 443–444
Steroid therapy, side effects and complications of, 654
Streptococcus pneumoniae
  CNS infections with, 170–171
  dual infection with legionellosis, 315
  humoral immune dysfunction and, 7
  opsonization of, 51
  in pulmonary infection epidemiologic history, 136, 137
Streptomycin, for mycobacterial infections, 241–242
Strongyloides stercoralis
  cellular immune dysfunction and, 6
  CNS infections with, 181–182
  as posttransplant infection, 563
  in pulmonary infection epidemiologic history, 135
  in strongyloidiasis, 295–298
Strongyloidiasis, 295
  clinical manifestations, 295–297
  diagnosis, 297
  with *Strongyloides stercoralis*, 295
  treatment, 297–298
Substitution, to strengthen host-defense, 62
Sulfonamide, *see also* Trimethoprim–sulfamethoxazole
  AIDS patients and
    fever due to, 390
    hypersensitivity to, 397
  for nocardiosis, 247
  for *P. carinii* pneumonia, 268
  for toxoplasmosis, 291
Superinfection, 156
  case study, 156–157
  and CMV infection, 357, 358
    in cardiac transplant patients, 632–633
    in renal transplant patients, 575–577
Supplementation, to strengthen host-defense, 62

Surgery, 649
  with adrenal insufficiency, 653–654
  CNS infection and, 168
  considerations in cardiac transplant patients, 643
  and diagnostic approach to infection, 649–653
  in febrile child with cancer, 462–463
  intraoperative considerations, 656–659
  postoperative management, 659–665
  preoperative preparation, 653–656
    antibiotics in, 655–656
  and wound-related sepsis prevention, 566–567
Surveillance criteria, for AIDS, 381–382
Surveillance culture, following bone marrow transplantation, 529, 531
Surveillance sites, and invasive fungus infection, 537
Syndrome of inappropriate antidiuretic hormone secretion (SIADH), in granulocytopenic child, 444
Syndrome(s): *see individually named syndromes*
Systemic lupus erythematosus (SLE)
  abdominal pain in patient with, 518–519
  altered mental state in patient with, 515–516
  immunologic abnormalities in, 508
  and infection
    as cause of death, 507
    as cause of morbidity, 506
    features, 514
    spectrum, 512
    susceptibility to, factors associated with, 511
  and infectious diseases, symptoms compared, 504
  pleuritic chest pain and fever in patient with, 516–518
  suppressed host-defense mechanisms in, 59
Systemic mycotic infection, 122–123

T-cell-mediated immunity, and herpesvirus infections, 351
T-cells
  defects, in congenital immunodeficiency syndromes
    combined with B-cell defects, 419–422
    pure, 422–423
  phenotypic profiles
    in AIDS, 386
    in ARC, 387
T-lymphocytes, 53
  in EBV infection, 361
  and macrophage interaction, 53
  testing for abnormalities, 408

T-lymphocytes (*Cont.*)
  thymus-derived. *see* Thymus-derived T-lymphocytes
  in VZV infections, 355
T4 molecule, viral attachment and, 385
TBI: *see* Total-body irradiation (TBI)
Temperature, *see also* Fever
  body, host-defense and, 55
  elevation pathway, 77
Tetracyclines
  for babesiosis, 279
  for legionellosis, 318
  in treatment of fever and septicemia, 105
Tetrahymena spp., 309
Thiabendazole, in strongyloidiasis therapy, 297–298
Thymosin, 418
Thymus-dependent immune system, infections and, 408
Thymus-derived T-lymphocytes
  CNS infection and, 167
  leukemia and, 469
Thymus transplantation
  fetal, 418
  to strengthen host-defense, 63
Ticks, transmittal of *Babesis* spp. by, 276
Torulopsis glabrata
  in bone marrow transplant patients, 539
  granulocytopenia and, 6
Total-body irradiation (TBI), 525
  and interstitial pneumonia incidence, 541
Total joint arthroplasty (TJA), 514
Toxoplasma gondii, *see also* Toxoplasmosis
  in cardiac transplant patients, 642–643
  cellular immune dysfunction and, 6–7
  CNS infections with, 181, 282
    in AIDS patients, therapy for, 399
Toxoplasmosis, 282–283
  in AIDS patients, 288–289
  in cardiac transplant patients, 642–643
  CNS involvement
    in AIDS patients, therapy for, 399
    diagnostic approach to, 290–291
  in compromised host, 286, 287–288
  congenital, 287
  diagnosis, 289–290
  following bone marrow transplantation, 550
  history, 283
  pathogenesis, 285–286
  prevention of, 292
  serodiagnostic tests for, 289–290
  signs and symptoms in immunologically intact patients, 286–287
  therapy for, 291–292
  and *Toxplasma* spp., 283–285

Transfer factor, 418
Transfusions
  blood: *see* Blood transfusions
  granulocyte: *see* Granulocyte
      transfusions
  of neutrophils for leukemia and lym-
      phoma patients, 490–494
Transient hypogammaglobulinemia, of
    infancy, 423
Transplantation: *see* Organ
    transplantation
Transpleural lung biopsy, in diagnosis
    of febrile pneumonitis syn-
    drome, 154
Transtracheal aspiration (TTA)
  in diagnosis of febrile pneumonitis
      syndrome, 151–152
  in diagnosis of *Legionella* pneu-
      monia, 315–316
  in diagnosis of *P. carinii* pneumonia,
      265
Trauma patients, postoperative care for,
    661–663
Trephine biopsy technique, in diagnosis
    of febrile pneumonitis syn-
    drome, 153
Trichinella spp., 283
Trichomonas vaginalis infection, metro-
    nidazole for, 282
Trichosporon spp.
  begelii, and fever in gran-
      ulocytopenic child, 445
  infection with, 207
Trimethoprim–sulfamethoxazole
  for babesiosis, 279
  for chronic infection prevention, 417
  for legionellosis, 318
  prophylactic
    and antimicrobial therapy com-
        pared, 20–21
    for bone marrow transplant pa-
        tients, 534, 546
    with ciprofloxacin, 24
    and control group compared, 19–
        20
    with erythromycin, 23
    and FRACON compared, 23
    against GvHD, 552
    for leukemia and lymphoma pa-
        tients, 487–488
    and nalidixic acid compared, 21–
        23
    with norfloxacin, 23–24
  as therapy for *P. carinii* pneumonia,
      264–265, 268–270
    in AIDS patients, 396–397
    dosage, 269
  in treatment of fever and septicemia,
      104–105
Trophozoites, of *T. gondii*, 283, 284
Trypanosoma spp.
  cruzi, 254
  lewisi, 254

TTA: *see* Transtracheal aspiration
    (TTA)
Tuberculin skin test, 223
Tuberculosis, *see also* Mycobacteria
  in AIDS patients, therapy for, 398
  extrapulmonary, 232–233
  mimicking cancer, 227–228
  occult miliary, 234–235
  pathogenesis, 224–226
  prevalence by neoplastic disease, 480
  prophylaxis for, 31
  pulmonary: *see* Pulmonary
      tuberculosis
  reactivation, 226, 230–231
  in renal transplant patient, 599–600
  skin testing for, 223–224
Tuftsin, as host-defense mechanism, 45
Tumors, in childhood: *see* Childhood
    cancer
Tzanck preparation, in VZV infection,
    252, 253

United States of America, AIDS inci-
    dence in, 382–383
  report cases by risk group, 384
Urinary leaks, prevention of, 566–567
Urinary tract candidiasis, 198
Urinary tract infection (UTI)
  with *Candida* spp., 198
  in cardiac transplant patients, 626
  in renal transplant patients, 588–591
UTI: *see* Urinary tract infection (UTI)

Vaccine, *see also* Immunization
  Bacillus Calmette–Guerin (BCG),
      236–237
  hepatitis B, 339–340
  Pneumococcus
    humoral immune dysfunction and,
        33–34
    in leukemia and lymphoma pa-
        tients, 494–495
  Pseudomonas aeruginosa, in leuk-
      emia and lymphoma patients,
      495–497
  VZV, 355–356
Vaccinia
  morbidity of, 372–373
  organ involvement by, 368
Vancomycin
  as empirical therapy after bone mar-
      row transplantation, 533
  prophylactic, for leukemia and lym-
      phoma patients, 487
Varicella–zoster immune globulin
    (VZIG), 355
  for granulocytopenic child, 444–445
Varicella–zoster virus (VZV) infection
  in cardiac transplant patients, 635
  case study, 351–352
  cellular immune dysfunction and, 6–
      7
  of CNS, 183

Varicella–zoster virus (VZV) infection
    (*Cont.*)
  diagnosis and therapy, 355–356
  epidemiology and patterns, 352–354
  following bone marrow transplanta-
      tion, 550–551
  pathogenesis, 354–355
  prophylaxis for, 32
  in renal transplant patients, 585–586
  vaccine against, 355–356
Vascular anastomotic-related infections,
    following liver transplanta-
    tion, 605–606
Vascular line-related infections, in liver
    transplant patients, 607
Ventilation, as support in *P. carinii*
    pneumonia, 271
Vidarabine, for CMV infection, 357,
    359
  following bone marrow transplanta-
      tion, 545
Viral hepatitis: *see* Hepatitis
Viruses, *see also* individually named
    viruses
  and antibody recovery in bone mar-
      row transplant patients, 526
  as cause of fever in granulocytopenic
      child, 444–445
  cellular immune dysfunction and, 6
  in renal transplant patients, 582
  and malignant disease relationship,
      583
  skin infection with, 117–118, 119
VZIG: *see* Varicella-zoster immune
    globulin (VZIG)
VZV: *see* Varicella–zoster virus (VZV)
    infection

Water supply, legionellosis and, 309–310
  environmental, 309
  prevention, 319
Wiskott–Aldrich syndrome
  in immunodeficiency syndromes,
      421–422
  life-threatening infection in, 410
Wound closure, 657–659
Wound hematoma, prevention of, 567
Wound infections
  in cardiac transplant patients, 625
  following liver transplantation, 606–
      607
  following renal transplantation, 566–
      568

X-linked immunodeficiency syndrome,
    EBV and, 360

ZIG: *see* Zoster immune globulin (ZIG)
ZIP: *see* Zoster immune plasma (ZIP)
Zoster immune globulin (ZIG), 354
Zoster immune plasma (ZIP), 354
Zygomycetes spp., CNS infections
    with, 180–181